Thieme

Edited by
Gheorghe M. Constantinescu

Illustrated Veterinary Anatomical Nomenclature

Former editions with the cooperation of
Gheorghe M. Constantinescu, Robert E. Habel†,
Anton Hillebrand, Wolfgang O. Sack†,
Oskar Schaller†, Paul Simoens, Nestor R. de Vos†

4th, revised edition

280 Plates including 1308 Illustrations

Georg Thieme Verlag
Stuttgart • New York

Bibliographical data of the German National Library
(Deutsche Nationalbibliothek)

The German National Library (Deutsche Nationalbibliothek) lists this publication in the German National Bibliography; detailed bibliographic information can be found on the Internet at http://dnb.d-nb.de.

Address of the editor:

Gheorghe M. Constantinescu, D.V.M., Ph.D.,
mult. Dr.h.c., EAVA (Hon.)
Professor Emeritus of Veterinary Anatomy
Department of Biomedical Sciences
College of Veterinary Medicine
University of Missouri-Columbia
Columbia, Missouri 65211-5120
U.S.A.

1st edition 1992
2nd edition 2007
3rd edition 2012

Georg Thieme Verlag KG
Rüdigerstraße 14, 70469 Stuttgart, Germany
www.thieme.com

Printed in Germany

Cover design: © Thieme
Illustration by: Gheorghe M. Constantinescu
Typesetting by: SOMMER media GmbH & Co. KG,
D-91555 Feuchtwangen
Printed by: CPI Druckdienstleistungen GmbH,
Ferdinand-Jühlke-Straße 7, 99095 Erfurt

ISBN 978-3-13-242517-0 1 2 3 4 5 6

Also available as eBook:
eISBN (PDF) 978-3-13-242518-7

Preface to the 4. edition

Prof. Dr. Dr. Oskar Schaller, the first and sole editor of the first two editions passed away after the previous edition was published. This edition is respectfully dedicated to him, in gratitude of his outstanding contribution to the international veterinary anatomical nomenclature, and veterinary anatomy in general.

The 6th edition of the N.A.V. has been released in November 2017, including more than 60 new and changed terms of structures. Therefore, the Georg Thieme publishing company asked me to update the 3rd edition of this book. (The previous editions have been published by Enke Verlag). No changes on the Osteology, Arthrology, Myology, Systema nervosum periphericum and autonomicum chapters are made. Most of the changes are updated in the chapters of Splanchnology, Angiology, and Systema nervosum centrale. A few changes are made in the chapters of Systema endocrinum and Termini generales. The term "Apparatus" has been replaced by "Systema", and the names of some structures have been updated to correspond with the detailed list of terms provided by the Nomina Histologica Veterinaria. All changes in this 4th edition are made to contribute to the harmonization of the three veterinary nomenclatures: gross anatomy, histology, and embryology.

The Editorial Committee of I.C.V.G.A.N. has a new member, Mario Pereira-Sampaio, the President of W.A.V.A. Several changes of the chairpersons of the subcommittees of I.C.V.G.A.N. from the 5th edition can be found in the 6th edition of the N.A.V. as follows: Termini generales, Partes and regiones corporis; Osteologia et Arthrologia; Systema nervosum centrale; Organa sensuum.

My gratitude goes to Thieme, especially to Ms. Désirée Schwarz, managing editor/project manager, who gave me the opportunity to revise and update the 4th edition of this book, and to her team.

Columbia, Missouri USA, March 26, 2018
Gheorghe M. Constantinescu

Preface to the 3. edition

The book published in 1992 was based on the 3rd edition of the Nomina Anatomica Veterinaria (N.A.V.), 1983. The present edition is updated from the last (5th) edition of the N.A.V., 2005, and revised in both text and figures. Updating the text was followed by updating the labels of the figures. In addition, some figures have been replaced by new and original drawings. The revision included some changes in the text, comments, and footnotes. It was a sustained and continuous work over one year and four months spent by myself as the sole editor including the new drawings, in addition to my duties as professor of veterinary anatomy, including teaching, scholar activity and participation in international meetings.

From the contributors to the first edition, Professors Wolfgang O. Sack and Nestor R. de Vos passed away. The veterinary anatomist community is grateful for their valuable contribution and the success of the book. The name of Prof. Dr. Anton Hillebrand, from the University Spiru Haret in Bucharest, Romania was added to the list of contributors. I am deeply grateful to the three colleagues who sent their comments on the first edition. They are Prof. Emeritus Dr. Alexander de Lahunta, from Cornell, Assoc. Prof. Dr. Brian L. Frappier, from the University of Columbia, Missouri, and Prof. Dr. Michael Stoffel from the University of Bern. I am also thankful to Assist. Prof. Dr. Ileana A. Constantinescu for proof reading and suggestions.

Many explanatory comments and footnotes are added for better understanding of the text.

In the footnotes the Nomina Anatomica Veterinaria is abbreviated as N.A.V., and the Nomina Anatomica as N.A. Many structures of the 1st edition were omitted from the 5th edition of the N.A.V. and they are mentioned in the footnotes.

Due to the limited space of the pages and as many as 8 footnotes were necessary to be added to some structures, the Publisher with the consent of the Editor decided to include the majority of footnotes in the text.

The International Committee on Veterinary Gross Anatomical Nomenclature (I.C.V.G.A.N.) has now a new Chairman and Secretary, and several new chairpersons of the Subcommittees, as follows:

Chairman: Prof. Hagen Gasse, Hannover, Germany. Secretary: Prof. Wim Van den Broek, Gent, Belgium

Termini generales, Partes et Regiones corporis: Prof. Yoshiharu Hashimoto, Sapporo, Japan, Chairman of the Subcommittee

Osteologia et Arthrologia: Prof. Karl-Dieter Budras, Berlin, Germany, Chairman of the Subcommittee

Myologia: Prof. Gheorghe M. Constantinescu, Columbia, Missouri, U.S.A., Chairman of the Subcommittee

Splanchnologia: Prof. A. S. Saber, Minoufia University, Egypt, Chairman of the Subcommittee

Angiologia: Prof. Paul Simoens, Gent, Belgium, Chairman of the Subcommittee

Integumentum commune: Prof. H. Bragulla, Berlin, Germany, Chairman of the Subcommittee

Systema nervosum centrale: Prof. Ignacio Salazar, Lugo, Spain, Chairman of the Subcommittee

Systema nervosum periphericum: Prof. Peter Sótonyi, Budapest, Hungary, Chairman of the Subcommittee

Organa sensuum: Prof. Heinz Augsburger, Zurich, Switzerland, Chairman of the Subcommittee

The names of all members of the Subcommittees are listed in the 5th edition of the N.A.V. A very interesting and educational History of I.C.V.G.A.N., the Procedure to change terms in the N.A.V., the Principles of the N.A.V., Hints for the user of the N.A.V., and a Brief Latin grammar for anatomists can be found in the 5th edition of the N.A.V. Those interested in the Illustrated Veterinary Anatomical Nomenclature are encouraged to read them before searching for an anatomical term.

A list of eponyms for Systema nervosum centrale is provided at the end of the book. These eponyms are used by neurologists, by neuroanatomists, by neurosurgeons, and by those especially interested in the Systema nervosum centrale.

In general, structures are symmetrical. The vertebral column and sternum, some cranial bones, several ligaments and muscles are nonsymmetrical. The latter are mentioned as such. Therefore, there is no need to use the plural for the symmetrical structures.

For some muscles the origin is mentioned by "O" (from "Origo = origin"), and the insertion by "T" (from "Terminatio = insertion"). However, there are some muscles with reversible action, the origin and insertion being interchangeable under different circumstances – such as the Biceps femoris, Semitendinosus, Semimembranosus, Gluteus medius, Psoas major, Psoas minor and the Triceps brachii muscles. In these cases the term "attachment" is preferable for both origin and insertion.

In the 5th edition of the N.A.V. a list of structures precedes each chapter from "Osteologia" to "Systema nervosum" (separate for the Systema nervosum centrale, Systema nervosum periphericum and Systema nervosum autonomicum). All these lists and other different terms were together subject to a special chapter in the 1st edition of this book, called "Termini generales", and I decided to leave them in the same place, with the necessary changes. The name of the chapter is now "Termini generales et peculiares".

Lastly, and paraphrasing John F. Kennedy, "I decided to take this responsibility not because it was easy, but because it was hard".

I cannot finish without sending my sincere and great thanks especially to Dr. Ulrike Arnold, Ms. Gesina Cramer and Dr. Sonja Ruffer from the MVS Medizinverlage Stuttgart GmbH & Co. KG, also to Ms. Uta Schödl (the copy editor), and to my wife, Ileana, for her understanding, moral support, constructive comments and encouragements.

Columbia, Missouri, U.S.A., January 2011
Gheorghe M. Constantinescu

Preface to the 1. edition

The *Nomina Anatomica Veterinaria* (N.A.V.) constitute the first internationally recognized list of terms serving the gross anatomy of the domestic animals, specifically the cat, dog, pig, ox, sheep, goat, and horse. The N.A.V. were first published in 1968 by the International Committee on Veterinary Anatomical Nomenclature (I.C.V.A.N.) which was appointed by the World Association of Veterinary Anatomists. The third edition appeared in 1983. The present work already includes the changes that have been approved for the fourth edition of the N.A.V. This was possible because the authors are either members or chairmen of subcommittees of the International Committee on Veterinary Gross Anatomical Nomenclature (I.C.V.G.A.N.).

The *Nomina Anatomica Veterinaria* are 6,545 Latin terms (synonyms and terms of structures present only in primates not counted) of which fewer than ten percent are explained in footnotes. Besides, the nine figures illustrating the list are all in the section on the central nervous system. Some terms appear repeatedly; ramus caudalis and tunica muscularis, for instance, 13 times each.

Similar circumstances with the *Nomina Anatomica* (N.A.) of human anatomy prompted Heinz Feneis in 1967 to publish an illustrated anatomical nomenclature with the original title of "Anatomisches Bildwörterbuch der Internationalen Nomenklatur". The book was well received and subsequently translated into several languages. It proved useful not only to students, teachers, and researchers of anatomy, but also in many other branches of medicine and biology.

The editor of the present *Illustrated Veterinary Anatomical Nomenclature* was Chairman of the International Committee on Veterinary Anatomical Nomenclature (I.C.V.A.N.) from 1965 to 1980 and soon recognized the need for an illustrated version similar to that of Feneis. He was fortunate in securing as authors outstanding veterinary anatomists who were active in matters of veterinary anatomical nomenclature and were members of the respective subcommittees of the International Committee on Veterinary Gross Anatomical Nomenclature (I.C.V.G.A.N.):

Parts and regions of the body: W. O. Sack, U.S.A., Chairman of the subcommittee;

Osteology and arthrology: O. Schaller, Austria, former Chairman of the subcommittee;

Myology: Begun by the late L. E. St. Clair, U.S.A., former Chairman of the subcommittee; continued by O. Schaller;

Splanchnology: R. E. Habel, U.S.A., Chairman of the subcommittee;

Angiology: Begun by N. R. de Vos, Belgium, former Chairman of the subcommittee; continued by P. J. Simoens, Belgium, present Chairman of the subcommittee;

Nervous system: Begun by R. C. McClure, U.S.A., Chairman of the subcommittee on Systema nervosum periphericum; continued by G. Constantinescu, U. S.A., member of the subcommittee;

Sense organs and integument: W. O. Sack, U.S.A., member of the subcommittee on Integumentum commune.

Moreover, O. Schaller was the Chairman and R. E. Habel a member of the Editorial Committee for the first edition of the N.A.V., and R. E. Habel was the Chairman and W. O. Sack was a member of the Editorial Committee for the third edition. The composition of the team of authors thus guarantees that the aims of the International Committee on Veterinary Gross Anatomical Nomenclature (I.C.V.G.A.N.) find expression in the present illustrated version of the list.

The arrangement of text and illustrations – similar to that of the "Feneis" – makes the book easy to use. The left (verso) pages contain numbered terms arranged as in the N.A.V., and each term is followed by a brief definition. The respective illustrations, labeled by numbers that correspond to those of the terms, are on the opposite page. The names of structures, their definition and depiction are therefore easy to find. An index lists all terms alphabetically.

The illustrations were produced by several artists of whom Lewis Sadler, Adrian Cornford, and William P. Hamilton are prominent medical illustrators. Dr. P. J. Simoens, who contributed the chapter on Angiologia, and Dr. G. M. Constantinescu, who contributed the chapter on Systema nervosum, drew most of the figures of those chapters themselves. A few drawings were adopted from other publications for which permission from the respective authors and publishers was obtained and indicated in the legends. The sources are listed under References. Obviously, in many cases the subject matter will be represented by illustrations similar to those in other books, although they were not copied.

I thank the Enke Verlag for publishing this book, but especially Mr. J. Niendorf, Dr. P. Kleiner, and Mr. D. Kosmidis who were directly involved in its production.

Vienna, October 1991
Oskar Schaller

Contents

Directions for the Use of the Book

The three ways for looking up a specific term are

1. to find it by reference to the body systems which are indicated at the top of each page,
2. by reference to the index, or
3. by consulting the relevant illustrations.

Terms of the index set in italics are embryologic terms. On the text pages different type faces indicate the hierarchy of terms. Official alternatives and explanatory additions are set in square brackets [ ]. Common anatomical variations are enclosed in parentheses ( ), except in Systema lymphaticum, where many of the lymph modes cited are variable in occurence. Terms for ontogenetic structures are designated by (ont).

The species of domestic animals considered in the N.A.V. are:

Oryctolagus	(or)		
Carnivora	(Car)	Ruminantia	(Ru)
Felis catus	(fe)	Bos taurus	(bo)
Canis familiaris	(ca)	Ovis aries	(ov)
Ungulata	(Un)	Capra hircus	(cap)
Sus scrofa domestica	(su)	Equus caballus	(eq)

The larger group designations are, of course, restricted in their meaning to the species of domestic mammals designated; for example, "Ungulata" includes only Sus scrofa domestica, Ovis aries, Capra hircus, Bos taurus and Equus caballus. The term Artiodactyla, used in the definitions, means Sus scrofa domestica and Ruminantia (Bos taurus, Ovis aries, Capra hircus), the term Carnivora means Felis catus and Canis familiaris. Oryctolagus (cuniculus) – the rabbit was introduced in the 5th edition of the N.A.V., 2005 as a new species, so far only in Osteologia, Arthrologia and Systema lymphaticum. When a species designation is listed after a term, it indicates that the structure occurs only in that species among domestic mammals. However, the absence of a species designation does not necessarily mean that the structure is present in all domestic mammals. In the nomenclature of the blood vessels and peripheral nerves it was often necessary to make separate lists for different species. Such lists begin with a heading that gives the species or order in capitals. At the end of the separate list, the nomenclature common to all species is resumed under the heading TERMINI COMMUNES, and the special terms under the heading TERMINI PECULIARES. The latter are listed for each chapter.

The following is a list of useful abbreviations and Latin terms:

abs. = absent
cum = with
dext. = the right (limb, part of the body, structure etc.), dexter (masc.), dextra (fem.), dextrum (neutr.)
sin. = the left (limb, part of the body, structure etc.), sinistrum (masc.), sinistra (fem.), sinistrum (neutr.)
esp. = especially
o = origo, origin
s = sive (or – this is not the symbol for the rabbit!)
T = Terminatio, insestion
vide = see

1 ***Linea mediana dorsalis***. Dorsal midline. Longitudinal line in the middle of the dorsal surface of head, neck, trunk, and tail. A C

2 ***Linea mediana ventralis***. Ventral midline. Longitudinal line in the middle of the ventral surface of head, neck, trunk, and tail. A C

3 ***Margo tricipitalis***. Formed by the caudal border of M. triceps brachii. B

4 ***Planum medianum***. Median plane, dividing the body in two symmetrical halves. B

5 ***Plana sagittalia [paramediana]***. Sagittal planes, parallel to the median plane. B

6 ***Plana transversalia***. Transverse planes, at right angles to the longitudinal axis of the body, limbs, or any other organ or part. B

7 ***Plana dorsalia***. Dorsal planes, parallel to the Dorsum (back) and corresponding surfaces of the head, neck, and tail, Dorsum manus, and Dorsum pedis. They are perpendicular to the median and transverse planes. B C

8 **Regiones capitis**. Regions on the surface of the head.

9 **Regiones cranii**. Cranial regions, regions on the dorsocaudal part of the head.

10 ***Regio frontalis***. Frontal region, over the frontal bone. In bo it extends caudally to the Regio occipitalis. D

11 ***Regio parietalis***. Parietal region, over the parietal bone. In bo the parietal bone is on the caudolateral surface of the head. D

12 ***Regio occipitalis***. Occipital region, over the occipital bone. D

13 ***Regio temporalis***. Temporal region, over the temporal bone and muscle. D

14 ***Fossa supraorbitalis***. Supraorbital fossa, the depression caudal to the Orbita and dorsal to the Arcus zygomaticus. D

15 ***Regio auricularis***. Auricular (ear) region. D

16 ***Regio cornualis***. Cornual (horn) region. C

17 **Regiones faciei**. Regions on the rostroventral or facial part of the head.

18 ***Regio nasalis***. Nasal region. D

19 *Regio dorsalis nasi*. Dorsal nasal region. D

20 *Regio lateralis nasi*. Lateral nasal region. D

21 *Regio naris*. Region surrounding the nostril. D

22 ***Regio oralis***. Oral region, surrounding the Rima oris. D

23 *Regio labialis superior*. Region of the upper lip. D

24 *Regio labialis inferior*. Region of the lower lip. D E

25 ***Regio mentalis***. Region of the chin. D E

26 ***Regio orbitalis***. Orbital region, outlined by the margin of the bony orbit. D

27 *Regio palpebralis superior*. Region of the upper eyelid. D

28 *Regio palpebralis inferior*. Region of the lower eyelid. D

29 ***Regio zygomatica***. Zygomatic region, over the Arcus zygomaticus, ventral and caudal to the Orbita. D

30 ***Regio infraorbitalis***. Infraorbital region, rostroventral to the Orbita. D

31 ***Regio articulationis temporomandibularis***. Region of the temporomandibular joint, caudal to the Regio zygomatica. D

32 ***Regio masseterica***. Masseteric region, over M. masseter. D E

33 ***Regio buccalis***. Buccal region, between Regio masseterica and Regio oralis. D E

34 ***Regio maxillaris***. Maxillary region, over the maxilla, between Regio buccalis and Regio nasalis. D

35 ***Regio mandibularis***. Mandibular region, over the Corpus mandibulae, ventral to the Regio buccalis. D E

36 ***Regio intermandibularis***. Intermandibular region, between the two mandibles, extending from the Regio mentalis to the Regio subhyoidea. E

37 ***Regio subhyoidea***. Subhyoid region, over the Basihyoideum, caudal to the Regio intermandibularis. E

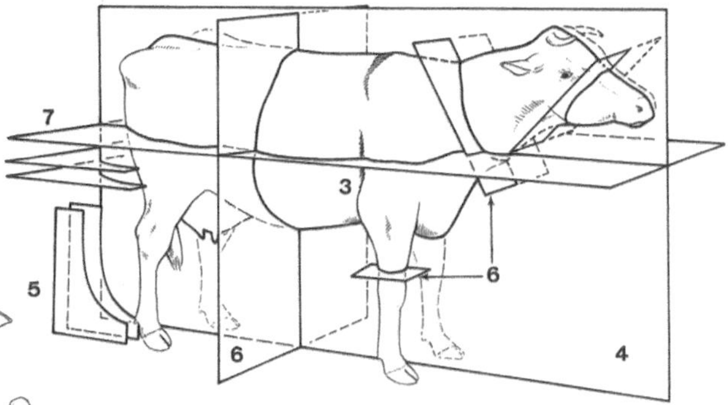

B Planes of the body (bo) (Dyce, Sack, Wensing)

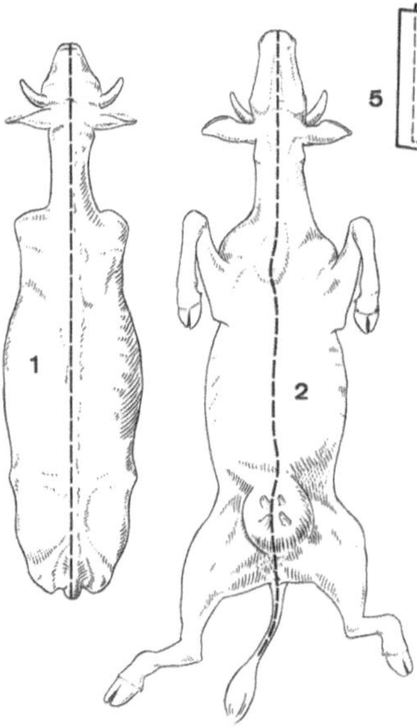

A Dorsal and ventral midlines (bo)

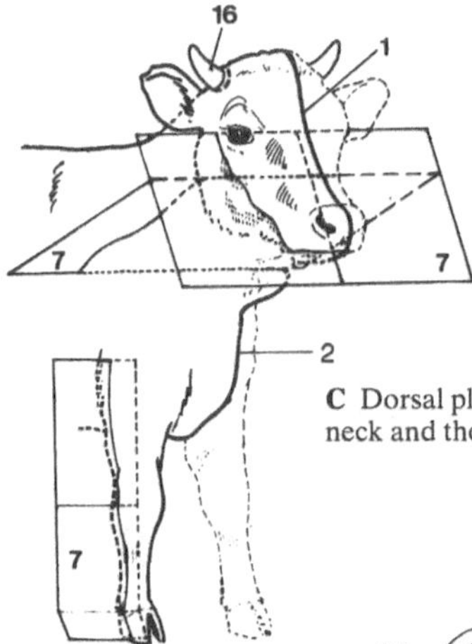

C Dorsal planes on head, neck and thoracic limb (bo)

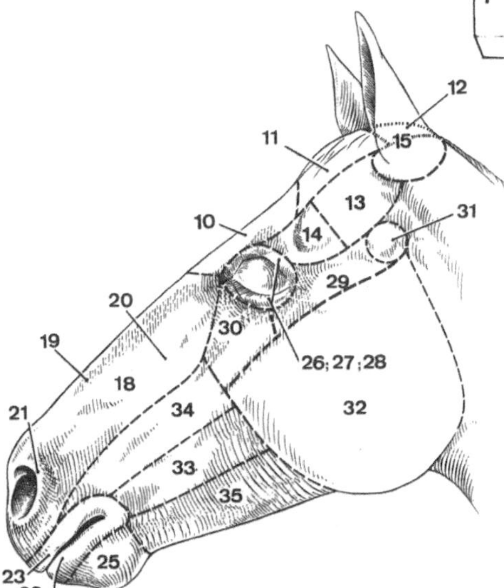

D Regions of the left lateral head (eq)

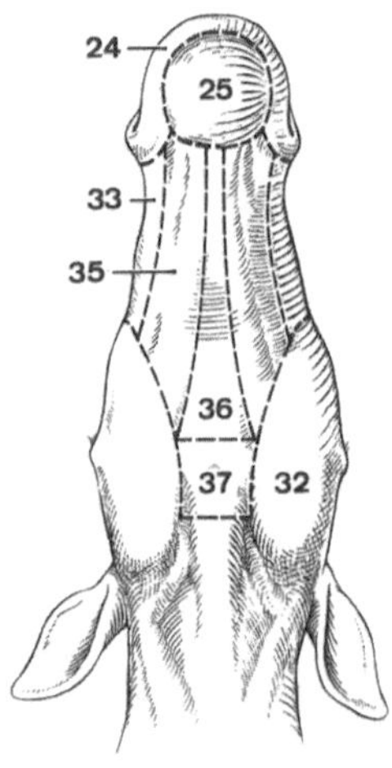

E Regions of the ventral head (eq)

1 **Regiones colli**. Neck regions.

2 ***Margo colli dorsalis***. Dorsal border of the neck, the crest in the horse. A B

3 ***Regio colli dorsalis***. Dorsal neck region. A B

4 ***Regio colli lateralis***. Lateral neck region. A B

5 ***Regio parotidea***. Parotid region, over the parotid gland at the cranial end of the neck. B

6 *Fossa retromandibularis*. Retromandibular fossa, the depression in the Regio parotidea, caudal to the mandible and ventral to the Ala atlantis. B

7 ***Regio retroauricularis***. Retroauricular region. B

8 ***Regio pharyngea***. Pharyngeal region, over the pharynx between Regio parotidea and Regio laryngea. B

9 ***Regio brachiocephalica***. Brachiocephalic region, over M. brachiocephalicus, ventral to Regio colli lateralis. A

10 ***Sulcus jugularis***. Jugular groove, the depression over V. jugularis externa, bounded dorsally by M. brachiocephalicus and ventrally by M. sternocephalicus. A B C

11 ***Fossa jugularis***. Jugular fossa, the depression at the caudal end of the Sulcus jugularis. C

12 ***Regio sternocephalica***. Sternocephalic region, over M. sternocephalicus ventral to the Sulcus jugularis. A B C

13 ***Regio prescapularis [prae-]***. Prescapular region, cranial to the scapula at the caudal end of the neck. A

14 ***Regio colli ventralis***. Ventral neck region, ventral to Regio sternocephalica, and consisting of Regio laryngea and Regio trachealis. B

15 *Regio laryngea*. Laryngeal region, on the ventral surface of the neck between Regio subhyoidea and Regio trachealis. B

16 *Regio trachealis*. Tracheal region, the wedge-shaped region over the trachea ventral to the Regio sternocephalica and caudal to Regio laryngea. B C

17 **Regiones pectoris**. Regions on the surface of the chest.

18 ***Regio presternalis [prae-]***. Presternal region, over M. pectoralis descendens, between Sulcus pectoralis lateralis and Sulcus pectoralis medianus. C

19 ***Sulcus pectoralis medianus***. Median pectoral groove. The groove between the right and the left M. pectoralis descendens. D

20 ***Sulcus pectoralis lateralis***. Lateral pectoral groove, between M. pectoralis descendens and M. brachiocephalicus; in the depth of the groove is the V. cephalica and the ramus deltoideus a. cervicalis superficialis. C

21 ***Regio sternalis***. Sternal region, over the sternum. A D

22 ***Regio mammaria thoracica***. Region of the thoracic mammary glands in Car and su. D

23 ***Regio scapularis***. Scapular region, over the scapula. A

24 *Regio cartilaginis scapulae*. Region of the scapular cartilage. A

25 *Regio supraspinata*. Supraspinatus region, over M. supraspinatus. A

26 *Regio infraspinata*. Infraspinatus region, over M. infraspinatus. A

27 *Regio acromialis*. Acromial region, over the acromion or over the ventral end of the Spina scapulae. A

28 ***Regio costalis***. Costal region, over the ribs excluding the costal cartilages. A

29 ***Regio cardiaca***. Cardiac region, over the heart caudal to the Margo tricipitalis. It can be enlarged by advancing the thoracic limb, to ease the approach to the auscultation and/or percussion of the heart. A

30 ***Arcus costalis***. Costal arch, formed by the Cartilagines costales of the asternal ribs and connecting the ventral end of the last rib with the sternum. A

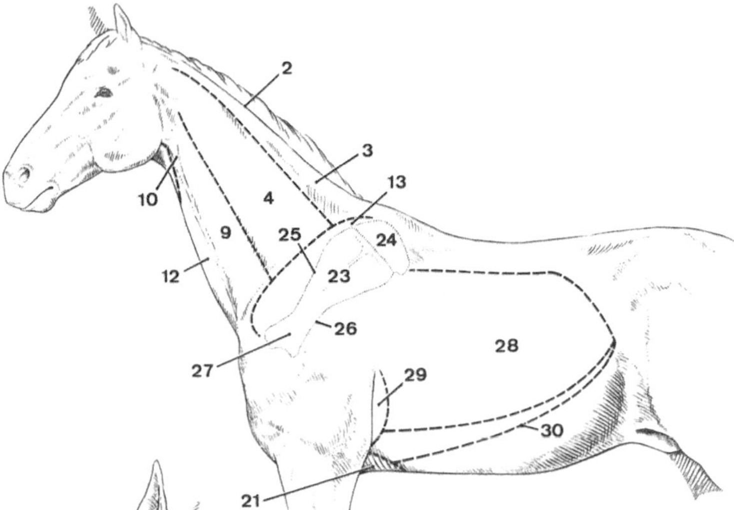

A Regions of the left lateral neck and thorax (eq)

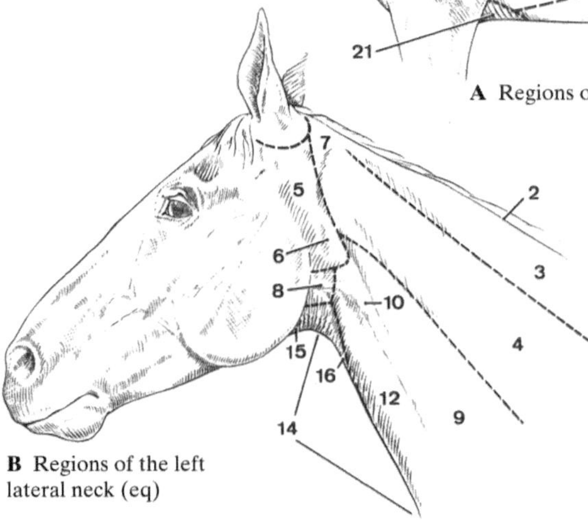

B Regions of the left lateral neck (eq)

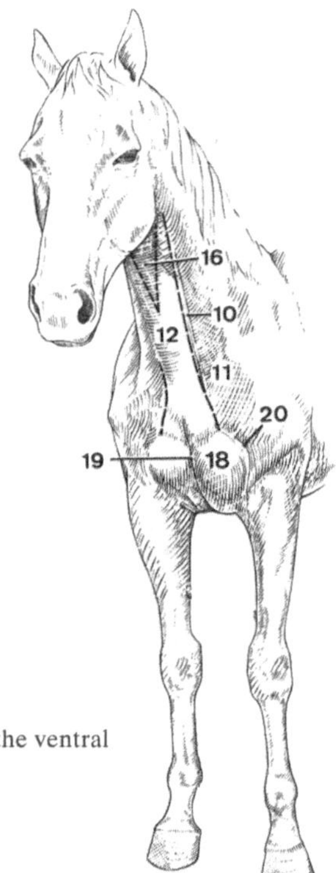

C Regions of the ventral neck and cranial thorax (eq)

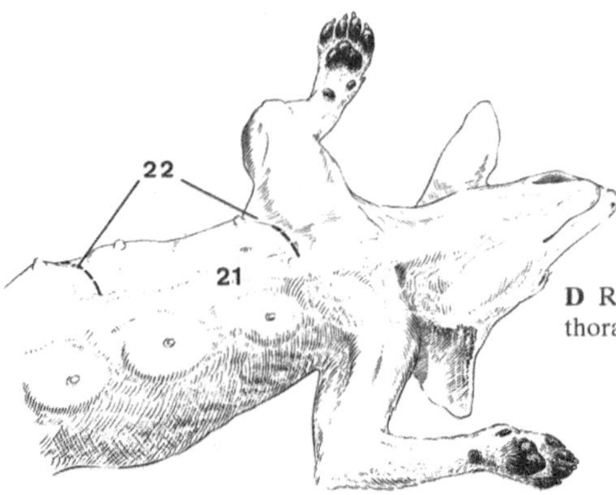

D Regions of the ventral thorax (ca)

1 **Regiones abdominis**. Regions on the surface of the abdomen.

2 ***Regio abdominis cranialis***. Cranial abdominal region, consisting of Regio hypochondriaca (dextra et sinistra) and Regio xiphoidea. B

3 *Regio hypochondriaca*. Hypochondriac region, the band of abdominal wall over the costal cartilages. A B

4 *Regio xiphoidea*. Xiphoid region, the ventral surface of the abdomen between the Arcus costales, extending to the level of the ventral end of the last rib. A B

5 ***Regio abdominis media***. Middle abdominal region, consisting of Regio abdominis lateralis (dextra et sinistra) and Regio umbilicalis. B

6 *Regio abdominis lateralis*. Lateral abdominal region, called the flank, extending to the level of the Tuber coxae. A (The flank is conventionally divided in the large mammals in three parts; in a dorsoventral order they are: the paralumbar fossa, [fossa or hole of the flank], the cord of the flank [attachment of muscular fibers of the internal abdominal oblique muscle on the last costochondral joint], and the slope of the flank. They are very important in assessing the topography of the abdominal viscera in the large mammals. The 5th ed. of the N. A. V. does not mention anything specific distal to the cord of the flank.)

7 **Fossa paralumbalis**. Paralumbar fossa, a depression bounded dorsally by the lumbar transverse processes, ventrally by the part of M. obliquus abdominis internus passing from the Tuber coxae to the last rib (conventionally called "the cord of the flank", see 6), and cranially by the last rib. A

8 **Regio plicae lateris**. Region of the fold of the flank. A

9 *Regio umbilicalis*. Umbilical region. B

10 ***Regio abdominis caudalis***. Caudal abdominal region, the ventral surface of the abdomen between the folds of the flank, and extending from the Regio abdominis media to the Pecten ossis pubis. B

11 *Regio inguinalis*. Inguinal region, lateral to the Regio pubica. In A it is located deep, out of reach from this perspective. A B C

12 *Regio pubica*. Pubic region, cranial to Os pubis, between right and left Regiones inguinales. B C

13 **Regio preputialis [prae-]**. Preputial region. C

14 ***Regio mammaria abdominalis***. Region of the abdominal mammary glands in Car and su. E

15 ***Regio mammaria inguinalis***. Region of the inguinal mammary glands in Car and su. E

16 ***Regio uberis***. Region of the udder. D E

17 **Regiones dorsi**. Regions on the surface of the back.

18 ***Regio vertebralis thoracis [Reg. dorsocostalis]***. Region of the thoracic vertebrae, extending from the Regio colli dorsalis to the Regio lumbalis. A

19 *Regio interscapularis*. Interscapular region, between the dorsal borders of the scapulae or of the Cartilagines scapulae. Owing to the length of the Processus spinales in large domestic mammals, it forms a high ridge, the withers. A

20 ***Regio lumbalis***. Lumbar region, over the lumbar vertebrae. A

21 **Regiones pelvis**. Regions on the surface of the pelvis.

22 ***Regio sacralis***. Sacral region, over the Os sacrum. A

23 ***Regio glutea [glutaea]***. Gluteal region, over the M. gluteus medius, caudal to the Regio tuberis coxae. A

24 ***Regio tuberis coxae***. Region of the Tuber coxae. A

25 ***Regio clunis***. The caudal end of the rump (part of the Pelvis dorsal to the level of the Tuber ischiadicum), lateral to the Radix caudae. A

26 ***Regio tuberis ischiadici***. Region of the Tuber ischiadicum. A F

27 ***Regio caudalis***. Tail region. A F

28 *Regio radicis caudae*. Region of the root of the tail. A

29 ***Regio perinealis***. Perineal region. F

30 *Regio analis*. Anal region, surrounding the anus. F

31 *Regio urogenitalis*. Urogenital region, ventral to the Regio analis and between the thighs. In the male of most species it extends to the caudal attachment of the scrotum, but, owing to the short distance between the scrotum and the anus in fe and su, includes the scrotum in these species. C F

32 ***Regio scrotalis***. Scrotal region. Its position in some species would justify the inclusion in Regiones pelvis. C

33 ***Regio supramammaria***. Supramammary region, in Ru and eq the region dorsal to the caudal attachment of the udder. F

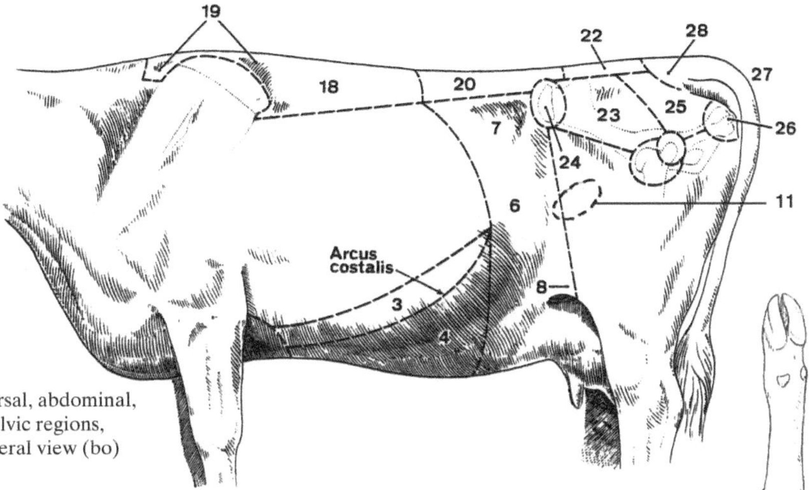

A Dorsal, abdominal, and pelvic regions, left lateral view (bo)

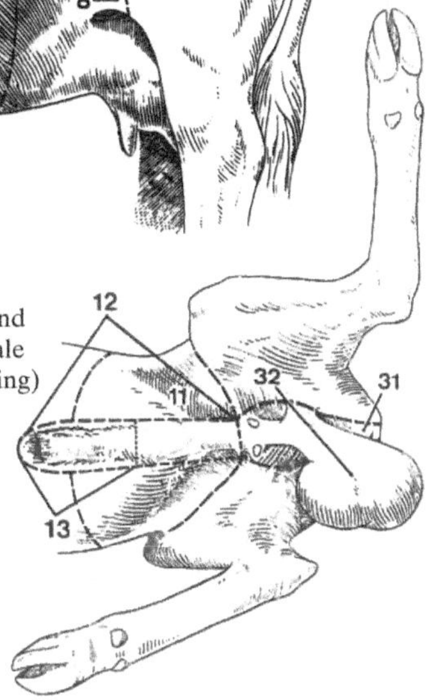

C Ventral abdominal and pelvic regions of the male (ov) (Dyce, Sack, Wensing)

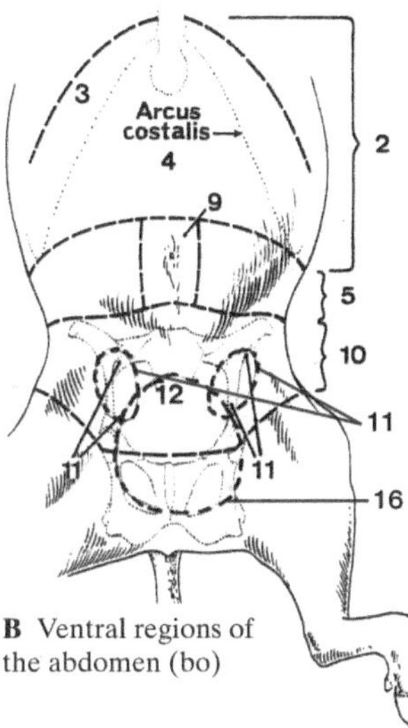

B Ventral regions of the abdomen (bo)

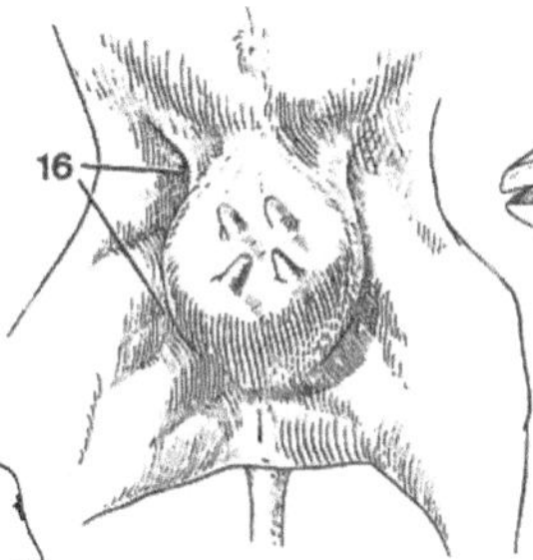

D Region of the udder, ventral view (bo)

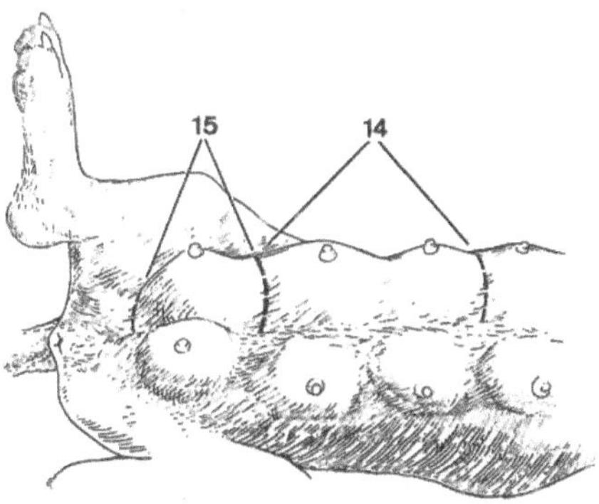

E Abdominal regions of the female, ventral view (ca)

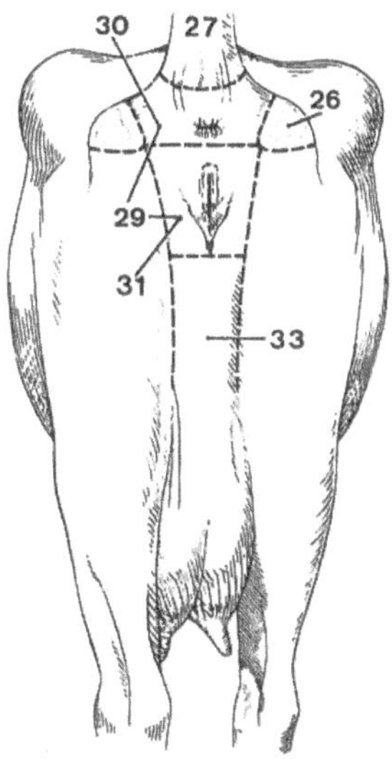

F Caudal regions of the pelvis (bo)

1 **Regiones membri thoracici**. Regions on the surface of the thoracic limb.

2 ***Regio articulationis humeri***. Shoulder joint region. A

3 ***Regio axillaris***. Axillary region. F

4 ***Fossa axillaris***. Axillary fossa, the depression between arm and thorax. F

5 ***Regio brachii***. Brachial region, on the arm distal to the Regio articulationis humeri. A F

6 ***Regio tricipitalis***. Triceps region, over Caput longum m. tricipitis brachii. A F

7 ***Regio cubiti***. Region of the elbow joint, distal to the Regio brachii. A F

8 ***Regio olecrani***. Olecranon region, distal to the Regio tricipitalis. A F

9 ***Regio antebrachii***. Antebrachial region. A F

10 ***Regio carpi***. Carpal region. A D F

11 ***Regio metacarpi***. Metacarpal region. A D

12 ***Regio metacarpophalangea***. Metacarpophalangeal region, the surface over the Articulatio metacarpophalangea. In the large animals it is also called the fetlock. A C D

13 ***Regio phalangis proximalis***. Proximal phalangeal region. D

14 ***Regio compedis***. Pastern region, part of the digit of Un between metacarpophalangeal joint and Regio coronalis. A C

15 ***Regio interphalangea proximalis***. Proximal interphalangeal region, surrounding the Articulatio interphalangea proximalis. D

16 ***Regio phalangis mediae***. Middle phalangeal region. D

17 ***Regio coronalis***. Coronal region, slightly raised band of skin that joins the narrower Regio compedis to the coronet (junction of skin and hoof). A C

18 ***Spatium interdigitale***. Interdigital space. C

19 **Regiones membri pelvini**. Regions on the surface of the pelvic limb.

20 ***Regio articulationis coxae***. Hip joint region. B

21 *Regio trochanterica*. Region over the Trochanter major. B

22 ***Regio femoris***. Region of the thigh. B

23 ***Regio genus cranialis***. Cranial stifle region. B

24 *Regio patellaris*. Region of the patella. B

25 ***Regio genus lateralis***. Lateral stifle region. B

26 ***Regio genus medialis***. Medial stifle region.

27 ***Regio poplitea***. Popliteal region, caudal to the stifle. B

28 ***Regio cruris***. Crural region. B

29 ***Regio tendinis calcanei communis***. Region of the common calcanean (Achile's) tendon. B

30 ***Regio tarsi***. Tarsal region. In the large animals it is also called the hock. B E

31 ***Regio calcanea***. Region over the calcaneus. B E

32 ***Regio metatarsi***. Metatarsal region. B E

33 ***Regio metatarsophalangea***. Metatarsophalangeal region, the surface over the Articulatio metatarsophalangea. Homologous to #12. B C E

34 ***Regio phalangis proximalis***. Proximal phalangeal region. E

35 ***Regio compedis***. Pastern region, part of the digit of Un between metatarsophalangeal joint and Regio coronalis. B C

36 ***Regio interphalangea proximalis***. Proximal interphalangeal region, surrounding the Articulatio interphalangea proximalis. E

37 ***Regio phalangis mediae***. Middle phalangeal region. E

38 ***Regio coronalis***. Coronal region, slightly raided band of skin that joins the narrower Regio compedis to the coronet (junction of skin and hoof). B C

39 ***Spatium interdigitale***. Interdigital space. C

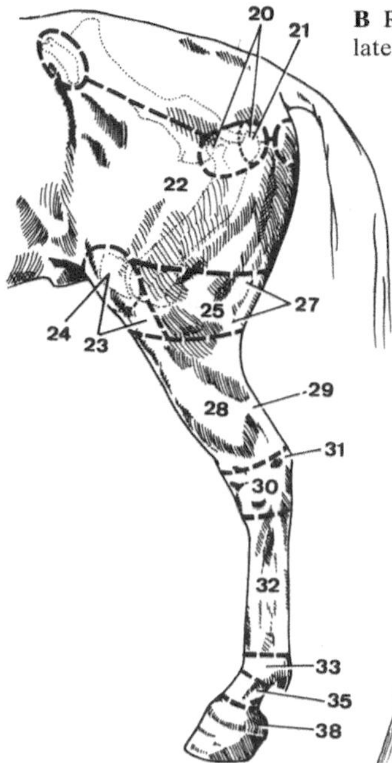

B Regions of the left pelvic limb, lateral view (eq)

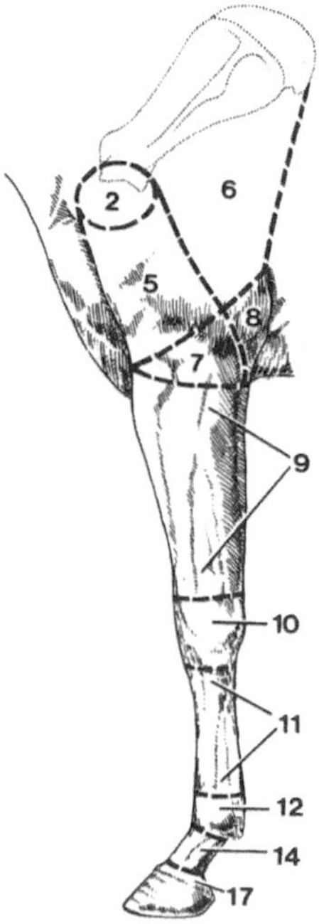

A Regions of the left thoracic limb, lateral view (eq)

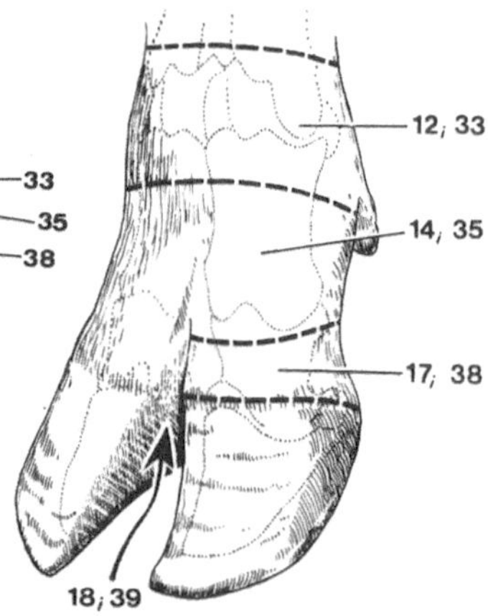

C Regions of the left digit, dorsolateral view (bo)

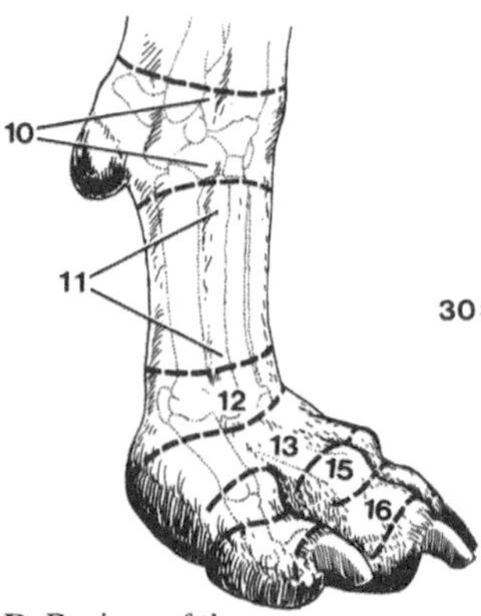

D Regions of the right manus, dorsolateral view (ca)

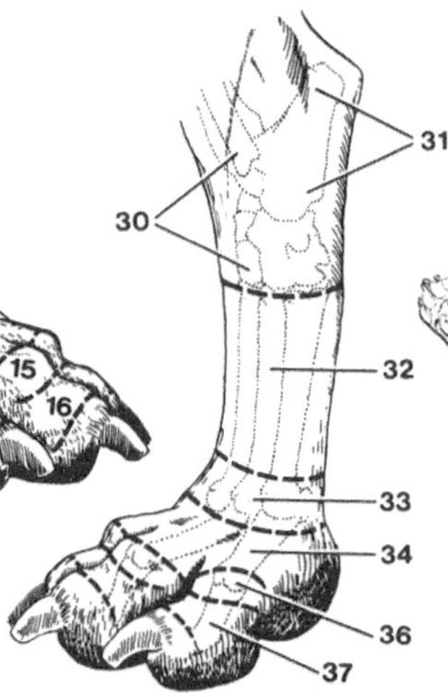

E Regions of the left pes, dorsolateral view (ca)

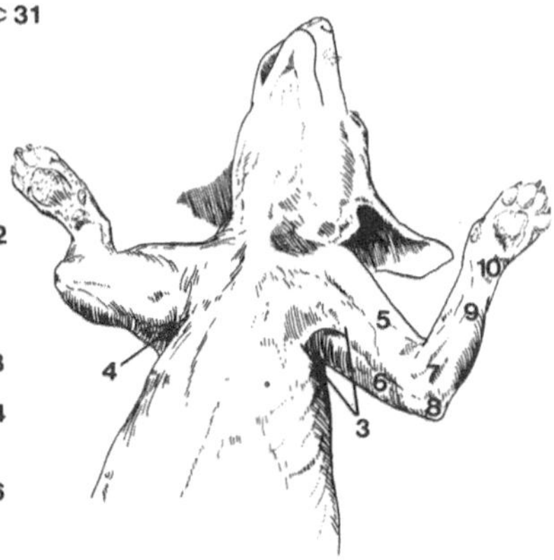

F Regions of the thoracic limb, medial view (ca)

1 **SKELETON AXIALE.** Axial skeleton, formed by Ossa cranii, Ossa faciei, Columna vertebralis, and Skeleton thoracis.

2 **CRANIUM.** Part of the skull that encloses the brain (formerly Neurocranium). A

3 ***Cavum cranii.*** Cranial cavity, encloses the brain with its membranes and vessels.

4 ***Pericranium.*** Periosteum on the external surface of the skull. B

5 ***Lamina externa.*** External lamina of cranial bones. B

6 ***Diploë.*** Spongiosa between Lamina externa and Lamina interna of the cranial bones. B

7 *Canales diploici.* Venous canals in the diploë. B

8 ***Lamina interna.*** Internal lamina of the cranial bones. B

9 *Sulcus sinus sagittalis dorsalis.* Groove for the dorsal sagittal sinus. C

10 *Tentorium cerebelli osseum.* Osseous shelf over the dorsal surface of the cerebellum in Car and eq, formed by Processus tentoricus of Os occipitale, Os interparietale and Ossa parietalia. C

11 *Eminentia cruciformis.* Cruciform elevation on the inner surface of the Calvaria in su and Ru with the Protuberantia occipitalis interna in the center. D

12 *Meatus temporalis.* Temporal meatus (passage), formed by Os temporale and Os parietale (except bo) for the Sinus temporalis, rudimentary in fe and su. C

13 *Canalis sinus transversi.* Canal for the transverse sinus in ca and eq in the Tentorium cerebelli osseum. C

14 *Foveolae granulares.* Pits for arachnoid granulations on the inner surface of the Calvaria. C

15 *Impressiones digitatae.* Shallow grooves accommodating the gyri of the brain. C

16 *Sulci venosi.* Grooves for veins on the inner surface of the cranial bones. C

17 *Sulci arteriosi.* Grooves for arteries on the inner surface of the cranial bones. C

18 ***(Ossa suturarum).*** Sutural bones, occasionally in the sutures of the skull. F

19 ***Calvaria.*** Roof of the cranium. A B C E F

20 *Vertex.* Highest part of Calvaria in the normal position of the head. A

21 *Frons.* Forehead. A

22 **Fossa frontalis.** Shallow depression on the external surface of the Ossa frontalia. A

23 **Protuberantia intercornualis***. Thick border, separating nuchal and frontal surfaces of the skull in bo. E

24 *Occiput**. Back part of the skull. A

25 ***Fossa temporalis.*** Temporal fossa, area surrounded by the Linea temporalis. A

26 ***Arcus zygomaticus****. Zygomatic arch, consisting of the Processus zygomaticus of the squamous part of the temporal bone and the Processus temporalis of the zygomatic bone. In some species also the Processus zygomaticus ossis frontalis. A

27 ***Fossa infratemporalis.*** Ventral extension of the Fossa temporalis. A

28 ***Basis cranii externa.*** External surface of the base of the skull. A

28a *Foramen jugulare.* Jugular foramen, between occipital and petrosal bones for passage of cranial nerves IX, X, and XI. Formerly called Foramen lacerum aborale. See 12.1.

29 *Foramen mastoideum.* Mastoid foramen, dorsolateral to the Foramen magnum, for blood vessels, absent in su. A

* Reminder: The structures followed by an asterisk are landmarks for physical examination and/or clinical approach.

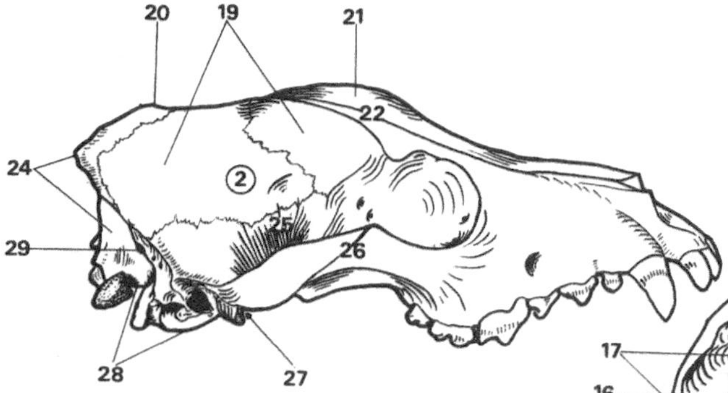

A Skull (ca)

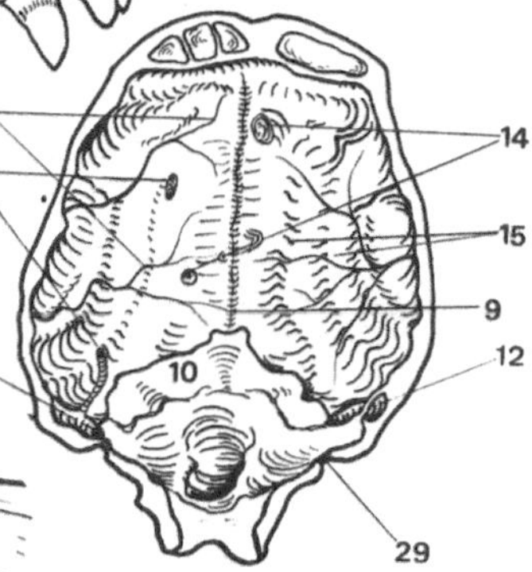

C Calvaria, interior aspect (ca)

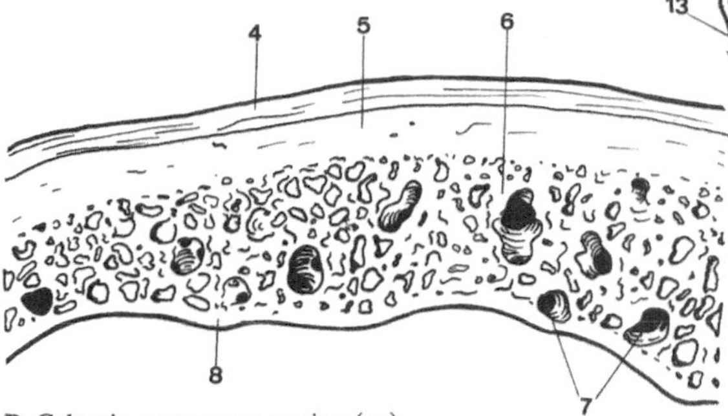

B Calvaria, transverse section (ca)

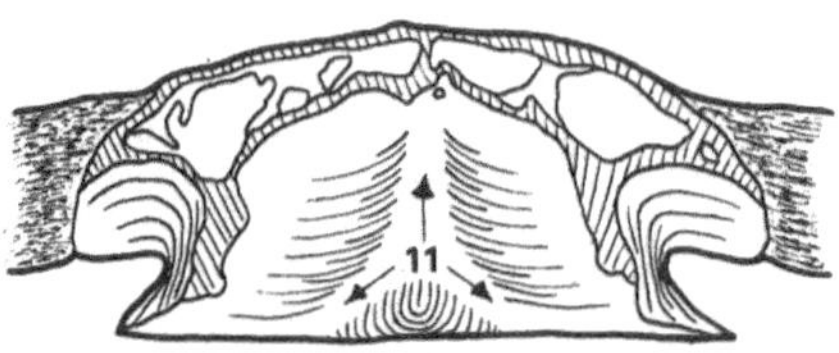

D Occiput, interior aspect (bo)

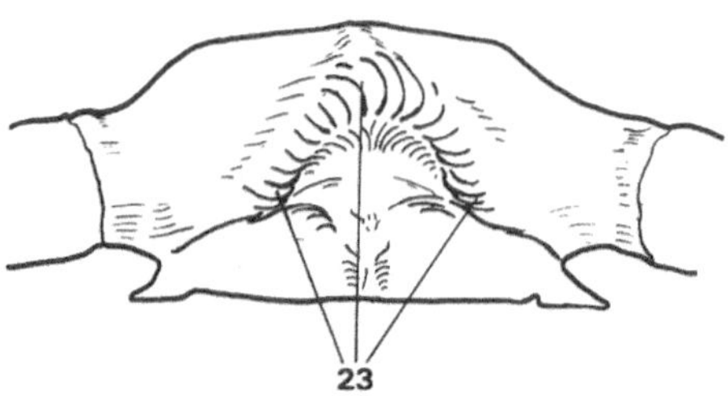

E Calvaria, caudal aspect (bo)

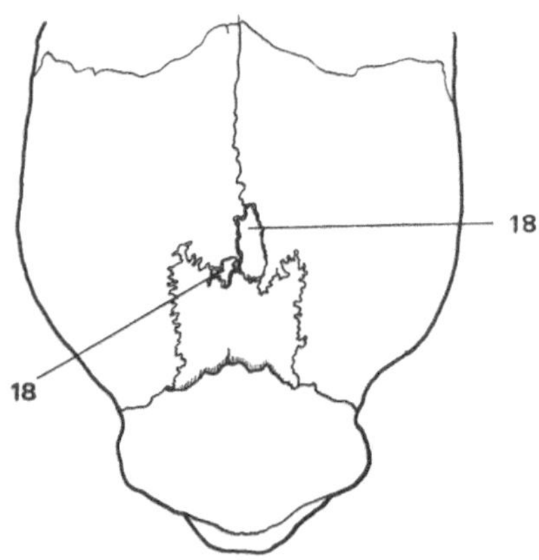

F Calvaria, dorsal aspect (eq, young)

1 *Foramen jugulare*. Jugular foramen, between occipital and petrosal bones for passage of cranial nerves IX, X, and XI. A B C (This structure is listed as 28a in the previous page after Basis cranii externa according to the 5th edition of the N. A. V.)

2 *Fissura sphenopetrosa* (Car). Sphenopetrosal fissure, between Pars petrosa of Os temporale and Os basisphenoidale. C

3 *Fissura sphenotympanica* (Car, Ru). Sphenotympanic fissure, between Pars tympanica of Os temporale and Os basisphenoidale. A

4 *Fissura petrooccipitalis* (Car, Ru). Petrooccipital fissure, between Pars petrosa of Os temporale and Os occipitale. C

5 *Fissura tympanooccipitalis* (Car, Ru, eq). Tympanooccipital fissure, between Pars tympanica of Os temporale and Os occipitale. A

6 *Canalis petrooccipitalis*. Petrooccipital canal, within the Fissura petrooccipitalis for passage of the Sinus petrosus ventralis in ca and Ru. A C

7 *Foramen lacerum*. Large opening with irregular border between Os temporale, basisphenoidale, and occipitale in su and eq (formerly Foramen lacerum orale). B

8 ***Basis cranii interna***. Internal surface of the base of the skull. D

9 *Fossa cranii rostralis*. Rostral cranial fossa, between the Lamina cribrosa and the Alae ossis presphenoidalis. D

10 **Fossae ethmoidales**. Ethmoidal fossae, for the Bulbi olfactorii. D

11 *Fossa cranii media*. Middle cranial fossa, from the caudal borders of the Alae ossis presphenoidalis to the Crista sphenooccipitalis and the Cristae partis petrosae of Os temporale. D

12 *Crista sphenooccipitalis*. Sphenooccipital crest. D

13 *Fossa cranii caudalis*. Caudal cranial fossa, from the Crista sphenooccipitalis and Cristae partis petrosae of Os temporale to the Foramen magnum. D

14 **Clivus**. Part of the Basis cranii interna between Dorsum sellae and Foramen magnum. D

15 ***Fonticuli cranii***. Membranous intervals between cranial bones in youngsters, called fontanelles. They ossify after birth at different ages depending on species. E (Four fontanelles are listed in the N.A., and up to 14 in Medical Dictionaries.)

16 *Fonticulus frontoparietalis*. Median space between Os frontale and parietale, existing for some time only in small breeds of dogs. E

17 *Fonticulus sphenoidalis*. Space between Os frontale, parietale, temporale, and presphenoidale. E

18 *Fonticulus mastoideus*. Space between Os parietale, occipitale, and temporale. E

19 **FACIES**. Part of the skull that encloses parts of Apparatus digestorius and respiratorius (formerly Splanchnocranium).

20 ***Fossa pterygopalatina***. Pterygopalatine fossa. Space between Processus pterygoideus of Os basisphenoidale and Maxilla. A B

21 ***Canalis palatinus major***. Greater palatine canal, formed by Os palatinum and Maxilla – in bo only by Os palatinum – for A. palatina major and N. palatinus major. A B

22 ***Foramen palatinum caudale***. Caudal opening of the Canalis palatinus major. A

23 ***Palatum osseum***. Osseous palate consisting of Processus palatinus of Ossa incisiva and Ossa maxillae, and Lamina horizontalis Ossa palatini. A B

24 *Foramen palatinum majus*. Rostral opening of the Canalis palatinus major. A B

25 *Fissura palatina*. Paramedian fissure in the rostral part of the osseous palate. The Canalis incisivus is accommodated in it. A B

26 *Canalis interincisivus*. Median canal betwen the Ossa incisiva in ca and eq. B

27 *Fissura interincisiva*. Median fissure between the Ossa incisiva in su and Ru. A

28 *Impressiones rugales*. Impressions on the ventral surface of the osseous palate, caused by Rugae palatinae in older swine and horses. B

29 *Torus palatinus*. Median longitudinal protuberance caudally, on the ventral surface of the osseous palate. A B

A Base of skull and hard palate (bo)

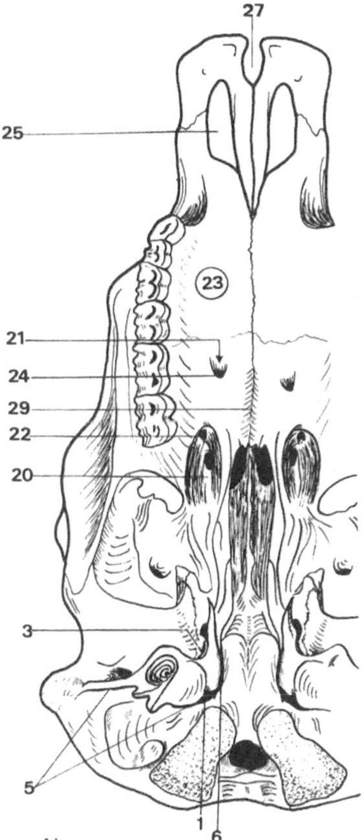

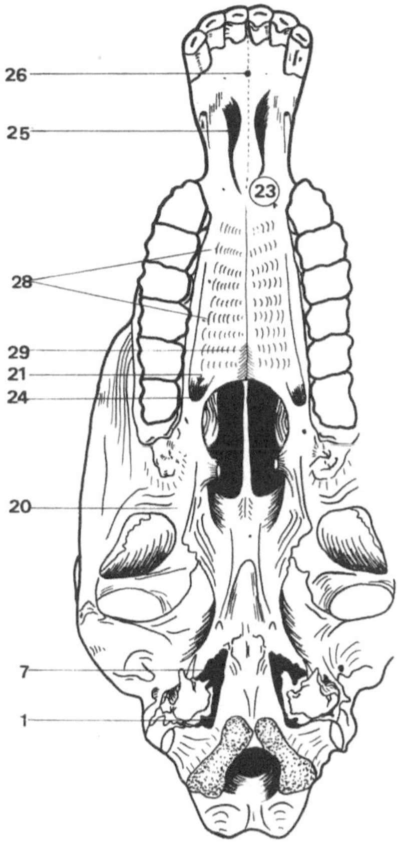

B Base of skull and hard palate (eq)

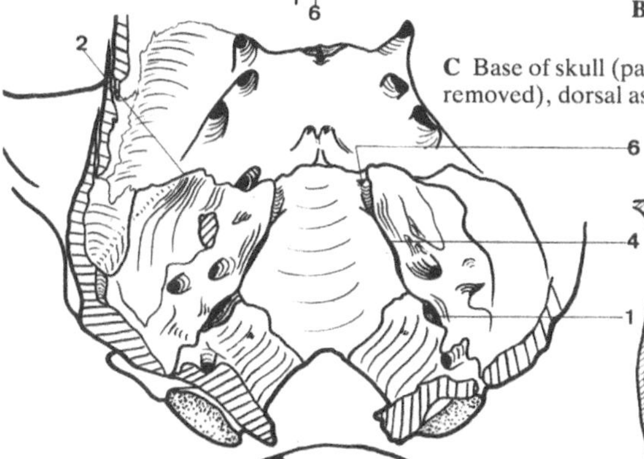

C Base of skull (part of the left petrosal bone removed), dorsal aspect (ca)

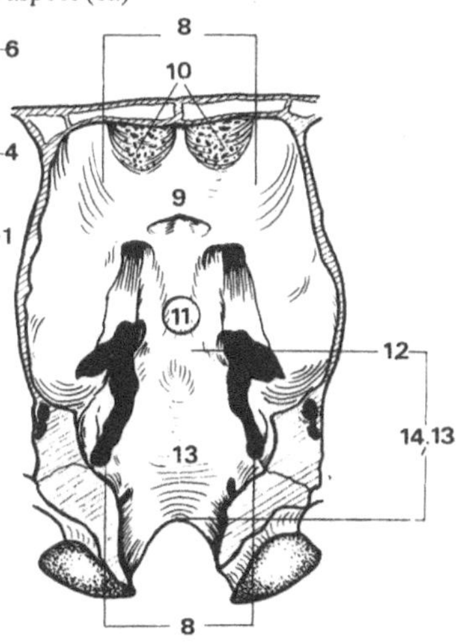

D Base of skull, dorsal aspect (eq)

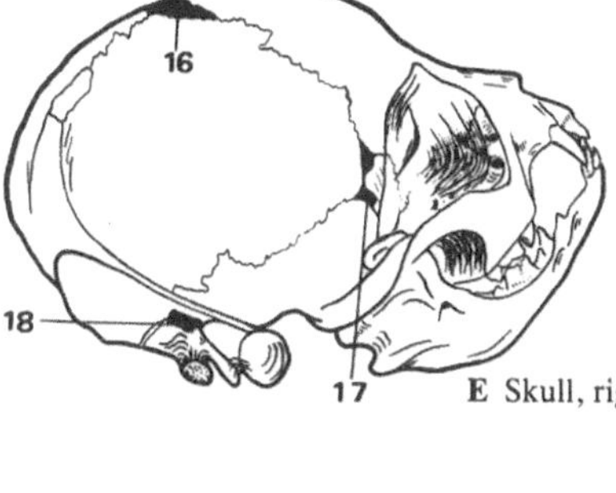

E Skull, right caudodorsal aspect (ca, newborn)

1 ***Cavum nasi***. Nasal cavity. A

2 *Septum nasi osseum*. Osseous nasal septum, composed of Vomer and Lamina perpendicularis ossis ethmoidalis. A

3 *Apertura nasi ossea*. Rostral opening of the nasal cavity in the skull. A

4 **Incisura nasoincisiva***. Nasoincisive notch, between nasal and incisive bones. B

5 *Meatus nasi dorsalis*. Dorsal nasal meatus, situated dorsal to the dorsal concha. A

6 *Meatus nasi medius*. Middle nasal meatus, between the dorsal and ventral conchae. A

7 *Meatus nasi ventralis**. Ventral nasal meatus, ventral to the ventral concha. A

8 *Meatus nasi communis*. Common nasal meatus, space between the nasal septum and the conchae. A

9 *Canalis nasolacrimalis*. Nasolacrimal canal, in the lateral wall of the nasal cavity for the nasolacrimal duct. C

10 *Meatus nasopharyngeus*. Caudal continuation of Meatus nasi ventralis. C

11 *Choanae*. The caudal openings of the nasal cavity. C

12 *Foramen sphenopalatinum*. Sphenopalatine foramen, opening of the nasal cavity into the Fossa pterygopalatina. C

13 *Recessus maxillaris*. In Car there is no Sinus maxillaris within the Maxilla; the Recessus is bounded medially by the Lamina orbitalis of the Os ethmoidale and laterally by the Maxilla and Os palatinum, in ca also by the Os lacrimale. It is very reduced in fe. C

14 *Fissura nasomaxillaris*. Fissure between Os nasale and Maxilla in ov, cap, and sometimes bo. B

15 *Fissura nasolacrimalis*. Fissure between Os nasale and Os lacrimale in Ru. B

16 ***Orbita****. Orbit. D E

17 *Aditus orbitae*. Orbital entrance. D E

18 *Margo orbitalis**. Orbital margin. E

19 **Margo supraorbitalis**. Supraorbital margin, dorsal part of the Margo orbitalis. D E

20 **Margo infraorbitalis**. Infraorbital margin, ventral part of the Margo orbitalis. D E

21 **Lig. orbitale**. Between Processus temporalis of the Os frontale and Os zygomaticum, forming the lateral part of the Margo orbitalis in Car and su, it is very short in fe. E

22 *Paries dorsalis*. Dorsal wall of the orbit. D E

23 *Paries ventralis*. Ventral wall of the orbit. D E

24 *Paries lateralis*. Lateral wall of the orbit. D

25 *Paries medialis*. Medial wall of the orbit. D E

26 **Foramen ethmoidale**. Ethmoidal foramen, in medial wall of orbit for like-named nerve and vessels. D

27 **Foramina ethmoidalia**. There are usually two Forr. ethmoidalia in ca. Sometimes one is situated rostral to, but often dorsal to the other. E

28 **Sulcus lacrimalis**. Groove in Os lacrimale, whose border is formed by the Processus frontalis of the maxilla in fe. F

29 **Fossa sacci lacrimalis**. Listed also under Orbita, because in fe it is formed not only by the Os lacrimale, but also by the Processus frontalis of the Maxilla. F

30 *Fissura orbitalis*. Orbital fissure, between the wings of the pre- and basisphenoids for nerves and vessels in Car and eq. E

31 *Foramen orbitorotundum* (or, su, Ru). Wide opening by fusion of Fissura orbitalis and Foramen rotundum. D

A Nasal cavity, rostral aspect (ca)

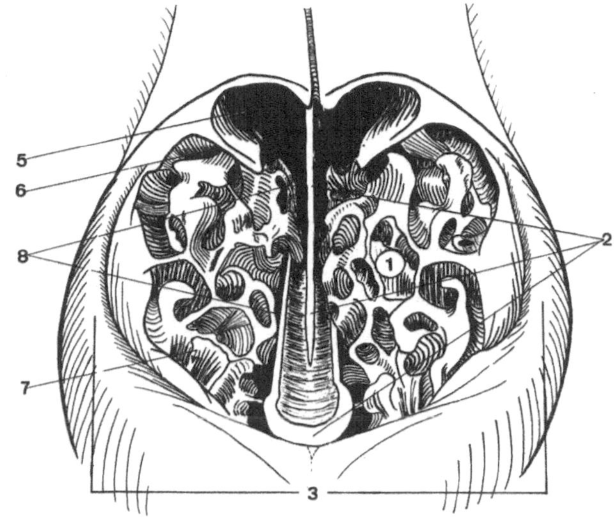

B Right facial bones (bo)

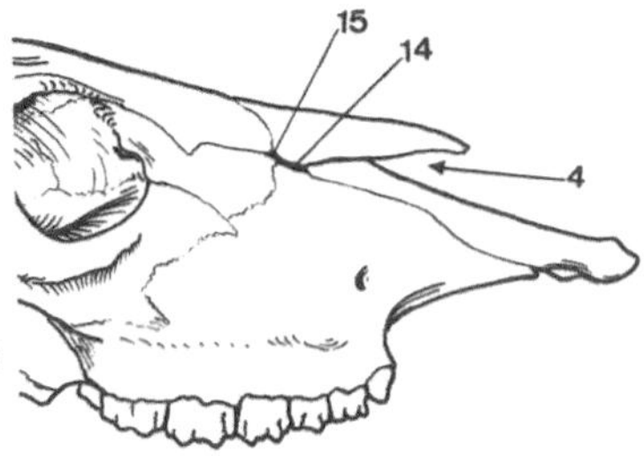

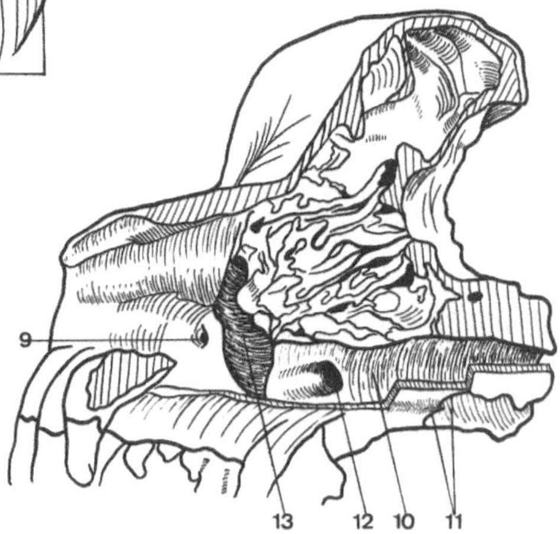

C Lateral wall of right half of nasal cavity (nasal conchae partly removed), rostromedial aspect (ca)

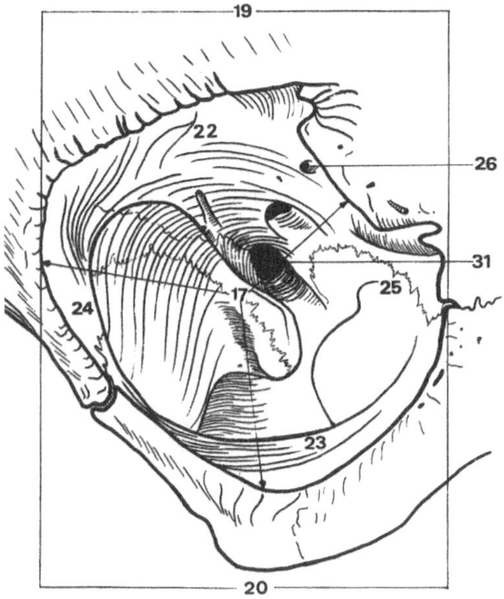

D Right orbit, rostrolateral aspect (bo)

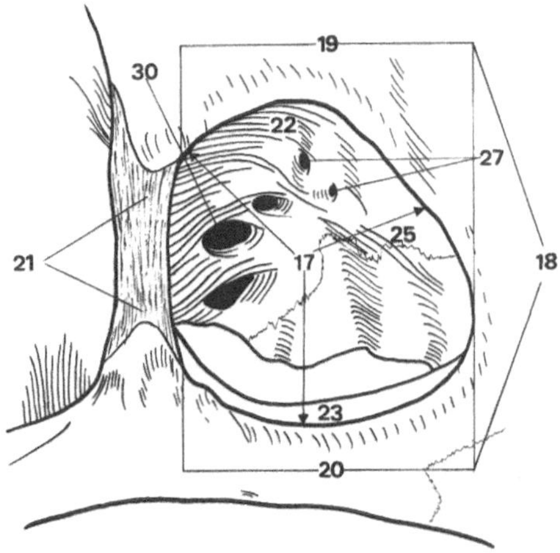

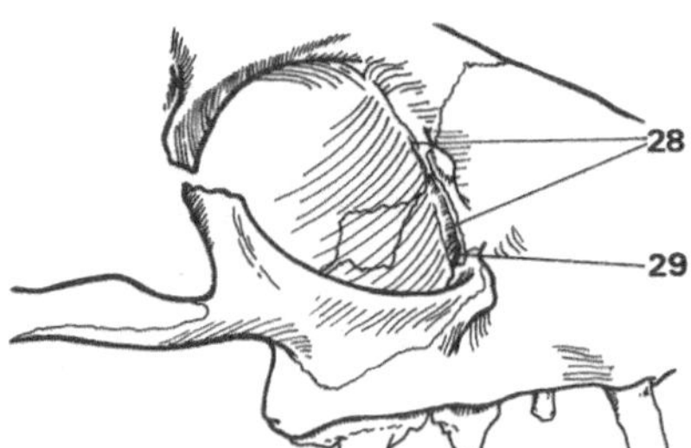

F Right orbit, lateral aspect (fe)

E Right orbit, rostrolateral (and dorsal) aspect (ca)

1 **OSSA CRANII.** Cranial bones.

2 ***Os occipitale.*** Occipital bone. A B C

3 ***Foramen magnum.*** Large foramen for the Medulla oblongata. A B C

4 *Tuberculum nuchale.* Tubercle on the dorsolateral border of the Foramen magnum in Car and su. A B

5 **Pars basilaris.** Basilar part of Os occipitale. A B C

6 ***Sulcus sinus petrosi ventralis.*** Groove for ventral petrosal sinus in Car and Ru. A

7 ***Tuberculum pharyngeum.*** Small median tubercle on the ventral surface of the Pars basilaris in Car. B

8 ***Tuberculum musculare.*** Paramedian tubercle on the ventral surface of the Pars basilaris. B

9 ***Impressio pontina.*** Impression for the Pons. C

10 ***Impressio medullaris.*** Impression for the Medulla oblongata. C

11 ***Sinus sphenoidalis.*** May excavate also Os occipitale in elder su. D

12 **Pars lateralis.** Lateral part of Os occipitale. A B C

13 ***Condylus occipitalis.*** Occipital condyle, for articulation with the atlas. B E

14 ***Processus jugularis.*** Process lateral to the Foramen jugulare, corresponding to a transverse process of a vertebra. A C E

15 *Processus paracondylaris**. The Processus jugularis projects laterally from the base of the Condylus occipitalis in man and domestic mammals. From this projects, in domestic mammals, an apophysis for muscular attachment (not homologous with Processus paramastoideus of man). A B C D E

16 ***Fossa condylaris dorsalis.*** Depression dorsal to the Condylus occipitalis. B E

17 ***Fossa condylaris ventralis.*** Depression ventral to the Condylus occipitalis. B

18 ***Canalis n. hypoglossi.*** Canal for the twelfth cranial nerve. A B C D

19 ***Canalis condylaris.*** Canal for the Sinus condylaris, absent in su and eq. A B

20 ***Incisura jugularis.*** Jugular notch, at the caudal border of Os occipitale for the Foramen jugulare. A C

21 *Processus intrajugularis.* Opposite to jugular process within the cranial cavity. A

22 **Squama occipitalis.** Dorsal part of Os occipitale. A B C

23 ***Margo mastoideus.*** Mastoid margin, connected with Os temporale. A B C

24 ***Margo parietalis.*** Parietal margin, connected with Ossa parietalia and Os interparietale. A B C

25 ***Processus interparietalis.*** Extends between Ossa parietalia, formed by prenatal fusion of Os interparietale with Squama occipitalis in ca. A B

26 ***Protuberantia occipitalis externa**.** Median protuberance on the external surface of the squama. Absent in su. B E

27 ***Crista occipitalis externa.*** Crest from Protuberantia occipitalis externa to Foramen magnum. B E

28 ***Crista nuchae.*** The sharp transverse crest on the external surface of the squama in or, Car, su and eq, which corresponds to the Linea nuchae of Ru. B D

29 ***Linea nuchae.*** Transverse line on the external surface of the squama in Ru. E

30 ***Crista sagittalis externa.*** Median sagittal crest on the dorsal surface of the squama in Car and eq. B

31 ***Linea temporalis**.** The border of the Fossa temporalis, to witch the Fascia temporalis is attached. The part on the Os frontale was formerly called Crista frontalis (externa), and the part on the Os parietale was called Crista parietalis. C E

32 ***Protuberantia occipitalis interna.*** In su and Ru. F

33 ***Crista occipitalis interna.*** Internal occipital crest. A

34 ***Processus tentoricus.*** Part of Tentorium cerebelli osseum in ca and eq. A

35 ***Foramen sinus sagittalis dorsalis.*** On the rostral surface of the Processus tentoricus in Car. The venous sagittal sinus joins the venous transverse sinus via this foramen. A

36 ***Impressio vermialis.*** Impression by Vermis cerebelli. A

37 ***Sulcus sinus transversi.*** Groove for the Sinus transversus. A

38 ***Sinus frontalis caudalis.*** Excavates also the squama in su and Ru. D

39 *Septum sinuum frontalium.* Separates the symmetrical frontal sinuses. D

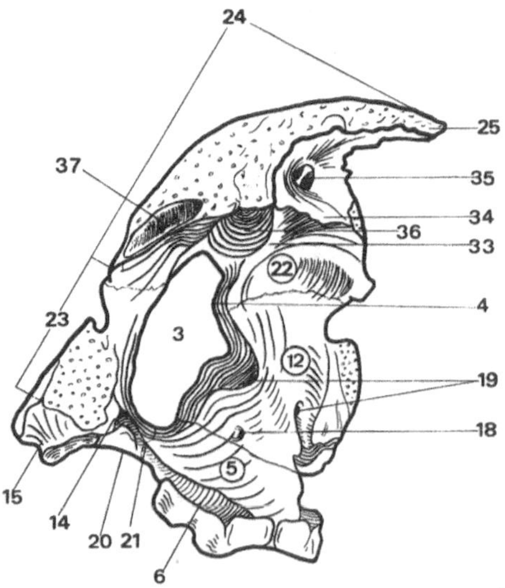

A Os occipitale, right rostral aspect (ca)

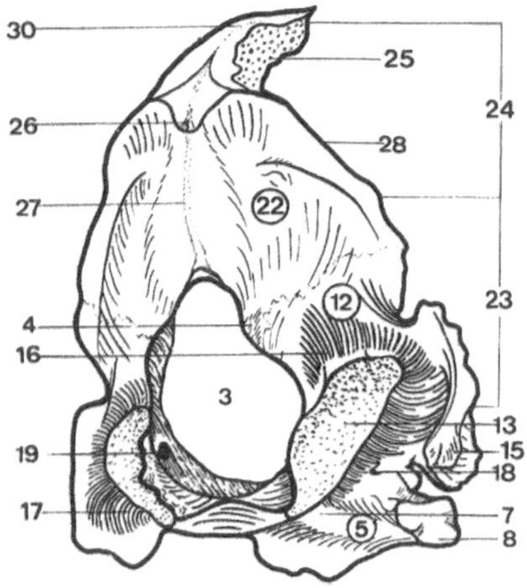

B Os occipitale, right caudal aspect (ca)

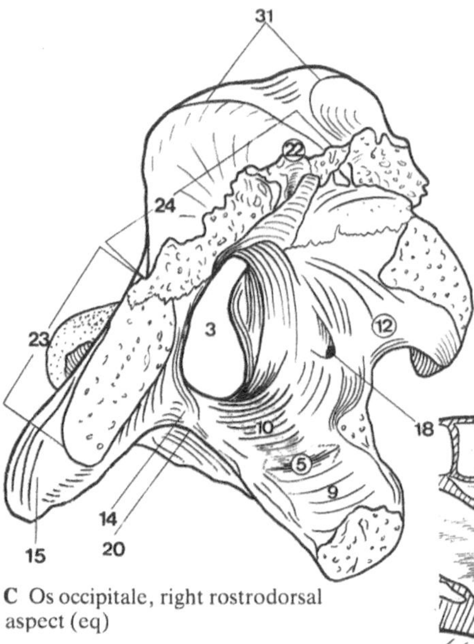

C Os occipitale, right rostrodorsal aspect (eq)

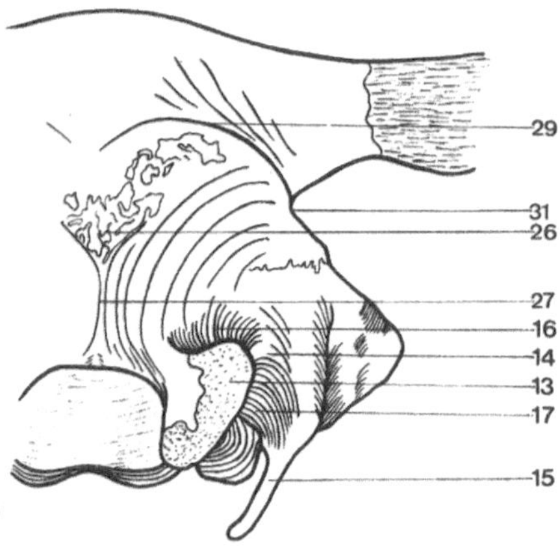

E Back of skull, right half, caudal aspect (bo)

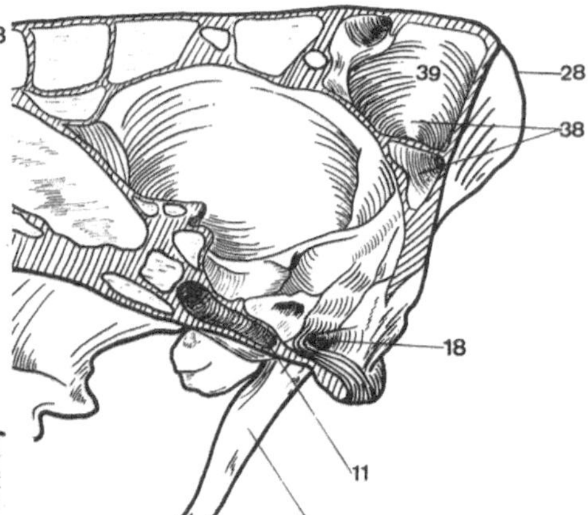

D Cranium, median section (Pars petrosa removed), right half (su)

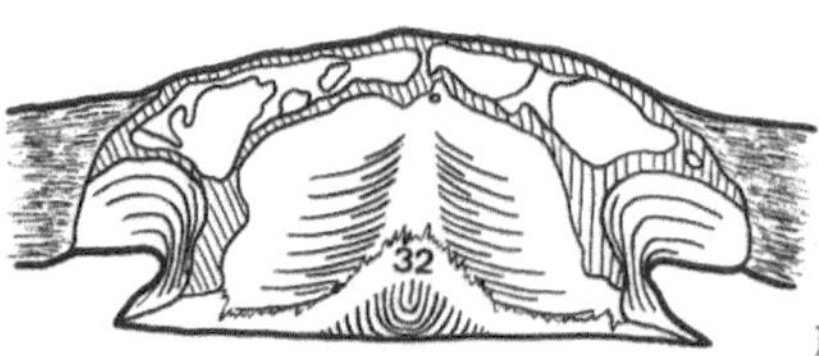

F Calvaria, interior aspect (bo)

1 **Os interparietale**. Interparietal bone, absent on the external surface in su, forms Processus interparietalis of Os occipitale in ca. A B

2 ***Processus tentoricus***. Part of the Tentorium cerebelli osseum in ca and eq. A

3 ***Crista sagittalis externa***. Median crest on the external surface in Car and eq. A

4 ***Linea temporalis***. Temporal line, attachment of the Fascia temporalis in Car and eq. A

5 ***Crista sagittalis interna***. Median crest on the rostral surface of the Processus tentoricus in ca and eq. A

6 ***Sulcus sinus transversi***. Groove for the transverse sinus in Car and eq. A

7 ***Sinus frontalis caudalis***. The frontal sinus may excavate also the Os interparietale in bo. B

8 *Septum sinuum frontalium*. Separates the symmetrical frontal sinuses. B

9 **Os basisphenoidale**. Basisphenoid bone. With the exception of the pig, the fusion between the basisphenoid and the presphenoid bones occurs at a later age. Therefore, they are considered as separate bones. C D E F

10 **Corpus**. Body, median part of Os basisphenoidale. C D E F G

11 ***Sella turcica***. Dorsal part of the body of the basisphenoid bone. C

12 *Fossa hypophysialis*. Central depression in the sella for the hypophysis. C D

13 *(Canalis craniopharyngeus)*. More or less rudimentary canal between pre- and basisphenoid bones in connection with the development of the Adenohypophysis. Remains in fe, sometimes in ca, cap, and eq, seldom in ov and bo. D

14 *Dorsum sellae*. Caudal wall of the Fossa hypophysialis, absent in eq. C G

15 *Processus clinoideus caudalis*. Process on each side of Dorsum sellae. G

16 ***Sulcus caroticus***. Groove for A. carotis interna in ca and eq. D

17 **Ala**. Wing, lateral part of Os basisphenoidale. C D E F G

18 ***Facies cerebralis***. Cerebral surface of the Ala, facing the brain. C D

19 *Fossa piriformis*. Depression for the caudal part of the Lobus piriformis. D

20 ***Facies temporalis***. Temporal surface, lateral surface of the Ala. E F

21 ***Facies maxillaris***. Maxillary surface, facing the Maxilla. C

22 ***Facies orbitalis***. Orbital surface, facing the Orbita. E F

23 ***Crista infratemporalis***. Ridge between the laterally and ventrally oriented surfaces of the Ala. E

24 ***Foramen rotundum***. Round foramen, connecting Cavum cranii and Fossa pterygopalatina, for N. maxillaris in Car and eq. D G

25 ***Incisura carotica***. Notch on the caudal border of the Ala for passage of A. carotis interna in ca and eq. D F

26 ***Fossa carotica***. Depression on the ventral surface of the Ala for the S-shaped segment of the A. carotis interna in eq. F

27 ***Foramen ovale***. For passage of the N. mandibularis in Car and Ru. E G H

28 ***Incisura ovalis***. Notch on the caudal border of the Ala for passage of N. mandibularis in su and eq. D F

29 ***Foramen spinosum***. For the passage of A. meningea media in Car. H

30 ***Incisura spinosa***. Notch on the caudal border of the Ala for passage of A. meningea media in su and eq. D F

31 ***Spina ossis sphenoidalis***. Laterocaudal tip of the Ala. D F

32 ***Sulcus n. ophthalmici*** (Car, eq). Groove for N. ophthalmicus. D

33 ***Sulcus n. maxillaris*** (Car, eq). Groove for N. maxillaris. D

34 ***Sulcus nn. ophthalmici et maxillaris*** (su, Ru). Groove for N. ophthalmicus and N. maxillaris. C

35 ***Sulcus tubae auditivae***. Groove for the Tuba auditiva on the ventral surface of the Ala, lateral to the root of Processus pterygoideus. E H

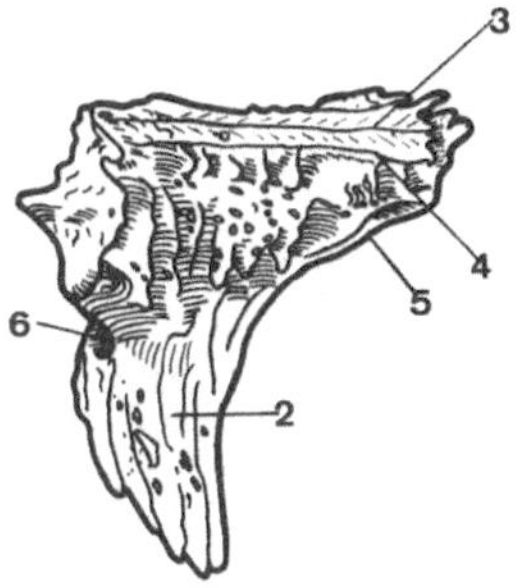

A Os interparietale, right dorsal aspect (eq)

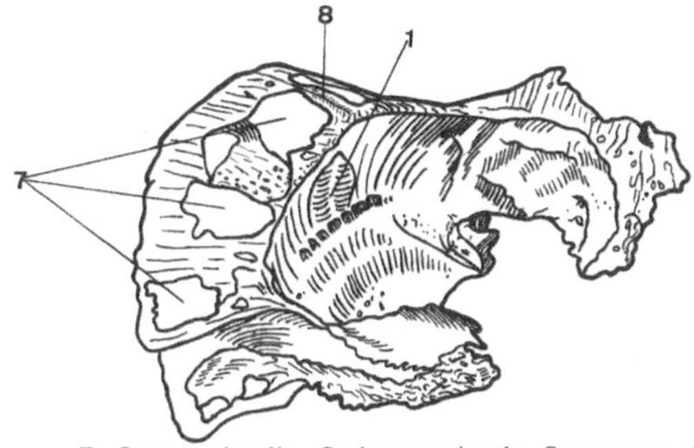

B Ossa parietalia, Os interparietale, Squama occipitalis, right rostrodorsal aspect (bo)

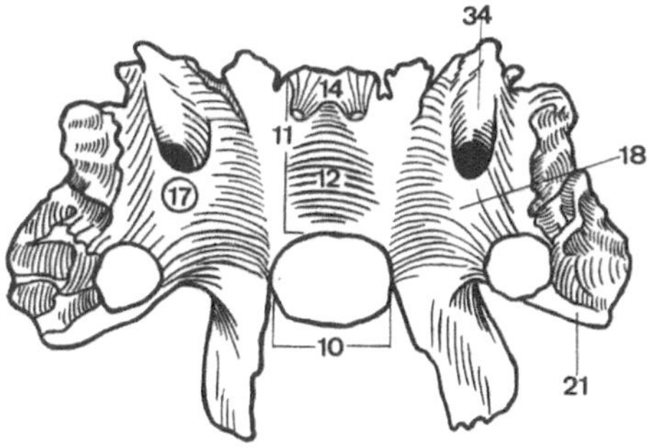

C Os basisphenoidale, rostrodorsal aspect (bo)

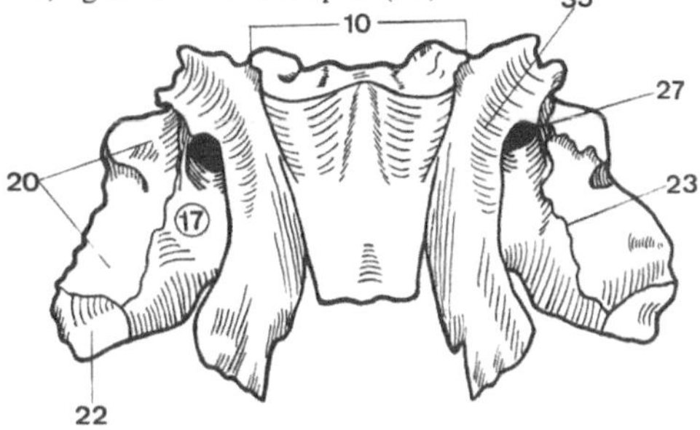

E Os basisphenoidale, ventral aspect (bo)

D Os basisphenoidale, rostrodorsal aspect (eq)

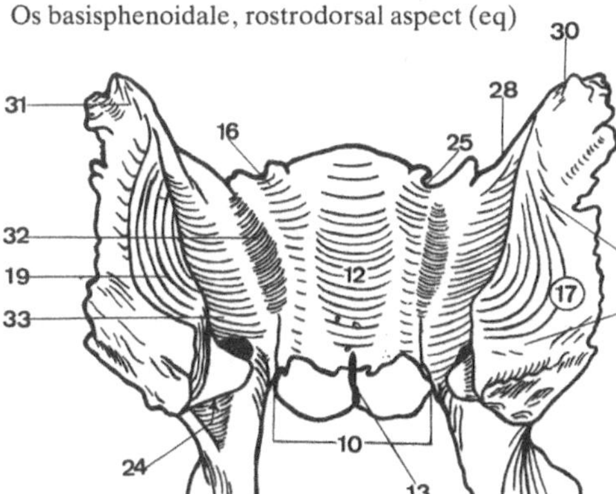

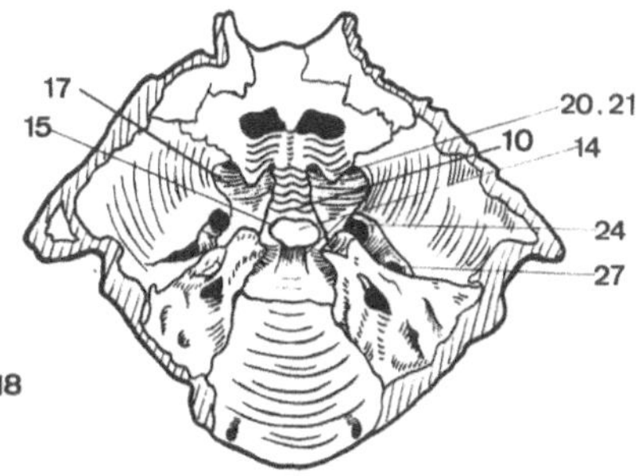

G Part of base of skull, dorsocaudal aspect (ca)

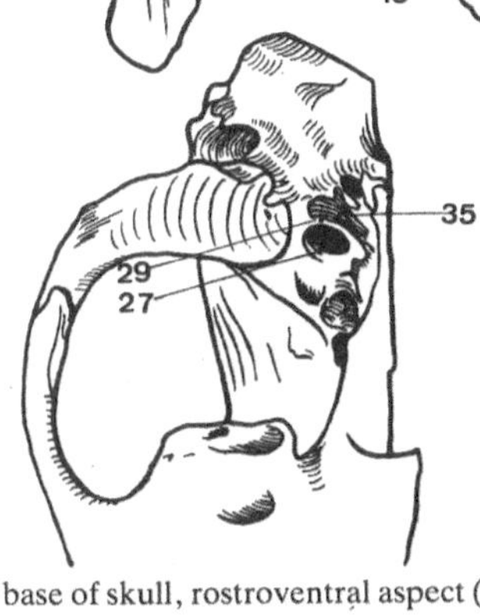

H Part of base of skull, rostroventral aspect (ca)

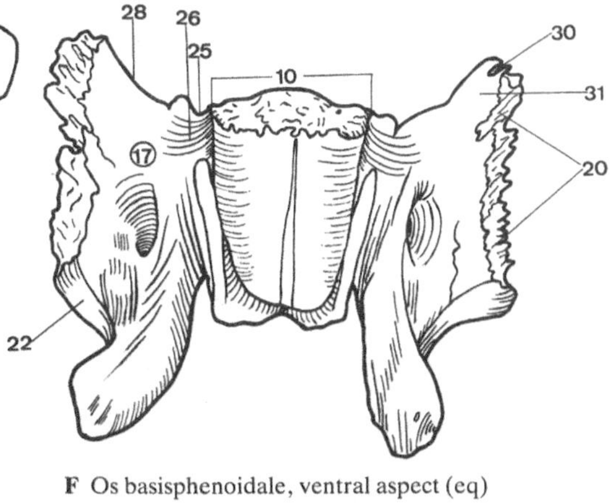

F Os basisphenoidale, ventral aspect (eq)

1 **Processus pterygoideus**. Pterygoid process of the basisphenoid. A B

2 ***Canalis alaris***. Perforates the Processus pterygoideus for passage of the A. maxillaris in ca and eq. A

3 ***Foramen alare rostrale***. Rostral opening of the Canalis alaris. A

4 ***Foramen alare caudale***. Caudal opening of the Canalis alaris. A B

5 ***Foramen alare parvum***. Small alar foramen, for A. temporalis profunda rostralis in eq. A

6 ***Crista pterygoidea***. Crest continuing the Processus pterygoideus dorsally as border of the Fossa pterygopalatina, absent in Car. A F

7 ***Fossa scaphoidea***. Depression on the caudal surface of the pterygoid process, dorsal to the Fossa pterygoidea in su, hardly distinguishable in eq. B F

8 ***Canalis pterygoideus***. Longitudinal canal through the base of Processus pterygoideus for N. canalis pterygoidei. B

9 ***Sulcus n. canalis pterygoidei***. Caudal continuation of Canalis pterygoideus between body and pterygoid process of the basisphenoid. B

10 **Sinus sphenoidalis**. Excavates in su also the basisphenoid. C

11 ***Septum sinuum sphenoidalium***. Does not completely separate right and left sinuses. C

12 **Os presphenoidale [prae-]**. Presphenoid bone. With the exception of the pig, the fusion between the basisphenoid and the presphenoid bones occurs at a later age. Therefore, they are considered as separate bones. D E

13 **Corpus**. Body, median part of Os presphenoidale. D

14 ***Jugum sphenoidale***. Raised flattened part of the presphenoid, overlying the entrance to the optic canals. D

15 ***Sulcus chiasmatis***. Chiasmatic groove, between the entrances to the right and left optic canals. D

16 ***Crista sphenoidalis***. Sphenoid crest. Median ridge on the rostral surface of the presphenoid for attachment of the Lamina perpendicularis of the ethmoid bone. E

17 ***Rostrum sphenoidale***. Extension of the body of the presphenoid. E

18 **Ala**. Wing, lateral part of Os presphenoidale. D E

19 ***Crista orbitosphenoidalis***. Caudal border of Jugum sphenoidale. D

20 ***Canalis opticus***. Canal for the optic nerve. C E

21 ***Processus clinoideus rostralis***. Process on the caudal border of the wing of the presphenoid. 19 G

22 **Sinus sphenoidalis**. Paired sphenoid sinus, may be absent in Ru. C E

23 ***Septum sinuum sphenoidalium***. Partition between right and left Sinus sphenoidalis, may be incomplete. C E

24 ***Apertura sinus sphenoidalis***. Opening of the Sinus sphenoidalis. C

25 **Os pterygoideum**. Pterygoid bone. B F

26 ***Incisura pterygoidea*** (su, ov, cap). Ventrocaudal notch between Os pterygoideum and Processus pterygoideus. F

27 ***Fossa pterygoidea***. Caudal depression between Os pterygoideum and Processus pterygoideus in su. F

28 ***Hamulus pterygoideus***. Hook-like process at the rostro-ventral end of the Os pterygoideum. B F

29 *Sulcus hamuli pterygoidei*. Groove on the lateral surface or rostral border of the Hamulus pterygoideus. F

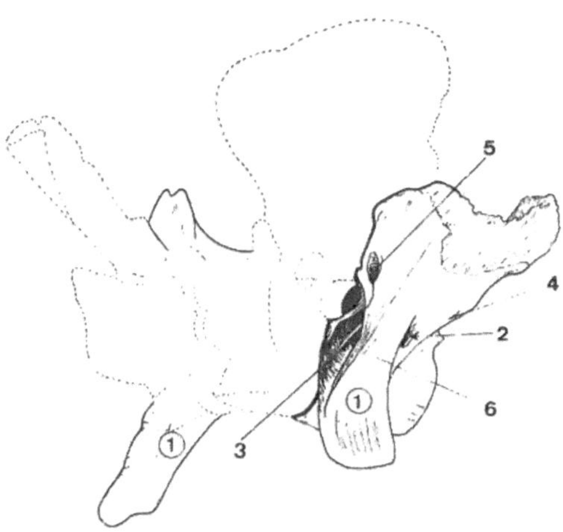

A Os basisphenoidale, left rostral aspect (eq)

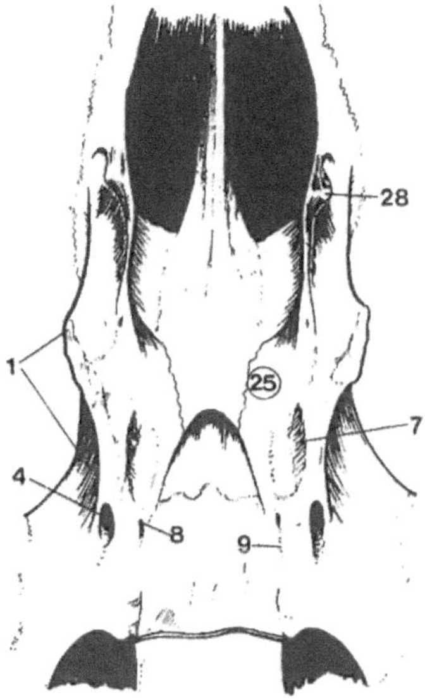

B Part of base of skull, ventral aspect (eq, young)

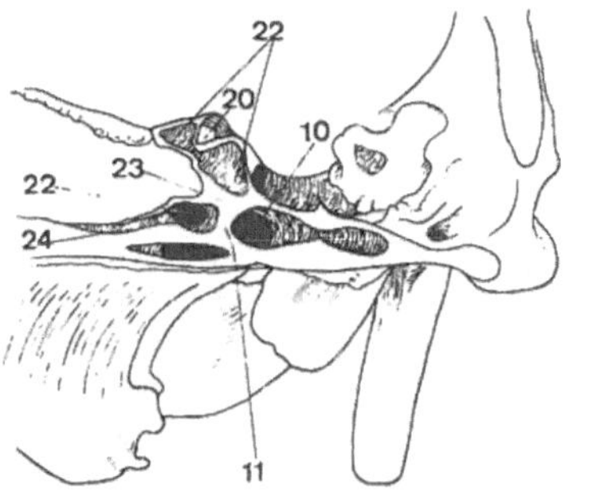

C Part of base of skull, paramedian section, left aspect (su)

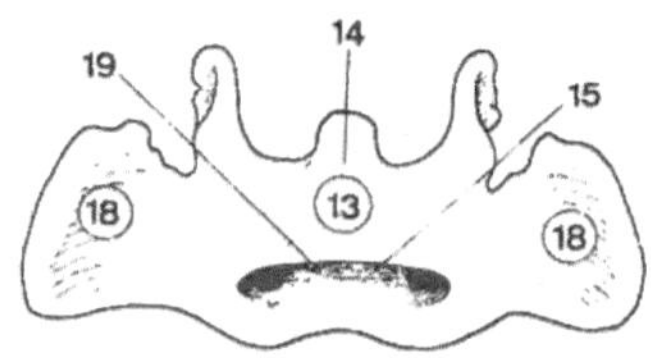

D Os presphenoidale, dorsal aspect (eq)

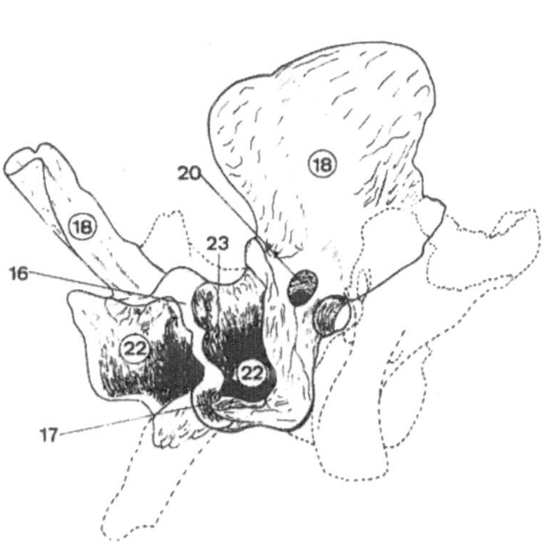

E Os presphenoidale, left rostral aspect (eq)

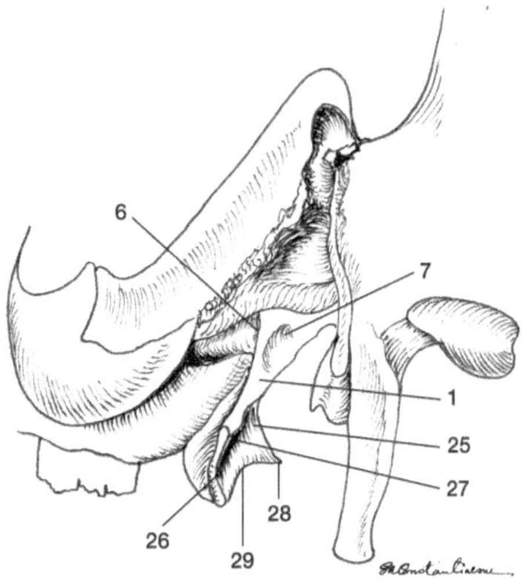

F Left Processus pterygoideus and Os pterygoideum, laterocaudal aspect (su)

1 **Os temporale.** Temporal bone. E

2 **Pars petrosa.** Petrous part of the Os temporale, petrosal bone. A B C D E

3 ***Facies occipitalis.*** Surface of the petrosal bone facing the Os occipitale. A

4 ***Processus mastoideus.*** Ventral process, caudal to the external auditory meatus. A B C

5 ***Sulcus a. meningeae caudalis.*** Groove on the lateral surface of the petrosal bone in eq, for the passage of a. meningea caudalis. B

6 ***Canalis facialis.*** Canal for N. facialis, originates in the internal acoustic meatus and terminates at the Foramen stylomastoideum. C

7 *Geniculum canalis facialis.* Sharp bend of the facial canal in a laterocaudal direction. C

8 ***Canaliculus chordae tympani.*** Narrow passage for the Chorda tympani between facial canal and tympanic cavity. C

9 ***Apex partis petrosae.*** Tip of the petrosal bone directed rostroventrally. D E

10 ***Facies rostralis partis petrosae.*** Rostral surface of the petrosal bone, directed rostroventrally. B D E

11 *Tegmen tympani.* Roof of the tympanic cavity. D E

12 *Canalis n. petrosi majoris.* Canal in the rostral wall of the petrosal bone for the N. petrosus major. E

13 *Canalis n. petrosi minoris.* Canal in the rostral wall of the petrosal bone for the N. petrosus minor. E

14 *Impressio n. trigemini.* Depression near the Apex partis petrosae for the Ganglion trigeminale in fe and Un. A C E

15 *Canalis n. trigemini.* Canal for Ganglion trigeminale in ca. D

16 ***Crista partis petrosae.*** Sharp crest in ca and eq (low in bo) between rostral and medial surfaces of the petrosal bone. A D E

17 *Sulcus sinus petrosi dorsalis.* Groove for the dorsal petrosal sinus in the Crista partis petrosae in Car and eq. D

18 ***Facies medialis partis petrosae.*** Medial surface of the petrosal bone. A C D

19 *Porus acusticus internus.* Opening of internal acoustic meatus. A C D

20 *Meatus acusticus internus.* Internal auditory canal. A D

21 *Fossa cerebellaris.* Large depression dorsal to the Meatus acusticus internus for the cerebellum. A

22 **Fossa subarcuata.** Deep depression dorsal to the Porus acusticus internus in Car. D

23 **Aqueductus [Aquae-] vestibuli.** Canal for the Ductus endolymphaticus. A

24 **Apertura externa aqueducti vestibuli.** External opening of Aqueductus vestibuli. A

25 ***Margo ventralis partis petrosae.*** Ventral border of petrosal bone. A C D

26 *Incisura jugularis.* Jugular notch, rostral border of the Os temporale for the Foramen jugulare. D

27 *Canaliculus cochleae.* Canal for the Ductus perilymphaticus. A

28 **Apertura externa canaliculi cochleae.** External opening of the Canaliculus cochleae. A

29 ***Facies ventralis partis petrosae.*** Ventral surface of the petrosal bone. C

30 *Canaliculus mastoideus.* Canal for Ramus auricularis n. vagi. A C

31 *Processus styloideus.* Cylindric process in Ru and eq, rough area in Car and su. B C

32 *Foramen stylomastoideum.* Opening of the Canalis facialis. B C

33 *Canaliculus tympanicus.* Small canal for N. tympanicus. A

34 *Fossula petrosa.* Small fossa for the Ganglion distale of N. glossopharyngeus. A

35 ***Cavum tympani.*** (vide Organum vestibulocochleare).

36 ***Fissura petrotympanica.*** Between Pars petrosa and Pars tympanica. A E

37 ***Fissura petrosquamosa.*** Between Pars petrosa and Pars squamosa. Found in cap, ov, su, eq, ossifies in the other species. E

38 ***Fissura tympanomastoidea.*** Between Pars tympanica and Pars mastoidea. A B

39 ***Fissura tympanosquamosa.*** Between Pars tympanica and Pars squamosa. Found in cap, ov, eq, ossifies in the other species. E

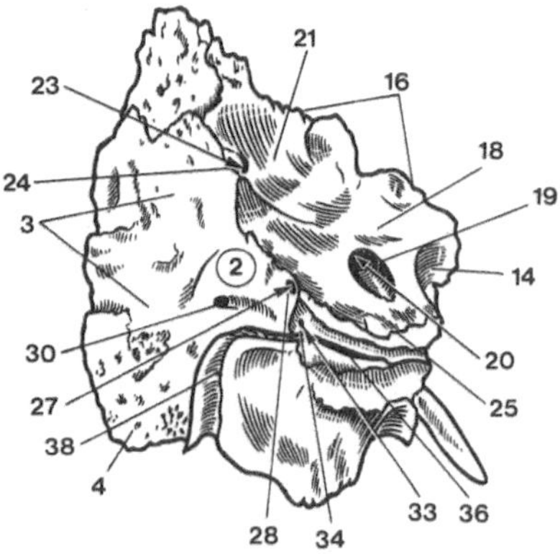

A Petrous and tympanic parts of left temporal bone, caudomedial aspect (eq)

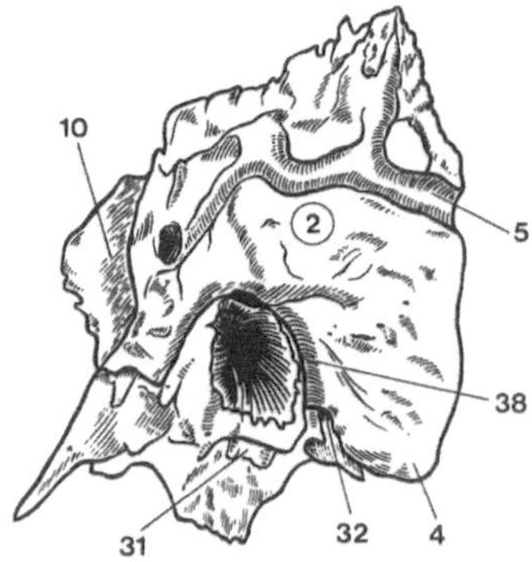

B Petrous and tympanic parts of left temporal bone, lateral aspect (eq)

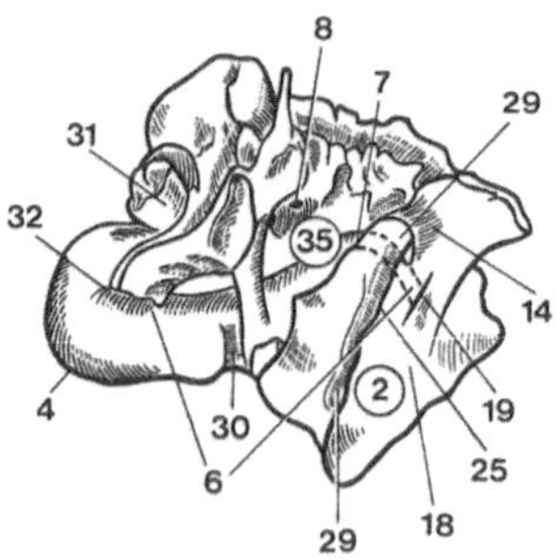

C Petrous and (part of) tympanic parts of right temporal bone (tympanic cavity open), ventral aspect (eq)

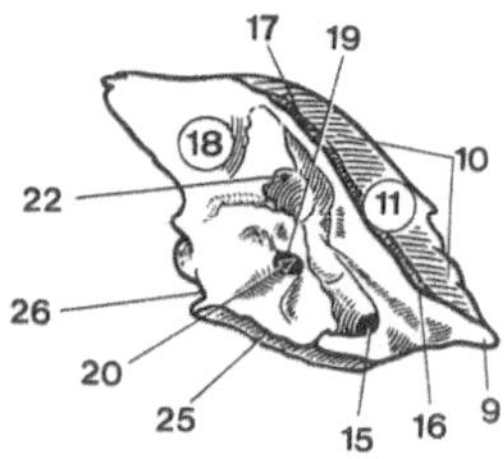

D Petrous part of left temporal bone, mediodorsal (and caudal) aspect (ca)

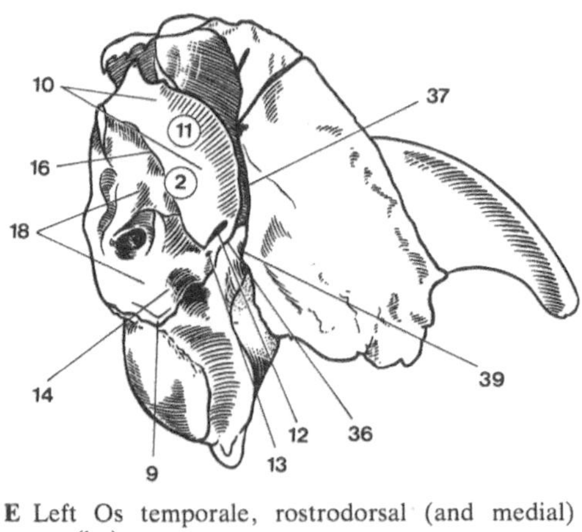

E Left Os temporale, rostrodorsal (and medial) aspect (bo)

1 **Pars tympanica**. Tympanic part of Os temporale. A B C

2 ***Anulus tympanicus***. Thin ring which almost completely surrounds the tympanic membrane. A

3 ***Sulcus tympanicus***. Groove in the Anulus tympanicus for attachment of the tympanic membrane. A

4 ***Meatus acusticus externus****. Osseous external acoustic meatus. B

5 ***Porus acusticus externus****. Opening of the osseus external acoustic meatus. B C

6 ***Vagina processus styloidei***. Sheath of the styloid process in Ru and eq. B

7 ***Processus muscularis***. Rostroventral process, long in Ru and eq, short in su and ca. A B

8 ***Bulla tympanica****. Ventral thin-walled extension enclosing part of the tympanic cavity. A

9 *Septum bullae*[1)]. Septum in the tympanic bulla in ca. A

10 ***Canalis caroticus***. Canal through the medial wall of the tympanic bulla for the A. carotis interna in ca. A

11 *Canaliculi caroticotympanici*. Small canals connecting Canalis caroticus and Cavum tympani in ca. A

12 ***Canalis musculotubarius***. Double canal leading into the tympanic cavity for the Tuba auditiva and the M. tensor veli palatini, formed by Pars tympanica in su and eq and additionally by Os basisphenoidale in Car and Ru. A

13 *Semicanalis m. tensoris veli palatini*. A

14 *Semicanalis tubae auditivae*. A

15 *Septum canalis musculotubarii*. Separates incompletely the lateral Semicanalis m. tensoris veli palatini and the medial Semicanalis tubae auditivae. A

16 **Pars endotympanica**. Forms in fe the large medial part of the Bulla tympanica. Does not ossify directly from connective tissue as the Pars tympanica, but is preformed in cartilage. C

17 ***Bulla tympanica****. In fe the larger medial part of the bulla is formed by the Pars endotympanica. C

18 *Septum bullae*[1)]*. Is formed in fe by the Pars tympanica and the Pars endotympanica. C

19 **Pars squamosa**. Squamous part of the Os temporale. C D

20 ***Margo parietalis***. Dorsal border adjoining the parietal bone. C D

21 ***Processus occipitalis***. Caudal process of the squamous part, forms a suture with the Os occipitale. C D

22 ***Margo frontalis***. Rostrodorsal border adjoining the frontal bone in su, bo, eq. D

23 ***Margo sphenoidalis***. Rostroventral border adjoining the sphenoid bones. D

24 ***Facies temporalis***. Temporal (external) surface. C D

25 ***Crista supramastoidea***. Ridge crossing the external surface transversely for attachment of Fascia temporalis. C D

26 ***Processus zygomaticus****. Forms part of the zygomatic arch. C D E

27 ***Fossa mandibularis***. Fossa for the condyle of the mandible. C D

28 *Facies articularis*. For the Caput mandibulae. C D

29 ***Tuberculum articulare***. Rounded eminence rostral to the Fossa mandibularis. C D

30 ***Processus retroarticularis***. Process caudal to Fossa mandibularis. C D

31 ***Foramen retroarticulare***. External opening of the Meatus temporalis (for Sinus temporalis), rudimentary in fe and su. D

32 ***Incisura tympanica***. Notch facing the Pars tympanica. D

33 ***Processus retrotympanicus***. Process caudal to Pars tympanica, absent in fe. D

34 ***Facies cerebralis***. Cerebral (internal) surface. E

35 *Crista tentorica*. The Tentorium cerebelli is attached to a crest of the Pars squamosa in su, ov and cap. E

36 ***Sinus frontalis caudalis***. Excavates also the Pars squamosa of the temporal bone in old su and bo. E

37 ***Sinus sphenoidalis***. Excavates also the Pars squamosa in old su. E

1) In ca the septum separates the tympanic cavity into a fundic part and a dorsal part, whereas in fe the septum separates the tympanic bulla in a dorsolateral and a ventromedial compartments; the septum has a surgical importance especially in Ventral bulla osteotomy and in Feline respiratory tract polyps.

A Pars tympanica of left temporal bone, rostrodorsal aspect (ca)

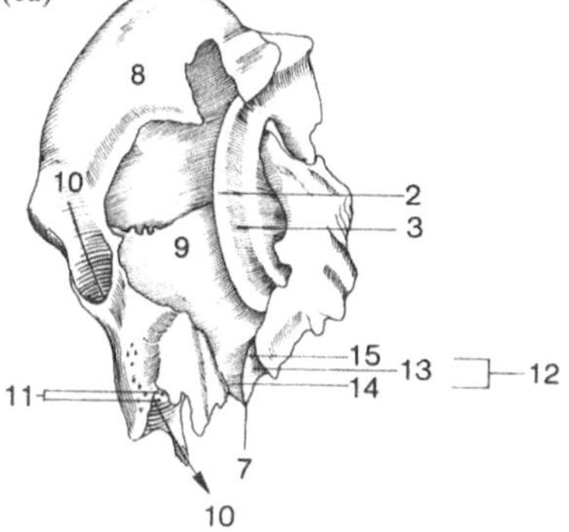

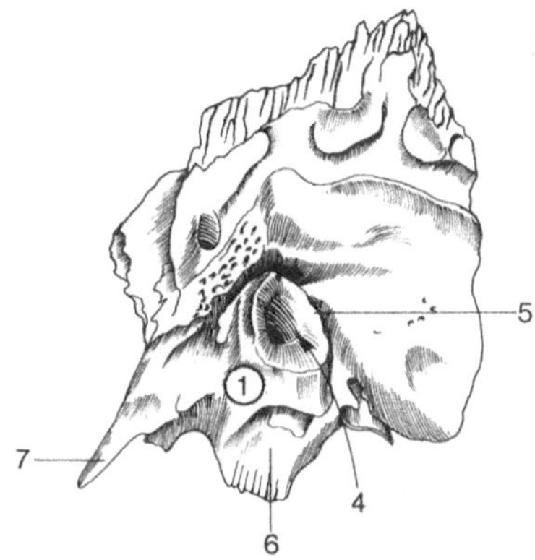

B Petrous and tympanic parts of left temporal bone, lateral aspect (eq)

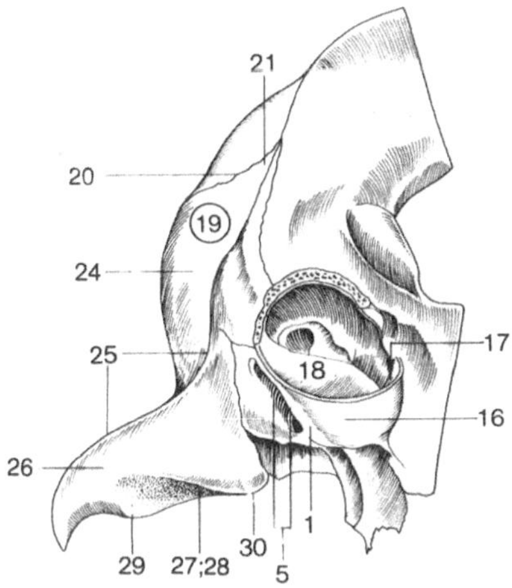

C Cranial bones (Bulla tympanica opened), caudoventral aspect (fe)

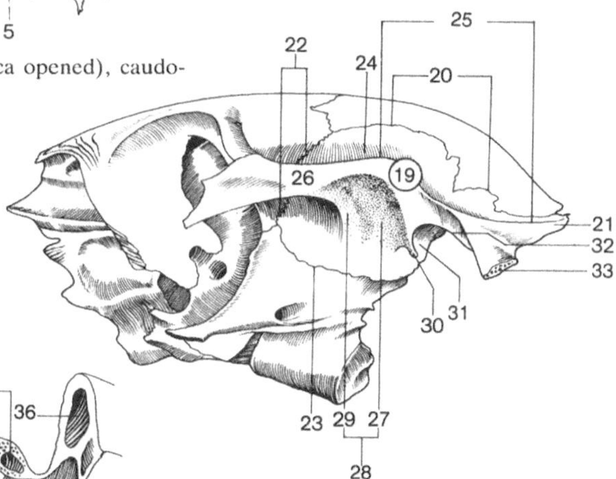

D Left cranial bones (eq)

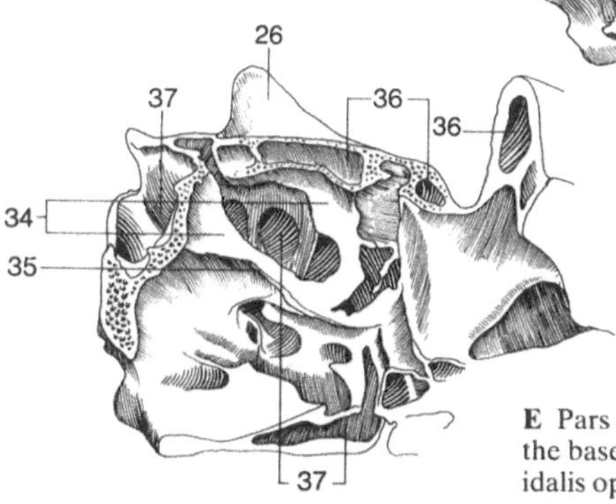

E Pars squamosa of left temporal bone and part of the base of skull (Sinus frontalis caudalis and sphenoidalis opened), dorsomedial aspect (su)

1 **Os parietale**. Parietal bone. A B C D E

2 ***Facies interna***. Internal surface. B D E

3 *(Crista sagittalis interna)*. Inconstant median ridge on the internal surface of Os parietale of eq. D

4 *Processus tentoricus*. Part of Tentorium cerebelli osseum in Car and eq. D

5 ***Facies externa***. External surface. A B C E

6 *Crista sagittalis externa**. External median crest in Car and eq. C

7 *Linea temporalis**. Border of the Fossa temporalis to which the Fascia temporalis is attached. C

8 *Tuber parietale*. More or less pronounced eminence on the external surface in Car and eq. A C

9 ***Margo occipitalis***. Border adjoining the Os occipitale. A B D

10 ***Margo squamosus***. Border adjoining the Os temporale. A B D

11 ***Margo sagittalis***. Median border. A B D E

12 ***Margo interparietalis***. Border adjoining Os interparietale, in ca Processus interparietalis. A B D

13 ***Margo frontalis***. Border adjoining the Os frontale. A B D

14 ***Angulus frontalis***. Rostrodorsal angle. A B D

15 ***Angulus occipitalis***. Dorsocaudal angle. A

16 ***Angulus sphenoidalis***. Rostroventral angle. A B D

17 ***Angulus mastoideus***. Ventrocaudal angle. A B D

18 ***Planum parietale***. Dorsal part of the external surface, medial to Linea temporalis, in dolichocephalic ca and in bo not existent. A E

19 ***Planum temporale***. Lateral part of the external surface, covered by the M. temporalis. A B

20 ***Planum nuchale***. Caudal part of the external surface in bo. B

21 ***Sulcus sinus sagittalis dorsalis***. Median groove for the Sinus sagitalis dorsalis. D

22 ***Sinus frontalis caudalis***. Excavates also the Os parietale in su and bo. E

23 *Septum sinuum frontalium*. Separates the symmetrical frontal sinuses. E

24 **Os frontale**. Frontal bone. A C E F

25 ***Squama frontalis***. Squama of the frontal bone. A F

26 *Facies externa*. External surface. A E F

27 **Tuber frontale**. Flat eminence on the external surface of Os frontale, visible especially in ca and bo. A C F

28 **Arcus superciliaris**. Elevation dorsal to the Margo supraorbitalis, especially in Ru. F

29 *Margo supraorbitalis*. Supraorbital margin. A C F

30 **Foramen supraorbitale***. Opening near the base of the Processus zygomaticus for passage of blood vessels and nerve in eq. A C

31 **Incisura supraorbitalis**. Notch in the Margo supraorbitalis sometimes present in ca.

32 **Canalis supraorbitalis**. Canal medial to the Margo supraorbitalis for passage of blood vessels and nerve in su and Ru. E F

33 *Sulcus supraorbitalis*. Groove from the opening of the Canalis supraorbitalis in rostral (su, Ru) and caudal (bo) directions. E F

34 ***Facies temporalis***. Temporal (lateral) surface. A

35 *Linea temporalis**. Border of the Fossa temporalis, to which the Fascia temporalis in attached. C F

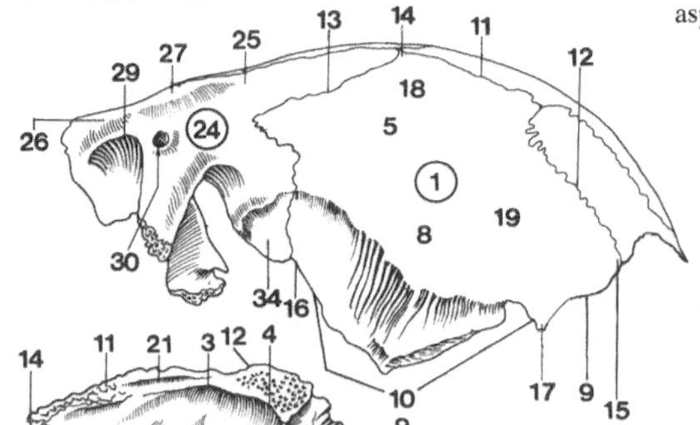

A Os parietale and Os frontale, caudolaterodorsal aspect (eq, young)

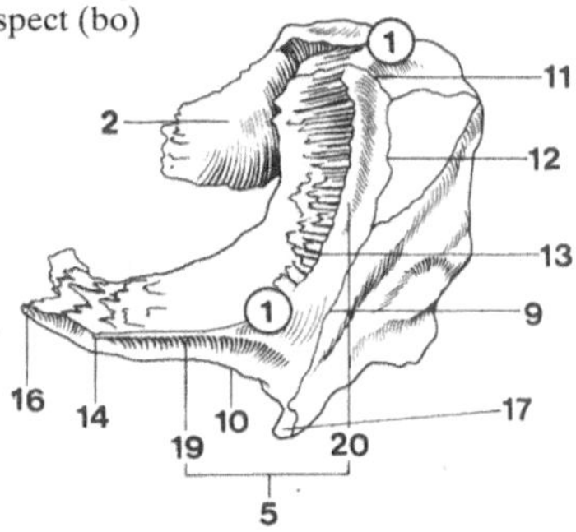

B Squama occipitalis, Os interparietale and Ossa parietalia, left and caudodorsal aspect (bo)

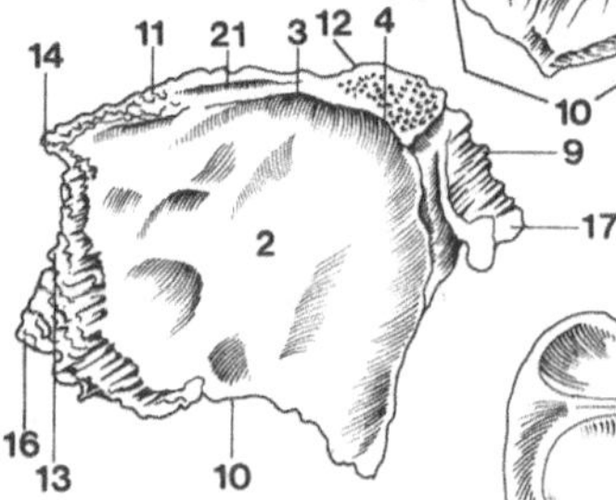

D Right Os parietale, ventromedial aspect (eq)

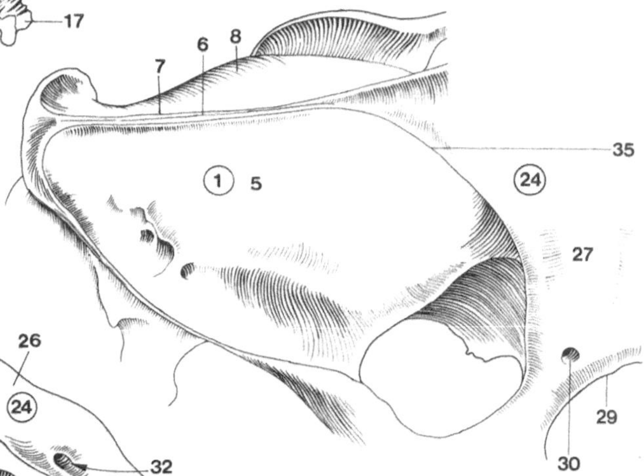

C Calvaria, right dorsal aspect (eq, old)

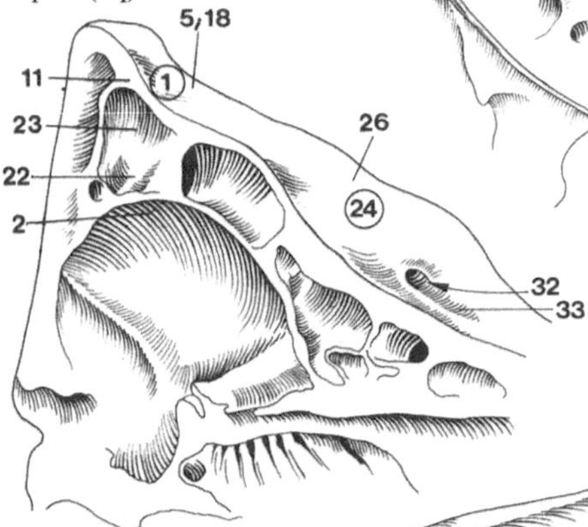

E Cranium, median section, rostromedial aspect, left half (su)

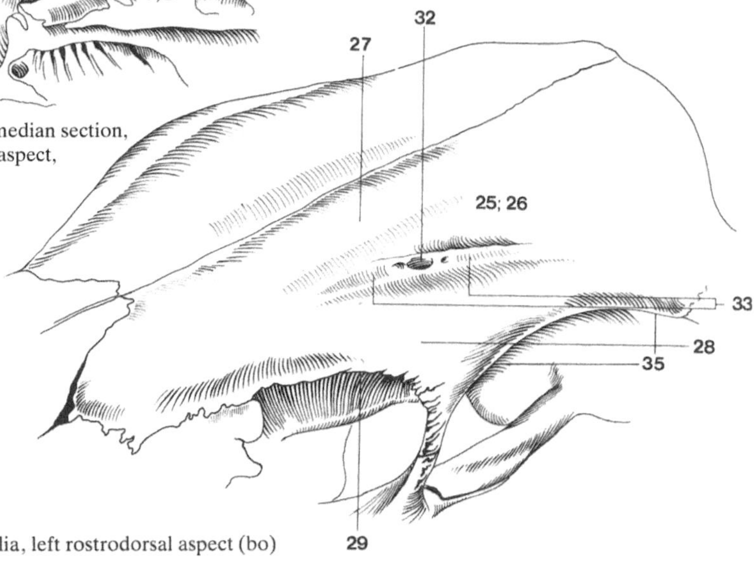

F Ossa frontalia, left rostrodorsal aspect (bo)

1 *Crista orbitotemporalis*. Crest between Pars orbitalis and Pars temporalis. B C

2 *Processus zygomaticus*. Lateral to the Orbita, connection with Os zygomaticum in Ru, Os temporale in eq, Lig. orbitale in Car and su. A B C

3 **Fossa glandulae lacrimalis**. Depression for the lacrimal gland in Ru and eq. A

4 ***Facies interna***. Internal surface, facing the brain. A D

5 *Crista frontalis*. Median crest on the internal surface for the attachment of Falx cerebri. A

6 *Sulcus sinus sagittalis dorsalis*. Groove in caudal continuation of the Crista frontalis for the Sinus sagittalis dorsalis. A

7 *Margo ethmoidalis*. Ethmoidal margin between internal surface and Pars nasalis, junction with the ethmoid bone. A D

8 ***Pars nasalis***. Rostral part of the frontal bone facing the nasal cavity. A D

9 *Margo nasalis*. Rostral border of the Pars nasalis. A B

10 ***Pars orbitalis***. Forms a part of the medial wall of the orbit. A

11 *Facies orbitalis*. Orbital surface, facing the Orbita. B C

12 **Fovea trochlearis**. Small depression for the attachment of trochlea serving the M. obliquus dorsalis. B C

13 **Foramen ethmoidale**. Opening in the Pars orbitalis, but on the border adjoining the ethmoid bone in eq. B

14 **Foramina ethmoidalia**. There are usually two foramina in the Pars orbitalis in ca. C D

15 **Crista orbitalis ventralis**. Crest which marks the junction between Orbita and Fossa pterygopalatina. C

16 *Incisura ethmoidalis*. Notch between right and left orbital parts into which the ethmoid bone is inserted. A

17 *Incisura sphenoidalis*. Notch between orbital and temporal parts into which the wing of the presphenoid is inserted in Ru and eq. A

17a *Incisura supraorbitalis caudalis* (or). Caudal supraorbital notch.

17b *Incisura supraorbitalis rostralis* (or). Rostral supraorbital notch.

18 ***Processus cornualis****. Supports the horn in horned Ru. B

19 *Corona processus cornualis*. Crown of the cornual process, an enlargement distal to its neck. B

20 *Collum processus cornualis*. Neck of the cornual process, a constriction of its base. B

21 ***Margo parietalis***. Border adjoining the Os parietale. A B D

22 ***Margo sagittalis***. Median border. A D

23 ***Sinus frontalis***. Frontal sinus in fe and eq. A

24 ***Sinus frontales***. Frontal sinuses in ca, su, and Ru. The plural indicates that there are more than one Sinus frontalis on each side. D

25 *Aperturae sinuum frontalium*. Openings of the frontal sinuses into the nasal cavity or the caudal maxillary sinus (eq). D

26 *Septa sinuum frontalium*. All septa between frontal sinuses. D

27 ***Processus septalis***. In Car, forms with the septal processes of the nasal bones a dorsal part of the Septum nasi. D

28 **Os ethmoidale**. Ethmoid bone. E F

29 ***Lamina cribrosa***. Cribriform plate, between the nasal cavities and the cranial cavity, perforated for the passage of Nn. olfactorii. E F

30 ***Crista galli***. Median ridge into the cranial cavity for attachment of Falx cerebri. E

31 ***Lamina perpendicularis***. Median plate forming the caudal part of the Septum nasi. E

32 ***Labyrinthus ethmoidalis***. Collective term for the Ethmoturbinalia. F

33 *Ethmoturbinalia*. Delicate scroll-like bones in the nasal cavity. F

34 **Ectoturbinalia**. Large ethmoturbinates, do not reach the nasal septum. F

35 **Endoturbinalia**. Small and numerous ethmoturbinates, reach the nasal septum. F

36 **Cellulae ethmoidales**. Exist in su and Ru. F

37 **Meatus ethmoidales**. Spaces between ethmoturbinates. F

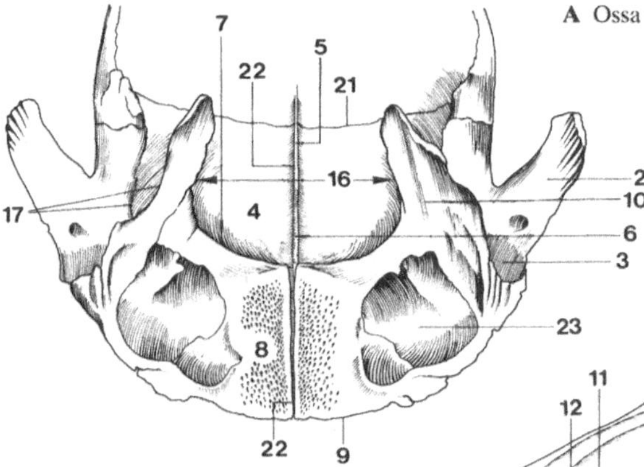

A Ossa frontalia, rostroventral aspect (eq)

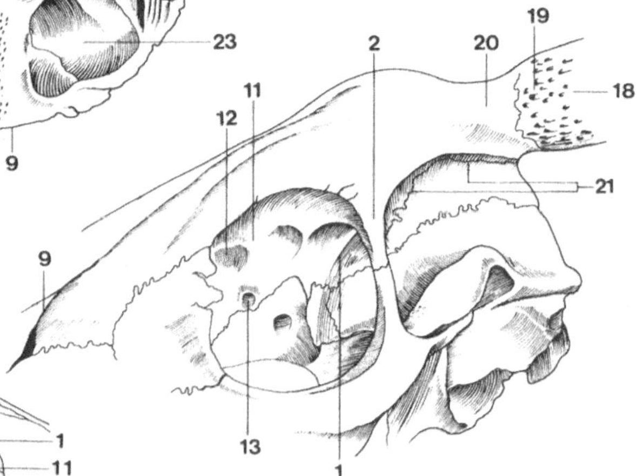

B Left cranial bones, rostrolateral aspect (bo)

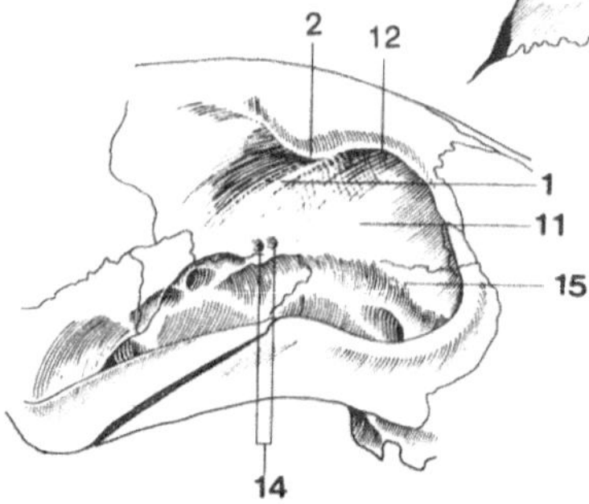

C Right orbit, lateral aspect (ca)

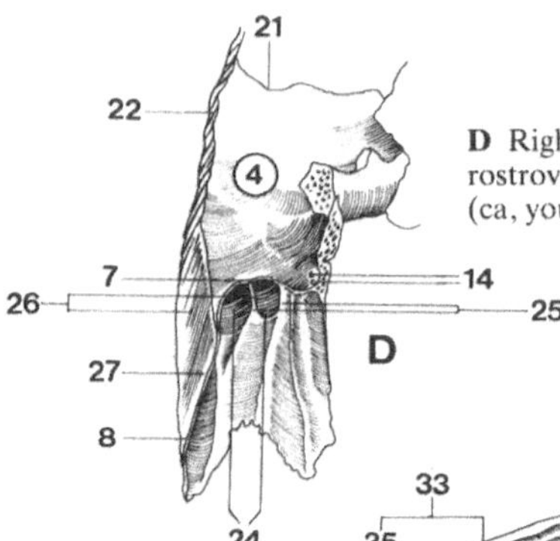

D Right Os frontale, rostroventral aspect (ca, young)

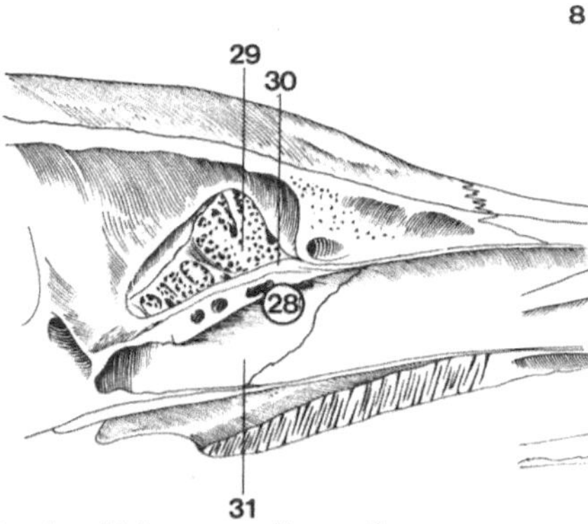

E Os ethmoidale, paramedian section, left (and dorsal) aspect (su)

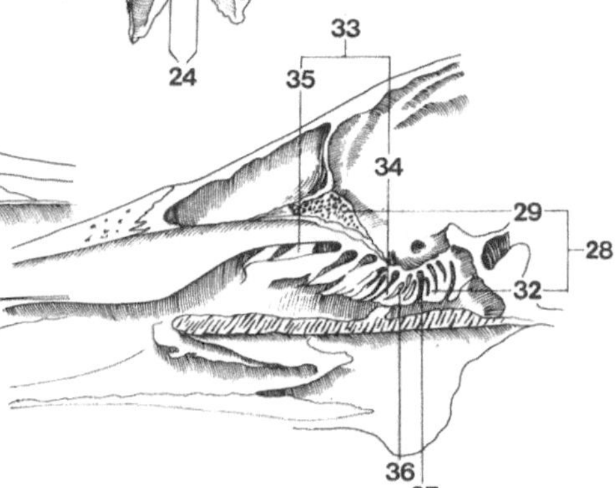

F Os ethmoidale, paramedian section, medial aspect, right half (su)

1 ***Lamina orbitalis***. Thin lateral plate, only in su and bo forming a part of the medial wall of the Fossa pterygopalatina, in Car the medial wall of the Recessus maxillaris. A D

2 ***Foramen ethmoidale***. Only in eq does the ethmoid take part in forming this foramen. B

3 ***Lamina tectoria***. Upper plate, forming the roof of the Labyrinthus ethmoidalis. B C

4 ***Lamina basalis***. Lower plate, forming the floor of the Labyrinthus ethmoidalis. C D

5 ***Concha nasalis dorsalis***. Dorsal nasal concha. B C

6 *Processus uncinatus*. Rostrodorsal end of Lamina orbitalis, detached from the nasal wall, partially closes the entrance to the Recessus maxillaris in Car. D

7 ***Concha nasalis media***. Middle nasal concha. C

8 **Vomer**. E

9 ***Sulcus vomeris [septalis]***. Dorsal groove containing the Cartilago septi nasi. E

10 ***Crista vomeris***. Ventral crest on the caudal part of the Vomer. E

11 ***Ala vomeris***. Wing-like lateral process on the caudal end of the Vomer. E

12 **OSSA FACIEI**. Facial bones.

13 **Os nasale**. Nasal bone. A C F G

14 ***Facies externa***. External surface. A F

15 *Sulcus supraorbitalis*. In su the Sulcus supraorbitalis extends onto the Os nasale. A F

16 ***Facies interna***. Internal surface. G

17 ***Processus septalis***. Sagittal crest for attachment of Cartilago septi nasi. G

18 ***Crista ethmoidalis***. Sagittal crest for attachment of Concha nasalis dorsalis. It continues onto the Os nasale. G

19 ***(Sinus frontalis)***. May excavate also the Os nasale in su, bo and eq. C

20 **Os lacrimale**. Lacrimal bone. A H I

21 ***Facies orbitalis***. Orbital surface, facing the Orbita. A H

22 ***Facies facialis***. Facial surface, rostral to the Orbita, small in ca, absent in fe. A

23 ***Facies nasalis***. Nasal (internal) surface. I

24 ***Incisura infratrochlearis****. Notch for passage of N. infratrochlearis. H

25 ***Processus frontalis***. Dorsal process into a notch of the Os frontale in ca. D

26 ***Processus lacrimalis caudalis****. Process on Margo supraorbitalis in Ru and eq. H

27 ***Processus lacrimalis rostralis***. Small process on Facies facialis in su and eq. A

28 ***Fossa lacrimalis externa***. On Facies orbitalis in su and ov. A

29 ***Fossa sacci lacrimalis***. Depression on Facies orbitalis for Saccus lacrimalis, absent in su. H

30 ***Foramen lacrimale***. Opening for the Ductus nasolacrimalis, absent in su. H

31 ***Foramina lacrimalia*** (su). Two openings on Facies facialis in su. A

32 ***Canalis lacrimalis***. Canal for the Ductus nasolacrimalis. I

33 ***Fossa m. obliqui ventralis***. Depression for muscle attachment. A H

34 ***Bulla lacrimalis***. Large thin-walled protuberance into the ventral part of the Orbita in Ru. H I

35 *Sinus maxillaris* (Ru). Extends also into the Bulla lacrimalis in Ru. I

36 ***Sinus lacrimalis*** (bo). Excavates the Os lacrimale except the Bulla lacrimalis, entrance from the Sinus maxillaris. I

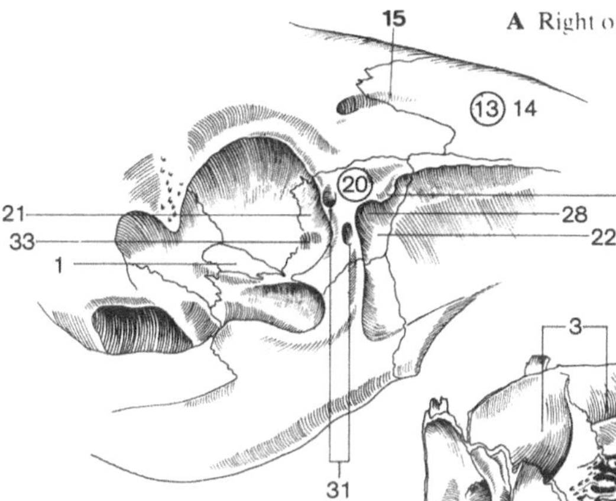

A Right orbit, dorsolateral aspect (su)

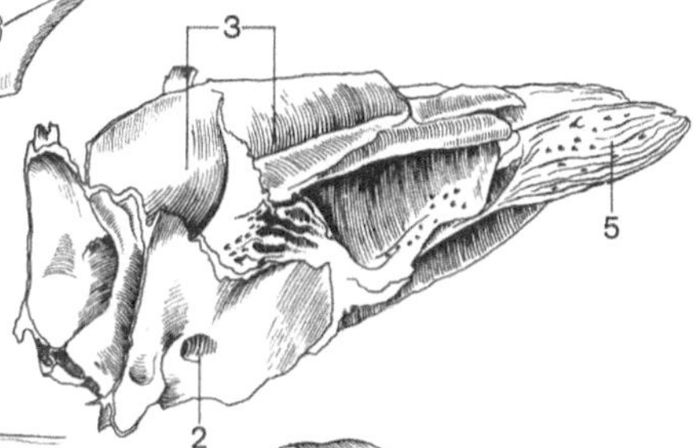

B Os ethmoidale, right dorsocaudal aspect (eq)

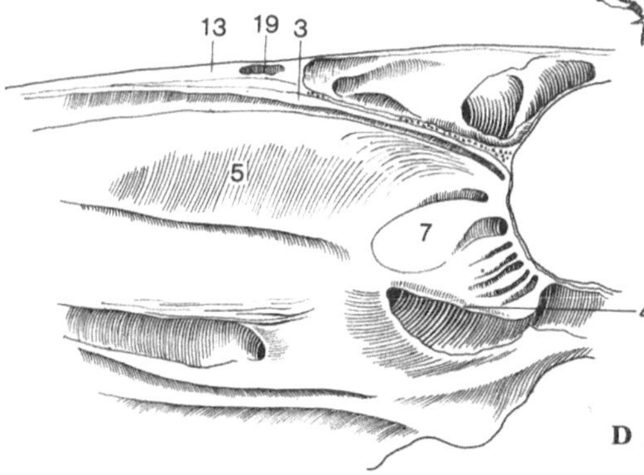

C Part of right half of nasal cavity, paramedian section, medial aspect (eq)

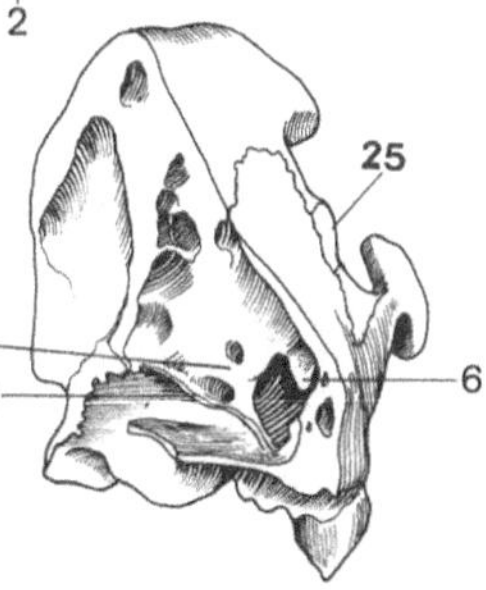

D Left facial bones, rostromedial aspect (ca)

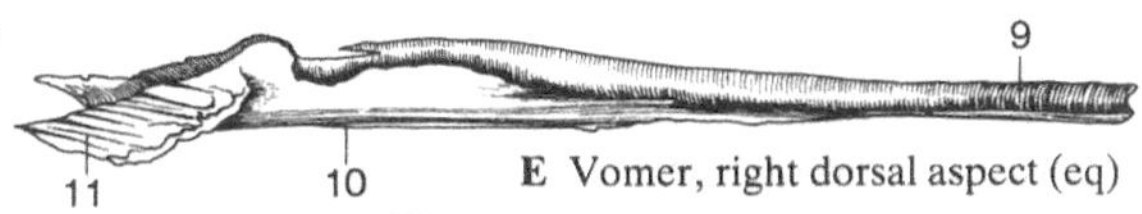

E Vomer, right dorsal aspect (eq)

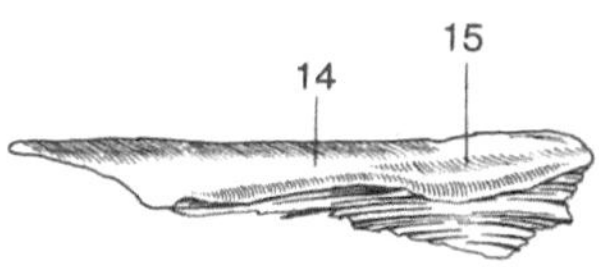

F Left Os nasale, dorsolateral aspect (su)

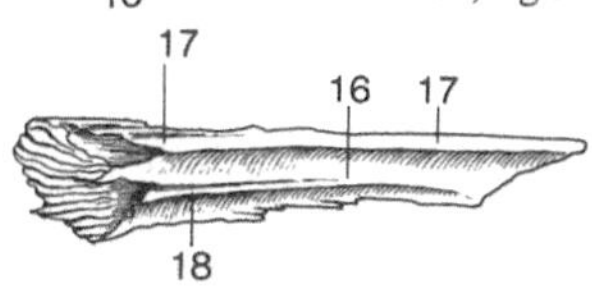

G Left Os nasale, ventromedial aspect (su)

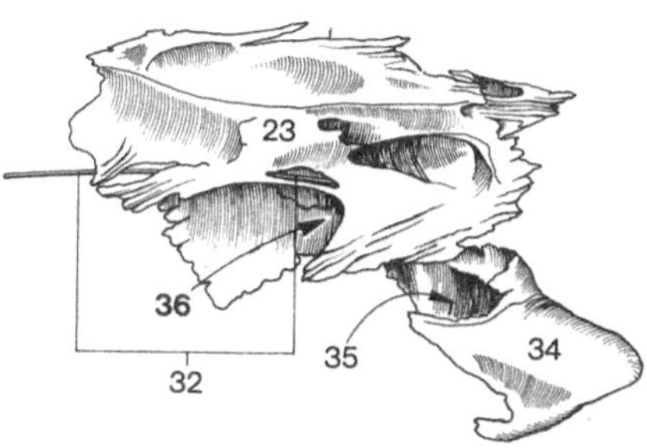

I Right Os lacrimale, medial aspect (bo)

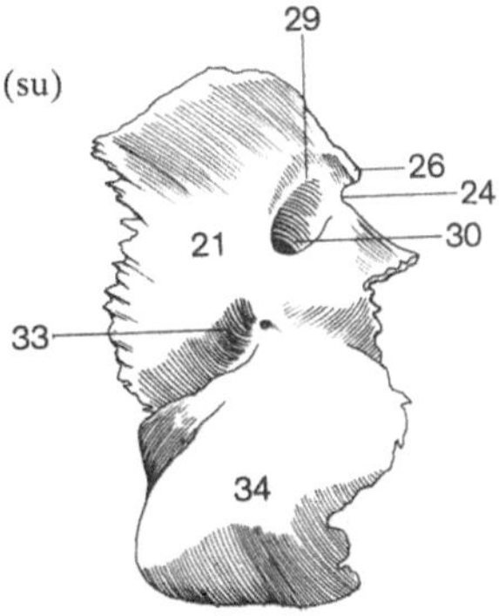

H Right Os lacrimale, caudal aspect (bo)

1 ***(Sinus lacrimalis)*** (su, ov, cap). In these species only occasionally as individual diverticulum of the nasal cavity, in other cases the Os lacrimale – except the Bulla – is excavated by a frontal sinus (see 3 and 4). B

2 *Apertura sinus lacrimalis*. Opening/communication of Sinus lacrimalis. B

3 ***(Sinus frontalis rostralis lateralis)*** (su). See 1. A

4 ***(Sinus frontalis lateralis)*** (ov, cap). See 1. B

5 ***Sinus maxillaris caudalis*** (eq). Excavates also the Os lacrimale. C

6 **Maxilla**. Principal bone of the upper jaw. A B C D E F

7 **Corpus maxillae**. Body of the maxilla. C D E F

8 ***Facies orbitalis***. Orbital surface, which in fe and to a lesser extent also in eq forms part of the wall of the orbit. D

9 ***Facies facialis***. Facial surface. C D E F

10 *Crista facialis**. Facial crest, for attachment of M. masseter. Incomplete in Ru, usually doesn't end at the Tuber faciale. C D E F

11 **Tuber faciale***. Sometimes isolated tuber at the rostral end where Crista facialis in Ru should be. E

12 *Foramen infraorbitale**. Rostral opening of the Canalis infraorbitalis. C D E F

13 *Canalis infraorbitalis*. Contains the N. infraorbitalis and accompanying blood vessels. C

14 *Canalis alveolaris*. Contains the nerves and blood vessels for Dentes incisivi, caninus, and premolares, absent in Ru. F

15 *Fossa canina*. Concavity dorsal to Crista facialis and Foramen infraorbitale in su. F

16 *Juga alveolaria*. Ridges caused by the underlying teeth. C D F

17 ***Facies pterygopalatina***. Caudal surface facing the Fossa pterygopalatina. D

18 *Foramina alveolaria*. Small openings for nerves and blood vessels for the molar teeth. D

19 *Canales alveolares*. Canals for all alveolar and dental branches of nerves and vessels to the molar teeth. D

20 *Tuber maxillae*. Prominence on the caudal end of maxilla. A C D E

21 *Foramen maxillare*. Caudal opening of the Canalis infraorbitalis. A

22 ***Facies nasalis***. Nasal (medial) surface. A B

23 *Sulcus lacrimalis*. Groove for the Ductus nasolacrimalis, rostral continuation of 24. A B

24 *Canalis lacrimalis*. Canal for the Ductus nasolacrimalis. A B

25 *Crista conchalis*. Ridge for the attachment of the Concha nasalis ventralis. A

26 *Hiatus maxillaris*. Wide opening into Sinus maxillaris after removal of Os ethmoidale and Concha nasalis ventralis. It is bounded solely by the Maxilla. A

27 ***Sulcus palatinus major***. Groove for greater palatine nerve and vessels, forms with Sulcus palatinus major of Os palatinum the Canalis palatinus major (except bo). A

28 ***Sinus maxillaris***. Maxillary sinus in su and Ru. A

29 ***Sinus maxillaris rostralis***. Smaller rostral maxillary sinus in eq. C

30 ***Sinus maxillaris caudalis***. Larger caudal maxillary sinus in eq. C

31 ***Septum sinuum maxillarium***. Septum between rostral and caudal maxillary sinuses in eq. C

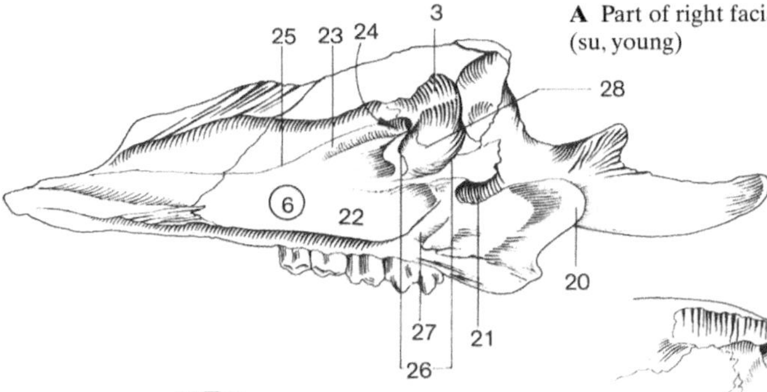

A Part of right facial bones, medial aspect (su, young)

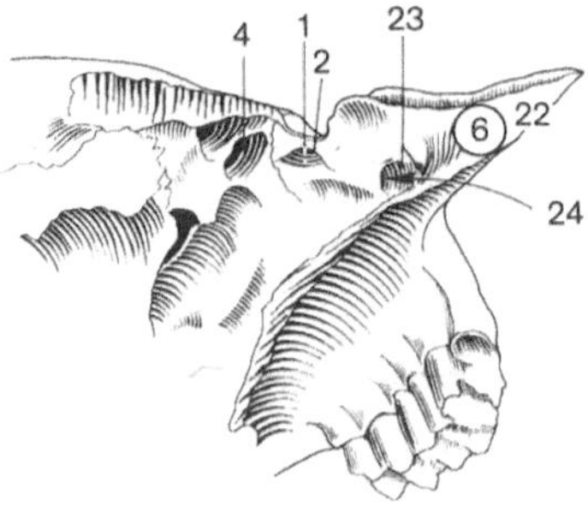

B Part of left facial bones, mediorostroventral aspect (cap)

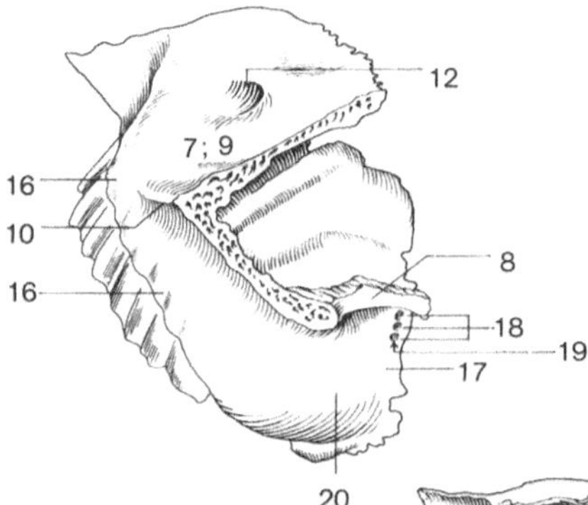

D Left maxilla, laterocaudal aspect (eq)

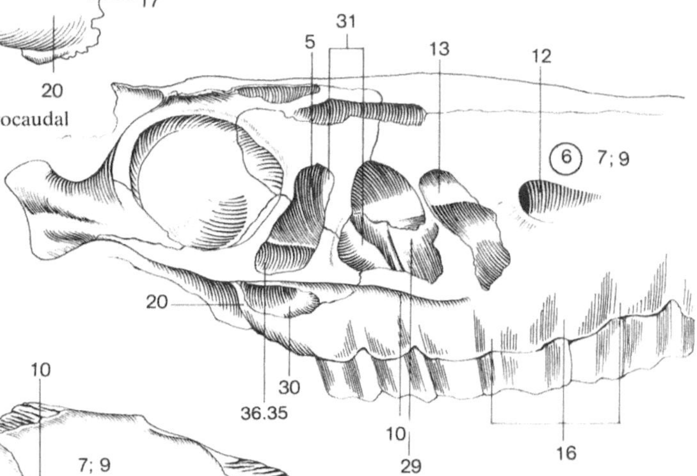

C Right facial bones (sinus opened), lateral aspect (eq)

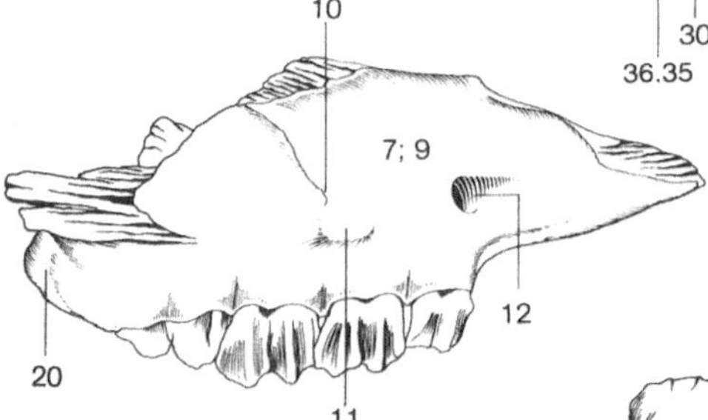

E Right maxilla, lateral aspect (bo)

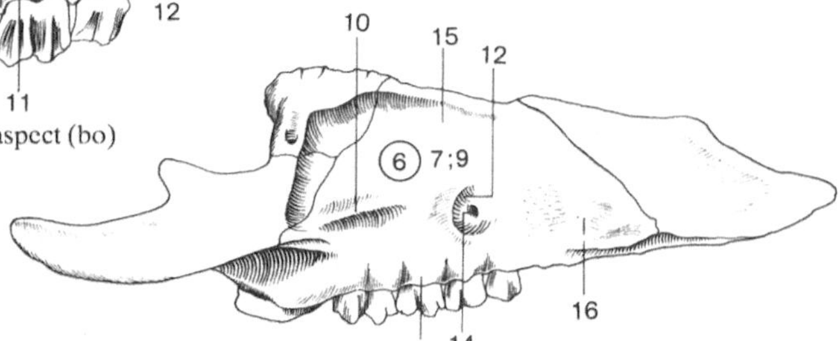

F Part of right facial bones, lateral aspect (su, young)

1 **Processus frontalis** (Car). Frontal process in Car. A

2 ***Crista ethmoidalis***. The line of attachment of the Concha nasalis dorsalis also runs across the maxilla in Car and su. A

3 **Processus zygomaticus.** Caudal process dorsolateral to the Tuber maxillae, adjoining the Os zygomaticum. A

4 **Processus palatinus.** Plate forming the largest portion of the hard palate. A B C D

5 ***Crista nasalis***. Median crest for attachment of Septum nasi (Vomer). A C

6 ***Sulcus palatinus***. Sagittal groove on the oral surface for the greater palatine nerve and vessels. B D

7 ***Foramen palatinum majus***. Rostral opening of Canalis palatinus, formed only by the maxilla in su and sometimes in ca. B

8 ***Sinus palatinus***. Excavates the Processus palatinus of the maxilla in Ru. C

9 *Septum sinuum palatinorum*. Septum between right and left palatine sinuses in Ru. C

10 **Processus alveolaris**. Ventral process presenting the alveoli for the teeth. D

11 ***Margo alveolaris****. Border of the Processus alveolaris presenting alveoli. D

12 ***Margo interalveolaris****. The rostral part of Processus alveolaris of maxilla does not present alveoli. Part of the Diastema. D

13 ***Alveoli dentales****. Cavities in the Processus alveolaris for the roots of the teeth. D

14 ***Septa interalveolaria***. Septa between the alveoli of neighboring teeth. D

15 *Septa interradicularia*. Septa between the chambers for the roots of one tooth. D

16 **Os conchae nasalis ventralis**. Ventral nasal conchal bone. A

17 **Os incisivum**. Incisive bone, rostral part of the upper jaw. B C D E

18 **Corpus ossis incisivi**. Body of the incisive bone. B C D E

19 ***Facies labialis***. Labial (external) surface, facing the upper lip. E

20 ***Facies palatina***. Palatine (internal) surface. B D E

21 **Processus alveolaris**. Process presenting the alveoli for the incisor teeth (except Ru). D E

22 ***Arcus alveolaris***. Arcuate border of the Processus alveolaris. D E

23 ***Alveoli dentalis****. Cavities in the Processus alveolaris for the roots fo the incisor teeth. D E

24 ***Septa interalveolaria***. Septa between alveoli. D E

25 ***Margo interalveolaris****. The caudal part of Processus alveolaris of Os incisivum does not present alveoli. Part of the Diastema. D E

26 ***Juga alveolaria***. Prominences on the external surface caused by the teeth. E

27 **Processus palatinus**. Thin plate forming the rostral portion of the hard palate. B C D E

28 **Processus nasalis**. Projects caudodorsally, forms part of the lateral wall of the nasal cavity. C E

29 **Os rostrale**. Forms the rostral end of the Septum nasi in su, sometimes in bo. F

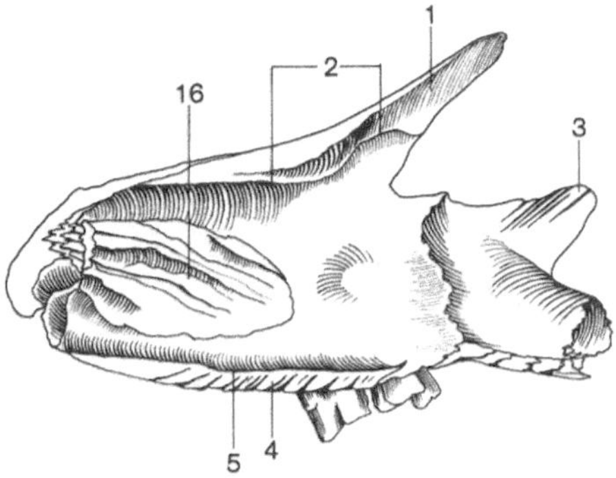

A Right maxilla, medial aspect (ca, young)

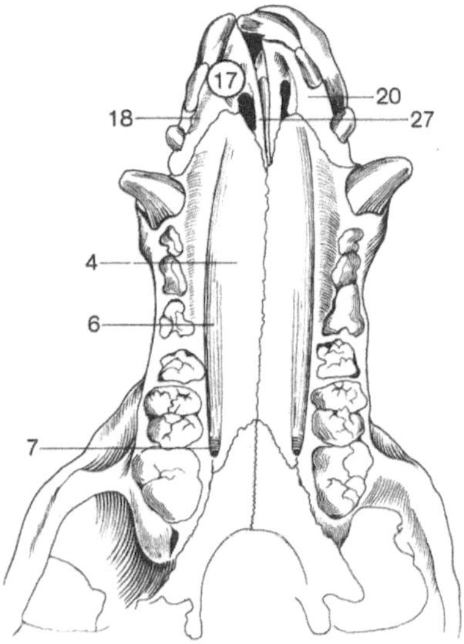

B Hard palate (su, young)

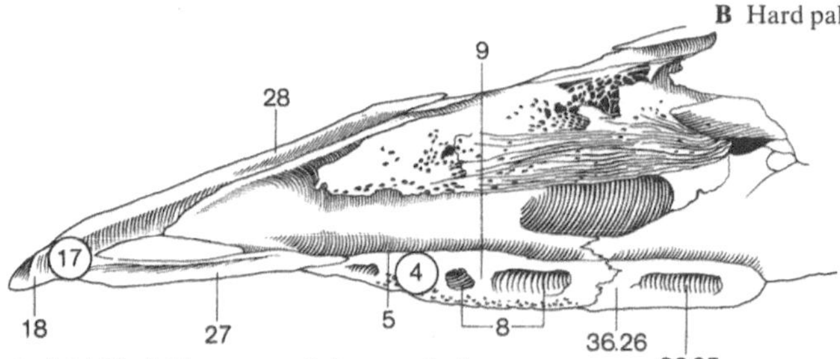

C Part of right facial bones, medial aspect (bo)

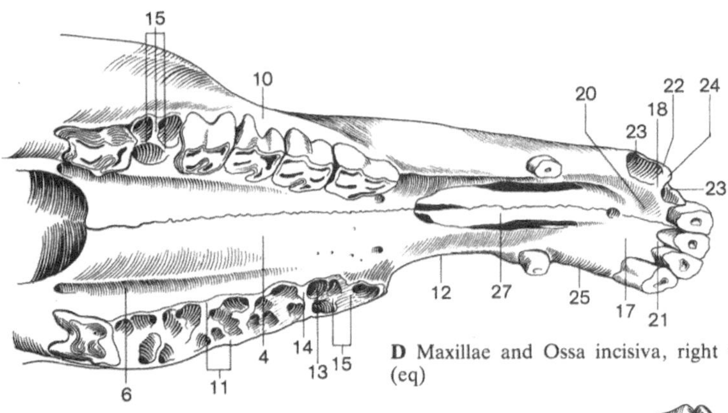

D Maxillae and Ossa incisiva, right ventral aspect (eq)

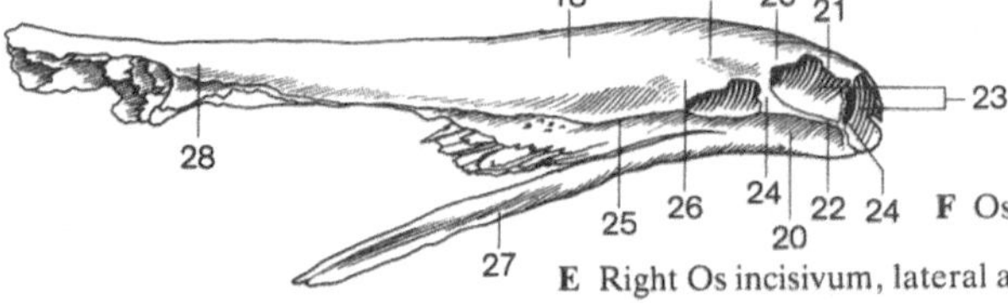

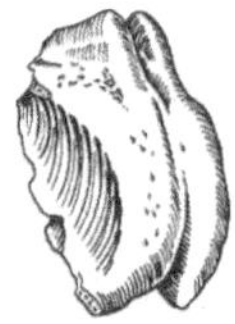

F Os rostrale, right rostral aspect (su)

E Right Os incisivum, lateral aspect (eq)

1 **Os palatinum**. Palatine bone. A B C D

2 **Lamina perpendicularis**. Perpendicular plate. A B C D

3 ***Facies nasalis***. Nasal (medial) surface. A C D

4 ***Facies maxillaris***. Maxillary (lateral) surface. B

5 ***Incisura sphenopalatina***. Notch present in bo and sometimes in eq, part of the Foramen sphenopalatinum. A B

6 ***Foramen sphenopalatinum***. Opening between Fossa pterygopalatina and Cavum nasi, in bo and sometimes in eq only partially formed by the Os palatinum. C

7 ***Sulcus palatinus major***. Groove for the greater palatine nerve and vessels, forms with Sulcus palatinus major of the maxilla the Canalis palatinus major (except in bo). B

8 ***Canalis palatinus major***. In bo this canal is formed only by the Os palatinum. A

9 ***Processus pyramidalis***. Caudoventral process, inserted between Processus pterygoideus of the basisphenoid and Os pterygoideum, well developed in su, absent in Car. B

10 ***Crista ethmoidalis***. Rostral continuation of Lamina sphenoethmoidalis in ca for attachment of an ectoturbinate. C

11 ***Lamina sphenoethmoidalis***. Plate detached from Facies nasalis, parallel to Pars horizontalis. The laminae of both sides separate the Meatus nasopharyngeus from the ethmoidal labyrinths, caudally adjoining the presphenoid, rostrodorsally united with Lamina basalis of the ethmoid bone. Absent in Ru, long in ca and su. C

12 ***Processus orbitalis***. Dorsal process to the medial wall of the orbit. B C

13 ***Processus sphenoidalis***. Caudomedial process to the body of the presphenoid. B C

14 *(Sinus sphenoidalis)*. May excavate the Processus sphenoidalis in su and eq. D

15 **Lamina horizontalis**. Horizontal plate, forms the caudal portion of the hard palate. A B C D

16 ***Facies nasalis***. Nasal (dorsal) surface. C

17 ***Facies palatina***. Palatine (ventral) surface. A B D

18 ***Margo liber***. Free (caudal) border. A B C D

19 ***Spina nasalis caudalis***. Median caudal spine on the caudal border in Car, su and occasionally eq. C

20 ***Canales palatini minores***. Canals for the minor palatine nerves and vessels in ca, su and bo. A

21 ***Foramen palatinum majus***. Rostral opening of Canalis palatinus major, in bo entirely formed by the Os palatinum. A

22 ***Foramina palatina minora***. Rostral openings of the Canales palatini minores in ca, su, and bo. A

23 ***Crista nasalis***. Median dorsal crest, sometimes absent in bo. A C D

24 ***(Crista palatina)***. Ridge on Facies palatina, occasionally present in su. D

25 **Sinus palatinus**. In the Pars perpendicularis in eq, in the Pars horizontalis in Ru. 35 C

26 ***Septum sinuum palatinorum***. Median septum between the palatine sinuses in bo. 35 C

27 **Os zygomaticum**. Zygomatic bone. D E F

28 ***Facies lateralis***. Lateral surface. E

29 ***Facies orbitalis***. Surface facing the orbit. E F

30 ***Processus temporalis****. Caudally directed process which forms the zygomatic arch with the Processus zygomaticus ossis temporalis. D E F

31 ***Processus frontalis***. Adjoining the Processus zygomaticus ossis frontalis in Ru, the Lig. orbitale in Car and su. D E F

32 ***Margo infraorbitalis***. Infraorbital margin, separates lateral and orbital surfaces. E F

33 ***Crista facialis***. Facial crest, continuation from maxilla. E

34 ***Sinus maxillaris***. Excavates also the Os zygomaticum in su and Ru. D F

35 ***Sinus maxillaris caudalis***. Excavates also the Os zygomaticum in eq. 33 C

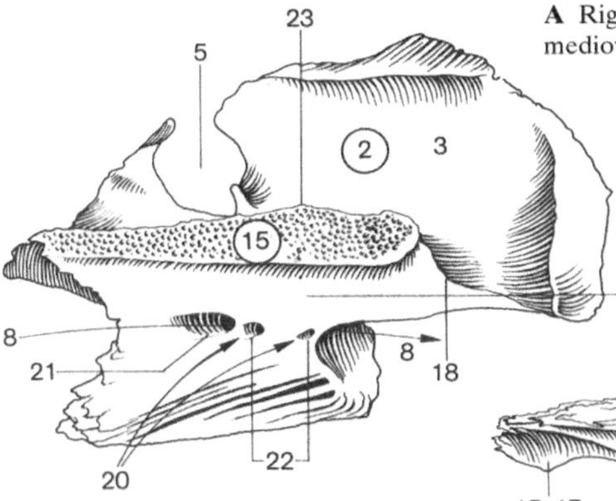

A Right Os palatinum, medioventral aspect (bo, young)

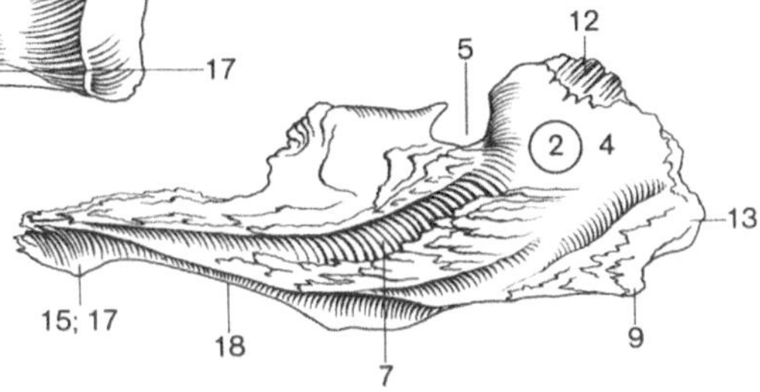

B Left Os palatinum, lateral aspect (eq)

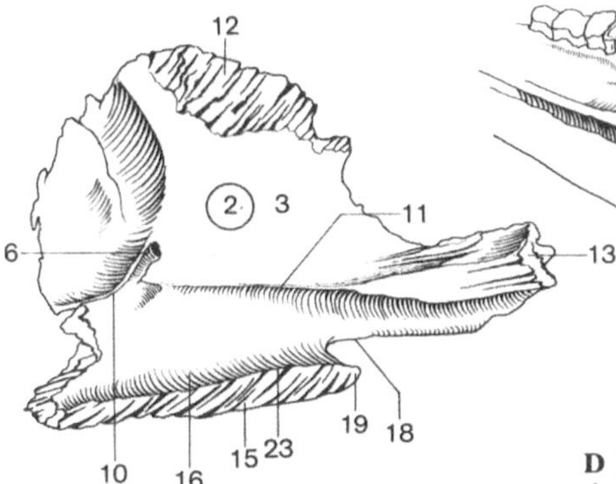

C Right Os palatinum, mediodorsal aspect (ca)

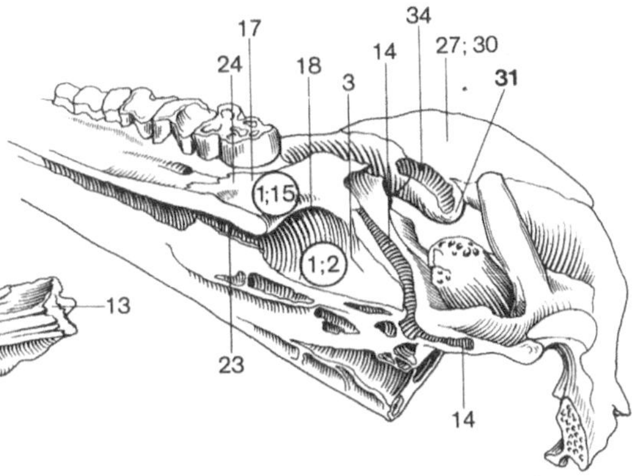

D Left Fossa pterygopalatina and part of the hard palate, Sinus sphenoidalis opened, caudoventromedial aspect (su)

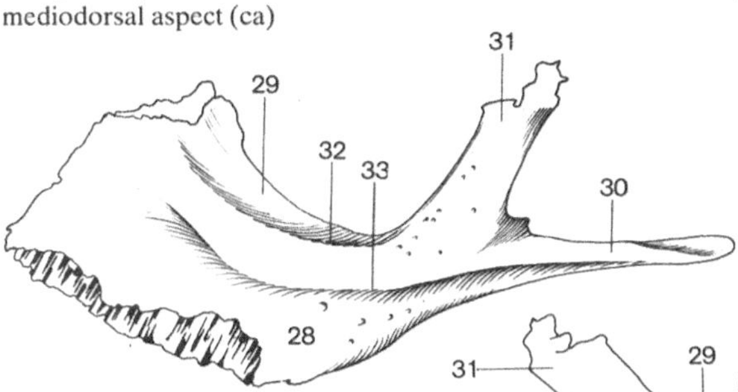

E Left Os zygomaticum, lateral aspect (bo)

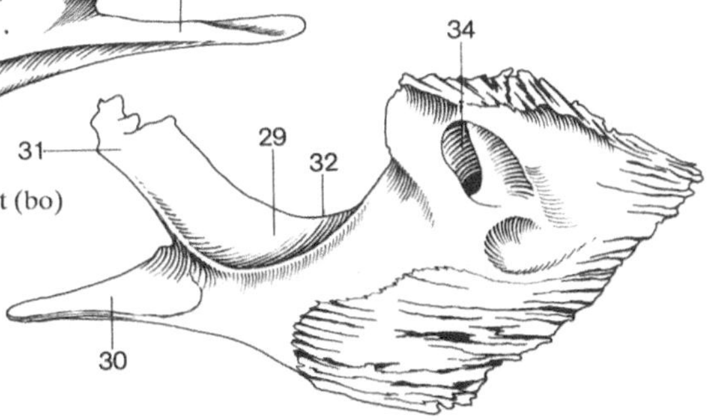

F Left Os zygomaticum, medial aspect (bo)

1 **Mandibula**. Mandible. Lower jaw bone. A B C D (The mandible is a paired bone as the result of fusion of two symmetrical bones, but usually it is called simply, the mandible.)

2 **Corpus mandibulae**. Body of mandible, presenting teeth. A B C D

3 ***Pars incisiva***. Rostral part with alveoli for incisor teeth. A B C D

4 *Arcus alveolaris**. Curved border of the Pars incisiva. A B D

5 *Canales alveolares*. Contain nerves and vessels for all incisor and canine teeth. A

6 ***Pars molaris***. Caudal part with alveoli for premolar and molar teeth. A B C D

7 *Margo alveolaris**. Dorsal border presenting alveoli. A B C D

8 *Margo ventralis*. Free ventral border. A B C D

9 **Incisura vasorum facialium***. Notch for facial vessels, absent in Car, ov, cap. A C D

10 *Foramen mentale**. Opening of Canalis mandibulae in Ru and eq. A

11 *Foramina mentalia**. Openings of Canalis mandibulae in Car. B

12 *Foramina mentalia lateralia**. Openings on the lateral surface of the mandible only in su. C

13 *Foramen mentale mediale*. Present only in su. C

14 ***Facies labialis***. Labial surface of Pars incisiva related to the lip. A B C

15 ***Facies buccalis***. Lateral surface of Pars molaris related to the cheek. A B C

16 ***Facies lingualis***. Lingual (internal) surface of the body of the mandible. D

17 *Linea mylohyoidea*. Line from which the M. mylohyoideus originates. C D

18 ***Alveoli dentales***. See 34.13. D

19 ***Septa interalveolaria***. See 34.14. D

20 *Septa interradicularia*. See 34.15. D

21 ***Juga alveolaria***. See 34.26. E

22 ***Margo interalveolaris****. Portion of dorsal border without alveoli, called also Diastema. A D

23 **Ramus mandibulae***. Dorsally directed caudal part of the mandible. A B C D

24 ***Angulus mandibulae****. Angle between body and ramus of the mandible. A B C D

25 *Processus angularis**. Caudoventral process in Car. B

26 ***Tuberositas m. sternomandibularis****. Insertion of M. sternocephalicus in eq (also called M. sternomandibularis). D

27 ***Fossa masseterica***. Depression on the lateral surface for M. masseter. B

28 ***Fossa pterygoidea***. Depression on medial surface for M. pterygoideus medialis. C D

29 ***Foramen mandibulae****. Dorsocaudal opening of the Canalis mandibulae on the medial surface. C D

30 *Canalis mandibulae*. Canal for N. alveolaris inf. A B C D

31 ***Sulcus mylohyoideus***. Groove rostroventral to Foramen mandibulae. C D

32 ***Processus coronoideus****. Process for the attachment of M. temporalis. A B C D

33 ***Incisura mandibulae****. Notch between coronoid and condylar processes. A B C D

34 ***Processus condylaris****. Condylar (articular) process. A B C D

35 *Caput mandibulae*. Articular head of Proc. condylaris. A B C D

36 *Collum mandibulae*. Neck of Processus condylaris. A B C

37 *Fovea pterygoidea*. Insertion of M. pterygoideus lateralis. C D

38 **Apparatus hyoideus [Os hyoideum]**. Hyoid apparatus [hyoid bone]. E

39 ***Basihyoideum [Corpus]****. Body, rostroventral part. E

40 *Processus lingualis**. Rostral process in Ru and eq. E

41 ***Ceratohyoideum [Cornu minus]***. Lesser horn. E

42 ***Thyrohyoideum [Thyreo-, Cornu majus]***. Greater horn. E

43 ***Epihyoideum***. Between Ceratohyoideum and Stylohyoideum, in su ligamentous. E

44 ***Stylohyoideum***. Between Epihyoideum and Tympanohyoideum. E

45 *Angulus stylohyoideus**. Angle of Stylohyoideum. E

46 ***Tympanohyoideum***. Between Stylohyoideum and Os temporale. E

A Left mandible, lateral aspect (bo)

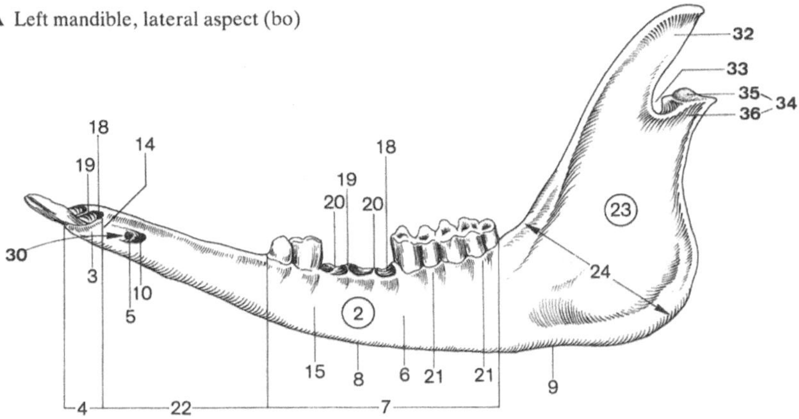

B Left mandible, lateral aspect (ca)

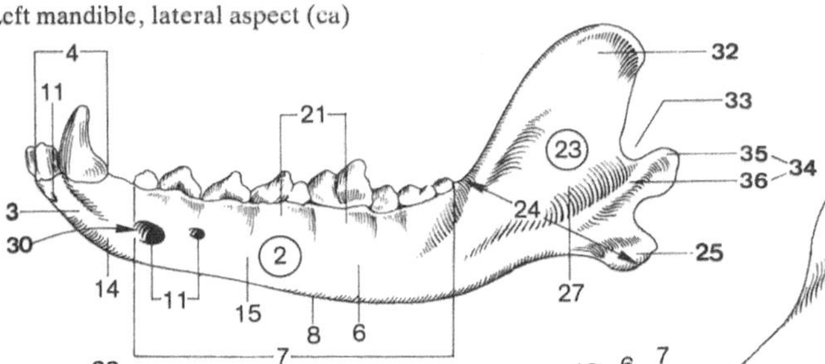

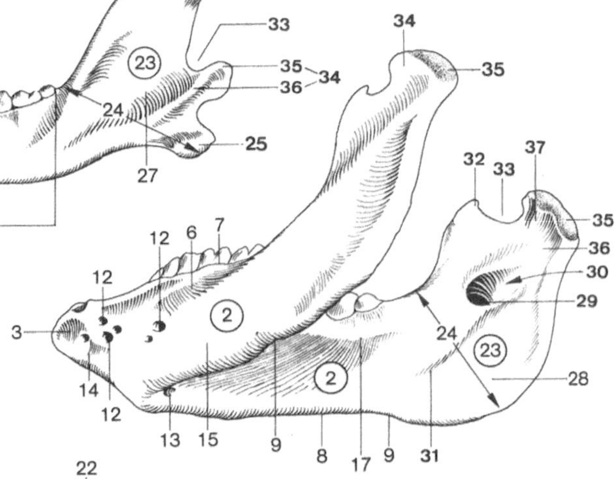

C Mandible, left caudoventral aspect (su)

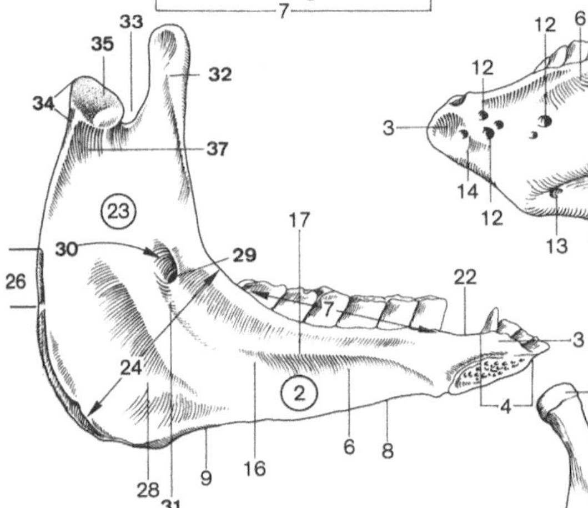

D Left mandible, caudomedial aspect (eq)

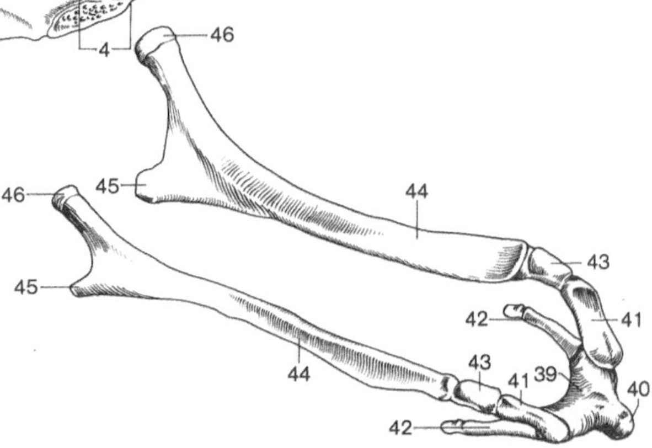

E Apparatus hyoideus, right dorsorostral aspect (bo)

1 **COLUMNA VERTEBRALIS.** Vertebral column. A

2 ***Corpus vertebrae.*** Body of vertebra. B

3 ***Extremitas cranialis [Caput vertebrae].*** Cranial extremity (head). B C

4 ***Extremitas caudalis [Fossa vertebrae].*** Caudal extremity. B

5 ***Crista ventralis.*** Ventral crest on the body of cervical, cranial and caudal thoracic, and lumbar vertebrae. B

6 ***Arcus vertebrae.*** Vertebral arch, forms the Foramen vertebrale dorsally and laterally. Each half (right or left) of an Arcus vertebrae consists of a ventral Pediculus, and a dorsal Lamina. C

7 *Pediculus arcus vertebrae.* Pedicle (root) of the arch, attached to the body. C

8 *Lamina arcus vertebrae.* Dorsal portion of vertebral arch. C

9 ***Foramen vertebrale.*** Formed by the vertebral arch and body. C

10 ***Canalis vertebralis.*** Vertebral canal, formed by the Foramina vertebralia, contains the spinal cord. B

11 ***Spatium interarcuale.*** Interval separating adjacent arches dorsally. B

12 ***Foramen intervertebrale.*** Opening between adjacent vertebrae for passage of a spinal nerve. B

13 ***Incisura vertebralis cranialis.*** Cranial notch on the Pediculus. B C

14 ***Incisura vertebralis caudalis.*** Caudal notch on the Pediculus. B

15 ***Foramen vertebrale laterale.*** Conversion of a large caudal notch into a foramen, esp. in thoracic vertebrae of bo, occasionally eq, often doubled in su. 43 D

16 ***Sulcus n. spinalis.*** Groove for spinal nerve on transverse process of fourth to sixth cervical vertebra in fe, su, and bo. C

17 ***Processus spinosus****. Spinous process. B C

18 ***Processus transversus.*** Transverse process. C

19 *Processus costalis**. The transverse process of a lumbar vertebra homologous to a rib. B

20 ***Processus articularis cranialis.*** Cranial articular process on the vertebral arch. B C

21 ***Processus articularis caudalis.*** Caudal articular process on the vertebral arch. B C

22 ***Processus accessorius.*** Between transverse and caudal articular process on caudal thoracic (Car and su), and lumbar (Car) vertebrae. B

23 ***Processus mamillaris.*** Between transverse and cranial articular process on thoracic and lumbar vertebrae. B

24 **Vertebrae cervicales.** Cervical vertebrae. A

25 ***Processus transversus.*** Transverse process. C

26 *Tuberculum ventrale.* Cranioventral branch of transverse process of third to fifth cervical vertebra. C 43 A B

27 *Lamina ventralis [vertebrae cervicalis VI].* Symmetrical rectangular plate, the enlargement of the Tuberculum ventrale. A

28 *Foramen transversarium.* Opening in transverse process for passage of vertebral vessels and nerve. C

29 *Tuberculum dorsale.* Caudodorsal branch of transverse process of third to sixth cervical vertebra. C

30 ***Fovea costalis caudalis [vertebrae cervicalis VII].*** For the head of the first rib. A

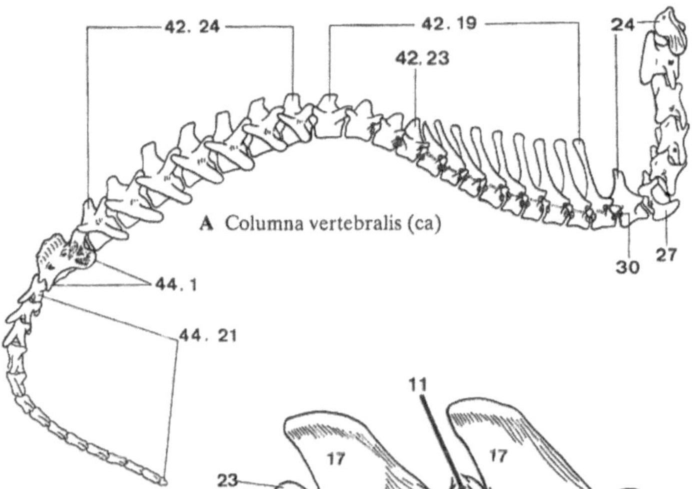

A Columna vertebralis (ca)

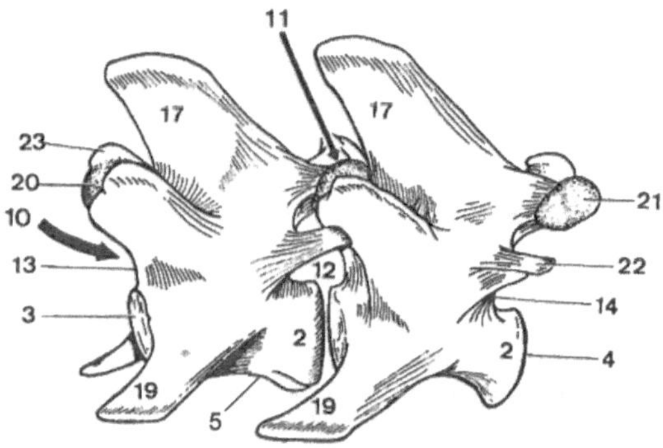

B Vertebrae lumbales II et III, left (and dorsal) aspect (ca)

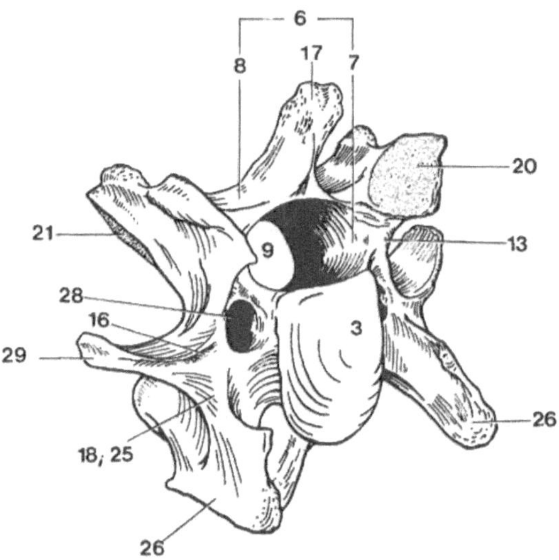

C Vertebra cervicalis IV, right cranial aspect (bo)

1 **Atlas**. First cervical vertebra, lacking a body. A B

2 ***Massa lateralis***. Lateral portion of the Atlas. A B

3 *Processus transversus [Ala atlantis]**. Transverse process (wing). A B

4 **Foramen alare**. Perforates the wing cranially for A. vertebralis, absent in Car. A

5 **Incisura alaris** (Car). Notch in the cranial border of the wing for A. vertebralis. B

6 *Fossa atlantis*. Concavity on ventral surface of the wing, esp. deep in eq, flat in Car. A

7 *Fovea articularis cranialis*. For articulation with the paired Condylus occipitalis. A

8 *Fovea articularis caudalis*. For articulation with Facies articularis of Axis. B

9 ***Arcus ventralis***. Ventral arch. It represents a small part of the body of the Atlas, the larger part being incorporated in the Dens and cranial articular surfaces of the Axis. A

10 *Fovea dentis*. Articular fovea for dens of axis on the dorsal surface of the ventral arch. B

11 *Tuberculum ventrale*. Ventral tubercle. Cranioventral branch of transverse process of third to fifth cervical vertebra. A B (This structure of the Atlas was omitted from the 5th edition of the N. A. V. It is listed for the rest of the Vertebrae cervicales on page 40.26. However, the ventral tubercle is also a structure of the atlas.)

12 ***Arcus dorsalis***. Dorsal arch. A B

13 *Tuberculum dorsale**. Dorsal tubercle, vestige of a spinous process. B

14 **Axis**. Second cervical vertebra. C

15 ***Dens***. Tooth-like cranial process of axis. C

16 *Apex*. Cranial extremity of the dens. C

17 *Facies articularis ventralis*. Ventral articular surface of the dens. C

18 *Facies articularis dorsalis*. Dorsal articular surface of the dens in Car and su. C

19 **Vertebrae thoracicae**. Thoracic vertebrae. 41 A

20 ***Fovea costalis cranialis***. Facet on the cranial extremity for the caudal part of the head of a rib. D

21 ***Fovea costalis caudalis***. Facet on the caudal extremity for the cranial part of the head of a rib. D

22 ***Fovea costalis processus transversi***. Articular facet on transverse process for the Tuberculum costae. D

23 ***Vertebra anticlinalis****. First vertebra in the caudal thoracic or lumbar region whose spinous process is perpendicular to the body. The spinous processes of the preceding vertebrae incline caudally. 41 A

24 **Vertebrae lumbales**. Lumbar vertebrae. 41 A

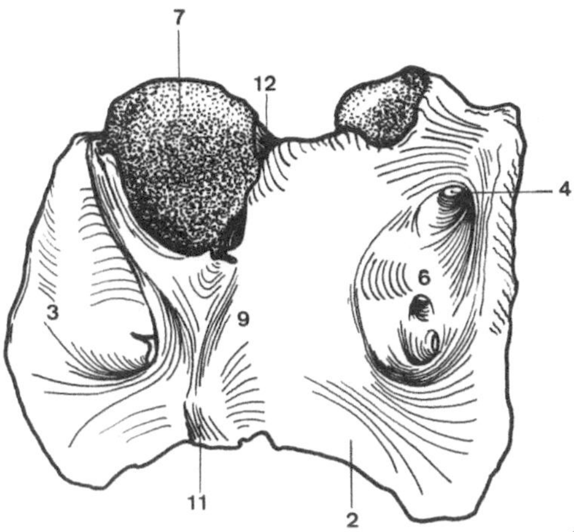

A Atlas, left ventral aspect (eq)

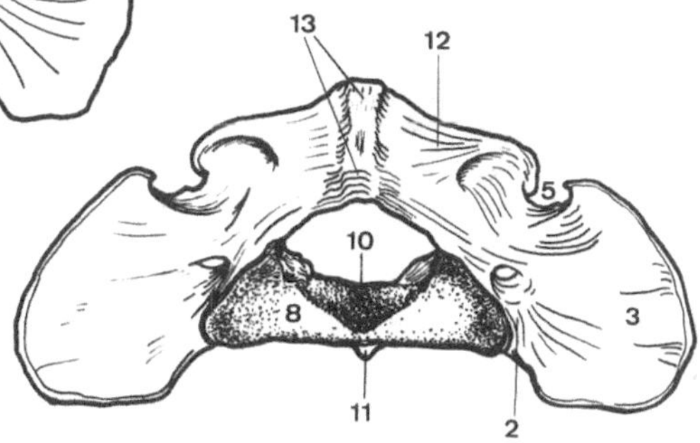

B Atlas, caudodorsal aspect (ca)

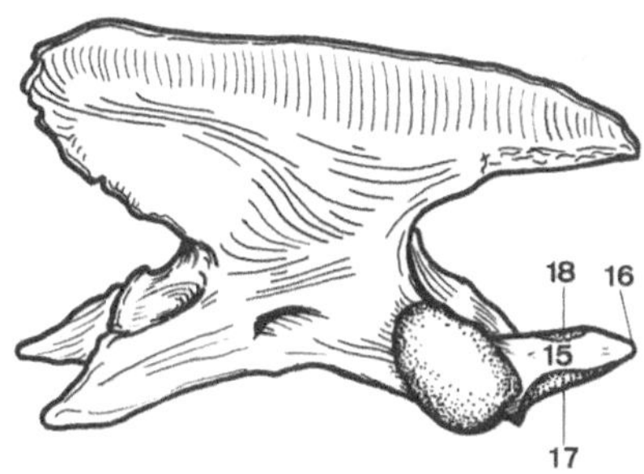

C Axis, right aspect (ca)

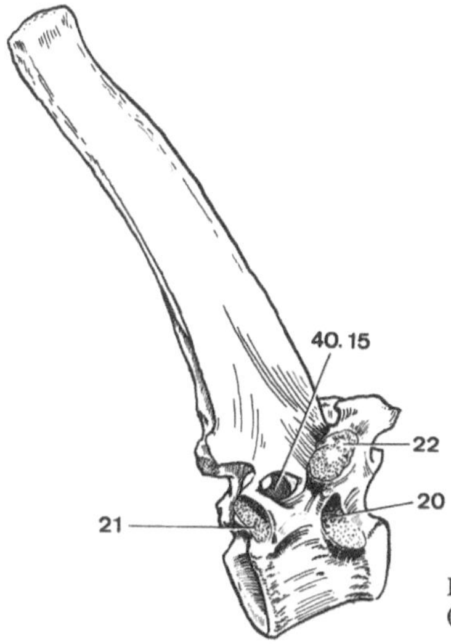

D Vertebra thoracica VIII, right (and caudal) aspect (eq)

1 **Os sacrum [Vertebrae sacrales].** Fused sacral vertebrae. A B C D

2 ***Basis ossis sacri.*** Base (cranial extremity) of sacrum. A B C D

3 *Processus articularis cranialis.* Articulates with the caudal articular process of the last lumbar vertebra. A C D

4 *Promontorium**. Ventral border of Basis ossis sacri projecting together with the intervertebral disc into the pelvic inlet. A B C

5 ***Pars lateralis.*** Lateral part, composed of fused transverse processes. A B D

6 *Ala sacralis.* Wing of sacrum, the elongated first (eq, bo) or first and second transverse processes. A B D

7 *Facies auricularis.* Auricular surface for articulation with the ilium. A

8 *Tuberositas sacralis.* Rough surface dorsal to the Facies auricularis for attachment of ligaments. A

9 ***Facies dorsalis.*** Dorsal surface. D

10 *Crista sacralis mediana**. Dorsal crest in bo, sometimes also in ov and cap, formed by the totally fused spinous processes. A C

11 *Crista sacralis intermedia.* Dorsolateral crest in bo formed by fusion of the articular processes. A

12 *Foramina sacralia dorsalia.* Openings for the exit of the dorsal branches of the sacral nerves. A D

13 *Crista sacralis lateralis.* Lateral crest formed by the fused transverse processes. A B

14 ***Facies pelvina.*** Pelvic (ventral) surface. B

15 *Foramina sacralia ventralia**. Openings for the exit of the ventral branches of the sacral nerves. B

16 *Lineae transversae.* Lines of fusion of the sacral vertebral bodies. B

17 ***Apex ossis sacri.*** Small caudal extremity of the sacrum. A B C

18 *Processus articularis caudalis.* Present only in Car and su. D

19 ***Canalis sacralis.*** Vertebral canal in the sacrum. C

20 ***Foramina intervertebralia.*** Openings between the arches of the sacral vertebrae for passage of the spinal nerves. C

21 **Vertebrae caudales [coccygeae].** Caudal [coccygeal] vertebrae. 41 A

22 ***Processus hemalis [haemalis].*** Paramedian ventral process in Car and Ru. E

23 ***Arcus hemalis [haemalis].*** Hemal arch, formed by fusion of right and left Processus hemales usually of the second and third caudal vertebrae in bo, in Car by the Processus hemales and attached Ossa arcus hemalis of one or more of the third to the eighth caudal vertebrae. E

24 *Os arcus hemalis [haemalis].* Separate paired bone attached to Processus hemalis in Car. Right and left bones may fuse to form a single V-shaped bone. E

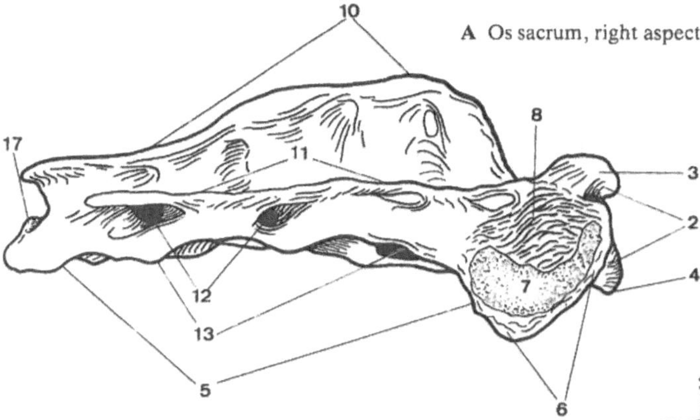

A Os sacrum, right aspect (bo)

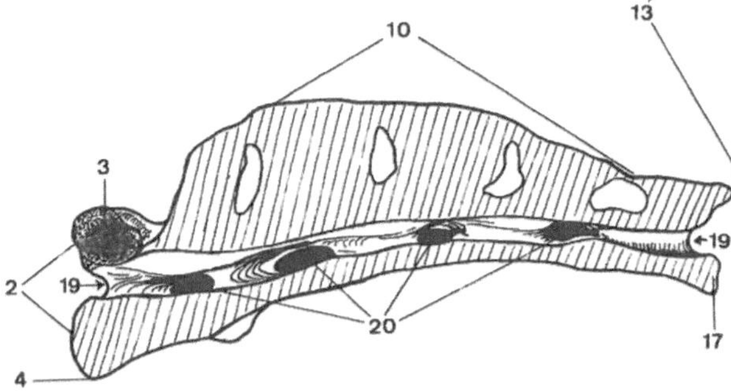

C Os sacrum, median section, right half (bo)

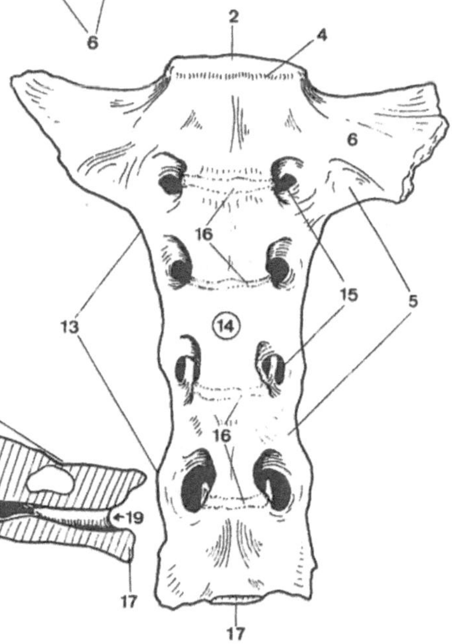

B Os sacrum, ventral aspect (bo)

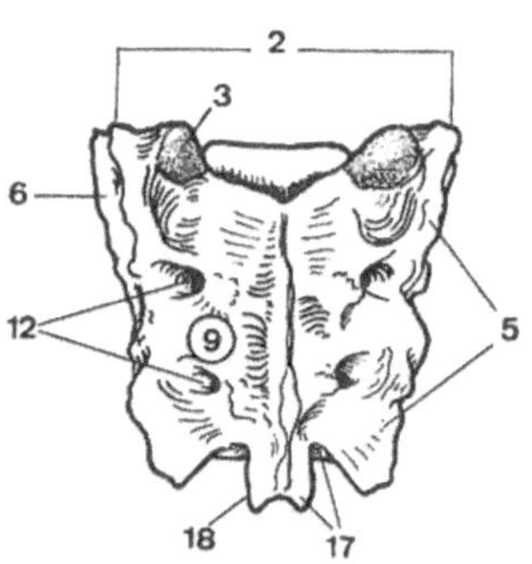

D Os sacrum, dorsal (and left) aspect (ca)

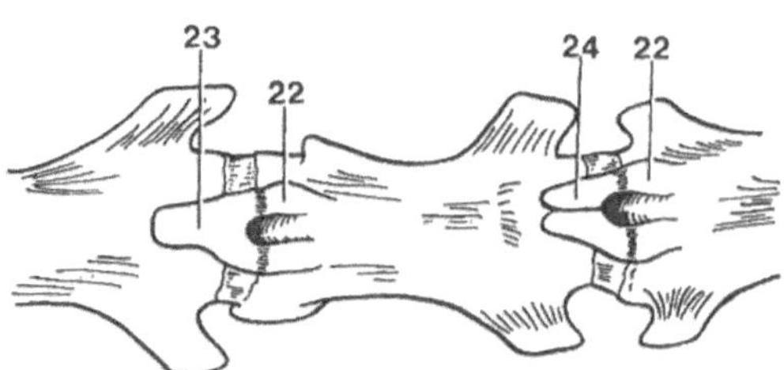

E Vertebrae caudales V, VI, VII, ventral aspect (fe)

1 **SKELETON THORACIS.** Bony thorax comprizing the thoracic vertebrae, ribs, and sternum. Sometimes called the thoracic cage. D

2 **Costae.** Ribs. D

3 ***Costae verae [sternales].*** Sternal ribs, connected directly with the sternum. D

4 ***Costae spuriae [asternales].*** Asternal ribs, indirectly connected to the sternum. D

5 *Costae fluctuantes.* Floating ribs, their ventral ends are free. D

6 ***Cartilago costalis*.*** Costal cartilage, the ventral part of the rib. D

7 ***Os costale.*** Bony dorsal part of the rib. D

8 *Caput costae.* Head of rib, articulates with two adjacent vertebral bodies. A B

9 **Facies articularis capitis costae.** Articular surface of the head of a rib. A B

10 **Crista capitis costae.** Crest of head of a rib, separates the two parts (cranial and caudal) of the Facies articularis. The crest is provided with a groove in the middle of it for attachment of the Lig. intercapitale. B

11 *Collum costae.* Neck of rib. Narrow portion extending lateral from the head. B

12 **Crista colli costae.** Crest on cranial border of the neck of the rib. B

13 *Corpus costae*.* Body (main part) of the rib. A

14 *Tuberculum costae.* Tubercle of the rib. Dorsal eminence between Collum and Corpus costae. A B

15 **Facies articularis tuberculi costae.** Articular surface of tubercle, articulates with the transverse process of a vertebra. A B

16 *Angulus costae.* Angle of the rib, accentuated point of the curvature near the Tuberculum costae. B

17 ***Tuberculum m. scaleni ventralis.*** Raised area on the cranial border of the first rib for the caudal attachment of M. scalenus ventralis, easily seen in su and eq. A

18 ***Tuberositas m. longissimi.*** Tuberosity for attachment of M. longissimus, always present in eq, often occurring in other species. B

19 ***Tuberositas m. iliocostalis.*** Tuberosity for attachment of M. iliocostalis, always present in eq, often occurring in other species. B

20 ***Sulcus costae.*** Costal groove, on medial surface near caudal border, for intercostal vessels and nerve. A B

21 ***Genu costae.*** Knee of rib, curvature near costochondral junction in Un, within the cartilage in Car. D

22 **Sternum.** C D

23 ***Manubrium sterni*.*** Cranial extremity of the sternum. C D

24 *Cartilago manubrii.* Cartilage of manubrium, absent or small in Ru. C D

25 ***Corpus sterni.*** Body of the sternum, between Manubrium and Processus xiphoideus. C D

26 *Crista sterni.* Cartilaginous ventral crest in eq. C

27 ***Sternebrae.*** Bony segments, united by intervening cartilages or fused by synostoses. They remain separate in some species of domestic mammals. C

28 ***Processus xiphoideus.*** Xiphoid process at caudal extremity of the sternum. C

29 ***Cartilago xiphoidea*.*** Xiphoid cartilage, caudal continuation of xiphoid process. C

30 ***Incisurae costales.*** Costal notches, depressions for costal cartilages. C

31 **Cavum thoracis.** Thoracic cavity. D

32 ***Apertura thoracis cranialis.*** Cranial thoracic aperture, thoracic inlet. D

33 ***Apertura thoracis caudalis.*** Caudal thoracic aperture, thoracic outlet. D

34 ***Sulcus pulmonalis.*** Dorsal part of thoracic cavity, lateral to the vertebral bodies. D

35 ***Arcus costalis*.*** Costal arch, formed by cartilages of the last sternal and the asternal ribs. D

36 ***Spatium intercostale*.*** Intercostal space. D

37 ***Angulus arcuum costalium.*** Angle between right and left costal arches. D

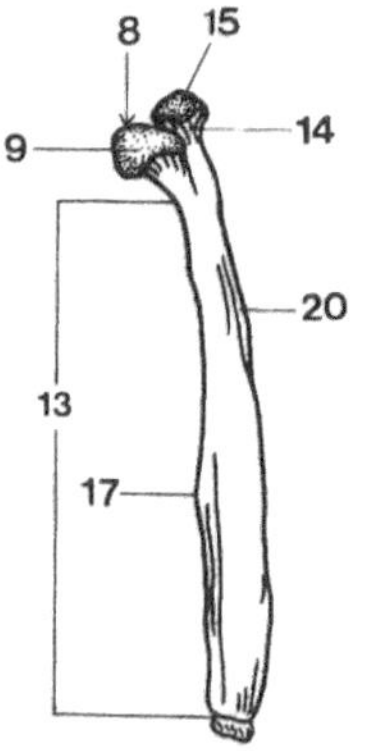

A Right 1st rib, medial aspect (eq)

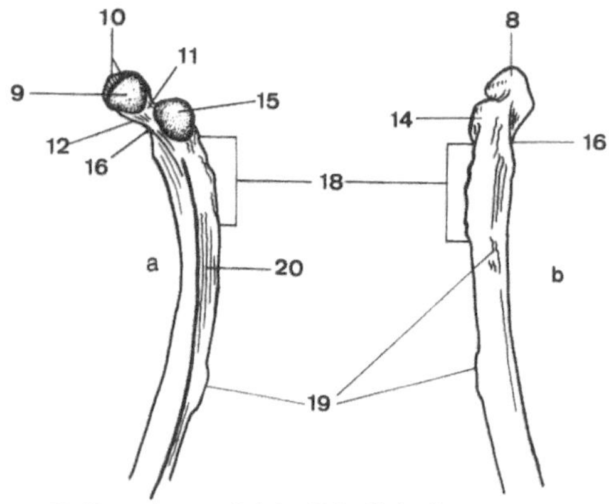

B Dorsal part of right 12th rib (eq)
a medial aspect
b lateral aspect

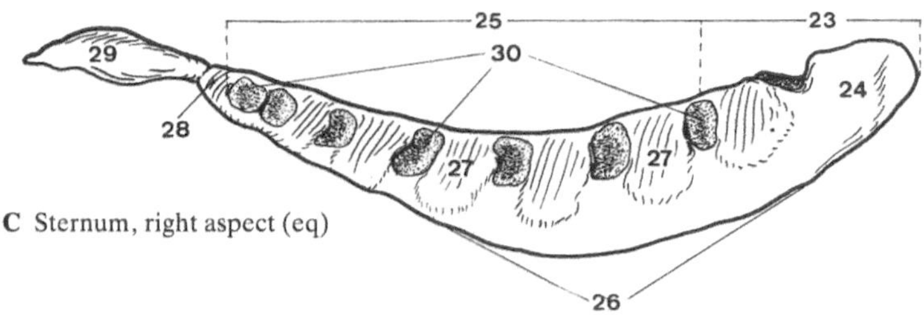

C Sternum, right aspect (eq)

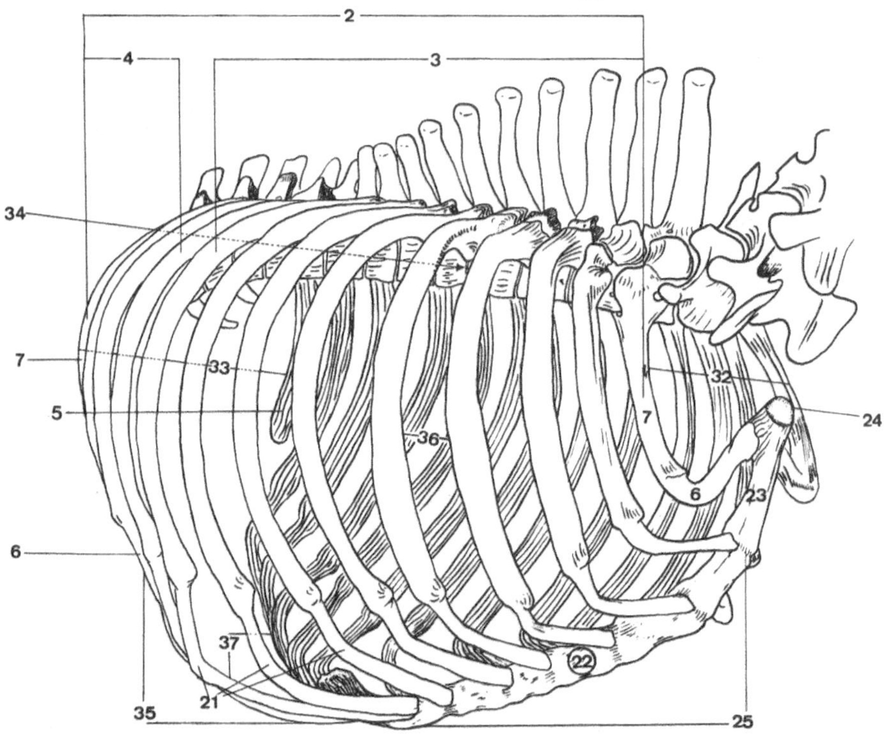

D Thorax, right cranioventral aspect (ca)

1 **SKELETON APPENDICULARE**. Appendicular skeleton.

2 **OSSA MEMBRI THORACICI**. Bones of thoracic limb. (There is a Foramen nutricium [or more] on the bones of the thoracic limb, very important in orthopaedic surgery, not listed in the 5th edition of the N. A. V.)

3 **Cingulum membri thoracici**. Shoulder girdle or thoracic Zonoskeleton, in mammals consisting of scapula and clavicle (or, fe, rudimentary in ca). The coracoid bone of birds is represented in mammals by the supraglenoid tubercle.

4 **Scapula**. Shoulder blade. A B C

5 ***Facies costalis [medialis]***. Costal (medial) surface, facing the ribs. C

6 *Facies serrata*. Surface for the origin (proximal attachment) of M. serratus ventralis. C

7 *Fossa subscapularis*. Concavity for origin of M. subscapularis. C

8 ***Facies lateralis***. Lateral surface. A B

9 *Spina scapulae**. Spine on lateral surface of the scapula. A B D

10 **Tuber spinae scapulae (su, eq)***. Tuber in the middle of Spina scapulae. B

11 *Fossa supraspinata*. Fossa cranial to Spina scapulae. A B

12 *Fossa infraspinata*. Fossa caudal to Spina scapulae. A B

13 ***Acromion****. Ventral end of Spina scapulae in Car and Ru. A D

14 *Processus hamatus* (or, Car). Ventral process of Acromion. A D

15 *Processus suprahamatus* (or, fe). Caudal process of Acromion. A

16 ***Margo dorsalis***. Dorsal border facing the vertebral column. A B C

17 ***Margo caudalis***. Caudal border facing the Regio tricipitalis. A B C

18 ***Margo cranialis***. Cranial border facing the neck. A B C

19 *Incisura scapulae*. Scapular notch on cranial border dorsal to Tuberculum supraglenoidale. A B C

20 ***Angulus caudalis****. Caudal angle. A B C

21 ***Angulus ventralis****. Ventral angle, bears the glenoid cavity. B C E

22 ***Angulus cranialis****. Cranial angle. A B C

23 ***Cavitas glenoidalis***. Glenoid cavity, for articulation with the humerus. C D E

24 *Incisura glenoidalis*. Craniomedial notch in the border of glenoid cavity in eq. E

25 ***Collum scapulae***. Neck of scapula, dorsal to the Angulus ventralis. B C

26 ***Tuberculum infraglenoidale***. Tubercle on the caudal border dorsal to the Angulus ventralis for origin of M. triceps brachii in ca and eq, and in fe, su, and eq for origin of M. articularis humeri. D

27 ***Tuberculum supraglenoidale***. Tubercle on ventral end of the cranial border for origin of M. biceps brachii. A B C

28 ***Processus coracoideus***. Medial process on Tuberculum supraglenoidale for origin of M. coracobrachialis. Small in domestic mammals. C E

29 ***Cartilago scapulae****. Scapular cartilage on dorsal border, small in Car. A C

30 **Clavicula** (or, fe). Clavicle in or, fe, rudimentary in ca. F

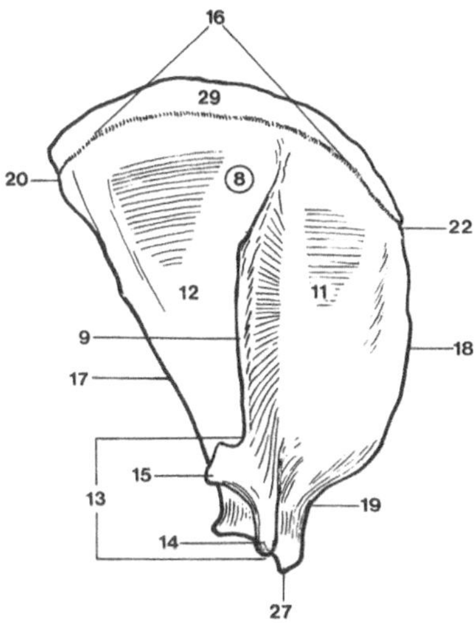

A Right scapula, lateral aspect (fe)

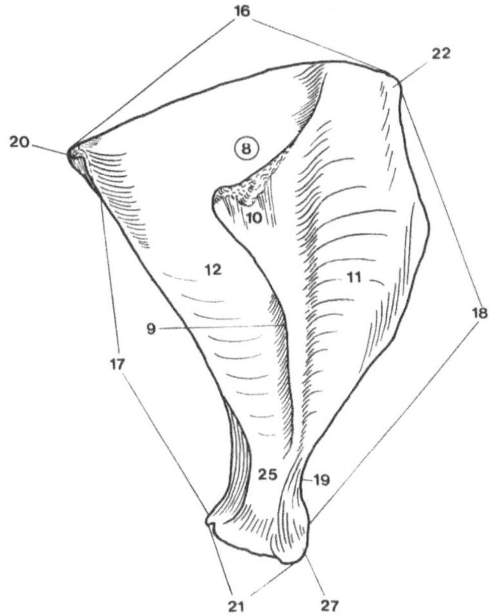

B Right scapula, lateral aspect (su)

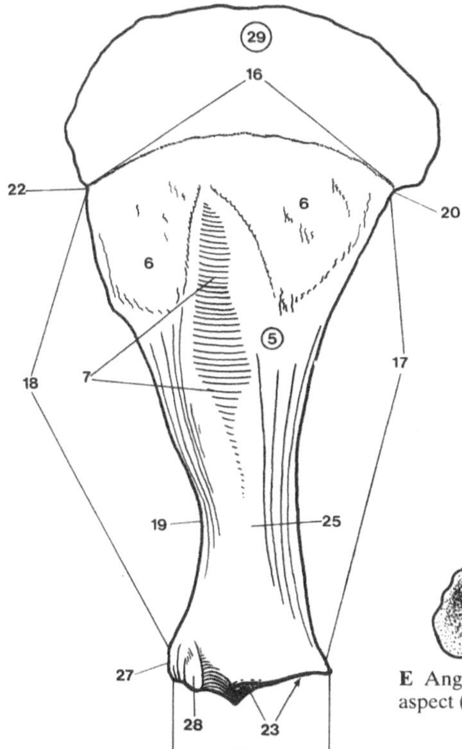

C Right scapula, medial aspect (eq)

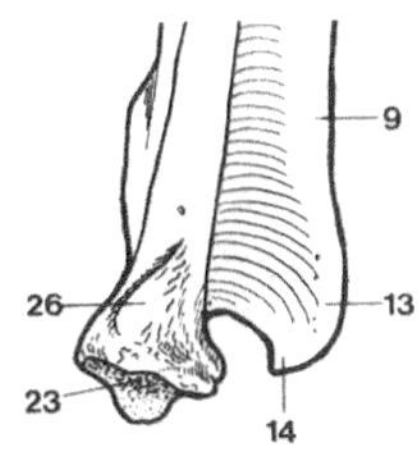

D Part of right scapula, caudal aspect (ca)

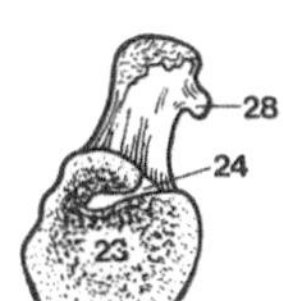

E Angulus ventralis of right scapula, cranioventral aspect (eq)

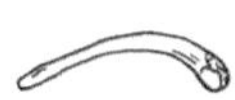

F Right clavicula, dorsal aspect (fe)

1 **Skeleton brachii.** Skeleton of the arm, or thoracic Stylopodium.

2 **Humerus.** A B

3 ***Caput humeri.*** Head of humerus. B C

4 ***Collum humeri.*** Neck of humerus. Between the head and the tubercles, and the body. B C

5 ***Tuberculum majus****. Greater tubercle, craniolateral on the proximal extremity of the humerus. A C

6 *Pars cranialis.* Cranial part of Tuberculum majus in Un. A B

7 *Pars caudalis.* Caudal part of Tuberculum majus in Un, area of insertion of the deep part of M. infraspinatus. A B

8 *Crista tuberculi majoris**. Crest of the greater tubercle running distally, up to Tuberositas deltoidea. Less visible in some species. A B

9 ***Tuberculum minus.*** Lesser tubercle, craniomedial on the proximal extremity of the humerus. A B C

10 *Pars cranialis.* Cranial part of Tuberculum minus in Ru and eq. A B

11 *Pars caudalis.* Caudal part of Tuberculum minus in Ru and eq. A B

12 *Crista tuberculi minoris.* Crest of lesser tubercle running distally, up to Tuberositas teres major. Less visible in some species. C

13 ***Sulcus intertubercularis.*** Intertubercular groove between the two tubercles. A C

14 *Tuberculum intermedium.* Intermediate tubercle in the Sulcus intertubercularis in eq, rudimentary in Ru. A B

15 ***Facies m. infraspinati.*** Area of insertion of the superficial part of M. infraspinatus in Un. A B

16 ***Tuberositas teres minor.*** Area of -insertion of M. teres minor. A

17 ***Linea m. tricipitis.*** Line of origin of Caput laterale m. tricipitis brachii. B

18 ***Corpus humeri****. Body of humerus. A B

19 *Facies cranialis.* Cranial surface. A

20 *Facies lateralis.* Lateral surface. A

21 *Facies caudalis.* Caudal surface. B

22 *Facies medialis.* Medial surface. A B

23 *Crista humeri.* Crest of humerus, running distomedially from Tuberositas deltoidea. A

24 *Tuberositas deltoidea**. Deltoid tuberosity, on the lateral surface for insertion of M. deltoideus. A B

25 *Sulcus m. brachialis.* Spiral groove in laterodistal direction for M. brachialis. A B

26 *Tuberositas teres major.* Teres tuberosity, area of termination of M. teres major and M. latissimus dorsi on the medial surface in Un. A B

27 *Crista supracondylaris lateralis.* Crest running proximomedially from Epicondylus lateralis. A B D

28 ***Condylus humeri.*** The whole distal end of the humerus except the epicondyles. A B D

29 *Capitulum humeri**. Present in Car, more distinctly in fe. In all species it looks like a segment of a cylinder (condyle). A D

30 *Trochlea humeri.* Pulley-like portion of distal end. A B D

31 *Fossa olecrani.* Deep depression on the caudal surface proximal to the trochlea. B

32 *Fossa coronoidea.* Depression on the cranial surface in fe, medial to Fossa radialis accommodating the Processus coronoideus medialis ulnae when the elbow is flexed. D

33 *Fossa radialis.* Radial fossa, proximal to the Trochlea humeri, opposite to the Fossa olecrani. A

34 *Epicondylus medialis.* Medial epicondyle. A B

35 *Epicondylus lateralis.* Lateral epicondyle. A B

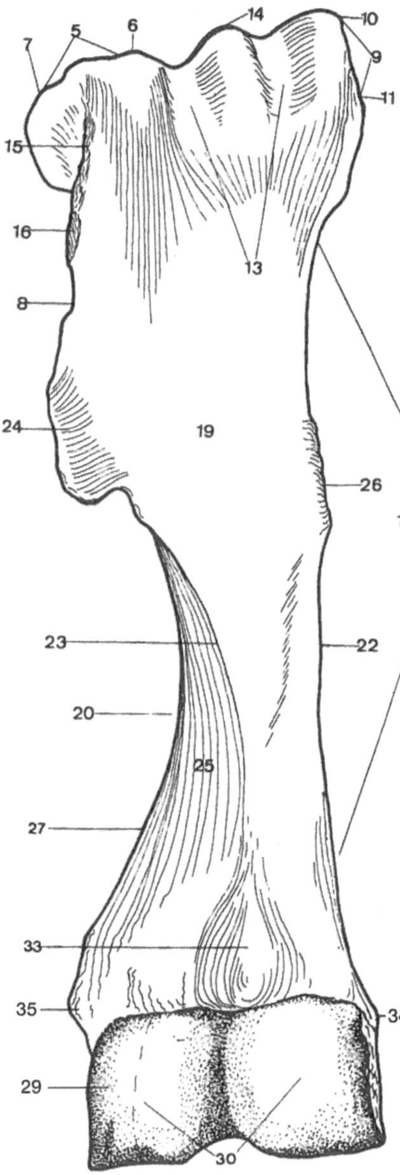

A Right humerus, cranial aspect (eq)

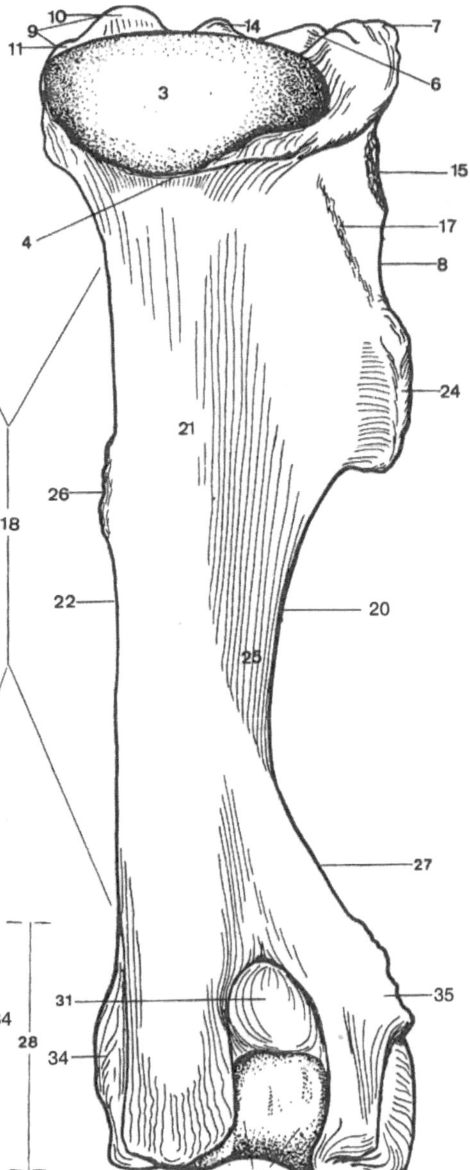

B Right humerus, caudal aspect (eq)

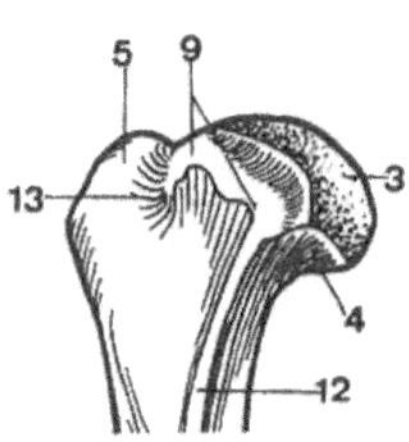

C Part of right humerus, medial aspect (ca)

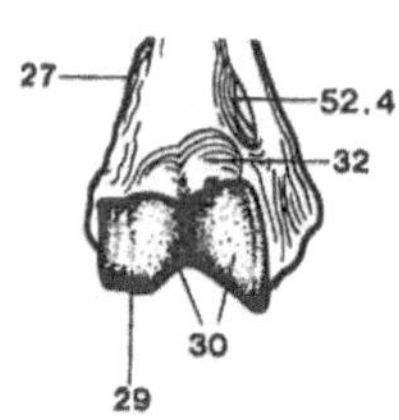

D Condylus of right humerus, cranial aspect (fe)

1 *Fossa radialis*. Depression on the cranial surface proximal to the trochlea accommodating the Caput radii when the elbow is flexed. A, 51 A

2 *Foramen supratrochleare* (ca). Opening between Fossa olecrani and Fossa radialis in ca and occasionally in su. A (There is an inconsistency regarding the species with the supratrochlear foramen: in the 5th edition of the N. A. V. it is listed only under ca [see page 22], whereas in the note 46 this structure is mentioned in Car [see page 30] [maybe a typo mistake?].)

3 ***Epicondylus medialis****. Medial nonarticular prominence of Condylus humeri. A, 51 A B

4 *Foramen supracondylare* (fe). Opening in Epicondylus medialis. 51 D

5 ***Epicondylus lateralis****. Lateral nonarticular prominence of Condylus humeri. A, 51 A B

6 **Skeleton antebrachii**. Skeleton of the forearm, or thoracic Zeugopodium.

7 **Radius**. The craniomedial bone of the forearm. B D

8 ***Caput radii***. Head of radius. B D

9 *Fovea capitis radii*. Fovea of head of radius, typical in or, Car, su. B D

10 *Circumferentia articularis*. Circumference for articulation with Incisura radialis ulnae in Car, reduced to two small caudal facets in Un. B

11 ***Collum radii***. Neck of radius. Between the head and the body. B D

12 *Tuberositas radii*. Radial tuberosity. Medially located, roughened area of the neck of the radius for insertion of the biceps brachii muscle. D

13 ***Corpus radii****. Body of the radius. B D

14 *Facies cranialis*. Cranial surface. Toward the distal end three grooves for tendons are obvious in bo and eq ; lateromedially they are : for the tendon of abductor pollicis longus m. (obliquely oriented), for the tendon of extensor carpi radialis m., and for the tendon of common digital extensor m., both vertical grroves. D

15 *Facies caudalis*. Caudal surface. B

16 *Crista transversa*. Transverse crest on the caudal surface, proximal to the trochlea. C

17 *Margo medialis*. Medial border. B D

18 *Margo lateralis*. Lateral border. B D

19 ***Trochlea radii***. Trochlea of radius, distal end. B C D

20 *Facies articularis carpea*. Surface for articulation with the carpal bones in Car. In Un it is provided with the negative aspect of the first row of carpal bones, depressions and prominences. B C D

21 *Processus styloideus*. Styloid process, distal extension of radius, located medially, except eq. B

22 *Processus styloideus medialis*. For sake of clarity in eq the process homologous to Processus styloideus of other species is designated “medialis”. C D

23 *Processus styloideus lateralis*. The lateral styloid process in eq appears to originate from the radius, although developmentally it belongs to the ulna. C D

24 *Incisura ulnaris*. Ulnar notch. Concave surface for articulation with the ulna in Car and su. B

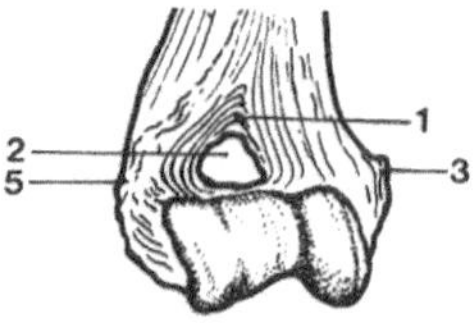

A Condylus of right humerus, cranial aspect (ca)

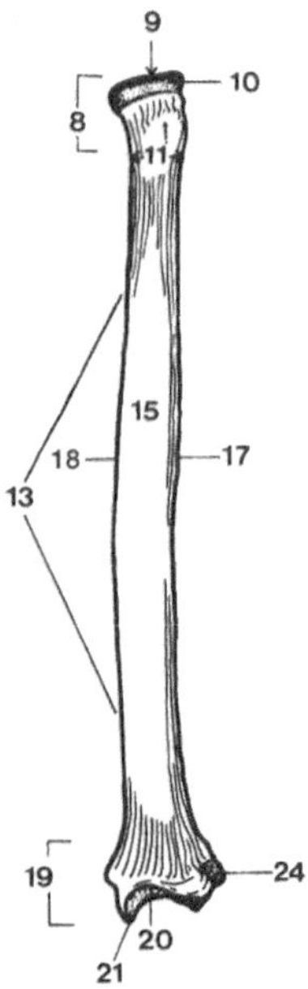

B Right radius, caudal aspect (ca)

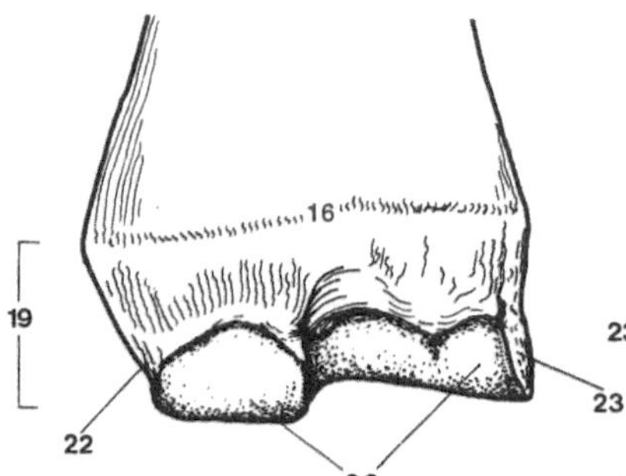

C Part of right radius, caudal aspect (eq)

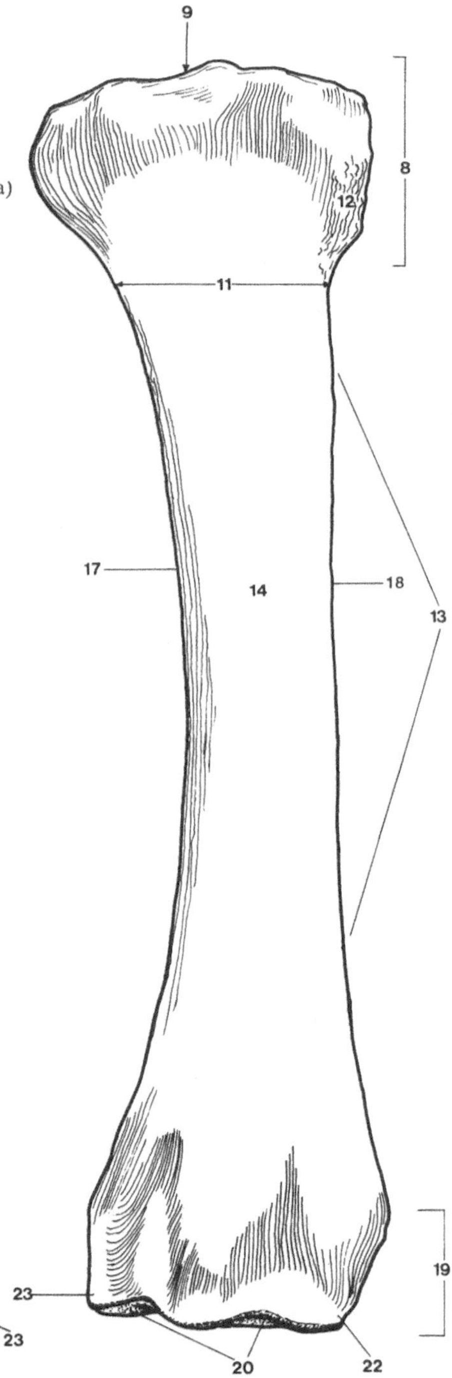

D Right radius, cranial aspect (eq)

1 **Ulna**. The caudolateral bone of the forearm. A C D E

2 ***Olecranon****. Proximal extremity of the ulna. A C D E

3 *Tuber olecrani**. Proximal tuberosity for attachment of M. triceps brachii. A B C D E

4 *Processus anconeus [anconaeus]*. Cranial process at the proximal end of Incisura trochlearis. A B C D E

5 ***Processus coronoideus medialis***. Craniomedial process at the distal end of Incisura trochlearis. It articulates with the Condylus humeri in Car. Greatly reduced in Un. A D E

6 ***Processus coronoideus lateralis***. Craniolateral process at the distal end of Incisura trochlearis, reduced in Car. A B C D E

7 ***Incisura trochlearis***. Trochlear notch, articulating with Trochlea humeri. A B C D

8 ***Incisura radialis***. Radial notch, between the coronoid processes, facing the Caput radii. A D

9 ***Corpus ulnae****. Body of the ulna, reduced in eq. A C D E

10 *Facies lateralis*. Lateral surface. A B C E

11 *Facies cranialis*. Cranial surface. D

12 *Facies medialis*. Medial surface. A E

13 *Margo interosseus*. Border for attachment of Membrana interossea only in Car. A

14 *Margo lateralis*. Lateral border in Un. D E

15 *Margo caudalis*. Caudal border. B C E

16 *Margo medialis*. Medial border. D E

17 ***Caput ulnae****. Head of the ulna, distal extremity, except in eq. A C

18 *Circumferentia articularis*. Circumference for articulation with Incisura ulnaris of radius in Car and su. A

19 *Processus styloideus**. Styloid process, distal extension of the ulna. A C

20 *Facies articularis carpea*. Surface for articulation with Os carpi ulnare. A

21 ***Spatium interosseum antebrachii***. Interosseous space between radius and ulna in eq. B

22 ***Spatium interosseum antebrachii proximale***. Proximal interosseus space between radius and ulna in Ru. C

23 ***Spatium interosseum antebrachii distale***. Distal interosseous space between radius and ulna in Ru. C

B Part of right radius and ulna, lateral aspect (eq)

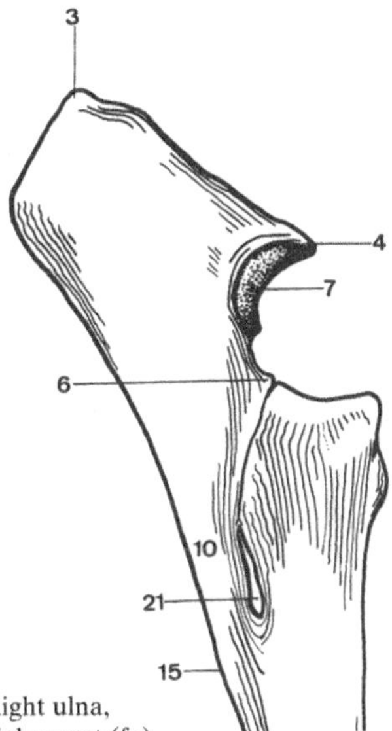

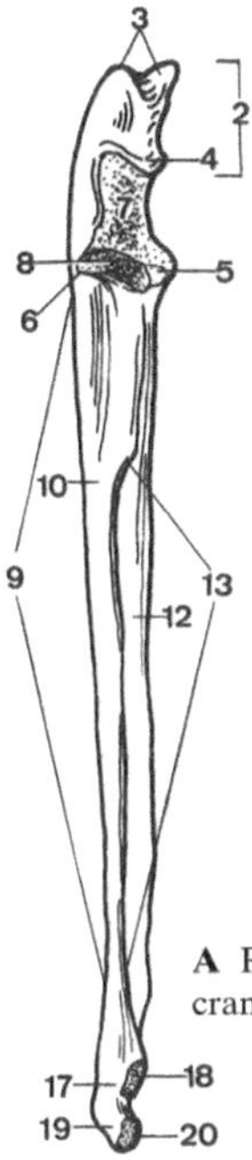

A Right ulna, cranial aspect (fe)

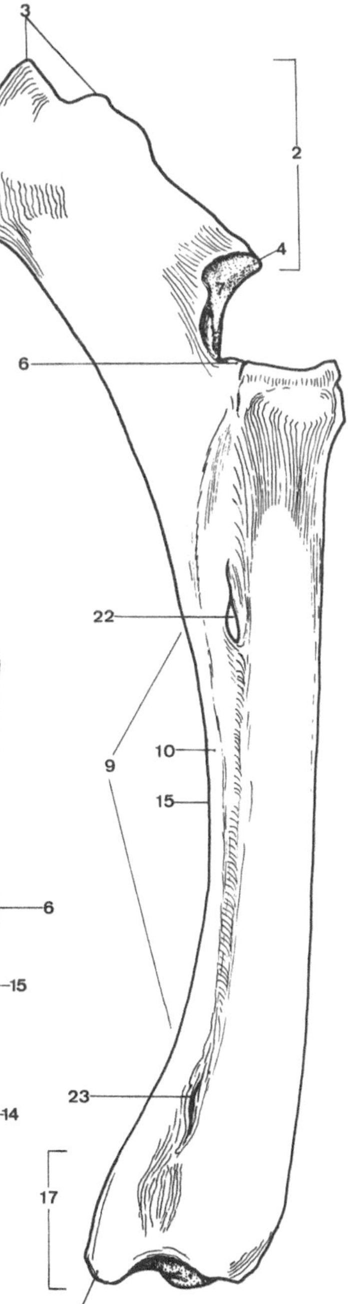

C Right radius and ulna, lateral aspect (bo)

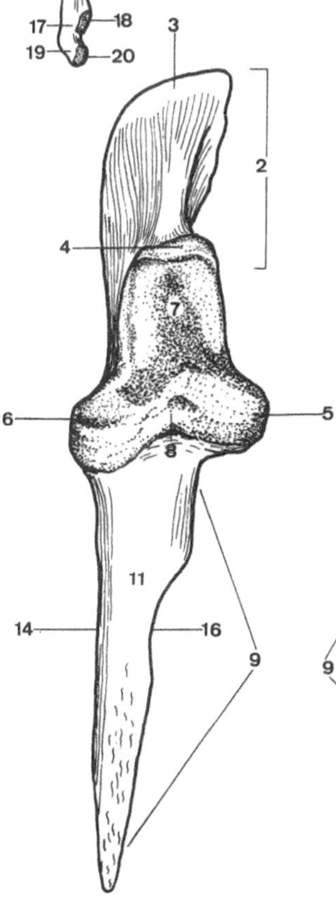

D Right ulna, cranial aspect (eq)

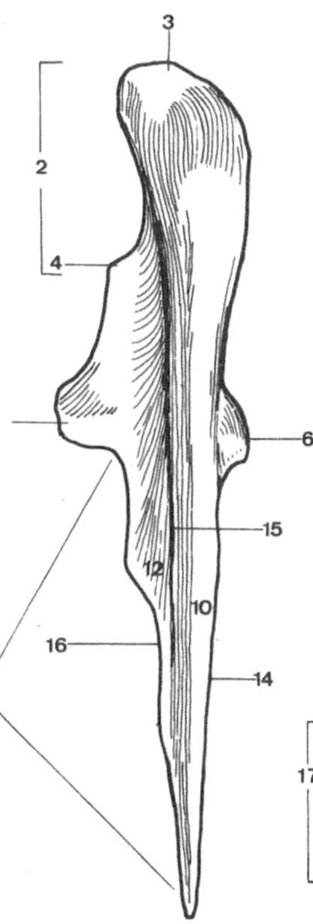

E Right ulna, caudal aspect (eq)

1 **Skeleton manus, Thoracic autopodium.**

2 **Ossa carpi*, Thoracic basipodium**. Carpal bones. A B C

3 ***(Os carpi centrale)***. The central carpal bone of Car is situated distal to the Os carpi intermedioradiale, proximal to the Os carpale II and Os carpale III, and fuses with the Os carpi intermedioradiale some weeks after birth.

4 ***Os carpi radiale [Os scaphoideum]***. Radial carpal [scaphoid] bone. C

5 ***Os carpi intermedium [Os lunatum]***. Intermediate carpal [lunate] bone. C

6 ***Os carpi ulnare [Os triquetrum]***. Ulnar carpal [triangular] bone. A B C

7 ***Os carpi accessorium [Os pisiforme]***. Accessory carpal [pisiform] bone. A B C

8 ***Os carpale I [Os trapezium]***. First carpal [trapezium] bone, absent in Ru and often in eq. A B

9 ***Os carpale II [Os trapezoideum]***. Second carpal [trapezoid] bone. A B

10 ***Os carpale III [Os capitatum]***. Third carpal [capitate] bone. A B

11 ***Os carpale IV [Os hamatum]***. Fourth carpal [hook like] bone. A B C

12 ***Os carpi intermedioradiale [Os scapholunatum]***. Fused radial and intermediate carpal bones in Car. A B

13 ***Os carpale II et III [Os trapezoideocapitatum]***. Fused second and third carpal bones in Ru. C

14 ***Sulcus carpi***. Carpal groove, formed by the palmar surface of radial and intermediate carpal bones and the medial surface of the accessory carpal bone, converted into the Canalis carpi for digital flexor tendons by the Retinaculum flexorum. A

15 ***Os sesamoideum m. abductoris digiti I [pollicis] longi***. Sesamoid bone on the medial side of the carpus in Car. A B

16 ***(Ossa sesamoidea palmaria)***. Variable sesamoid bones on the palmar surface of the carpus in Car. A

17 **Ossa metacarpalia I–V***. Metacarpal bones I–V, or thoracic Metapodium. A B D E

18 ***Basis***. Base, the proximal end. A B D E

19 *Facies articularis*. Articular surface. D E

20 ***Corpus***. Body. A B D E

21 *Facies dorsalis*. Dorsal surface. B E

22 **Tuberositas ossis metacarpalis III.** Tuberosity at the base of the third metacarpal bone for insertion of M. extensor carpi radialis (brevis in Car). E

23 *Facies palmaris*. Palmar surface. A D

24 *Margo medialis*. Medial border. D E

25 *Margo lateralis*. Lateral border. D E

26 ***Caput***. Head, the distal end. A B D E

27 ***Os metacarpale III et IV*** (Ru). Fused third and fourth metacarpal bones. D, E (There is a metacarpal bone V in Ru, rudimentary, on the palmar aspect of the base of metacarpal bone IV, and looking similar to a canine tooth [Barone 1999, p. 559, Planche 307].)

28 *Sulcus longitudinalis dorsalis*. Dorsal longitudinal groove. E

29 *Sulcus longitudinalis palmaris*. Palmar longitudinal groove. D

30 *Canalis metacarpi proximalis*. Proximal metacarpal canal. D E

31 *Canalis metacarpi distalis*. Distal metacarpal canal. D E

32 *Incisura intercapitalis*. Former intertrochlear notch dividing the distal ends (head) in Ru. D E

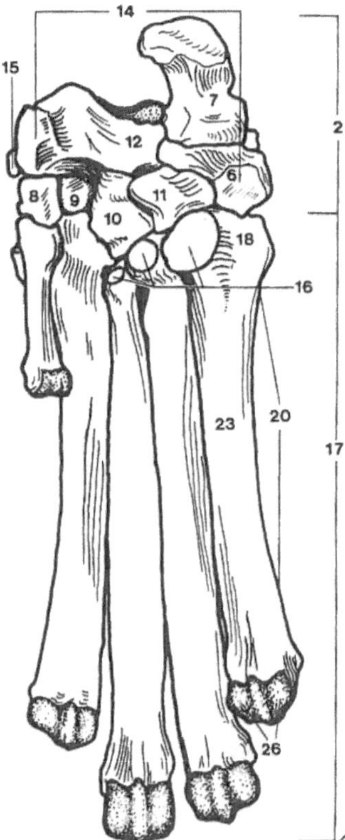

A Right carpal and metacarpal bones, palmar aspect (ca)

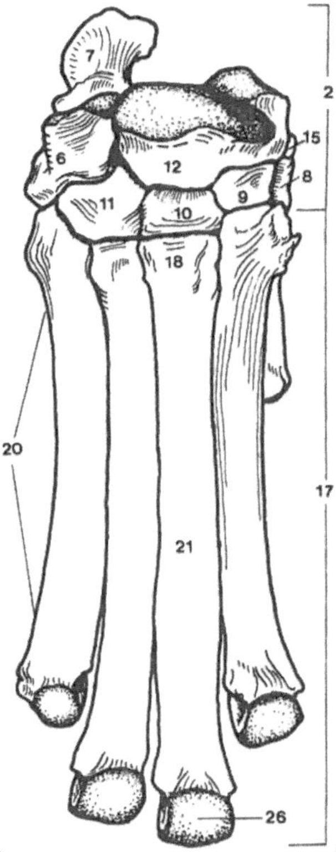

B Right carpal and metacarpal bones, dorsal aspect (ca)

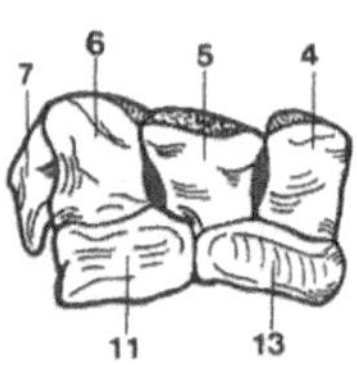

C Right carpal bones, dorsal aspect (bo)

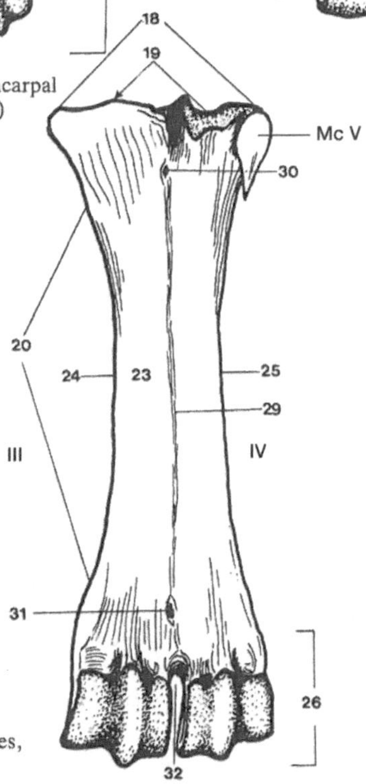

D Right metacarpal bones, palmar aspect (bo)

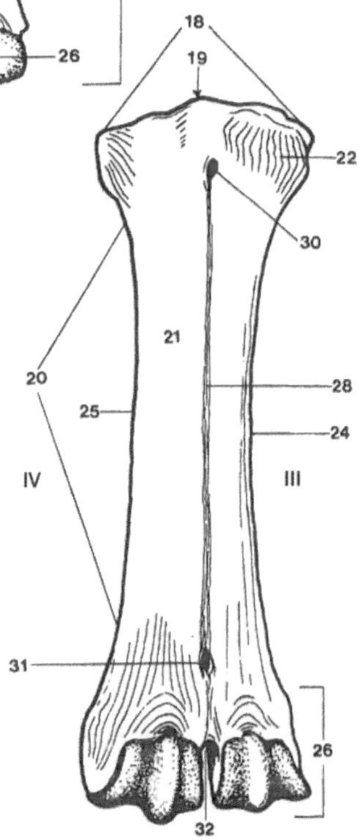

E Right metacarpal bones, dorsal aspect (bo)

1 **Ossa digitorum manus**. Digital bones of the manus, or thoracic Acropodium. To assist in the naming of the ligaments of the joints, the terms Os compedale, Os coronale, and Os ungulare (Un) or unguiculare (Car) are introduced as alternate terms. A

2 ***Phalanx proximalis [Os compedale]***. Proximal phalanx. A B

3 *Basis phalangis proximalis**. Base of proximal phalanx, proximal end. A B

4 **Fovea articularis**. Articular fovea. B

4a **Eminentia palmaris medialis***. Prominent structures of the Phalanx proximalis where the medial parts of the collateral ligaments of the fetlock joint as well as the medial short sesamoid ligaments insert. B

4b **Eminentia palmaris lateralis***. Same as above, on the lateral side. B

5 *Corpus phalangis proximalis**. Body of proximal phalanx. A B

6 **Trigonum phalangis proximalis**. Triangular rough area on the palmar surface in eq. B

7 *Caput phalangis proximalis**. Head of proximal phalanx, distal end. A B

8 ***Phalanx media [Os coronale]***. Middle phalanx. A C

9 *Basis phalangis mediae**. Base of middle phalanx, proximal end. A C

10 **Fovea articularis**. Articular fovea. C

11 **Processus extensorius***. Extensor process in Ru and eq, dorsally. C

12 **Tuberositas flexoria**. Thickened palmar border for passage of deep digital flexor tendon in Ru and eq over the middle scutum. C

13 *Corpus phalangis mediae**. Body of middle phalanx. A C

14 *Caput phalangis mediae*. Head of middle phalanx, distal end. A C

15 ***Phalanx distalis [Os unguiculare, Os ungulare]***. Distal phalanx. A D E

16 *Facies articularis*. Articular surface. D

17 **Facies articularis sesamoidea**. Part of articular surface articulating with Os sesamoideum distale. D

18 *Facies parietalis*. Parietal surface. D

18a **Facies axialis**. Axial surface in Car, su and Ru. 61 A

18b **Sulcus parietalis axialis**. Parietal groove on the axial side.

18c **Foramen axiale**. Axial foramen in su and Ru. 61 A

18d **Margo dorsalis**. Dorsal border, except in eq. 61 A

18e **Facies abaxialis**. Abaxial surface in Car, su, and Ru.

18f **Sulcus parietalis abaxialis**. Parietal sulcus on the abaxial side.

18g **Foramen abaxiale**. Abaxial foramen in Car, su and Ru.

18h **Pars medialis**. Medial part.

19 **Sulcus parietalis medialis**. Medial parietal groove in eq. D

20 **Processus palmaris medialis**. Medial palmar process in eq. D E

20a **Foramen processus palmaris medialis**. Foramen of medial palmar process. May transform into the notch.

20b **Incisura processus palmaris medialis**. Notch of medial palmar process.

20c **Pars dorsalis**. Dorsal part.

20d **Pars lateralis**. Lateral part.

21 **Sulcus parietalis lateralis**. Lateral parietal groove in eq. D

22 **Processus palmaris lateralis**. Lateral palmar process in eq. D E

22a **Foramen processus palmaris lateralis**. Variable foramen of palmar process. May transform into the notch. D

22b **Incisura processus palmaris lateralis**. Variable notch of palmar process.

23 ***Processus unguicularis***. Ungual (distal) process in Car. 61 B C

24 ***Facies solearis***. Sole surface. E

25 *Tuberculum flexorium*. Eminence, present in Ru and Car and faintly in su, on which the deep digital flexor tendon ends. A, 61 A

26 *Facies flexoria*. Flexor surface for insertion of deep digital flexor tendon in su and eq. E

27 *Linea semilunaris*. Semilunar line in eq, separating Facies flexoria from Planum cutaneum. E

28 *Planum cutaneum*. Corresponds to the sole of the hoof in Un. E

29 *Sulcus solearis medialis*. Medial solear groove in eq. E

30 *Sulcus solearis lateralis*. Lateral soelar groove in eq. E

30a *Foramen soleare axiale*. Axial solear foramen in Car. 61 B C

30b *Foramen soleare abaxiale*. Abaxial solear foramen in Car. 61 B

31 *Foramen soleare mediale*. Medial solear foramen in eq. E

32 *Foramen soleare laterale*. Lateral solear foramen in eq. E

33 *Canalis solearis*. Solear canal within the Phalanx distalis in eq. E

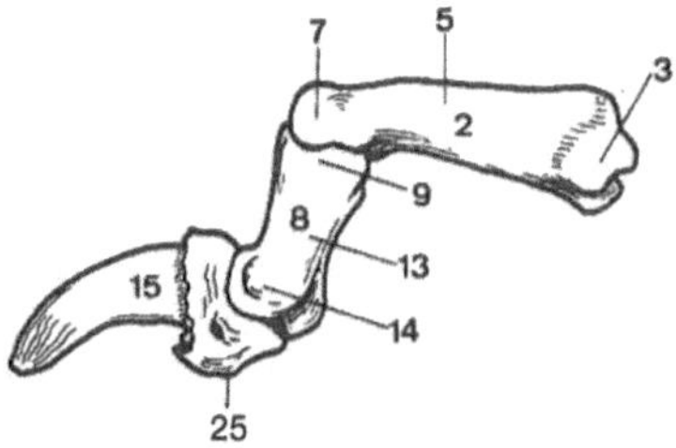

A Bones of the right fourth digit, axial aspect (ca)

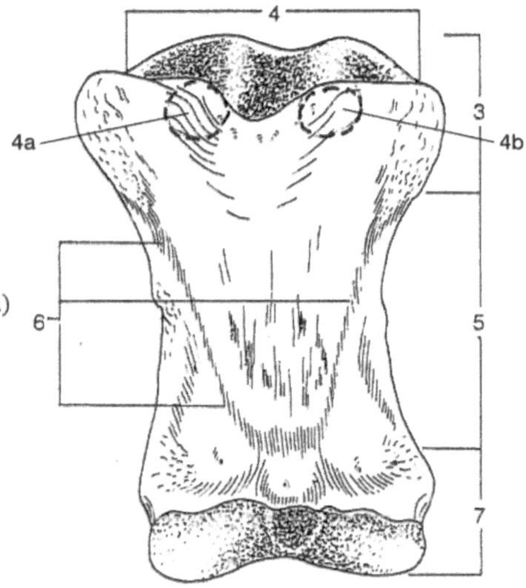

B Phalanx proximalis of right digit, palmar aspect (eq)

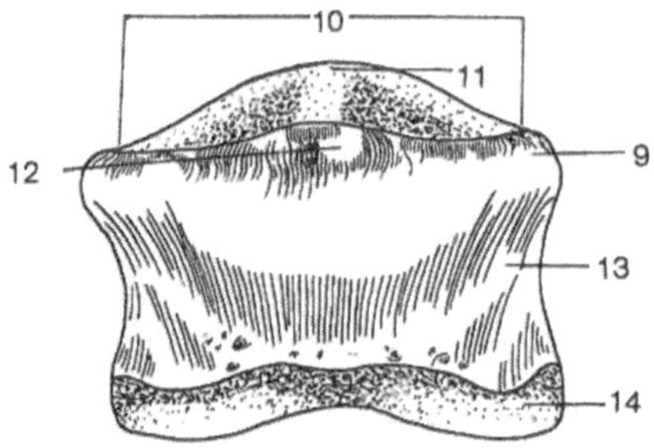

C Phalanx media of right digit, palmar aspect (eq)

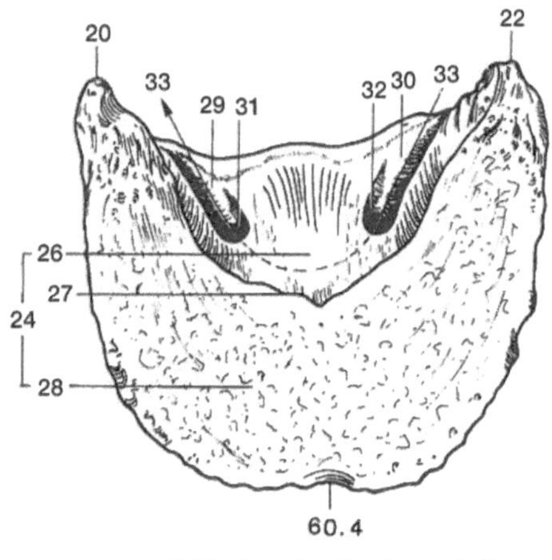

E Phalanx distalis of right digit, distal aspect (eq)

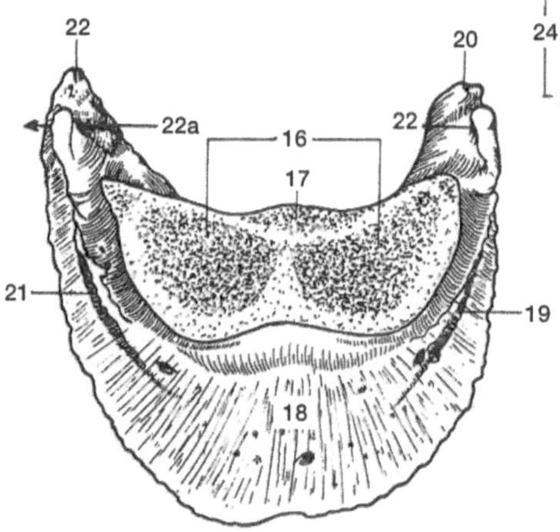

D Phalanx distalis of right digit, proximal aspect (eq)

1 ***Margo coronalis***. Coronary (proximal) border. A C D

1a *Crista unguicularis*. Ungual crest in Car, shelf at base covering the root of the claw. B C

1b *Sulcus unguicularis*. Ungual groove in Car, contains the root of the claw. C

2 **Processus extensorius**. Extensor process, attachment of common digital extensor tendon. A D

3 *Margo solearis*. Solear (distal) border. A D

4 **(Crena marginis solearis)**. Shallow middorsal notch of Margo solearis in eq. 59 E

5 *Apex*. Distal end of Margo dorsalis in Car, su, and Ru. A B

6 ***Cartilago ungularis medialis****. Medial cartilage of hoof in eq. D

7 ***Cartilago ungularis lateralis****. Lateral cartilage of hoof in eq. D

8 ***Ossa sesamoidea proximalia****. Two proximal sesamoid bones, palmar to distal end of each Os metacarpale. E

9 *Facies articularis*. Articular (dorsal) surface. E

10 *Facies flexoria*. Flexor (palmar) surface for the deep digital flexor tendon. E

11 *Facies m. interossei*. Axial, or abaxial (in eq medial, or lateral) surface for attachment of M. interosseus. E

12 ***Os sesamoideum distale***. Distal sesamoid bone, palmar to the distal end of Phalanx media, in Car replaced by cartilage. F G (The distal sesamoid bone is called "navicular bone" by the clinicians in Equine Medicine and Surgery, see: navicular disease, navicularthritis etc.)

13 *Facies flexoria*. Flexor (palmar) surface for the deep digital flexor tendon. F

14 *Facies articularis*. Articular (dorsal and small distal) surface. G

15 *Margo proximalis*. Proximal border. F

16 *Margo distalis*. Distal border, attachment of Lig. sesamoideum distale impar. G (In eq is called "navicular ligament" by the clinicians, see 12.)

17 ***Ossa sesamoidea dorsalia***. Dorsal sesamoid bones in ca, sometimes replaced by cartilage. H

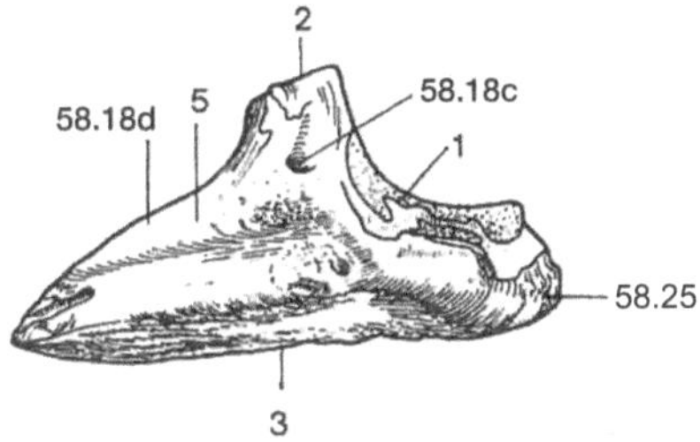

A Phalanx distalis of right fourth digit, axial aspect (bo)

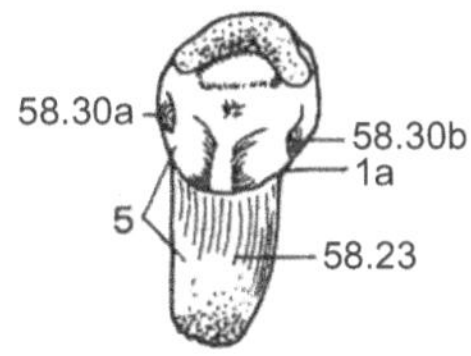

B Phalanx distalis of left third digit, proximal aspect (ca)

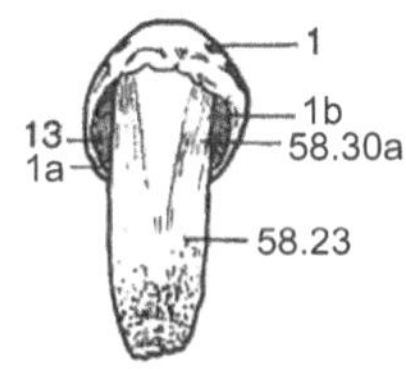

C Phalanx distalis of left third digit, dorsodistal aspect (ca)

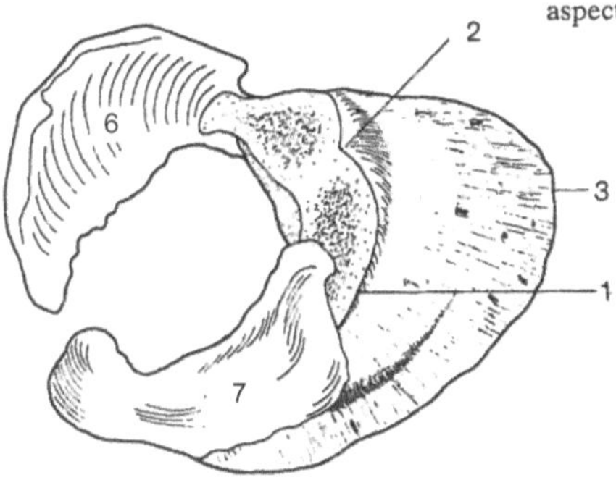

D Phalanx distalis and hoof cartilages of right digit, proximolateral aspect (eq)

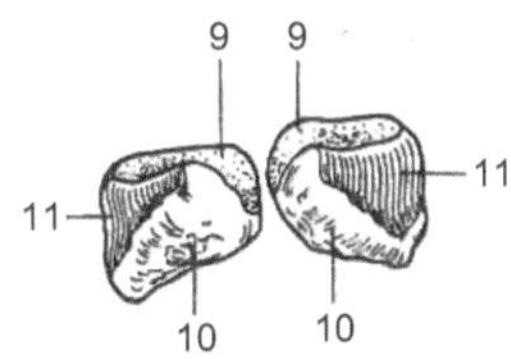

E Proximal sesamoid bones of right digit, proximal aspect (eq)

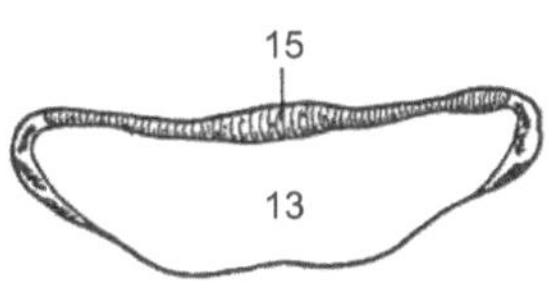

F Distal sesamoid bone of right digit, proximopalmar aspect (eq)

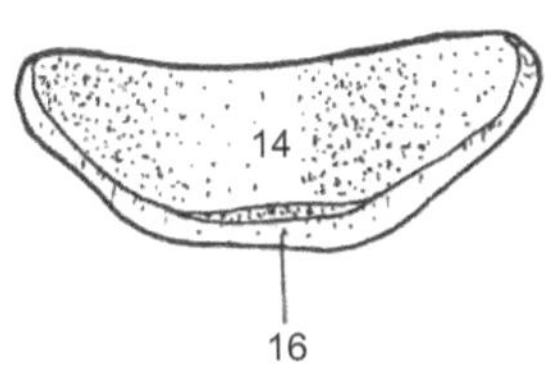

G Distal sesamoid bone of right digit, distodorsal aspect (eq)

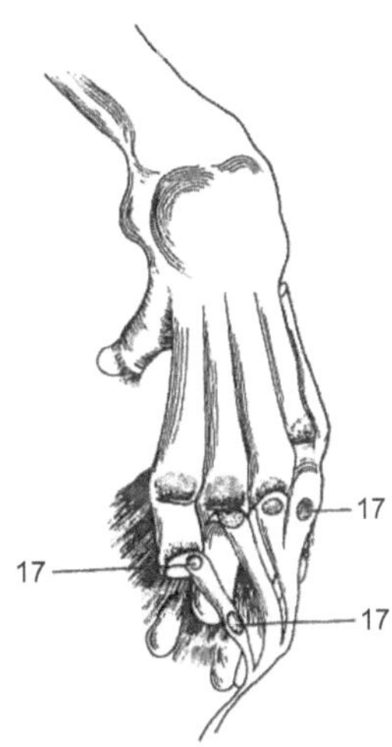

H Bones of the right manus, dorsal aspect (ca)

1 **OSSA MEMBRI PELVINI**. Bones of pelvic limb. (There is a Foramen nutricium [or more] on the bones of the pelvic limb, very important in orthopaedic surgery, not listed in the 5th edition of the N. A. V.)

2 **Cingulum membri pelvini**. Pelvic girdle, or pelvic Zonoskeleton.

3 **Os coxae**. Hip bone, composed of ilium, ischium and pubis. A B C

4 ***Acetabulum***. Socket of the hip joint. A B

5 *Margo acetabuli*. Acetabular rim. A

6 *Fossa acetabuli*. Deep part of the acetabulum for attachment of Lig. capitis ossis femoris. A B

7 *Incisura acetabuli*. Acetabular notch, interruption of Facies lunata, facing the Foramen obturatum. A B

8 *Facies lunata*. Moon-shaped articular surface. In Ru consists of two parts, as follows. A B

9 **Pars major**. In Ru the major part of Facies lunata. A

10 **Pars minor**. In Ru the minor part of Facies lunata. The two parts are separated by a rough area free of cartilage. A

11 ***Spina ischiadica***. Elevation between Incisura ischiadica major and minor, formed by ilium and ischium. A B C D

12 ***Foramen obturatum***. Large opening bounded by pubis and ischium. A B C

13 **Os ilium**. A B C

14 ***Corpus ossis ilii***. Body of ilium, constricted caudoventral part. A B C D

15 *Area lateralis m. recti femoris*. Because they are eminences in Car, the points of origin of M. rectus femoris are no longer called Foveae, but Areae, a neutral term. A B

16 *Area medialis m. recti femoris [Spina iliaca ventralis caudalis]*. See above. B C

17 ***Ala ossis ilii***. Wing of ilium, wide craniodorsal part. A B C D

18 *Spina alaris*. Prominence at the ventral border of the wing in Car, ov, and cap. B C

19 *Crista iliaca**. Iliac crest, dorsocranial border of ilium. A B C D

20 **Tuber coxae***. Coxal tuber, lateroventral projection of the wing. A B C D

21 Spina iliaca ventralis cranialis. Cranioventral angle of Tuber coxae in Car, ov, and cap. B C

22 Labium internum. Internal lip in Ru and eq, border of the area of origin of M. iliacus. A

23 Labium externum. External lip in Ru and eq, border of the area of origin of M. gluteus medius. A D

24 **Tuber sacrale***. Sacral tuber, dorsomedial projection of the wing. A B C D

25 Spina iliaca dorsalis cranialis. Prominence at the cranial end of Tuber sacrale in Car, ov, and cap. B C

26 Spina iliaca dorsalis caudalis. Prominence at the caudal end of Tuber sacrale in Car, ov, and cap. B C

27 *Facies glutea [glutaea]*. External surface of the wing. A B D

28 **Lineae gluteae [glutaeae]**. Lines at the borders of fields of attachments of Mm. glutei.

29 **Linea glutea [glutaea] ventralis**. Line between the fields of M. gluteus medius, (accessorius) (Barone, 1999, p. 640, Planche 359) and profundus in Car, accessorius and profundus in bo and eq. A B D

30 **Linea glutea [glutaea] caudalis**. Borderline of the field of M. gluteus profundus. A B

30a **Linea glutea dorsalis (or).**

31 **Linea glutea [glutaea] accessoria** (bo, eq). Line between the fields of M. gluteus medius and accessorius. D

32 *Facies sacropelvina*. Internal surface of the wing. C

33 **Facies iliaca**. Iliac surface, craniolateral part of Facies sacropelvina. C

34 **Facies auricularis**. Ear-shaped surface for articulation with the sacrum. C

35 **Tuberositas iliaca**. Roughened area craniodorsal to the Facies auricularis for attachment of sacroiliac ligaments. C

36 ***Linea arcuata***. Ventromedial border of Corpus ossis ilii, part of Linea terminalis. C

37 *Tuberculum m. psoas minoris*. Absent in ca. 65 E

38 ***Incisura ischiadica major***. Greater sciatic (ischiatic) notch between Tuber sacrale and Spina ischiadica. A B D

D Left Os ilium, lateral aspect (eq)

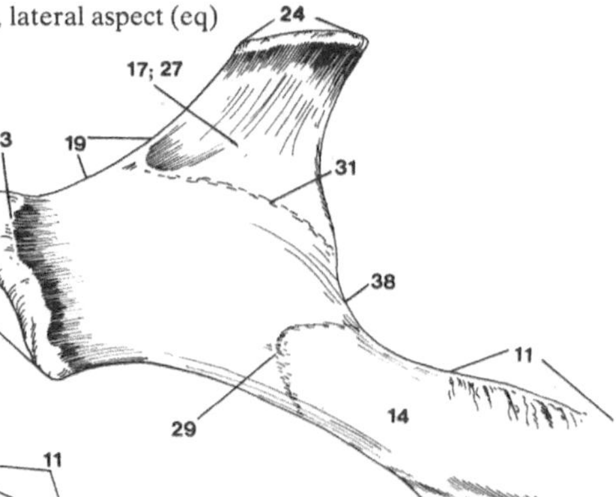

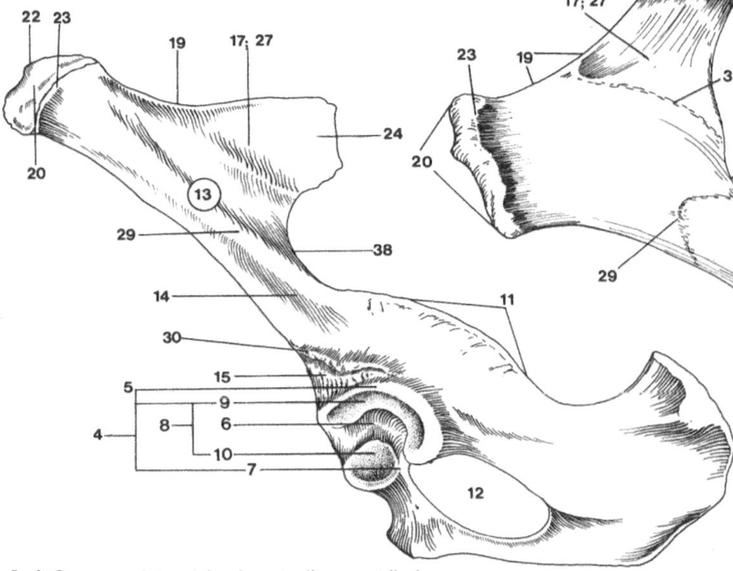

A Left Os coxae, lateral (and ventral) aspect (bo)

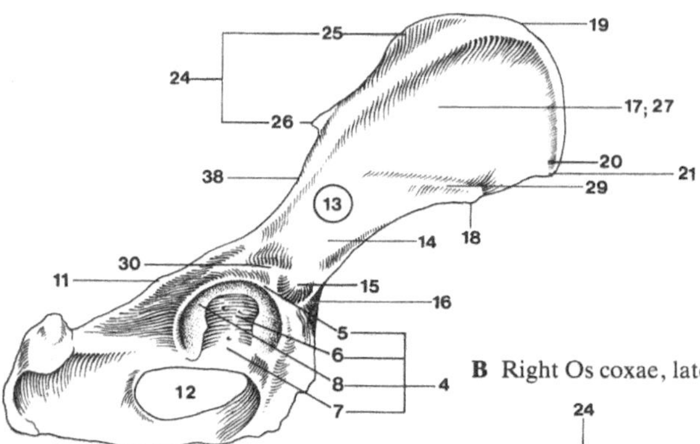

B Right Os coxae, lateral (and ventral) aspect (ca)

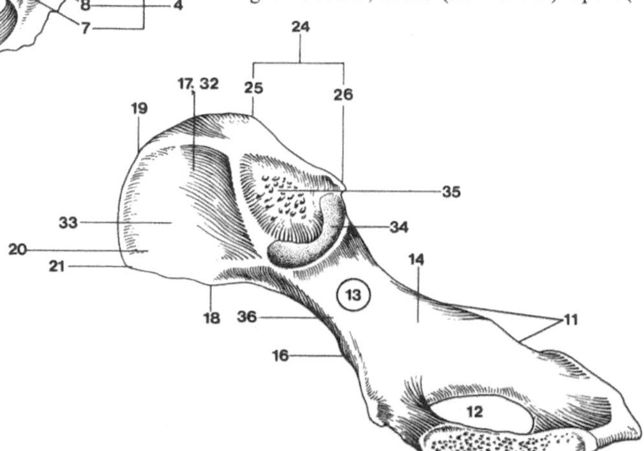

C Right Os coxae, medial (and dorsal) aspect (ca)

1 **Os ischii**. Ischium, or ischial bone. A B C E

2 ***Corpus ossis ischii***. Body of ischium, lateral to Foramen obturatum. A B C E

3 ***Tabula ossis ischii***. Tabula of ischium, caudal to Foramen obturatum. A B C E

4 ***Ramus ossis ischii***. Branch of ischium, medial to Foramen obturatum, fused cranially with Ramus caudalis ossis pubis. A B C E

5 *Facies symphysialis*. Surface facing the Symphysis pelvina. E

6 ***Tuber ischiadicum****. Ischial (ischiatic) tuber, caudolateral extremity of the ischium. A B C E (Tricuspid in bo)

7 ***Incisura ischiadica minor***. Lesser ischiatic notch, between Spina ischiadica and Tuber ischiadicum. B E

8 **Os pubis**. Pubis, or pubic bone. A B C E

9 ***Corpus ossis pubis***. Body of pubis. A C

10 ***Ramus cranialis ossis pubis***. Cranial branch of pubis, cranial to Foramen obturatum. A B

11 ***Ramus caudalis ossis pubis***. Caudal branch of pubis, medial to Foramen obturatum, fuses caudally with Ramus ossis ischii. A B

12 *Facies symphysialis*. Surface facing the Symphysis pelvina. E

13 ***Pecten ossis pubis***. Sharp cranial border of Ramus cranialis ossis pubis. A B C

14 ***Eminentia iliopubica***. Eminence at the lateral end of Pecten ossis pubis. A C E

15 ***Tuberculum pubicum dorsale***. Dorsal median tubercle in the male, esp. eq. B

16 ***Tuberculum pubicum ventrale***. Ventral paramedian tubercle. C

17 ***Sulcus obturatorius***. Groove on the pelvic floor craniolateral to the Foramen obturatum for the passage of N. obturatorius, vulnerable during parturition in cows. B

18 ***Sulcus ligamenti accessorii ossis femoris*** (eq). Groove for the accessory ligament of the head of femur on the ventral surface of Ramus cranialis ossis pubis. C

19 **Pelvis**. Composed of Os sacrum and right and left Os coxae. D E

20 ***Arcus ischiadicus****. Ischial (ischiatic) arch, formed by the caudal borders of right and left Tabula ossis ischii between right and left Tuber ischiadicum. C

21 ***Crista symphysialis***. Median crest on the ventral surface of Symphysis pelvina in bo. A

22 ***Cavum pelvis***. Pelvic cavity, between Apertura pelvis cranialis and caudalis. D

23 ***Linea terminalis***. Circular line from the Promontorium, across Ala ossis sacri, along Linea arcuata and Pecten ossis pubis. D

24 ***Apertura pelvis cranialis****. Cranial pelvic aperture, bordered by the Linea terminalis. D

25 ***Apertura pelvis caudalis****. Caudal pelvic aperture, bordered by Os sacrum, Lig. sacrotuberale (ca) or Lig. sacrotuberale latum in the large animals, and Arcus ischiadicus. E

26 ***Axis pelvis***. Center of all median diameters between pelvic surface of the sacrum and the pelvic symphysis. E

27 ***Solum pelvis osseum****. Floor of the pelvic cavity, formed by the Ossa pubis and Ossa ischii. B C

28 ***Diameter conjugata***. Line from the Promontorium to the cranial end of the Symphysis pelvina. E

29 ***Diameter transversa***. Greatest transverse diameter of Apertura pelvis cranialis. D

30 ***Diameter verticalis***. Line from the cranial end of the Symphysis pelvina to the pelvic surface of sacrum or a caudal vertebra, perpendicular to the Solum pelvis osseum. E

31 ***Inclinatio pelvis***. Angle between Diameter conjugata and Diameter verticalis. E

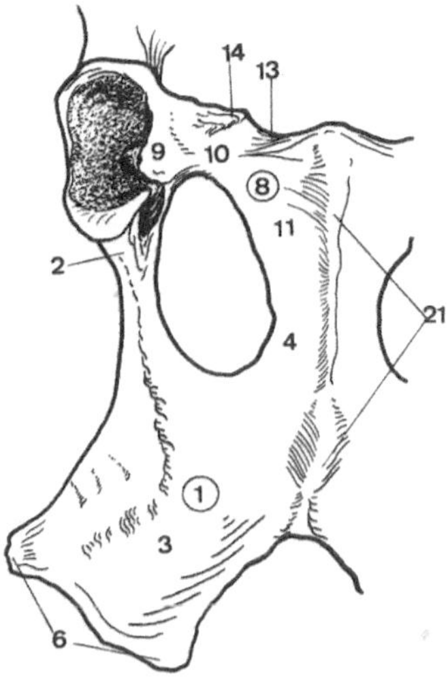

A Right Os ischii and Os pubis, ventral aspect (bo masc)

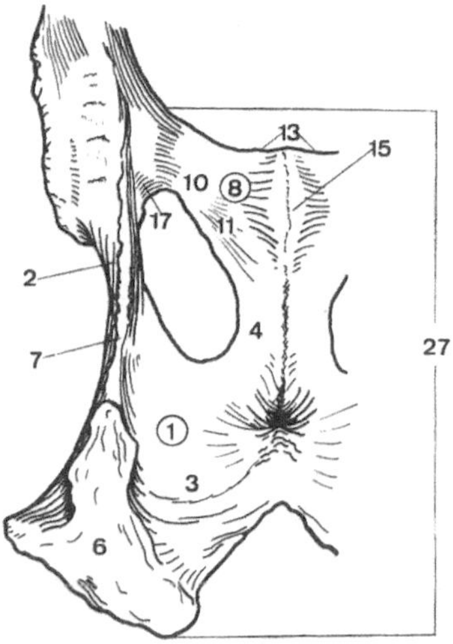

B Left Os ischii and Os pubis, dorsal aspect (eq)

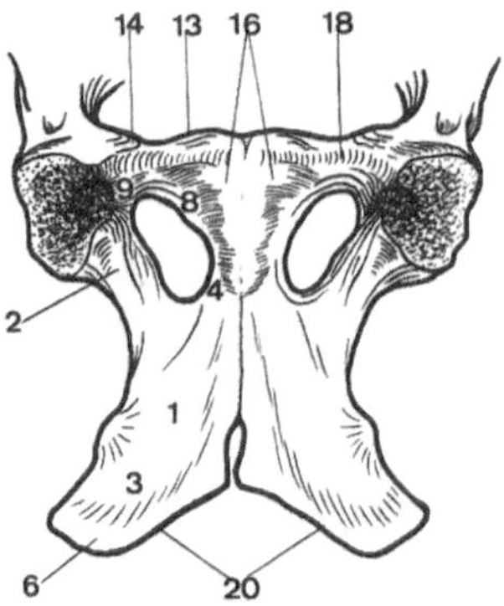

C Solum pelvis osseum, ventral aspect (eq)

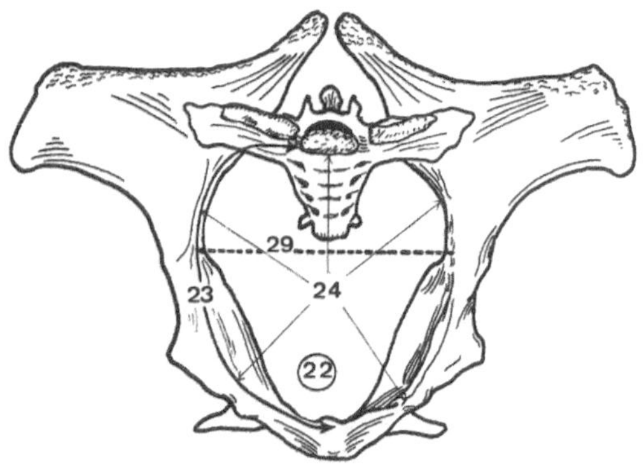

D Pelvis, cranial aspect (eq)

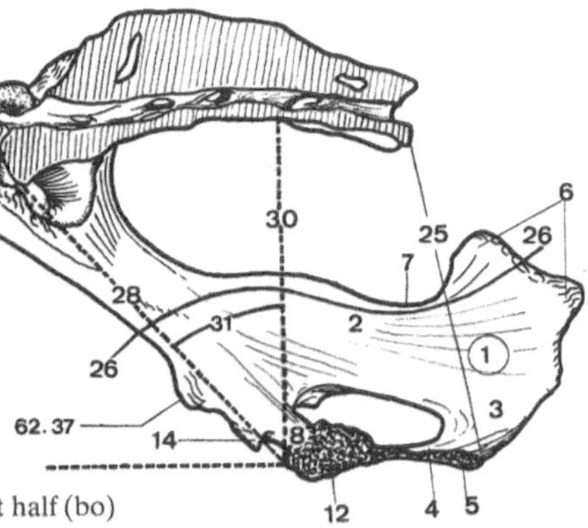

E Pelvis, median section, right half (bo)

1 **Skeleton femoris**. Skeleton of the thigh, or pelvic Stylopodium (including the patella).

2 **Os femoris [Femur]**. A B

3 ***Caput ossis femoris***. Head of femur. A B C

4 *Fovea capitis*. Fovea of head, attachment of Lig. capitis ossis femoris, and in eq in addition, the Lig. accessorium ossis femoris . A B C

5 ***Collum ossis femoris***. Neck of femur, between Caput and Corpus. B C

6 ***Trochanter major****. Greater trochanter, proximolateral extremity, attachment of Mm. glutei medius, accessorius and profundus. There is a horizontal crest separating the greater trochanter from the body of the femur in bo, for the attachment of m. vastus lateralis[1)]. A B C

7 *Pars cranialis*. Cranial part, eq. There is a prominent crest on the lateral aspect of Pars cranialis for the insertion of the M. gluteus accessorius[1)]. A B

8 *Pars caudalis*. Caudal part, eq. A B

9 *Incisura trochanterica**. Notch between cranial and caudal parts in eq. A B

10 *Fossa trochanterica*. Deep notch at the caudal surface, medial to the root of Trochanter major. B C

11 ***Trochanter minor***. Lesser trochanter, medial eminence for attachment of M. iliopsoas. A B C

12 ***Linea intertrochanterica***. Line on the cranial surface, running from Trochanter minor to Caput, absent in su. A

13 ***Crista intertrochanterica***. Crest on the caudal surface, continuation of the medial border of Trochanter major. B C

14 ***Corpus ossis femoris***. Body of femur. A B

15 ***Trochanter tertius***. Third trochanter well developed in eq, absent in su and Ru, lateral protuberance for attachment of M. gluteus superficialis. A B

16 *Facies aspera*. Rough caudal surface for attachment of adductor muscles. B C

17 **Labium laterale**. Lateral border of Facies aspera. B C

18 **Labium mediale**. Medial border of Facies aspera. B C

19 *Tuberositas glutea [glutaea]*. Rough area at the proximal end of Labium laterale in Car, attachment of M. gluteus superficialis. C

20 *Tuberositas m. bicipitis*. Attachment of biceps femoris muscle in eq. B

21 *Fossa supracondylaris*. Depression proximal to Condylus lateralis, deep in eq. shallow in Ru and su, attachment of M. flexor digitorum/digitalis superficialis. B

22 *Tuberositas supracondylaris lateralis*. Rough area proximal to Condylus lateralis, in Car and su, lateral to Fossa supracondylaris, attachment of Caput laterale m. gastrocnemii. B E

23 *Tuberositas supracondylaris medialis*. Rough area proximal to Condylus medialis, attachment of Caput mediale m. gastrocnemii. B E

24 *Facies poplitea*. Popliteal surface, smooth part of the caudal surface, proximal to the condyles. B E

25 ***Condylus medialis****. Medial condyle for articulation with the tibia. B E

26 *Facies articularis sesamoidea medialis*. Facet for the medial sesamoid bone of M. gastrocnemius in Car. E

27 *Epicondylus medialis**. Medial nonarticular elevation on Condylus medialis. A B D E

28 ***Condylus lateralis****. Lateral condyle for articulation with the tibia. B E

29 *Facies articularis sesamoidea lateralis*. Facet for lateral sesamoid bone of M. gastrocnemius in Car. E

30 *Epicondylus lateralis**. Lateral nonarticular elevation on Condylus lateralis. A B D

31 *Fossa extensoria**. Small depression between Condylus lateralis and Trochlea, origin of Mm. extensor digitorum/digitalis longus and fibularis tertius. D

32 *Fossa m. poplitei*. Depression lateral on Condylus lateralis. The origin of M. popliteus. B D

33 ***Fossa intercondylaris***. Large and deep depression between the condyles. B E

34 ***Linea intercondylaris***. Caudal ridge at the proximal end of Fossa intercondylaris. B E

35 ***Trochlea ossis femoris****. For articulation with patella, consisting of a medial and a lateral ridge. A D

36 *Tuberculum trochleae ossis femoris*. Medial eminence on the proximal end of the medial ridge of the trochlea in eq. A

1) The editor suggests this crest to be named "Crista trochanterica lateralis". Barone called it the crest of the greater trochanter (1999, p. 642, Planche 360).

A Right femur, cranial aspect (eq)

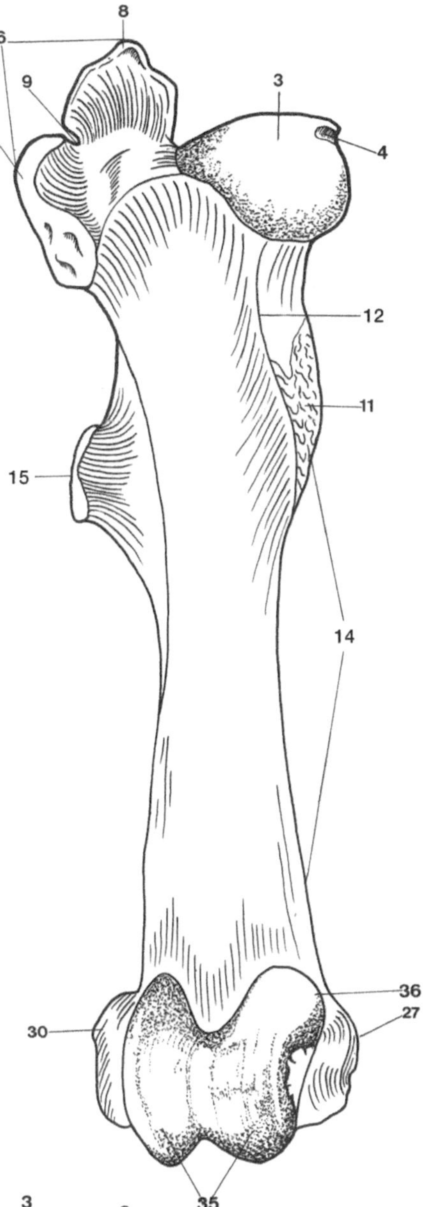

B Right femur, caudal aspect (eq)

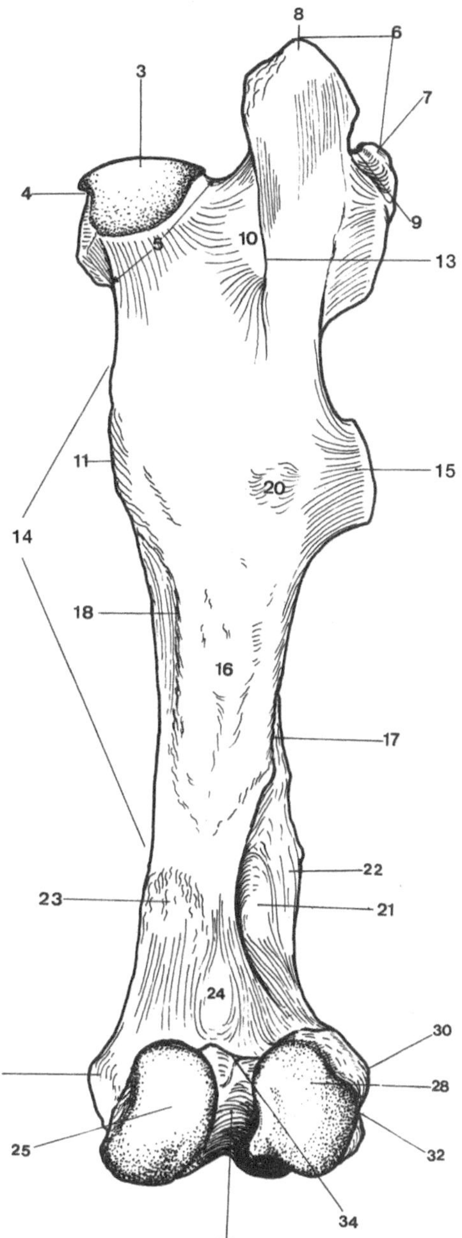

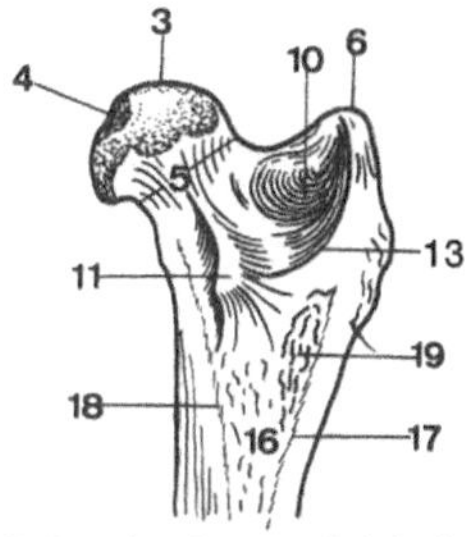

C Proximal part of right femur, mediocaudal aspect (ca)

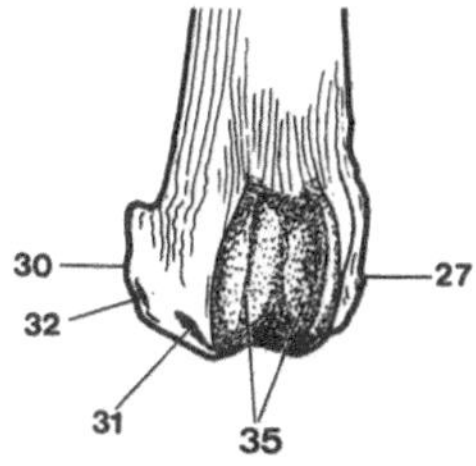

D Distal part of right femur, cranial (and lateral) aspect (ca)

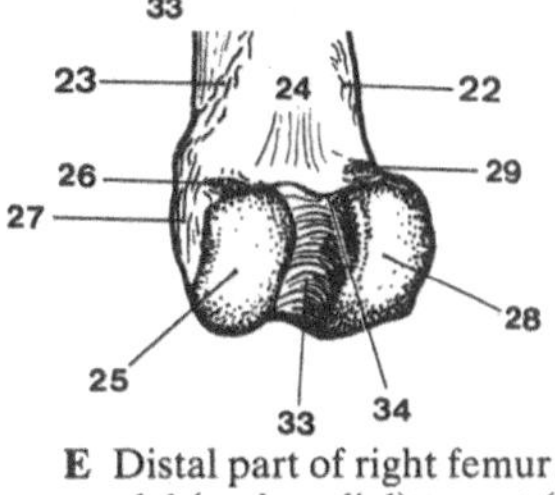

E Distal part of right femur, caudal (and medial) aspect (ca)

1 **Ossa sesamoidea m. gastrocnemii**. Two sesamoid bones in the heads of M. gastrocnemius in Car. A (These bones are often called "fabellae" in Veterinary medicine.)

2 **Os sesamoideum m. poplitei**. Sesamoid bone in the tendon of M. popliteus in Car. A

3 **Patella***. Knee cap. B C

4 ***Basis patellae***. Base of the patella, somewhat wider proximal part. B

5 ***Apex patellae***. Distal tip of the patella. B C

6 ***Facies articularis***. Articular surface, facing the femur. B

7 ***Facies cranialis***. Cranial surface. C

8 ***Processus cartilagineus***. Medial process in bo and eq, partly cartilaginous. B C

9 **Skeleton cruris**. Skeleton of the crus, or pelvic Zeugopodium.

10 **Tibia**. D E

11 ***Facies articularis proximalis***. Proximal articular surface. D E

12 ***Condylus medialis****. Medial condyle for articulation with the medial condyle of the femur. D E

13 ***Condylus lateralis****. Lateral condyle for articulation with the lateral condyle of the femur. D E

14 *Facies articularis fibularis*. Surface for articulation with Caput fibulae, except Ru. E

15 ***Incisura poplitea***. Popliteal (caudal) notch on the proximal extremity of the tibia. D

16 ***Area intercondylaris cranialis****. Two rough areas cranial to Eminentia intercondylaris for attachment of menisci. D

17 ***Area intercondylaris centralis****. Rough depression in the center of the Eminentia intercondylaris for attachment of Lig. cruciatum craniale. D

18 ***Area intercondylaris caudalis****. Rough area caudal to Eminentia intercondylaris for attachment of Lig. cruciatum caudale and Meniscus medialis. D E

19 ***Eminentia intercondylaris****. Proximal eminence between the two condyles. D E

20 *Tuberculum intercondylare mediale*. Medial tubercle of the Eminentia intercondylaris. D E

21 *Tuberculum intercondylare laterale*. Lateral tubercle of the Eminentia intercondylaris. D E

22 ***Sulcus extensorius****. Craniolateral groove on the proximal extremity of tibia for Mm. extensor digitorum/digitalis longus and fibularis tertius. D

23 ***Corpus tibiae***. Body of tibia. E

24 *Tuberositas tibiae**. Cranial elevation on the proximal extremity for attachment of Lig. patellae. D E

25 **Sulcus tuberositatis tibiae***. Groove on the Tuberositas tibiae in su and eq for attachment of the patellar ligament in su, intermediate patellar ligament in eq. D

26 *Facies medialis**. Craniomedial surface. D

27 *Facies caudalis*. Caudal surface. E

28 **Linea m. poplitei**. Mediodistally oriented border of the field of attachment of M. popliteus separating it from the M. flexor digitorum/digitalis lateralis. E

A Right stifle joint, caudal aspect (ca)

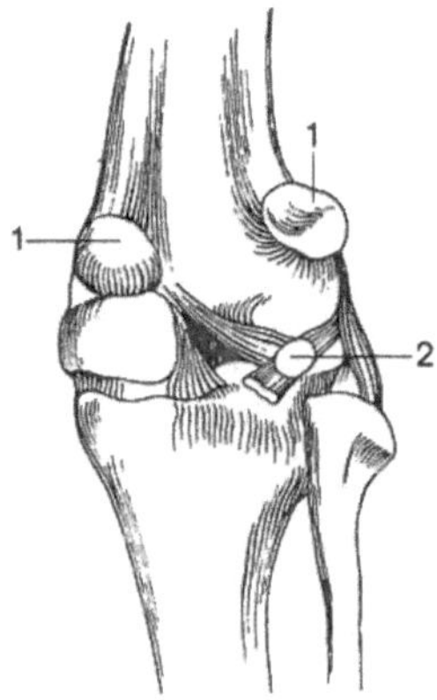

B Left patella, caudal aspect (eq)

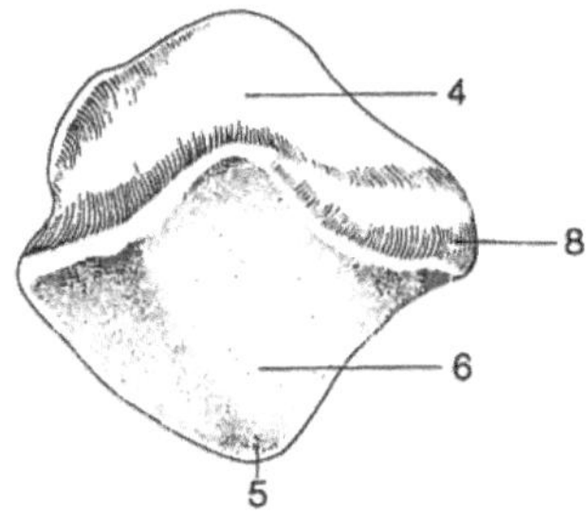

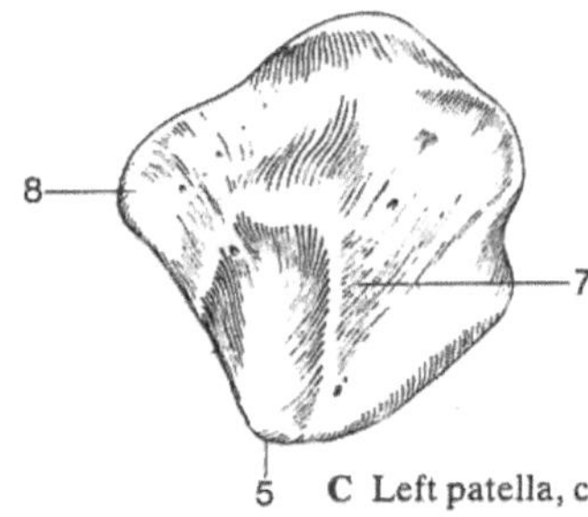

C Left patella, cranial aspect (eq)

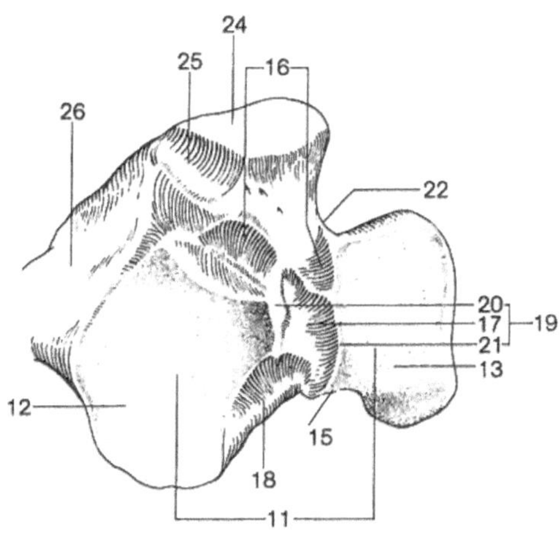

D Right tibia, proximal (and medial) aspect (eq)

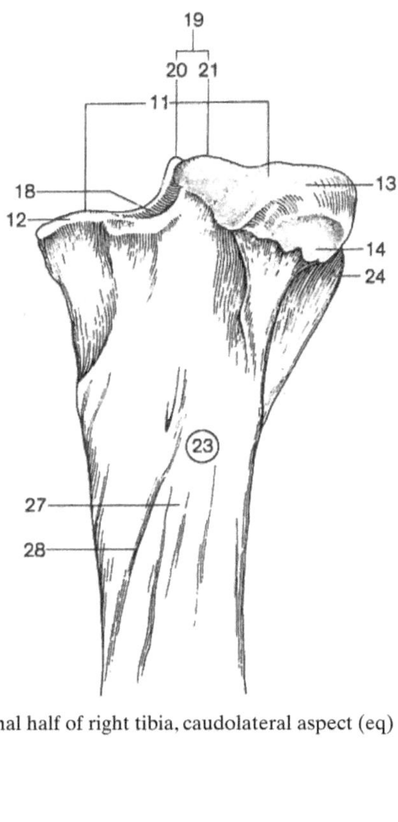

E Proximal half of right tibia, caudolateral aspect (eq)

1 *Facies lateralis*. Craniolateral surface. A

2 *Margo cranialis**. Cranial border, formerly Crista tibiae. A

3 *Margo medialis**. Medial border. A

4 *Margo lateralis [Margo interosseus]*. Lateral border facing fibula in Car, su and partly eq, attachment of Membrana interossea. A

5 ***Cochlea tibiae***. Distal articular surface, facing the talus. A B D

6 ***Malleolus medialis****. Nonarticular prominence medial to cochlea. A B D

7 *Sulcus malleolaris*. Flat groove in the caudal part of Malleolus medialis for the tendon of M. flexor digitorum/digitalis medialis (and M. tibialis caudalis in Car). B D

8 ***Incisura fibularis***. Fibular notch on lateral surface of distal extremity in Car, su, and Ru, facet for fibula. D

9 ***Malleolus lateralis*** (eq)*. Part of tibia, nonarticular prominence lateral to cochlea. A B

10 *Sulcus malleolaris**. Flat groove in eq, for the tendon of M. extensor digitalis lateralis B

11 **Fibula**. C D

12 ***Caput fibulae****. Head of fibula, proximal extremity, rudimentary and fused with tibia in Ru. C

13 *Facies articularis capitis fibulae*. Articular surface of fibular head in Car, su, and eq. C

14 ***Collum fibulae***. Neck of fibula. C

15 ***Corpus fibulae***. Body of fibula, usually absent in Ru, rudimentary in eq. C D

16 *Margo interosseus*. Interosseous border on the medial surface in su, fused with Margo cranialis in Car, attachment of Membrana interossea. C

17 *Margo medialis*. Present in su and in the proximal half of the fibula in Car. C

18 *Margo lateralis*. Present in su and on the proximal half of the fibula in Car. C

19 *Margo cranialis*. Present in Car, su, and eq. C D

20 *Margo caudalis*. Present on the distal part of the fibula in su and Car. D

21 *Facies medialis*. Medial surface, faces the tibia. It is present on the Fibula in su, and on the proximal half of the Fibula in Car. C

22 *Facies lateralis*. Lateral surface. It is present on the Fibula in su, and on the proximal half of the Fibula in Car. D

23 *Facies caudalis*. Caudal surface in the proximal half of the fibula of Car, narrow in su, between Margo medialis and lateralis. C

24 ***Malleolus lateralis*** (Car, su). Distal extremity of the fibula in Car and su, separate bone in Ru (see 29), part of tibia in eq. C D

25 *Facies articulares malleoli*. Articular surfaces in Car, su and Ru for tibia, talus, and calcaneus. C D E

26 *Sulcus malleolaris*. Groove on the lateral surface in Un. In su and Ru for the tendon of M. extensor digitorum lateralis and M. fibularis longus, in eq for the tendon of M. extensor digitalis lateralis. In Car there are two sulci: one on the lateral surface for the tendon of M. fibularis longus, and the other one on the caudal border which allowes passage to the tendons of M. extensor digitorum lateralis and M. fibularis brevis. E

27 *Sulcus tendinis m. fibularis [peron.] longi*. Groove on the lateral surface in Car for the tendon of M. fibularis longus. D

28 *Sulcus tendinum mm. extensoris digitorum lateralis et fibularis [peron.] brevis*. Groove on the caudal side for tendons of M. extensor digitorum lateralis and M. fibularis brevis in Car. D

29 ***Os malleolare*** (Ru)*. Crown-shaped bone on the laterodistal end of Tibia in Ru. E

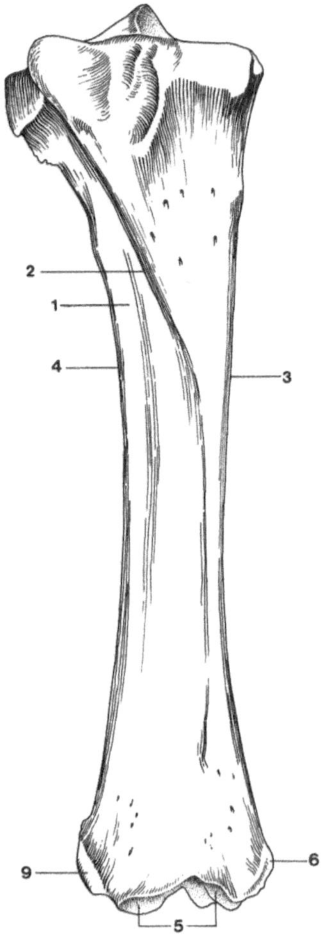

A Right tibia, cranial aspect (eq)

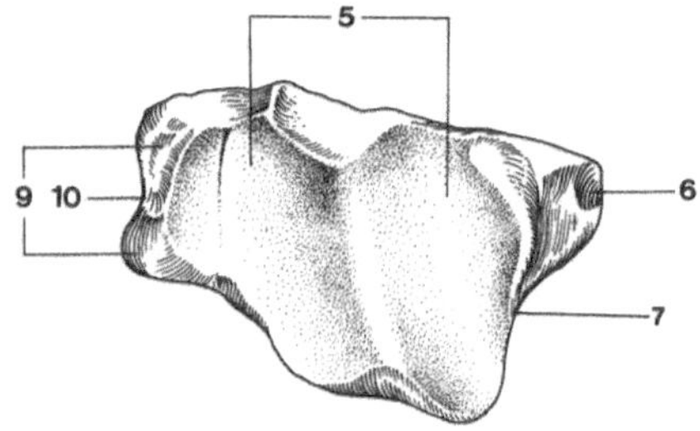

B Right tibia, distal aspect (eq)

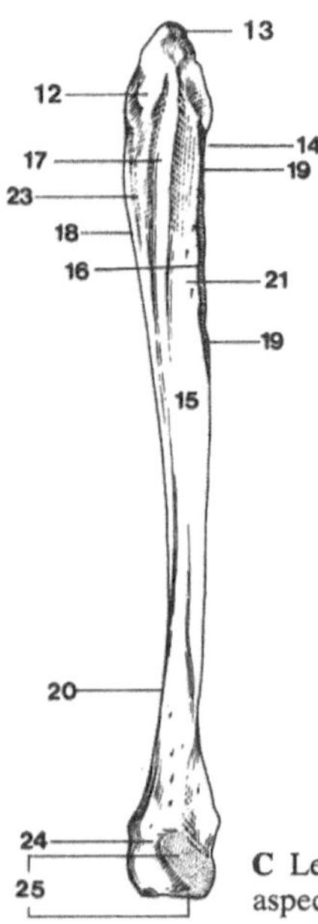

C Left fibula, caudomedial aspect (su)

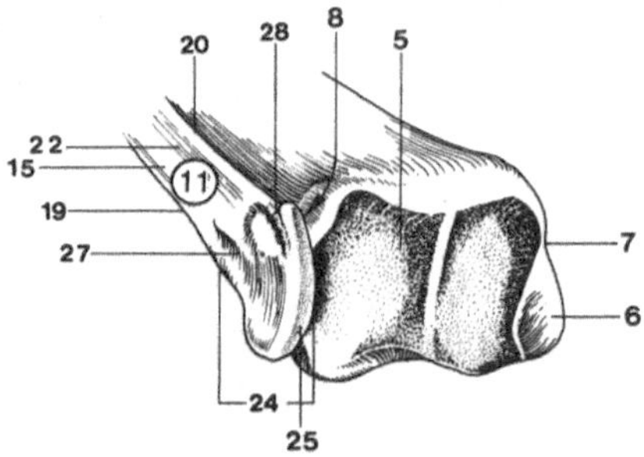

D Left tibia and fibula, distocaudolateral aspect (ca)

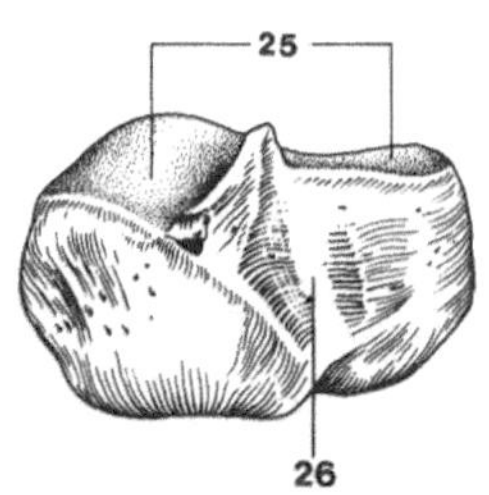

E Right Malleolus lateralis, lateral aspect (bo)

1 **Skeleton pedis**. Skeleton of the pes, or pelvic Autopodium.

2 **Ossa tarsi**. Tarsal bones, or pelvic Basipodium. A B C

3 ***Talus***. A B C D

4 *Caput tali*. Head of talus in Car, articulates with Os tarsi centrale. D

5 *Collum tali*. Neck of talus, distinct in Car, absent in eq. D

6 *Corpus tali*. Body of talus. A B D

7 **Trochlea tali***. Proximal part for articulation with the tibia in eq, tibia and fibula in Car. C D (There is a third trochlea in Ru, for articulation with the calcaneus; the editor suggests to call it “Trochlea tali plantaris”.)

8 **Trochlea tali proximalis**. Proximal part for articulation with tibia and fibula in su and Ru. A B

9 *Facies articulares calcaneae*. Articular surfaces for calcaneus, located plantarly. D

10 *Sulcus tali*. Proximodistally running groove between plantar articular surfaces in Car and eq. D

11 *Tuberculum tali**. Medial tubercle in eq for the attachment of the Lig. tarsometatarseum dorsale. C

12 *Facies articularis navicularis*. Distal articular surface for Os tarsi centrale in Car and eq. D

13 *Trochlea tali distalis*. Distal part for articulation with Os tarsi centrale and tarsale IV in su and Ru. A B

14 ***Calcaneus***. A B C E

15 *Tuber calcanei**. Point of the hock. A B C E

16 *Processus coracoideus*. Dorsal process at the root of Tuber calcanei. E

17 *Sustentaculum tali*. Medial projection with an articular surface for the talus. C E

18 **Sulcus tendinis m. flex. digit. lateralis**. Groove for tendon on the plantar surface of the Sustentaculum tali, tendon bound down by the Retinaculum flexorum. C

19 *Sulcus calcanei*. Proximodistally running groove between the dorsal articular surfaces in Car and eq. E

20 *Sinus tarsi*. Space between talus and calcaneus. C D E

21 *Facies articulares talares*. Articular surfaces for talus, located dorsally. E

22 *Facies articularis cuboidea*. Distal articular surface for Os tarsale IV. A C E

23 *Facies articularis malleolaris*. Articular surface for Malleolus lateralis, in Ru for the Os malleolare. B

24 ***Os tarsi centrale [Os naviculare]****. Central tarsal [navicular] bone. A C

25 ***Os tarsale I [Os cuneiforme mediale]***. First tarsal [medial cuneiform] bone. A

26 ***Os tarsale II [Os cuneiforme intermedium]***. Second tarsal [intermediate cuneiform] bone. A

27 ***Os tarsale III [Os cuneiforme laterale]***. Third tarsal [lateral cuneiform] bone. A

28 ***Os tarsale IV [Os cuboideum]****. Fourth tarsal [cuboid] bone. A C

29 *Sulcus tendinis m. fibularis [peron.] longi*. Lateroplantar groove for this tendon. A B

30 ***Os tarsale I et II [Os cuneiforme mediointermedium]****. Fused first and second tarsal bones in eq. C

31 ***Os tarsale II et III [Os cuneiforme intermediolaterale]***. Fused second and third tarsal bones in Ru. B

32 ***Os centroquartale [Os naviculocuboideum]***. Fused central and fourth tarsal bones in Ru. B

33 ***Canalis tarsi***. Vascular canal for the perforating tarsal vessels in Un between third and fourth tarsal bones, in su additional canal between talus and calcaneus. A C

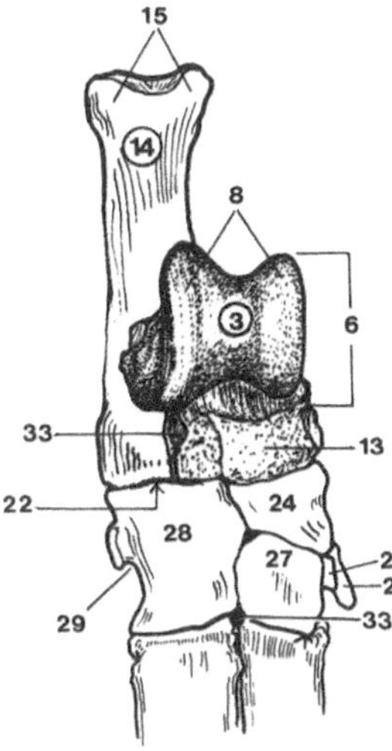

A Right tarsal bones, dorsal aspect (su)

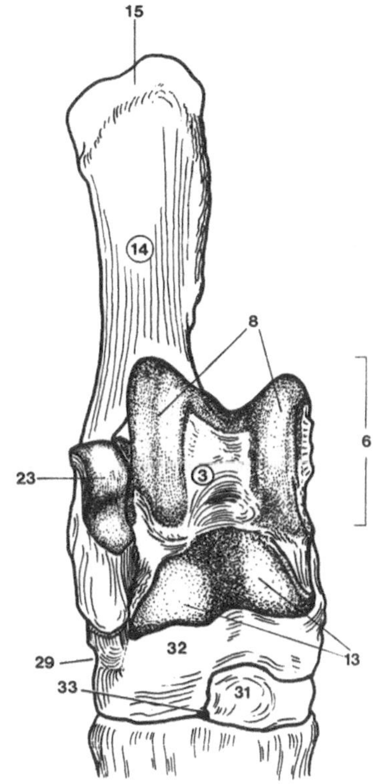

B Right tarsal bones, dorsal aspect (bo)

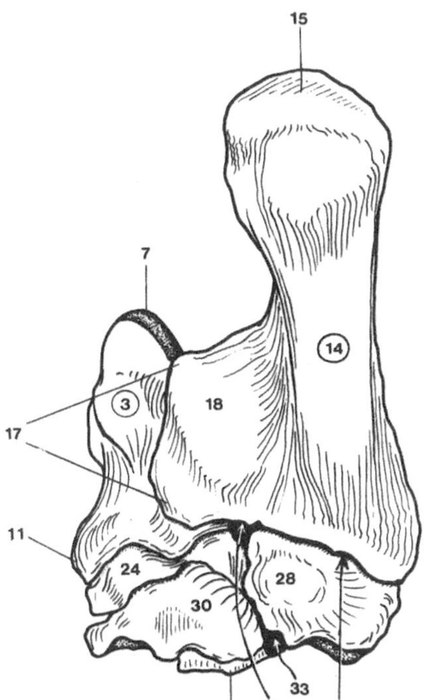

C Right tarsal bones, plantar aspect (eq)

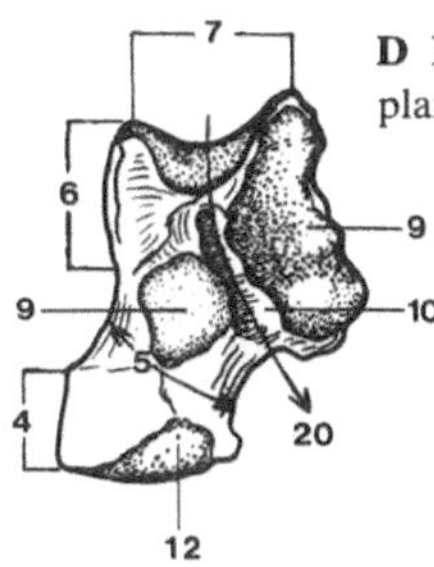

D Right talus, plantar aspect (ca)

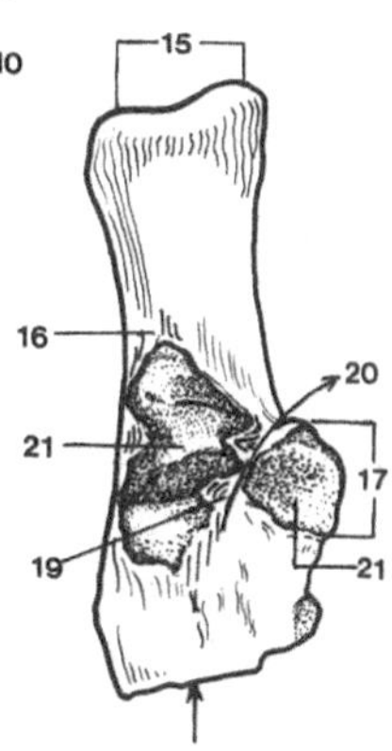

E Right calcaneus, dorsal aspect (ca)

1 **Ossa metatarsalia I–V**, or pelvic Metapodium. A B

2 ***Basis****. Base, the proximal end. A B C D

3 *Facies articularis tarsea*. Articular surface. C D

4 ***Corpus***. Body. A B C D

5 *Facies dorsalis**. Dorsal surface. B D

6 *Tuberositas ossis metatarsalis III**. Dorsal tuberosity at the base of the third metarsal bone for tendinous insertions in su, Ru and eq. D

7 *Facies plantaris*. Plantar surface. A C

8 *Facies medialis**. Medial surface. C

9 *Facies lateralis**. Lateral surface. D

10 ***Caput****. Head, the distal end. A B C D

11 ***Os metatarsale III et IV*** (Ru)*. Fused third and fourth metatarsal bones. C D

12 *Sulcus longitudinalis dorsalis*. Dorsal longitudinal groove. D

13 *Sulcus longitudinalis plantaris*. Plantar longitudinal groove. C

14 *Canalis metatarsi proximalis*. Proximal metatarsal canal. C D

15 *Canalis metatarsi distalis*. Distal metatarsal canal. C D

16 *Incisura intercapitalis**. Former intertrochlear notch, dividing the distal ends (the heads) in Ru. C D

17 ***Os sesamoideum metatarsale***. Plantar sesamoid bone in su and Ru, articulating with the base of Os metatarsale III. C

18 **Ossa digitorum pedis, Pelvic acropodium***. Digital bones of pes. (vide Ossa digitorum manus, sed.) See Ossa digitorum manus.

19 ***Eminentia plantaris medialis***. Medial plantar process in eq. E

20 ***Eminentia plantaris lateralis***. Lateral plantar process in eq. E

20a ***Processus plantaris medialis***. Medial plantar process. E

20b ***Processus plantaris lateralis***. Lateral plantar process. E

21 *Foramen processus plantaris*. Variable foramen of plantar process. E

22 *Incisura processus plantaris*. Variable notch of plantar process. E

A Left metatarsal bones, plantar aspect (ca)

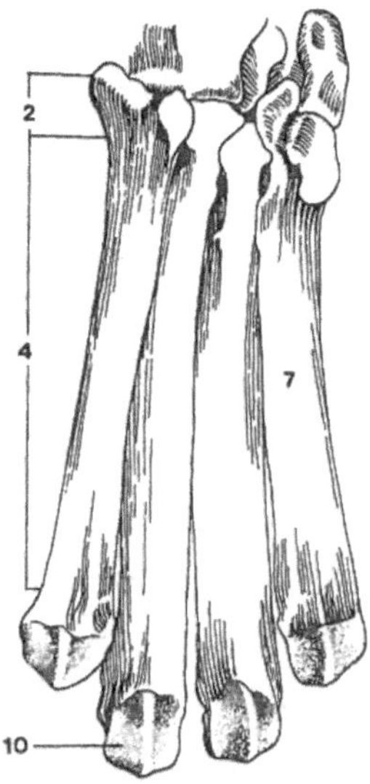

B Left metatarsal bones, dorsal aspect (ca)

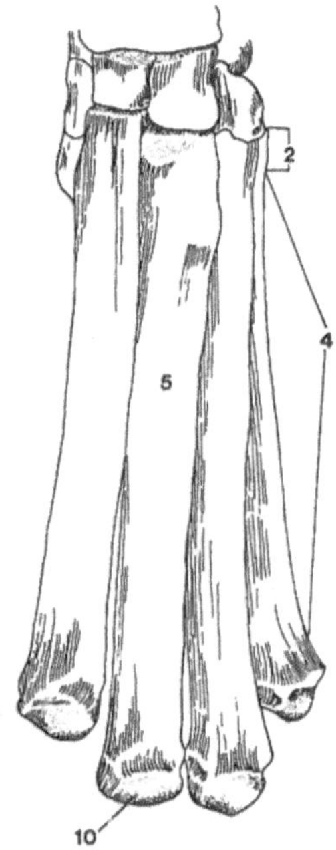

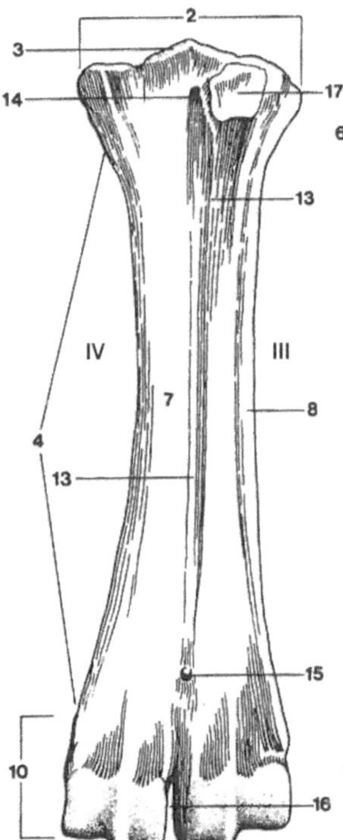

C Left metatarsal bones, plantar aspect (bo)

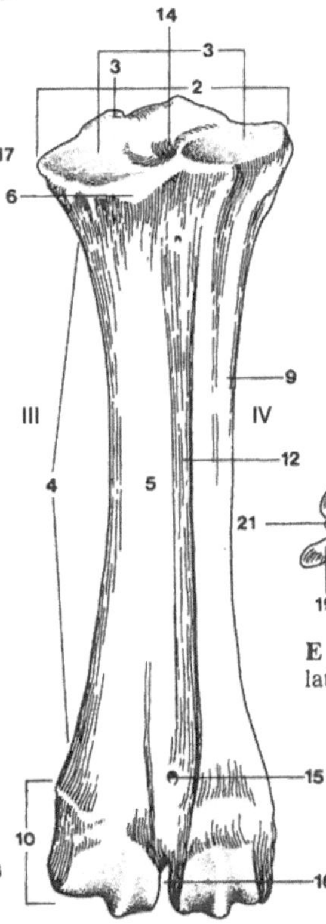

D Left metatarsal bones, dorsal aspect (bo)

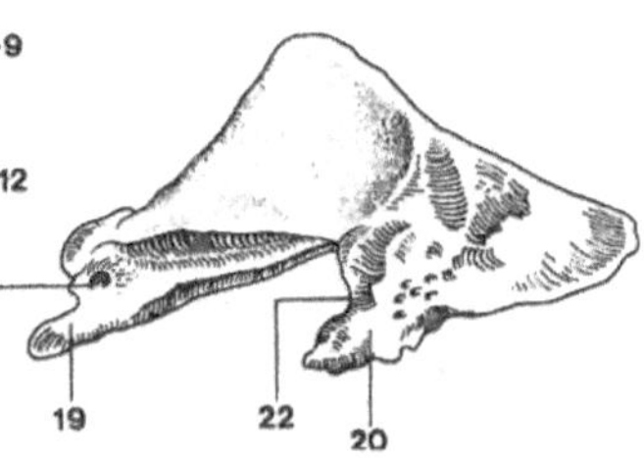

E Phalanx distalis of right hind digit, lateroplantar aspect (eq)

1 **SUTURAE CAPITIS.** Skull sutures.

2 ***Sutura coronalis.*** Coronal suture, between frontal and parietal bones. A B C

3 ***Sutura sagittalis.*** Sagittal suture, between right and left parietal bones. A

4 ***Sutura lambdoidea.*** Lambdoid suture, between parietal bones and occipital (and interparietal) bone. A B

5 ***Sutura occipitointerparietalis.*** Between occipital and interparietal bones in fe, Ru, and eq, persistent only in fe and ov. A

6 ***Sutura occipitosquamosa.*** Between occipital bone and squama temporalis. A B C D

7 ***Sutura occipitomastoidea.*** Ventral continuation of the Sutura occipitosquamosa. A C D

8 ***Sutura occipitotympanica.*** Between occipital bone and tympanic (endotympanic in fe) part of temporal bone, absent in eq. C D

9 ***Sutura sphenofrontalis.*** Between frontal and sphenoid bones. B D

10 ***Sutura sphenoethmoidalis.*** Between presphenoid and ethmoid bones, in Car and eq only inside the skull. B D

11 ***Sutura sphenosquamosa.*** Between basisphenoid (and presphenoid in eq) and squama temporalis. B C D

12 ***Sutura sphenoparietalis.*** Between basisphenoid and parietal bone in Car, ov, and cap. C

13 ***Sutura sphenopalatina.*** Between sphenoid and palatine bones. B C D

14 ***Sutura pterygopalatina.*** Between pterygoid and palatine bones. B C

15 ***Sutura pterygosphenoidalis.*** Between pterygoid and sphenoid bones. C

16 ***Sutura squamosa.*** Squamosal suture, between parietal and temporal bones. A B C D

17 ***Sutura interfrontalis.*** Between right and left frontal bones. A

18 ***Sutura squamosomastoidea.*** Between squamous and petrous parts of the temporal bone. A D

19 ***Sutura squamosofrontalis.*** Between squama temporalis and frontal bones in su, older bo, and eq. A B

20 ***Sutura frontonasalis.*** Between frontal and nasal bones. A D

21 ***Sutura frontoethmoidalis.*** Between frontal and ethmoid bones, in Car and eq only inside the skull. B D

22 ***Sutura frontomaxillaris.*** Between frontal bone and maxilla in Car and su. B

23 ***Sutura frontolacrimalis.*** Between frontal and lacrimal bones. A B C

24 ***Sutura frontozygomatica.*** Between frontal and zygomatic bones in Ru, Processus zygomaticus of temporal bone in eq, at the lateral wall of the Orbita. A

25 ***Sutura frontopalatina.*** Between frontal and palatine bones in Car and eq. C

26 ***Sutura zygomaticomaxillaris.*** Between zygomatic bone and maxilla. A B

27 ***Sutura vomeropalatina.*** Between Ala vomeris and Pars perpendicularis of palatine bone, in ca and su also the ventral border of vomer and Pars horizontalis of palatine bone. C D

28 ***Sutura vomeromaxillaris.*** Between ventral border of vomer and Processus palatinus of right and left maxilla. D

29 ***Sutura vomeroincisiva.*** Between vomer and Processus palatinus of right and left incisive bones. D

30 ***Sutura vomerosphenoidalis.*** Between Ala vomeris and presphenoid. C

31 ***Sutura vomeroethmoidalis.*** Between Sulcus vomeris and Pars perpendicularis of ethmoid bone, also between Ala vomeris and Lamina basalis of the ethmoid bone in Car and su. D

32 ***Sutura ethmoidomaxillaris.*** Between maxilla and Laminae basalis and orbitalis of ethmoid bone. B

33 ***Sutura ethmoidonasalis.*** Between nasal bone and Lamina tectoria of ethmoid bone. D

34 ***Sutura sphenomaxillaris.*** Between Processus pterygoideus of basisphenoid and maxilla in su. B

35 ***Sutura temporozygomatica.*** Between temporal and zygomatic bones on the Arcus zygomaticus. A

* Reminder: The structures followed by an asterisk are landmarks for physical examination and/or clinical approach.

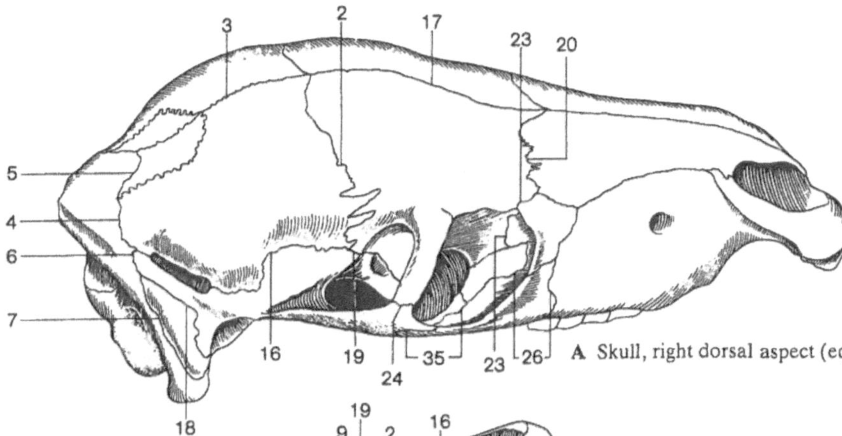

A Skull, right dorsal aspect (eq, young)

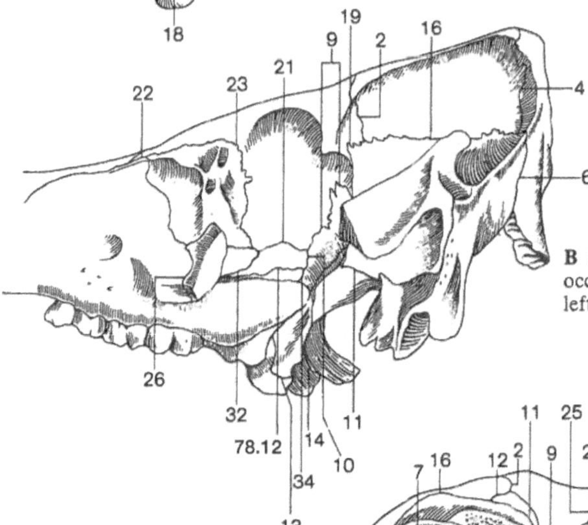

B Skull (zygomatic arch, and part of the occipital and pterygoid bones removed), left aspect (su)

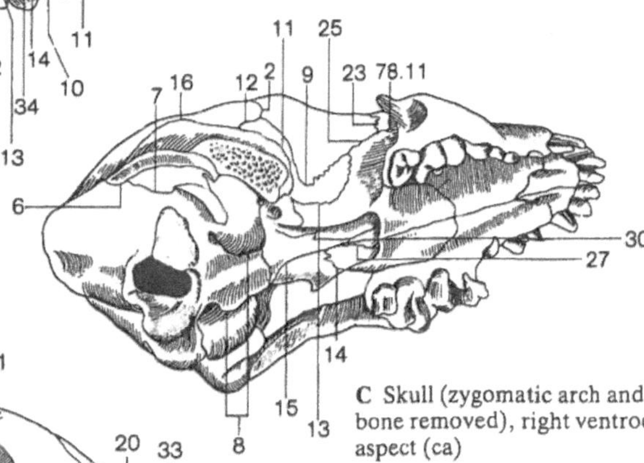

C Skull (zygomatic arch and pterygoid bone removed), right ventrocaudal aspect (ca)

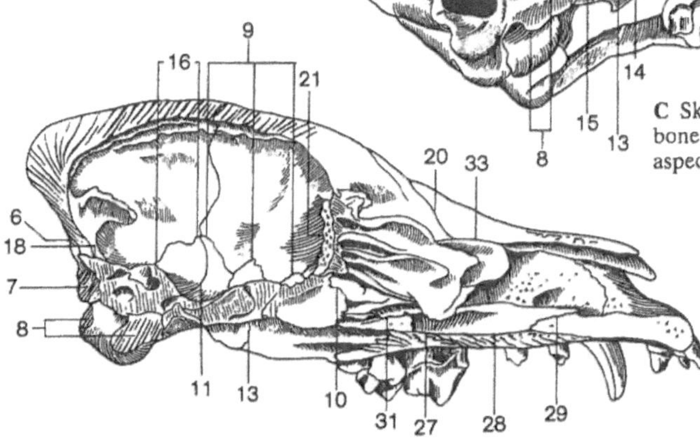

D Skull, paramedian section (occipital and pterygoid bones removed), left medial aspect (ca)

1 ***Sutura internasalis***. Between right and left nasal bones. A

2 ***Sutura nasomaxillaris***. Between nasal bone and maxilla in Car, su, and eq, sometimes in bo. There is a Fissura nasomaxillaris in ov, and cap, sometimes in bo. A

3 ***Sutura nasoincisiva***. Between nasal and incisive bones in Car, su, and eq. A

4 ***Sutura lacrimomaxillaris***. Between lacrimal bone and maxilla. A B

5 ***Sutura lacrimoconchalis***. Between lacrimal and ventral nasal conchal bones in su and Ru. B

6 ***Sutura lacrimozygomatica***. Between lacrimal and zygomatic bones, absent in fe. A

7 ***Sutura nasolacrimalis***. Between nasal and lacrimal bones in eq. There is a Fissura nasolacrimalis in Ru. A

8 ***Sutura interincisiva***. Median suture between the bodies of right and left incisive bones in Car and eq. A

9 ***Sutura maxilloincisiva***. Between maxilla and incisive bone. A B C

10 ***Sutura palatomaxillaris***. Between Pars perpendicularis of palatine bone and maxilla in the Fossa pterygopalatina. B C

11 ***Sutura palatolacrimalis***. Between palatine and lacrimal bones in Car. 77 C

12 ***Sutura palatoethmoidalis***. Between palatine bone and ethmoid, superficially in the Fossa pterygopalatina only in su and bo. 77 B

13 ***Sutura palatina mediana***. Between the two halves of the hard palate, except the rostral part in su and Ru. C

14 ***Sutura palatina transversa***. Between Processus palatinus of maxilla and Pars horizontalis of palatine bone. B C

15 **SYNCHONDROSES CRANII**. Cartilaginous joints of the skull. Most of them disappear by progressive ossification.

16 ***Synchondrosis sphenooccipitalis***. Between basisphenoid and occipital bones. C D

17 ***Synchondrosis sphenopetrosa***. Between basisphenoid and petrosal bones in Car. Remains in the adult as fissure in the macerated skull, contains then fibrocartilage. D

18 ***Synchondrosis petrooccipitalis***. Between petrosal and occipital bones in Car and Ru. Remains in the adult as fissure in the macerated skull, contains then fibrocartilage. D

19 ***Synchondrosis intersphenoidalis***. Between pre- and basisphenoid bones. C D

20 ***(Synchondrosis intraoccipitalis squamolateralis)***. Between Pars lateralis and Squama occipitalis. E

21 ***(Synchondrosis intraoccipitalis basilateralis)***. Betwen Pars basilaris and Squama occipitalis. D E

22 **Articulatio temporomandibularis***. Synovial joint between the Ramus mandibulae and the Pars squamosa of the temporal bone. F

23 ***Capsula articularis***. Joint capsule.

24 *Membrana synovialis dorsalis*. Between Os temporale and Discus articularis. F

25 *Membrana synovialis ventralis*. Between Discus articularis and Mandibula. F

26 ***Discus articularis***. Disk in the temporomandibular joint, dividing it into two completely separated compartments. F

27 ***Lig. laterale***. Ligament on the lateral surface of the joint capsule. F

28 ***Lig. caudale***. Elastic ligament from Processus retroarticularis to Collum mandibulae in eq (and Ru). F

29 **Articulatio temporohyoidea**. Attachment of Apparatus hyoideus to Os temporale. F

30 **Articulatio intermandibularis**. Median connection of the bodies of right and left halves of the mandible, in adult su and eq replaced by a synostosis. G

31 ***Synchondrosis intermandibularis***. The smaller part of Articulatio intermandibularis is formed by cartilage. G

32 ***Sutura intermandibularis***. The larger part of Articulatio intermandibularis is formed by connective tissue. G

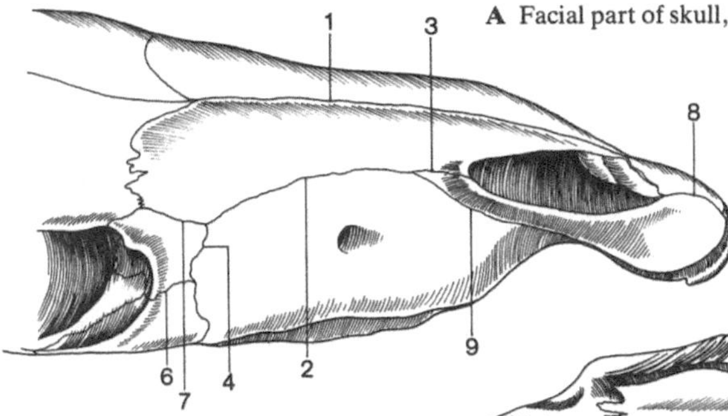

A Facial part of skull, right dorsal aspect (eq, young)

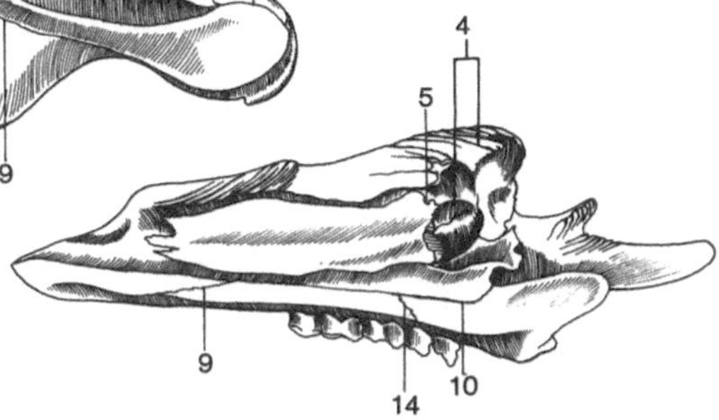

B Right maxilla, incisive, lacrimal and ventral turbinate bones, medial aspect (su)

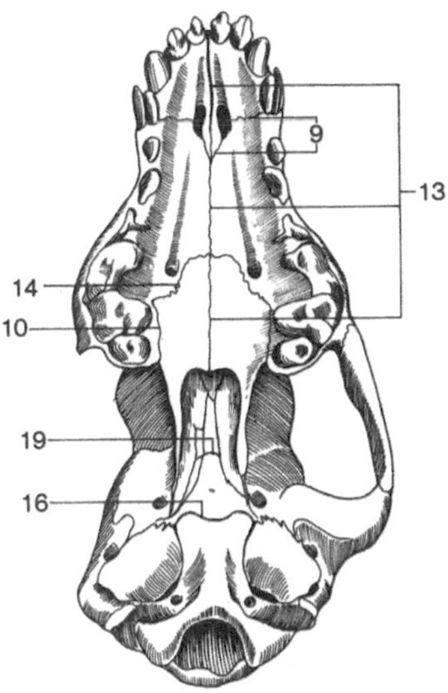

C Hard palate and base of skull (ca)

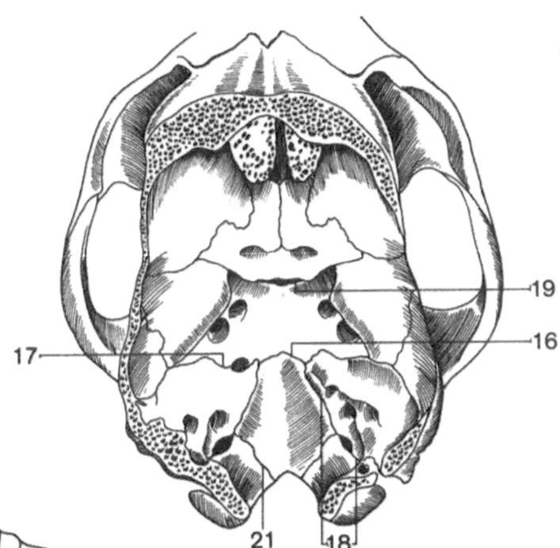

D Base of skull (part of left petrosal bone removed), dorsal aspect (ca)

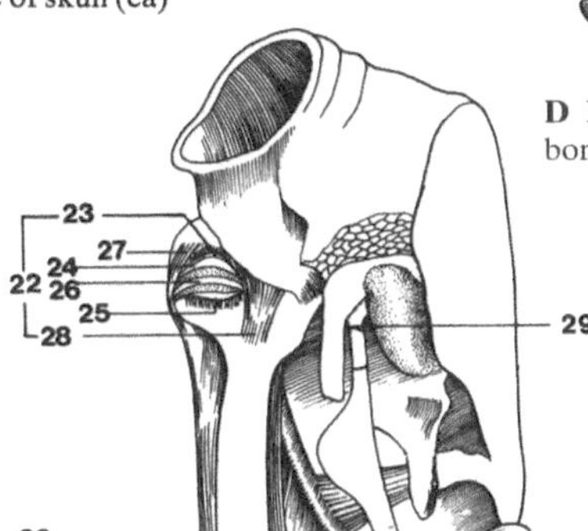

F Right temporomandibular and temporohyoid joints, caudomedial aspect (eq)

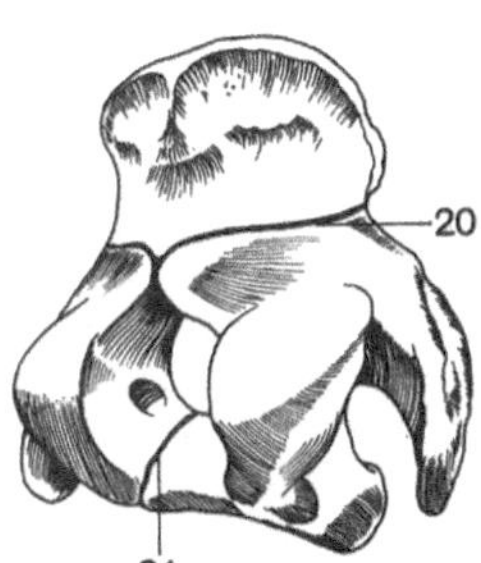

E Os occipitale, right caudal aspect (eq, young)

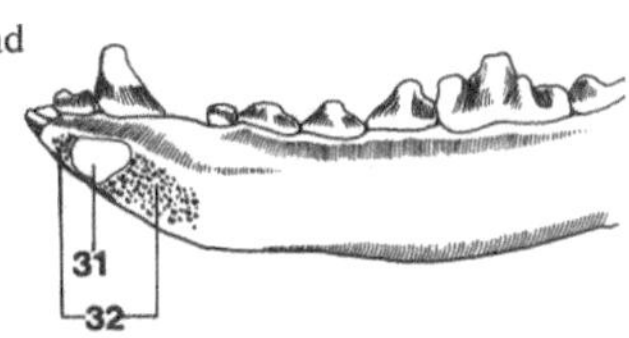

G Articulatio intermandibularis, median section, right half (ca)

1 **ARTICULATIONES COLUMNAE VERTEBRALIS, THORACIS ET CRANII.** Joints of the vertebral column, thorax, and skull.

2 ***Symphysis intervertebralis.*** B

3 *Discus intervertebralis.* Intervertebral disc, connecting adjacent vertebral bodies. A B D

4 **Anulus fibrosus.** Fibrous ring around the nucleus pulposus. A B

5 **Nucleus pulposus***. Soft, but noncompressible substance in the center of the intervertebral disc, susceptible to herniate inside of Canalis vertebralis. A B

6 *Lig. longitudinale ventrale.* Connects the ventral surfaces of the vertebral bodies from 7th thoracic vertebra to sacrum. B

7 *Lig. longitudinale dorsale.* Connects the dorsal surfaces of the vertebral bodies. A B

8 ***Ligg. flava.*** Yellow elastic ligaments connecting the vertebral arches. A

9 ***Articulationes processuum articularium.*** Joints between articular processes of the cervical, thoracic, lumbar vertebrae, and between the last lumbar vertebra and the sacrum. A C D

10 *Capsula articularis.* Joint capsule. A C

11 ***Ligg. intertransversaria.*** Between transverse processes of lumbar vertebrae. B D

12 ***Ligg. interspinalia.*** Between spinous processes, absent in Car. C

13 ***Lig. supraspinale.*** Attached to the tips of the spinous processes of thoracic and lumbar vertebrae. C

14 ***Lig. nuchae.*** Nuchal ligament. Modified elastic continuation of Lig. supraspinale in ca, Ru, and eq. C

15 *Funiculus nuchae.* From Protuberantia occipitalis externa in Ru* and eq*, from spinous process of axis in ca to spinous processes of thoracic vertebrae. C

16 *Lamina nuchae.* From spinous processes of cervical vertebrae to Funiculus nuchae in Ru and eq. C

17 ***Articulationes intertransversariae lumbales.*** Synovial joints in eq between transverse processes of Vertebrae lumbales V et VI, often also between IV et V. D

18 ***Articulatio lumbosacralis.*** Joint between last lumbar vertebra and sacrum. D

19 *Lig. iliolumbale.* Lamina from transverse processes of last (Car, su, ov, cap), last two (bo) or last 3–4 (eq) lumbar vertebrae to Crista iliaca. D

20 *Articulatio intertransversaria lumbosacralis.* Synovial joint between the transverse process of Vertebra lumbalis VI and Ala ossis sacri in eq. D

21 **Articulatio atlantooccipitalis***. Joint between atlas and occipital bone. C E F G

22 ***Capsula articularis.*** E F G

23 *Membrana atlantooccipitalis ventralis.* Ventral thickening of the capsule. E

24 ***Membrana atlantooccipitalis dorsalis.*** Connects Arcus dorsalis of atlas and occipital bone. E G

25 ***Lig. laterale.*** From Ala atlantis to occipital bone. E F G

26 **Articulatio atlantoaxialis.** Joint between atlas and axis. C E F G

27 ***Capsula articularis.*** E F G

28 ***Membrana atlantoaxialis dorsalis.*** Connection between Arcus dorsalis of atlas and arch of axis. E

29 ***Lig. atlantoaxiale dorsale.*** Elastic ligament between Tuberculum dorsale of atlas and Processus spinosus of axis. E

30 ***Membrana tectoria.*** From the dorsal surface of the body of the axis to the ventral border of the Foramen magnum, also attached inside the atlas. G

31 ***Lig. transversum atlantis*** (or, Car, su). From one side of the atlas to the other, dorsal to the dens. F

32 ***Lig. longitudinale dentis.*** In Ru and eq from the dorsal surface of the dens to the inner surface of Arcus ventralis of the atlas. G

33 ***Lig. apicis dentis*** (or, Car, su, Ru). From the Apex of the dens to the Pars basilaris of the occipital bone. G

34 ***Ligg. alaria*** (or, Car, su). From lateral border of dens to Condylus occipitalis (or, Car) or internal aspects of the Condylus occipitalis (su). F

35 ***Lig. atlantoaxiale ventrale.*** From Tuberculum ventrale of atlas to Crista ventralis of axis in Ru and eq. E

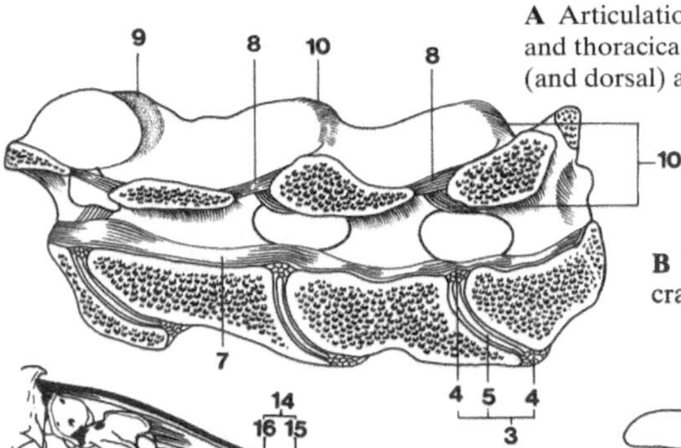

A Articulations of the last Vertebrae cervicales (on the left side) and thoracica I (on the right side), median section, right medial (and dorsal) aspect (eq)

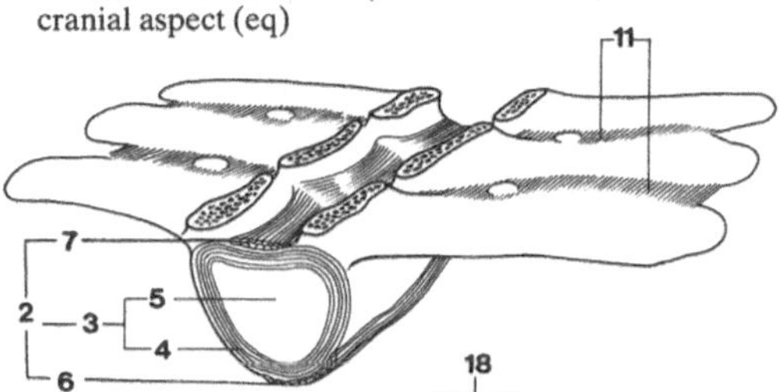

B Vertebrae lumbales (arches removed), left dorso-cranial aspect (eq)

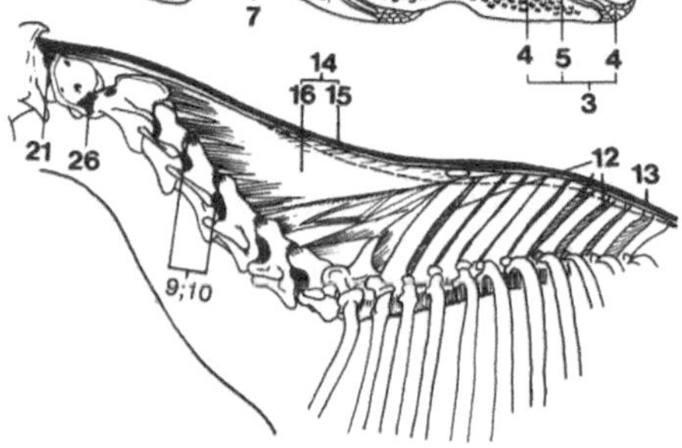

C Ligamentum nuchae, left aspect (eq)

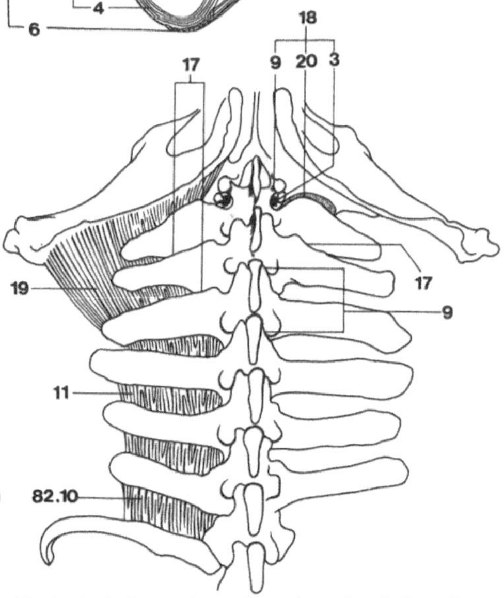

D Articulations of the Vertebrae lumbales, dorso-cranial aspect (eq)

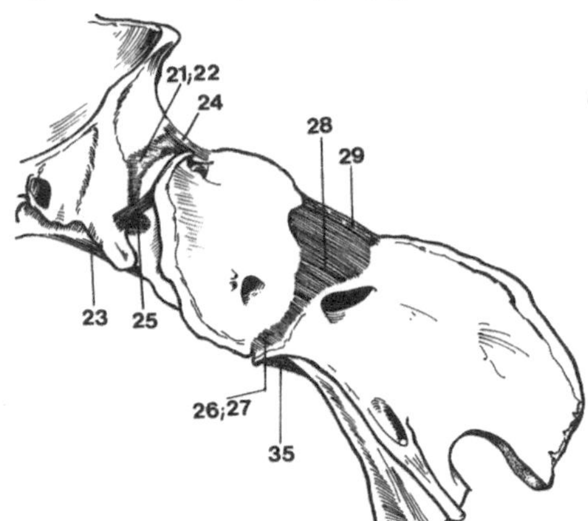

E Articulations of atlas and axis, left aspect (eq)

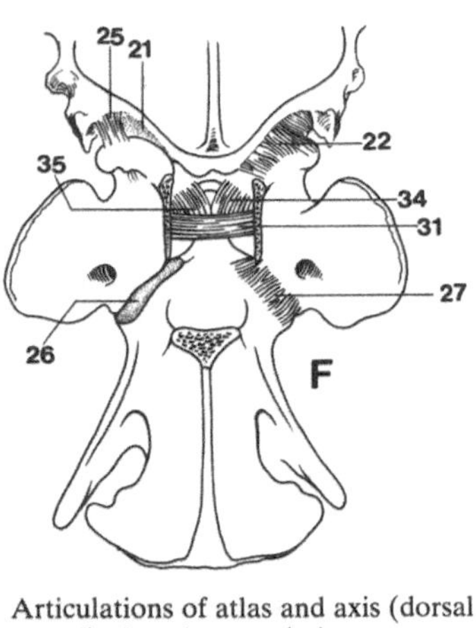

F Articulations of atlas and axis (dorsal arch of atlas removed), dorsal aspect (ca)

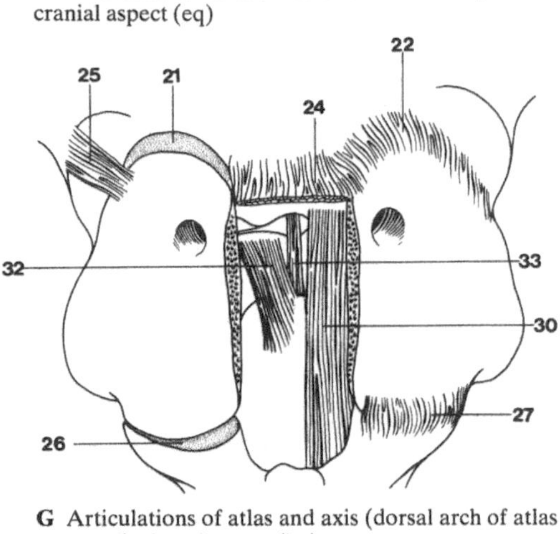

G Articulations of atlas and axis (dorsal arch of atlas removed), dorsal aspect (bo)

1 **Articulationes costovertebrales.** Joints between ribs and thoracic vertebrae. A B

2 **Articulatio capitis costae.** Joint between the head of a rib and the bodies of two adjacent vertebrae and intervertebral disc. A B

3 ***Capsula articularis.*** Joint capsule. B

4 ***Lig. capitis costae radiatum.*** Radiates from the ventral surface of the head of a rib to the bodies of two adjacent vertebrae. A B

5 ***Lig. capitis costae intraarticulare.*** From the Crista capitis costae to the dorsal surfaces of two adjacent vertebrae and the intervertebral disc. A

6 *Lig. intercapitale.* Part of Lig. capitis costae intraarticulare which connects the heads of ribs of the same segment. A

7 **Articulatio costotransversaria.** Joint between Tuberculum costae and transverse process of the thoracic vertebra caudal to the rib. A B

8 ***Capsula articularis.*** Joint capsule. A B

9 ***Lig. costotransversarium.*** Between neck of rib and transverse process of the thoracic vertebra caudal to the rib. A

10 ***Lig. lumbocostale.*** Between last rib and transverse process of the first lumbar vertebra, of different thickness according to species and individual. 81 D

11 **Articulationes sternocostales.** Joints between Cartilagines costales and sternum. C E

12 ***Capsula articularis.*** Jont capsule. C E

13 ***Ligg. sternocostalia radiata.*** Radiating from Cartilago costalis to sternum, especially on the dorsal surface. C

14 ***Lig. sterni.*** Fiber bundles on the dorsal surface of the sternum in bo and eq. C

15 ***Membrana sterni.*** Ligamentous tissue on the ventral surface of the sternum in su and Ru. D

16 ***Ligg. costoxiphoidea.*** Fibers from the last Costa vera (first Costa spuria in eq) to Processus xiphoideus. E

17 ***Membrana intercostalis externa.*** Continuation of Mm. intercostales externi at the ventral end of the intercostal space. Well developed only in bo and eq. E

18 ***Membrana intercostalis interna.*** Continuation of Mm. intercostales interni at the ventral end of the intercostal space. Well developed only in eq and especially in bo. E

19 **Synchondroses sternales.** Cartilaginous joints betwen parts of the sternum. E

20 ***Synchondrosis manubriosternalis.*** Cartilaginous joint between Manubrium and Corpus sterni in young domestic mammals; in adult only in Car, eq, and sometimes cap. E

21 ***Synchondroses intersternebrales.*** Cartilaginous joints between Sternebrae, ossify in su and Ru. D E

22 ***Synchondrosis xiphosternalis.*** Cartilaginous joint between Corpus sterni and Processus xiphoideus, ossifies in su and Ru. E

23 **Articulatio synovialis manubriosternalis.** Synovial joint between Manubrium and Corpus sterni in adult su, bo, ov, and sometimes cap. D

24 ***Capsula articularis.*** Joint capsule. D

25 ***Lig. sternocostale intraarticulare.*** Within the joint cavity, between right and left second ribs and sternum in su, bo, ov and sometimes cap. D

26 **Articulationes costochondrales*.** Between osseous and cartilaginous parts of the ribs. C D

27 **Articulationes intrachondrales.** Synovial joints within the cartilage of 2nd to 5th ribs in su, 2nd to 10th in Ru. Occur sometimes in older ca. D

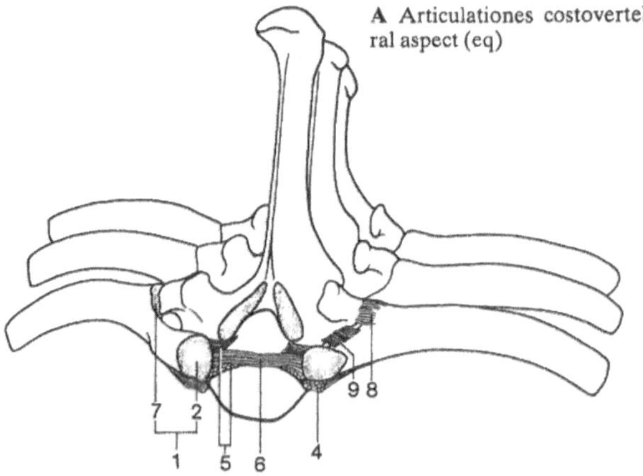

A Articulationes costovertebrales, craniodorsolateral aspect (eq)

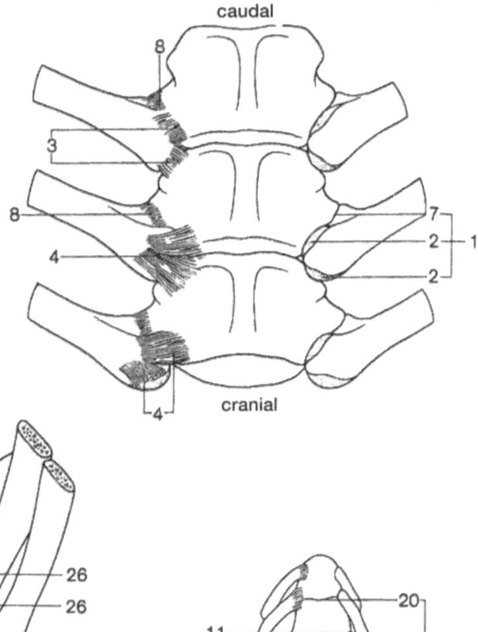

B Articulationes costovertebrales, ventral aspect (eq)

C Articulationes sternocostales, dorsal aspect (eq)

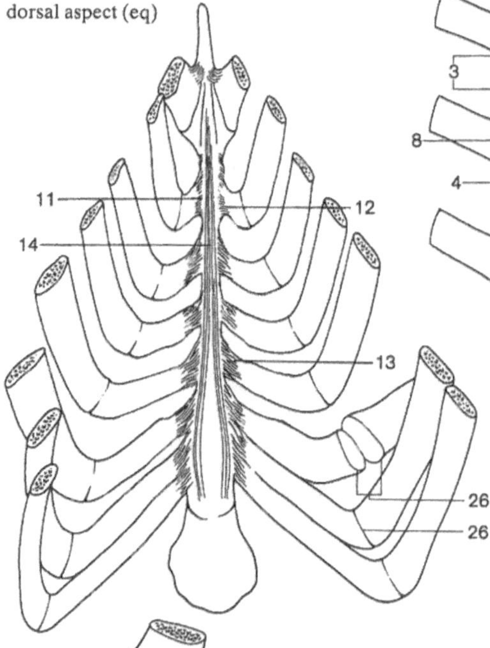

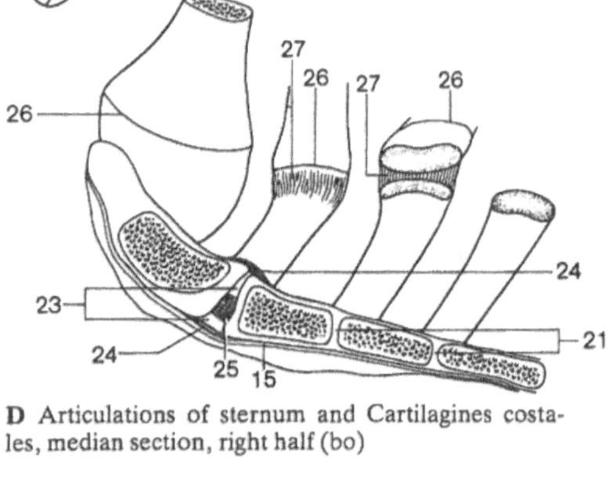

D Articulations of sternum and Cartilagines costales, median section, right half (bo)

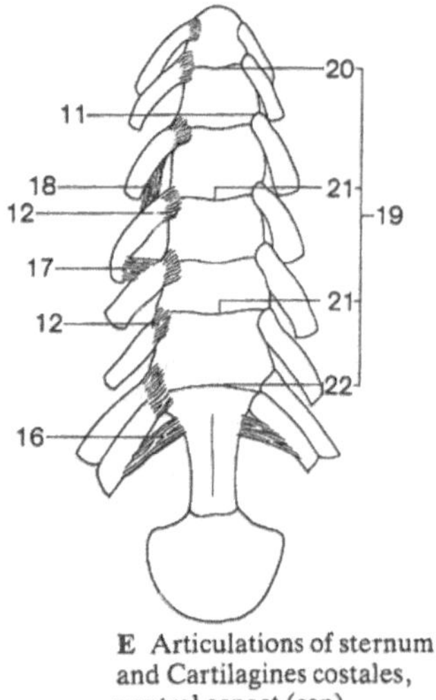

E Articulations of sternum and Cartilagines costales, ventral aspect (cap)

1 **ARTICULATIONES MEMBRI THORACICI.** Joints of the thoracic limb.

2 **Articulatio humeri***. Shoulder joint. Between scapula and humerus. A B

3 ***Capsula articularis.*** Joint capsule, surrounds the entire joint. A B

4 ***Labrum glenoidale.*** Glenoid labrum. Fibrocartilaginous rim enlarging and deepening the Cavitas glenoidalis. A

5 ***Lig. coracohumerale.*** Thickend part of capsule between Tuberculum supraglenoidale and the bases of Tuberculum majus and Tuberculum minus in Un. B

6 ***Ligg. glenohumeralia.*** Thickend parts in the lateral and medial walls on the inner surface of the capsule in ca (laterally and medially) and eq (cranially). A

7 **Articulatio cubiti***. Elbow joint. Between humerus, radius, and ulna. C D E

8 ***Articulatio humeroulnaris.*** Between humerus and ulna. C D E

9 ***Articulatio humeroradialis.*** Between humerus and radius. C D E

10 ***Capsula articularis.*** Joint capsule, the fibrous layer only on the cranial aspect (the flexion angle of the joint). C E (In ca it is reinforced cranially by a ligament unofficially known as the oblique ligament.)

11 ***Lig. collaterale cubiti mediale****. From Epicondylus medialis to radius, in Car and su also to ulna[1)]. D

12 ***Lig. collaterale cubiti laterale****. From Epicondylus lateralis to radius, in Car, su, and Ru also to ulna[1)]. E

13 ***Lig. olecrani.*** Elastic ligament from the medial border of Fossa olecrani to olecranon in Car. D E

14 **Articulatio radioulnaris proximalis.** Joint between Circumferentia articularis radii and Incisura radialis ulnae. C E

15 ***Lig. anulare radii.*** Encircles the head of radius, is attached to the edges of the Incisura radialis ulnae in Car. C E

16 ***Membrana interossea antebrachii.*** Connects radius and ulna as a membrane only in Car; ossifying connective tissue in Un. C D E

17 ***Lig. interosseum antebrachii.*** Connects radius and ulna in the proximal half of Spatium interosseum in Car, lateral to Membrana interossea antebrachii. E

18 **Articulatio radioulnaris distalis.** Joint between Incisura ulnaris radii and Circumferentia articularis ulnae in Car and su. F G

19 ***Capsula articularis.*** Joint capsule. F

20 ***Lig. radioulnare.*** Cranial fibers at the distal ends of radius and ulna in Car. F

21 **Articulationes manus.** Joints of the manus. This term is the heading for all joints of the hand.

22 **Articulatio carpi.** Carpal joint, includes the joints between forearm, carpal and metacarpal bones. F G (The dorsal and palmar joint capsules are not listed in the 5th edition of the N. A. V. as they should have been.)

23 ***Lig. collaterale carpi laterale.*** Extends from Processus styloideus ulnae to Os carpi ulnare in Car, also to Os carpale IV and ossa metacarpalia in Un, with superficial and deep distinct fascicles. F G

24 ***Lig. collaterale carpi mediale.*** Extends from Processus styloideus radii to Os carpi intermedioradiale in Car, also to Os carpale II and ossa metacarpalia in Un, with superficial and deep distinct fascicles. F G

25 **Articulatio antebrachiocarpea.** Joint between the distal parts of radius and ulna and the proximal row of carpal bones. F

26 ***Articulatio radiocarpea.*** Between radius and the first (proximal) row of carpal bones. F G

27 ***Articulatio ulnocarpea.*** Between ulna and the first row of carpal bones. F

28 ***Capsula articularis.*** Joint capsule. G

29 ***Lig. radiocarpeum dorsale.*** Dorsal fibers from radius to Os carpi ulnare (su also intermedium), absent in eq. F

30 ***Lig. radiocarpeum palmare.*** Palmar fibers from radius to Os carpi radiale (eq), intermedium (Car), and ulnare (su, Ru). G

31 ***Lig. ulnocarpeum palmare.*** Palmar fibers from Processus styloideus ulnae to Os carpi radiale, intermedium, in bo ulnare. G

32 **Articulationes intercarpeae.** Joints between carpal bones of one row. F G

33 ***Ligg. intercarpea dorsalia.*** Dorsal ligaments between carpal bones. F

34 ***Ligg. intercarpea palmaria.*** Palmar ligaments between carpal bones. G

35 ***Ligg. intercarpea interossea.*** Interosseous fibers between carpal bones of one row of carpal bones. G

36 **Articulatio mediocarpea.** Joint between proximal and distal rows of carpal bones. F G

37 ***Capsula articularis.*** Joint capsule. F There are no individual fibrous joint capsules for each joint in most species; they are part of the common dorsal and palmar joint capsules of Articulatio carpi.

38 ***Lig. carpi radiatum.*** Palmar fibers diverging from Os carpale III. F G

1) In eq they consist of twisted fibers and are responsible for the spring-like flexion and extension of the joint, after the muscles initiate the motion; these ligaments are muscle energy savers (Ghetie and Riga, 1944/1945).

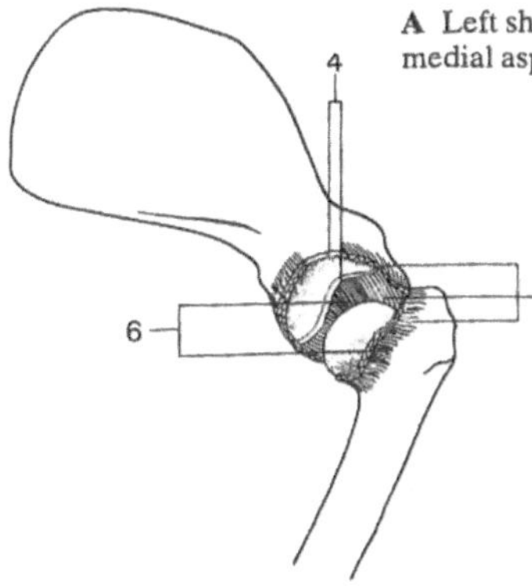

A Left shoulder joint (opened), medial aspect (ca)

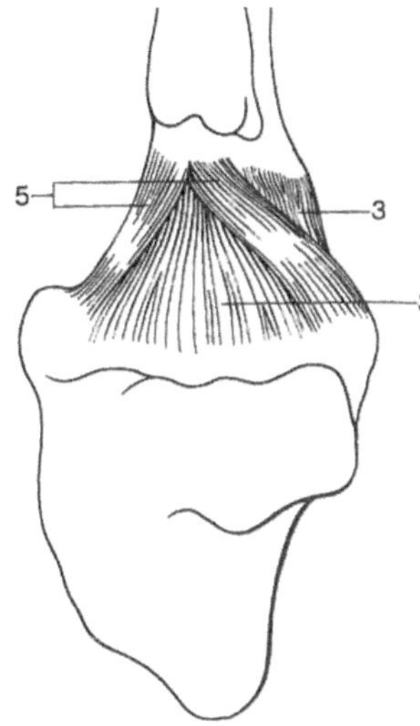

B Right shoulder joint, cranial aspect (eq)

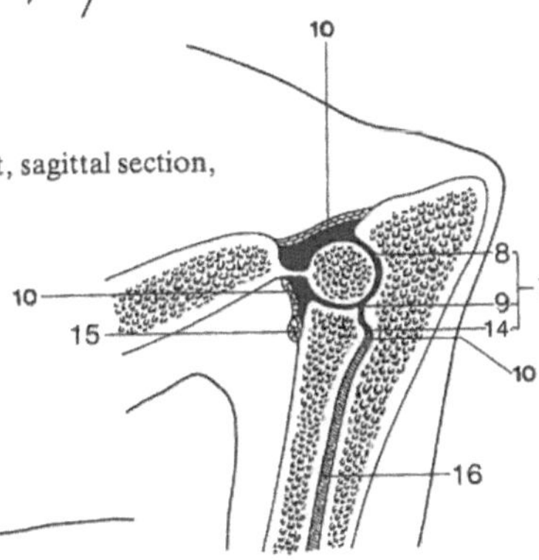

C Left elbow joint, sagittal section, lateral aspect (ca)

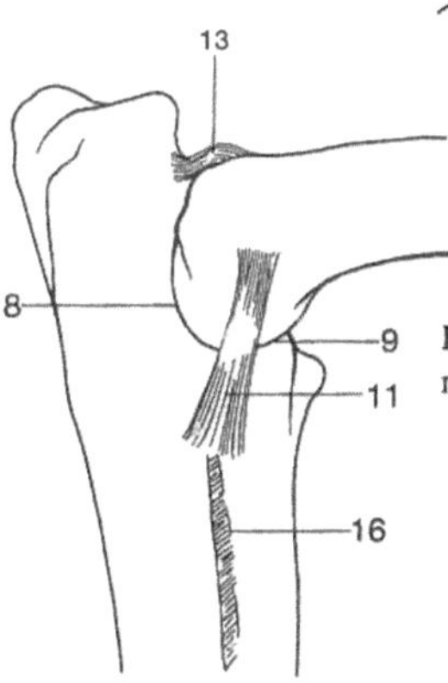

D Left elbow joint, medial aspect (ca)

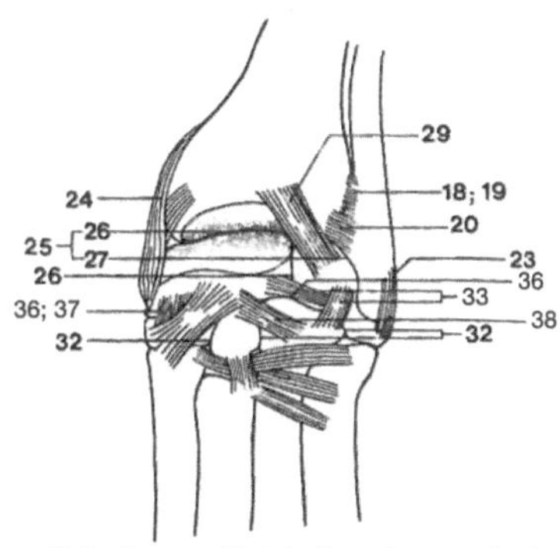

F Left carpal joint, dorsal aspect (ca)

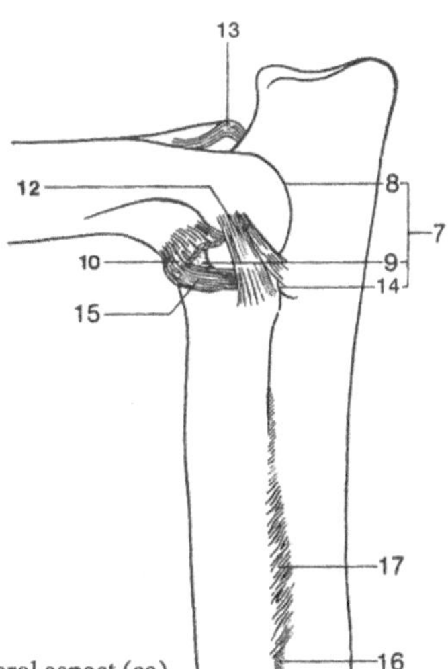

E Left elbow joint, lateral aspect (ca)

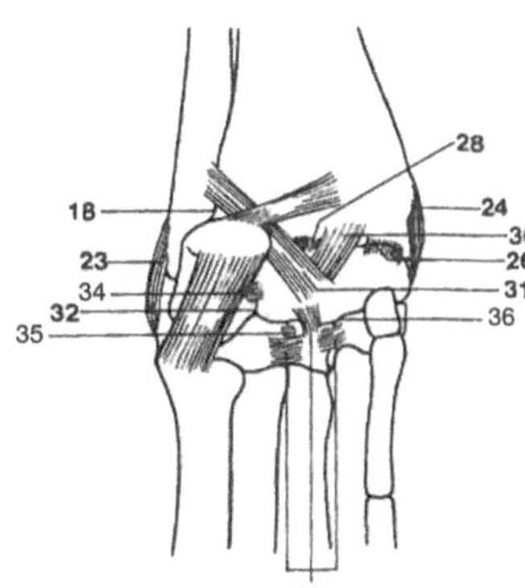

G Left carpal joint, palmar aspect (ca)

1 **Articulatio ossis carpi accessorii [ossis pisiformis]**. Joint between Os carpi accessorium and Os carpi ulnare, in Car also ulna, in eq radius. A B

2 ***Capsula articularis***. Joint capsule between Os carpi accessorium on one side, and the Os carpi ulnare and Caput ulnae/Processus styloideus ulnae (Processus styloideus lateralis), depending on species, on the other side. A

3 ***Lig. accessorioulnare [pisoulnare]***[1]. From Os carpi accessorium to ulna (eq radius). A

4 ***Lig. accessoriocarpoulnare [pisotriquetrum]***[1]. From Os carpi accessorium to Os carpi ulnare. A

5 ***Lig. accessorioquartale [pisohamatum]***[1]. From Os carpi accessorium to Os carpale IV. A

6 ***Lig. accessoriometacarpeum [pisometacarpeum]***[1]. From Os carpi accessorium to metacarpus. A B (It is clinically the most important ligament in bo and eq, landmark for a nerve block anesthesia.)

7 ***Canalis carpi***. Canal between the proximal row of carpal bones and Retinaculum flexorum. B (In Ru and eq it has a deep compartment [the proper or deep carpal canal], and a superficial carpal canal. In Ru through the proper carpal canal glide together the deep digital flexor tendon and the deep tendon of the superficial digital flexor muscle, and through the superficial carpal canal the superficial tendon of the superficial digital flexor and the tendon of the flexor carpi radialis muscles. In eq through the proper carpal canal glide together the tendons of the digital flexor muscles, whereas through the superficial carpal canal only the tendon of the flexor carpi radialis muscle.)

8 **Articulationes carpometacarpeae**. Joints between distal carpal and proximal metacarpal bones. A B

9 ***Capsulae articulares***. Joint capsules. A B (There are no individual fibrous joint capsules for each joint in most species; they are part of the common dorsal and palmar joint capsules of Articulatio carpi.)

10 ***Ligg. carpometacarpea dorsalia***. Dorsal fibers between carpal and metacarpal bones. A

11 ***Ligg. carpometacarpea palmaria***. Palmar fibers between carpal and metacarpal bones. B

12 **Articulationes intermetacarpeae**. Joints between bases of the metacarpal bones. A B

13 ***Capsulae articulares***. Joint capsules. A B

14 ***Ligg. metacarpea dorsalia***. Dorsal fibers between bases of metacarpal bones. A

15 ***Ligg. metacarpea palmaria***. Palmar fibers between bases of metacarpal bones. B

16 ***Ligg. metacarpea interossea***. Interosseous fibers between the bases of metacarpal bones. B

17 ***Spatia interossea metacarpi***. Spaces between metacarpal bones. B

18 **Articulationes metacarpophalangeae***. Joints between metacarpal bones and proximal phalanges. C D E F (In Un it is called the fetlock joint.)

19 ***Capsulae articulares***. Joint capsules around the joints except the palmar sides. C E

20 *Recessus dorsales*. Proximally directed dorsal pouch of each joint capsule. C

21 *Recessus palmares*. Proximally directed palmar pouch of each joint capsule. C

22 ***Ligg. collateralia***. Two collateral ligaments of each joint. D E F

23 ***Ligg. palmaria***. Containing transverse fibers they are attached to the proximal sesamoid bones, but extend beyond them in Un, especially proximally, serving as a fibrocartilaginous bearing surface for the digital flexor tendons. This fibrocartilage forms the Scutum proximale (vide Myologia). C D E F

24 ***Ligg. sesamoidea collateralia***. Each connects a sesamoid bone to metacarpus and Phalanx proximalis. D E F

25 ***Lig. metacarpointersesamoideum***. Elastic ligament of eq with two proximal attachments to Os metacarpale III and ending in the Lig. palmare. D

26 ***Lig. intersesamoideum interdigitale***. Between the axial sesamoid bones of the third and fourth digits in Ru. F

27 ***Lig. sesamoideum rectum***. From sesamoid bones to the middle phalanx in eq. Called also the superficial or "Y" ligament. C D

28 ***Ligg. sesamoidea obliqua***. From the sesamoid bones to the Phalanx proximalis in eq, lateral, medial, and deep to Lig. sesamoideum rectum, "V"-shaped. Called also the middle or "V" ligament. D

29 ***Ligg. sesamoidea brevia***. Short fibers from the distal border of a sesamoid bone to Phalanx proximalis in Un, on both sides of Ligg. cruciata. E F

30 ***Ligg. sesamoidea cruciata***. Crossing fibers from the distal borders of the sesamoid bones to the Phalanx proximalis, in Un between the Ligg. brevia. Called also the "X" ligaments. E F

31 ***Ligg. phalangosesamoidea interdigitalia*** (bo). Between Phalanx proximalis of one digit and axial sesamoid bone of the other. F

32 ***Lig. metacarpeum transversum profundum***. Connects the palmar annular ligaments of adjacent digits in Car and su which bind down the digital flexor tendons. B

33 ***Lig. interdigitale proximale***. Short but thick ligament between the proximal halves of Phalanges proximales of digits III and IV in Artiodactyla. F

1) These ligaments should be called "pisi-...", and not "piso-...", because the name comes from Os pisiforme, and not pisoforme ("i" versus "o").

A Right carpal joint, lateral aspect (eq)

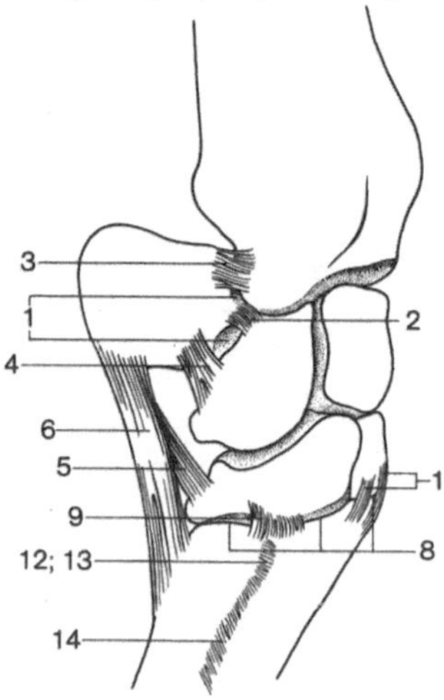

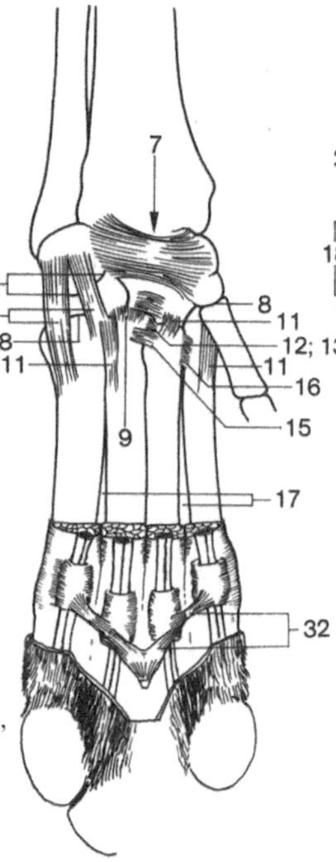

B Left carpal joint, palmar aspect (ca)

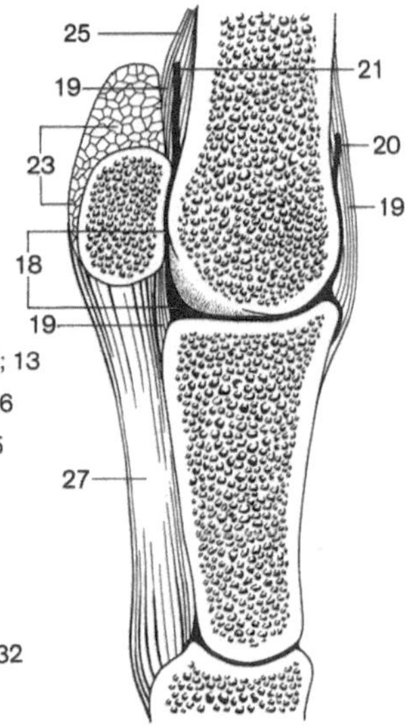

C Metacarpophalangeal joint, sagittal section, right aspect (eq)

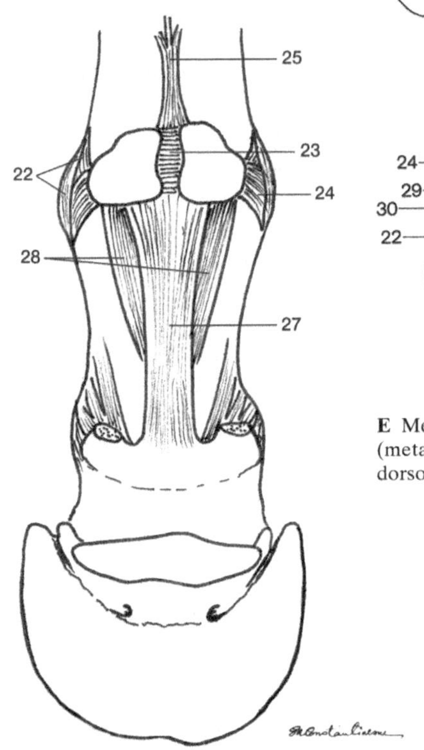

D Metacarpophalangeal joint, palmar aspect (eq)

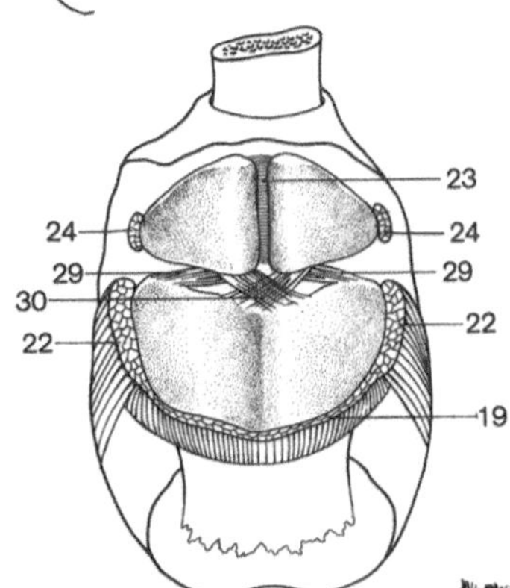

E Metacarpophalangeal joint (metacarpal bone removed), dorsoproximal aspect (eq)

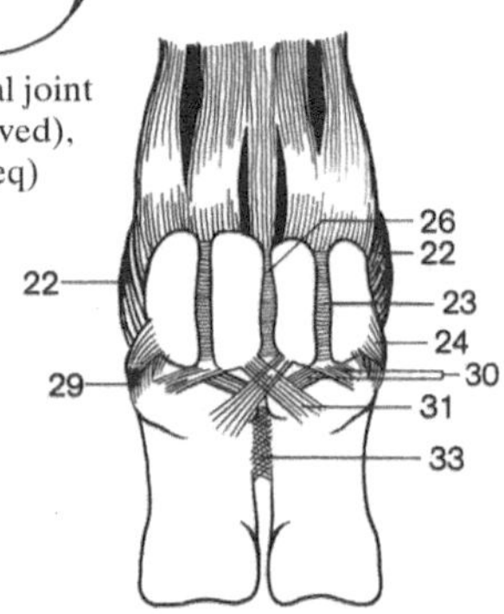

F Metacarpophalangeal joints, palmar aspect (bo)

1 **Articulationes interphalangeae proximales manus***. Joints between proximal and middle phalanges. A B C D E (called pastern joint in Un)

2 ***Capsulae articulares***. Joint capsules, with the fibrous layers only on the dorsal sides. A

3 *Recessus dorsales*. Proximally directed dorsal pouch of each joint capsule. A

4 *Recessus palmares*. Proximally directed palmar pouch of each joint capsule. A

5 ***Ligg. collateralia***. Two collateral ligaments of each joint. B D E

5a *Lig. collaterale commune axiale*. This ligament occurs in Ru and extends on the axial surface from the distal end of the proximal phalanx and the proximal end of middle phalanx to the distal phalanx. It is dorsal to the other collateral ligaments.

6 ***Ligg. palmaria***. From the proximopalmar border of the Phalanx media to the palmar aspect of Phalanx proximalis. On the third and fourth digits of su and Ru three, in eq six palmar ligaments attached to the Phalanx proximalis. C D E

7 **Articulationes interphalangeae distales manus**. Joints between middle and distal phalanges. A B C D E (called coffin joint in Un)

8 ***Capsulae articulares***. Joint capsules, with the fibrous layers only on the dorsal sides. A

9 *Recessus dorsales*. Proximally directed dorsal pouch of each joint capsule. A

10 *Recessus palmares*. Proximally directed palmar pouch of each joint capsule. A

11 ***Ligg. collateralia***. Two collateral ligaments of each joint. B D E

11a *Lig. collaterale commune axiale*. This ligament occurs in Ru and extends on the axial surface from the distal end of the proximal phalanx and the proximal end of middle phalanx to the distal phalanx. It is dorsal to the other collateral ligaments.

12 ***Ligg. dorsalia***. Two elastic dorsal ligaments of each joint from Phalanx media to Phalanx distalis in Car, one dorsoaxial in su and Ru. D

13 ***Ligg. interdigitalia distalia***. Connect digits immediately proximal to the Spatium interdigitale in su and Ru, between Phalanx media and Phalanx distalis. D

14 ***Ligg. sesamoidea collateralia***. Connect the Os sesamoideum distale to Phalanx media in Ru, and to the lateral and medial borders of Phalanx proximalis in eq. B C D E

15 ***Lig. sesamoideum distale impar***. Connects the Os sesamoideum distale and the Phalanx distalis in eq. A C F (In eq it may be called Lig. sesamoideum distale [distal navicular ligament], since there are no axial and/or abaxial ligaments in this species.)

16 ***Lig. sesamoideum distale axiale***. Connects the Os sesamoideum distale and the Phalanx distalis in Ru. D

17 ***Lig. sesamoideum distale abaxiale***. Connects the Os sesamoideum distale and the Phalanx distalis in Ru. D

18 ***Ligg. chondrocompedalia***[1]. Extend from Cartilago ungularis to Phalanx proximalis. E F

19 ***Ligg. chondrocoronalia***[1]. Extend from Cartilago ungularis to Phalanx media. E

20 ***Ligg. chondrosesamoidea***[1]. Extend from Cartilago ungularis to Os sesamoideum distale. B C

21 ***Ligg. chondroungularia collateralia***[1]. Extend from Cartilago ungularis to the Processus palmaris phalangis distalis of the same side (medial or lateral). B E

22 ***Ligg. chondroungularia cruciata***[1]. Extend from Cartilago ungularis of one side to that of the other side and to the opposite Processus palmaris phalangis distalis. F

1) The ligaments extending from the Cartilago ungularis are called "chondro" plus the name of the bone to which they are attached (the names of the phalanges within square brackets – see Osteologia).

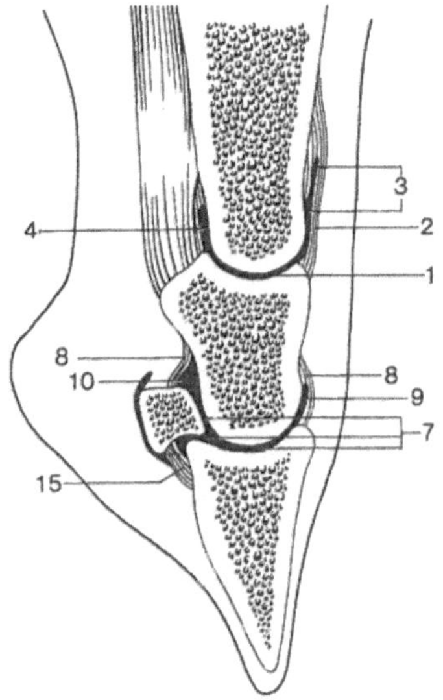

A Interphalangeal joints, sagittal section, right aspect (eq)

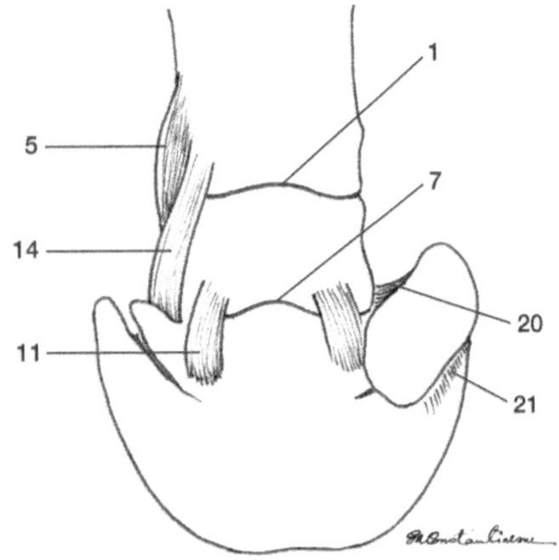

B Interphalangeal joints of right digit, dorsal aspect (eq)

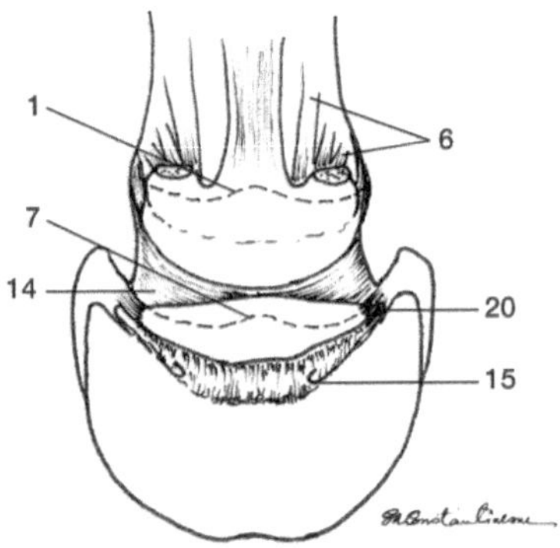

C Interphalangeal joints of right digit, palmar aspect (eq)

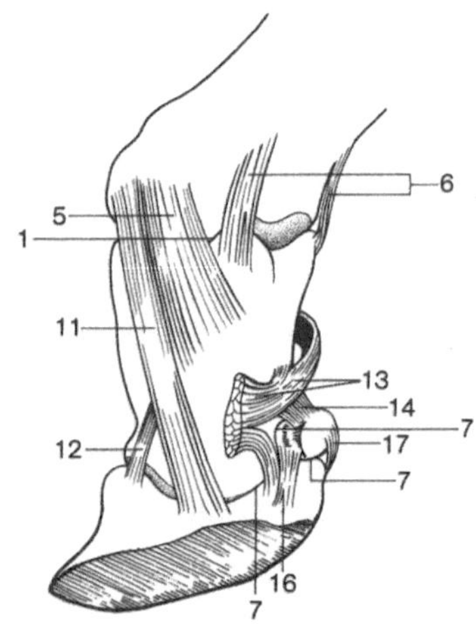

D Interphalangeal joints of right digit, axiopalmar aspect (bo)

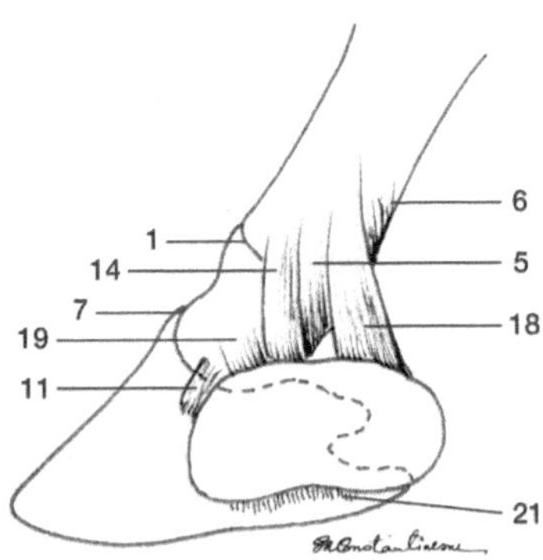

E Ligaments of right lateral hoof cartilage, lateral aspect (eq)

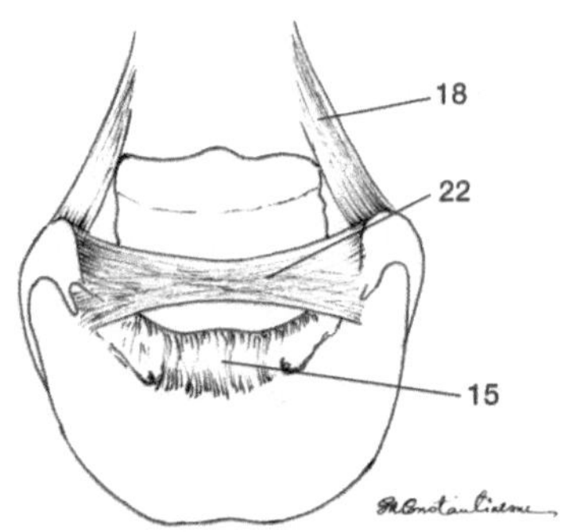

F Ligaments of right lateral hoof cartilage, mediopalmar aspect (eq)

1 **ARTICULATIONES MEMBRI PELVINI.** Joints of the pelvic limb.

2 ***Membrana obturatoria.*** Closes the Foramen obturatum in eq. A E

3 ***Canalis obturatorius.*** Canal for the obturator vessels (except Artiodactyla) and nerve in the craniolateral part of Foramen obturatum. A E

4 ***Lig. sacrotuberale*** (ca). Strong ligament from Os sacrum and first Vertebra caudalis to Tuber ischiadicum. B

5 ***Lig. sacrotuberale latum (lig. sacroischiadicum).*** Sacrosciatic (Sacroischiatic) ligament, from Os sacrum (Un) and first Vertebra caudalis (su, eq) to Spina ischiadica and Tuber ischiadicum. A C

6 ***Foramen ischiadicum majus.*** Greater sciatic (ischiatic) foramen, between Incisura ischiadica major, Os sacrum and Lig. sacrotuberale latum in Un. A C

7 ***Foramen ischiadicum minus.*** Lesser sciatic (ischiatic) foramen, between Incisura ischiadica minor and Lig. sacrotuberale (latum in Un). B C

8 **Articulatio sacroiliaca.** Sacroiliac joint. Between sacrum and ilium. A B

9 ***Ligg. sacroiliaca ventralia.*** Ventral fibrous lamina from Ala sacralis to Os ilium. A

10 ***Ligg. sacroiliaca interossea.*** From Tuberositas sacralis to Tuberositas iliaca. A

11 ***Ligg. sacroiliaca dorsalia.*** Superficial dorsal fibrous structures between sacrum and ilium. B C

12 **Symphysis pelvina.** Pelvic symphysis, may gradually ossify earlier (eq) or later. A B E

13 ***Symphysis pubica.*** Pubic symphysis. A B E

14 ***Symphysis ischiadica.*** Ischiadic symphysis, does sometimes not ossify. A B E

15 ***(Lig. pubicum craniale).*** Transverse fibers connecting right and left Pecten ossis pubis, occasionally only in ca. Called also prepubic ligament.

16 ***Lig. arcuatum ischiadicum.*** Transverse fibers in the Arcus ischiadicus. A E

17 ***Lamina fibrocartilaginea intercoxalis.*** Median fibrocartilaginous structure between right and left Os coxae. A B E

18 **Articulatio coxae***. Hip joint. Between Os coxae and Os femoris. B D E

19 ***Capsula articularis.*** Joint capsule. B D E

20 *Zona orbicularis.* Reinforcement in the dorsal part of the capsule, parallel to Margo acetabuli, especially in ca. B

21 *Lig. iliofemorale.* Reinforcement in the cranial part of the capsule. D

22 *Lig. ischiofemorale.* Reinforcement in the caudal part of the capsule in Car, esp. fe, and su. B

23 *Lig. pubofemorale.* Reinforcement in the ventral part of the capsule in su.

24 ***Labrum acetabulare.*** Acetabular labrum. Fibrocatilaginous rim enlarging and deepening the acetabulum. C E

25 *Lig. transversum acetabuli.* Bridges Incisura acetabuli. C E

26 ***Lig. capitis ossis femoris.*** Ligament of head of femur. Between Fossa acetabuli and Fovea capitis. Carries blood vessels. E

27 ***Lig. accessorium ossis femoris*** (or, eq). From Tendo prepubicus through Incisura acetabuli to Fovea capitis. E

A Pelvis, ventral aspect (eq)

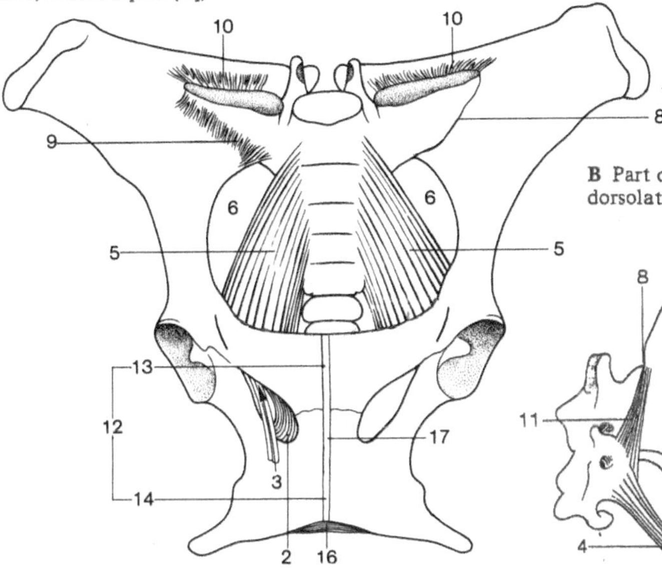

B Part of pelvis and right hip joint, dorsolateral aspect (ca)

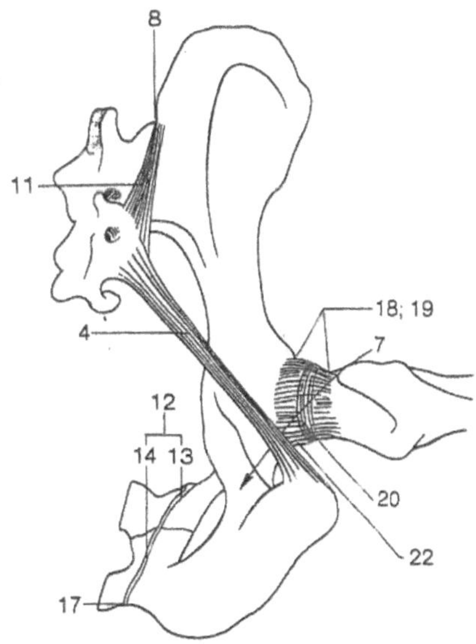

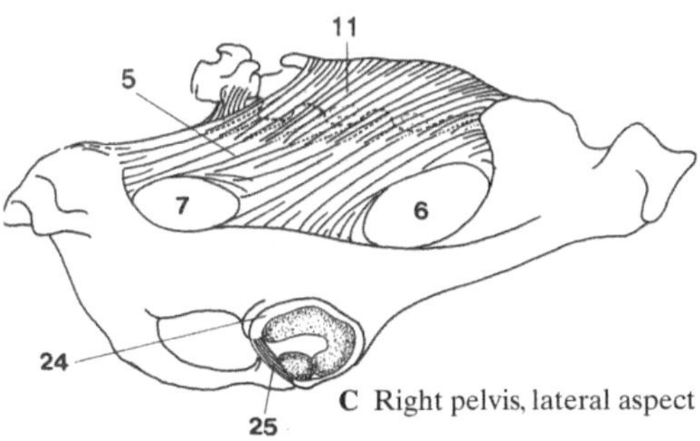

C Right pelvis, lateral aspect (bo)

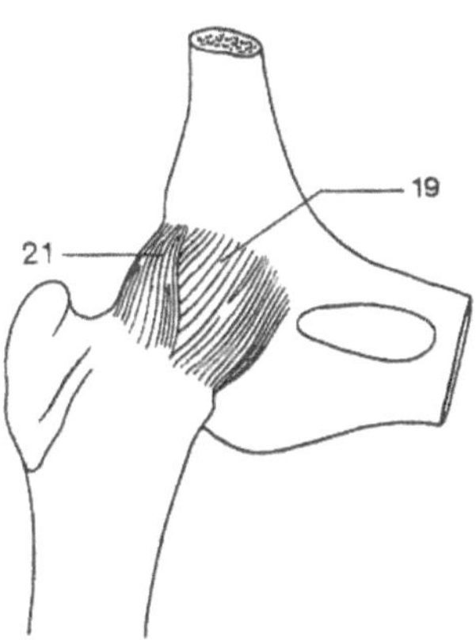

D Right hip joint, cranioventral aspect (ca)

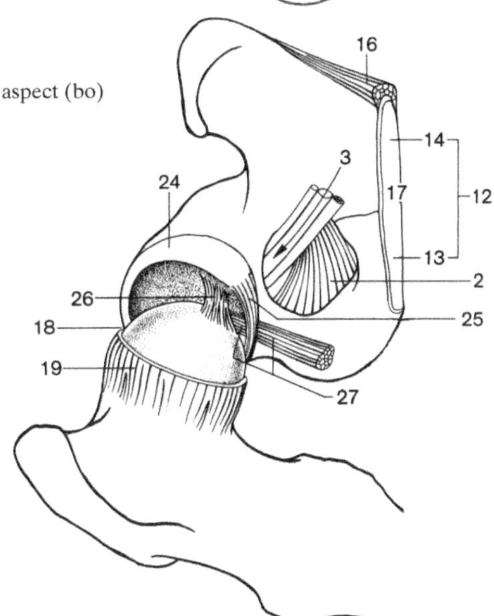

E Left hip joint (opened), caudoventral aspect (eq)

1 ***Articulatio genus****. Stifle joint.

2 **Articulatio femorotibialis**. A B C D

3 ***Capsula articularis***. Joint capsule. A

4 ***Meniscus lateralis***. Semilunar fibrocartilage between the lateral condyles of femur and tibia. B C D

5 *Lig. meniscofemorale*. From Meniscus lateralis to the inner surface of the medial femoral condyle, caudal to Lig. cruciatum caudale. B

6 ***Meniscus medialis***. Semilunar fibrocartilage between the medial condyles of femur and tibia. B C D

7 ***Lig. transversum genus***. Transverse ligament of stifle, connects menisci cranially, especially in ca and su. C

7a *Lig. meniscotibiale*. From Meniscus lateralis to the caudal border of lateral tibial condyle. B (This ligament should have been listed in the 5th edition of the N. A. V. as #5a, because it is a ligament of the lateral meniscus, and not subsequent to Lig. transversus genus or to the medial meniscus.)

8 ***Ligg. cruciata genus***. Cruciate ligaments of stifle. C

9 *Lig. cruciatum craniale*. From the inner surface of Condylus lateralis femoris to Area intercondylaris centralis tibiae. C

10 *Lig. cruciatum caudale*. From the inner surface of Condylus medialis femoris to Area intercondylaris caudalis tibiae. B C

11 ***Lig. collaterale laterale***. From Epicondylus lateralis femoris to Caput fibulae and tibia. A B C D

12 ***Lig. collaterale mediale***. From Epicondylus medialis femoris to tibia, fuses with the medial meniscus in the dog. A B C D

13 ***Lig. popliteum obliquum***. Reinforcement of the caudal wall of the joint capsule running in a lateroproximal-mediodistal direction. A

14 **Articulatio femoropatellaris***. A B C D

15 ***Capsula articularis***. Joint capsule. A C

16 ***Fibrocartilagines parapatellares***. Most developed in ca. C

17 ***Lig. patellae****. Patellar ligament, from Apex patellae to Tuberositas tibiae, except bo, eq (see 18, 21, 24). B C

18 ***Lig. patellae intermedium****. Intermediate patellar ligament in bo and eq. D

19 ***Retinaculum patellae mediale***. Reinforcement of the capsule medial to the patella, in bo and eq also in distal direction to Tuberositas tibiae. D

20 *Lig. femoropatellare mediale*. From medial border or Processus cartilagineus (bo, eq) of patella to femur or Os sesamoideum m. gastrocnemii (Car). A B C D

21 *Lig. patellae mediale**. Medial patellar ligament in bo and eq. A D

22 ***Retinaculum patellae laterale***. Reinforcement of the capsule lateral to the patella, in bo and eq also in distal direction to Tuberositas tibiae. D

23 *Lig. femoropatellare laterale*. From lateral border of patella to femur or Os sesamoideum m. gastrocnemii (Car). D

24 *Lig. patellae laterale**. Lateral patellar ligament in bo and eq. D

25 ***Corpus adiposum infrapatellare***. Infrapatellar fat pad, between Stratum fibrosum and Stratum synoviale of the capsule. A

26 **Articulatio tibiofibularis proximalis**. Joint between head of fibula and tibia, absent in Ru. A B C

27 ***Capsula articularis***. Joint capsule. A

28 ***Lig. capitis fibulae craniale***. Cranial ligament of fibular head to tibia. C

29 ***Lig. capitis fibulae caudale***. Caudal ligament of fibular head to tibia. B

30 ***Membrana interossea cruris***. Membrane connecting tibia and fibula. A B C

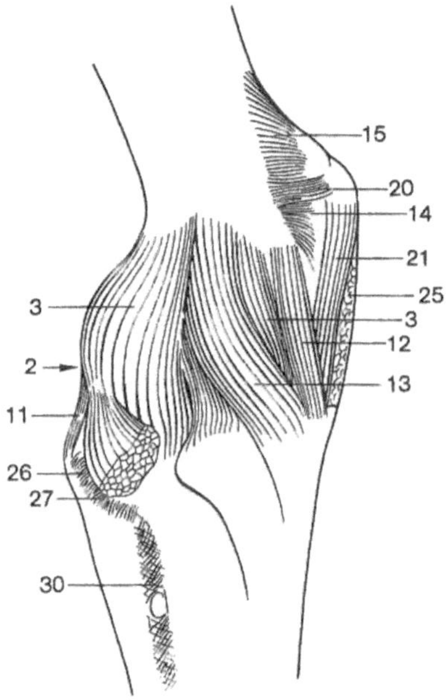

A Left stifle joint, mediocaudal aspect (eq)

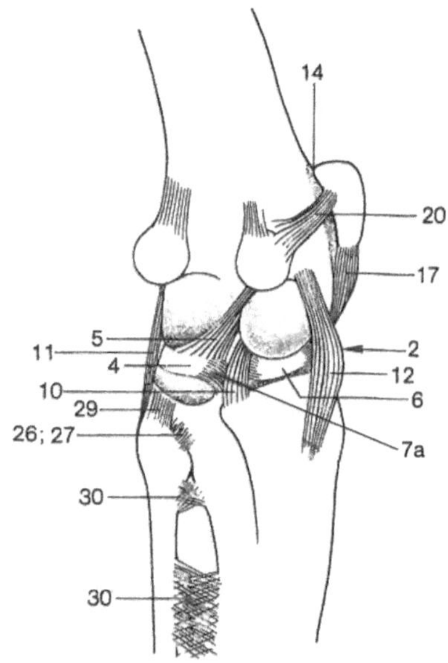

B Left stifle joint, mediocaudal aspect (ca). (The joint capsule has been removed)

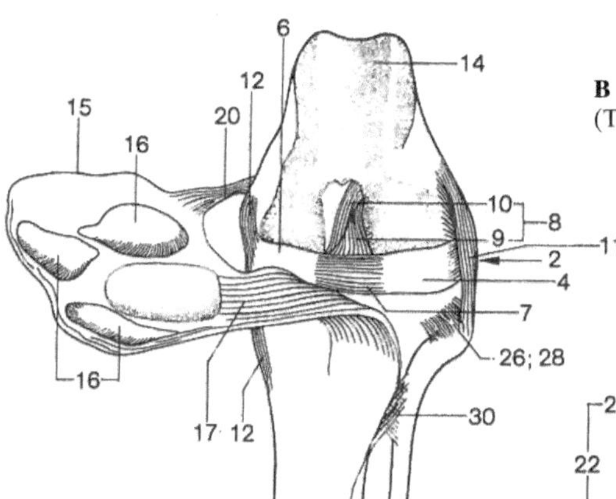

C Left stifle joint (opened), cranial aspect (ca)

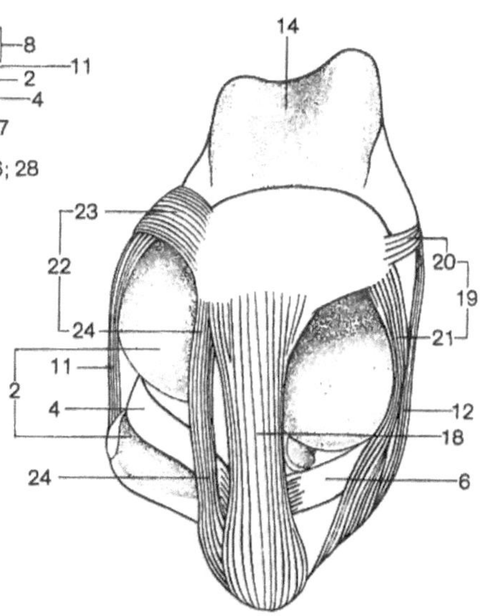

D Right stifle joint (opened), cranial aspect (eq)

1 **Articulatio tibiofibularis distalis**. Distal joint between tibia and fibula, absent in eq. A

2 ***Capsula articularis***. Joint capsule. A

3 ***Lig. tibiofibulare craniale***. Cranial ligament between the distal ends of tibia and fibula. A D

4 ***Lig. tibiofibulare caudale***. Caudal ligament between the distal ends of tibia and fibula. B

5 **Articulationes pedis**. Joints of the pes. This is the heading for all joints of the foot. Articulatio tarsi includes the joints between the Skeleton cruris, the Ossa tarsi, and the Ossa metatarsalia. The proximal joint is termed Articulatio tarsocruralis because in domestic mammals, except the horse, both Talus and Calcaneus articulate with the Skeleton cruris.

6 **Articulatio tarsi***. Tarsal joint, includes the joints between crural, tarsal and metatarsal bones. A B C D E

7 ***Lig. collaterale tarsi mediale****. Consists of the following parts. A B C (In eq it consists of twisted fibers and is responsible for the spring-like extension of the joint, after the extensor muscles of the hock initiate the motion; this ligament is a muscle energy saver [Ghetie and Riga 1943].)

8 *Lig. collaterale tarsi mediale longum*[1)]. Extends from the tibia to the distal tarsal bones and the metatarsus, in fe only to the Os tarsi centrale. A B C

9 *Lig. collaterale tarsi mediale breve*. Collective term for the short parts of the Lig. collaterale tarsi mediale. C (In eq there is a shortest and deepest part *[Lig. collaterale tarsi mediale profundum]* [Constantinescu and Constantinescu 2004], also called *Fasciculus accessorius* by Barone 1999a.)

10 **Pars tibiotalaris**. Part connecting Malleolus tibiae and talus. C

11 **Pars tibiocalcanea**. Part connecting Malleolus tibiae and calcaneus. C

12 **Pars tibiocentralis [tibionavicularis]**. Part connecting Malleolus tibiae and Os tarsi centrale in su and Ru. A B

13 ***Lig. collaterale tarsi laterale****. Consists of the following parts. A B D E (In eq it consists of twisted fibers and is responsible for the spring-like flexion of the joint, after the flexor muscles of the hock initiate the motion; this ligament is a muscle energy saver [Ghetie and Riga 1943].)

14 *Lig. collaterale tarsi laterale longum* [1)]. Extends from the fibula (in eq Malleolus lateralis of the tibia) to the Os tarsale IV and the metatarsus, in fe only to the calcaneus. A B D E

15 *Lig. collaterale tarsi laterale breve*. Collective term for the short and deep part of the Lig. collaterale tarsi laterale. B D E

16 **Pars talofibularis**. Part connecting Malleolus fibulae and talus in Car.

17 **Pars tibiotalaris**. Part connecting Malleolus lateralis tibiae and talus in eq. E

18 **Pars calcaneofibularis**. Part connecting Malleolus fibulae and calcaneus. A B D

19 **Pars tibiocalcanea**. Part connecting Malleolus lateralis tibiae and calcaneus in eq. E

20 **Pars calcaneometatarsea**. Part connecting calcaneus and metatarsus in Car and su, plantar to Lig. collaterale laterale longum. B D

21 **Articulatio tarsocruralis**. Most proximal joint of Articulatio tarsi, between tibia, fibula (except eq), talus and calcaneus (except eq). A B C D E

22 ***Capsula articularis***. Joint capsule. C D

23 ***Lig. talofibulare plantare***. Short ligament from Malleolus fibulae to the plantar surface of the talus, abesent in eq, strong in su and Ru. B D

24 ***Lig. tibiotalare plantare*** (or, su). From Malleolus tibiae to the plantar surface of the talus. C

25 **Articulationes intertarseae**. Joints between tarsal bones.

26 **Articulatio talocalcaneocentralis [talocalcaneonavicularis]**. Joint between talus, calcaneus and Os tarsi centrale [naviculare], in su and Ru also Os tarsale IV. A C E

27 **Articulatio talocalcanea**. Joint between talus and calcaneus. A B C E

28 ***Capsula articularis***. C

29 ***Lig. talocalcaneum laterale***. From talus to the lateral surface of the calcaneus, double in su. A D E

30 ***Lig. talocalcaneum plantare***. From Sustentaculum tali to the plantar surface of the talus, absent in Ru, double in eq. B C

31 **Articulatio calcaneoquartalis [calcaneocuboidea]**. Joint between calcaneus and Os tarsale quartum [cuboideum]. A B D E

32 ***Capsula articularis***. B

1) These are the most superficial fascicles of the collateral ligaments of the hock joint.

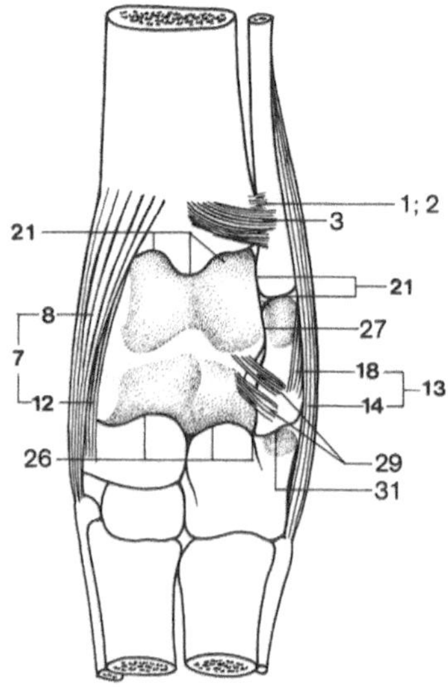

A Left tarsal joint, dorsal aspect (su) (Schreiber)

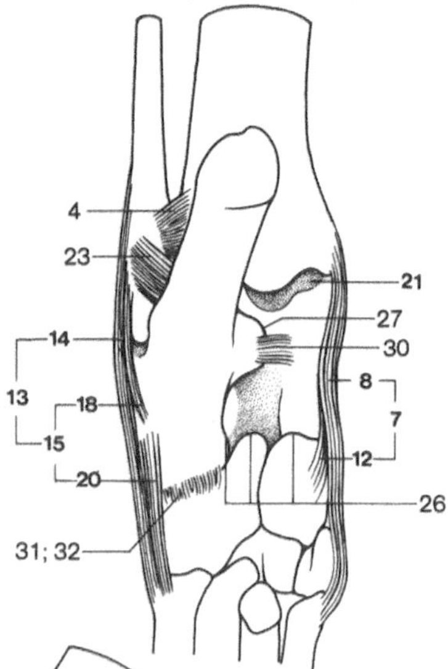

B Left tarsal jont, plantar aspect (su) (Schreiber)

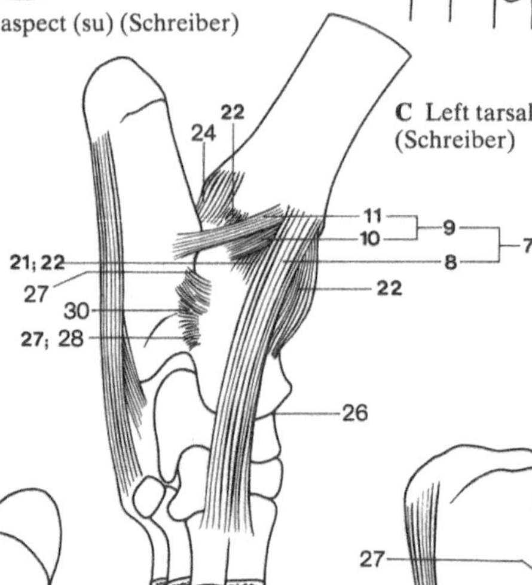

C Left tarsal joint, medial aspect (su) (Schreiber)

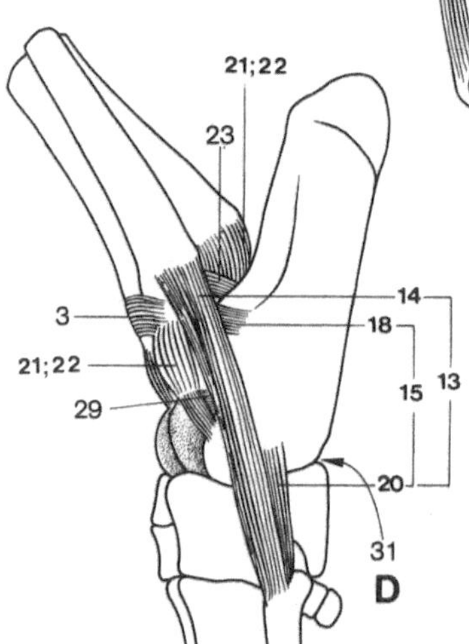

D Left tarsal joint, lateral aspect (su) (Schreiber)

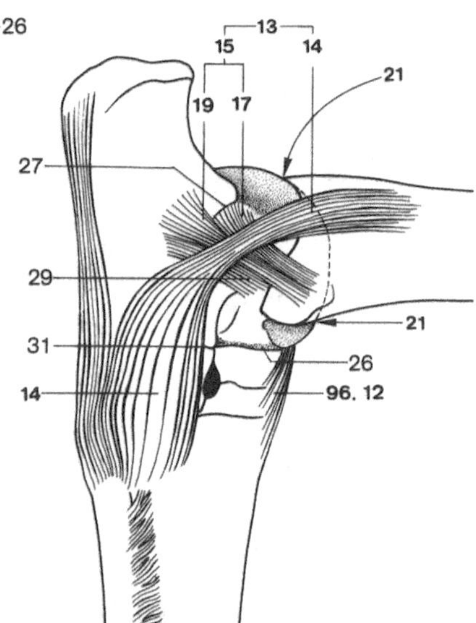

E Right tarsal joint, lateral aspect (eq)

1 **Articulatio centrodistalis [cuneonavicularis].** Joint between Os tarsi centrale and the distal tarsal bones. A B C D E

2 ***Capsula articularis.*** Joint capsule. A B C E

3 ***Ligg. tarsi interossea.*** Interosseous tarsal ligaments.

4 *Lig. talocalcaneum interosseum.* Between talus and calcaneus. It consists of three ligaments: interosseous, lateral, and plantar (absent in bo). E

5 *Lig. talocentrale [talonaviculare] interosseum* (eq). Between talus and central tarsal bone. E

6 *Lig. centrodistale [cuneonaviculare] interosseum.* Between central tarsal bone and third tarsal bone (T_3). E

7 *Lig. calcaneoquartale [calcaneocuboideum] interosseum.* Between calcaneus and fourth tarsal bone (T_4). E

8 *Lig. centroquartale [cuboideonaviculare] interosseum.* Between central tarsal bone and T_4. E

9 *Lig. quartodistale [cuneocuboideum] interosseum.* Between T_4 and T_3. E

10 *Ligg. interdistalia [intercuneiformia] interossea.* Between T_3 and T_2, or T_{1+2} (eq). E

11 ***Ligg. tarsi dorsalia.*** Dorsal tarsal ligaments.

12 *Lig. talocentrodistometatarseum [talonaviculocuneometatarseum].* Dorsal tarsometatarsal ligament In eq. From the medial surface of talus (Tuberculum in eq) in distodorsolateral direction, absent in Car. A C, 95 E

13 *Ligg. interdistalia [intercuneiformia] dorsalia.* Dorsal ligaments between T_3 and T_2, or T_{1+2} (eq). A

14 *Lig. quartodistale [cuneocuboideum] dorsale.* Dorsal ligament between T_4 and T_3. A D

15 *Lig. centroquartale [cuboideonaviculare] dorsale.* Dorsal ligament between central tarsal bone and T_4. A D

16 *Lig. calcaneocentrale [calcaneonaviculare] dorsale.* Dorsal ligament between calcaneus and central tarsal bone.

17 *Lig. calcaneoquartale [calcaneocuboideum] dorsale.* Dorsal ligament between calcaneus and T_4. A D

18 *Ligg. centrodistalia [cuneonavicularia] dorsalia* (Car). Occurs also in su. Dorsal ligaments between central tarsal bone and T_3 and T_2 or T_{1+2} (eq). A

19 ***Ligg. tarsi plantaria.*** Plantar tarsal ligaments.

20 *Lig. plantare longum**. Long plantar ligament. On the plantar surface of calcaneus, Os tarsale IV, and metatarsus. B C D

21 *Lig. calcaneoquartale [calcaneocuboideum] plantare.* Plantar ligament between calcaneus and T_4. D

22 *Lig. calcaneocentrale [calcaneonaviculare] plantare.* Plantar ligament between calcaneus and central tarsal bone. Plantar tarsometatarsal ligament in eq. B C

23 *Ligg. centrodistalia [cuneonavicularia] plantaria.* Plantar ligaments between central tarsal bone and T_3. B

24 *Lig. centroquartale [cuboideonaviculare] plantare.* Plantar ligament between central tarsal bone and T_4. B

25 *Ligg. interdistalia [intercuneiformia] plantaria.* Plantar ligaments between T_3 and T_2, or T_{1+2} (eq). B

26 *Lig. quartodistale [cuneocuboideum] plantare.* Plantar ligament between T_4 and T_3. B

27 **Articulationes tarsometatarseae.** Joints between distal tarsal and metatarsal bones. A B E

28 ***Capsulae articulares.*** Joint capsules. A B E

29 ***Ligg. tarsometatarseae dorsalia.*** Dorsal tarsometatarsal ligaments. A D

30 ***Ligg. tarsometatarseae plantaria.*** Plantar tarsometatarsal ligaments. B

31 ***Ligg. tarsometatarseae [cuneometatarsea] interossea.*** Interosseous tarsometatarsal ligaments, former ligaments between tarsal bones 1–4 and metatarsal bones. E

32 **Articulationes intermetatarseae.** Joints between the bases of the metatarsal bones. A B E

33 ***Capsulae articulares.*** Joint capsules. A B

34 ***Ligg. metatarseae interosseae.*** Fibers between the bases of the metatarsal bones. E

35 ***Ligg. metatarseae dorsalia.*** Dorsal fibers between the bases of the metatarsal bones. A

36 ***Ligg. metatarseae plantaria.*** Plantar fibers between the bases of the metatarsal bones. B

37 ***Spatia interossea metatarsi.*** Spaces between the metatarsal bones. A

38 **Articulationes metatarsophalangeae.** (vide Articulationes membri thoracici, sed) Recessus plantares, Ligg. plantaria, Lig. metatarsointersesamoideum, and Lig. metatarseum transversum profundum.

39 **Articulationes interphalangeae pedis.** (vide Articulationes membri thoracici, sed) Recessus plantares and Ligg. plantaria.

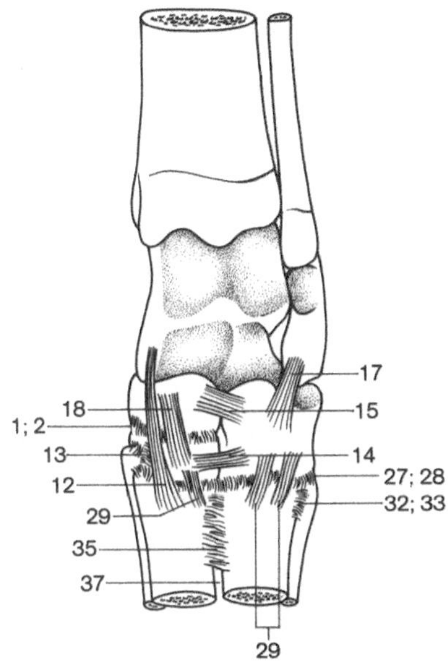

A Left tarsal joint, dorsal aspect (su)

B Left tarsal joint, plantar aspect (su)

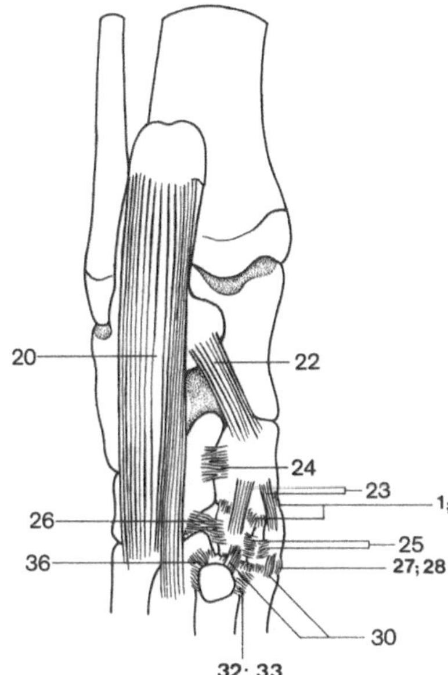

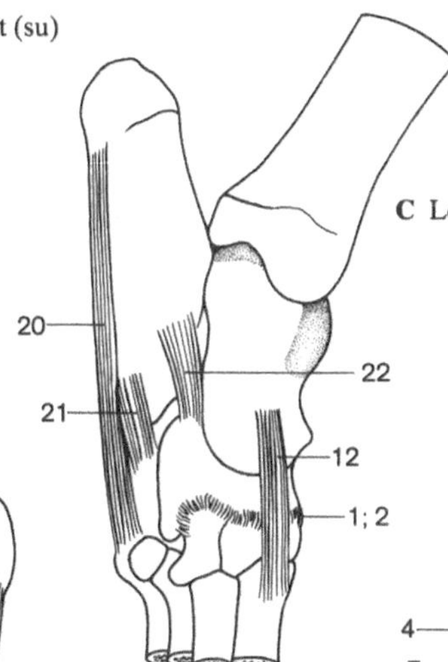

C Left tarsal joint, medial aspect (su)

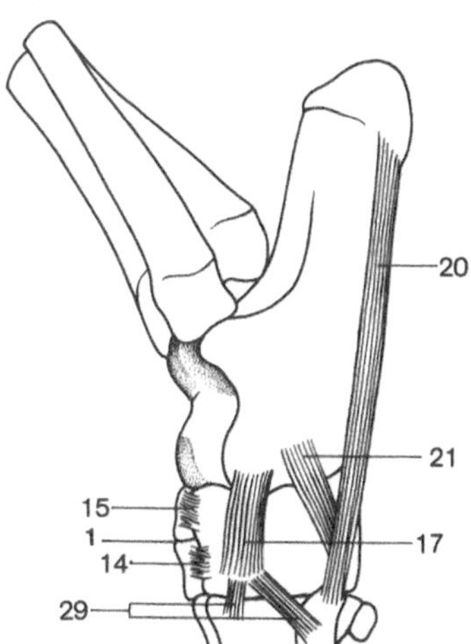

D Left tarsal joint, lateral aspect (su)

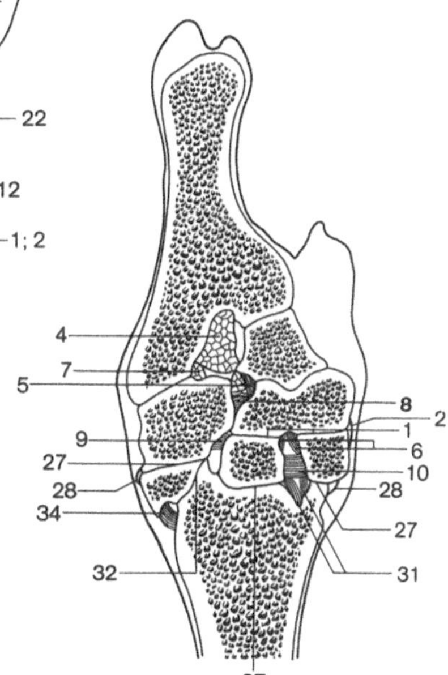

E Right tarsal joint, dorsal section, dorsal aspect (eq)

1 **MUSCULI CUTANEI***. Muscles located in specific regions of body moving the skin. The list of cutaneous muscle is not complete; other cutaneous muscles are listed topographically.

2 ***M. cutaneus trunci***. Covers lateral part of trunk caudal to shoulder and arm. Forms fold of flank. Dips medial to arm with M. pectoralis profundus. A

3 *M. cutaneus omobrachialis*. Continuation of M. cutaneus trunci in Ru and eq lateral to shoulder and arm. May be separated from M. cutaneus trunci in bo. A

4 *M. preputialis [prae-] cranialis*. Forms ring around Ostium preputiale. C

5 *M. preputialis [prae-] caudalis*. Along penis in preputial wall caudal to ostium in Ru, sometimes in su. C

6 *M. supramammarius cranialis* (Car). Slip associated with ventral edge of M. cutaneus trunci. Passes deep to mammary glands. B

7 *M. supramammarius caudalis* (Car). Fibers in inguinal region deep to, and between mammary glands. B

8 ***M. sphincter colli superficialis***. Transverse fibers ventral in neck from sternum to mandible in Car, rudimentary in su. D

9 ***Platysma***. From nuchal area to Angulus oris in Car and su. D

10 *M. cutaneus colli*. In the ventral neck lying obliquely over Sulcus jugularis, in Un. A

11 *M. cutaneus faciei*. Continuation of M. cutaneus colli to Regio masseterica in Ru and eq, part of platysma in Car and su. A

12 ***M. sphincter colli profundus***. Deep to platysma, ventral to ear in masseteric and parotid regions, in Car. D

13 **MUSCULI CAPITIS**. Muscles of head.

14 ***M. rectus capitis ventralis***. From Arcus ventralis atlantis to Pars basilaris ossis occipitalis. Flexes atlantooccipital joint. E

15 ***M. rectus capitis dorsalis major***. Dorsal to atlantoaxial articulation and atlas. From Processus spinosus axis to Squama occipitalis. Extends atlanto-occipital joint. Has a superficial and a deep part in bo and eq. E

16 ***M. rectus capitis dorsalis minor***. Deep to preceeding muscle. From Tuberculum dorsale atlantis to Squama occipitalis. Extends atlanto-occipital joint. E

17 ***M. rectus capitis lateralis***. From lateral part of Arcus ventralis atlantis to Processus paracondylaris. Flexes atlantooccipital joint laterally and ventrally. E

18 ***M. obliquus capitis cranialis***. Fibers run obliquely caudomedially dorsal to atlantooccipital joint from cranial edge of Ala atlantis to Squama occipitalis. Extends and flexes atlantooccipital joint laterally. E

19 ***M. obliquus capitis caudalis***. Fibers run obliquely craniolaterally dorsal to atlas and axis from Processus spinosus and articularis caudalis of axis to dorsal surface of Ala atlantis. Rotates atlantoaxial joint. E

20 ***M. splenius capitis***. Cranial continuation of M. splenius cervicis. Fibers run craniolaterally to insert on Squama occipitalis. Elevates head. F (In the 5th edition of N.A.V. this muscle was moved under Musculi colli [page 40] by error or typo mistake.)

21 ***M. longus capitis***. Lies ventrolaterally along cervical transverse processes. From Processus transversi of cervical vertebrae 3–6 to cranial portion of Pars basilaris ossis occipitalis. Flexes head and neck. E F

* Reminder: The structures followed by an asterisk are landmarks for physical examination and/or clinical approach.

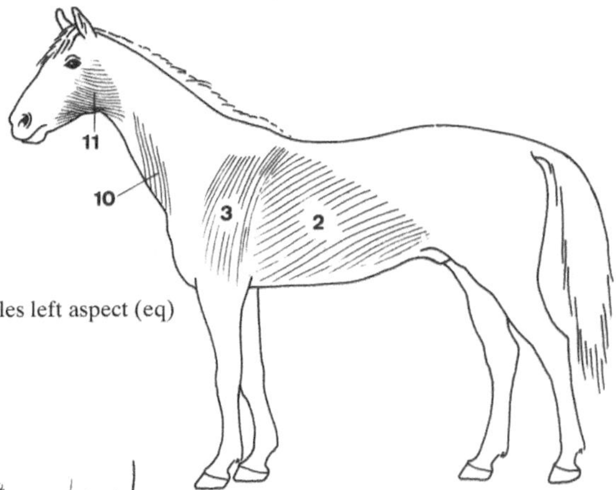

A Cutaneous muscles left aspect (eq)

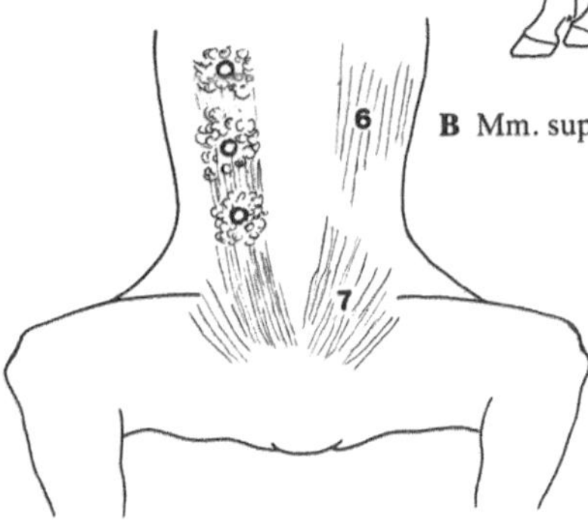

B Mm. supramammarii (fe)

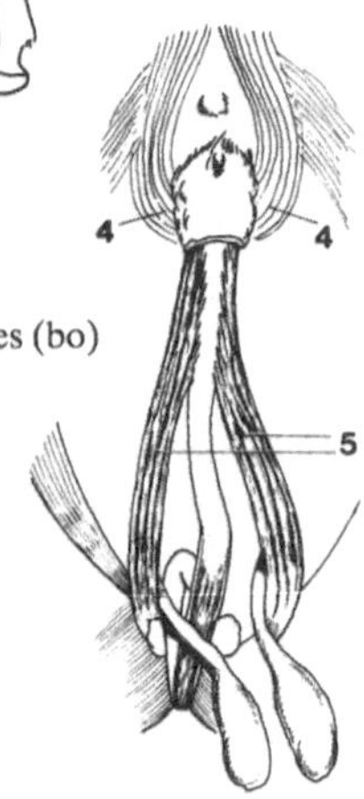

C Mm. preputiales (bo)

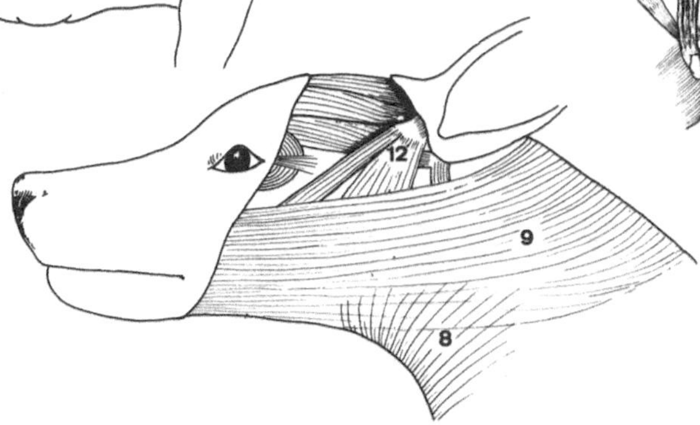

D Cutaneous muscles of left head and neck (ca)

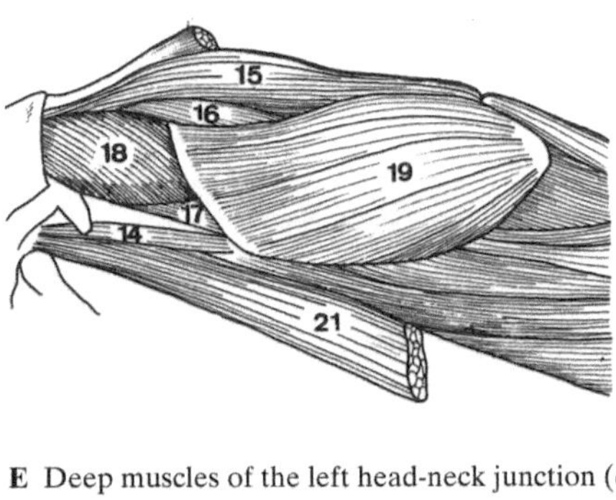

E Deep muscles of the left head-neck junction (eq)

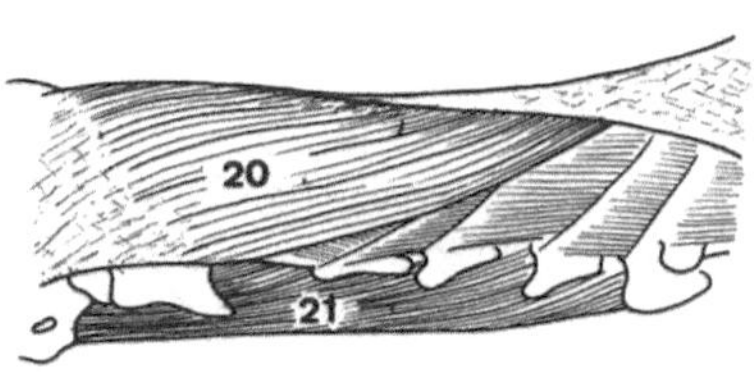

F Left M. splenius and M. longus capitis (ca)

1 ***M. frontalis.*** Cutaneous muscle which lies over frontal bone and M. temporalis in Car, su, and Ru. A C

2 ***M. occipitalis.*** Lies in Car over occipital and parietal bones and M. temporalis, partly covered by M. interscutularis. C

3 ***M. lateralis nasi.*** Small fiber groups ventral and dorsal along Incisura nasoincisiva and caudal portion of nostril in Ru and eq (four parts in eq). Assists in dilating nostril. A D

4 ***M. dilatator naris apicalis.*** Transverse fibers from median line to nostril in Ru and eq. Dilates nostril. D

5 ***M. orbicularis oculi.*** Sphincter of eyelids. A C

6 *Pars palpebralis.* Part within eyelid. A C

7 *Pars orbitalis.* Part encroaching upon orbit. A C

8 ***M. levator anguli oculi medialis.*** Rostrolaterally directed from frontal bone to medial portion of upper eyelid. Lifts medial portion of upper eyelid. C

9 ***M. retractor anguli oculi lateralis.*** From Fascia temporalis (Car) to lateral ocular angle, in bo continuation of M. frontoscutularis. A C

10 ***M. malaris.*** Cutaneous fibers directed ventrally from region of medial ocular angle. A

11 ***Mm. auriculares rostrales.*** From skull rostral to ear. Cartilago scutiformis is in the midst of group. A B (These are the so-called "muscles of attention".)

12 *Mm. scutuloauriculares superficiales.* Several muscles forming superficial group from Cartilago scutiformis to Concha auriculae. Turn Incisura intertragica rostrally. A B

13 *Mm. scutuloauriculares profundi.* Major and minor muscles from ventral surface of Cartilago scutiformis to Eminentia conchae. Turn Incisura intertragica caudally. B

14 *M. frontoscutularis.* From Linea temporalis in caudal direction to Cartilago scutiformis. Pulls Cartilago scutiformis rostrally. A B C

15 *M. zygomaticoscutularis.* Lateral to the preceeding muscle. From Processus zygomaticus ossis frontalis to Cartilago scutiformis. Pulls Cartilago scutiformis rostrally. A B

16 *M. zygomaticoauricularis.* From Arcus zygomaticus to Concha auriculae. Turns Incisura intertragica rostrally. A B

17 ***Mm. auriculares dorsales.*** From dorsal median line to Cartilago scutiformis or Concha auriculae. B (very well developed in Morgan horses)

18 *M. interscutularis.* Transverse fibers from dorsal median line (Car, eq), Linea temporalis (su, Ru, eq) to Cartilago scutiformis. B

19 *M. parietoscutularis.* Deep to Mm. inter- et cervicoscutularis. Detaches from M. parietoauricularis to insert on Cartilago scutiformis. B

20 *M. parietoauricularis.* Strap-like. Deep to Mm. inter- and cervicoscutularis. From parietal bone to Concha auriculae. Raises concha. B

21 ***Mm. auriculares caudales.*** From Nucha to Cartilago scutiformis or Concha auriculae. B (These are the so-called "muscles of wickedness".)

22 *M. cervicoscutularis.* Caudal to M. interscutularis from Linea temporalis to caudal portion of Cartilago scutiformis. A B

23 *M. cervicoauricularis superficialis.* Straplike. From Crista nuchae or Funiculus nuchae (Ru) to Concha auriculae. Raises concha. A B

24 *M. cervicoauricularis medius.* Caudal and deep to preceeding muscle. Turns Incisura intertragica laterally. B

25 *M. cervicoauricularis profundus.* Deep to preceeding muscle. Turns Incisura intertragica laterally. B

26 ***Mm. auriculares ventrales.*** In parotid region. Depress Concha auriculae. A

27 *M. styloauricularis.* Slips over Meatus acusticus externus cartilagineus. Courses from Mandibula or Pars tympanica ossis temporalis to Concha auriculae. A

28 *M. parotidoauricularis [parotideo-].* Runs dorsally over Gl. parotis to Concha auriculae. A

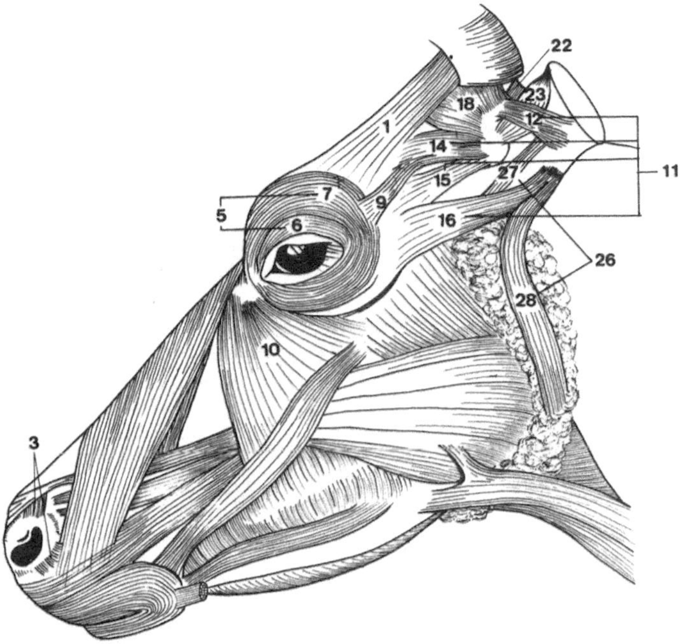

Muscles of the head, left aspect (bo)

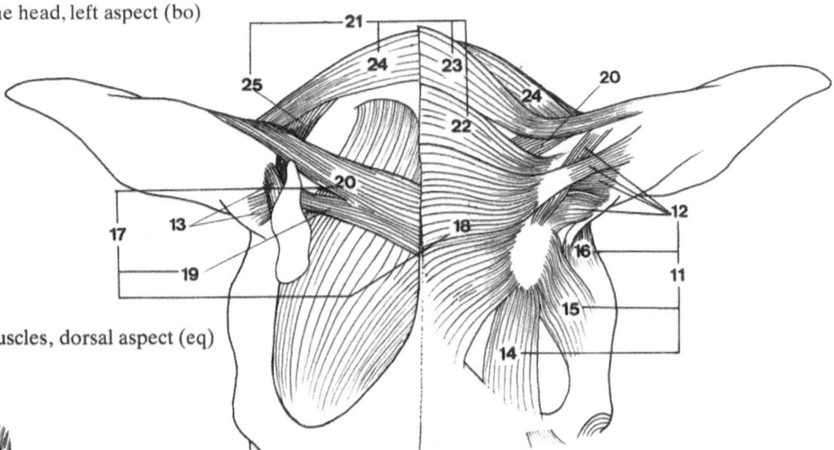

Auricular muscles, dorsal aspect (eq)

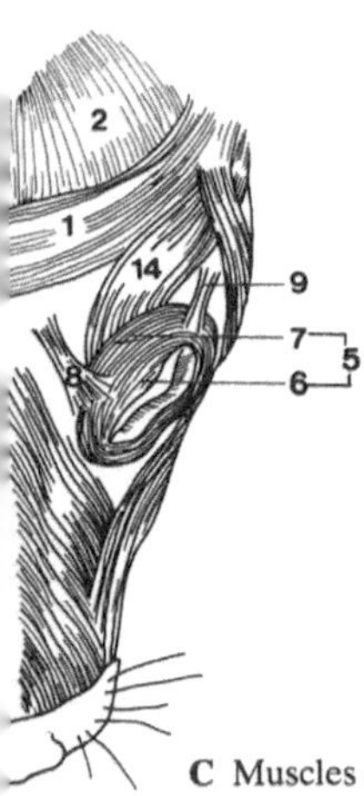

C Muscles of the head, dorsal aspect (ca)

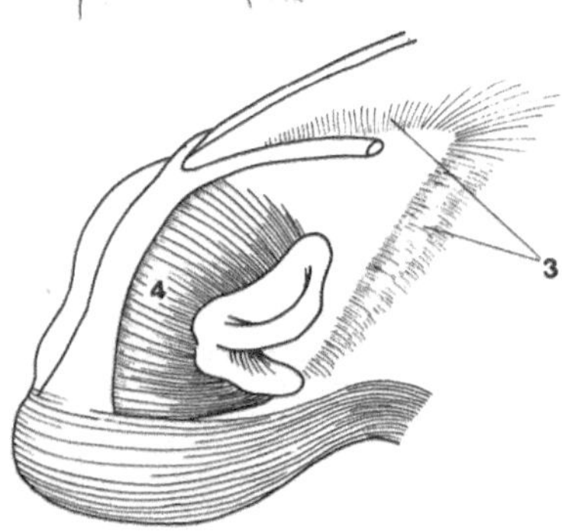

D Muscles of the nose, left rostrolateral aspect (eq)

1 ***M. incisivus superior***[1]. Radiating fibers in upper lip. Raises upper lip. C

2 ***M. incisivus inferior***[1]. Radiating fibers in lower lip. Depresses lower lip. C

3 ***M. orbicularis oris***. Sphincter of mouth. B C

4 *Pars marginalis*. Part near Rima oris. B C

5 *Pars labialis*. Main part within lips. B C

6 ***M. depressor anguli oris***. Part of Platysma (M. cutaneus faciei) at, and depresses the angle of mouth. A B C

7 ***M. zygomaticus***. Strap-like muscle running from area of Crista facialis (Un) or Cartilago scutiformis (Car) to angle of mouth deep to Platysma. Retracts angle of mouth. A B C

8 ***M. levator nasolabialis***. Flat muscle arising rostral to Orbita, inserting in upper lip and nostril. Raises upper lip and dilates nostril. A B C

9 ***M. levator labii superioris***. Arises ventral to preceeding muscle and courses rostrally deep to it. In eq tendon joints that of other side to insert in upper lip as an aponeurosis. In other species tendon spreads out and attaches also to Ala nasi lateralis. Raises upper lip. A B C

10 ***M. caninus***. Ventral to preceeding muscle. Perforates M. levator nasolabialis or is deep to its labial portion. Inserts on upper lip in Car, nostril in eq, both in su and Ru. Dilates nostril and raises upper lip. A B C

11 ***M. depressor labii superioris*** (su, Ru). Arises with, but lies ventral to preceeding muscle. Inserts with M. orbicularis oris. B

12 ***M. depressor labii inferioris***. Lies along Corpus mandibulae to insert in lower lip. Not present in Car. A B

13 ***M. buccinator***. Muscle of cheek. A B C

14 *Pars buccalis*. Attaches along molar areas of maxilla and mandible. Fibers pass toward each other in an acute angle to form raphe of insertion. A B C

15 *Pars molaris*. Deep to preceeding part. Longitudinal fibers which extend caudally on to Ramus mandibulae. A C

16 ***M. mentalis***. From lateral part of Corpus mandibulae to lower lip. Stiffens lower lip. A

17 ***M. masseter***. Large lateral muscle of mastication. Raises mandible to close mouth. A B

18 *Pars superficialis*. From zygomatic arch to caudal and ventral portion of mandible. Fibers course ventrocaudally. A B

19 *Pars profunda*. Smaller, deeper portion. Fibers more vertical. A B

20 ***M. temporalis***. Occupies entire Fossa temporalis from which it originates. Fibers converge to insert on Processus coronoideus mandibulae. Raises mandible to close mouth. A

21 ***M. pterygoideus lateralis***. Smallest muscle of mastication. From Crista pterygoidea to Fovea pterygoidea mandibulae and Discus articularis. Draws mandible rostrally, and laterally. D

22 ***M. pterygoideus medialis***. Large medial muscle of mastication. From pterygoid, basisphenoid, palatine bones and Fossa pterygopalatina to Fossa pterygoidea mandibulae. Raises mandible to close mouth. D

23 ***M. digastricus***. Two-bellied muscle which opens jaws. From Processus paracondylaris to Pars molaris of Corpus mandibulae. Tendon occurs between two bellies, in Car intermediate tendon is represented by tendinous intersection. D

24 *Venter rostralis*. Rostral belly, from intermediate tendon to mandible. D

24a *Tendo intermedius* (Ru, eq). Between the rostral and caudal bellies. This tendon is represented in rudimentary form in Car, usually called the "tendinous intersection". D

25 *Venter caudalis*. Caudal belly, from Processus paracondylaris to intermediate tendon. A D

26 **Pars occipitomandibularis**. Detaches from Venter caudalis and inserts on Ramus mandibulae in eq, or. It does not attach to the intermediate tendon. A D

1) developed in suckling animals

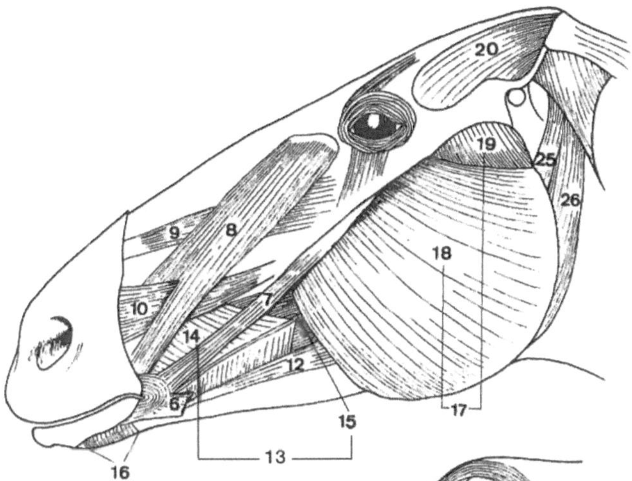

A Muscles of the head, left aspect (eq)

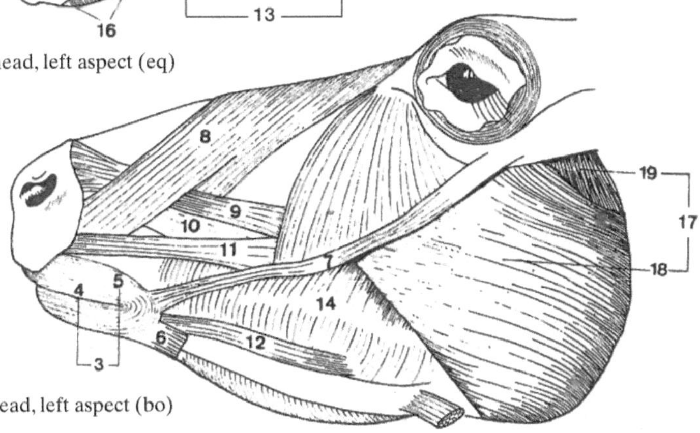

B Muscles of the head, left aspect (bo)

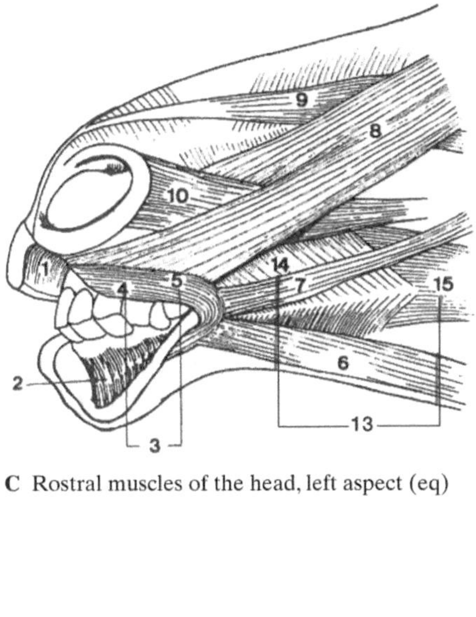

C Rostral muscles of the head, left aspect (eq)

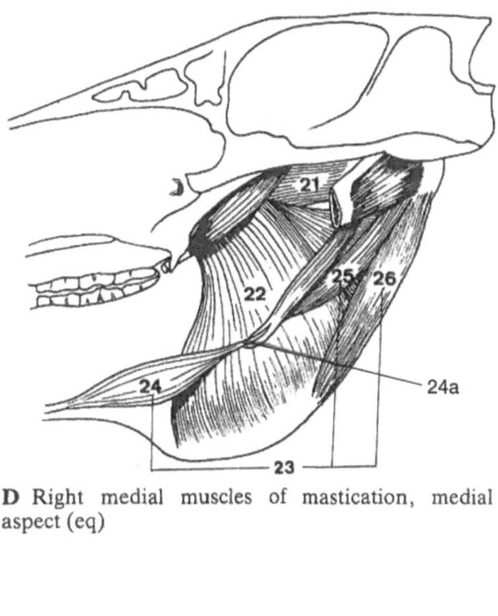

D Right medial muscles of mastication, medial aspect (eq)

1 ***Fascia buccopharyngea***[1]. Lies on M. buccinator and continues over mandible to Mm. constrictores pharyngis. A

2 ***Fascia masseterica***[1]. Covers M. masseter. A

3 ***Fascia parotidea***[1]. Continues from Fascia masseterica to cover parotid region. A

4 ***Fascia temporalis***. Covers M. temporalis. A

5 *Lamina superficialis*. Spreads over zygomatic arch to join Fascia parotidea. A

6 *Lamina profunda*. Attaches ventrally to zygomatic arch. A

7 **MUSCULI COLLI**. Muscles primarily in neck plus those associated with hyoid apparatus.

8 ***M. splenius cervicis***. Continuous with M. splenius capitis, M. splenius cervicis is absent in Car. Inserts on transverse processes of cervical vertebrae after arising from Ligamentum nuchae and Fascia thoracolumbalis. Extends neck and draws it laterally. E

9 ***M. brachiocephalicus***. Parts radiate from Intersectio clavicularis. Extends shoulder joint, pulls head and neck laterally and ventrally. B C E

10 *M. cleidobrachialis [Pars clavicularis m. deltoidei]*. Lies on cranial surface of arm. From Intersectio clavicularis to Crista humeri. In the domestic mammals the reduction of the clavicle to a rudiment makes the homologue of the human Pars clavicularis m. deltoidei an integral part of M. brachiocephalicus. B C E

11 *M. cleidocephalicus*. Lies on lateral surface of neck. From Intersectio clavicularis to parts of head (and neck in Car). B C

12 **Pars mastoidea**[2]*. Ventral part of M. cleidocephalicus from intersection to mastoid process. In bo it inserts also on the muscular tubercle of the occipital bone. B C

13 **Pars occipitalis** (su, Ru) [2]. Dorsal part. To Crista nuchae (su), Linea nuchae and Lig. nuchae (Ru). C

14 **Pars cervicalis** (Car)[2]. Dorsal part. To dorsal fibrous raphe of cranial portion of neck. B

15 *Intersectio clavicularis*. Between M. cleidobrachialis and M. cleidocephalicus, cranial to shoulder joint, difficult to demonstrate in bo (and eq). Clavicula is present in fe. B C (In the horse the clavicular intersection separates the cleidobrachialis muscle from both cleidomastoideus and omotransversarius – read cleidotransversarius [in eq only].)

15a ***M. omotransversarius***. From ventral part of Spina scapulae and Fascia brachii to the transverse processes of cranial cervical vertebrae. In eq connected with M. brachiocephalicus. Draws shoulder cranially. C E (In eq it is attached to the clavicular intersection, side by side with the M. cleidomastoideus, and it is called by some anatomists M. cleidotransversarius [Ghetie 1971, Constantinescu and Constantinescu 2004].)

16 ***M. sternocephalicus***. From sternum to Ramus mandibulae in eq, to mastoid process in su and ov, consists of two parts in other species. Flexes head and neck. B C E

17 *Pars mandibularis* (bo, cap, eq). Inserts on Fascia masseterica, in bo also on Corpus mandibulae, and in eq on the caudal border of Angulus mandibulae. C (In eq it is also called M. sternomandibularis since it is the only sternocephalicus M.)

18 *Pars mastoidea* (Car, bo, cap) [3]. Deep or ventral part. Inserts on mastoid process, and in bo also on the muscular tubercle of the occipital bone. B C

19 *Pars occipitalis* (Car)[3]. Dorsal part. Inserts on occipital bone. B

20 ***M. longus colli***. Many bundles which lie ventral to vertebral column in cervical and cranial thoracic parts. Flexes neck. D

21 ***M. scalenus ventralis*** (Un). From transverse processes of C3–C6 (su also C1 and C2) to the middle portion of first rib. Not present in Car. D

22 ***M. scalenus medius***. From transverse processes of C6 and C7 to the dorsal portion of first rib. D

23 ***M. scalenus dorsalis*** (Car, su, Ru). Lateral to M. scalenus medius, the dorsal portion of M. scalenus ventralis, and the cranial ribs. Absent in eq and mostly in ov, sometimes in cap, where it is differently shown on individual basis. From transverse processes of (C2, C3) C4–C6 to ribs 2–4, in Car additionally to ribs 8 or 9. Scaleni are inspiratory and flex neck. D

24 ***M. serratus ventralis cervicis***. Cervical part of large, serrated, fan-shaped muscle. From transverse processes of caudal cervical vertebrae to Facies serrata scapulae. Supports trunk. It is homologous to M. levator scapulae of man. See 107 F

[1] deep to Platysma and Sphincter colli profundus in ca

[2] In clinics they are called "M. cleido-"mastoideus, occipitalis, cervicalis.

[3] In clinics they are called M. sternomastoideus and M. sternooccipitalis.

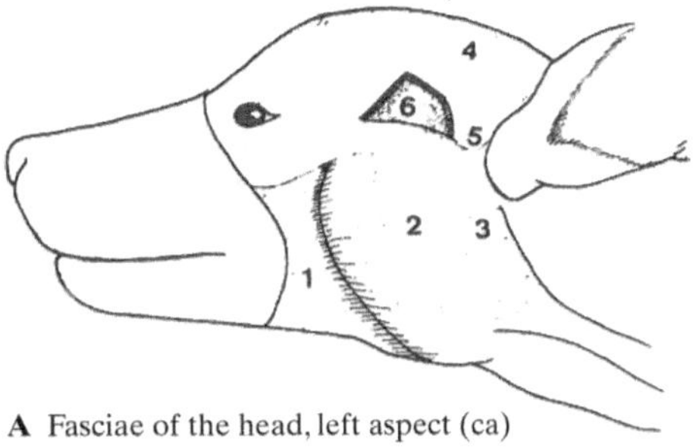

A Fasciae of the head, left aspect (ca)

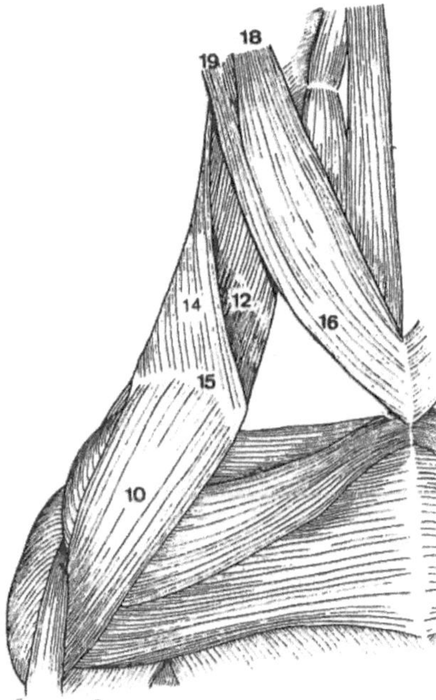

B Right M. brachiocephalicus and M. sternocephalicus, ventral aspect (ca)

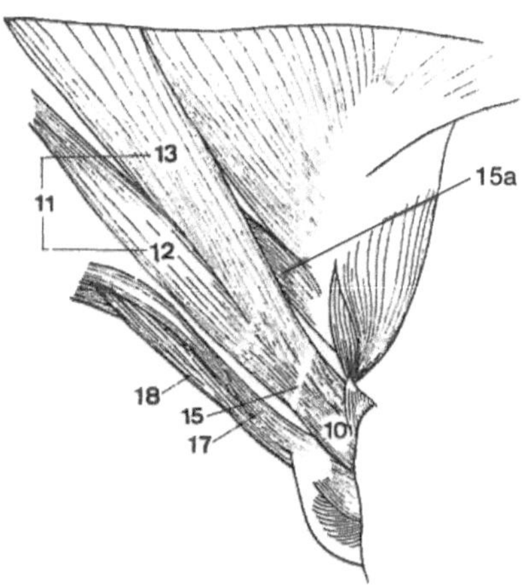

C M. brachiocephalicus and M. sternocephalicus, left aspect (bo)

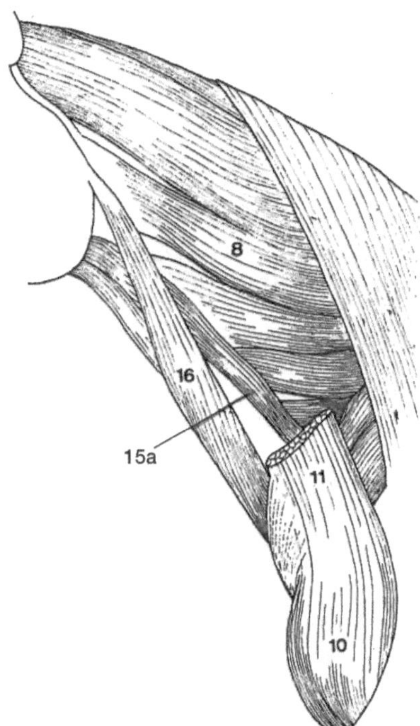

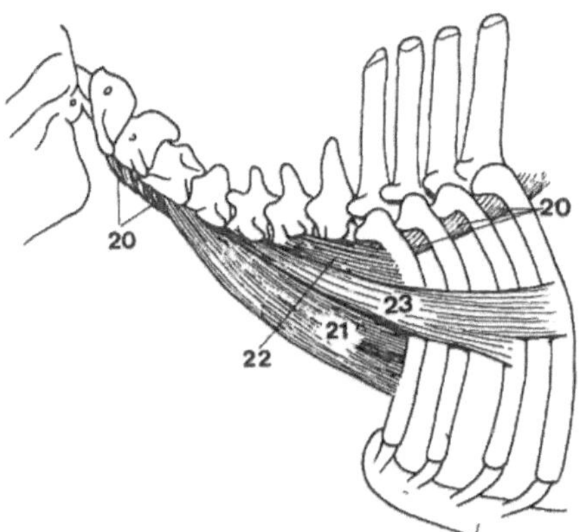

D Deep muscles of the neck, left aspect (bo)

E Muscles of the neck, left aspect (bo)

1 **Mm. hyoidei**. Muscles associated with hyoid apparatus. A B D

2 ***M. stylohyoideus***. Small muscle from stylohyoid to basihyoid, superficial to M. digastricus. Raises basihyoid. In eq the tendon is split by the passage of the intermediate tendon of the M. digastricus. A D

3 ***M. mylohyoideus***. Transverse fibers throughout intermandibular space. From Linea mylohyoidea of mandible to median raphe and basihyoid. Raises floor of oral cavity. A B

4 ***M. geniohyoideus***. Deep to preceeding muscle. From the rostromedial end of the body of mandible to basihyoid. Draws hyoid rostrally. A

5 ***M. sternohyoideus***. From Manubrium sterni to basihyoid. Pulls basihyoid caudally. A B C

6 ***M. omohyoideus***. From subscapular fascia in su and eq, from fascia lateral to middle cervical vertebrae in Ru, passing obliquely, deep to V. jugularis externa, to basihyoid. Retracts hyoid. Not present in Car. B

7 ***M. sternothyroideus [-thyreoideus]***. With and lateral to M. sternohyoideus. To thyroid cartilage. Draws larynx caudally. A B

8 ***M. thyrohyoideus [thyreo-]***. Short flat muscle from insertion of M. sternothyroideus to thyrohyoid. Draws hyoid caudally and larynx rostrally. A

9 ***M. occipitohyoideus****. Small muscle from paracondylar process of the occipital bone to stylohyoid. Moves stylohyoid caudally. A

10 ***M. ceratohyoideus***. Fills triangle between thyro- and ceratohyoids. Reduces angle. D

11 ***M. hyoideus transversus***. Small unpaired band between cerato- or epihyoids. D

12 **Fascia cervicalis**. Fascia of neck. Collective term for connective tissue layers of neck. E

13 ***Lamina superficialis***. From parotid to brachial fascia, deep to cutaneous muscles. Encloses Mm. sterno-, cleidocephalicus, and trapezius. E

14 ***Lamina pretrachealis [prae-]***. Layer ventral to, and surrounding and protecting trachea and esophagus. Encloses the caudal hyoid muscles. E

15 ***Vagina carotica***. Connective tissue sheath for A. carotis communis and associated structures. E

16 ***Lamina prevertebralis [prae-]***. Deep layer ventral to M. longus colli, dorsal to esophagus and trachea. E

17 **MUSCULI DORSI**. Extrinsic muscles of thoracic limb and epaxial muscles.

18 ***M. trapezius***. Broad, triangular muscle of neck and withers. Two continuous parts. Elevates and rotates scapula. C

19 *Pars cervicalis*. From median fibrous raphe of neck in Car and su, from Lig. nuchae in Ru and eq to Spina scapulae. C

20 *Pars thoracica*. From Lig. supraspinale over withers to dorsal third of Spina scapulae. C

21 ***M. omotransversarius***. C (It was moved to 104.15a according to the N.A.V. 5th edition).

22 ***M. latissimus dorsi***. Flat triangular muscle caudal to scapula. From superficial layer of Fascia thoracolumbalis to Tuberositas teres major (Un), Crista tuberculi minoris (Car) of humerus. Flexes shoulder joint. C

23 ***M. rhomboideus thoracis***. Deep to M. trapezius. Fibers course ventrally from spinous processes of cranial thoracic vertebrae to Margo dorsalis scapulae and medial side of Cartilago scapulae. Elevates scapula. F

24 ***M. rhomboideus cervicis***. From dorsal median raphe of neck (Car, su) or Lig. nuchae (Ru, eq) to Angulus cranialis scapulae and Margo dorsalis scapulae, cranial to M. rhomboideus thoracis. F

25 ***M. rhomboideus capitis*** (Car, su). Separates as narrow slip at cranial origin of M. rhomboideus cervicis. F (There is a M. rhomboideus atlantis in su [Constantinescu 1996].)

26 ***M. serratus ventralis cervicis***. F (It was moved to 104.24 according to the N.A.V. 5th edition).

27 ***M. serratus dorsalis caudalis***. From Fascia thoracolumbalis. Bundles course cranioventrally to attach to caudal ribs. Expiratory. C

28 ***M. serratus dorsalis cranialis***. Flat, serrated muscle from Fascia thoracolumbalis to cranial ribs. Fibers course caudoventrally. Inspiratory. F

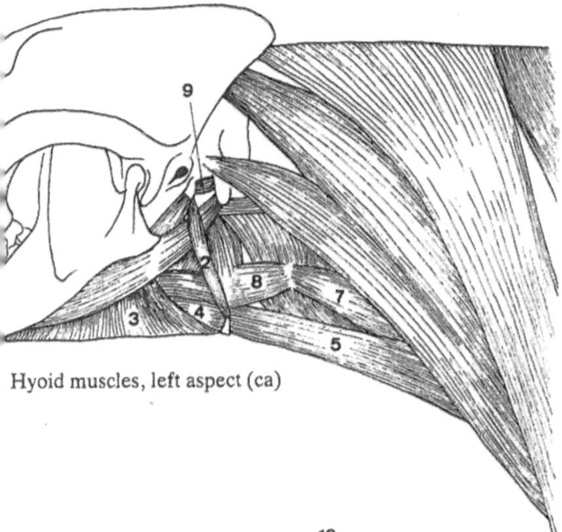

Hyoid muscles, left aspect (ca)

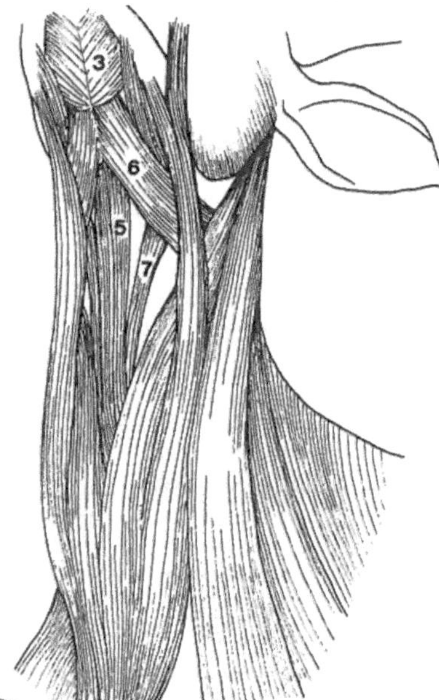

B Hyoid muscles, left ventral aspect (bo)

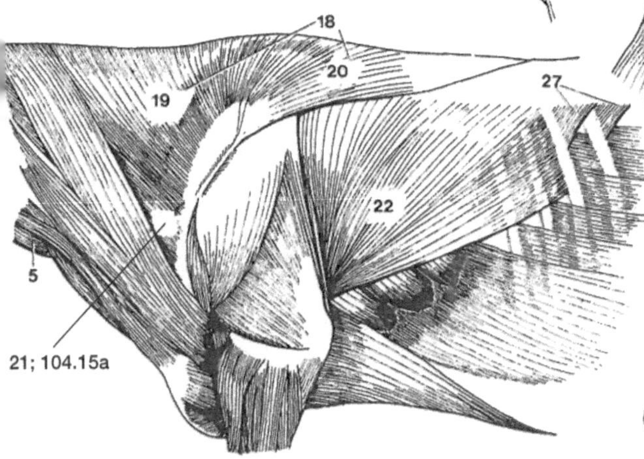

Superficial muscles of the back, left side (bo)

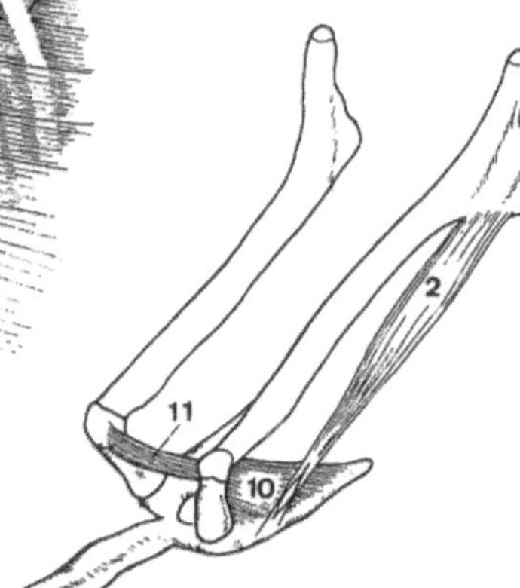

D Hyoid muscles, left rostral aspect (eq)

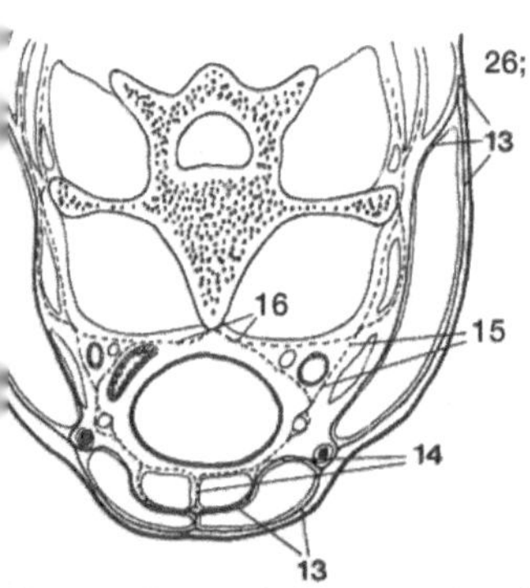

Fasciae of the neck, transversal section (eq)

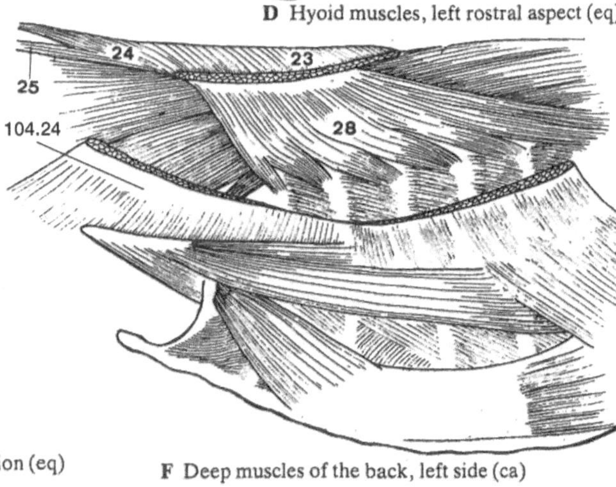

F Deep muscles of the back, left side (ca)

1 **M. erector spinae**. Epaxial muscles on dorsal surface of vertebral column and ribs. Extends vertebral column. A

2 ***M. iliocostalis***. Narrow longitudinal muscle mass. Tendons run cranioventrally over several segments. A

3 *M. iliocostalis lumborum*. Lateral portion of muscle mass dorsal to lumbar transverse processes. A

4 *M. iliocostalis thoracis*. Lateral to M. longissimus thoracis. Continuation forward of M. iliocostalis lumborum. Tendinous bundles course as far forward as last cervical transverse process. A

5 *M. iliocostalis cervicis*. Forward continuation of the preceding muscle as a narrow strip to last 3–4 cervical transverse processes. 111 E

6 ***M. longissimus***. Forms major portion of epaxial muscle mass. Bundles course cranioventrally several segments. Total extent from ilium to skull. A

7 *M. longissimus lumborum*. From Os ilium to continue as M. longissimus thoracis. A

8 *M. longissimus thoracis*. Bundles end as tendinous leaves. Continues as M. longissimus cervicis. A

9 *M. longissimus cervicis*. Bundles turn ventrally to insert on last few cervical transverse processes. A

10 *M. longissimus atlantis*. Parallel to, but ventral to M. longissimus capitis. Attaches to Ala atlantis. A

11 *M. longissimus capitis*. Cranially directed long muscle arising medial to M. longissimus cervicis to cross atlas and insert on mastoid process. A

12 ***M. spinalis***. Detaches from medial side of M. longissimus thoracis and travels forward near thoracic vertebral spinous processes to cervical vertebral spinous processes, in eq only to middle of neck. A B C

13 *M. spinalis thoracis*. Attaches to thoracic vertebral spinous processes and continues forward as M. spinalis cervicis. C

14 *M. spinalis cervicis*. Medial to Mm. multifidi to attach to cervical vertebral spinous processes. C

15 **M. transversospinalis**. Collective term for the following muscles.

16 ***M. semispinalis***. Closely associated with, but lateral to M. spinalis. Extends vertebral column and head. M. spinalis, M. semispinalis thoracis, and M. semispinalis cervicis are associated in one mass in Car and Ru. C

17 *M. semispinalis thoracis*. Bundles detach from Processus mamillares and course over lateral face of M. spinalis to dorsal portion of Processus spinosi. Continues as M. semispinalis cervicis. C

18 *M. semispinalis cervicis*. Fuses with M. spinalis cervicis in Car and Ru, absent in su and eq. C

19 *M. semispinalis capitis*. Distinct mass of two parts which arises between M. spinalis thoracis and M. longissimus thoracis. A

20 **M. biventer cervicis**. Dorsomedial division. From Fascia thoracolumbalis or thoracic vertebral transverse processes. Courses superficial to Mm. multifidi to insert on Os occipitale. A

21 **M. complexus**. Ventrolateral division which arises from cervical vertebral articular processes and inserts lateral to M. biventer cervicis on Os occipitale. A

22 ***Mm. multifidi***. Continous deep series of muscle bundles which course dorsocranially over several segments in lumbar, thoracic, and cervical region. Originate from mamillary, transverse, or articular processes to terminate on spinous processes. Extend vertebral column. B D

22a *Mm. multifidi laterales*. Lateral fascicles.

22b *Mm. multifidi mediales*. Medial fascicles.

22c *Mm. multifidi profundi*. Deep fascicles.

23 ***Mm. rotatores***. Long and short muscle bundles deep to Mm. multifidi in cranial thoracic region. Long bundles go dorsocranially from transverse to spinous processes, short are more vertical. Rotate vertebral column. D

24 **Mm. interspinales**. From caudal cervical to cranial lumbar regions between spinous processes. Lumbar fibers are deep to Mm. multifidi. D

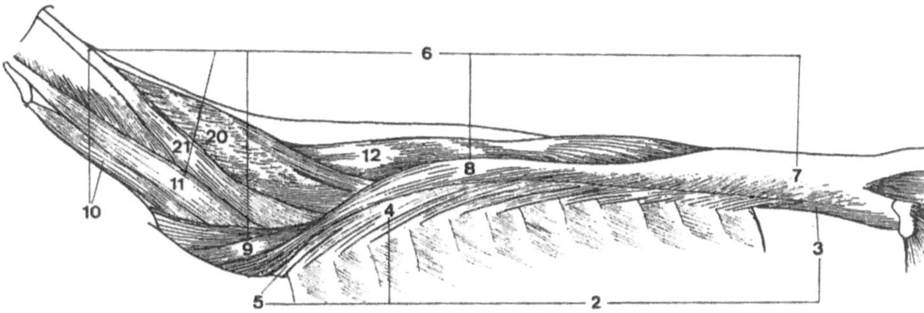

A Deep muscles of the back, left aspect (bo)

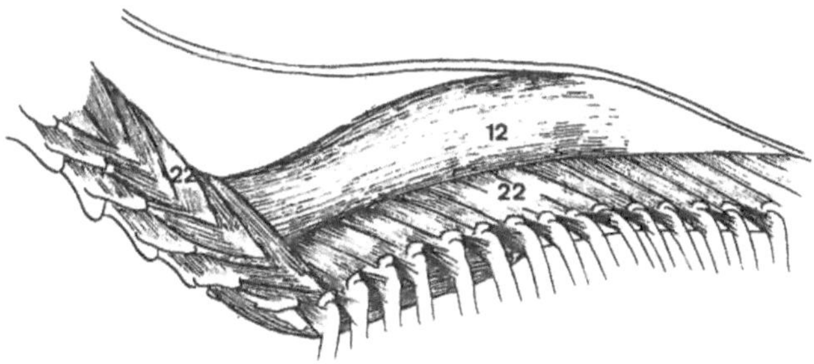

B Deep muscles of the back, left aspect (eq)

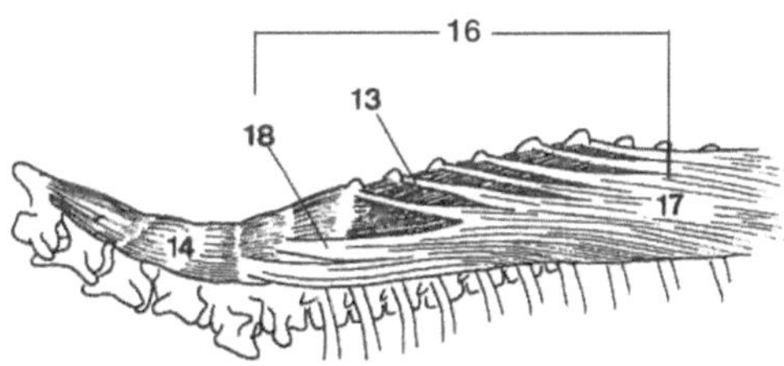

C Deep muscles of the back, left aspect (ca)

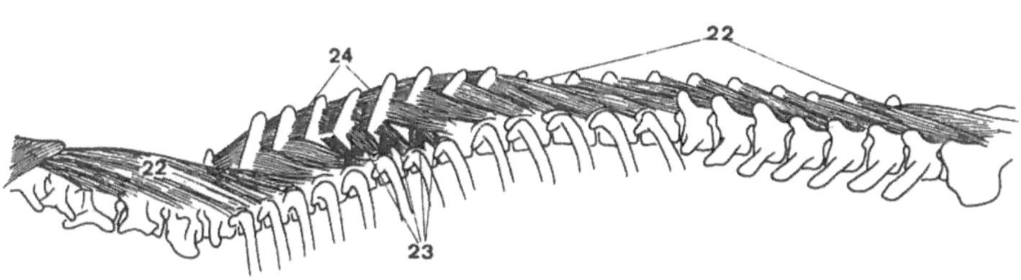

D Short back muscles, left aspect (ca)

1 **Mm. intertransversarii**. Between transverse, or articular and transverse, or mamillary and transverse processes. A B

2 ***Mm. intertransversarii lumborum***. Medial bundles run ventrocranially from Proc. mamillares to Proc. transversi (or accessorii), lateral lie between transverse processes. A

3 ***Mm. intransversarii thoracis***. Present in caudal thoracic region as continuation of medial lumbar group. A

4 ***Mm. intertransversarii dorsales cervicis***. Bundles run horizontally between cranial articular processes. B

4a *Mm. intertransversarii medii cervicis*. Bundles run cranioventrally from a cranial articular process to the caudal end of the transverse process skipping one vertebra in a cranial direction (C_5 to C_3 for example). B

5 ***Mm. intertransversarii ventrales cervicis***. Bundles run horizontally between caudal ends of two consecutive transverse processes. B

6 ***Fascia thoracolumbalis***. Fascia covering M. erector spinae. Divided into superficial layer which gives origin to M. latissimus dorsi, and deep layer which dips deep to scapula. M. splenius and Mm. serrati dorsales arise from it. C

7 *Lig. dorsoscapulare*. Extends in eq from spinous processes Th2–Th5 to the medial surface of scapula dorsal to termination of M. serratus ventralis, elastic. The aponeuroses of Mm. splenius, semispinalis capitis and serratus dorsalis cranialis, as well as elastic fibers from the Lig. supraspinale and of the Fascia thoracolumbalis contribute to the Lig. dorsoscapulare, important structure of the passive, suspensory or stay apparatus of the body in eq. C

8 ***Fascia nuchae***. Dorsal continuation of investment of neck.

9 **MUSCULI THORACIS**. Muscles of thoracic wall.

10 ***Mm. pectorales superficiales***. Run transversely from cranial half of sternum to humerus and Fascia antebrachii. Adduct thoracic limb. D E

11 *M. pectoralis descendens**. Cranial portion. From Manubrium sterni to distal end of Crista humeri. D E

12 *M. pectoralis transversus**. Broad origin along sternum. Fibers travel laterally to terminate on Crista humeri (Car) or Fascia antebrachii lamina superficialis (Un). D E

13 ***M. pectoralis profundus [M. pectoralis ascendens]****. Arises along sternum deep to M. pectoralis superficialis and from pectoral fascia caudal to Cartilago xiphoidea. Narrows to ascend to fascia and Tubercula humeri. Adducts thoracic limb and draws it caudally. D

14 ***M. subclavius***. From the 1st (–4th) costal cartilage. Swings dorsolaterally to deep face of M. brachiocephalicus (su, Ru) and/or cranial to M. supraspinatus (su, eq). Especially prominent in su and eq where it was formerly called M. pectoralis cleidoscapularis, and considered as a part of M. pectoralis profundus. In Ru it is small, in Car not present. Originating from the first costal cartilage, this muscle should not be confused in Ru with the fleshy termination of M. pectoralis profundus on M. supraspinatus. E

15 ***Fascia pectoralis***. Fascia covering pectoral muscles. D

16 ***M. serratus ventralis thoracis***. From ribs of cranial half of thorax to caudal part of Facies serrata. Supports thorax between thoracic limbs. D E

17 ***Mm. levatores costarum***. At proximal ends of intercostal spaces. From transverse process of each vertebra caudolaterally to succeeding rib. Inspiratory. F

18 ***Mm. intercostales externi***. Occupy intercostal spaces superficially from ventral extent of M. levatores costarum to costochondral junction. Fibers run caudoventrally. Inspiratory. E F

19 ***Mm. intercostales interni***. Throughout length of intercostal and interchondral spaces. Fibers run cranioventrally. Expiratory. F

20 *Mm. subcostales*. Muscle bundles at vertebral ends of caudal ribs deep to Mm. intercostales interni. Directed cranioventrally across several ribs, especially ribs 9–11 in Car. F

21 ***M. retractor costae***. Flat group of fibers coursing cranioventrally from first lumbar transverse process to proximal portion of last rib. F

22 ***M. transversus thoracis***. On deep surface of ventral thoracic wall. From sternum to costochondral junction of sternal ribs. In general muscle bundles are transversely oriented. Expiratory. G

23 ***M. rectus thoracis***. Flat muscle from first rib to course caudoventrally over several ribs to origin of M. rectus abdominis. Inspiratory. E

24 ***Fascia endothoracica***. Connective tissue layer between Pleura parietalis and thoracic wall. Continuation of Lamina prevertebralis fasciae cervicalis. G

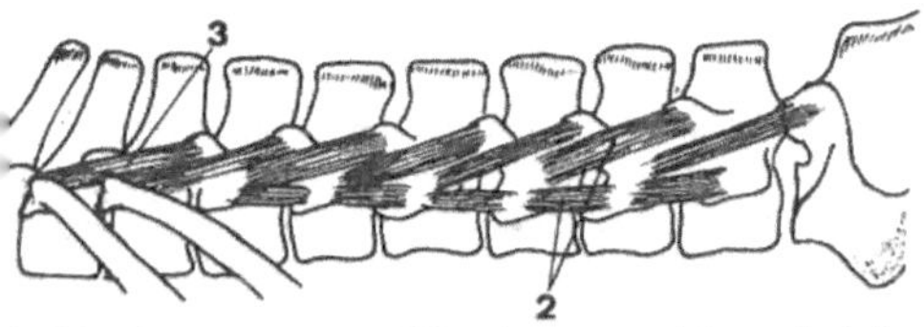

A Mm. intertransversarii lumborum and thoracis, left aspect (bo)

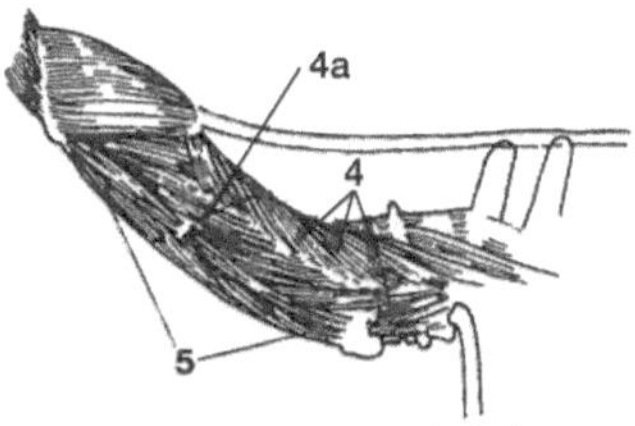

B Mm. intertransversarii of the neck, left aspect (ca)

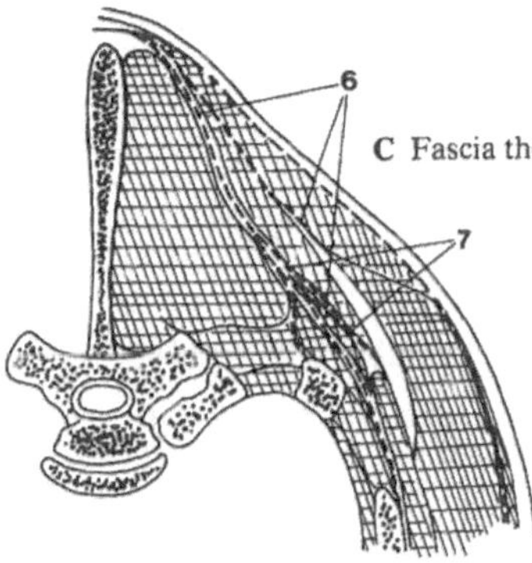

C Fascia thoracolumbalis, transverse section (eq)

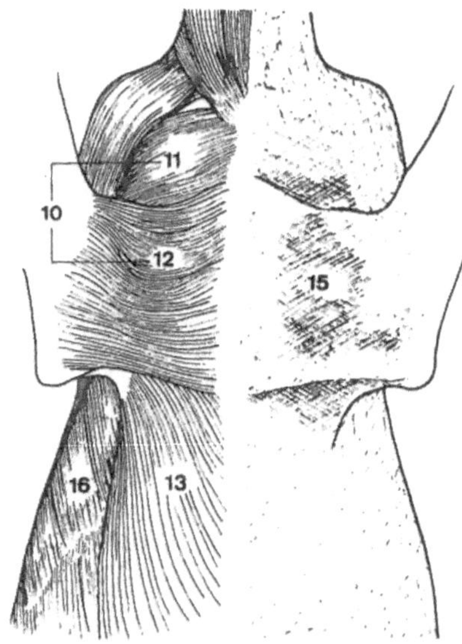

D Muscles and fascia of the thorax, ventral aspect (eq)

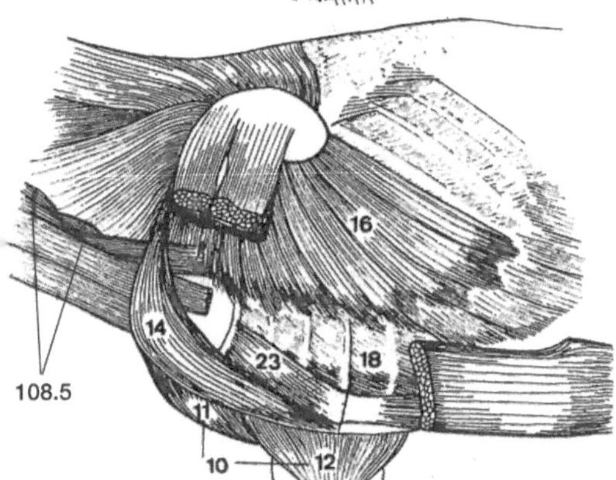

E Muscles of the thorax, left aspect (eq)

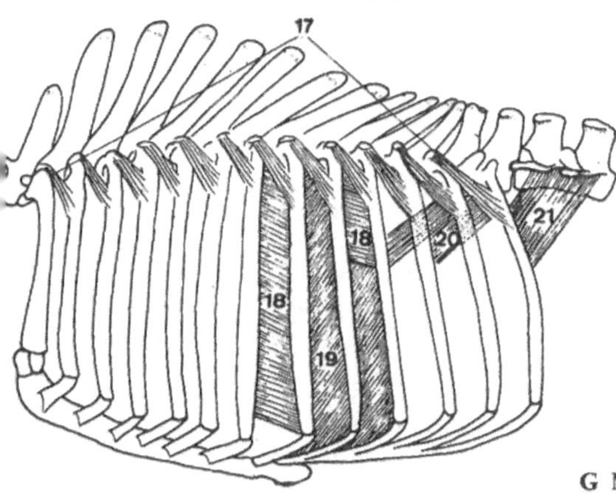

F Muscles of the ribs, left side (bo)

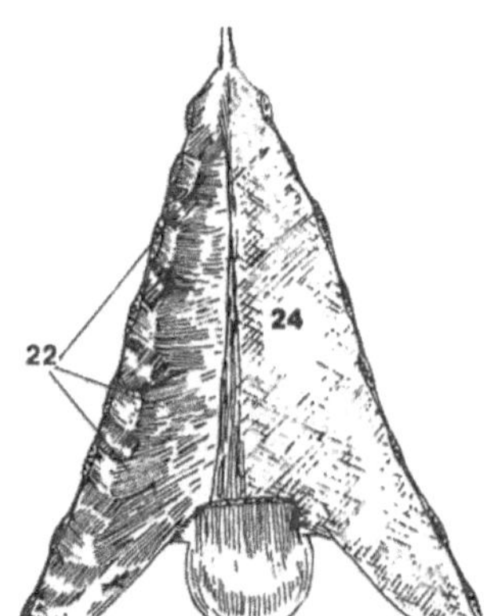

G M. transversus thoracis and Fascia endothoracia, dorsal aspect (eq)

1 **Diaphragma**. Musculotendinous partition between thoracic and abdominal cavities. Muscle of inspiration. A

2 ***Pars lumbalis***. Two crura from cranial lumbar vertebral bodies to spread out in diaphragm. A D

3 *Crus dextrum*. Larger crus, arising by long tendon from lumbar vertebrae to spread out surrounding esophagus. A

4 *Crus sinistrum*. Smaller crus. A

5 ***Pars costalis***. Arises from caudal ribs. Fibers course to Centrum tendineum. A D

6 ***Pars sternalis***. Continuation of Pars costalis arising from sternum and Cartilago xiphoidea. A D

7 ***Hiatus aorticus***. Opening between crural tendons at vertebral bodies. A D

8 ***Hiatus esophageus [oesophageus]***. Opening in cranioventral portion of Crus dextrum. A D

9 ***Centrum tendineum***. Tendinous sheet between Pars sternalis, costalis, and lumbalis. A D

10 ***Cupula diaphragmatis***. Most cranial portion of diaphragm. D

11 ***Foramen venae cavae***. Opening in Centrum tendineum for passage of V. cava caudalis. A D

12 ***Arcus lumbocostalis***. Ventral to psoas muscles where crura turn laterally toward Pars costalis. A

13 **MUSCULI ABDOMINIS**. Muscles of abdominal wall. Act to increase intraabdominal pressure.

14 ***M. rectus abdominis***. Lies parallel to ventral midline. Arises by flat tendon from sternum and costal cartilages, terminates on Os pubis as the major component of Tendo prepubicus. B C

15 *Intersectiones tendineae*. Sheets of fibrous tissue transversely placed across M. rectus abdominis. B C

15a *Anulus venae mammariae*. For passage of V. epigastrica cranialis superficialis, in Ru known as the milk well.

16 *Vagina m. recti abdominis*. Rectus sheath, formed by aponeuroses of abdominal muscles as they course to Linea alba. C

17 **Lamina externa**. Formed by aponeuroses of M. obliquus externus abdominis and M. obliquus internus abdominis. Cranial to Os pubis, aponeurosis of M. transversus abdominis joins Lamina externa in Car. B C

18 **Lamina interna**. Formed by aponeurosis of M. transversus abdominis. In Car, ov, and cap M. obliquus internus abdominis sends an aponeurotic sheet to Lamina interna cranial to umbilicus. C

19 **Linea arcuata**. Caudal border of aponeurosis of M. transversus abdominis. C

20 ***M. obliquus externus abdominis***. Fibers course obliquely ventrocaudally to form aponeurosis which expands in inguinal region. Arises from lateral surface of ribs and Fascia thoracolumbalis (except Ru). B C

21 *Arcus inguinalis [Lig. inguinale]*. Thickened caudal portion of aponeurosis of M. obliquus externus abdominis from Tuber coxae to Eminentia iliopubica. 115 A

22 ***M. obliquus internus abdominis***. Courses ventrocranially to form aponeurosis. Fibers closer to midline in inguinal region where they cover lateral border of M. rectus abdominis and turn caudally. From Fascia thoracolumbalis (except eq) and Tuber coxae. B C

23 *M. cremaster*. Caudal detachment of fibers from M. obliquus internus abdominis to Funiculus spermaticus. B

24 ***M. transversus abdominis***. Forms aponeurosis at lateral border of M. rectus abdominis. From medial surface of ribs and Fascia thoracolumbalis. A C

25 ***M. quadratus lumborum***. Longitudinal fibers ventral to bodies of last thoracic vertebrae and lumbar vertebral transverse processes. Dorsal to psoas muscles. A

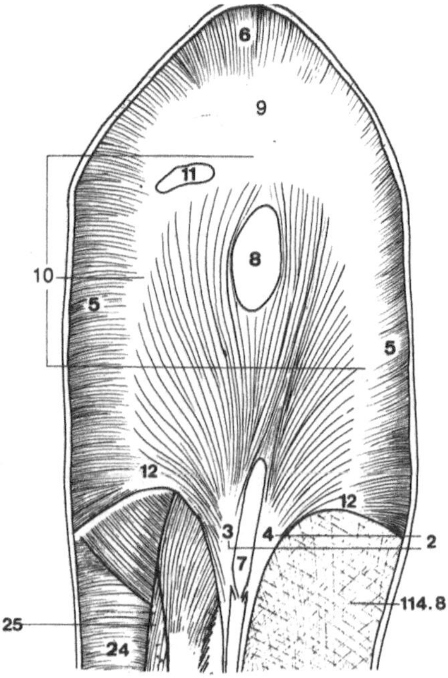

A Diaphragma, caudoventral aspect (ca)

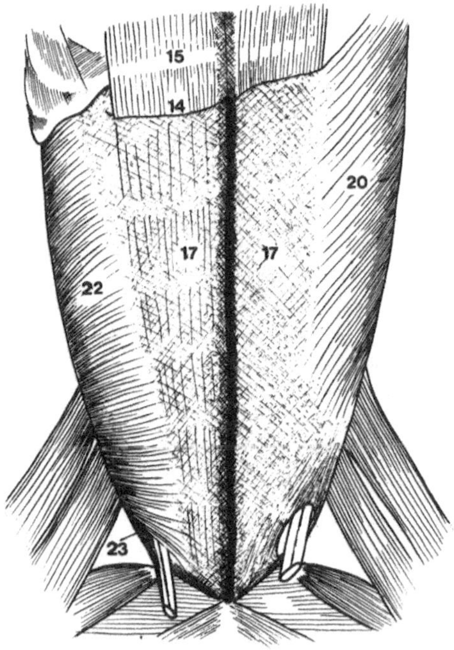

B Abdominal muscles (ca)

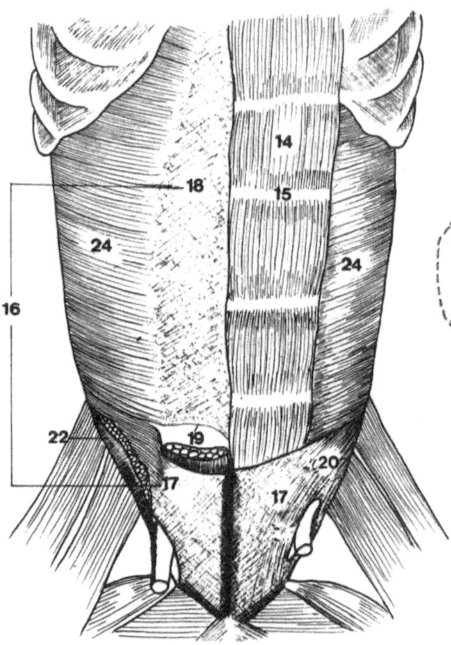

C Abdominal muscles (ca)

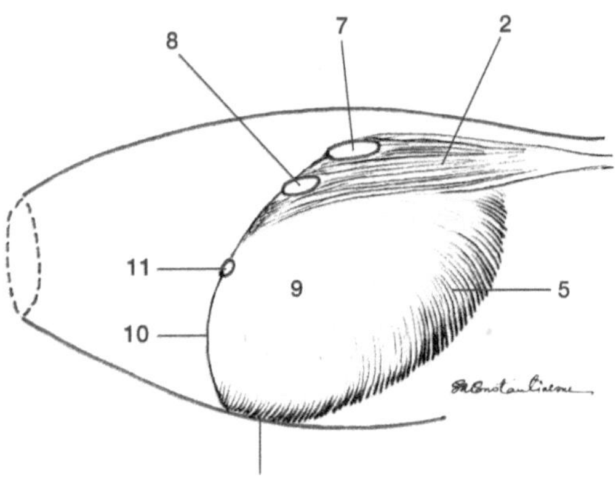

D Diaphragma, left lateral aspect (schematic)

1 ***Tunica flava abdominis***. Modified fascia as elastic sheet over M. obliquus externus abdominis in Un. It also provides the Laminae mediales of Apparatus suspensorius mammarius, very developed in the cow (see Integumentum commune p. 560). A

2 ***Linea alba***. White fibrous line of attachment of aponeuroses on ventral midline from Cartilago xiphoidea to Os pubis. A 217 B

3 *Anulus umbilicalis**. Widening of Linea alba representing closed umbilicus. A

4 *Lig. fundiforme penis*. Lateral elastic strands from Linea alba and fascia to preputium. C

5 *Tendo prepubicus [prae-]**. Complex of tendons, mainly of Mm. pectinei and Mm. recti abdominis attached to Rami craniales ossium pubis. A

6 ***Lig. suspensorium penis***. Median fibrous strands from the caudal part of Symphysis pelvina to penis. C

7 ***Lig. suspensorium clitoridis***. Median fibrous strands from the caudal part of Symphysis pelvina to clitoris.

8 ***Fascia transversalis***. Layer of abdominal wall outside peritoneum as far dorsal as tips of lumbar transverse processes. 113 A

9 **Canalis inguinalis [Spatium inguinale]**. Area between superficial and deep inguinal rings, these including. B

10 ***Anulus inguinalis profundus***. Obliquely oriented dorsoventrally and lateromedially abdominal entrance to the inguinal canal, bounded by the caudal border of M. obliquus internus abdominis and the Arcus inguinalis, lateral to M. rectus abdominis. B

11 ***Anulus inguinalis superficialis****. Slit or oval opening in aponeurosis of M. obliquus externus abdominis in inguinal region. A B

12 *Crus mediale*. Aponeurosis forming the craniomedial border of Anulus inguinalis superficialis. A B

13 *Crus laterale*. Aponeurosis forming the caudolateral border of Anulus inguinalis superficialis. A B

14 *Fibrae intercrurales*. Fibrous strands between Crus mediale and Crus laterale reinforcing craniolateral end of Anulus inguinalis superficialis. A

15 ***Lamina femoralis***. Sheet of aponeurosis of M. obliquus externus from Crus laterale of Anulus inguinalis superficialis to medial surface of the thigh and forming the Laminae laterales of Apparatus suspensorius mammarius, very developed in the cow (see Integumentum commune p. 560). A

16 **MUSCULI CAUDAE [COCCYGIS]**. Muscles of tail. D

17 ***M. coccygeus***. Arises from Spina ischiadica. Part of Diaphragma pelvis, it inserts laterally on transverse processes of first few coccygeal vertebrae. Depresses tail; singly also flexes tail laterally. D

18 ***M. sacrocaudalis [-coccygeus] ventralis medialis***. Medial of two ventral longitudinal muscles. Consists of short segments continuing caudally from last sacral vertebra. D

19 ***M. sacrocaudalis [-coccygeus] ventralis lateralis***. Arises from last lumbar vertebra (Car) and sacrum. Segments become tendinous. D

20 ***M. sacrocaudalis [-coccygeus] dorsalis medialis***. Continues caudally from Mm. multifidi at last lumbar vertebra. Composed of substantial segments. D

21 ***M. sacrocaudalis [coccygeus] dorsalis lateralis***. Arises between M. longissimus and Mm. multifidi as far forward as 1st lumbar vertebra. Consists of long bundles, in Car tendinous on the tail. D

22 ***Mm. intertransversarii ventrales caudae [coccygis]***. Ventral to transverse processes. Begin caudal to sacrum, are segmented.

23 ***Mm. intertransversarii dorsales caudae [coccygis]***. Dorsal to ventral group. Begin at sacrum but may not reach tip of tail. D

24 ***Fascia caudae [coccygis]***. Invests the tail, sends intermuscular septa to vertebrae especially in midline and investing Mm. intertransversarii. D

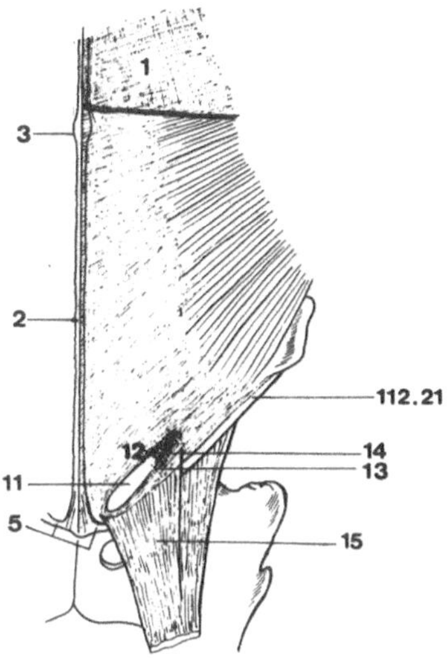

A Left side of ventral abdominal wall, ventral aspect (eq)

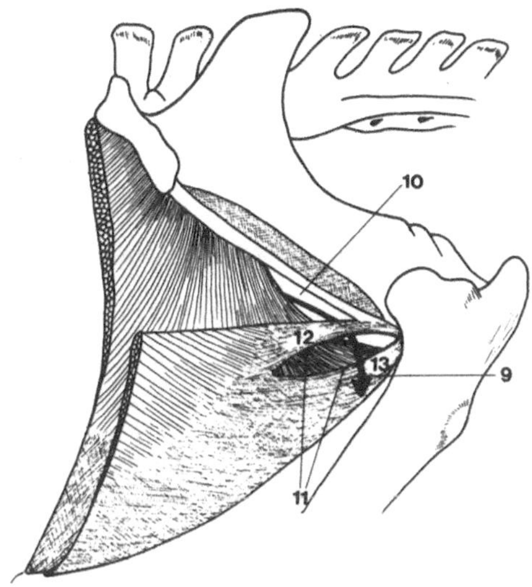

B Left Canalis inguinalis, lateral aspect (eq)

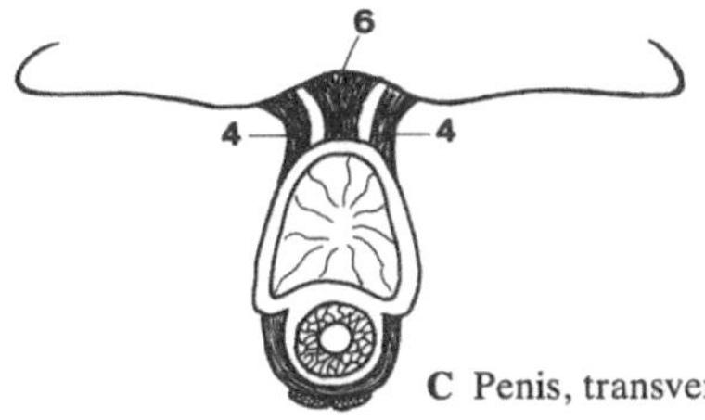

C Penis, transverse section (eq)

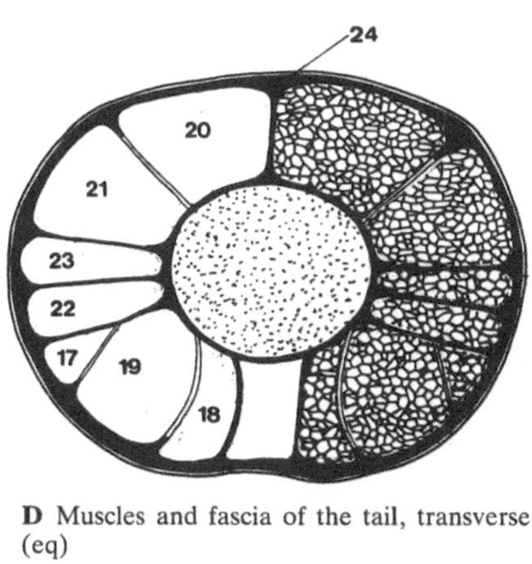

D Muscles and fascia of the tail, transverse section (eq)

1 **MUSCULI MEMBRI THORACICI**. Muscles of thoracic limb.

2 ***M. deltoideus***. Lateral muscle of shoulder. Divided origin, two parts are blended in eq, as there is no acromion. Flexes shoulder joint. A E

3 *Pars scapularis*. From Spina scapulae to Tuberositas deltoidea. A C

4 *Pars acromialis*. From acromion to Tuberositas deltoidea. A C

5 *Pars clavicularis [M. cleidobrachialis]*. In domestic mammals the reduction of the Clavicula makes the Pars clavicularis m. deltoidei to a part of M. brachiocephalicus. A (see 104.10)

6 ***M. supraspinatus***. Occupies Fossa supraspinata. Passes over cranial part of shoulder joint to Tuberculum majus, in Un also minus. Extends shoulder joint. A B C E F

7 ***M. infraspinatus****. Occupies Fossa infraspinata. Crosses lateral part of shoulder joint to roughened area of Tuberculum majus humeri. Acts as lateral collateral ligament of shoulder joint. A C E

8 ***M. teres minor***. Small round muscle from caudal border of scapula. Along caudal border of M. infraspinatus to terminate distal to it on humerus. Flexes shoulder joint. A C E

9 ***M. teres major***. From proximal part of caudal border of scapula to terminate with M. latissimus dorsi on Tuberositas teres major (Un) or Crista tuberculi minoris (Car). Flexes shoulder joint. A B C D F

10 ***M. subscapularis***. Occupies Fossa subscapularis. Inserts on caudal portion of Tuberculum minus. Acts as medial collateral ligament of shoulder joint. B C D F

11 ***M. articularis humeri*** (fe, su, eq). Small muscle over caudal surface of shoulder joint capsule. B

12 ***M. coracobrachialis***. Arises by tendon from Processus coracoideus to terminate around Tuberositas teres major, depending on species. Extends and adducts shoulder joint. B D F

13 ***M. biceps brachii***. From Tuberculum supraglenoidale. Passes distally through Sulcus intertubercularis to terminate on Tuberositas radii and fascia. Extends shoulder joint and flexes elbow joint. Tendon runs within full length of biceps from very strong tendon of origin which acts to fix shoulder joint. A B C D

13a ***Retinaculum transversum***. Strong transverse connective tissue band which binds down the tendon of the M. biceps brachii in Car, su, and Ru.

14 *Lacertus fibrosus*. Fibrous connection of M. biceps brachii with proximal tendon of M. extensor carpi radialis on medial surface. Especially developed in eq as part of passive, suspensory or stay apparatus of the thoracic limb. B

15 ***M. brachialis***. Occupies Sulcus m. brachialis. Crosses cranial surface of elbow to terminate near biceps on radius and ulna. Flexes elbow joint. A B E F

16 ***M. triceps brachii***. Caudal to humerus and shoulder joint. Consists of three or four heads which converge to terminate on olecranon. Extends elbow joint and acts as a propulsor of the limb. A

17 *Caput longum**. Only head arising from caudal border of scapula. Also flexes shoulder joint. A C D

18 *Caput laterale**. Arises from Linea m. tricipitis, in Car also on Crista humeri. A E

19 *Caput mediale*. From humerus caudal to Tuberositas teres major (Crista tuberculi minoris in Car). B F

20 *Caput accessorium*. Deep to other heads. Arises distal to Caput humeri. Absent in eq. A E F

21 ***M. anconeus [anconaeus]***. From humerus lateral to Fossa olecrani to olecranon. Extends elbow joint. A E F

22 ***M. tensor fasciae antebrachii***. Lies on medial surface of triceps. Arises from M. latissimus dorsi (Car, Ru, eq) and caudal border of scapula (su, Ru, eq) to terminate on olecranon and Fascia antebrachii lamina profunda. Extends elbow joint and flexes shoulder joint (except Car). B

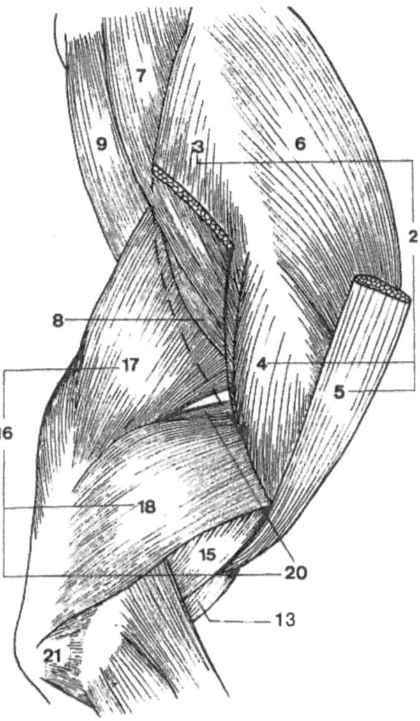

A Muscles of right shoulder and arm, lateral aspect (ca)

B Muscles of left shoulder and arm, medial aspect (eq)

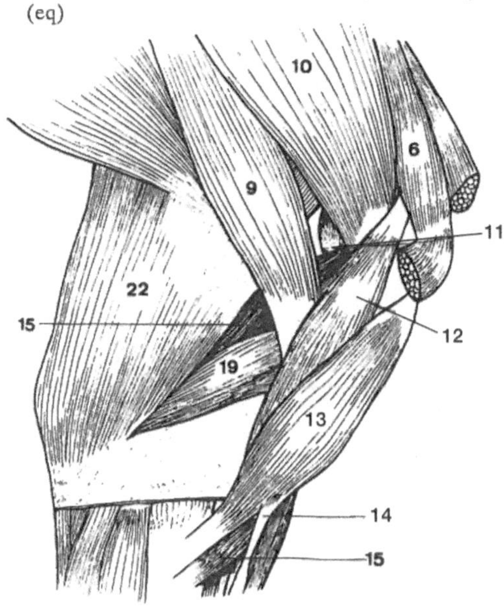

C Left scapula, lateral aspect (ca)

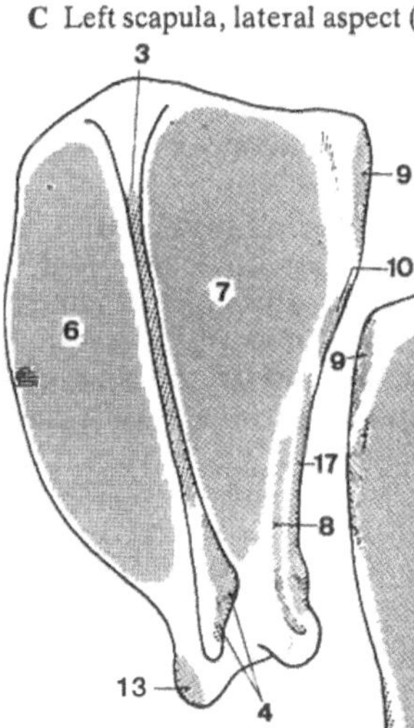

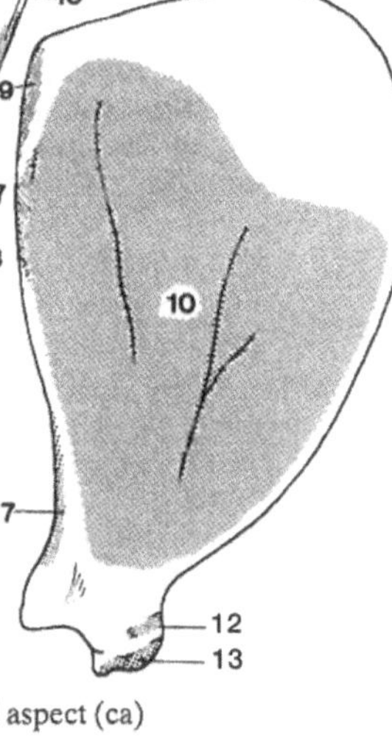

D Left scapula, medial aspect (ca)

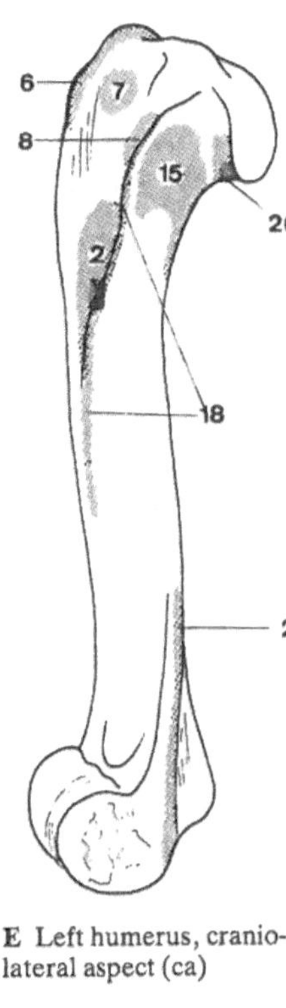

E Left humerus, craniolateral aspect (ca)

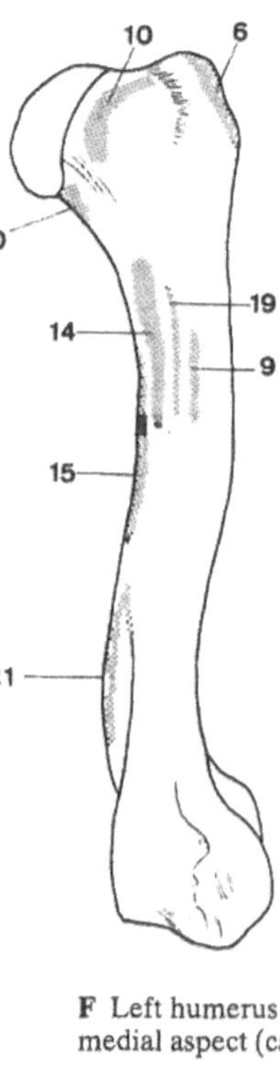

F Left humerus, medial aspect (ca)

1 ***M. pronator teres.*** From Epicondylus medialis humeri to medial surface of radius. Pronates radioulnar joints. Tendinous or not present in eq. C D

2 ***M. flexor carpi radialis.*** Next caudal from Epicondylus medialis to Basis of Os metacarpale II (Car, eq), III (Car, su, Ru). A C

3 ***M. flexor carpi ulnaris.*** Most caudal of flexor group. The two heads do not unite in Car. Flexes carpal joint. A B

4 *Caput humerale.* From Epicondylus medialis to Os carpi accessorium. Deep to M. flexor digitorum superficialis in Car. A B

5 *Caput ulnare.* From medial side of olecranon to Os carpi accessorium. A B C D

6 ***M. flexor digitorum [digitalis] superficialis***[1)]*. From Epicondylus medialis. Tendon divides for major digits. Each divides for passage of deep flexor tendon and terminates on middle scutum. Flexes carpal and proximal phalangeal joints. A C

7 *Ligamentum accessorium**. From distal portion of radius to superficial digital flexor tendon in eq. Part of passive, suspensory or stay apparatus of the thoracic limb. A

8 *Manica flexoria.* The sleeve formed by each tendon of M. flexor digitorum superficialis or the tendon of M. flexor digitalis superficialis in eq, around the corresponding tendon of M. flexor digitorum/digitalis profundus at the level of the Articulatio metacarpophalangea. A

9 ***M. flexor digitorum [digitalis] profundus***[1)]*. Deep in flexor group. Three heads with combined tendon which divides to terminate on flexor surface of each distal phalanx. Flexes carpal and phalangeal joints. A E

10 *Caput humerale.* Contains bulk of muscle. From Epicondylus medialis. A E

11 *Caput radiale.* A small slip from middle portion of caudal radius. C D E

12 *Caput ulnare.* Arises along ulna, mostly tendinous in eq. A D E

13 *Ligamentum accessorium**. Fibrous continuation of palmar carpal ligaments to deep digital flexor tendon in eq. Part of passive, suspensory or stay apparatus of the thoracic limb. A (Formerly termed Caput tendineum of the deep digital flexor tendon, it is still called "distal check ligament" in eq, the alternative of the accessory ligament of the deep digital flexor muscle.)

13a *Lamina transversa.* This is a connective tissue attachment (with an abundance of elastic fibers) of the tendon of M. Flexor digitorum/digitalis profundus to the palmar surface of Phalanx media in Ru and eq. It separates the Vagina synovialis tendinum digitorum manus from the Bursa podotrochlearis manus. 135 F

14 ***Mm. interflexorii.*** In Car longitudinal bundle from palmar surface of M. flexor digitorum profundus at carpus. Thin tendons to superficial digital flexor tendons. In su and Ru additional connection between superficial and deep digital flexor at antebrachium. Absent in eq. E

15 ***M. pronator quadratus.*** Transverse fibers between radius and ulna in Car. D E

16 ***M. brachioradialis.*** In Car as slender muscle on cranial surface of M. extensor carpi radialis, often absent in ca. Supinates antebrachium. B C D

17 ***M. extensor carpi radialis.*** Most cranial major muscle of extensor group. From Crista supracondylaris lateralis humeri to Tuberositas ossis metacarpalis III in Un, metacarpals II and III in Car. Extends carpal joint. A B C

18 ***M. extensor carpi radialis longus.*** Medial division in fe, medial tendon in ca, inserts on metacarpal II. B F

19 ***M. extensor carpi radialis brevis.*** Lateral division in fe, lateral tendon in ca. Inserts on metacarpal III. The Mm. extensor carpi radialis longus and extensor carpi radialis brevis are separate in fe, and partially fused in ca. B F

20 ***M. extensor digitorum [digitalis] communis***[1)]. Arises caudodistal to M. extensor carpi radialis. Tendon crosses dorsal surface of carpus to divide for Processus extensorius of distal phalanx of digitis II–IV (Car, su), III (eq), all phalanges of digits III and IV (Ru). In Ru separated medial portion is formed for digit III, in su there are three portions. Extends carpal and phalangeal joints. B F

20a *Caput accessorium* (Ru, eq) is a vestige of the former "Muscle of Thiernesse".

21 ***M. extensor digitorum [digitalis] lateralis.*** Lies caudolateral to preceding muscle, but arises from radius and ulna. Tendon terminates on proximal phalanx in eq, goes to all phalanges of digit IV in Ru, IV, V in su, III–V in ca, and II–V in fe. Extends carpal and phalangeal joints of corresponding digits. B F

21a *Caput accessorium* (ov, cap, eq) is a vestige of, and formerly called the "Muscle of Phillips".

22 ***M. extensor carpi ulnaris [M. ulnaris lateralis].*** Most caudolateral of extensor group. From Epicondylus lateralis. Tendon attaches on Os carpi accessorium, but sends tendon on to lateral metacarpal bone. Lies so far caudal that it acts as a carpal flexor. B

1) In eq both flexors of the digits should be called "digitalis", because of a single digit.

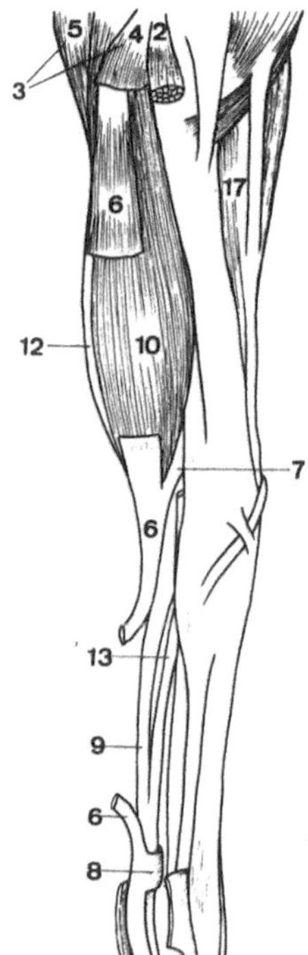

A Muscles of the left forearm, medial aspect (eq)

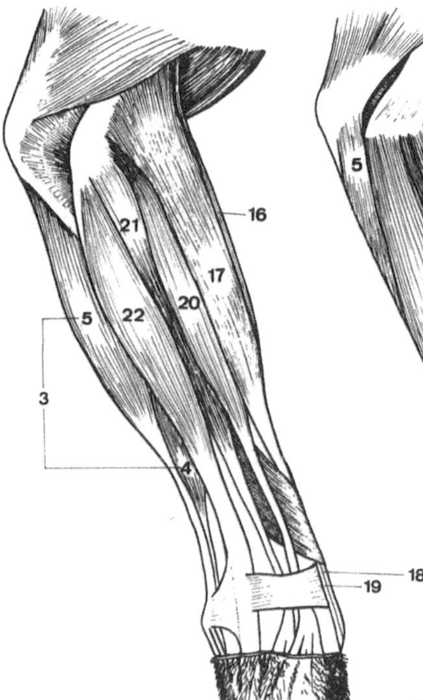

B Muscles of the right forearm, lateral aspect (ca)

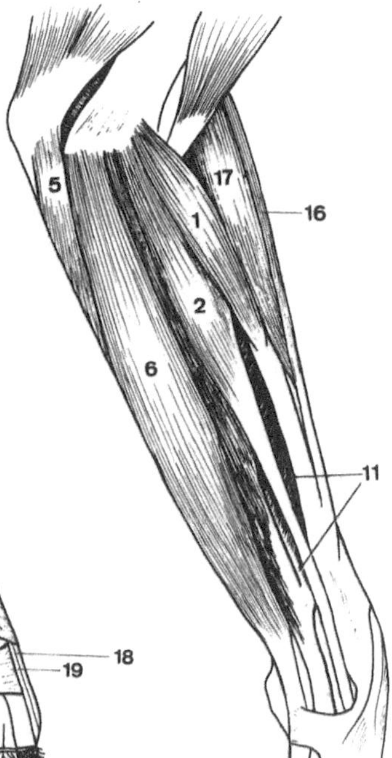

C Muscles of the left forearm, medial aspect (ca)

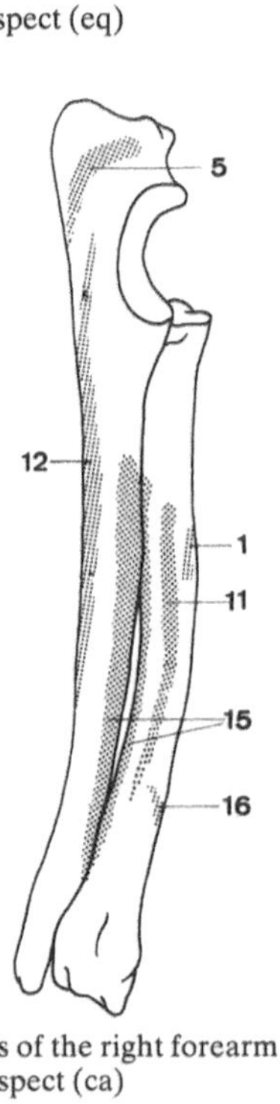

D Bones of the right forearm, medial aspect (ca)

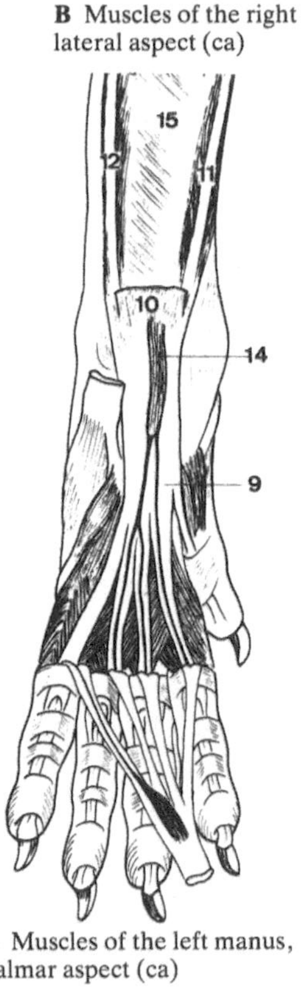

E Muscles of the left manus, palmar aspect (ca)

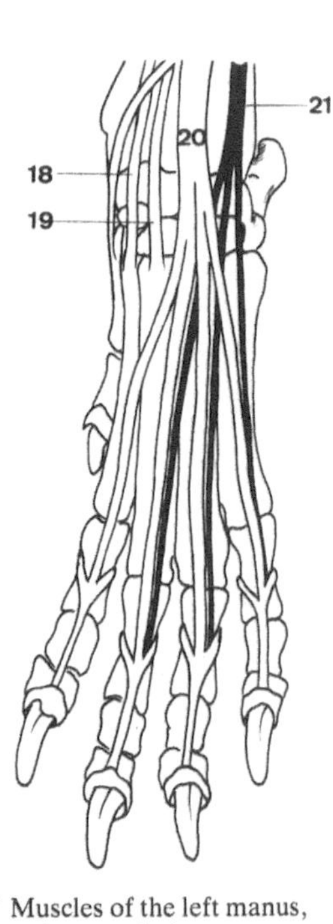

F Muscles of the left manus, dorsal aspect (ca)

1 ***M. supinator***. Deep to carpal and digital extensors. From Epicondylus lateralis humeri to proximal fourth of radius. Supinates antebrachium. Present in Car, rudimentary in su. A F

2 ***M. abductor digiti I [pollicis] longus [M. extensor carpi obliquus]***. From radius (Un) or radius and ulna (Car) obliquely to basis of metacarpal I (Car), II (su, eq), III (Ru). Abducts digit I (Car), extends digit I (Car) and carpus. E F

3 ***M. extensor digiti I [pollicis]***. Present in Car, it is combined with M. extensor digiti II. From middle of ulna between digital extensors to distal end of metacarpal I. E F

4 ***M. extensor digiti II***. Combined with preceding, tendon to common digital extensor tendon of digit II. E F

5 ***M. flexor digitorum brevis***. Small muscle on deep surface of M. flexor digitorum superficialis in Car. Tendons end on digit V (ca), digits III–V (fe). C

6 ***M. abductor digiti I [pollicis] brevis***. Small slip from Retinaculum flexorum to proximal sesamoids or proximal phalanx of digit I in Car. B C

7 ***M. flexor digiti I [pollicis] brevis***. Lateral to preceding muscle in Car. From Retinaculum flexorum to proximal phalanx of digit I. B C

8 ***M. adductor digiti I [pollicis]***. Lateral muscle of digit I in Car. B C

9 ***M. abductor digiti II***. Small muscle of su from Retinaculum flexorum to abaxial side of proximal phalanx of digit II. D

10 ***M. flexor digiti II***. Lateral to preceding in su. D

11 ***M. adductor digiti II***. From Retinaculum flexorum between M. interosseus II and M. adductor digiti V in Car and su. Inserts on proximal phalanx of digit II. B D

12 ***M. abductor digiti V***. From Os carpi accessorium to abaxial side of proximal phalanx of digit V in Car and su. B C D

13 ***M. flexor digiti V***. Small bundle of fibers medial to preceding with which it inserts in Car and su. B C D

14 ***M. adductor digiti V***. From Retinaculum flexorum. Descends medial to M. interosseus IV to axial side of proximal phalanx of digit V in Car and su. B D

15 ***Mm. lumbricales***. Muscle fibers between tendons of M. flexor digitorum profundus which run obliquely laterally to insert on proximal phalanges of digits II–V (fe), III–V (ca). Best developed in Car in which they insert on the proximal phalanges, absent in su and Ru, rudimentary in eq in which they insert on the palmar annular ligament. Flex metacarpophalangeal joints. C

16 ***Mm. interossei****. On palmar surface of metacarpal bones except I. Fibers of each divide distally to attach to proximal sesamoids and go on each side of metacarpophalangeal joints to join common extensor tendon. Tendinous in eq and Ru. Support metacarpophalangeal joints. The M. interosseous medius in eq is also called suspensory ligament and is part of the passive (stay) apparatus. There is only one interosseous muscle (III) in eq, two fused interossei muscles (III and IV) in Ru. B D

17 ***Fascia axillaris lateralis***. Covers lateral muscles of shoulder.

17a ***Fascia axillaris medialis***. Covers medial muscles of shoulder.

18 ***Fascia brachii***. Investment of muscles of arm with intermuscular septa. G

18a *Lamina superficialis.*

18b *Lamina profunda.*

19 ***Fascia antebrachii***. Investment of muscles of antebrachium. H

19a *Lamina superficialis.*

19b *Lamina profunda.*

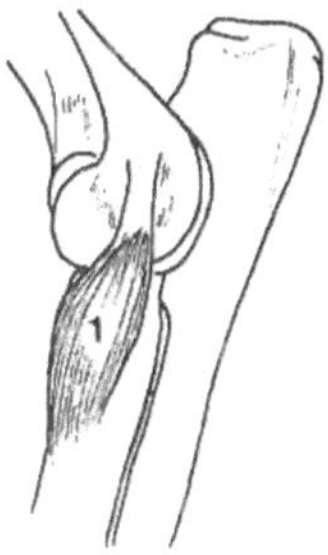

A Left M. supinator, lateral aspect (ca)

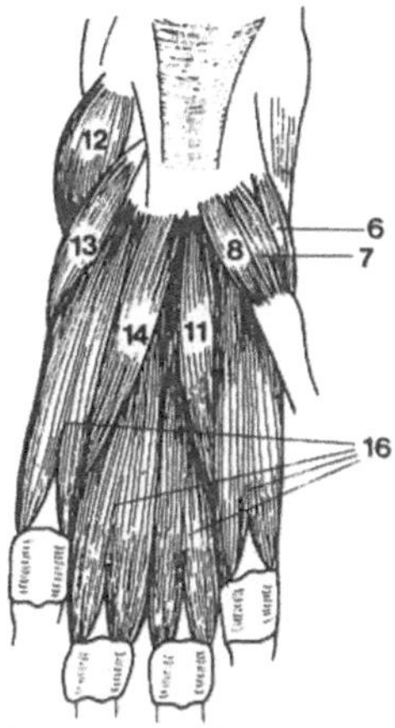

B Muscles of the left manus, palmar aspect (ca)

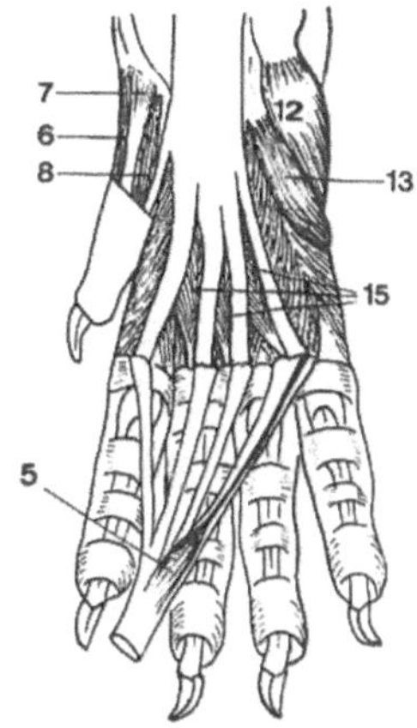

C Muscles and tendons of the right manus, palmar aspect (ca)

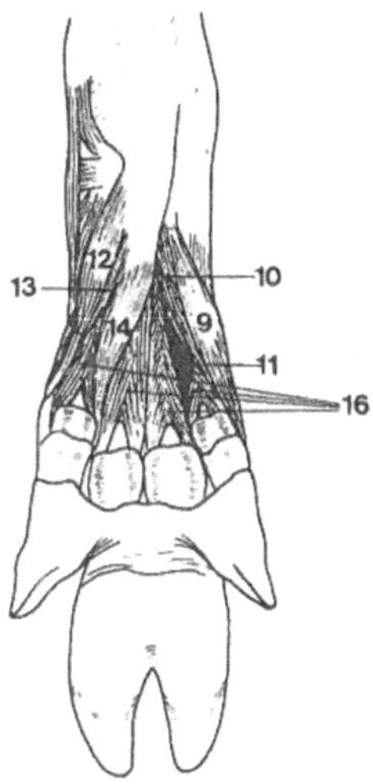

D Muscles of the left manus, palmar aspect (su)

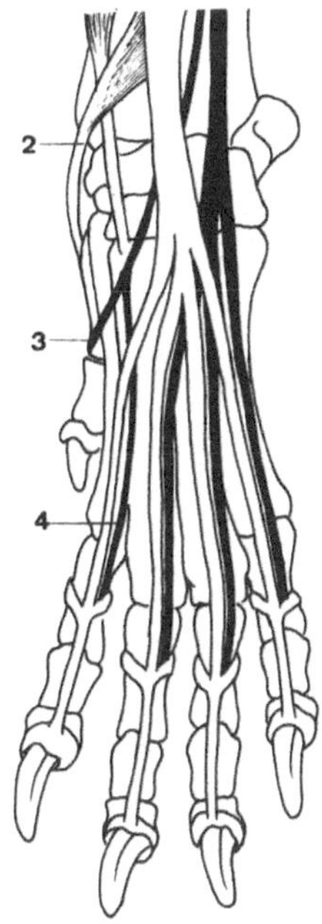

E Tendons of the left manus, dorsal aspect (ca)

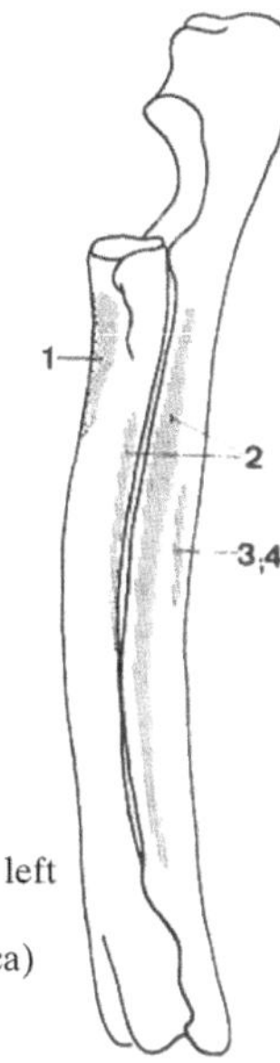

F Bones of the left forearm, lateral aspect (ca)

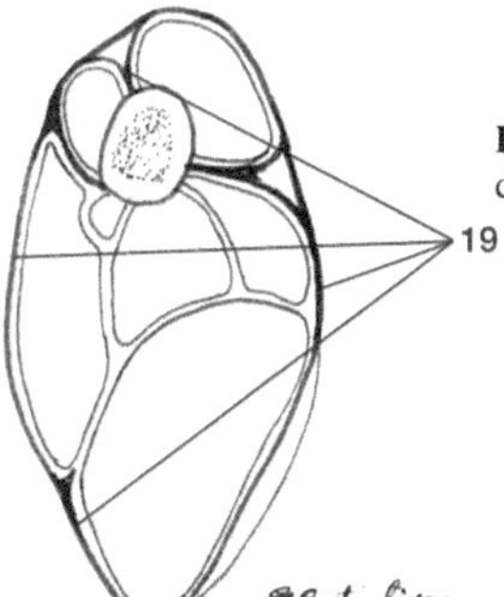

G Right arm, transverse section, proximal surface (ca) (modified and redrawn from R. Barone)

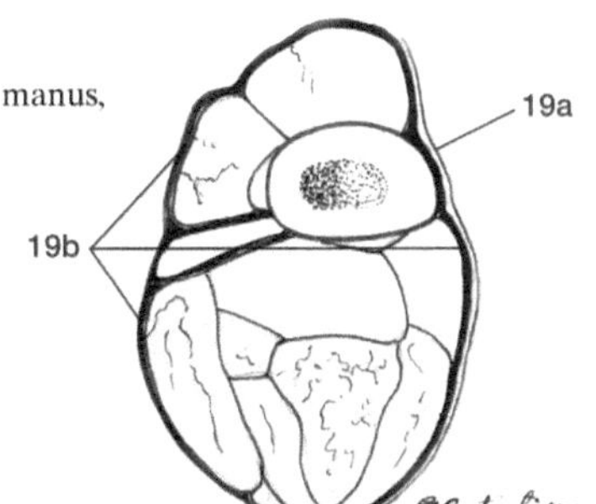

H Left forearm, transverse section, proximal surface (eq)

1 ***Fascia dorsalis manus.*** Retains and invests dorsal tendons of manus. D

2 *Retinaculum extensorum.* Fascial bands stretching transversely across dorsal surface of carpus retaining extensor tendons. A

3 ***Fascia palmaris manus****. Retains and invests palmar structures of manus. D

4 *Retinaculum flexorum.* Especially thick transverse fascial bands from medial carpal bones to Os carpi accessorium forming Canalis carpi. Double in Ru and eq resulting in two carpal canals: superficial and deep (proper). B

5 ***Canalis carpi.*** Canal between the proximal row of carpal bones and Retinaculum flexorum. See above and 86.7

6 ***Fascia digiti****. Superficial and deep layer, the latter forms anular ligaments. C E

7 ***Lig. metacarpeum transversum superficiale [Lig. annulare palmare]*** *. Thickening of fascia of metacarpophalangeal area on palmar surface, transversely oriented. Consists of superficial and deep part in Ru and eq. It is usually called palmar annular ligament by anatomists and clinicians. C E F

8 ***Vaginae fibrosae digitorum manus.*** Transverse and crossed fibers of digital fascia on palmar side. C

9 *Pars annularis vaginae fibrosae [Lig. annulare digiti].* Strong part with transverse fibers. There is a proximal (9) and a distal (9a) annular ligament. The proximal ligament has in eq proximal and distal symmetrical attachments on Phalanx proximalis and is not separated from the palmar annular ligament. C E

10 *Pars cruciformis vaginae fibrosae.* Thin part with crossed fibers. However in eq the proximal Pars cruciformis is strong and forms with the two symmetrical attachments of the proximal digital annular ligament a quadrilateral sheet. The distal Pars cruciformis forms with the two symmetrical attachments of the distal digital annular ligament a crescenting fibrous sheet in eq. C E

11 ***Scutum proximale.*** Fibrocartilaginous palmar surface of Lig. palmare, providing gliding surface for the digital flexor tendons. F

12 ***Scutum medium.*** Fibrocartilaginous plate that covers the palmar surface of the proximal part of Phalanx media, and also extends proximal to it, providing gliding surface for deep digital flexor tendons. The superficial digital flexor tendons attach to it. There are several Vincula tendinum at fetlock in bo and eq between the common tendon sheath, and manica flexoria dorsally. F

13 ***Scutum distale.*** Fibrocartilaginous plate that covers the palmar surface of Os sesamoideum distale. It also extends proximal to the bone attaching to the palmar surface of the middle phalanx, and laterally intermingles with the navicular collateral ligaments. The distal scutum provides gliding surface for each deep digital flexor tendon. F

14 ***Vaginae synoviales tendinum digitorum manus.*** Digital synovial tendon sheath around superficial and deep digital flexor tendons of each digit from distal portion of metacarpus to middle of Phalanx media. See 134.17

15 *Vincula tendinum.* Supporting vascular fibers from deep digital flexor tendon to the middle of Lig. sesamoideum rectum in eq. A vinculum tendinis was also found in the digital synovial tendon sheath of the pelvic limb in bo. F

16 **MUSCULI MEMBRI PELVINI.** Muscles of pelvic limb.

17 ***M. iliopsoas.*** Muscle composed of M. psoas major and M. iliacus, caudal attachment on Trochanter minor. Flexes and supinates hip joint. G

18 ***M. iliacus.*** From Trochanter minor to Facies iliaca (the long part) and Corpus ossis ilii (the short part). Grooved ventrally for M. psoas major. G

19 *M. psoas major*[1]. From Trochanter minor to ventral surface of lumbar vertebral bodies and transverse processes, reaching also the last two thoracic vertebrae and ribs. Increases on size cranially. G

20 ***M. psoas minor***[1]. On ventromedial surface of M. psoas major. Fleshy attachments to lumbar and 3–4 caudal thoracic vertebral bodies. Long tendon of attachment on Tuberculum m. psoas minoris of ilium (Linea arcuata in ca). G

[1] Both muscles act as flexors of the thigh, flexors of the vertebral column, and in rearing, as muscles with reversible action, which exchange the origin with the insertion; reason that “attachments” is a proper term for both “origin” and “insertion”.

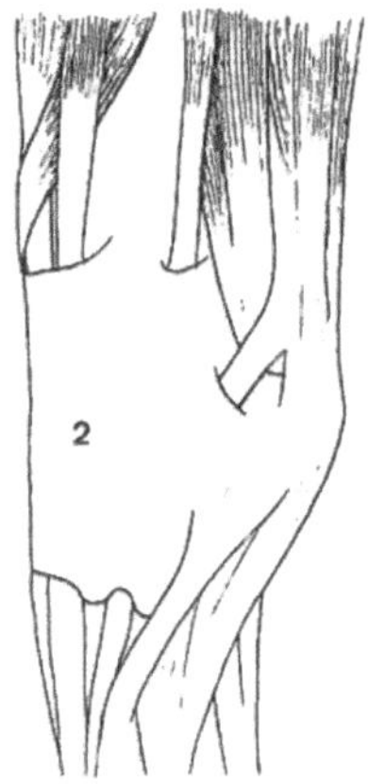

A Left Retinaculum extensorum, dorsolateral aspect (eq)

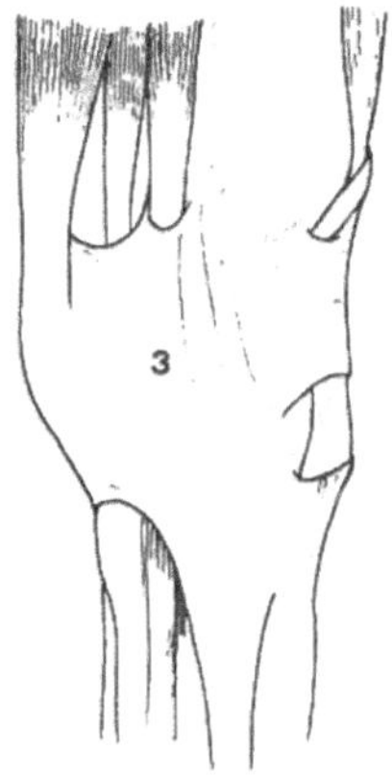

B Left Retinaculum flexorum, medial aspect (eq)

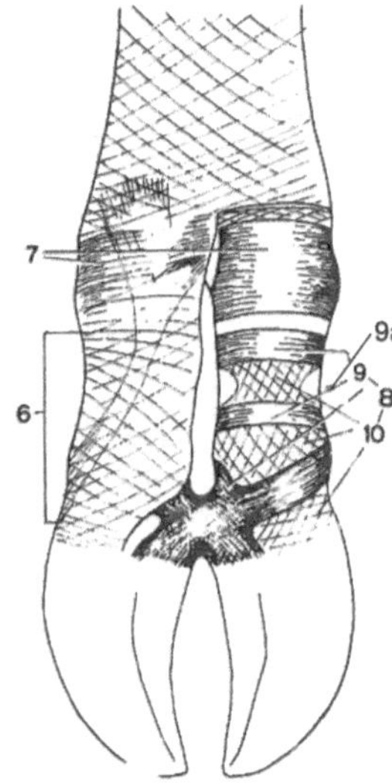

C Fasciae of the digits, palmar aspect (bo)

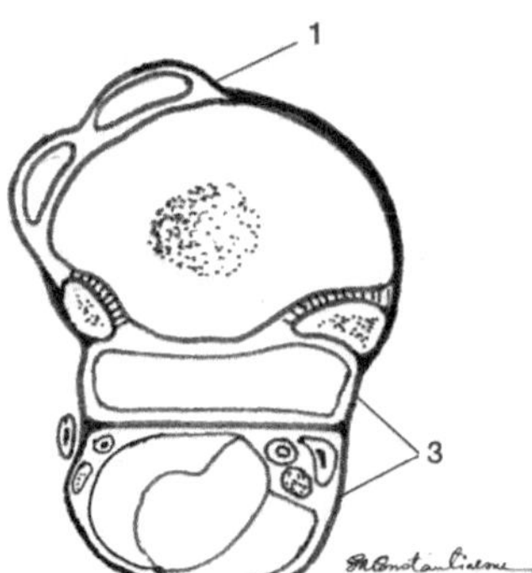

D Left metacarpus, transverse section, proximal surface (eq)

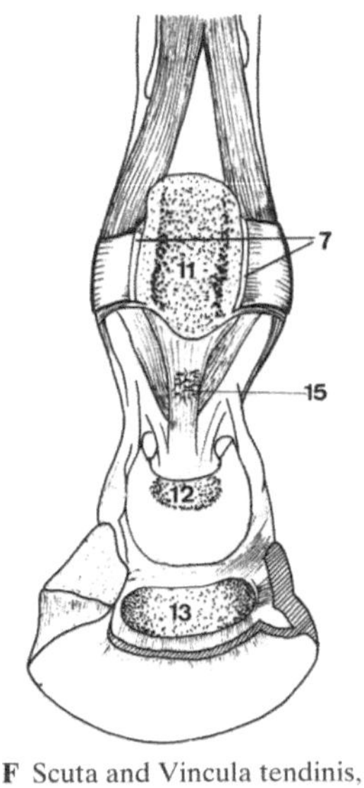

F Scuta and Vincula tendinis, palmar aspect (eq)

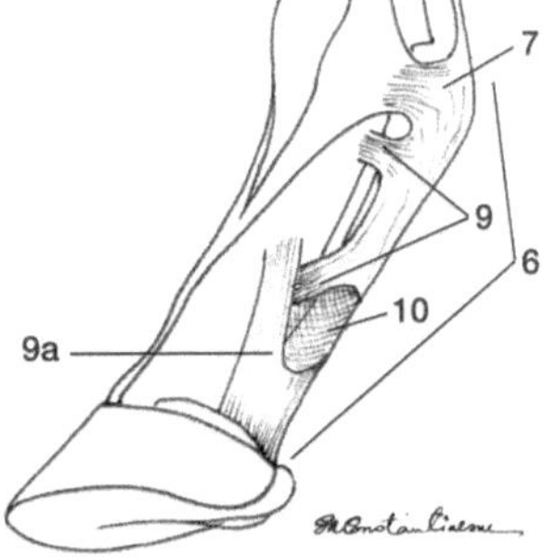

E Fascia of the digit, palmar aspect (eq)

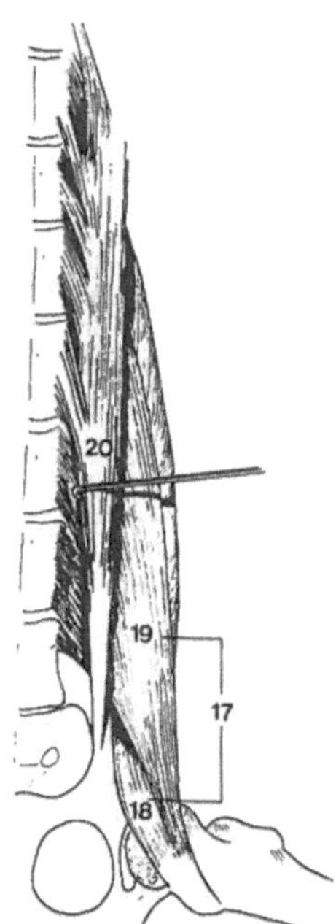

G Left Mm. iliopsoas and psoas minor, ventral aspect (ca)

1 ***M. gluteus [glutaeus] superficialis.*** On caudal surface of M. gluteus medius. From Fascia glutea and Os sacrum to Tuberositas glutea (Car) or Trochanter tertius (eq). Incorporated with M. gluteobiceps in su and Ru. Has cranial head originating with M. tensor fasciae latae in eq. Extends hip joint in Car, flexes in eq. A F G

2 ***M. gluteofemoralis [glutaeo-].*** Caudal to M. gluteus superficialis in fe. From first few caudal vertebrae to superficial layer of fascia lata. It was formerly called M. caudofemoralis or M. abductor cruris cranialis. Extends and abducts hip joint. A

3 ***M. gluteobiceps [glutaeobiceps].*** Fusion of M. gluteus superficialis and cranial portion of M. biceps femoris in su and Ru. Extends hip joint. B

4 ***M. gluteus [glutaeus] medius.*** Large muscle of hip. Cranial attachment on Facies glutea of ilium and in Un M. longissimus. Caudal attachment on Trochanter major. Extends hip jointand acts in propulsion. In eq it acts also and rearing. A B E F G (see foot note on page 122)

5 *M. gluteus [glutaeus] accessorius*. Deep portion of M. gluteus medius in Un. D (Barone mentioned this muscle in Car, as it is intimately fused with the M. gluteus medius, but their tendons attached to the Trochanter majus are easily separable, and also part of their muscular components [1999, p. 861].)

6 ***M. gluteus [glutaeus] profundus.*** Deep gluteal muscle. Attaches to shaft of ilium and Spina ischiadica. Terminates on cranial portion of Trochanter major in Car, su and eq, distal to it in Ru. Abducts hip joint. C D E G

7 ***M. tensor fasciae latae****. Fan-shaped muscle from Tuber coxae to Fascia lata. Flexes hip joint and tenses Fascia lata. A B

8 ***M. piriformis.*** Deep to caudal portion of M. gluteus medius in Car. From Os sacrum and Lig. sacrotuberale (ca) to Trochanter major. In Un it is part of M. gluteus medius (incompletelly separable from each other) and inserts on Crista intertrochanterica. Easy to identify by their different direction of fibers and attachments (M. piriformis attaches to Crista intertrochanterica). Extends hip joint. C

9 ***M. obturatorius internus.*** From internal surface of ischium, pubis and in eq shaft of ilium. Tendon over Incisura ischiadica minor to Fossa trochanterica. The term should be used to refer only to the muscle in Car and eq, innervated by a branch of N. ischiadicus. Supinates hip joint. C F

10 ***Mm. gemelli.*** Twin muscles from lateral border of ischium to Fossa trochanterica. Supinate hip joint. C E F

11 ***M. quadratus femoris.*** From ventral surface of ischium, inserts distal to Fossa trochanterica, Supinates hip joint. C F

12 ***M. sartorius.*** From Fascia iliaca (Un) and Corpus ossis ilii (su) or Tuber coxae (Car) to medial side of proximal portion of tibia by Fascia cruris. Flexes hip joint, adductor in Un. A E

13 *Pars cranialis* (ca). C

14 *Pars caudalis* (ca). C

15 ***M. articularis coxae*** (Car, eq). Small muscle deep to M. rectus femoris across hip joint. D E G

16 ***M. quadriceps femoris.*** Large group cranial in thigh. Four heads converge upon patella and terminate by means of patellar ligaments onto Tuberositas tibiae. Extends stifle joint. C D

17 *M. rectus femoris*. Arises from areas cranial to acetabulum. Also flexes hip joint. C D E

18 *M. vastus lateralis*. Arises from proximal portion of craniolateral surface of Os femoris, from Trochanter major in Ru. C D F G

19 *M. vastus intermedius*. Arises from cranial surface of Os femoris. D G

20 *M. vastus medialis*. Arises along medial surface of Os femoris. D F G

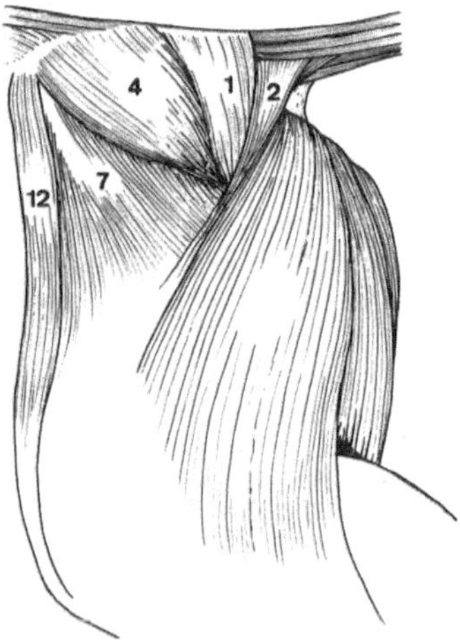

A Muscles of the left hip and thigh, lateral aspect (fe)

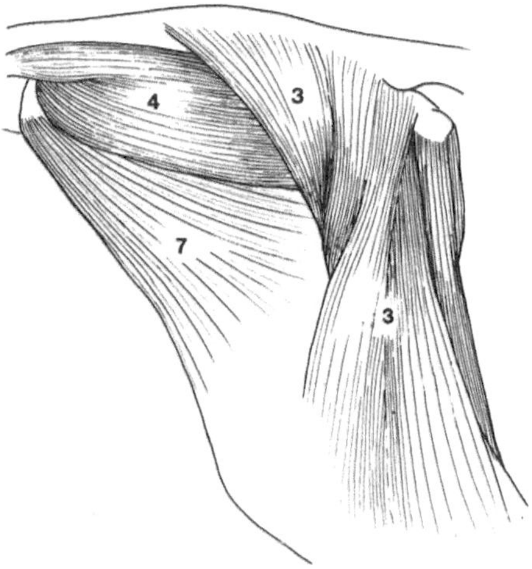

B Muscles of the left hip and thigh, lateral aspect (cap)

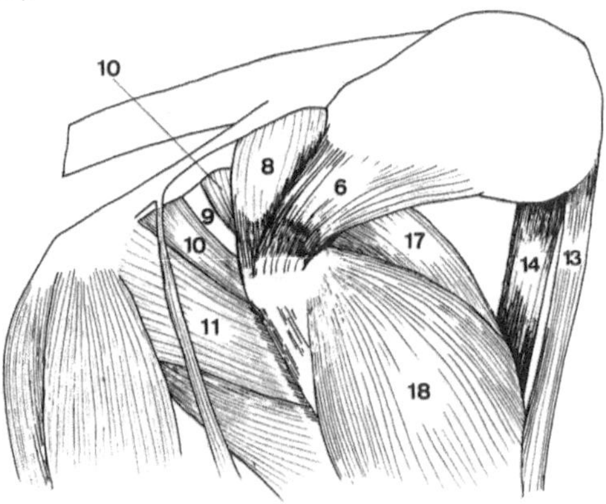

C Deep muscles of the right hip and thigh, lateral aspect (ca)

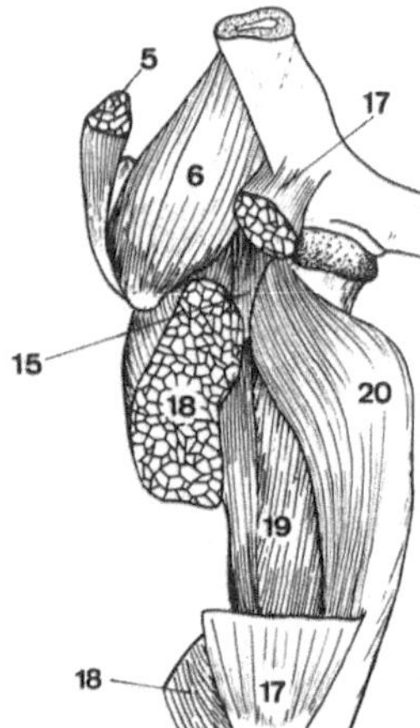

D Deep muscles of the right hip and thigh, cranial aspect (eq)

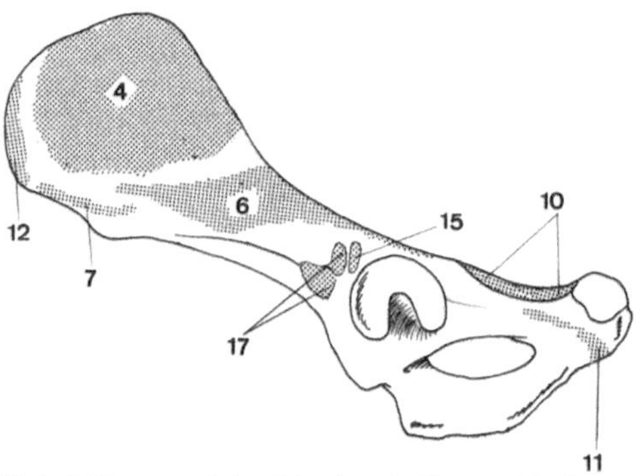

E Left Os coxae, lateral (and ventral), aspect (ca)

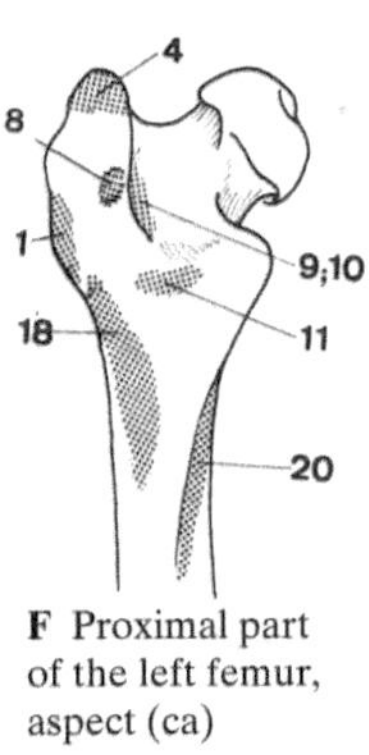

F Proximal part of the left femur, aspect (ca)

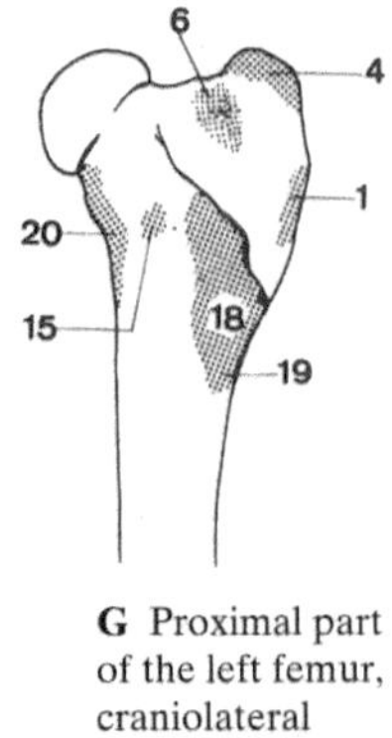

G Proximal part of the left femur, craniolateral aspect (ca)

1 ***M. articularis genus*** (Car, bo). Small muscle deep to termination of M. quadriceps femoris. Tenses stifle joint capsule. B

2 ***M. pectineus***. From contra- and ipsilateral Pecten ossis pubis and Eminentia iliopubica to Labium mediale of Facies aspera ossis femoris. C

3 ***M. gracilis***. Flat superficial adductor of thigh. From Symphysis pelvina by Tendo symphysialis to Fascia cruris on medial surface of proximal portion of the crus. C

4 *Tendo symphysialis*. Median tendon of origin of Mm. graciles and Mm. adductores. C

5 ***M. adductor***. Undivided as in su, Ru, or consists of as many as three portions. B E

6 *M. adductor longus*. Small fusiform muscle of fe which arises from pubis to terminate on Labium mediale of Facies aspera ossis femoris. In other species part of M. pectineus. E

7 *M. adductor brevis*. Usually (except fe, eq and often ca) united with magnus. Represents proximal portion. B

8 *M. adductor magnus*. Usually (except fe, eq and often ca) united with brevis. From Tendo symphysialis, Ramus caudalis ossis pubis, and Ramus ossis ischii to Facies aspera, in eq also Condylus medialis femoris. B

9 ***M. obturatorius externus***. From ventral surface of pelvis. Tendon courses laterally to terminate in Fossa trochanterica. E

10 *Pars intrapelvina*. Arises from dorsal surface of floor of pelvis in Artiodactyla. Passes through Foramen obturatum to join main portion of M. obturatorius externus. C

11 ***M. biceps femoris****. Arises by two heads from Os sacrum (eq), Ligamentum sacrotuberale latum, Tuber ischiadicum. Fused with M. gluteus superficialis in su and Ru. Attachments spread out lateral to Fascia lata, Fascia cruris, and Tendo calcaneus communis. Extends hip joint and flexes stifle joint in free limb, extends hip, stifle, and tarsal joints when bearing weight, acting therefore in propulsion. In eq it acts also in rearing[1)]. A

12 ***M. abductor cruris caudalis*** (Car). Long, narrow, and thin strap-like muscle deep to M. biceps femoris. Theoretically abducts limb. B

13 ***M. semitendinosus****. Arises from Tuber ischiadicum, descends over M. gastrocnemius to attach on medial surface of proximal portion of tibia and Tendo calcaneus communis. Has cranial attachment from Lig. sacrotuberale latum in su and eq. Extends hip and flexes stifle joint in free limb, extends hip, stifle, and tarsal joints when bearing weight, acting therefore in propulsion. In eq it acts also in rearing[1)]. A B C

14 ***M. semimembranosus****. From Tuber ischiadicum, cranial attachment from Lig. sacrotuberale latum in eq. Distal attachments on medial condyles of femur and tibia (except su and eq). Is divided longitudinally in Car, su, and Ru. Extends and adducts hip joint and the stifle joint acting also in propulsion except su, eq. In eq acts also in rearing[1)]. A B C

15 ***M. tibialis cranialis***. From Facies lateralis tibiae. Terminates medially on tarsal and metatarsal bones. Flexes tarsal joint. D F G

16 ***M. extensor digitorum [digitalis] longus***[2)]*. From Fossa extensoria femoris. Tendon splits to terminate on Phalanx distalis of each digit. Has a medial portion with an independent tendon to digit III in Ru (attached also on Phalanx proximalis and Phalanx media), II and III in su. Flexes tarsal, extends stifle and phalangeal joints. D F G

17 ***M. fibularis [peroneus, peronaeus] tertius***. Tendinous in eq, well developed in Artiodactyla and little in Car. From Fossa extensoria to terminate on proximal part of metatarsus. Extends stifle and flexes tarsal joints. Part of reciprocal and stay apparatus in eq. G

18 ***M. extensor digiti I [hallucis] longus*** (Car, su, ov). Delicate muscle from fibula to mediodistal portion of metatarsus. Weak flexor of tarsal joint. F

19 ***M. fibularis [peroneus, peronaeus] longus***. Arises from Condylus lateralis tibiae and Caput fibulae. Tendon passes over lateral surface of tarsus to terminate on plantar side of medial tarsal or metatarsal bones. Absent in eq. Flexes tarsal joints, pronator in Car. D

20 ***M. extensor digitorum [digitalis] lateralis***[2)]*. Arises from proximal portion of fibula, in Ru of tibia. Terminates by uniting with long extensor tendon in eq, of digit V in Car, inserts independentlyon digits IV and V in su, IV in Ru attached on all three phalanges. Extends phalangeal joints of corresponding digitis. D G

21 ***M. fibularis [peroneus, peronaeus] brevis***. Terminates on Basis ossis metatarsalis V in Car. Weak flexor of tarsal joint. D

1) see foot note on page 122

2) In eq both flexors of the digit should be called "digitalis", because the horse is monodactyle.

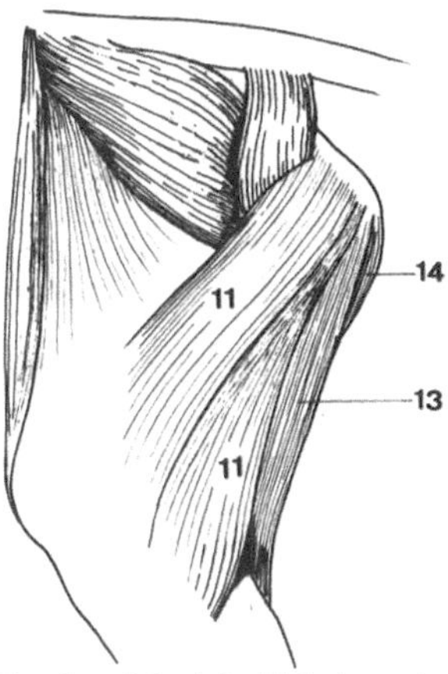

A Muscles of the left thigh, lateral aspect (ca)

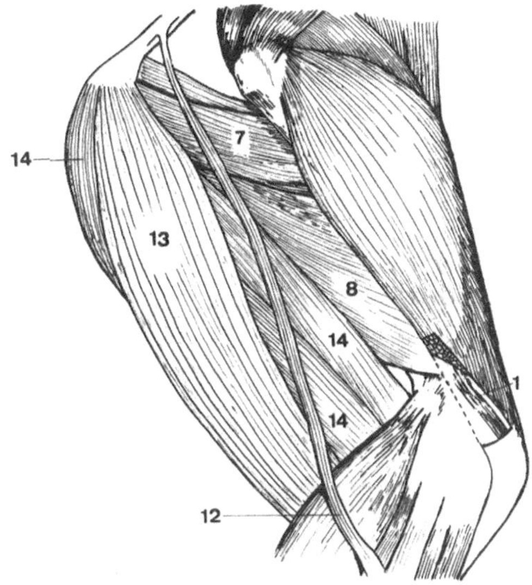

B Muscles of the right thigh, lateral aspect (ca)

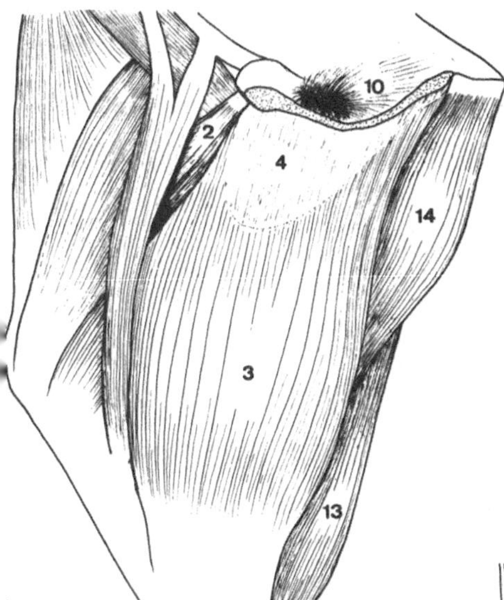

C Muscles of the right thigh, medial aspect (bo)

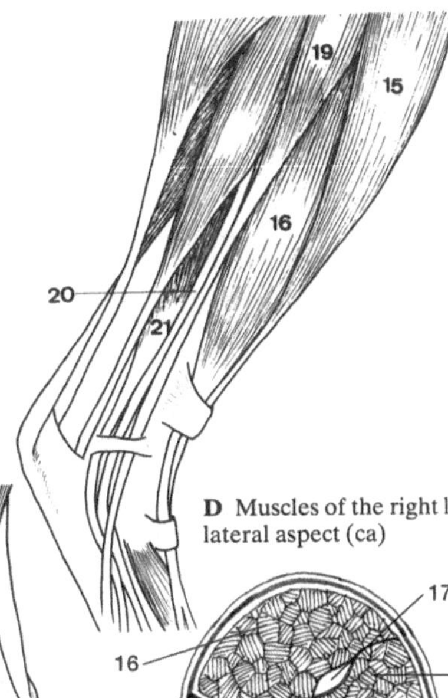

D Muscles of the right leg, lateral aspect (ca)

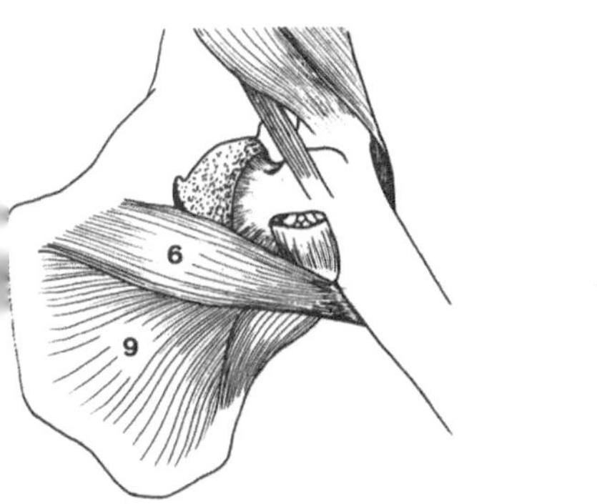

E Left M. adductor longus and M. obturatorius externus, medioventral aspect (fe)

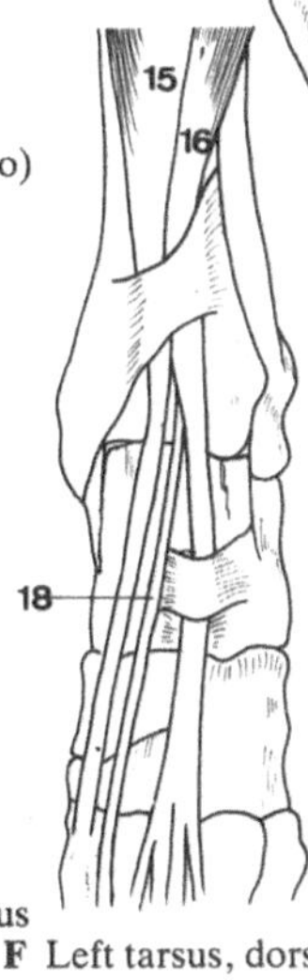

F Left tarsus, dorsal aspect (ca)

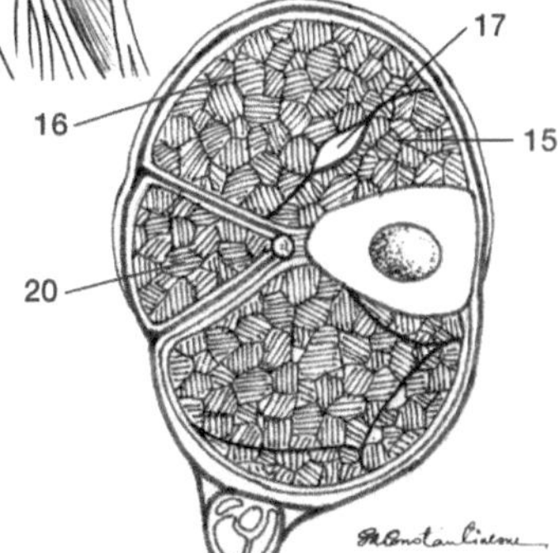

G Left leg, transverse section, proximal surface (eq)

1 ***M. triceps surae***. Two heads of M. gastrocnemius and M. soleus. Flexes stifle and extends tarsal joints. (There is no M. soleus in ca).

2 *M. gastrocnemius*. Consists of two heads, terminates by long tendon on Tuber calcanei. A B

3 **Caput laterale**. From Tuberositas supracondylaris lateralis femoris. B

4 **Caput mediale**. From Tuberositas supracondylaris medialis femoris. A

5 *M. soleus*. From fibula (lateral tibial condyle in Ru) to join tendon of Caput laterale m. gastrocnemii. Not present in ca. B

6 ***Tendo calcaneus communis****. Combined tendons of Mm. triceps surae, flexor digitorum/digitalis superficialis, biceps femoris, and semitendinosus, bound intimately and surrounded by Lamina propria fasciae cruris. Attaches to Tuber calcanei. B

7 ***M. flexor digitorum [digitalis] superficialis****. Arises from Fossa supracondylaris femoris. Tendon winds the tendon of M. gastrocnemius in a mediocaudal direction and attaches to Tuber calcanei in its way to the digit(s). Descends to digits and inserts on middle scutum. Mostly tendinous in eq. Flexes stifle and phalangeal joints, extends tarsal joints. Part of reciprocal and stay apparatus in eq. A B D F

8 *Manica flexoria*. The sleeve formed by each tendon of M. flexor digit. superficialis around the corresponding tendon of M. flexor digit. profundus at the level of Articulatio metatarsophalangea. In Ru the sleeve is formed for each digit by the tendon of M. flexor digit. superficialis and the corresponding tendon of the interosseous muscle. B

9 ***M. popliteus***. Triangular muscle arising by tendon from Fossa poplitea. Terminates on Facies caudalis tibiae as far as Linea poplitea. Flexes and pronates stifle joint. A C

10 ***Mm. flexores digitorum [digitales] profundi***. The tendons of Mm. flexores digit. lateralis and medialis (in Un also M. tibialis caudalis) unite to deep flexor tendon. This divides to terminate on flexor surface of each distal phalanx. Extend tarsal and flex phalangeal joints. A

11 *M. flexor digitorum [digitalis] lateralis*. Main portion of deep flexors. Originates caudal on tibia and except Ru, fibula. Descends over Sustentaculum tali. A B C

12 *M. flexor digitorum [digitalis] medialis*. Arises between M. flexor digit. lateralis and M. popliteus. Long tendon joins deep flexor tendon distal to tarsus. A C

13 *M. tibialis caudalis*. Small head of deep digital flexor except Car. In Car the tendon of this muscle has an independent termination on the medial surface of the tarsus and does not contribute to the formation of the (common) deep digital flexor tendon. A C

14 *Tendo communis*. Common tendon of Mm. flexores digit. profundi. A B D F

15 *Lig. accessorium*. Fibrous continuation of plantar tarsal ligament to deep digital flexor tendon in eq. Part of passive, suspensory or stay apparatus of the pelvic limb. B (Formerly termed Caput tendineum of the deep digital flexor tendon, it is still called "distal check ligament", the alternative of the accessory ligament of the deep digital flexor muscle.)

16 ***Mm. interflexorii***. 2 (ca) or 3 (fe) bundles from plantar surface of deep digital flexor tendon to superficial digital flexor tendons. D

17 ***M. extensor digitorum [digitalis] brevis****. From tarsus to tendons of M. extensor digit. longus (in eq also lateralis). B

18 ***M. abductor digiti I [hallucis]***. Lies medial on plantar surface of metatarsus if digit I is present in ca. E

19 ***M. flexor digiti I [hallucis] brevis***. Middle muscle on plantar surface of metatarsus if digit I is present in ca. E

20 ***M. adductor digiti I [hallucis]*** . Medial muscle on plantar surface of metatarsus if digit I is present in ca. E

21 ***M. abductor digiti II***. Small muscle in su from plantar surface of tarsus to proximal phalanx of digit II. F

22 ***M. adductor digiti II***. From plantar tarsal ligaments to axial side of proximal phalanx of digit II in Car and su. E F

23 ***M. abductor digiti V***. From lateral part of tarsus to proximal phalanx of digit V in su. F

24 ***M. adductor digiti V***. From plantar tarsal ligaments to axial side of proximal phalanx of digit V in Car and su. E F

25 ***M. flexor digitorum [digitalis] brevis***. From deep surface of superficial digital flexor tendon to area of metatarsophalangeal joints, esp. in fe. D

26 ***M. quadratus plantae [M. flexor accessorius]***. From calcaneus to deep digital flexor tendon in ca. D

27 ***Mm. lumbricales***. From tendons of M. flexor digitorum profundus to proximal phalanges of digits III, IV, V in Car. Rudimentary in eq. D

28 ***Mm. interossei***. On plantar surface of Ossa metatarsalia to proximal sesamoids. The M. interosseous medius in eq is also called suspensory ligament and is part of the passive (stay) apparatus. There is only one interosseous muscle (III) in eq, two interossei muscles fused (III and IV) in Ru. See 120.16 D

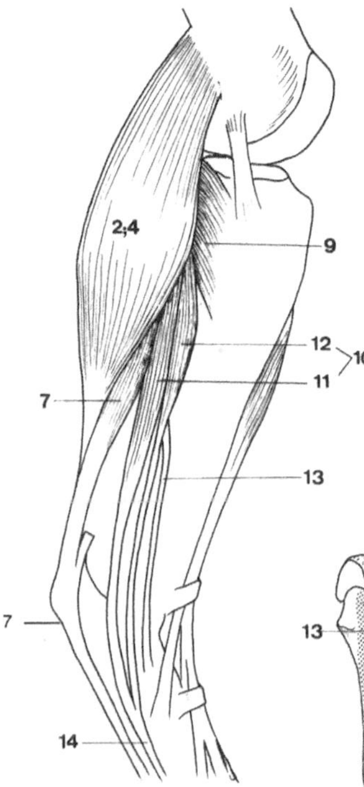

A Muscles of the left leg, medial aspect (ca)

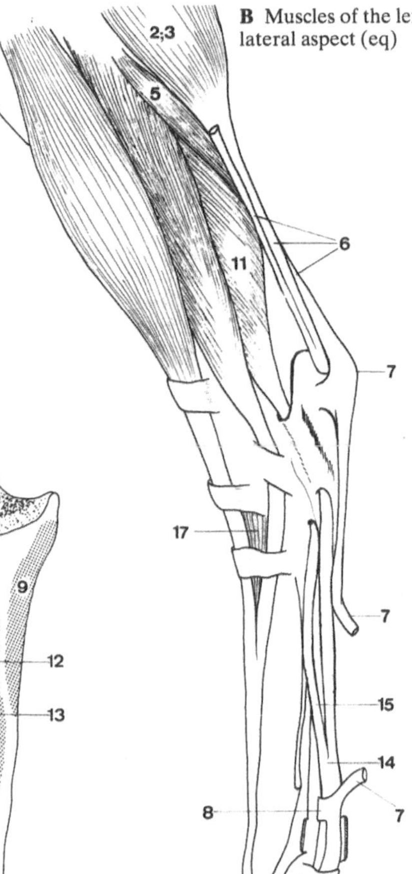

B Muscles of the left leg, lateral aspect (eq)

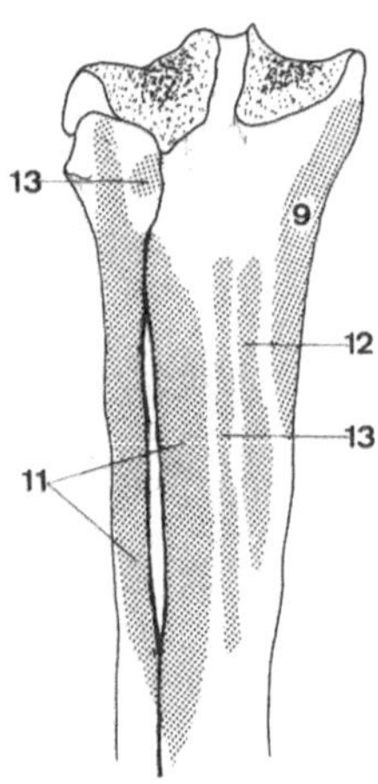

C Bones of the left leg, caudal aspect (ca)

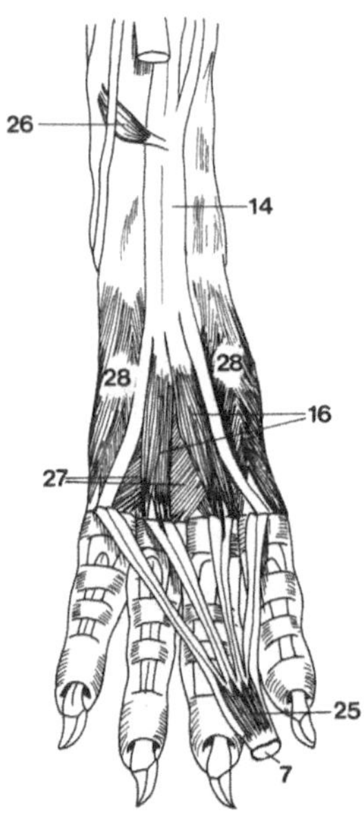

D Left plantar muscles, plantar aspect (ca)

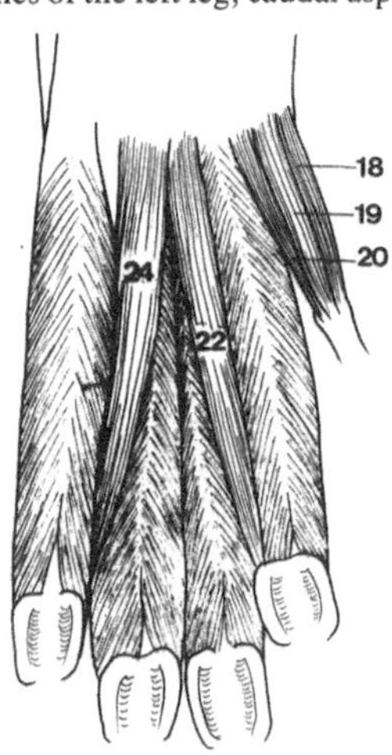

E Left plantar muscles, plantar aspect (ca)

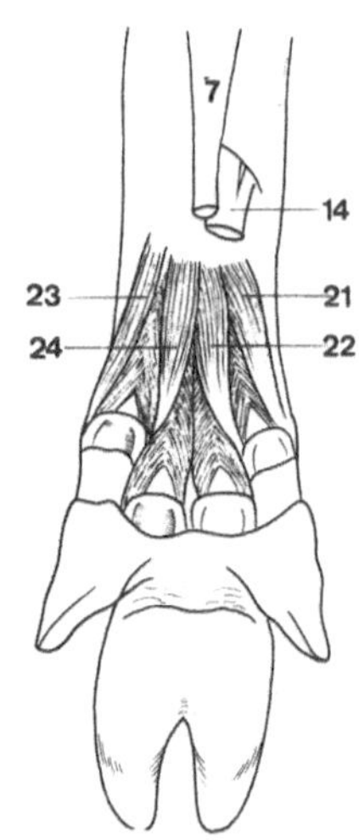

F Left plantar muscles, plantar aspect (su)

1 ***Fascia glutea [glutaea].*** Thick deep fascia, continuation of Fascia thoracolumbalis over M. gluteus medius. Gluteal muscles partially arise from it. A

2 ***Fascia lata.*** Continuous with Fascia glutea over lateral surface of thigh and over the crus with different names. Insertion of M. tensor fasciae latae. A

2a *Lamina superficialis.* Covers intimately the caudolateral muscles of the thigh and becomes the superficial lamina of crural fascia.

2b *Lamina profunda.* Insinuates under the caudolateral muscles of the thigh and becomes the deep lamina of crural fascia.

3 ***Fascia iliaca.*** Associated with iliac and psoas muscles. Dorsal continuation of Fascia transversalis. B

4 ***Lacuna musculorum.*** Compartment for passage of Mm. iliopsoas and sartorius between Os ilium and Arcus inguinalis. B

5 ***Lacuna vasorum.*** Space between Arcus inguinalis and Os ilium for passage of femoral vessels. Caudomedial to Lacuna musculorum. B

6 *Anulus femoralis.* Ring of entrance of vessels from abdominal cavity into Canalis femoralis at Arcus inguinalis. B

7 *Septum femorale.* Connective tissue across entrance into Canalis femoralis. Part of Lamina femoralis. B

8 ***Trigonum femorale.*** Triangle between M. sartorius cranially and M. pectineus caudally, M. iliopsoas deep, and Lamina femoralis superficially, for passage of vessels. B

9 ***Canalis femoralis.*** Canal in medial area of femur containing femoral vessels, and deep inguinal lymph nodes in eq. B

10 ***Fascia cruris.*** Fascia of leg. Gives attachment to muscles of thigh, binds down muscles of leg sending intermuscular septa. C

10a *Lamina superficialis.* Surrounds the cranial muscles of the crus.

10b *Lamina profunda.* Surrounds the deep muscles of the caudal crus.

10c *Lamina propria.* Surrounds the entire crus and forms the retinacula.

11 ***Retinaculum extensorum crurale.*** Transverse reinforcement of Lamina propria fasciae cruris binding down M. extensor digit. longus, M. tibialis cranialis, and M. fibularis tertius. D E F

12 ***Retinaculum extensorum tarsale.*** Tarsal retaining band from the same fascia as above, binding down M. extensor digitorum longus, absent in Ru. D E F

13 ***Retinaculum extensorum metatarsale.*** Metatarsal retaining band from the same fascia as above in Ru and eq, binding down long and lateral digital extensor tendons, and M. extensor digitorum/digitalis brevis. D

14 ***Retinaculum mm. fibularium [peronei].*** Retaining band binding down Mm. fibularis and extensor digitorum lateralis at tarsus in Car. E

15 ***Retinaculum flexorum.*** Plantar retaining band binding down Mm. flexores digit. profundi at tarsus. F

16 ***Fascia dorsalis pedis.*** Retains and invests dorsal tendons of pes. G

17 ***Fascia plantaris****. Retains and invests plantar structures of pes. G

18 ***Fascia digiti****. See 122.6

19 ***Lig. metatarseum transversum superficiale [Lig. annulare plantare]*** *. See 122. 7

20 ***Vaginae fibrosae digitorum pedis.*** See 122.8

21 *Pars annularis vaginae fibrosae [Lig. annulare digiti].* See 122.9

22 ***Pars cruciformis vaginae fibrosae.*** See 122.10

23 ***Scutum proximale.*** See 122.11

24 ***Scutum medium.*** See 122.12

25 ***Scutum distale.*** See 122.13

26 ***Vaginae synoviales tendinum digitorum pedis.*** See 122.14

27 *Vincula tendinum.* See 122.15

A Fasciae of the left hip and thigh (bo)

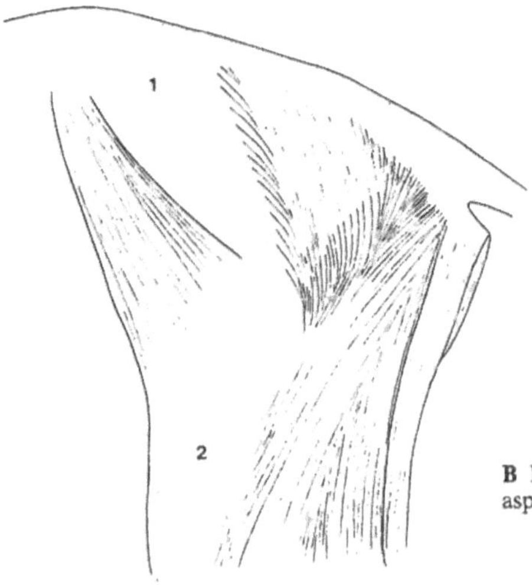

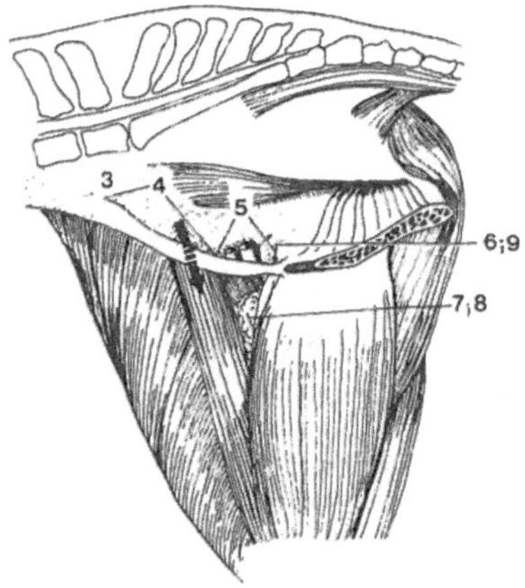

B Pelvis (median section) and right thigh, medial aspect (eq)

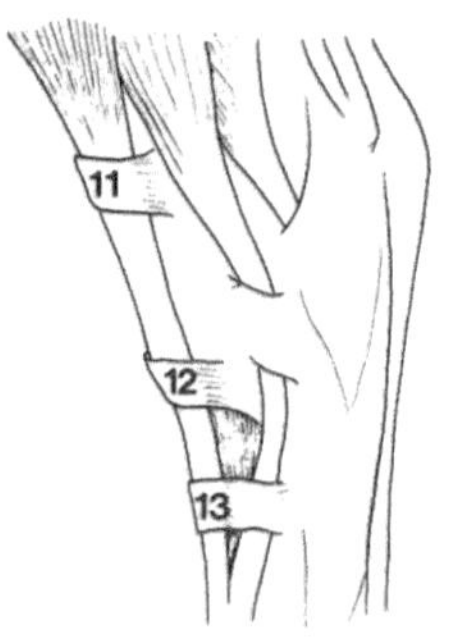

D Left tarsus, lateral aspect (eq)

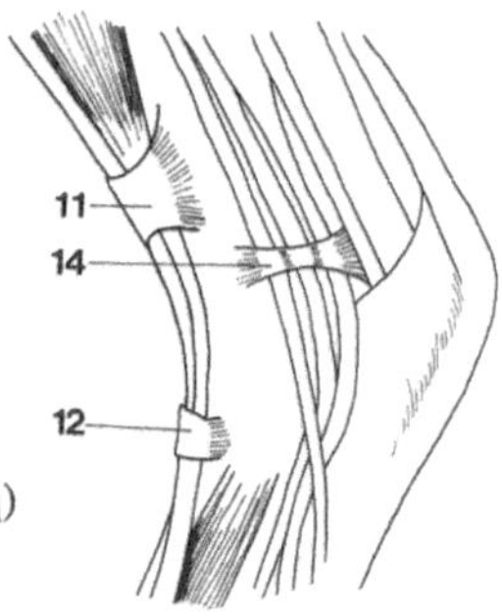

E Left tarsus, lateral aspect (ca)

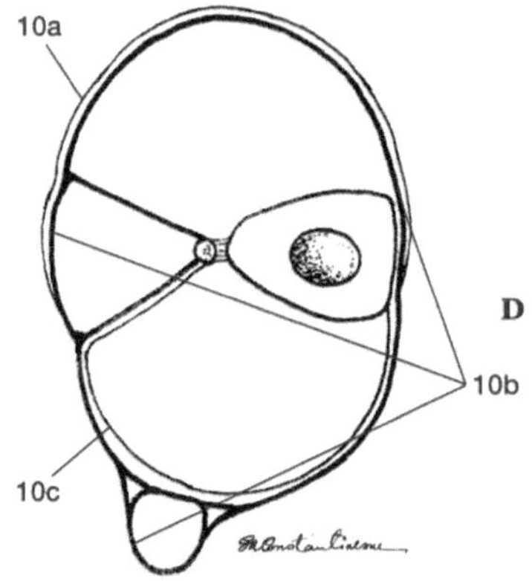

C Left leg, transverse section, proximal surface (eq)

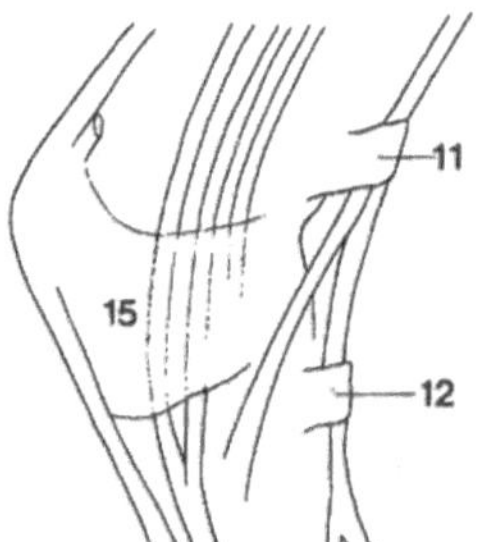

F Left tarsus, medial aspect (ca)

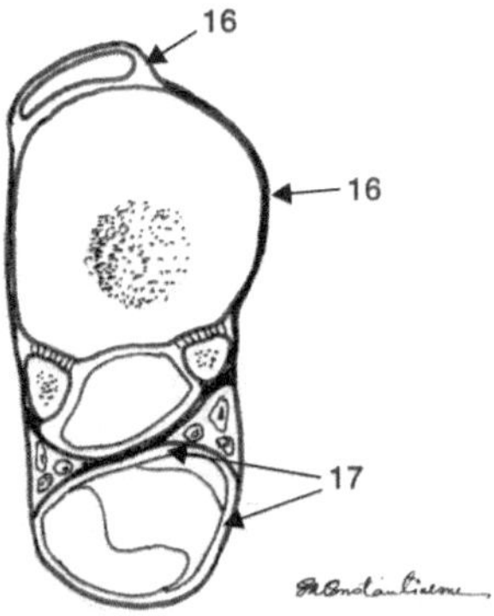

G Left metatarsus, transverse section, proximal surface (eq)

1 **Bursae et vaginae synoviales capitis, colli et trunci**. Synovial bursae and tendon sheaths of the head, neck and trunk.

2 ***Vag. synovialis m. obliqui dorsalis.*** Synovial sheath around tendon of M. obliquus dorsalis bulbi where it contacts trochlea. See Mm. bulbi (muscles of the eyeball).

3 ***B. m. tensoris veli palatini.*** Bursa for tendon of M. tensor veli palatini where it surrounds Hamulus pterygoideus. A

4 ***Vag. tendinis m. digastrici.*** Synovial sheath around intermediate tendon of M. digastricus where it perforates tendon of insertion of M. stylohyoideus in eq. A

5 ***B. subligamentosa supraspinalis**.** Bursa between Ligamentum nuchae and the spines of 2nd, 3rd, and 4th thoracic vertebrae in eq. B

6 ***B. subligamentosa nuchalis cranialis**.** Bursa between Ligamentum nuchae and Mm. recti dorsales over Tuberculum dorsale of atlas in eq, inconstant. B

7 ***B. subligamentosa nuchalis caudalis**.** Bursa between Ligamentum nuchae and spine of axis in eq (and ca), inconstant. B

8 **Bursae et vaginae synoviales membri thoracici**. Synovial bursae and tendon sheaths of the thoracic limb. Many listed bursae are inconstant.

9 ***B. subcutanea prescapularis [prae-]*** (eq). Bursa between skin and Tuber spinae scapulae. C

10 ***B. subdeltoidea.*** Bursa under Pars acromialis as it passes over tendon of M. infraspinatus in Car and bo. D

11 ***B. subtendinea m. coracobrachialis.*** Bursa under tendon of origin medial to shoulder joint in Un. E

12 ***Vag. synovialis m. coracobrachialis.*** Synovial sheath around tendon of origin in Car. F

13 ***B. subtendinea m. infraspinati**.** Bursa between tendon of insertion and Pars caudalis of Tuberculum majus humeri. B

14 ***B. subtendinea m. supraspinati*** (su). Bursa between M. supraspinatus and Tuberculum majus humeri. E

15 ***B. subtendinea m. subscapularis.*** Bursa under tendon of insertion as it passes over shoulder joint, only recess of joint capsule in Car. F

16 ***B. subtendinea m. teretis majoris*** (su). Bursa deep to tendon of insertion occurs sometimes also in ca. E

17 ***B. subtendinea m. teretis minoris.*** Bursa between tendon of insertion and humerus just caudal and distal to that of M. infraspinatus in Un. B

18 ***Vag. synovialis intertubercularis.*** In Car, su, and ov the tendon of M. biceps brachii is provided with synovial tendon sheath as it passes through Sulcus intertubercularis humeri. E F

19 ***B. intertubercularis**.** In cap, bo, and eq there is a synovial bursa for M. biceps brachii. B

20 ***B. subcutanea olecrani.*** Bursa between skin and olecranon. C

21 ***B. intratendinea olecrani.*** Bursa between tendons of insertion of Caput mediale and Caput longum m. tricipitis on olecranon. G

22 ***B. subtendinea m. tricipitis brachii.*** Bursa between tendon of insertion and olecranon. G

23 ***B. bicipitoradialis.*** Bursa between radius and insertion of M. biceps brachii. G

24 ***B. subtendinea m. brachialis.*** Bursa beneath tendon of insertion of M. brachialis on radius. G

25 ***B. subcutanea precarpalis [prae-].*** Bursa deep to skin on dorsal surface of carpus in Ru and eq. C

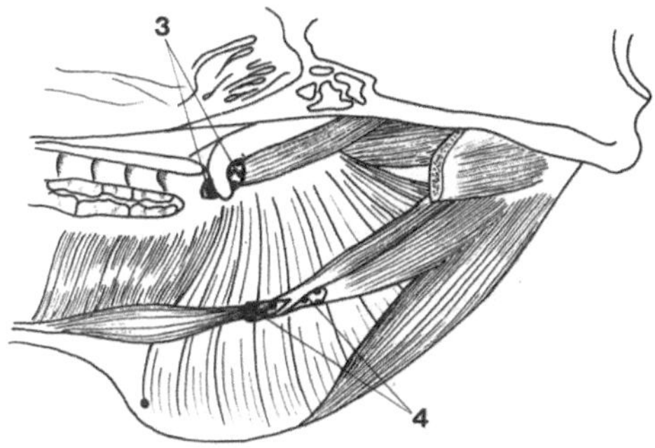

A B. m. tensoris veli palatini and synovial sheath of M. digastricus, right side, medial aspect (eq)

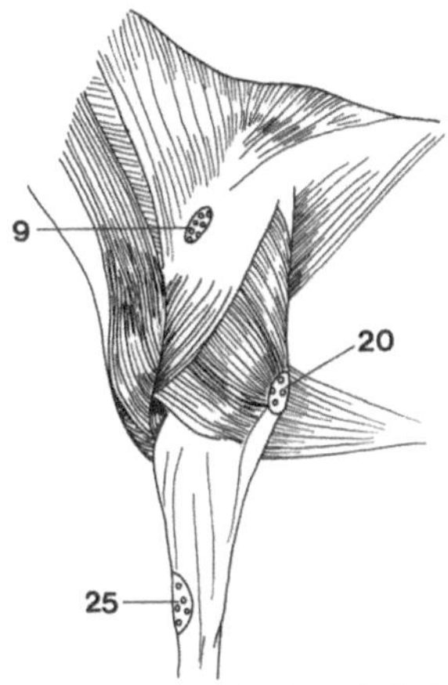

C Subcutaneous bursae of the thoracic limb (eq)

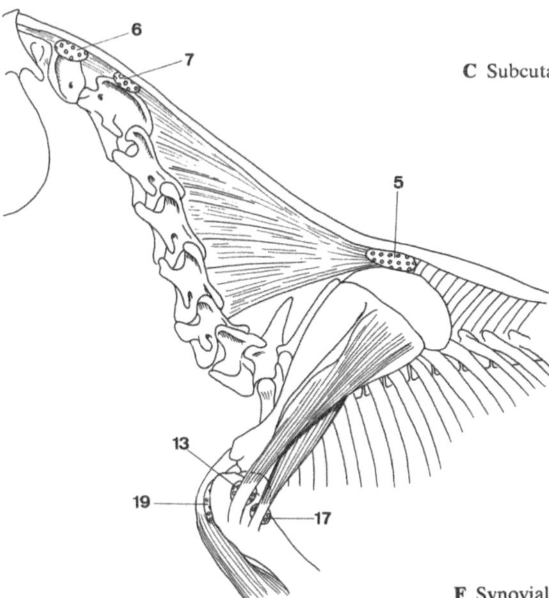

B Bursae of the neck and left shoulder (eq)

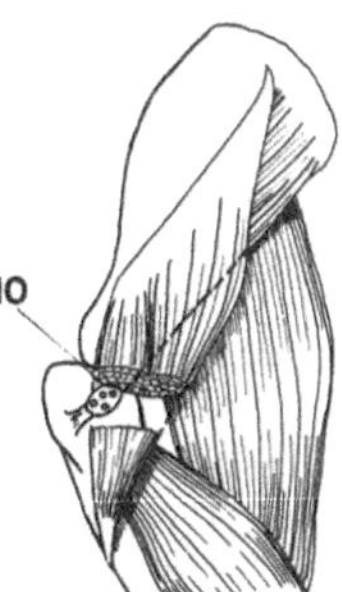

D Left B. subdeltoidea, lateral aspect (ca)

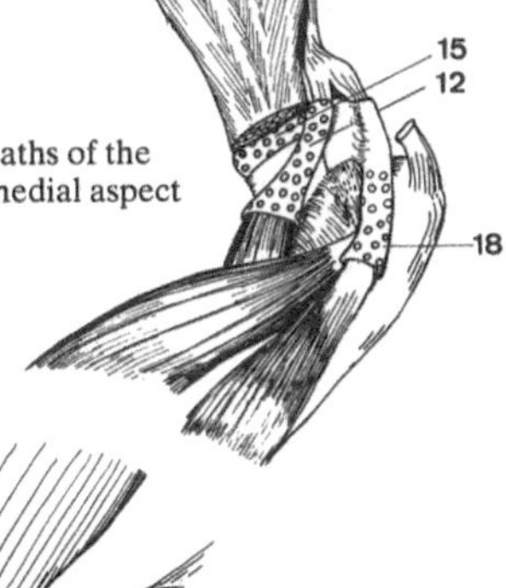

F Synovial sheaths of the left shoulder, medial aspect (ca)

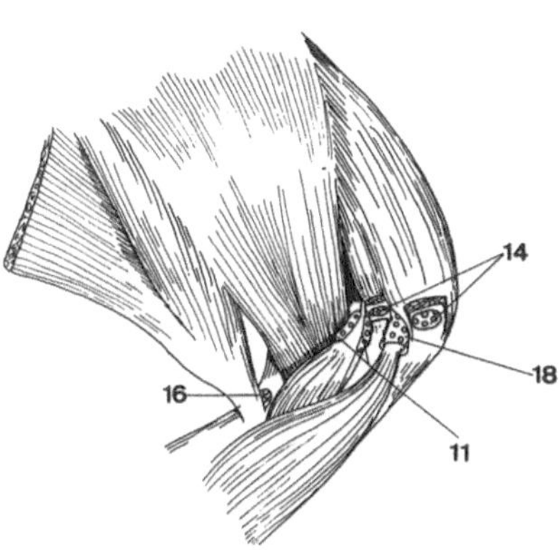

E Bursae of the left shoulder, medial aspect (su)

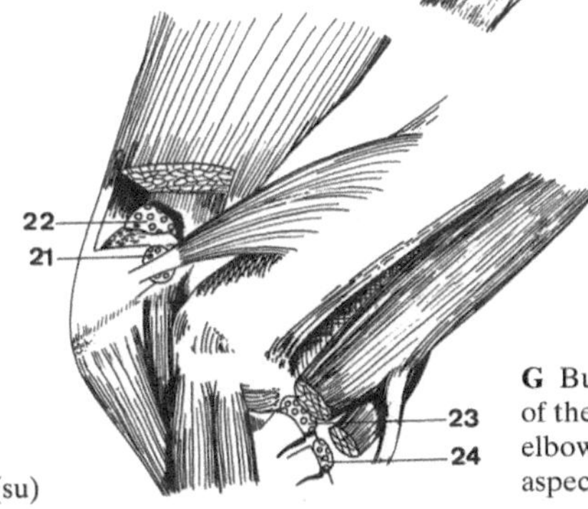

G Bursae of the left elbow, medial aspect (eq)

1 ***Vag. tendinis m. abductoris digiti I [pollicis] longi [m. extensoris carpi obliqui]***. Synovial sheath around tendon of insertion over dorsomedial surface of carpus. B C

2 ***B. subtendinea m. abductoris digiti I [pollicis] longi [m. extensoris carpi obliqui]*** (bo, eq). Subtendinous bursa, distal to the synovial sheath, close to the attachment of the tendon. C

3 ***Vag. tendinis m. extensoris carpi radialis***. Synovial sheath around tendon or tendons (Car) of insertion crossing medial part of cranial surface of radius and dorsal surface of carpus. A B C

4 ***Vag. tendinis m. extensoris digit. communis***. Synovial sheath around tendon or tendons crossing cranial surface of radius and dorsal surface of carpus. A B

5 ***Vag. tendinis m. extensoris dig. lateralis manus***. Synovial sheath around tendon or tendons crossing lateral surface of carpus, in su in most cases two sheaths. A B

6 ***Vag. tendinis m. extensoris carpi ulnaris [m. ulnaris lateralis]***. Synovial sheath around long tendon of insertion over lateral surface of carpus in eq. A

7 ***B. subtendinea m. extensoris carpi ulnaris [m. ulnaris lateralis]***. Bursa deep to long tendon of insertion over lateral surface of carpus in su and Ru, over ulna in Car. B

8 ***B. subtendinea m. extensoris carpi radialis***. Bursa under insertion at dorsal surface of proximal end of metacarpus in Ru and eq. B C

9 ***Vag. tendinis m. flexoris carpi radialis***. Synovial sheath around tendon of insertion as it crosses medial portion of palmar surface of carpus. C

10 ***Vag. synovialis communis mm. flexorum***. Synovial sheath common to both digital flexor tendons in the deep (proper) carpal canal and proximal and distal to it in eq. A

11 ***B. subtendinea m. flexoris digit. profundi***. Bursa deep to tendons in the carpal canal in Car, su, and in the deep (proper) carpal canal in Ru. C

12 ***Bb. m. flexoris digit. superficialis***. Bursae under two tendons of M. flexor digit. superficialis in Ru (in the deep and the superficial carpal canals), one for superficial tendon in su. C

13 ***Vag. tendinis m. flexoris carpi ulnaris*** (Car). Synovial tendon sheath around tendon of insertion at Os carpi accessorium. E

14 ***B. subtendinea m. extensoris digit. communis*** (Ru, eq). Bursa between tendon of medial portion of M. extensor digit. communis and dorsal side of medial metacarpophalangeal joint in Ru, and tendon of M. extensor digit. communis and metacarpophalangeal joint in eq. D F

15 ***B. subtendinea m. extensoris digit. lateralis manus*** (Ru, eq). Bursa between tendon of M. extensor digit. lateralis and dorsal side of lateral metacarpophalangeal joint in Ru and tendon of M. extensor digit. lateralis and metacarpophalangeal joint in eq. A D

16 ***Vag. distalis tendinum m. extensoris digit. communis*** (Ru). Synovial sheath begins proximal to metacarpophalangeal joints, divides for the both tendons to Phalanx distalis of 3rd and 4th digit. D

17 ***Vag. synovialis tendinum digitorum manus****. Synovial sheaths common to deep and superficial flexor tendons to each digit in manus. A E F

18 ***Bb. subtendineae mm. interosseorum manus***. Bursa under each tendon as it crosses side of metacarpophalangeal joint on way to common digital extensor tendon in eq. A

19 ***Bb. podotrochleares manus****. Bursa between deep digital flexor tendon and distal sesamoid bone for each digit in Un. F

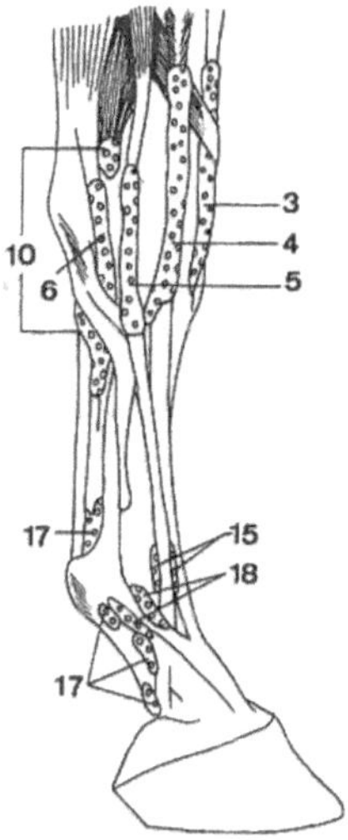

A Bursae and synovial sheaths of the right manus, lateral aspect (eq)

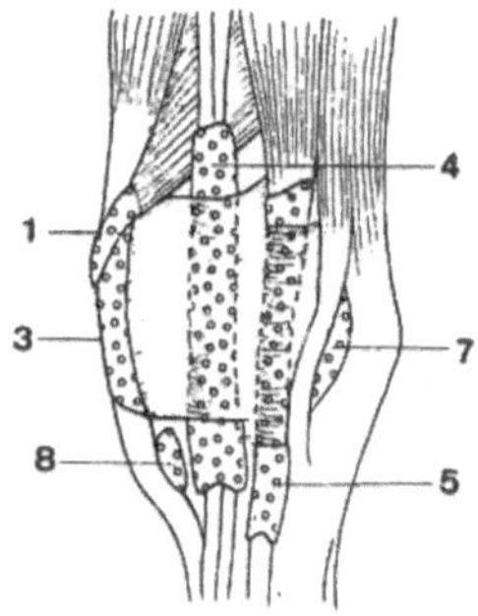

B Bursae and synovial sheaths of the left carpus, dorsolateral aspect (bo)

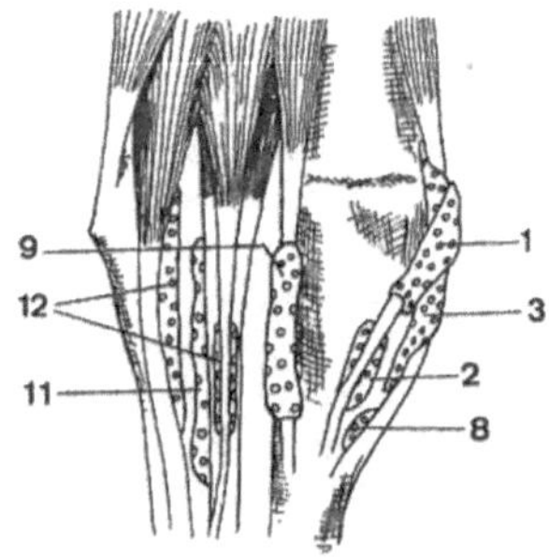

C Bursae and synovial sheaths of the left carpus, medial aspect (bo)

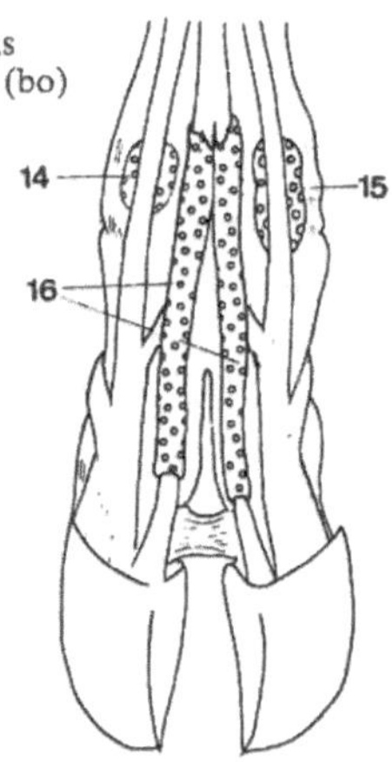

D Bursae and synovial sheaths of the left digits, dorsal aspect (bo)

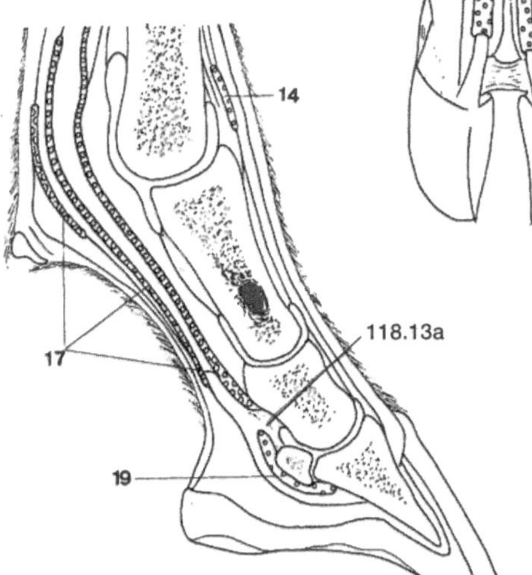

F Bursae and synovial sheaths of the digit, sagittal section (eq)

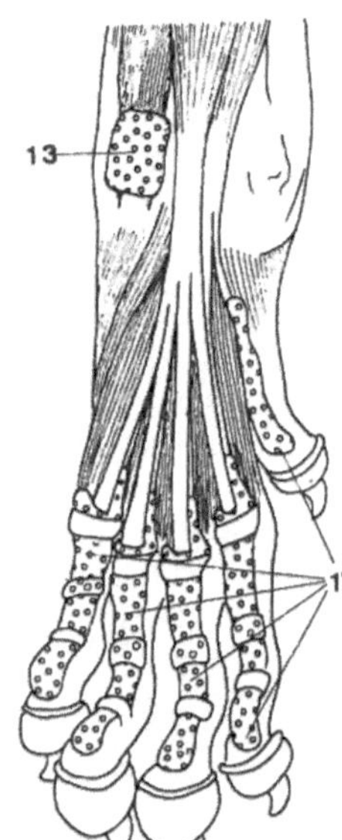

E Synovial sheaths of the left manus, palmar aspect (ca)

1 **Bursae et vaginae synoviales membri pelvini**. Synovial bursae and tendon sheaths of the pelvic limb. Many listed bursae are inconstant.

2 ***B. subcutanea trochanterica***. Bursa between skin and muscles over Trochanter major in eq. A

3 ***B. subcutanea iliaca [coxalis]***. Bursa between skin and Tuber coxae. A

4 ***B. subcutanea ischiadica***. Bursa between skin and M. semitendinosus over Tuber ischiadicum in eq, skin and Tuber in bo (and ca). A

5 ***B. trochanterica m. glutei [glutaei] superficialis***. Bursa between tendon of insertion and Trochanter tertius in eq, Trochanter major in ca. C

5a ***B. trochanterica m. glutei [glutaei] medii***. In su and Ru 2 or 3 bursae cranial to greater trochanter, in eq deep to tendon of insertion of this muscle on caudal part of greater trochanter.

6 ***Bb. trochantericae m. glutei [glutaei] accessorii*** (eq). Bursa deep to tendon of M. gluteus accessorius on Pars cranialis of Trochanter major. B

7 ***B. trochanterica m. glutei [glutaei] profundi***. Bursa under insertion of muscle. E

8 ***B. ischiadica m. obturatorii interni*** (Car, eq). Bursa between muscle and Incisura ischiadica minor. F

9 ***B. ischiadica m. obturatorii externi*** (su, Ru). Bursa between Pars intrapelvina and lateral edge of Foramen obturatum. B

10 ***B. subtendinea m. obturatorii interni*** (Car, eq). Bursa in Fossa trochanterica as tendon inserts. F

11 ***B. subtendinea m. obturatorii externi*** (su, Ru). Bursa in Fossa trochanterica as tendon inserts. B

12 ***B. trochanterica m. bicipitis femoris***. Bursa deep to muscle as it passes over Trochanter major. E

13 ***B. ischiadica m. semitendinosi***. Bursa deep to muscle as it passes over Tuber ischiadicum in eq. A

14 ***B. m. recti femoris***. Bursa between origin of muscle and Os ilium, in ca also between muscle and distal third of Corpus ossis femoris. F

15 ***B. subtendinea iliaca***. Bursa deep to tendon of insertion of M. iliopsoas in bo (and ca). E

16 ***B. subcutanea prepatellaris [prae-]***. Bursa between skin and Lamina superficialis fasciae latae. A

17 ***B. subfascialis prepatellaris [prae-]***. Bursa deep to Lamina superficialis fasciae latae. C F

18 ***Bb. subtendineae prepatellares [prae-]***. Bursae deep to tendons of insertion of components of M. quadriceps femoris. C D

19 ***B. infrapatellaris proximalis*** (eq). Bursa between Lig. patellae intermedium and patella. C

20 ***B. infrapatellaris distalis***. Bursa between Lig. patellae and tibia. C

21 ***B. subcutanea tuberositatis tibiae***. Bursa between skin and Tuberositas tibiae. A

22 ***B. subtendinea m. semitendinosi***. Bursa deep to tendon of attachment of muscle on tibia. D

23 ***B. subtendinea m. bicipitis femoris distalis***. Bursa under attachment of muscle as it passes over Condylus lateralis femoris in Ru, on its insertion to lateral portion of patella in eq. C

24 ***Recessus subpopliteus***. Synovial extension beneath tendon of origin of M. popliteus over Condylus lateralis tibiae. C

25 ***Recessus subextensorius***. Synovial extension beneath tendon of origin of M. extensor digitorum longus and M. fibularis tertius (except Car) as it passes through Sulcus extensorius tibiae. C

26 ***B. subcutanea malleoli lateralis***. Bursa beneath skin over Malleolus lateralis tibiae. A

27 ***B. subcutanea malleoli medialis***. Bursa beneath skin over Malleolus medialis tibiae. A

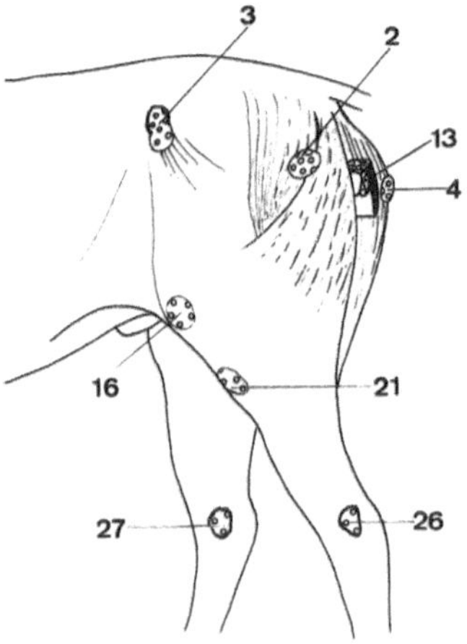

A Subcutaneous bursae of the pelvic limb (eq)

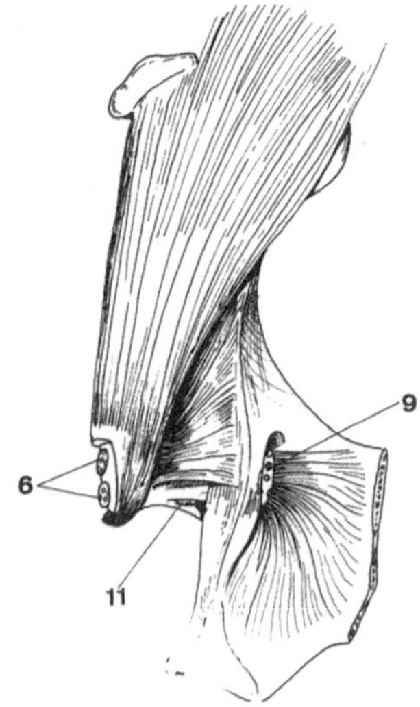

B Bursae of the left hip, dorsal aspect (bo)

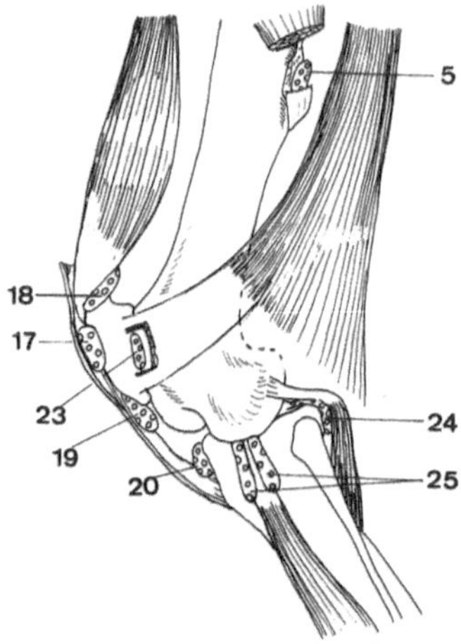

C Bursae and recesses of the left stifle, lateral aspect (eq)

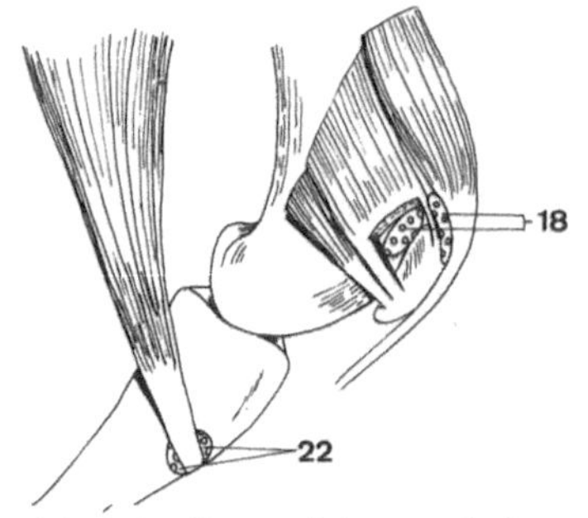

D Bursae of the left stifle, medial aspect (eq)

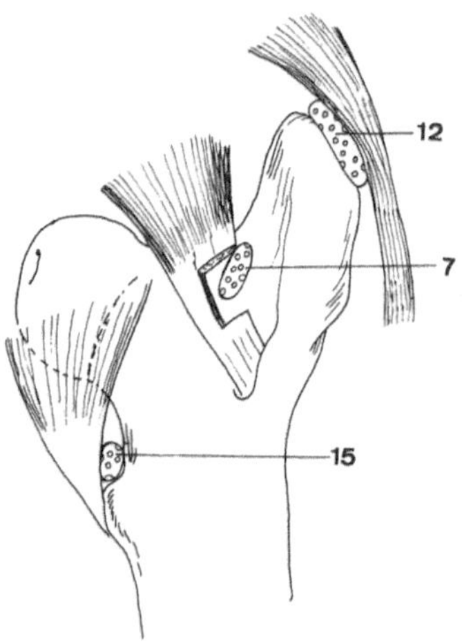

E Bursae of the left thigh, cranial aspect (bo)

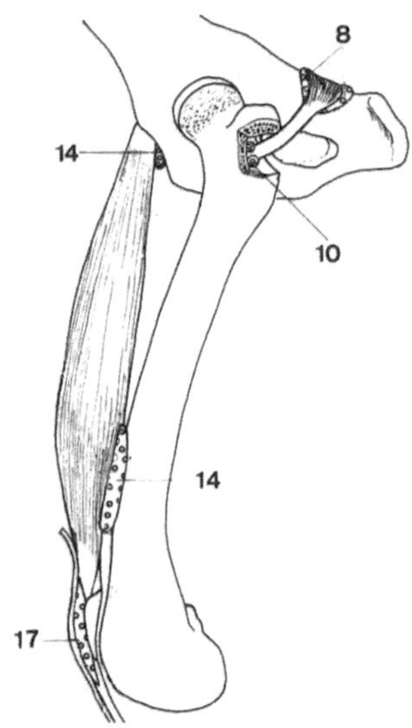

F Bursae of the left thigh and stifle, lateral aspect (ca)

1 ***Vag. tendinis m. tibialis cranialis.*** Synovial sheath around tendon of insertion on dorsomedial surface of tarsus. Fuses with 2 and 3 in su and Ru. B C

2 ***Vag. tendinis m. fibularis [peron.] tertii*** (su, Ru). Synovial sheath around tendon of insertion on dorsal surface of tarsus. Fuses with 1 and 3. D

3 ***Vag. tendinum m. extensoris digit. longi.*** Synovial sheath around tendons descending over dorsal surface of tarsus. Fuses with 1 and 2 in su and Ru. A D

4 ***Vag. tendinis m. extensoris digit. lateralis pedis.*** Synovial sheath around tendon as it crosses dorsolateral surface of tarsus, includes M. peroneus brevis in Car. A D

5 ***Vag. tendinis m. tibialis caudalis*** (ca). Synovial sheath around tendon of insertion on medial surface of tarsus. B

6 ***Vag. tendinis m. flexoris digit. medialis.*** Synovial sheath around tendon as it descends on medial surface of tarsus. May be continuous distally with 7 in su and eq. B C

7 ***Vag. tendinis m. flexoris digit. lateralis.*** Synovial sheath of tendon on plantar surface of tarsus, includes M. tibialis caudalis in Un. May be continuous distally with 6 in su and eq. B C

8 ***Vag. tendinis m. fibularis [peron.] longi lateralis.*** Synovial sheath around tendon of insertion as it crosses lateral side of tarsus. A D

9 ***B. subtendinea m. fibularis [peron.] brevis*** (Car). Bursa between tendon of insertion and distal portion of lateral surface of tarsus. A

10 ***B. subtendinea m. tibialis cranialis.*** Bursa between the tendon of insertion and distal medial portion of tarsus. B C

11 ***B. subcutanea calcanea.*** Bursa between skin and M. flexor digit. superficialis over Tuber calcanei. C

12 ***B. calcanea subtendinea m. flexoris digit. superficialis.*** Bursa deep to tendon over M. gastrocnemius and Tuber calcanei. Fuses often with 13 in eq. A B C D

13 ***B. tendinis calcanei.*** Bursa deep to Tendo calcaneus of M. triceps surae. Fuses often with 12 in eq. A B C

14 ***Vag. tendinis m. fibularis [peron.] longi plantaris.*** Synovial sheath around distal part of tendon of insertion as it becomes plantar in Ru, recess of joint capsule in Car and su. A

15 ***B. subtendinea m. fibularis [peron.] longi*** (su, Ru). Bursa between terminal tendon and distal part of plantar surface of tarsus, recess of joint capsule. D

16 ***B. subtendinea m. extensoris digit. longi*** (Ru, eq). See 134.14

17 ***B. subtendinea m. extensoris digit. lateralis pedis*** (Ru). See 134.15, but exists only in Ru.

18 ***Vag. distalis tendinum m. extensoris digit. longi*** (Ru). See 134.16

19 ***Vagg. synoviales tendinum digitorum pedis.*** See 134.17

20 ***Bb. subtendineae mm. interosseorum pedis.*** See 134.18

21 ***Bb. podotrochleares pedis.*** See 134.19

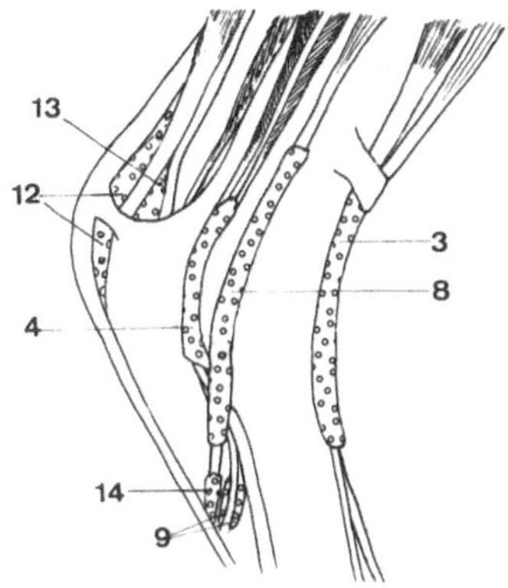

A Bursae and synovial sheaths of the right tarsus, lateral aspect (ca)

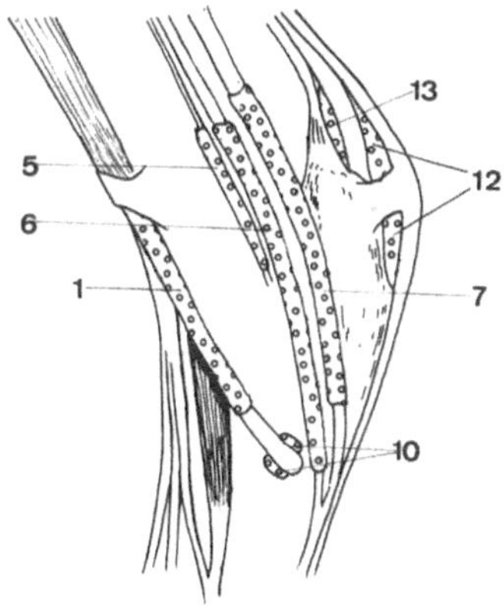

B Bursae and synovial sheaths of the right tarsus, medial aspect (ca)

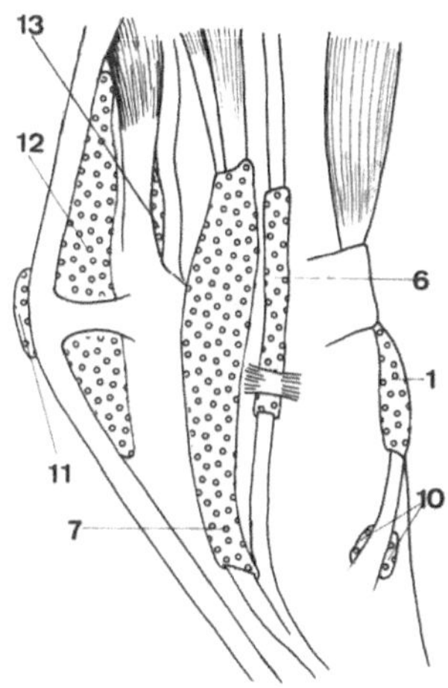

C Bursae and synovial sheaths of the left tarsus, medial aspect (bo)

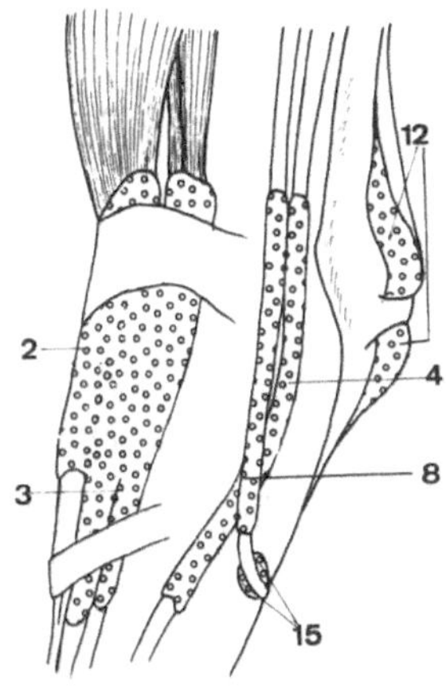

D Bursae and synovial sheaths of the left tarsus, dorsolateral aspect (bo)

1 **SYSTEMA DIGESTORIUM**.

2 **CAVUM ORIS**. Oral cavity. C

3 ***Vestibulum oris***. Space between the teeth and lips and cheeks. C D F

4 *Rima oris*. Mouth opening, slit between the lips. Ends at anguli oris. A

5 *Labia oris*. Lips. A

6 **Labium superius**. Upper lip. A D

7 **Philtrum**. Median groove from the nasal septum to the upper lip. A

8 **Labium inferius**. Lower lip. A E

9 *Angulus oris*. The end of rima oris – symmetrical. A E

10 *Bucca*. Cheek. A

11 **Corpus adiposum buccae**. Buccal fat pad, on the M. buccinator at the rostral border of the M. masseter. B

11a **Organum juxtaorale**. This ductless and encapsulated epithelial cord is found in man, cat, dog, pig, and ox between M. temporalis and M. buccinator. It is grossly demonstrable in man only. (This information is taken from the N.A.V. 5th edition, 2005. The structure is not listed in the N.A. However, it is listed in the Terminologia Anatomica of the Federative Committee on Anatomical Terminology 1998.)

12 ***Cavum oris proprium***. Cavity enclosed by the teeth and limited caudally by the Arcus palatoglossus. C F

13 *Palatum*. Palate, partition separating the nasal cavity and nasopharynx from the oral cavity and oropharynx. C

14 **Palatum durum**. Hard palate, supported by bone. C D

15 **Palatum molle [Velum palatinum]**. Soft, caudal part of the palate. C

16 **Raphe [Rhape] palati**. Median line of junction of the halves of the palate. D

17 *Recessus sublingualis lateralis*. Symmetrical space under the tongue. F

18 **Tunica mucosa oris**. Mucous membrane lining the oral cavity. Stratified squamous epithelium, penetrated by the ducts of many submucosal glands.

19 ***Frenulum labii superioris***. Median fold of mucous membrane between the upper lip and the gingiva. G

20 ***Frenulum labii inferioris***. Median fold of mucous membrane between the lower lip and the gingiva. E

21 ***Gingiva***. Gum, the mucous membrane attached to the teeth and alveolar bone. C E

22 *Margo gingivalis*. Border of gum around the tooth. C E

23 *Papilla gingivalis [interdentalis]*. Small mucosal elevation between teeth. C E

24 *Sulcus gingivalis*. Groove between gingiva and tooth. C E

25 ***Caruncula sublingualis***. Flattened projection rostrolateral to the Frenulum linguae. The Ductus mandibularis and (except in eq) the Ductus sublingualis major open there. E F

26 ***Tonsilla sublingualis***. Lymphatic follicles in the vicinity of the Caruncula sublingualis. F

27 ***Plica sublingualis***. Fold of mucous membrane on the floor of the mouth lateral to the Frenulum linguae. It ends at the Caruncula sublingualis. E F

28 ***Organum orobasale***. Rudimentary epithelial cords or ducts extending into the Lamina propria from pits or grooves behind the lower central incisors. E F

29 ***Papilla parotidea***. Small elevation of the buccal mucosa at the orifice of the Ductus parotideus opposite the 2–5 upper cheek teeth, depending on species (fe 2nd PM; ov, cap, eq 3rd PM; ca, su 3rd or 4th PM, bo 2nd M; PM=premolars, M=molars). G

30 ***Papilla zygomatica*** (Car). Short fold of buccal mucosa extending caudally from the Papilla parotidea and bearing the orifices of the Ductus glandulae zygomaticae opposite the upper molars. G

31 ***Rugae palatinae***. Transverse ridges of the mucosa on the hard palate. C D

32 ***Pulvinus dentalis***. Dental pad, a tough plate of oral mucous membrane which takes the place of the missing upper incisors in Ru. C D

33 ***Papilla incisiva***. Elevation of mucous membrane at the rostral end of the Raphe palati. It conceals the orifices of the Ductus incisivi. D

34 ***Papillae labiales*** (ca, Ru). In ca, on margin of lower lip. In Ru, sharp, cornified, inside the lips. C D E G

35 ***Papillae buccales*** (Ru). Projections of the buccal mucosa covered by cornified epithelium. C

36 ***Plica pterygomandibularis***. Dorsoventral fold of mucous membrane between the palate and the mandible behind the last molars. G

* Reminder: The structures followed by an asterisk are landmarks for physical examination and/or clinical approach.

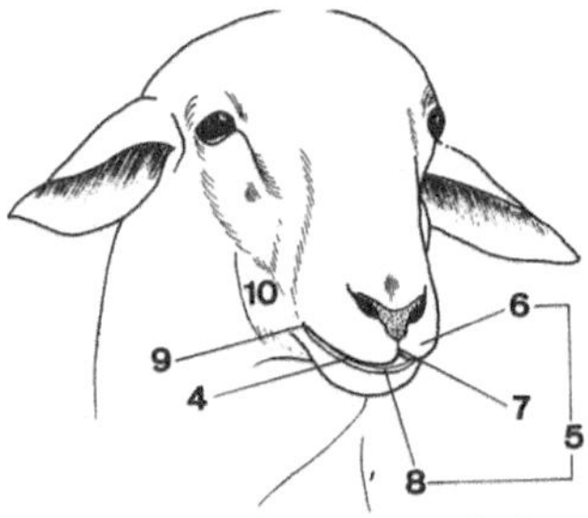

A Oral region, right rostral aspect (ov)

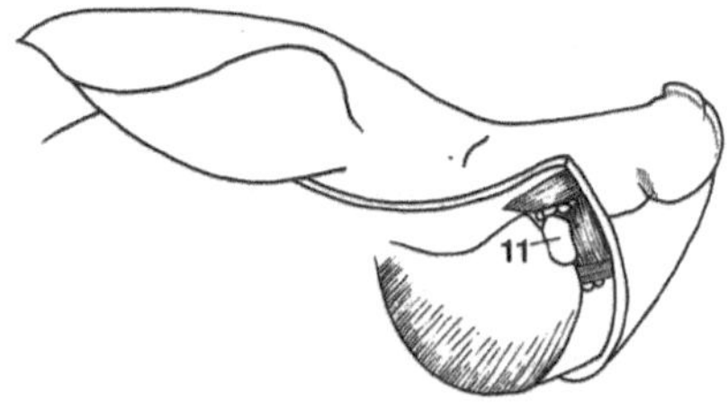

B Buccal region (cutaneous muscles removed) (su)

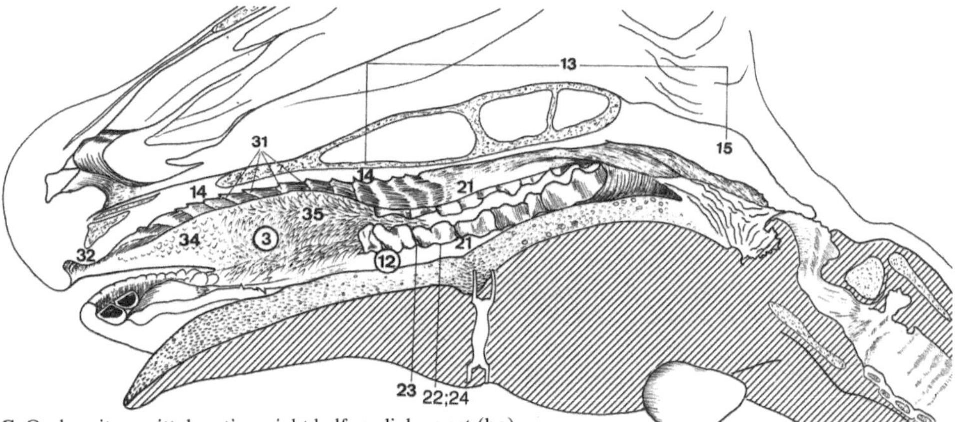

C Oral cavity, sagittal section, right half medial aspect (bo)

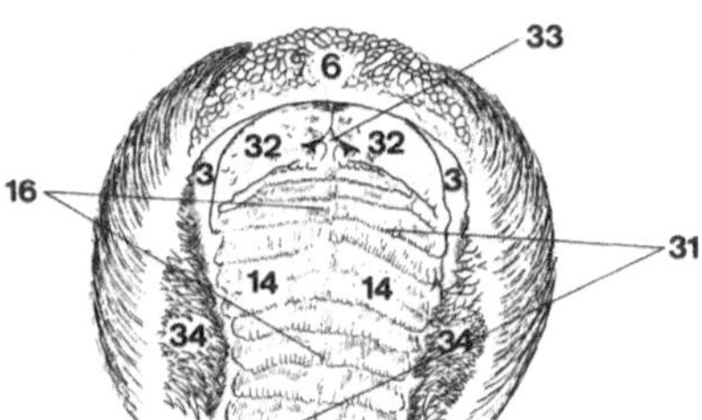

D Hard palate and upper lip (bo)

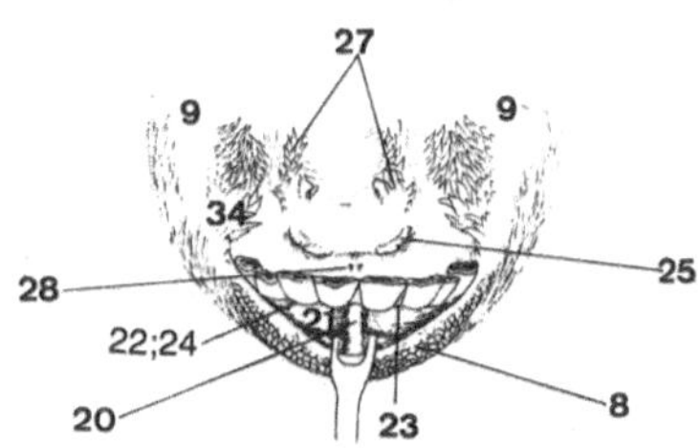

E Sublingual recess and lower lip (bo)

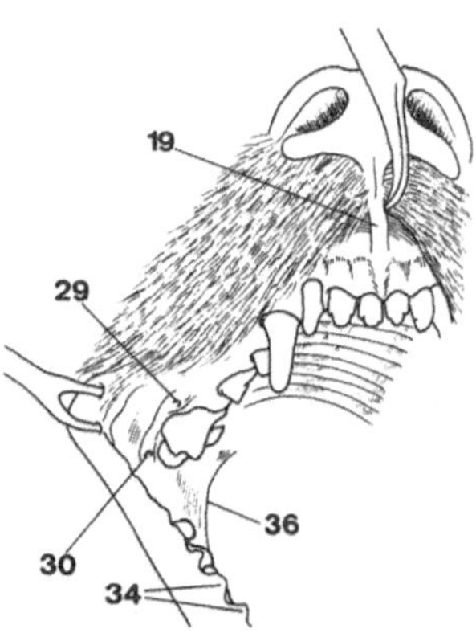

G Right oral vestibule (ca)

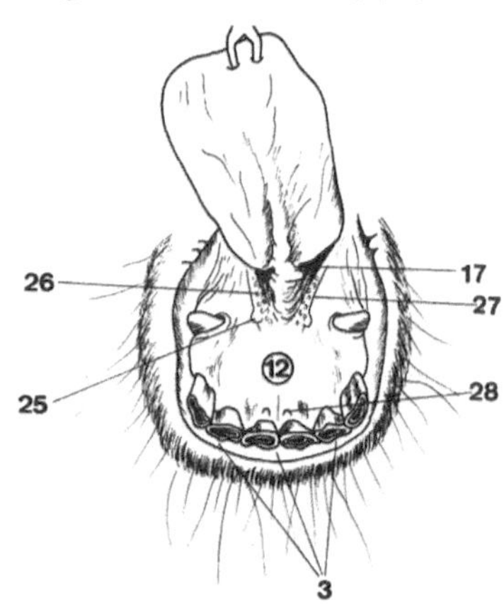

F Sublingual recess and lower lip (eq)

1 **Glandulae oris**. Glands of the mouth, oral glands.

2 **Glandulae salivariae minores**. Smaller salivary glands.

3 ***Gll. labiales***. Glands of the lips. A

4 ***Gll. buccales***. Glands of the cheeks.

5 *Gll. buccales dorsales*. Extend from the angle of the mouth to M. masseter. One layer is superficial to M. buccinator, along the A. labialis superior. Another layer is covered by the superficial part of M. buccinator. Represented by Gl. zygomatica in Car. C

6 *Gl. zygomatica*. A major salivary gland of Car, medial to the zygomatic arch and in contact with the periorbita and the M. pterygoideus medialis. E

7 **Ductus glandulae zygomaticae major**. Main duct of Gl. zygomatica. It opens on a papilla opposite the upper first molar. E

8 **Ductus glandulae zygomaticae minores**. Two to four minor ducts of Gl. Zygomatica open caudal to the main duct. E

9 *Gll. buccales intermediae* (Ru). Along the dorsal border of the A. labialis inferior between the two layers of M. buccinator. C

10 *Gll. buccales ventrales*. Extend from the angle of the mouth to M. masseter, ventral to A. labialis inferior and covered, except for the caudal part, by M. buccinator. C

11 ***Gll. molares***. Molar glands, the caudal continuation of the Gll. buccales ventrales deep to M. masseter. C

12 ***Gll. palatinae***. Palatine glands on the oropharyngeal side of the soft palate; they occur also on the nasopharyngeal side and in the hard palate of Car, ov and cap. A

13 ***Gll. linguales***. Lingual glands, mainly on root and margins of the tongue. A

14 *Gll. gustatoriae*. Taste glands, whose ducts discharge into the grooves of the Papillae vallatae. D

15 *Gl. lingualis apicalis*. Apical lingual gland, in the musculature of the ventral surface of the apex of tongue in ov. B

16 ***Gl. paracaruncularis*** (cap, eq). Paracaruncular gland, group of small glands near Caruncula sublingualis, in cap continuous with the Gl. sublingualis. A

17 **Glandulae salivariae majores**. Larger salivary glands.

18 **Gl. sublingualis monostomatica**. It extends along the Ductus mandibularis between M. digastricus and M. masseter medial to the mandible. In Car the caudal part is in contact with the Gl. mandibularis. It is absent in eq. E

19 ***Ductus sublingualis major***. Duct of the monostomatic sublingual gland. It accompanies the Ductus mandibularis and opens on or near the Caruncula sublingualis. E

20 **Gl. sublingualis polystomatica**. Series of small salivary glands with separate ducts, in the submucosa on the floor of the mouth, along the Ductus mandibularis. E

21 ***Ductus sublinguales minores***. Ducts of the polystomatic sublingual gland. They open along the Plica sublingualis.

22 **Gl. mandibularis**. Mandibular gland, covered wholly or in part, depending on the species, by the Gl. parotis. C E

23 ***Ductus mandibularis***. Runs along the floor of the mouth to the Caruncula sublingualis. E

24 **Gl. Parotis**. Parotid gland, the most superficial and, except in bo, the largest salivary gland, related dorsally to the base of the ear. C E

25 ***Pars superficialis***. Part of the gland superficial to the N. facialis. C

26 ***Pars profunda***. Deep to the N. facialis. C

27 ***Gl. parotis accessoria***. Small glands may occur along the duct. C

28 ***Ductus parotideus***. Runs across the lateral surface of M. masseter in Car and ov, ventral to M. masseter in su, bo, cap, eq. It ends at the Papilla parotidea. C E

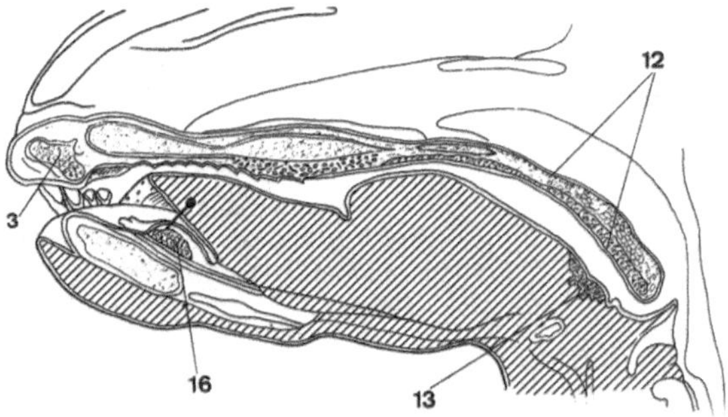

A Oral cavity, sagittal section, right half medial aspect (cap)

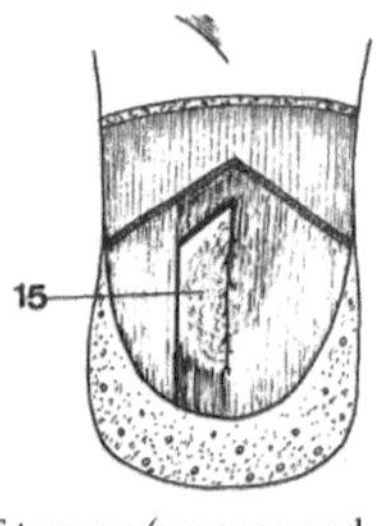

B Tip of tongue (mucosa and superficial musculature removed), ventral surface (ov)

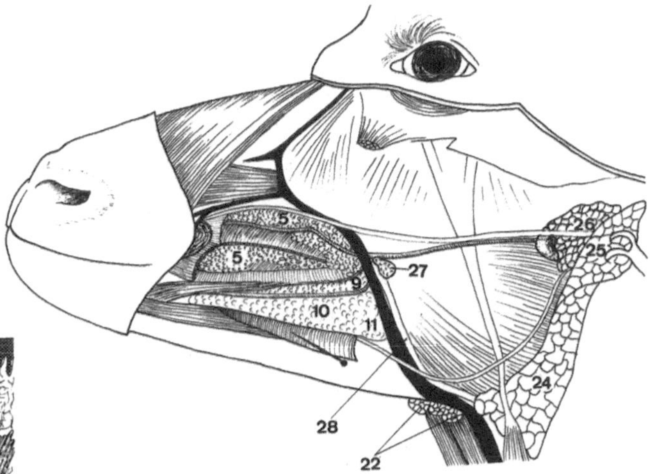

C Head, lateral dissection (cap)

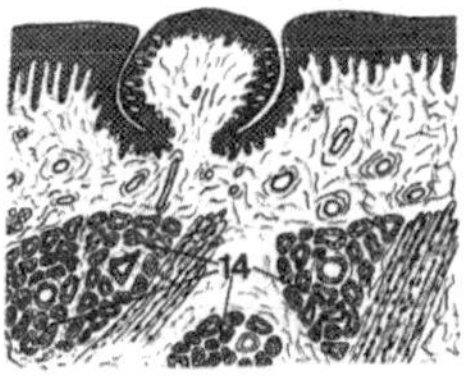

D Vallate papilla, histological section

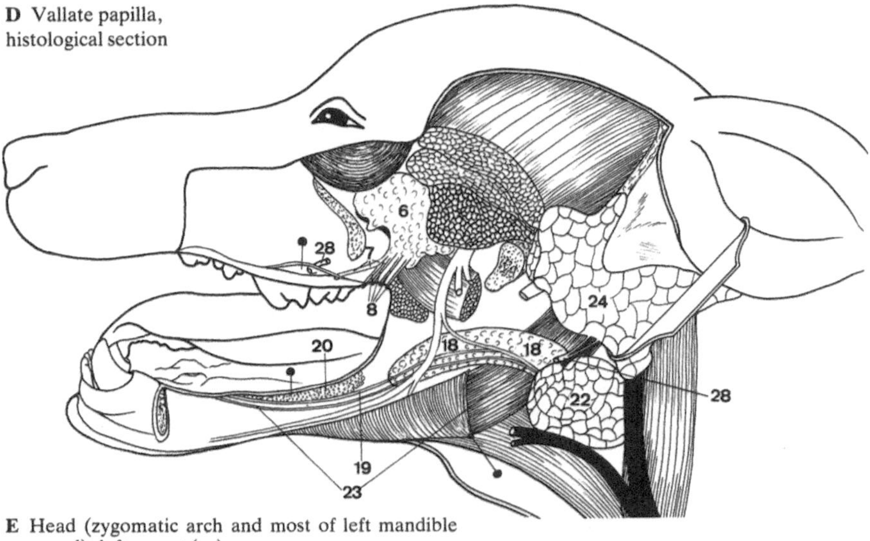

E Head (zygomatic arch and most of left mandible removed), left aspect (ca)

1 **Dentes**. Teeth.

2 **Corpus dentis**. Body of the tooth, applied to hypsodont teeth, in which corona and cervix cannot be distinguished. It includes all of the tooth except the root. The part covered by enamel is not homologous to the Corona dentis (anatomical crown) as defined for the brachidont tooth. A

3 **Corona dentis**. Crown of brachydont tooth, covered by enamel and demarcated from the root by the neck. E F

4 *Cuspis [coronae] dentis*. Cusp, one of the main projections on the occlusal surface; it may be pointed or rounded. E

5 **Apex cuspidis**. The tip of a dental cusp. E

6 *Tuberculum [coronae] dentis*. Tubercle, a secondary projection of the crown not on the occlusal surface, present on the lingual surface of some incisors of fe and bo. B

7 *Infundibulum dentis*. Invagination of enamel and cementum on the occlusal surface of incisors (su, eq), premolars, and molars (Ru, eq). A D

8 *Plica enameli*. Enamel fold, an infolding from the side of a premolar or molar. C

9 *Crista enameli*. Enamel crest, a free occlusal edge of one of the enamel layers of a worn tooth. C

10 **Corona clinica**. Clinical crown, the free part of the tooth that projects from the gingiva. A

11 **Cervix dentis**. Neck of the tooth, constriction between crown and root. E F

12 **Radix dentis**. Root of the tooth. It is not covered by enamel. A E F

13 *Apex radicis dentis*. The tip of a dental root. E F

14 **Radix clinica**. Clinical root, the part of the tooth that is concealed by the gingiva and alveolus. A

15 **Facies occlusalis**. Occlusal surface. It meets the teeth of the opposite jaw. D

16 **Facies vestibularis [facialis]**. Outer surface, directed toward the Vestibulum oris. D

17 **Facies lingualis**. Inner surface, directed toward the tongue. D

18 **Facies contactus**. Each tooth, except the last molar (and species specific the first premolar and/or the corner incisor), has two contact surfaces, which are related to the adjacent teeth in the same dental arch. D

19 *Facies mesialis*. Mesial surface, on the central incisor (I_1) next to the median plane, on other teeth directed toward the central incisor. D

20 *Facies distalis*. The opposite surface from the Facies mesialis. D

21 **Cingulum**. Ridge on the lingual surface of the crown near the neck, connecting the Cristae marginales. It occurs on the incisors of ca and Ru. F

22 **Crista marginalis**. Marginal crest, a ridge on each contact border of the lingual surface of the crown of incisor and canine teeth in ca and Ru. F

23 **Margo incisalis**. Occlusal border of the incisor teeth. F

24 **Cavum dentis [pulpare]**. Cavity of the tooth that contains the pulp. A

25 *Cavum coronale dentis*. Cavity contained in the crown. G

25a **Cornu cavitatis dentis**. Cornu cavitatis dentis is a prolongation of the dental pulp cavity extending toward the cusp of a tooth. The enclosed dental pulp is designated as the "dental pulp horn" in veterinary dentistry.

26 *Canalis radicis dentis*. Root canal. G

27 **Foramen apicis dentis**. Orifice of the root canal. A G

27a **Cornu cavitatis dentis**. Prolongation of the dental pulp cavity extending toward the cusp of a tooth. The enclosed dental pulp is designated as the "dental pulp horn" in veterinary dentistry.

28 **Pulpa dentis**. Pulp of the tooth. A

29 *Pulpa coronalis*. Pulp in the crown. G

30 *Pulpa radicularis*. Pulp in the root canal. G

31 **Papilla dentis** (ont). (This structure was omitted from the 5th edition of the N. A. V., because it is an ontogenetic term.)

32 **Dentinum**. Dentin, the main substance of the tooth, a calcified collagenous matrix permeated by the processes of odontoblasts. A C G

33 **Enamelum**. Enamel, the hard white substance covering the dentin in the crown or the body of the tooth. A G

34 **Cementum**. Cement, bone-like substance that covers the root. In hypsodont teeth it also covers the Corpus dentis and fills the infundibula and plicae. A C G

35 **Periodontium**. Connective tissue that attaches the tooth and gingiva to the alveolus. A

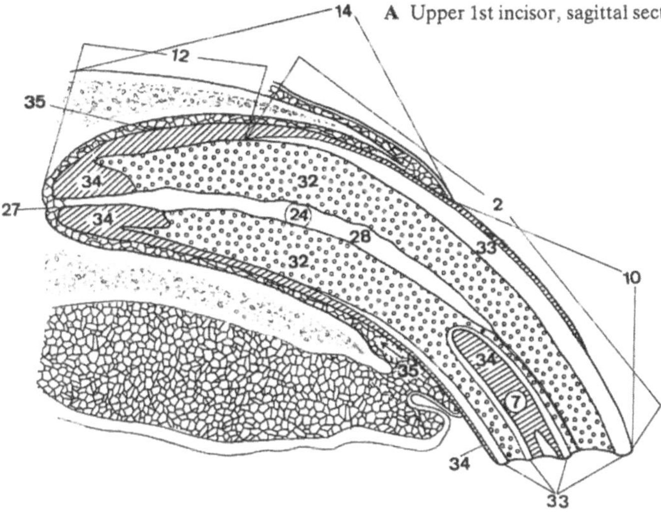

A Upper 1st incisor, sagittal section (eq)

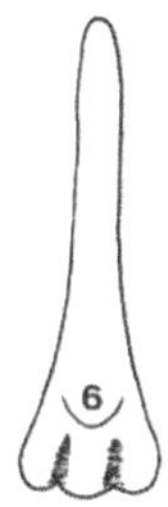

B Upper 2nd incisor, lingual surface (fe)

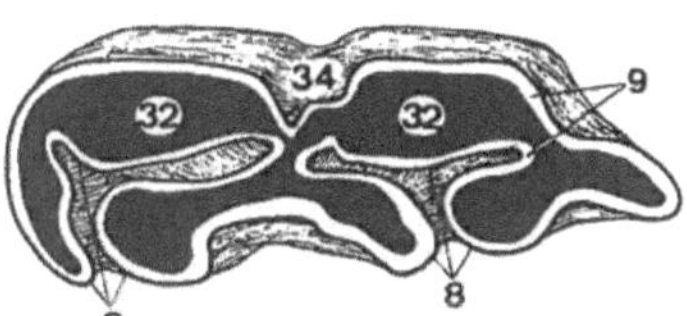

C Lower 2nd molar, occlusal surface (eq)

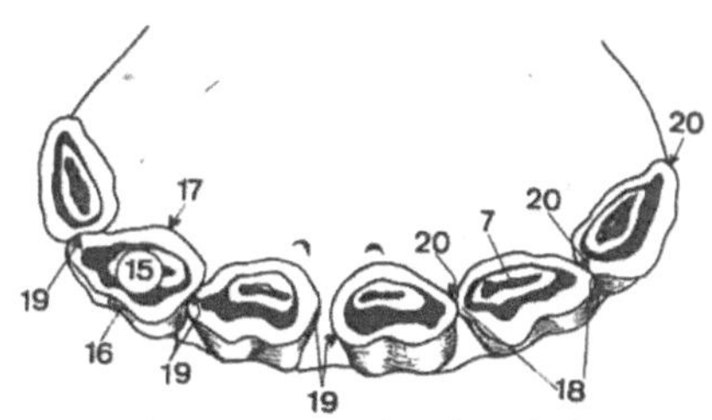

D Lower incisors, occlusal surfaces (eq)

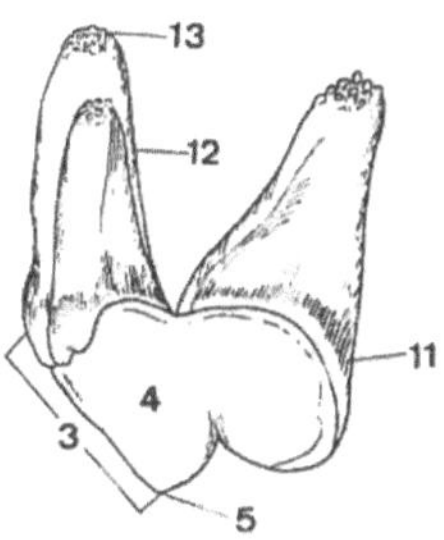

E Upper right 4th premolar (sectorial tooth), lingual surface (ca)

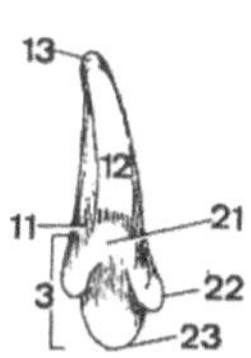

F Right upper 2nd incisor, lingual surface (ca)

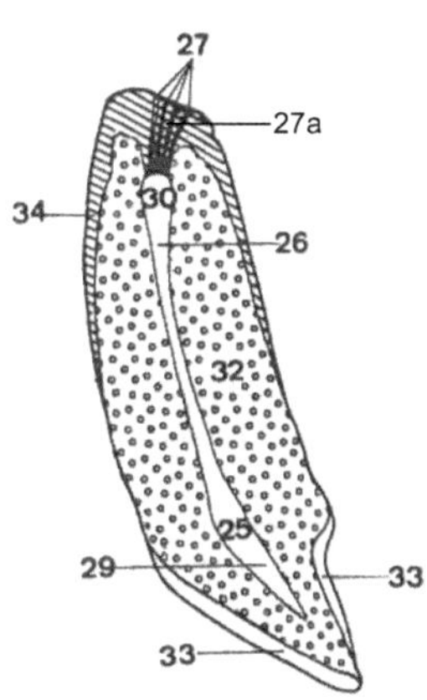

G Upper incisor, sagittal section (ca)

1 ***Arcus dentalis superior***. Arch formed by all of the upper teeth. A

2 ***Arcus dentalis inferior***. Arch formed by all of the lower teeth. A

3 ***Diastema***. Space between two adjacent teeth in the same dental arch. B

4 ***Dentes incisivi*** (I). Incisors, the first three teeth on either side of the median plane, called central, intermediate and corner incisors. In Ru a fourth tooth has the form of an incisor, but it is a migrated canine tooth incorporated into the row of incisors. Therefore, in Ru there are first and second intermediate incisors. A

5 ***Dentes canini*** (C). Canine teeth, curved pointed tooth between incisors and premolars. Absent in Ru. A (5 – left side, 5a – right side canine teeth)

6 ***Dentes premolares [prae-]*** (PM). The first four cheek teeth in the full eutherian dentition. They are rostral to the molars. All except the first are preceded by deciduous teeth. A (Eutheria is a subclass of mammals – except Monotremes and Marsupials –, having a placenta through which the fetus is nourished.)

7 *Dens lupinus* (eq). Wolf tooth, the first premolar, which is rudimentary and inconstant. B

8 ***Dentes molares*** (M). Molars, the last three teeth in each jaw, one or two can be missing. They are not preceded by deciduous teeth. A

9 ***Dens sectorius*** (Car). Sectorial tooth, the largest cutting tooth in each jaw, the last upper premolar and the first lower molar. A

10 ***Dentes decidui*** (Di, Dc, Dp). Milk teeth. They are replaced by the permanent incisors, canines and premolars.

11 ***Dentes permanentes***. Permanent teeth.

12 **Lingua**. Tongue. C F

13 ***Corpus linguae***. Body of the tongue, between apex and root. C

14 ***Radix linguae***. Root of the tongue, the part caudal to the vallate papillae. G

15 ***Apex linguae***. Tip of the tongue. C

16 ***Dorsum linguae***. Dorsal part of the tongue. C

17 ***Torus linguae*** (Ru). Prominence of the dorsum caudal to the Fossa linguae in bo. D

18 ***Fossa linguae*** (bo). Deep pit on the dorsum rostral to the torus. D

19 ***Facies ventralis linguae***. Ventral surface. C

20 *Plica fimbriata*[1]. Found in man, not in domestic mammals.

21 ***Margo linguae***. Margin of the tongue. D

22 ***Tunica mucosa linguae***. Mucous membrane of the tongue.

23 ***Frenulum linguae***. Ventral median fold that attaches the tongue to the floor of the mouth. Double in su and bo. C

24 ***Papillae linguales***. The lingual papillae cover the dorsal surface of the tongue.

25 *Papillae filiformes*. Thread-like cornified epithelial processes in fe and Un with a mechanical role, connective tissue core projects into the papilla in ca. D F

26 *Papillae conicae*. Large conical mechanical papillae with a connective tissue core. D

27 *Papillae fungiformes*. Mushroom-shaped elevations of the Tunica mucosa. They bear taste buds. C D F

28 *Papillae lentiformes*. Large lens-shaped mechanical papillae. D

29 *Papillae vallatae*. Flat papillae surrounded by a circular groove, the inner wall of which bears taste buds. D F G

30 *Papillae foliatae*. Parallel folds of Tunica mucosa at the caudal end of the margin of the tongue. The walls of the intervening grooves bear taste buds. Absent in Ru. C G

31 *Papillae marginales*. Present in newborn Car and su. E

32 ***Sulcus medianus linguae***. Median dorsal groove. F

33 ***Ductus thyroglossus [thyreo-]*** (ont)[1].

34 ***Tonsilla lingualis***. Lymphatic follicles (bo, eq) and tonsillar papillae (su). G

35 *Folliculi linguales*. Rounded elevations of the mucosa, each formed by the lymphatic tissue surrounding a crypt (Fossula tonsillaris). G

36 *Papillae tonsillares* (su). Conical papillae containing lymphatic nodules on the root of the tongue. H

1) These structures were omitted from the 5th edition of the N. A. V., because they are ontogenetic terms.

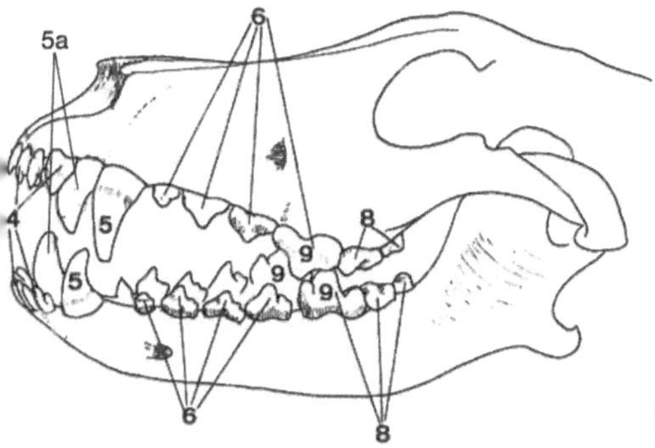

Dental arches (ca)

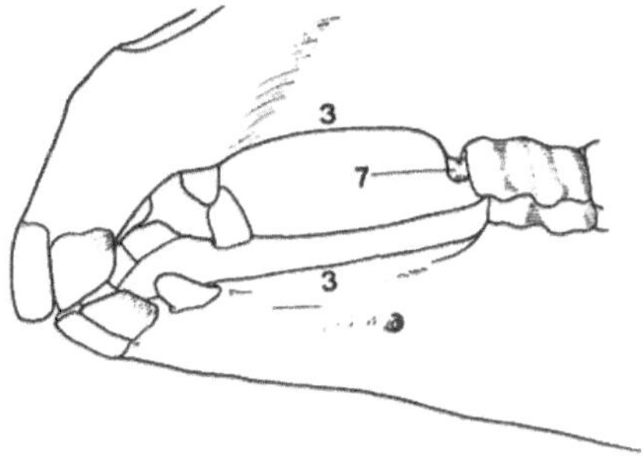

B Incisors, canine teeth and 1st and 2nd premolars (eq)

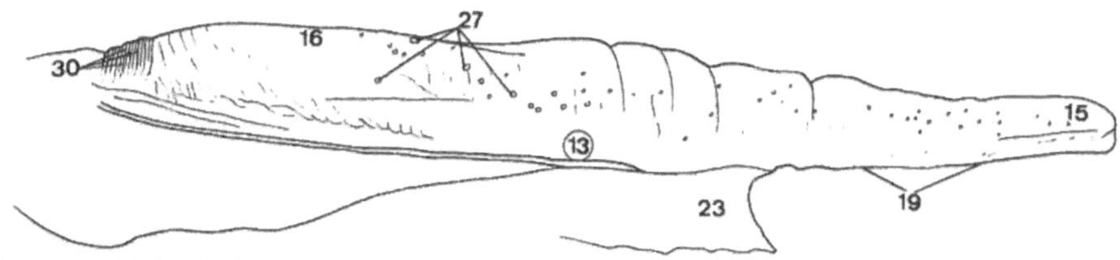

Tongue, right side (eq)

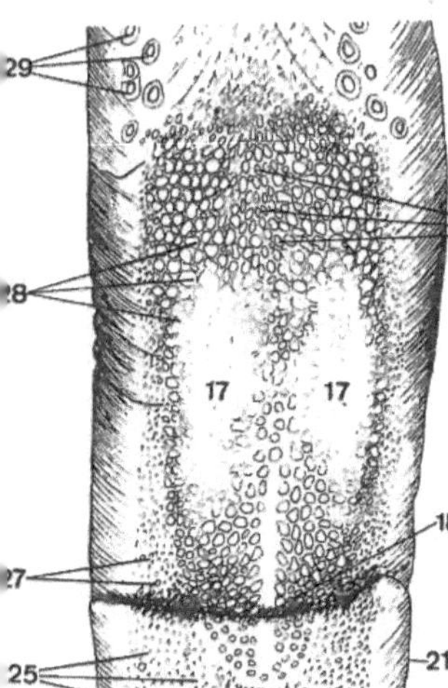

Part of dorsum of tongue (bo)

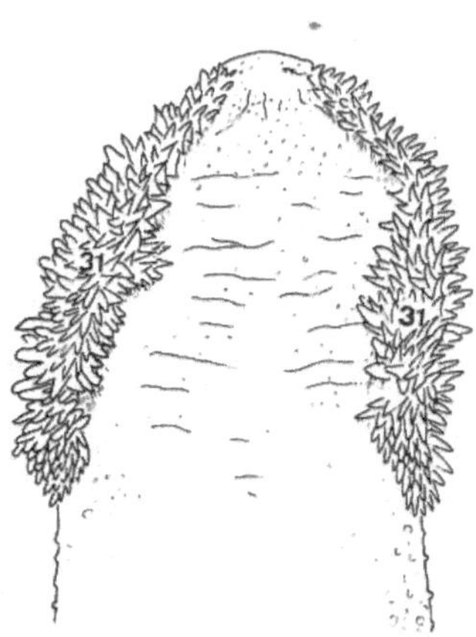

E Tip of tongue, dorsal surface (su, newborn) (Habermehl)

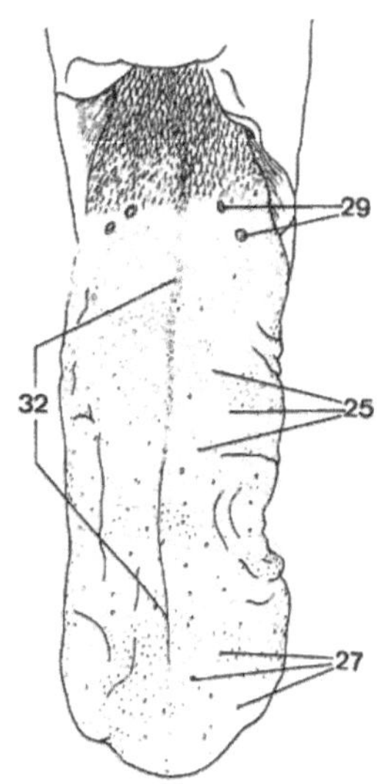

F Dorsum of tongue (ca)

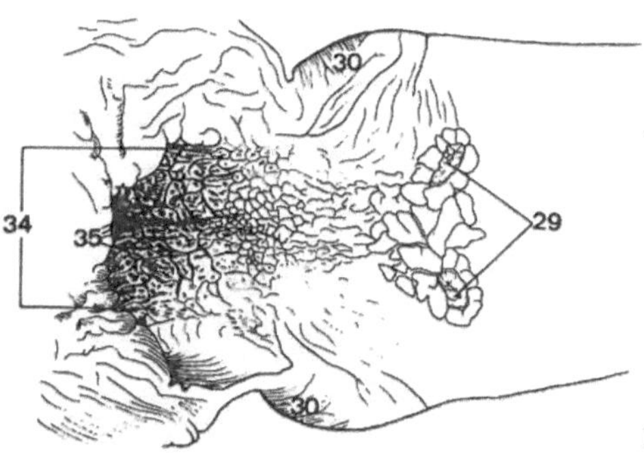

Root of tongue (eq)

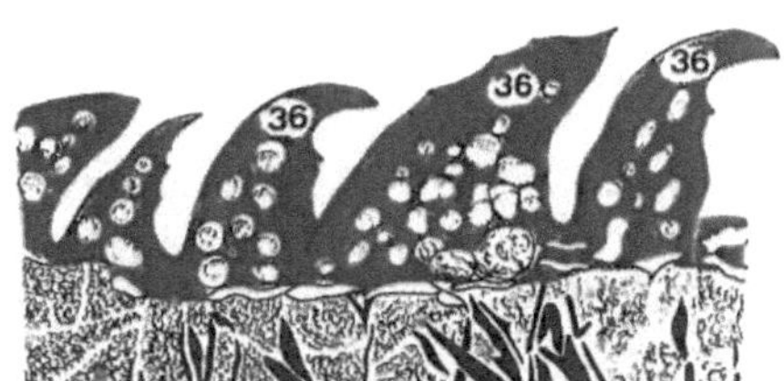

H Tonsillar papillae, histological section (su) (Vollmerhaus)

1 ***Septum linguae***. Sheet of connective tissue in the median plane. B

2 ***Lyssa*** (Car). The rostral part is a fusiform median structure in the submucosa of the ventral surface of the tongue. It consists of a collagenous sheath enclosing fat, striated muscle, and chondroid cells. It is continued caudally between the Mm. genioglossi by a fibrous cord. A

3 ***Cartilago dorsi linguae*** (eq). Palpable median dorsal thickening of the lamina propria. It contains isolated chondroid and fat cells. B

4 ***Aponeurosis linguae***. Dense layer of connective tissue which covers the musculature of the tongue and to which the muscles are attached. On the dorsum it is fused with the Lamina propria mucosae. B

5 **Musculi linguae**. Muscles of the tongue.

6 ***M. genioglossus***. It consists of a tendon ventrally, and muscle fibers oriented rostrally, dorsally, and caudally. O: Pars incisiva mandibulae. T: Enters the tongue ventrally, parallel to the median plane, as far back as the hyoid bone. Its primary action is to protrude the tongue. A E

7 ***M. hyoglossus***. O: Os hyoideum. T: Enters the tongue between M. genioglossus medially and M. styloglossus laterally. It retracts and depresses the tongue. A E

8 ***M. styloglossus***. O: Ventral end of lateral aspect of Stylohyoideum. T: Apex linguae. It is the most lateral of the extrinsic muscles and serves to retract the tongue or turn the apex to one side. A E

9 ***M. lingualis proprius***. Intrinsic musculature of the tongue. B

10 *Fibrae longitudinales superficiales*. Superficial longitudinal fibers. B

11 *Fibrae longitudinales profundae*. Deep longitudinal fibers. Occur in eq. B

12 *Fibrae transversae*. Transverse fibers. B

13 *Fibrae perpendiculares*. Perpendicular fibers. B

14 **PHARYNX**. Musculomembranous cross way of the respiratory and digestive tracts between the oral and nasal cavities rostrally, and the esophagus and larynx caudally.

15 **Cavum pharyngis**. Divided into nasal, oral, and laryngeal parts. The parts of the pharynx in domestic mammals do not correspond to those in man, because of the long soft palate and the more obtuse cervicocephalic angle in the domestic mammals.

16 ***Pars nasalis pharyngis***. The part caudodorsal to the soft palate. It extends from the choanae to the Ostium intrapharyngeum. C

17 *Fornix pharyngis*. The most dorsal part of the cavity. C

18 *Septum pharyngis* (su, Ru). Membranous continuation of the Septum nasi in the fornix. C

19 *Tonsilla pharyngea*. On the caudodorsal wall of the nasopharynx, in su and Ru on the Septum pharyngis. C

20 ***Folliculi tonsillares***. Occur in su and eq. A tonsillar follicle is composed of lymphatic tissue surrounding a crypt with its orifice (the tonsillar fossula). C

21 *Ostium pharyngeum tubae auditivae*. Pharyngeal opening of the auditory tube. C D

22 *Torus tubarius**. Swelling caudodorsal to the Ostium tubae, caused by the medial lamina of the cartilage of the auditory tube. D

23 *Torus levatorius**. Low ridge running rostroventrally from the Ostium pharyngeum tubae to the soft palate, and caused by the M. levator veli palatini. D

24 *Tonsilla tubaria*. Tubal tonsil, occurs at the Ostium pharyngeum tubae in su and Ru. C

25 *Recessus pharyngeus*. Niche at the caudodorsal angle of the nasopharynx in Un. Absent in Car. D

26 *(Bursa pharyngea)*. Median dorsal epithelial pouch. Inconstant vestige occurring only in eq, either as a tubular extension of Recessus pharyngeus or as an independent evagination. D

27 *Diverticulum pharyngeum*. Median caudal blind sac formed by the mucous membrane of the nasopharynx dorsal to the esophagus in su only. It has nothing to do with the Bursa pharyngea. C

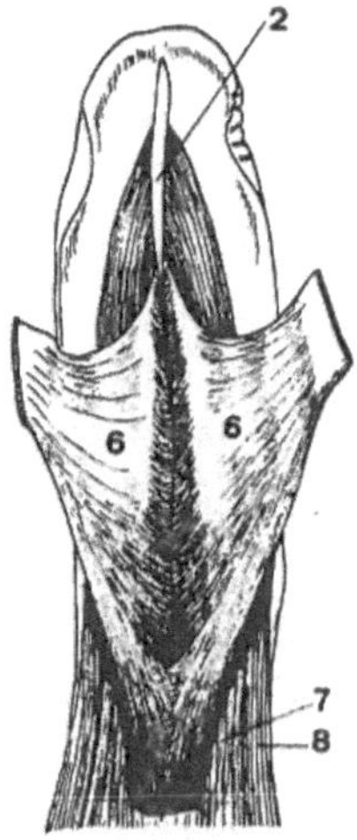

A Tongue (geniohyoid muscles and part of mucosa removed, symmetrical genioglossal muscles separated), ventral aspect (ca)

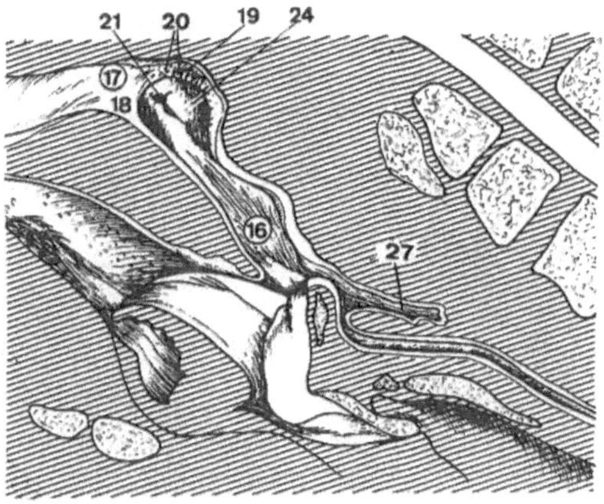

C Pharynx, paramedian section, right half medial aspect (su)

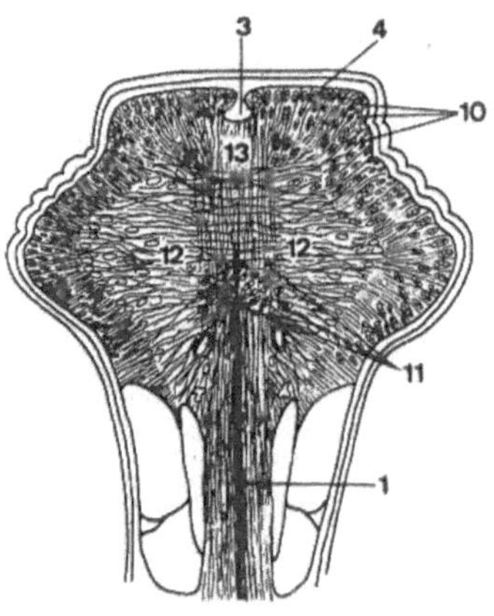

B Tongue, transverse section (eq)

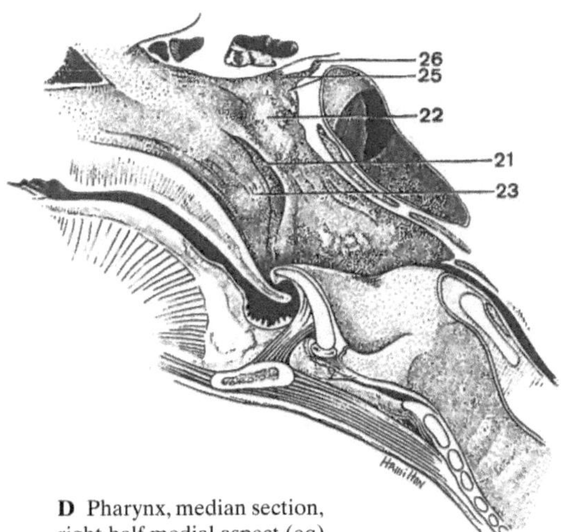

D Pharynx, median section, right half medial aspect (eq)

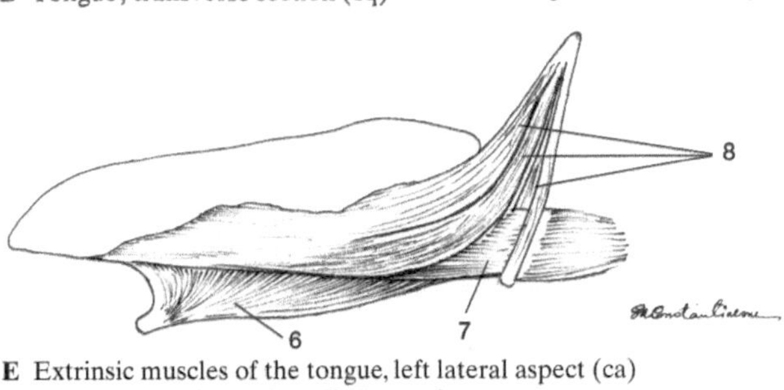

E Extrinsic muscles of the tongue, left lateral aspect (ca) (modified and redrawn from R. Barone)

1 ***Ostium intrapharyngeum***. Passage between Pars nasalis and Pars laryngea pharyngis. It is formed by the free border of the soft palate and the right and left Arcus palatopharyngeus. A

2 ***Palatum molle [Velum palatinum]***. Soft palate. A D

3 *Uvula [palatina]* (su). Short median projection on the free border of the soft palate. A

4 *Arcus palatoglossus*. Symmetrical ridge or fold of mucosa extending from the soft palate to the tongue at the boundary between mouth and pharynx. A D

5 *Arcus palatopharyngeus*. Symmetrical mucosal fold extending from the free border of the soft palate around the Ostium intrapharyngeum. They meet on the caudal wall of the pharynx. A D

6 ***Isthmus faucium***. Orifice between Cavum oris and Pars oralis pharyngis, bounded by Arcus palatoglossi, soft palate, and tongue. A D

7 ***Pars oralis pharyngis***. Extends from the Arcus palatoglossi to the base of the epiglottis. The cavity corresponding to the posterior part of the human Pars oralis is cut off by the long soft palate and belongs to the Pars nasalis. A

8 *Fauces*. Part of the oropharynx just caudal to Arcus palatoglossi, bounded laterally by Tonsilla palatina and the surrounding structures. In domestic mammals the Pars oralis pharyngis consists mainly of the Fauces. D (singular FAUX, plural FAUCES)

9 **Tonsilla palatina**. The tonsil related to the lateral attachment of the soft palate between Arcus palatoglossus and palatopharyngeus muscle. It does not occur in su. D

10 **Folliculi tonsillares**. A tonsillar follicle is a crypt, its orifice (the fossula), and its surrounding lymphatic tissue (Lymphonoduli). B

11 **Fossulae tonsillares**. A tonsillar fossula is the orifice of a follicle. It opens on the mucosa or into a tonsillar sinus. B

12 **Cryptae tonsillares**. A tonsillar crypt is a blind epithelial tubule extending inward from a fossula tonsillaris. B

13 **Lymphonoduli [Noduli lymphatici]**. A tonsillar follicle contains lymphonoduli. B

14 **Sinus tonsillaris**. Deep, narrowmouthed cavity in the palatine tonsil of Ru. B

15 **Capsula tonsillaris**. Tonsillar capsule. B

16 **Plica semilunaris**. Fold of mucosa from the ventral surface of the lateral part of the soft palate in Car. It forms the medial wall of the Fossa tonsillaris. D

17 **Fossa tonsillaris**. Depression containing the palatine tonsil in Car. D

18 **Fossa supratonsillaris**. Dorsal part of Fossa tonsillaris in fe.

19 *Tonsilla veli palatini* (su, eq). Mass of follicles on the oral surface of the soft palate. A C

20 *Tonsilla paraepiglottica* (fe, su, ov, cap). On the Plica aryepiglottica in fe, lateral to base of epiglottis in su, ov, cap. C

21 **Sulcus tonsillaris (su)**. Deep groove in the Tonsilla paraepiglottica. C

22 *Vallecula epiglottica**. Depression between the tongue and the epiglottis and between Plica glossoepiglottica mediana and lateralis. C, D

23 **Plica glossoepiglottica mediana**. Median fold from the tongue to the epiglottis. C

24 **Plica glossoepiglottica lateralis**. Lateral fold from the tongue to the epiglottis. C

25 ***Pars laryngea pharyngis***. Part of the pharynx ventral to the Ostium intrapharyngeum. It extends from the base of the epiglottis to the esophagus. A D

26 *Recessus piriformis*. Channel between epiglottis, Plica aryepiglottica and arytenoid cartilage medially, and Membrana thyrohyoidea and thyroid cartilage laterally. C

27 *Vestibulum esophagi [Pars esophagea, oesophagea]*. Part of the laryngopharynx between the arytenoid cartilages and the beginning of the esophagus. A D

28 *Limen pharyngoesophageum [-oesophageum]* (Car). Interior boundary between pharynx and esophagus, formed by a circular fold in fe, by a glandular thickening in ca. D

29 ***Fascia pharyngobasilaris***. Pharyngeal fascia that attaches to the Basis cranii. D

30 ***Tela submucosa***. Layer of loose connective tissue and fat under the Tunica mucosa. D

31 ***Tunica mucosa***. Covered by pseudostratified columnar epithelium in the Pars nasalis, by stratified squamous epithelium in the other parts. D

32 ***Gll. pharyngeae***. Pharyngeal glands. D

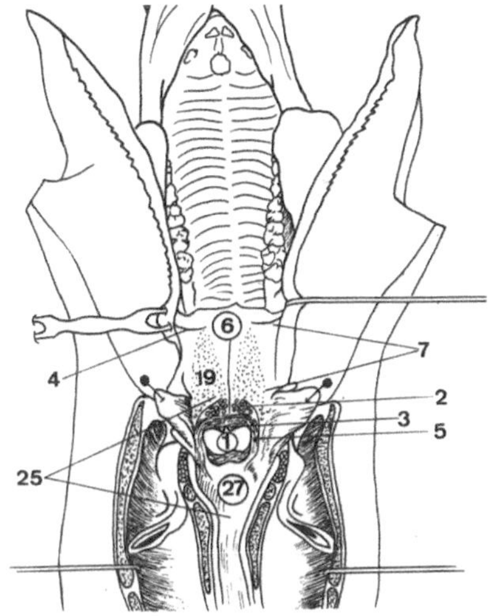

A Palate (tongue and larynx bisected and retracted, esophagus opened), ventral aspect (su)

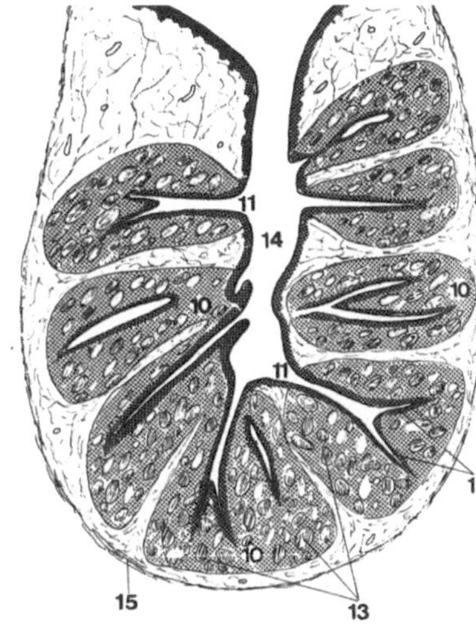

B Palatine tonsil, histological section (bo)

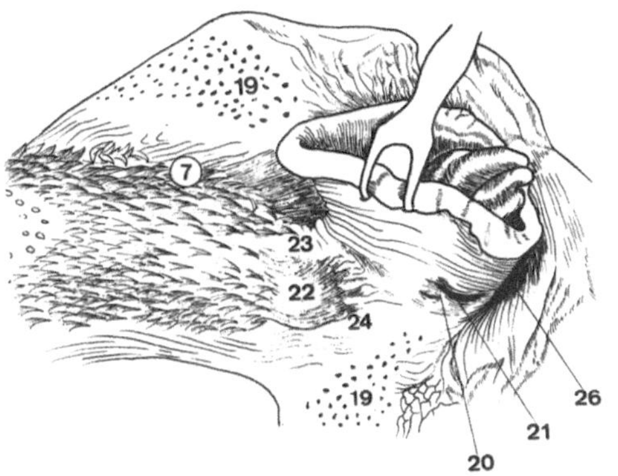

C Pars oralis and Pars laryngea of pharynx (soft palate bisected and retracted), dorsolateral aspect (su)

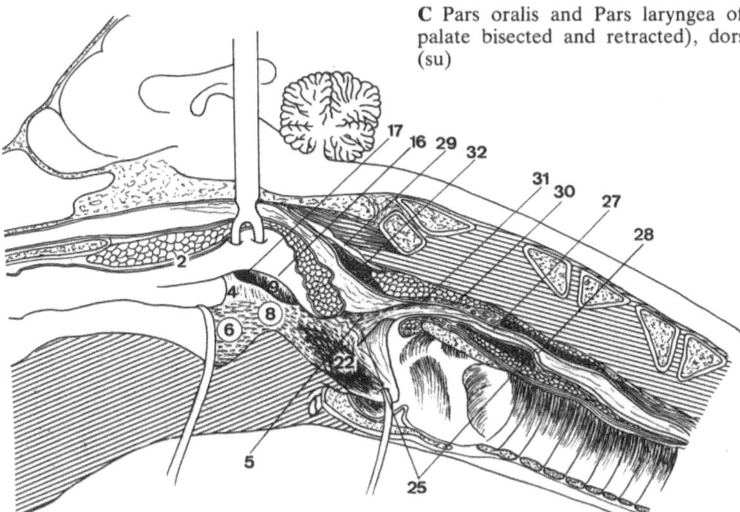

D Pharynx (tongue and epiglottis retracted), median section, right half medial aspect (ca)

1 **Tunica muscularis pharyngis**. The muscular coat of the pharynx is composed of the following striated muscles.

2 ***Raphe [Rhaphe] pharyngis***. Median dorsal line of termination of the pharyngeal constrictors. A

3 ***Mm. constrictores pharyngis rostrales***. M. palatopharyngeus is an important part of the Tunica muscularis pharyngis, although it is listed as a muscle of the soft palate. Functionally it is one of the rostral constrictors of the pharynx.

4 *M. pterygopharyngeus*. O: Os pterygoideum and Aponeurosis palatina, except eq (Os pterygoideum only). T: Raphe pharyngis. It is also a rostral constrictor of the pharynx. A B

5 *M. stylopharyngeus rostralis*. O: distal half of the medial aspect of the Stylohyoideum. T: Raphe pharyngis. Occurs in Ru and occasionally in eq. It is a rostral constrictor of the pharynx in Ru. A

6 ***M. stylopharyngeus caudalis***. O: proximal half of the medial aspect of the Stylohyoideum. Passes between the rostral constrictors and the M. hyopharyngeus. T: wall of pharynx, in bo mainly attached to the thyroid cartilage. Dilator of the pharynx, in bo elevator of the larynx. This is the only M. stylopharyngeus in species other than Ru. A B

7 ***M. hyopharyngeus [M. constrictor pharyngis medius]***. O: Ceratohyoideum and Thyrohyoideum. T: Raphe pharyngis. It is the sole middle constrictor of the pharynx. A B E

8 ***Mm. constrictores pharyngis caudales***.

9 *M. thyropharyngeus [thyreo-]*. O: Linea obliqua on the thyroid cartilage. T: Raphe pharyngis. A D E

10 *M. cricopharyngeus*. O: cricoid cartilage. T: Raphe pharyngis. A D E

11 ***Spatium retropharyngeum***. Dorsocaudal space to the pharynx. A

12 ***Spatium lateropharyngeum***. Lateral space to the pharynx.

13 **Musculi palati et faucium**. Muscles of the palate and fauces.

14 ***Aponeurosis palatina***. Tendinous lamina in the rostral part of the soft palate, attached to Os palatinum. B

15 ***M. levator veli palatini***. O: Pars tympanica ossis temporalis (Processus muscularis), in eq also cartilage of the auditory tube. Raises the soft palate. T : soft palate, to unite with the contralateral muscle. A B

16 ***M. tensor veli palatini***. O: Pars tympanica ossis temporalis (Processus muscularis). T: Aponeurosis palatina. A

17 ***M. palatinus***. O: Lamina horizontalis ossis palatini; in eq Aponeurosis palatina. T: blends with the M. palatopharyngeus. Shortens the soft palate. B

18 ***M. palatopharyngeus***. O: palatine aponeurosis, M. palatinus. T: Raphe pharyngis. Sphincter of the nasopharynx and Ostium intrapharyngeum. See 3 B D

19 **CANALIS ALIMENTARIUS**. Esophagus, stomach, and intestines.

20 **ESOPHAGUS [OESOPHAGUS]**. Tube extending from the pharynx to the stomach.

21 ***Pars cervicalis***. The part from the pharynx to the first rib. C

22 ***Pars thoracica***. The part from the first rib to the diaphragm. C

23 ***Pars abdominalis***. The short part between the diaphragm and the stomach. C

24 ***Tunica adventitia***. Outer coat of connective tissue. F

25 ***Tunica muscularis***. Straited muscle, except a caudal segment of smooth muscle in fe, su and eq. D F

26 *Tendo cricoesophageus [-oesophageus]*. Attaches the esophageal musculature to the cricoid and arytenoid cartilages. D

27 *M. esophageus [oesophageus] longitudinalis dorsalis*. Dorsal longitudinal esophageal muscle. E

28 *M. esophageus [oesophageus] longitudinalis lateralis*. O: larynx (Car, Ru) or pharynx (su, eq). T: lateral surface of the esophagus. D E

29 *M. esophageus [oesophageus] longitudinalis ventralis*. O: cricoesophageal tendon. E

30 ***M. bronchoesophageus [-oesophageus]***. Smooth muscle fibers from the main left bronchus to the esophagus[1].

31 ***M. pleuroesophageus [-oesophageus]*** (ca). Smooth muscle tract between the esophagus and the left mediastinal pleura[1].

32 ***Tela submucosa***. Layer of loose connective tissue and fat under the Tunica mucosa.

33 ***Tunica mucosa***. Covered by stratified squamous epithelium. F

34 *Lamina muscularis mucosae*. Incomplete in domestic mammals. F

35 ***Gll. esophageae [oesophageae]***. Mucous glands in the submucosa. In fe, Ru, eq restricted to the cranial end. F

[1] The definitions are taken from the "Pocket Atlas of Human Anatomy" by Feneis and Dauber 2000. Barone (1976) considers that the names of these two muscles are a little abusive, because their muscle fibers vary with species and individuals.

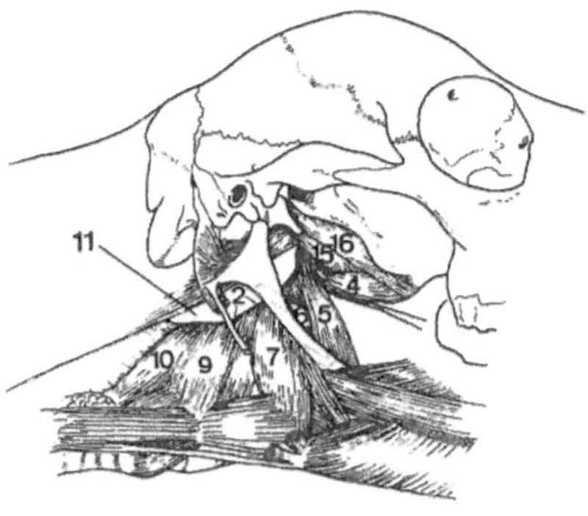

A Pharyngeal muscles, right side (ov) (Habel)

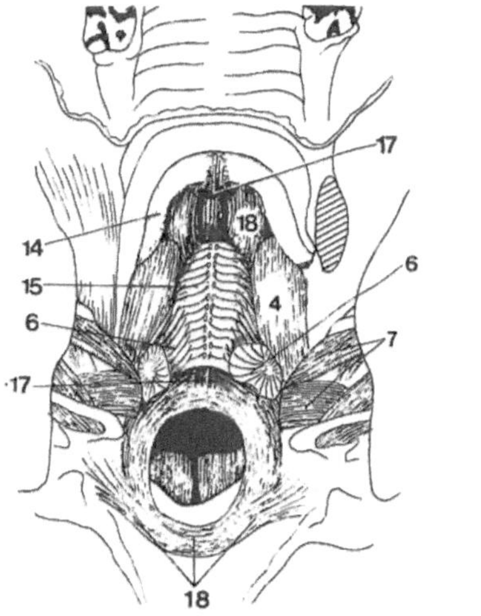

B Muscles of the soft palate (left pterygoid muscles removed), ventral aspect (su)

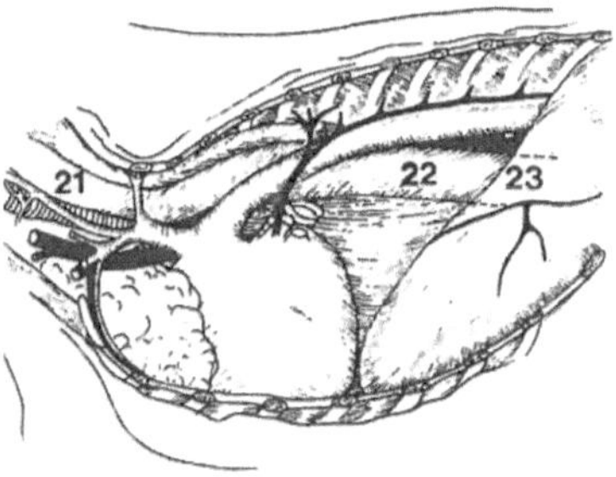

C Thoracic cavity and base of neck, left side (ov) (Habel)

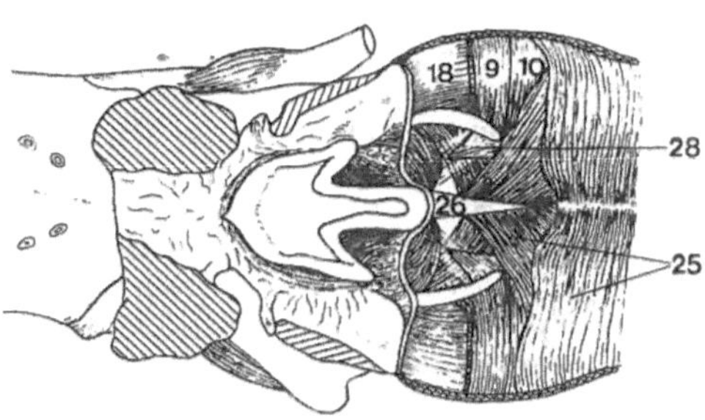

D Muscles of pharynx and esophagus opened dorsally (ca)

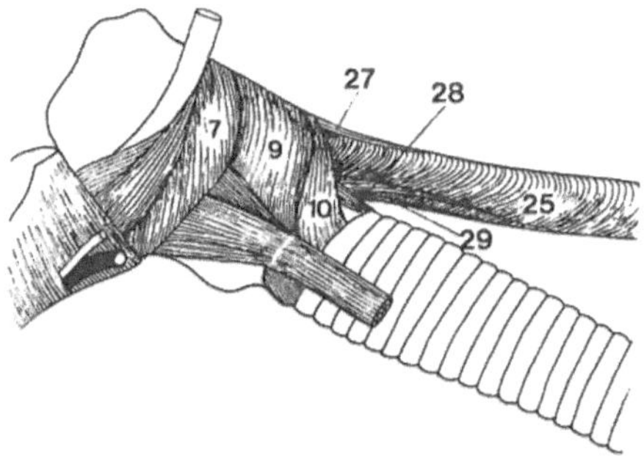

E Muscles of pharynx and esophagus, left side (cap)

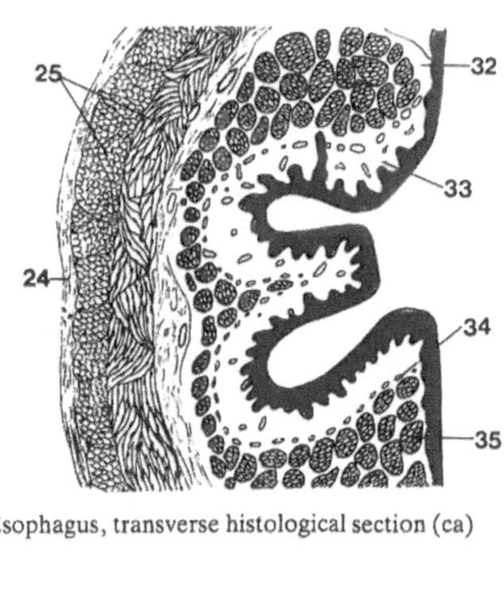

F Esophagus, transverse histological section (ca)

1 **VENTRICULUS [GASTER]**. Stomach. It is divided into four compartments in Ru.

2 ***Facies parietalis***. Surface that faces the abdominal wall and liver. A B

3 ***Facies visceralis***. Surface that faces the intestines. C

4 ***Curvatura ventriculi major***. Greater curvature. A

5 ***Curvatura ventriculi minor***. Lesser curvature. A

6 *Incisura angularis*. Notch on the Curvatura minor between Corpus ventriculi and Pars pylorica. A B

7 ***Pars cardiaca***. Region around the esophageal opening. A B

8 *Ostium cardiacum*. Opening between the esophagus and the stomach. C

9 ***Incisura cardiaca***. Cardiac notch between esophagus and fundus. A

10 ***Fundus ventriculi***. Blind sac on the left of the cardiac part. The term is derived from the depth of this part of the human stomach as seen from an abdominal incision. The fundus is lined by proper gastric glands, except su (cardiac glands) and eq (nonglandular). A

11 *Saccus cecus [caecus] ventriculi* (eq). Blind sac, the large Fundus ventriculi of eq. Saccus cecus, Pars cardiaca and the adjacent part of the Corpus ventriculi of eq are lined by stratified squamous epithelium. B

12 *Diverticulum ventriculi* (su). Flattened conical pouch of the fundus. It projects caudally and to the right and is lined by cardiac glands. C

13 ***Corpus ventriculi***. Main part of the stomach, between the fundus and Pars pylorica. It is lined by Glandulae gastricae [propriae]. A B

14 *Sulcus ventriculi*. Gastric groove. It extends along the inside of the Curvatura minor from the cardiac orifice to the pylorus. C. In Ru the Sulcus ventriculi is divided by the Ostium reticuloomasicum and Ostium omasoabomasicum into three segments: Sulcus reticuli, Sulcus omasi, and Sulcus abomasi. See 158.7, .19, .31.

15 ***Pars pylorica***. Pyloric part of the stomach, between Incisura angularis and Pylorus. A

16 *Antrum pyloricum*. First, wider portion of the Pars pylorica. A B

17 *Canalis pyloricus*. Second, short narrow segment of the Pars pylorica, just before the pylorus. A B

18 ***Pylorus***. Distal constriction of the stomach containing the sphincter. A

19 *Ostium pyloricum*. Opening between the stomach and the duodenum. C

20 *Torus pyloricus* (su, Ru). Protuberance in the pylorus formed by the circular muscle at the end of the Curvatura minor, fat, and the mucous membrane. C

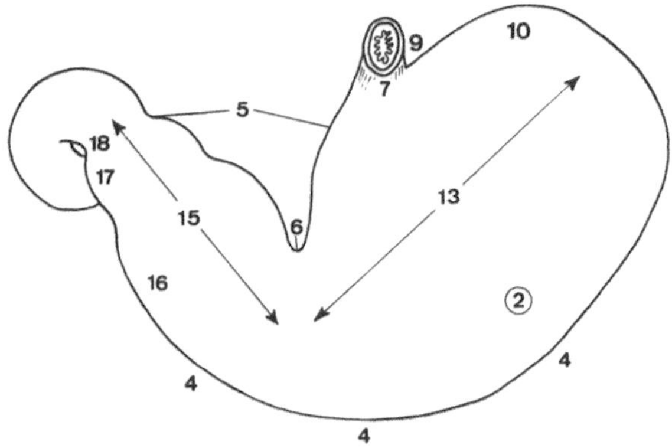

A Stomach, parietal surface (ca)

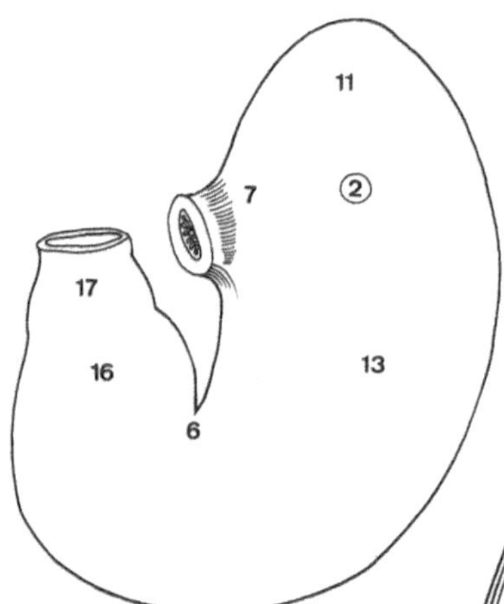

B Stomach, parietal surface (eq)

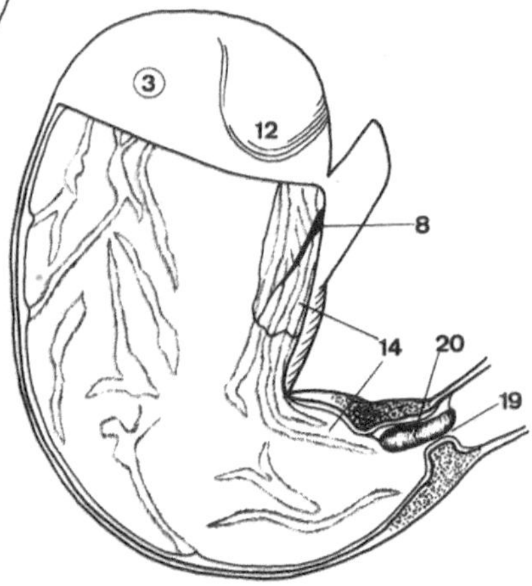

C Stomach (most of the visceral wall removed), visceral aspect (su)

1 **Proventriculus**. Forestomach in Ru, divided into three compartments: Rumen, Reticulum, and Omasum.

2 ***Ruminoreticulum***. Term often employed to indicate the morphological and physiological unity of the two compartments. C

3 **Rumen**. Largest compartment of the ruminant stomach. A B C

4 ***Facies parietalis***. Surface facing the body wall to the left and ventrally. A

5 ***Facies visceralis***. Surface facing the intestines, to the right. B

6 ***Curvatura dorsalis***. Dorsal curvature. A

7 ***Curvatura ventralis***. Ventral curvature. B

8 ***Extremitas cranialis***. Cranial end, adjacent to the Reticulum. A

9 ***Extremitas caudalis***. Caudal end, the blind sacs. A

10 ***Atrium ruminis [Saccus cranialis]***. Lies between Reticulum and Saccus ventralis (Recessus ruminis). It is morphologically and functionally distinct from the dorsal sac. A C

11 ***Saccus dorsalis***. The dorsal sac is dorsal to the longitudinal grooves. A C

12 *Saccus cecus [caecus] caudodorsalis*. Caudodorsal blind sac. A C

13 ***Saccus ventralis***. The ventral sac is ventral to the longitudinal grooves. A C

14 *Recessus ruminis*. Cranial end of the ventral sac. A C

15 *Saccus cecus [caecus] caudoventralis*. Caudoventral blind sac. A C

16 ***Sulcus cranialis***. Cranial groove between Atrium and Recessus ruminis. A (The sulci [sing. sulcus] are external grooves, which correspond inside to muscular prominences such as pillars or pilae [sing. pila] and mucosal folds or plicae [sing. plica].)

17 ***Sulcus caudalis***. Separates the caudodorsal from the caudoventral blind sac. A B

18 ***Sulcus longitudinalis dexter***. Right longitudinal groove. B

19 ***Sulcus accessorius dexter***. Right accessory groove, dorsal to the right longitudinal groove. B

20 ***Insula ruminis***. Island of the rumen, elliptical area enclosed by the right longitudinal and accessory grooves. B C

21 ***Sulcus longitudinalis sinister***. Left longitudinal groove. A

22 ***Sulcus accessorius sinister***. Left accessory groove, a dorsal branch of the left longitudinal groove. A

23 ***Sulcus coronarius dorsalis***. Dorsal coronary groove, limits the caudodorsal blind sac. A B

24 ***Sulcus coronarius ventralis***. Ventral coronary groove, limits the caudoventral blind sac. A B

25 ***Pila cranialis***. Cranial pillar, a muscular prominence projecting into the cavity of the rumen between Atrium and Recessus ruminis. C

26 ***Pila caudalis***. Caudal pillar, between the caudodorsal and caudoventral blind sacs. C

27 ***Pila longitudinalis dextra***. Right longitudinal pillar. C

28 ***Pila accessoria dextra***. Right accessory pillar, dorsal to the right longitudinal pillar. C

29 ***Pila longitudinalis sinistra***. Left longitudinal pillar, corresponding to the Sulcus longitudinalis sinister.

30 ***Pila accessoria sinistra***. Dorsal branch of the left longitudinal pillar, corresponding to the Sulcus accessorius sinister.

31 ***Pila coronaria dorsalis***. Left dorsal coronary pillar, limits the caudodorsal blind sac. C

32 ***Pila coronaria ventralis***. Left ventral coronary pillar, limits the caudoventral blind sac. C

33 ***Ostium intraruminale***. Opening between the dorsal and ventral sacs. It is bounded by the cranial, caudal, and longitudinal pillars. C

34 ***Sulcus ruminoreticularis***. Ruminoreticular groove. A

35 ***Plica ruminoreticularis***. Ruminoreticular fold. C

36 ***Ostium ruminoreticulare***. Opening between rumen and reticulum. C

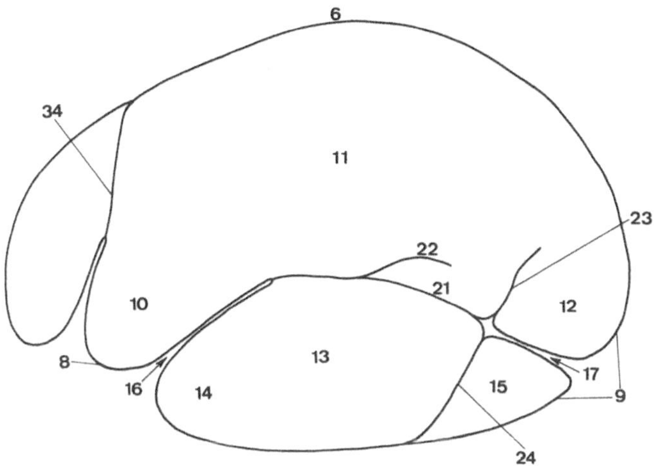

A Rumen and reticulum, left side (bo)

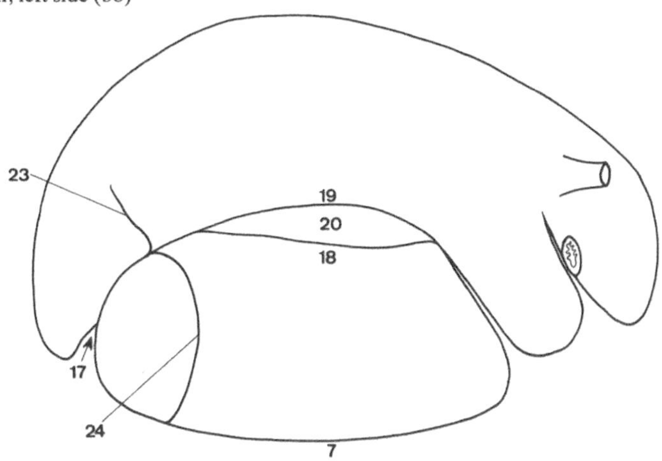

B Rumen and reticulum, right side (bo)

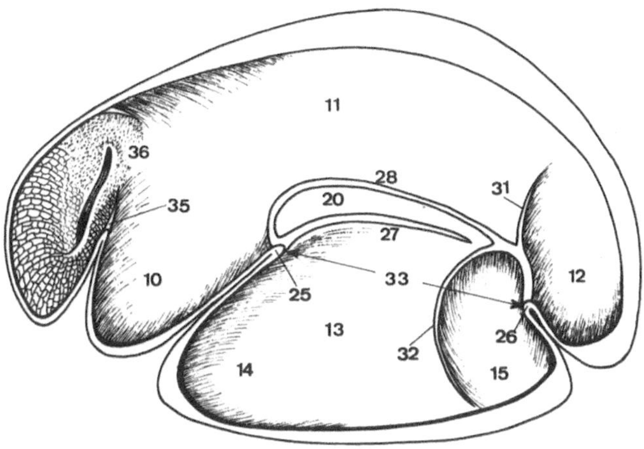

C Rumen and reticulum, interior viewed from the left (bo)

1 **Reticulum.** Most cranial compartment of the ruminant stomach, named for its network of honeycomb-like mucosal crests. A

2 ***Facies diaphragmatica.*** Surface in contact with the diaphragm. B

3 ***Facies visceralis.*** Surface toward the rumen. B

4 ***Curvatura major.*** The greater curvature courses on the left side and ventrally. B

5 ***Curvatura minor.*** The lesser curvature faces to the right and caudally and is connected to the omasum. A

6 ***Fundus reticuli.*** Rounded ventral portion. A

7 ***Sulcus reticuli.*** The reticular groove extends from the cardiac orifice to the reticuloomasal orifice along the inside of the lesser curvature. B

8 *Fundus sulci reticuli.* Floor of the reticular groove, between the labia. B

9 *Labium dextrum.* Right lip (at the cardiac orifice). The right lip overlaps the left one in a X-shaped crossing. B

10 *Labium sinistrum.* Left lip (at the cardiac orifice). B

11 ***Ostium reticuloomasicum.*** Opening from the reticulum to the omasum. B C

12 **Omasum.** Third compartment of the ruminant stomach. A C

13 ***Corpus omasi.*** Body of the omasum, between the Curvatura and the Basis. A

14 ***Facies parietalis.*** Side facing the liver. A

15 ***Facies visceralis.*** Side facing the rumen.

16 ***Curvatura omasi.*** Faces dorsally, caudally, and to the right. A

17 ***Basis omasi.*** The base faces cranially and to the left and is attached to the reticulum and to the abomasum. It contains the Sulcus omasi. A

18 ***Collum omasi.*** The neck is attached to the reticulum and contains the Ostium reticuloomasicum. A

19 ***Sulcus omasi.*** Short segment of the Sulcus ventriculi in the omasum. It extends from the Ostium reticuloomasicum to the Ostium omasoabomasicum. C

20 ***Canalis omasi.*** Part of Sulcus ventriculi, it is formed by the Sulcus and the free borders of the Laminae omasi. C

21 ***Pila omasi.*** The transverse muscular pillar at the abomasal end of the Sulcus omasi. C

22 ***Sulcus omasoabomasicus.*** External groove between omasum and abomasum. A

23 ***Ostium omasoabomasicum.*** C

24 **Abomasum.** Glandular part of the ruminant stomach. A B C

25 ***Facies parietalis.*** Side facing the abdominal wall. A

26 ***Facies visceralis.*** Side facing the Rumen. C

27 ***Curvatura major.*** Greater curvature oriented ventrally. B

28 ***Curvatura minor.*** Lesser curvature oriented dorsally. A

29 ***Fundus abomasi.*** Dilation cranial and to the left of the Ostium omasoabomasicum. B

30 ***Corpus abomasi.*** Body of the abomasum. A C

31 ***Sulcus abomasi.*** Part of Sulcus ventriculi, it is the groove between mucosal folds along the inside of the lesser curvature. 163 B

32 ***Pars pylorica.*** Pyloric part. A C

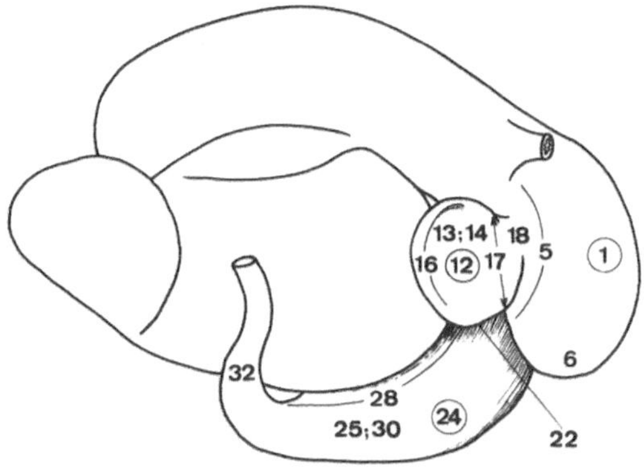

A Stomach, right side (ov)

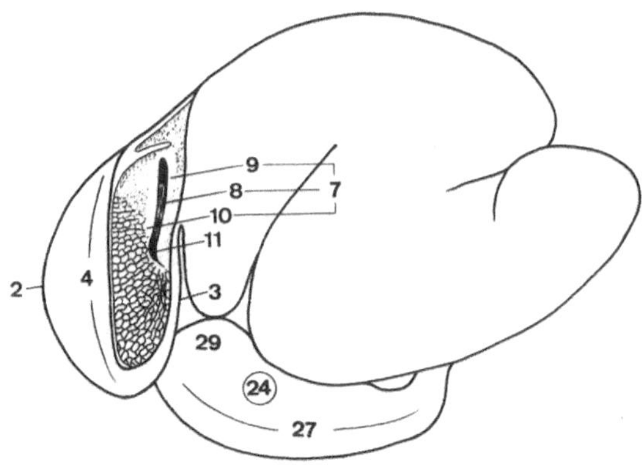

B Stomach, left side (part fo the wall of the reticulum removed) (ov)

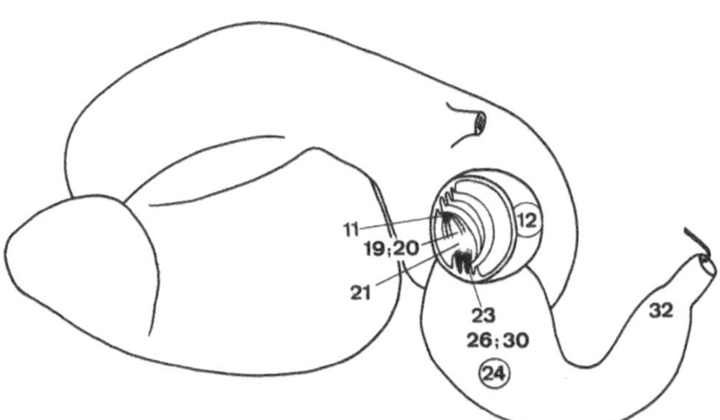

C Stomach, right side (omasum and abomasum drawn cranially and to the right, part of visceral wall of omasum removed) (ov)

1 **Paries ventriculi**. Wall of the stomach.

2 ***Tunica serosa***. Serous membrane. It is composed of mesothelium and a layer of connective tissue. D

3 ***Tela subserosa***. Layer of loose connective tissue and fat under the Tunica serosa. D

4 ***Tunica muscularis***. Main muscular coat. A D

5 *Stratum longitudinale*. Outer, longitudinal layer. It is incomplete. A

6 *Fibrae ruminoreticuloabomasicae*. Sheets of superficial muscle connecting the Reticulum, Atrium ruminis, Saccus ventralis, and Fundus abomasi on the left side. B

7 *Fibrae obliquae externae*. On the parietal and visceral surface of the fundus and cardiac portion of the corpus, the external muscle fibers are oblique. A

8 *Stratum circulare*. Middle, circular, and most extensive layer. A C

9 **M. sphincter pylori**. The thickened circular muscle at the pylorus. A

10 *Fibrae obliquae internae*. Internal oblique fibers that spread out from the Pars cardiaca toward the Curvatura major. A C

11 **Ansa cardiaca**. Cardiac loop, tract of internal oblique fibers that passes from one side of the Sulcus ventriculi on the other around the Ostium cardiacum. In Ru it forms the longitudinal musculature of the lips of the Sulcus reticuli. C

12 *M. sphincter cardiae*. Muscle around the Ostium cardiacum, formed by the Ansa cardiaca and the Stratum circulare. C

13 *M. sphincter reticuloomasicus*. Reticuloomasal sphincter, formed by fibers from the lips of the Sulcus reticuli and by the circular muscle. C

14 ***Tela submucosa***. Loose connective tissue under the mucous membrane. D

15 ***Tunica mucosa***. Mucous membrane. In Car it is entirely glandular, in Un it presents a Pars glandularis and a Pars nonglandularis. D E F G H I

16 *Pars glandularis*. Glandular part of the Tunica mucosa. D H

17 **Plicae gastricae**. Folds of the mucous membrane, generally longitudinal. H

18 *Lamina muscularis mucosae*. Thin sheet of smooth muscle forming the deepest layer of the mucous membrane, gives off bundles into the Lamina propria. D E F G

19 *Areae gastricae*. Gastric fields of 1–5 mm in diameter, bounded by a network of Sulci gastrici. D

20 *Sulci gastrici*. Grooves between Areae gastricae. D

21 *Plicae villosae*. Microscopic projections between the Foveolae gastricae in the Pars pylorica. G

22 *Foveolae gastricae*. Microscopic gastric pits, into which glands open. D E F G

23 *Glandulae cardiacae*. Cardiac glands. In su they occupy the fundus, the diverticulum, and part of the corpus. In other species they are limited to a narrow zone at the beginning of the Pars glandularis. E

24 **Glandulae gastricae [propriae]**. Proper gastric glands, characterized by zymogenic and parietal cells. They line Corpus and in Car also Fundus ventriculi, in Ru Corpus and Fundus abomasi. F

25 *Glandulae pyloricae*. Pyloric glands, found in the Pars pylorica. G

26 *Lymphonoduli [Noduli lymphatici] gastrici*. Gastric lymph nodules. E

27 ***Pars nonglandularis***. Nonglandular part of the Tunica mucosa, covered by stratified squamous epithelium in Un. H

28 ***Margo plicatus*** (su, eq). Sinuous thick border between the nonglandular and glandular parts. H

29 ***Papillae ruminis***. Finger-, tongue-, or leaf-shaped projections of the mucous membrane, about 1 cm long. I

30 ***Cellulae reticuli***. Cells of the reticulum, 4-, 5-, or 6-sided recesses enclosed by Cristae reticuli resembling a honeycomb. I

31 ***Cristae reticuli***. Reticular crests, permanent folds of the mucous membrane. I

32 ***Papillae reticuli***. The conical papillae on the crests and in the cells of the reticulum. I

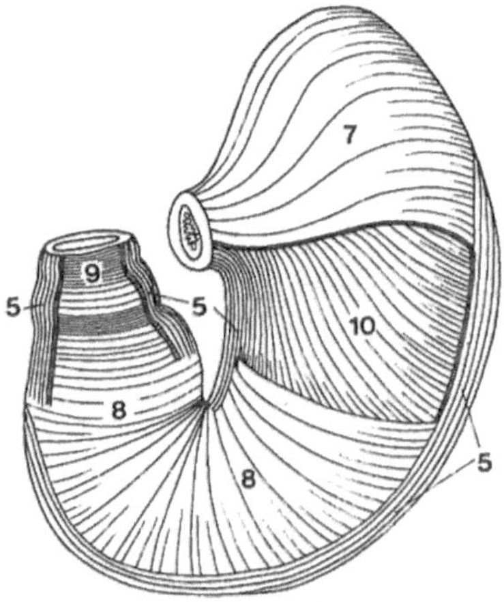

A Stomach musculature (parts of longitudinal, circular, and external oblique layers removed) eeq)

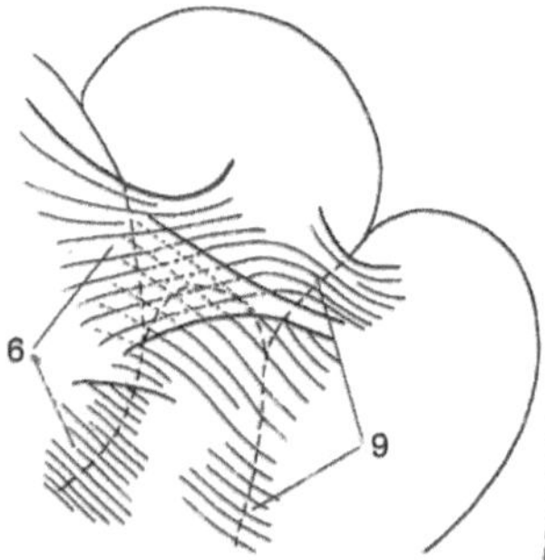

B Parts of ruminant stomach, left side (reticulum left, ventral sac of rumen right, atrium above, fundus of abomasum below) (Hofmann)

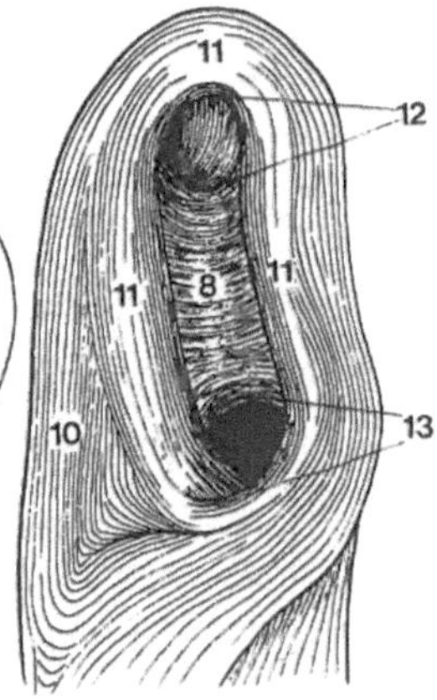

C Musculature of the reticular groove (bo)

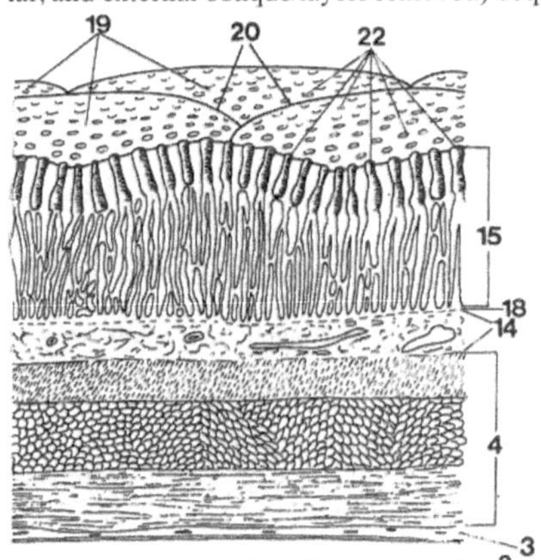

D Glandular stomach wall, stereoscopic

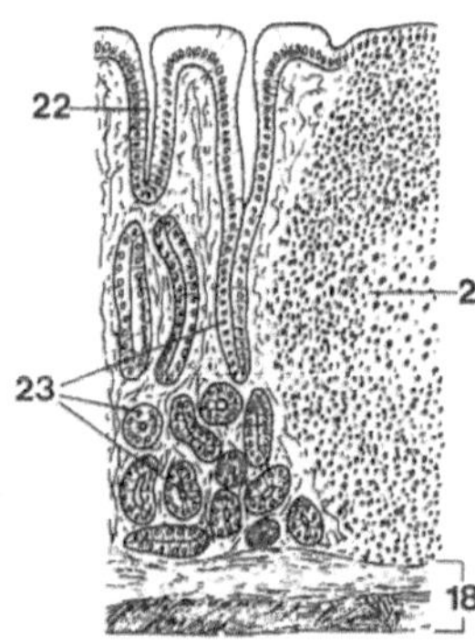

E Cardiac glands (su)

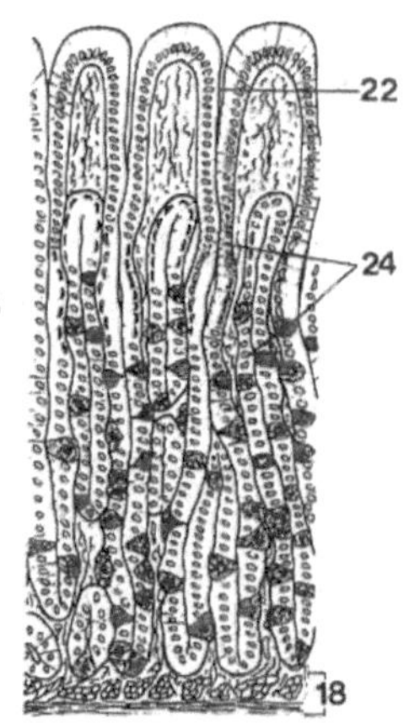

F Proper gastric glands (ca)

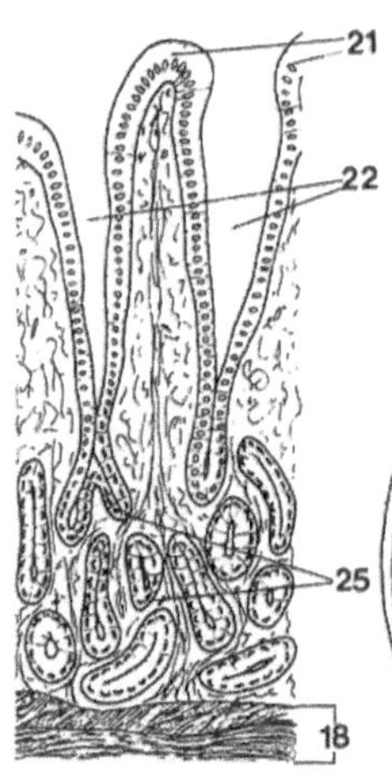

G Pyloric glands (ca)

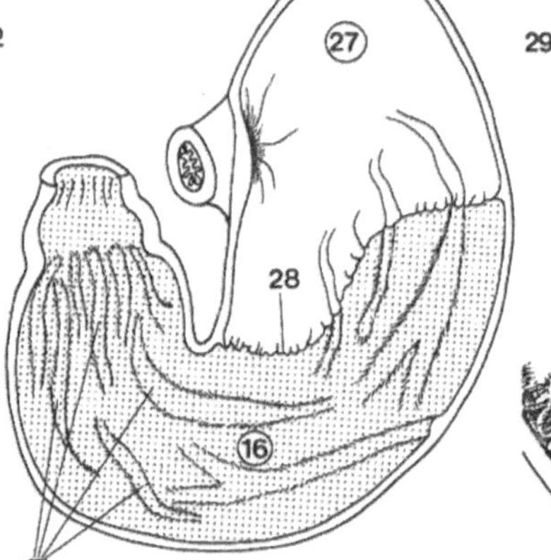

H Gastric mucosa (parietal wall removed) (eq)

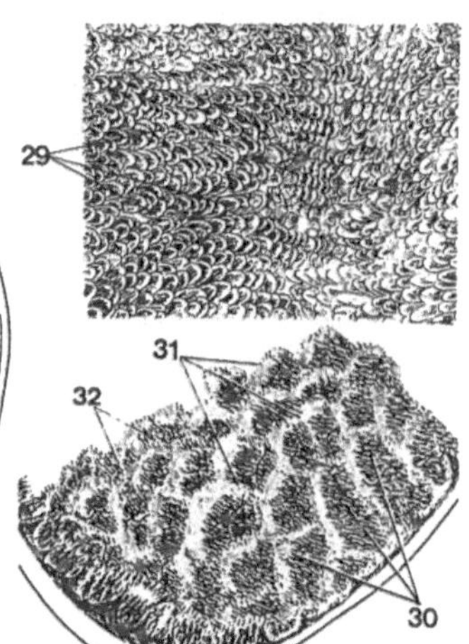

I Mucosa of rumen (above), and reticulum (below) (ov)

1 ***Papillae unguiculiformes*** (Ru). Long, curved, sharp, claw-shaped projection in and near the Ostium reticuloomasicum. A

2 ***Laminae omasi***. Flat parallel folds of mucous membrane extending from the Curvatura omasi toward the Sulcus omasi. There are up to four intercalated different sizes of the folds (there are only three in cap, for example). A

3 *Recessus interlaminares*. Narrow spaces between the laminae. A

4 ***Papillae omasi***. Omasal papillae, large on the reticular ends and smaller on the abomasal ends of the laminae. A

5 ***Vela abomasica***. Folds of mucous membrane on both sides of the Ostium omasoabomasicum. B

6 ***Plicae spirales abomasi***. Large mucosal folds in the fundus and corpus. They extend obliquely toward the Curvatura major and Pars pylorica. B

7 **INTESTINUM TENUE**. Small intestine, the duodenum, jejunum, and ileum.

8 ***Tunica serosa***. Serous membrane, composed of mesothelium and a layer of connective tissue. C

9 ***Tela subserosa***. Layer of loose connective tissue under the Tunica serosa. C

10 ***Tunica muscularis***. Main muscular coat. C

11 *Stratum longitudinale*. Outer, longitudinal layer. C

12 *Stratum circulare*. Inner, circular layer. C

13 ***Tela submucosa***. Loose connective tissue under the Tunica mucosa. C

14 ***Tunica mucosa***. The mucous membrane is glandular and bears villi covered by columnar epithelium. C

15 *Lamina muscularis mucosae*. Thin sheet of smooth muscle forming the deepest layer of the mucous membrane. It sends bundles into the villi. C

16 *Plicae circulares*. Circular folds of mucosa and submucosa. D, E

17 *Villi intestinales*. Minute projections of the mucous membrane. They are about 1 mm long and give the mucosal surface a velvet-like appearance. C

18 *Gll. intestinales*. Intestinal glands. C

19 *Lymphonoduli [Noduli lymphatici] solitarii*. Solitary lymph nodules, 0.15–1.5 mm in diameter. C

20 *Lymphonoduli [Noduli lymphatici] aggregati*. Aggregated lymph nodules, plaques of lymphatic tissue. D

21 **Duodenum**. Part of the small intestine from the Pylorus to the Flexura duodenojejunalis. F

22 ***Pars cranialis***. Part of the duodenum between the pylorus and the Flexura duodeni cranialis. F

23 *Ampulla duodeni*. Duodenal bulb, a dilation of the Pars cranialis. F

24 *Ansa sigmoidea* (Un). S-shaped loop, the double curvature of the Pars cranialis in Un only. F

25 ***Flexura duodeni cranialis***. Cranial flexure between Pars cranialis and Pars descendens. F

26 ***Pars descendens***. Descending part, running caudally on the right side. F

27 ***Flexura duodeni caudalis***. Caudal flexure between Pars descendens and Pars transversa. F

28 ***Pars transversa [Pars caudalis]***. Transverse part. F

29 ***Pars ascendens***. Ascending part, running cranially from the Pars transversa to the Flexura duodenojejunalis. F

30 ***Flexura duodenojejunalis***. The flexure is marked by an abrupt lengthening of the mesentery. F

31 ***Papilla duodeni major***. Projection of the duodenal mucosa bearing the opening of the Ductus choledochus and of the Ductus pancreaticus if present. E

32 ***Papilla duodeni minor***. Projection of the duodenal mucosa bearing the opening of the Ductus pancreaticus accessorius if present. E

33 ***Gll. duodenales***. Duodenal glands. Branched, tubuloalveolar mucous glands in the submucosa. According to species they may occupy a short initial part of the duodenum or extend far beyond it. C

34 **Jejunum**. Part of the small intestine between duodenum and ileum. The mesojejunum is attached to the lesser curvature. F

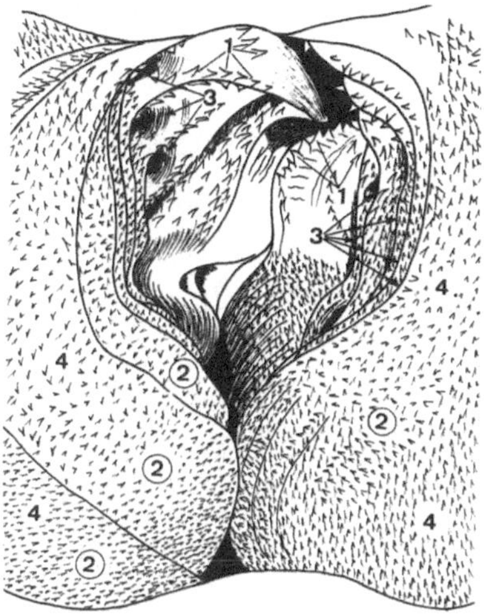

A Omasal groove (opened by cutting parallel to the laminae) (ov)

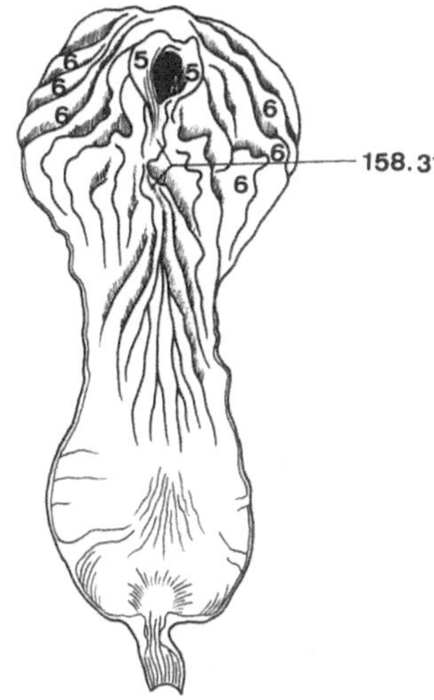

B Abomasum (opened along the greater curvature) (ov)

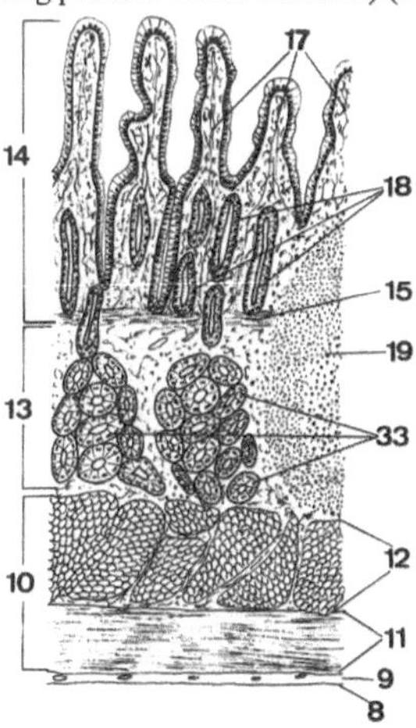

C Duodenum, histological section (bo)

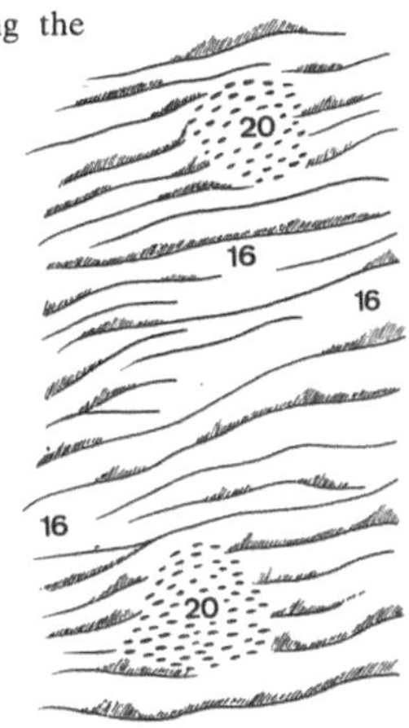

D Jejunal mucosa (eq)

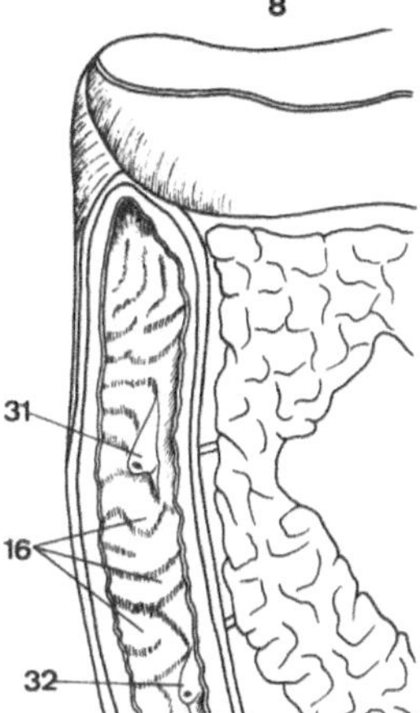

E Descending duodenum (opened ventrally) (ca)

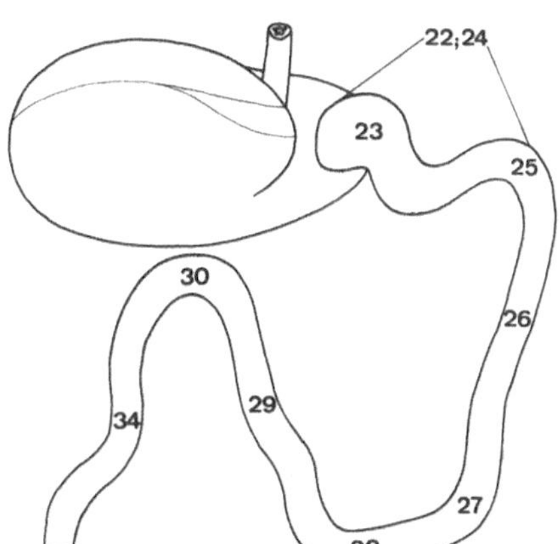

F Stomach and duodenum, dorsal aspect (eq)

1 **Ileum**. Defined in verterinary anatomical literature as the short terminal part of the small intestine to which the Plica ileocecalis is attached to the major curvature. The mesoileum is attached to the opposite side, on the lesser curvature. D

2 ***M. sphincter ilei***. Circular muscular fibers around the terminal ileum. It is not present in eq. The entire muscle coat of ileum in eq may be regarded as a functional ileal sphincter in conjunction to the venous network of Papilla ilealis. C (Schummer 1953, cited by Nickel et al. 1979, p. 187)

3 ***Papilla ilealis****. Projection of the end of the ileum into the lumen of the large intestine. B E (Here is the site for ileal intussusception in the horse.)

4 *Ostium ileale*. Opening of the ileum. B C

5 ***Frenulum papillae ilealis***. Fold of Tunica mucosa of the large intestine attached to the Papilla ilealis. B

6 **INTESTINUM CRASSUM**. Large intestine: the cecum, colon, rectum, and Canalis analis.

7 ***Tunica serosa***. Serous membrane, composed of mesothelium and a layer of connective tissue. A

8 ***Tela subserosa***. Layer of loose connective tissue under the serosa. A

9 ***Tunica muscularis***. Main muscular coat. A

10 *Stratum longitudinale*. Outer, longitudinal layer. A

11 *Stratum circulare*. Inner, circular layer. A

12 ***Tela submucosa***. Loose connective tissue under the Tunica mucosa. A

13 ***Tunica mucosa***. Mucous membrane. It is glandular, but does not bear villi. A

14 *Lamina muscularis mucosae*. Thin sheet of smooth muscle forming the deepest layer of the mucous membrane. It sends bundles between the glands. A

15 *Gll. intestinales*. Intestinal glands. A

16 *Lymphonoduli [Noduli lymphatici] solitarii*. Solitary lymph nodules, 0.15–1.5 mm in diameter. A

17 *Lymphonoduli [Noduli lymphatici] aggregati*. Aggregated lymph nodules, elongated plaques of lymphatic tissue. B

18 **Cecum [Caecum]***. Blind intestine. It opens freely into the Colon at the Ostium ileale, except in eq, where the junction is at the Ostium cecocolicum.

19 ***Basis ceci [caeci]***. Dorsal dilation of the Cecum in eq. The part cranial to the Papilla ilealis develops from the first part of the embryonic Colon. Although the part of Basis ceci cranial to Papilla ilealis develops from the first part of the embryonic colon, it is conventionally included in the Basis ceci. D E

20 ***Corpus ceci [caeci]***. Body of the cecum. D E

21 ***Apex ceci [caeci]***. Apex of the cecum. D

22 ***Curvatura ceci [caeci] major***. Greater curvature of the cecum. D

23 ***Curvatura ceci [caeci] minor***. Lesser curvature of the cecum. D

24 ***Teniae ceci [Taeniae caeci]***. Bands of the cecum in su and eq. The longitudinal layer of the Tunica muscularis is thickened to form the bands and is thin elsewhere.

25 *Tenia [Taenia] dorsalis**. Dorsal band, absent in su. In eq the attachment of the ileocecal fold. D

26 *Tenia [Taenia] ventralis*. Ventral band. D

27 *Tenia [Taenia] medialis*. Medial band. D

28 *Tenia [Taenia] lateralis**. Lateral band. In eq the attachment of the cecocolic fold. E

29 ***Haustra ceci [caeci]*** (sing. haustrum). Sacculations of the cecum between, and caused by the Teniae (which are slightly shorter than the cecum), and between grooves separating them from each other. The grooves correspond inside to the Plicae semilunares. D E

30 ***Plicae semilunares ceci [caeci]***. Semilunar folds of the cecum mucosa formed by contraction of the wall between haustra. They correspond on the outside surface to the grooves separating the haustra.

31 ***Ostium cecocolicum [caeco-]****. Opening from the cecum to the colon. E F (Here is one of the impaction sites in the horse.)

32 ***Valva cecocolica [caeco-]*** (eq). Cecocolic valve, formed by two mucosal folds. E

33 ***M. sphincter ceci [caeci]***. Sphincter of the cecum, the muscle around the Ostium cecocolicum except eq. F

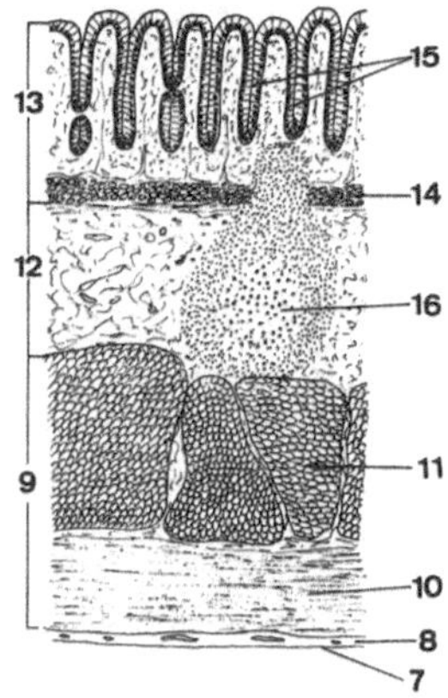

A Colon, histological section

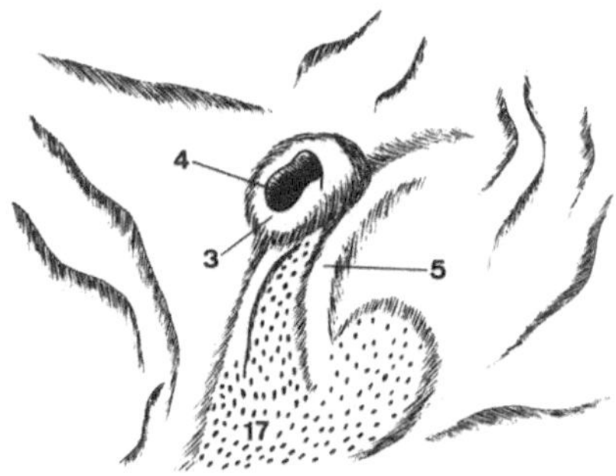

B Ileal papilla (ov)

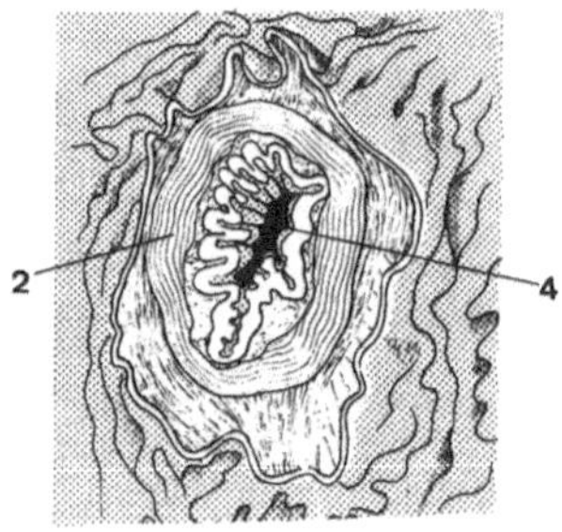

C Ileal papilla (mucosa removed) (eq)

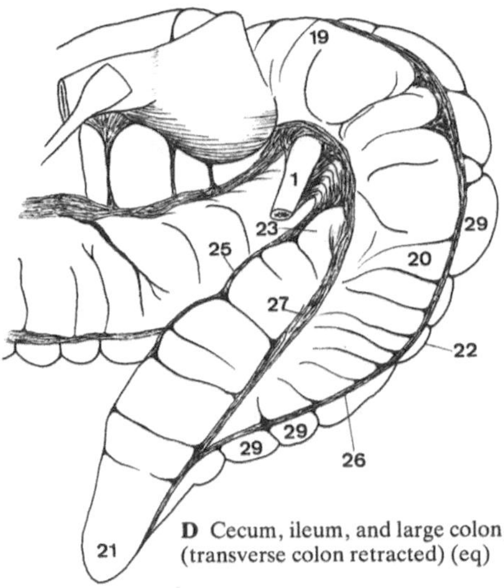

D Cecum, ileum, and large colon, left side (transverse colon retracted) (eq)

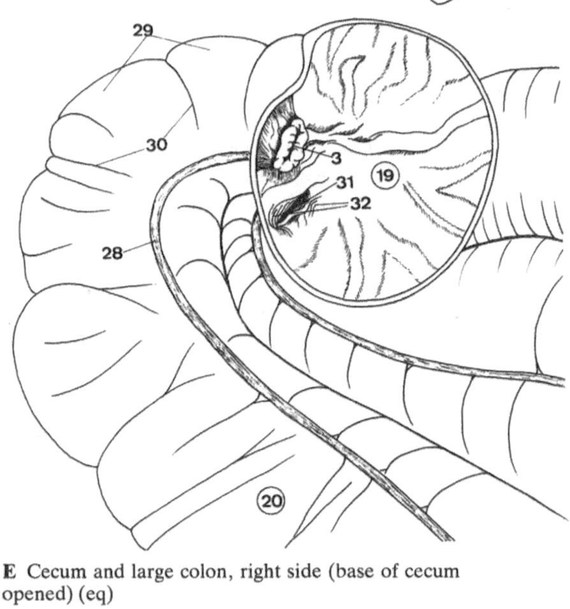

E Cecum and large colon, right side (base of cecum opened) (eq)

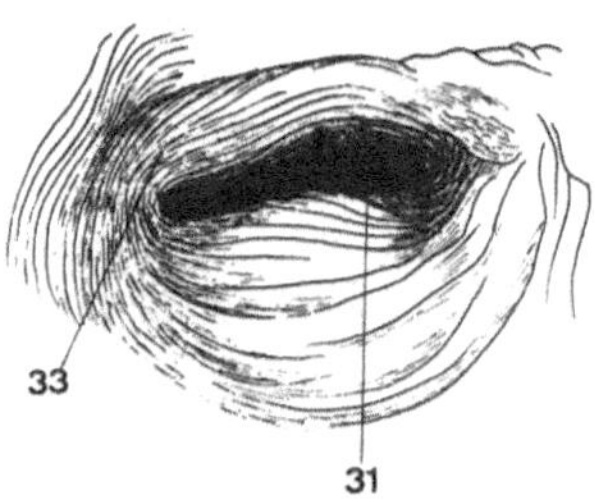

F Cecal sphincter (mucosa removed) eq)

1 **Colon**. Part of the large intestine from the cecum to the rectum.

2 ***Colon ascendens***. Ascending colon, extends from the cecum to the Colon transversum. A B C

3 *Colon crassum* (eq). Large colon. It is a loop formed by the Colon ventrale and the Colon dorsale, which bends around to the left side. C

4 **Collum coli**[1)]*. Neck of the colon, the origin of the right ventral colon. C

5 **Colon ventrale dextrum***. Right ventral colon. It extends from the cecum to the Flexura sternalis, and has haustra and four teniae (two mesocolic, medial and lateral, dorsally, and two free teniae, medial and lateral, distally). C

6 **Flexura sternalis [diaphragmatica ventralis]**. Sternal flexure, positioned horizontally. C

7 **Colon ventrale sinistrum***. Left ventral colon, extends from the Flexura sternalis to the Flexura pelvina; has haustra and four teniae, similar to those of the right ventral colon. C

8 **Flexura pelvina**[1)]*. Pelvic flexure, positioned vertically and ingesta advances in a ventrodorsal direction. C

9 **Colon dorsale sinistrum***. Left dorsal colon, extends from the Flexura pelvina to the Flexura diaphragmatica. It is smooth and has one tenia for the mesocolic attachment of the ascending mesocolon and corresponds to the right colic A, V., nerves and colic lymph nodes. C

10 **Flexura diaphragmatica [dorsalis]**. Diaphragmatic flexure, positioned horizontally. C

11 **Colon dorsale dextrum***. Right dorsal colon, the terminal part of the Colon crassum. It joins the Colon transversum and has haustra and three teniae. C (There is only one mesocolic tenia ventrally in the Colon dorsale dextrum, corresponding to the right colic A., V., nerves and colic lymph nodes, where the ascending mesocolon attaches. Dorsally two free teniae are provided.)

12 **Ampulla coli***. Dilation of the Colon dorsale dextrum, which abruptly diminishes in diameter[1)] and continues with the Colon transversum. C

13 *Ansa proximalis coli* (Ru). Proximal loop of the colon, the first part of the Colon ascendens, S-shaped, continued by the Ansa spiralis. B

14 *Ansa spiralis coli* (su, Ru). Spiral loop. It is coiled on the left side of the mesentery in a vertical position. B

15 **Gyri centripetales**. In-going coils in which the ingesta move toward the Flexura centralis. B

16 **Flexura centralis**. Central flexure where the last in-going coil is continuous with the first out-going coil. B

17 **Gyri centrifugales**. Out-going coils in which the ingesta moves away from the Flexura centralis toward the Ansa distalis. B

18 *Ansa distalis coli* (su, Ru). Distal loop of the colon, the last part of the Colon ascendens. B

19 ***Flexura coli dextra***. Right flexure of the colon. It connects the Colon ascendens to the Colon transversum. A

20 ***Colon transversum***[1)]*. The transverse colon passes from right to left, cranial to the cranial mesenteric artery, joining the right and left colic flexures. A B C

21 ***Flexura coli sinistra***. Left flexure of the colon, connects the Colon transversum to the Colon descendens. A

22 ***Colon descendens; [Colon tenue]*** (eq). Descending colon, extends from the Flexura coli sinistra to the rectum. A B C 217 B

23 ***Colon sigmoideum***. Sigmoid colon, an S-shaped curve just cranial to the rectum in bo. B

24 ***Teniae [Taeniae] coli****. Bands of the colon in su and eq, formed by longitudinal muscle. There are two in su. In eq the left dorsal colon has one; the right dorsal colon, three; and the ventral colon, four.

25 *Tenia [Taenia] mesocolica lateralis*. Lateral mesocolic band in eq. This is dorsally oriented in the ventral colon of the horse (both right and left) and is concealed into the attachment of the ascending mesocolon. C

26 *Tenia [Taenia] mesocolica medialis*. Medial mesocolic band in eq. This is also dorsally oriented in the ventral colon of the horse and corresponds to the right colic branch A., V., nerves and colic lymph nodes. C

27 *Tenia [Taenia] libera lateralis*. Lateral free band. Ventrally oriented in the ventral colon and dorsally oriented in the right dorsal colon of the horse. C

28 *Tenia [Taenia] libera medialis*. Medial free band. Similar to the previous tenia. C

29 ***Haustra coli***. Sacculations of the colon between Teniae and between Plicae semilunares in su and eq. C

30 ***Plicae semilunares coli***. Semilunar folds of the colon mucosa formed by contraction of the wall between haustra. They correspond on the outside surface to the grooves separating the haustra. C

31 ***Appendices epiploicae***. Pendant fat bodies covered by peritoneum, attached along the Teniae coli. C

cont. p. 168 ►

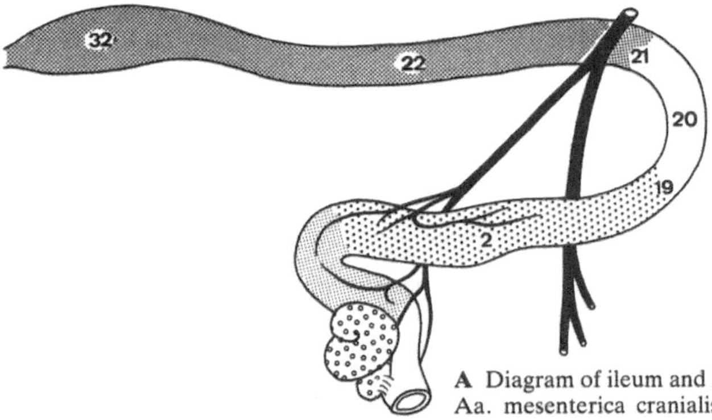

A Diagram of ileum and large intestine in relation to Aa. mesenterica cranialis and ileocolica, right side (ca)

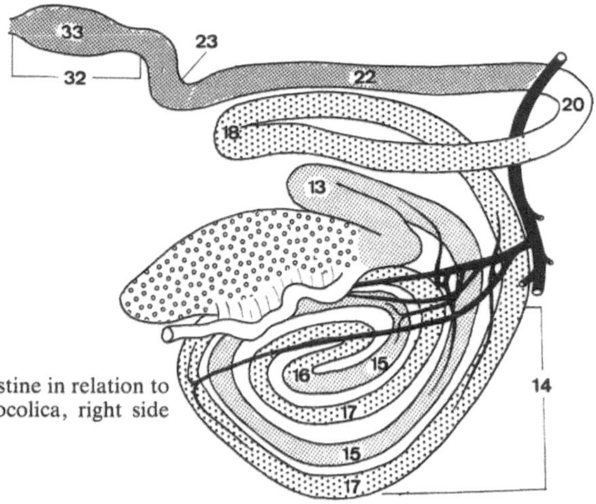

B Diagram of ileum and large intestine in relation to Aa. mesenterica cranialis and ileocolica, right side (bo)

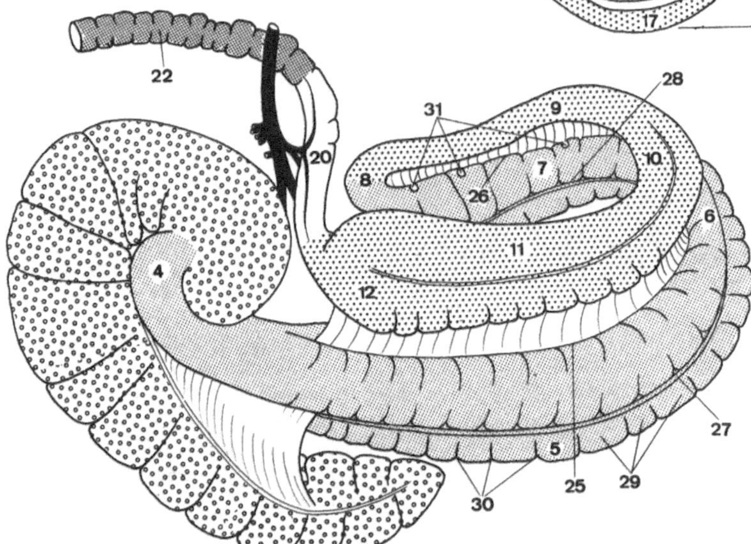

C Large intestine and A. mesenterica cranialis, right side, (left parts of large colon shortened) (eq)

32 **Rectum**. Pelvic part of the large intestine, terminates at the Canalis analis. A B

33 ***Ampulla recti***. Enlargement of the terminal part. Absent in fe, ov, cap. B

1) These are potential impaction sites in the horse.

---

1 ***Tunica adventitia***. Connective tissue covering the retroperitoneal part of the rectum. C

2 ***M. rectococcygeus***. Consists of agglomerated longitudinal muscle fibers to the roof of rectum. O: caudal vertebrae 2–7, depending on species. T: rectum. B

3 ***M. rectourethralis***. O: rectum. T: male urethra; female vestibule and Labia pudendi. B

4 ***Plicae transversales recti***. Temporary constrictions in Ru.

5 ***Columae rectales***. Rectal columns in Ru, short longitudinal folds of mucosa extending cranially from the Linea anorectalis.

6 **Canalis analis**. Anal canal, the terminal segment of the intestine, lined by stratified squamous epithelium. A

7 ***M. sphincter ani internus***. Internal anal sphincter, smooth muscle continuous with the Stratum circulare of the rectum. B C

8 ***Junctio anorectalis***. Anorectal line, between rectal mucosa with simple columnar epithelium, and anal canal with stratified squamous epithelium. A

9 ***Zona columnaris ani*** (ca, su). Columnar zone of the anus, lined by stratified squamous noncornified epithelium. A C

10 *Columnae anales*. Anal columns, short longitudinal folds of mucosa extending caudally from the Linea anorectalis, absent in fe, Ru and eq. A

11 *Sinus anales*. Anal sinuses, the grooves between the columnae. A

12 *Gll. anales*. Anal glands, tubulo-alveolar, in the submucosa or outside the M. sphincter ani internus. C

13 ***Zona intermedia***. Intermediate zone, lined by stratified squamous noncornified epithelium, between Zona columnaris and Linea anocutanea, narrow in ca. A C

14 ***Junctio anocutanea***. Anocutaneous line, boundary between mucous membrane and skin. A

15 ***Zona cutanea***. Cutaneous zone, cornified epidermis, skin glands, and hairs. A C

16 *Sinus paranalis* (Car). Paranal sinus, lateral cutaneous pouch between Canalis analis and M. sphincter ani externus. C

17 **Gll. sinus paranalis**. Glands of the paranal sinus, Gll. apocrinae and Gll. sebaceae. C

18 *Gll. circumanales* (ca). Circumanal glands, lobules composed of large polyhedral cells, derived from sebaceous glands, but have no ducts. C

19 ***M. sphincter ani externus*** (vide Perineum). C

20 ***Anus***. Terminal orifice of the intestine. B

21 **HEPAR**. Liver.

22 ***Facies diaphragmatica***. Diaphragmatic surface. E

23 *Area nuda*. Bare spot, not covered by Tunica serosa. E

24 *Sulcus venae cavae*. Groove for the V. cava caudalis. E

25 ***Facies visceralis***. Visceral surface, in contact with the stomach. D

26 *Fossa vesicae felleae*. Fossa for the gall bladder. D

27 *Fissura lig. teretis*. Fissure for the round ligament. D

28 *Lig. teres hepatis*. Round ligament of the liver, vestige of the V. umbilicalis. D

29 *Sulcus venae umbilicalis* (ont)[1].

30 *Fossa ductus venosi* (ont)[1].

31 *Porta hepatis*. Hilus of the liver. D

32 *Tuber omentale* (Car). Omental tuber, prominence of the visceral surface of the left lateral lobe. D

33 *Impressio esophagea [oesophagea]*. Esophageal impression on the Margo dorsalis. 171 A

34 *Impressio gastrica*. Impression of the stomach on the left lobe in species with a simple stomach. 171 A

35 *Impressio reticularis*. Impression of the reticulum on the left lobe. In fig. 171 B the liver is positioned with the long axis horizontally, rotated 90 degrees clockwise, whereas in the nature it is almost vertical with the left lobe pointing ventrally. This explains the position of reticular impression on the upper left corner of the figure (in situ in the lower left corner of the liver). 171 B

1) These structures were omitted from the 5th edition of the N. A. V., because they are ontogenetic terms.

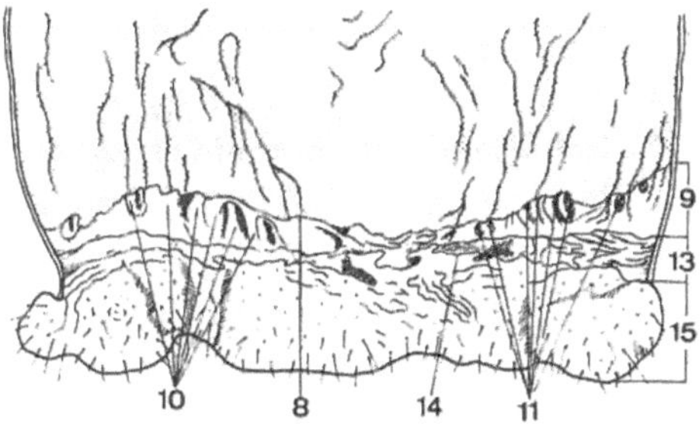

A Anal canal (opened dorsally) (su)

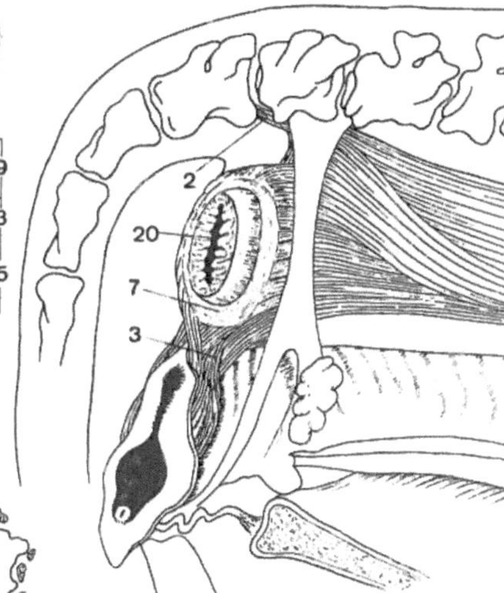

B Perineum (bo) (Geiger)

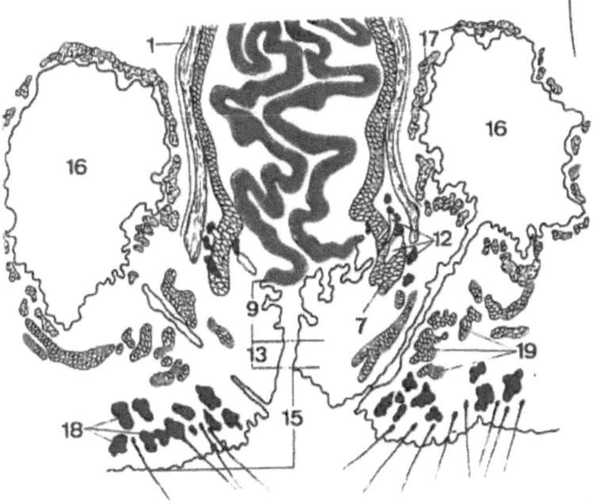

C Anal canal (ca) (Gerisch and Neurand)

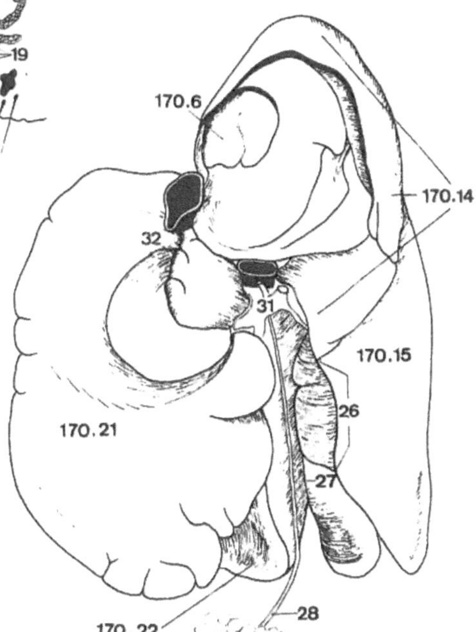

D Liver, visceral surface (ca)

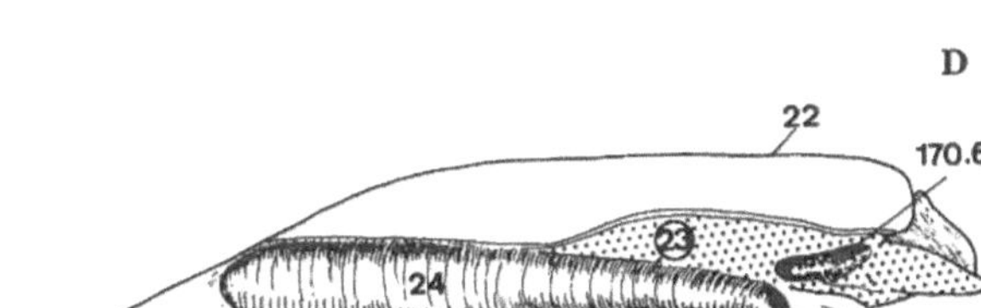

E Liver, dorsal border (adrenal gland reflected) (bo)

1 *Impressio omasica*. Omasal impression, occupies a large part of the visceral surface. See explanation on page 168.35 B

2 *Impressio duodenalis*. Duodenal impression, ventral and to the right of the porta. A

3 *Impressio colica*. Colic impression, on the right ventral part of the visceral surface in eq, made by the sternal and diaphragmatic flexures of the ascending colon. A

4 *Impressio cecalis [caecalis]* (eq). Cecal impression, on the right lobe. A

5 *Impressio renalis*. Renal impression, on the right lobe and caudate process, absent in su. A

6 *Impressio adrenalis [supra-]*. Impression by the right adrenal gland on the Lobus/Processus caudatus. 169 D

7 ***Margo dorsalis***. Dorsal border, in Ru almost median. B

8 ***Margo dexter***. Right border, in Ru dorsocaudal. B

9 ***Margo sinister***. Left border, in Ru cranioventral. B

10 ***Margo ventralis***. Ventral border, in Ru on the right side of the body. B

11 *Incisurae interlobares*. Interlobar notches. A

12 *Incisura lig. teretis*. Notch for the round ligament. B

13 ***Lobus hepatis dexter***. Right lobe of the liver in Ru and eq. B

14 ***Lobus hepatis dexter lateralis***. Right lateral lobe in Car and su. 169 D

15 ***Lobus hepatis dexter medialis***. Right medial lobe in Car and su. 169 D

16 ***Lobus quadratus***. Quadrate lobe, between Fossa vesicae felleae and Incisura lig. teretis (except in eq in which it is located between the Lobus hepatis dexter and Lobus hepatis sinister medialis). B

17 ***Lobus caudatus***. Caudate lobe, dorsal to the Porta hepatis. B

18 *Processus papillaris*. Papillary process, projection of the Lobus caudatus into the Vestibulum bursae omentalis in Car and Ru. B

19 *Processus caudatus*. Caudate process, elongated right projection from the visceral surface of the Lobus caudatus. B

20 ***Lobus hepatis sinister***. Left lobe of the liver of Ru. B

21 ***Lobus hepatis sinister lateralis***. Left lateral lobe of the liver of Car, su, eq. 169 D

22 ***Lobus hepatis sinister medialis***. Left medial lobe of Car, su, eq, between left lateral lobe and Incisura lig. teretis. 169 D

23 ***(Appendix fibrosa hepatis)***. Fibrous appendage, vestige of an atrophied portion at the caudal end of the right lobe in old eq. A

24 ***Lobuli hepatis***. Hepatic lobules, histological units of the liver, about 1 mm in diameter and 2 mm long. There is a discrete yet visible polyhedral design on the liver surface starting one month after birth in pigs. C

25 ***Tunica serosa***. Serous membrane. B

26 ***Tela subserosa***. Layer of loose connective tissue and fat under the Tunica serosa. B

27 ***Tunica fibrosa***. Fibrous coat, the connective tissue on the outer surface of the liver between the parenchyma and the Tela subserosa. B

28 ***Capsula fibrosa perivascularis***. Fibrous perivascular sheath (of Glisson), ensheathing bile ducts, branches of hepatic artery and portal vein within the liver. A C

29 ***Arteriae interlobulares***. Between the Lobuli hepatis. C

30 ***Venae interlobulares***. Branches of the portal vein between the Lobuli hepatis. C

31 ***Venae centrales***. Terminal branches of the hepatic veins in the Lobuli hepatis. C

32 ***Ductuli interlobulares***. Interlobular bile ductules. C

33 ***Ductuli biliferi***. Biliferous ductules.

34 ***Ductus hepaticus communis***. Common hepatic duct, from the junction of the right and left hepatic ducts to the entry of the cystic duct; absent in Car. B (In Car the right and the left hepatic ducts open separately into the cystic duct, which then becomes the bile duct or Choledochus.)

35 *Ductus hepaticus dexter*. Right hepatic duct or ducts draining the right part of the liver. B

36 *Ductus hepaticus sinister*. Left hepatic duct or ducts draining the left part of the liver. B

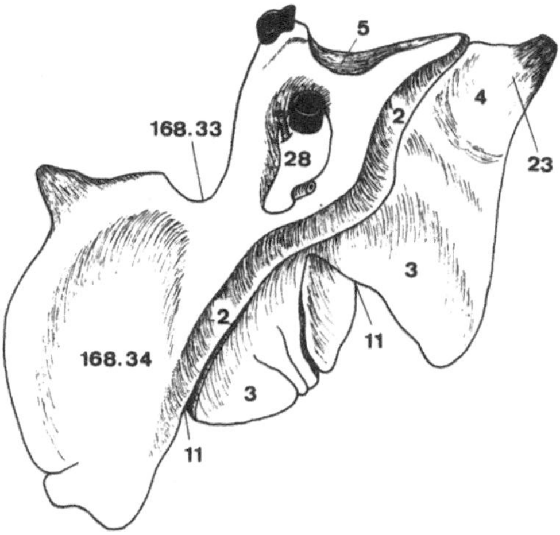

A Liver, visceral surface (eq)

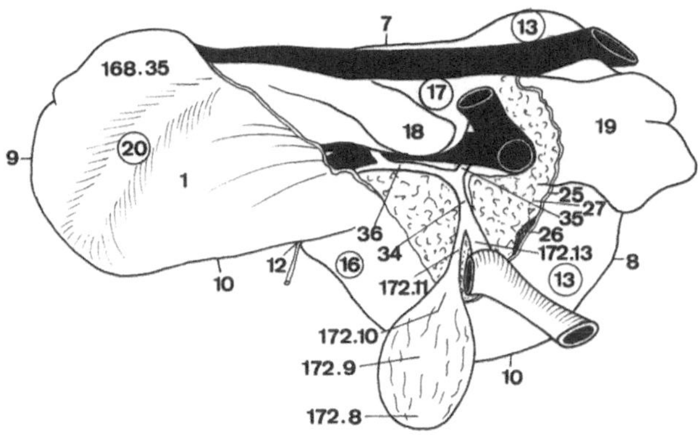

B Liver, visceral surface (rotated clockwise 90 degrees) (bo)

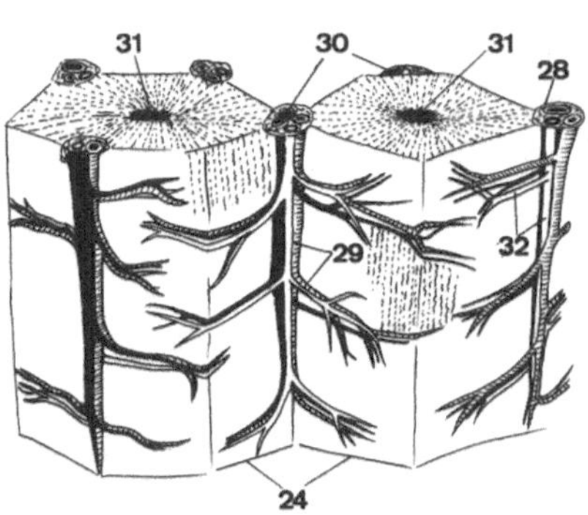

C Lobuli hepatis, stereoscopic

1 **Vesica biliaris [Vesica fellea].** Gall bladder.

2 ***Tunica serosa vesicae felleae.*** Serous membrane of the gall bladder. A

3 ***Tela subserosa vesicae felleae.*** Loose connective tissue under the serosa. A

4 ***Tunica muscularis vesicae felleae.*** Muscular coat of the gall bladder. A

5 ***Tunica mucosa vesicae felleae.*** Mucous membrane of the gall bladder, covered by simple columnar epithelium. A

6 *Plicae tunicae mucosae vesicae felleae.* Folds of the mucous membrane. A

7 *Gll. vesicae felleae.* Glands of the gall bladder, numerous tubular glands in the body in Ru, rare and restricted to the neck in Car and su. A

8 ***Fundus vesicae felleae.*** Bottom of the gall bladder, the blind end. 171 B

9 ***Corpus vesicae felleae.*** Body of the gall bladder. 171 B

10 ***Collum vesicae felleae.*** Neck of the gall bladder. 171 B

11 ***Ductus cysticus.*** Duct of the gall bladder. It joins the Ductus hepaticus communis to form the Ductus choledochus. 171 B

12 ***Ductus hepatocystici.*** Hepatocystic ducts, pass directly from the liver into the gall bladder, variably in Car, Ru.

13 **Ductus choledochus.** Common bile duct, formed by the union of cystic and common hepatic ducts and ending on the Papilla duodeni major. C 171 B (In Car there is no common hepatic duct, therefore the choledocus is called bile duct, and not common bile duct.)

14 ***M. sphincter ductus choledochi.*** Terminal thickening of the circular muscle of the Ductus choledochus. C

15 ***Ampulla hepatopancreatica.*** Short common terminal duct formed by the bile and pancreatic ducts in the Papilla duodeni major (fe, eq). In ov, cap the bile and pancreatic ducts unite before they reach the duodenum. B

16 *M. sphincter ampullae hepatopancreaticae [M. sphincter ampullae].* A tract of muscle fibers passes around the ampulla (fe), or the common hepatopancreatic duct (ov, cap), or the terminal parts of both ducts (ca, eq). C

17 **PANCREAS.** Large digestive gland associated with the stomach, and the cranial and descending parts of the duodenum. D E F

18 ***Lobus pancreatis dexter.*** Right lobe, in the Mesoduodenum descendens. D E F

19 *Processus uncinatus* (Ru). Hooked process, extends medially from the right lobe around the caudodorsal surface of the portal vein. D

20 ***Corpus pancreatis.*** Body, the middle part, in contact with the cranial part of the duodenum. E F

21 *Tuber omentale.* Ventral prominence of the Corpus pancreatis in the Bursa omentalis. D

22 ***Lobus pancreatis sinister.*** Left lobe, on the visceral surface of the stomach, in Ru dorsal to the rumen. D E F

23 ***Incisura pancreatis*** (Car, Ru). Notch for the portal vein in the Margo caudalis. D E

24 ***Anulus pancreatis*** (su, eq). Ring of the pancreas around the portal vein. F

25 ***Facies ventralis.*** Ventral surface. D E F

26 ***Facies dorsalis.*** Dorsal surface.

27 ***Margo cranialis.*** Cranial border. E F

28 ***Margo caudalis.*** Caudal border. E F

29 ***Margo dexter.*** Right border. E F

30 ***Margo sinister.*** Left border. E F

31 ***Ductus pancreaticus.*** Pancreatic duct, opening on the Papilla duodeni major, main duct in fe, ov, cap, eq, absent in su, bo. C D E F

32 *M. sphincter ductus pancreatici.* Sphincter of Ductus pancreaticus. C

33 ***Ductus pancreaticus accessorius.*** Opening on the Papilla duodeni minor, the largest duct in ca, the only one in su and bo. E F

34 *M. sphincter ductus pancreatici accessorii.* Sphincter of Ductus pancreaticus accessorius.

35 ***(Pancreas accessorium).*** Accessory pancreas, reported in ca.

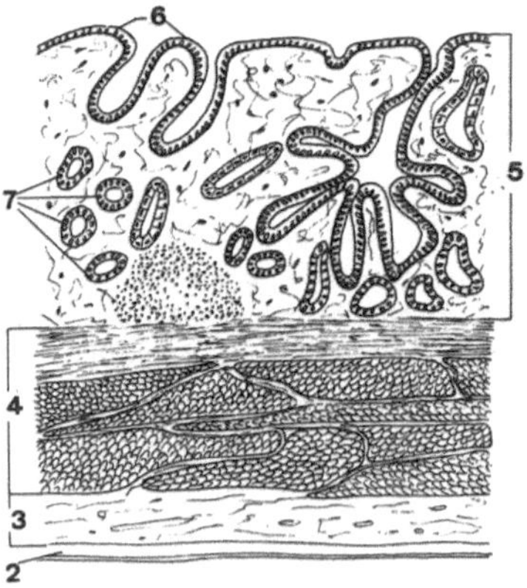

A Gall bladder, histological

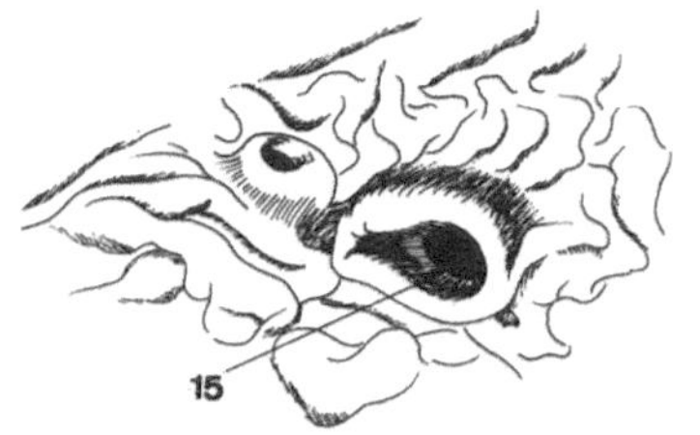

B Major and minor duodenal papillae (eq)

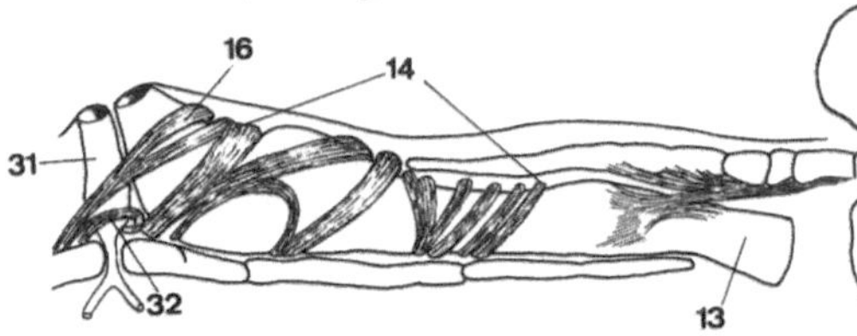

C Major duodenal papilla (ca) (Eichorn and Boyden)

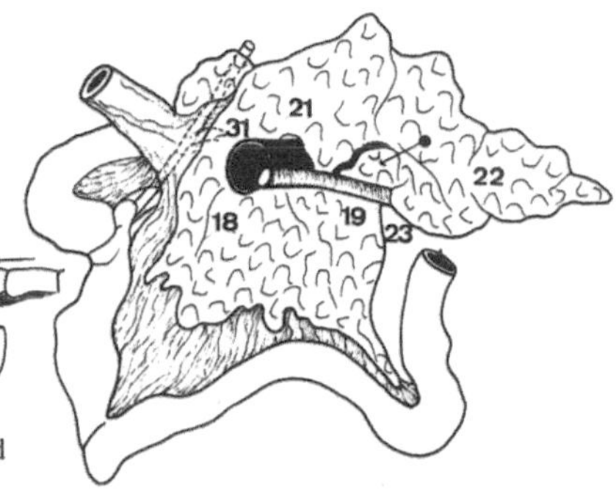

D Pancreas and duodenum, ventral surface (ov)

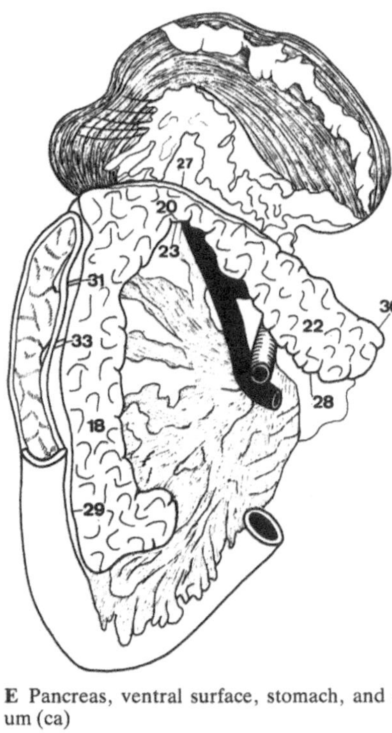

E Pancreas, ventral surface, stomach, and duodenum (ca)

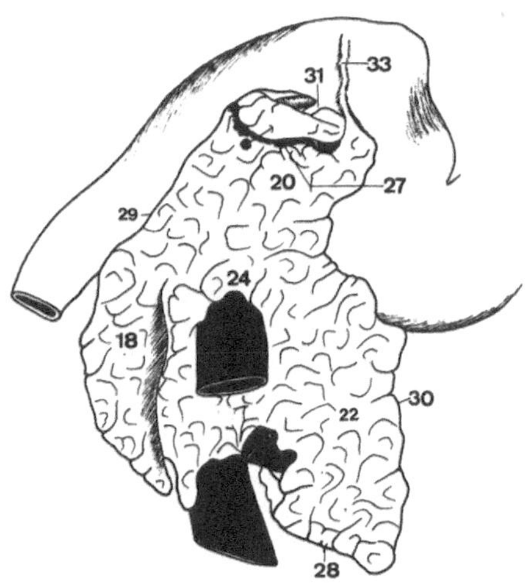

F Pancreas, ventral surface, pylorus, and duodenum (eq)

1 **SYSTEMA RESPIRATORIUM.**

2 **NASUS EXTERNUS.** External nose, the part of the face rostral to the frontal region and dorsal to the infraorbital, buccal, and oral regions. A

3 ***Radix nasi.*** Root of the nose, the caudal end of the external nose. A

4 ***Dorsum nasi.*** Dorsal surface of the nose. A

5 ***Apex nasi.*** Tip of the nose. A

6 ***Alae nasi.*** The two wings of each Naris (nostril), which takes different positions depending on species and even breeds in ca . A B D

7 ***Pars mobilis septi nasi.*** Mobile rostral part of nasal septum. F

8 ***Rostrum.*** Snout in su. B

9 ***Planum nasale*** (Car)[1]. Zone of hairless and nonglandular skin on the Apex nasi. A

10 *Areae.* Polygonal fields about 1 mm in diameter, separated by grooves. A

11 *Sulci.* Grooves between areae. A

12 ***Planum rostrale*** (su)[1]. Skin of the snout-disk, hairless except for sparse, short tactile hairs. B

13 *Areae.* Fields about 2 mm in diameter separated by grooves. B

14 *Sulci.* Faint grooves in the upper half of the planum. B

15 *Foveolae.* Pits into which the glands open. B

16 *Glandulae.* Large serous glands in the subcutaneous tissue.

17 ***Planum nasolabiale*** (bo) [1]. Hairless skin of the nose and upper lip. C

18 *Areae.* Fields about 2–4 mm in diameter, separated by grooves. C

19 *Sulci.* Grooves between areae. C

20 *Foveolae.* Pits into which glands open. C

21 *Glandulae.* Large serous glands in the subcutaneous tissue. C

22 ***Planum nasale*** (ov, cap)[1]. Narrow zone of bare skin between the nares and along the free border of the alae. D

23 *Areae.* Fields about 2 mm in diameter. D

24 *Sulci.* Grooves between areae. D

25 *Foveolae.* Pits into which glands open. D

26 *Glandulae.* Large serous glands in the subcutaneous tissue.

27 ***Cartilagines nasi externi.*** Cartilages of the external nose. E F

28 *Cartilago nasi lateralis dorsalis**. Dorsal lateral nasal cartilage, lateral expansion from the dorsal border of the septal cartilage. E F (During intubation in the dog, the tracheal tube is sutured to this cartilage.)

29 *Cartilago nasi lateralis ventralis.* Ventral lateral nasal cartilage, lateral expansion from the ventral border of the septal cartilage; absent in eq. F

30 *Cartilago alaris.* Alar cartilage of eq, comma-shaped, with the broad part (Lamina) within the upper medial wing of the nostril and the narrow part (Cornu) ventral to the nostril, lying on the incisive bone. E

31 **Cornu** (eq). Horn of the alar cartilage. E

32 **Lamina** (eq). Plate of the alar cartilage. E

33 *Cartilago nasalis accessoria lateralis.* Lateral accessory cartilage, attached in Car to the ventral lateral cartilage; in su to the rostral bone; in Ru to the dorsal lateral cartilage. F 34 Cartilago nasalis accessoria medialis. Medial accessory cartilage in the alar fold. E

34 *Cartilago nasalis accessoria medialis.* Medial accessory cartilage in the alar fold. E

1) In healthy individuals they should be humid and cold.

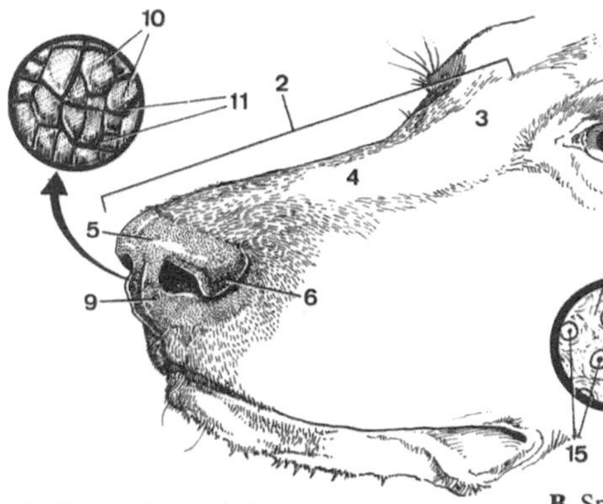

A External nose (ca)

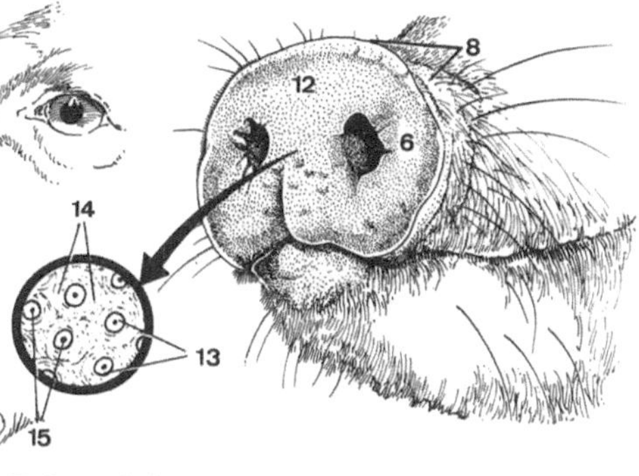

B Snout (su)

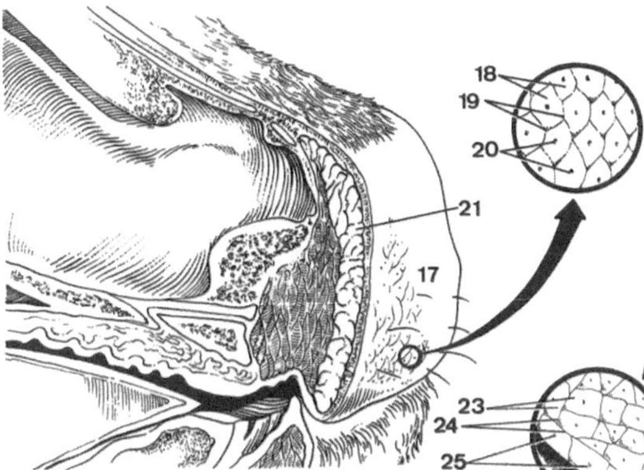

C Nose, sagittal section, left half, rostromedial aspect (bo)

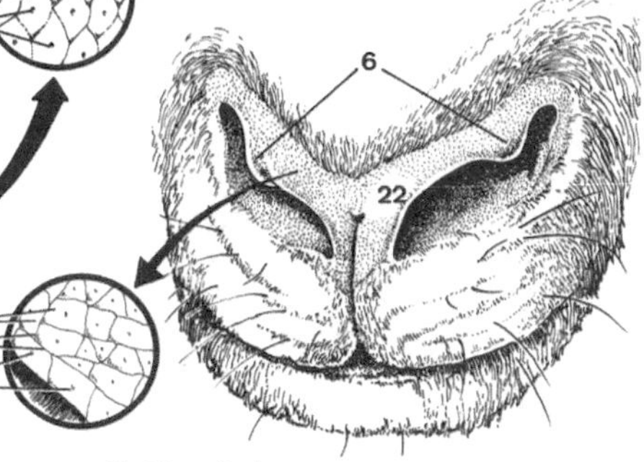

D Nose (ov)

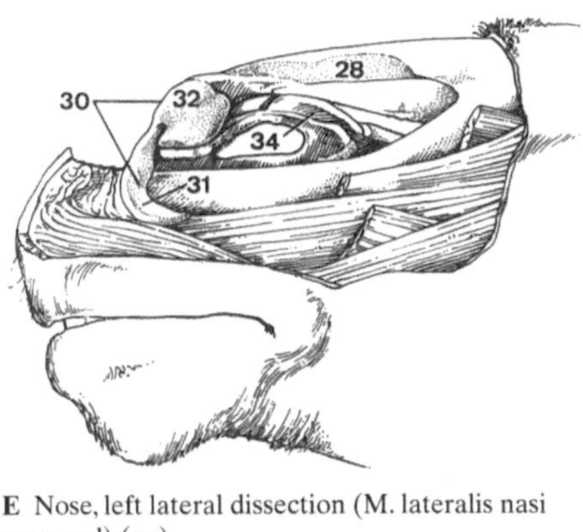

E Nose, left lateral dissection (M. lateralis nasi removed) (eq)

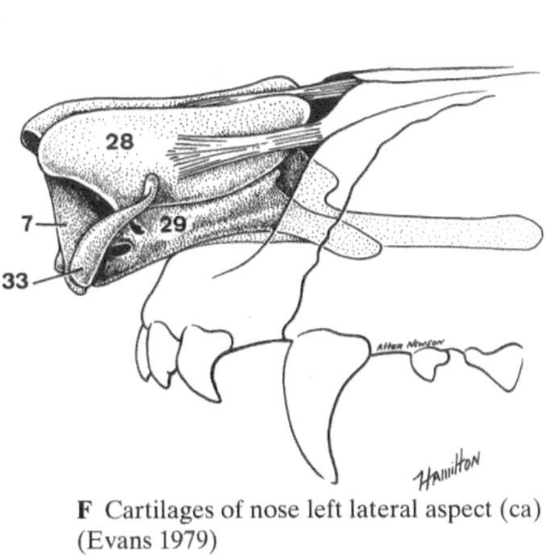

F Cartilages of nose left lateral aspect (ca) (Evans 1979)

1 **CAVUM NASI**. Nasal cavity. D

2 ***Nares***. Nostrils. The two symmetrical openings of the nose (sing. Naris). A

3 *Sulcus alaris*. Alar groove, at the caudolateral angle of the nostril between the ala and the lateroventral border in Car, Ru. A

4 *Diverticulum nasi* (eq). Cutaneous blind sac extending from the dorsal angle of the nostril to the caudal end of the Incisura nasoincisiva. Its opening is called the false nostril. It lies on the periosteal membrane filling the space between the Os nasale and Processus nasalis ossis incisivum. B

5 ***Choanae***. Openings between the two compartments of the nasal cavity and the nasopharynx. C

6 ***Septum nasi***. Nasal septum, separating the nasal cavity into the right and left compartments. C

7 *Cartilago septi nasi*. Cartilage of the nasal septum. C

8 **Processus caudalis**. Caudal process of the cartilage, extending into the angle between Vomer and Lamina perpendicularis of the ethmoid. C

9 *Pars membranacea*. Membranous part, between the rostral end of the cartilage and the skin between the nares. The dog has another membranous part in the plane of the osseous nasal aperture, where a large defect in the septal cartilage provides mobility of the rostral portion. C

10 *Pars ossea*. Osseous part, composed of Lamina perpendicularis of the ethmoid, Vomer, and in su and bo (if present) Os rostrale. C (This structure is listed as “Septum nasi osseum” on page 14.2.)

11 ***Organum vomeronasale***. Vomeronasal organ, a tubular organ of special sense on the floor of the nasal cavity next to the septum. It extends caudally from the rostral end of the Fissura palatina to a transverse plane that varies with species from the third incisor (su) to the fourth premolar (ov). C

12 *Ductus vomeronasalis*. Epithelial tube, blind caudally and opening rostrally into the Ductus incisivus. The medial wall is composed in large part of neurosensory epithelium with axons forming the N. vomeronasalis. C

13 *Cartilago vomeronasalis*. Incomplete cartilaginous cylinder partially surrounding the Ductus vomeronasalis and associated glands, vessels, and nerves. It is connected to the nasal cartilages. C

14 ***Ductus incisivus***. Incisive duct, formerly Ductus nasopalatinus. It extends rostroventrally from the nasal cavity through the Fissura palatina to the oral cavity, where it opens in the groove beside the Papilla incisiva, except in eq, in which the ventral end is blind. The Ductus incisivus receives the Ductus vomeronasalis. C

15 ***Vestibulum nasi***. Vestibule of the nose, rostral part of the nasal cavity, lined by stratified squamous epithelium. B D

16 ***Limen nasi***. Boundary between stratified squamous epithelium of the vestibule and respiratory epithelium of the rest of the nasal cavity. B D

17 ***Ostium nasolacrimale***. Orifice of the nasolacrimal duct. B D

18 ***Plica alaris***. Alar fold, a fold of Tunica mucosa supported by the medial accessory cartilage and extending from the rostral end of the ventral concha to the Ala nasi. B D

19 ***Plica recta***. Straight fold of Tunica mucosa from the dorsal concha to the nostril. It originates as dorsal and ventral branches from the end of the concha in eq. D

20 ***Plica basalis***. Basal fold of Tunica mucosa. In eq it runs rostroventrally from the ventral concha to the floor of the nasal cavity and contains the nasolacrimal duct. In the other species it begins ventral to the ventral concha and runs rostrally to join the rostal end of the alar fold. B D

21 ***Plica obliqua*** (Car). The oblique fold extends rostroventrally from the straight fold to the lateral side of the alar fold. It contains, near the straight fold, the orifice of the duct of the lateral nasal gland. D

22 ***Plicae parallelae*** (Car). Parallel folds on the dorsolateral wall of the vestibule. They extend rostrodorsally from the oblique fold. D

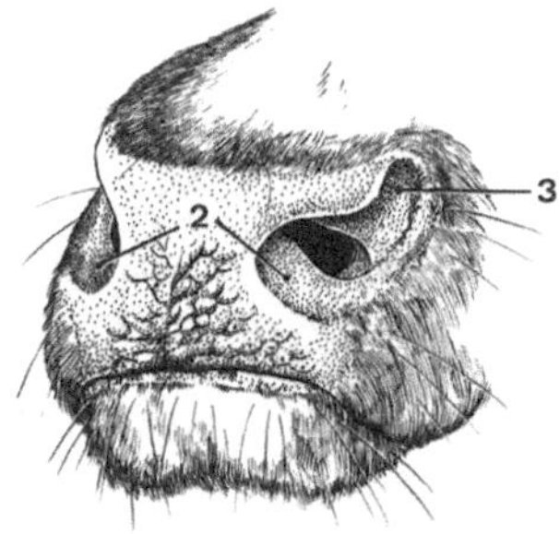

A Nostrils (bo)

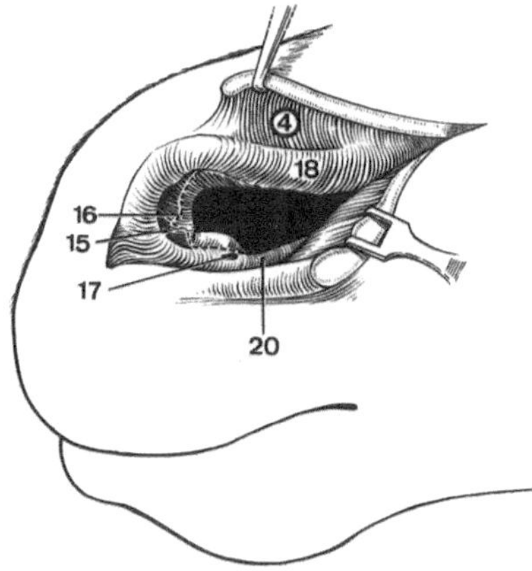

B Nasal vestibule and diverticulum left aspect (eq)

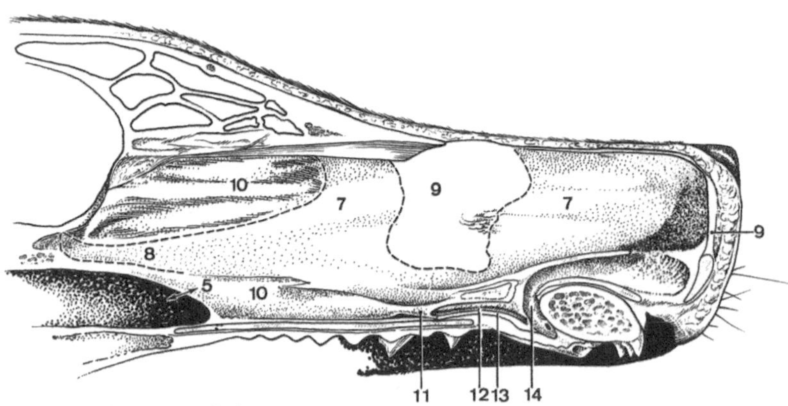

C Nasal septum right aspect (ca)

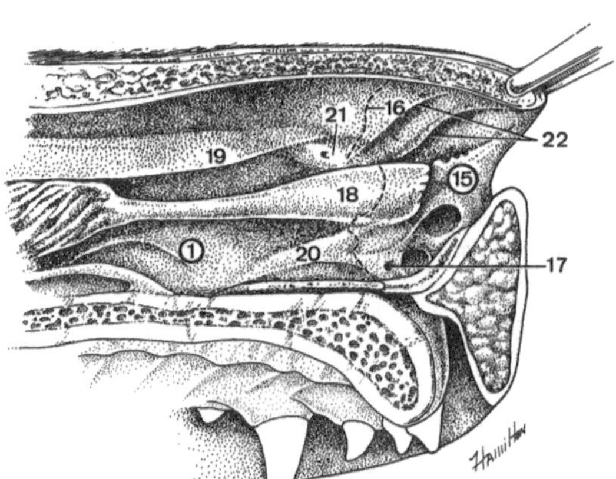

D Rostral part of left nasal cavity medial aspect (ca)

1 ***Concha nasalis dorsalis***. Dorsal nasal concha, attached to ethmoid and nasal bones, not homologous to Concha nasalis superior of man. A B

2 *Septum conchae dorsalis* (eq). Septum of the dorsal concha, transverse partition between rostral and caudal part. A

3 *Pars rostralis*. Rostral part of the concha. A

4 *Pars caudalis*. Caudal part of the concha. A

5 ***Concha nasalis media***. Middle nasal concha, wedged between the caudal ends of the dorsal and ventral conchae and the ethmoidal conchae. It is the largest ethmoidal concha. A

6 ***Conchae ethmoidales***. The ethmoidal conchae form the labyrinth in the caudal end of the nasal cavity. A

7 ***Concha nasalis ventralis***. Ventral nasal concha, attached to the maxilla. A B E

8 *Septum conchae ventralis* (eq). Septum of the ventral concha, partition between the rostral and caudal parts. A

9 *Pars rostralis*. Rostral part of the concha. A

10 *Pars caudalis*. Caudal part of the concha. A

11 *Pars dorsalis* (su, Ru). Dorsal part of the ventral concha, rolled dorsally. E

12 *Pars ventralis* (su, Ru). Ventral part of the ventral concha, rolled ventrally. E

13 ***Tunica mucosa nasi***. Mucous membrane lining the nasal cavity. E

14 *Regio respiratoria*. Respiratory region, covered by pseudostratified columnar ciliated epithelium with goblet cells. A D

15 *Regio olfactoria*. Olfactory region, on the caudal parts of the ethmoidal conchae and adjacent nasal septum. It is covered by olfactory epithelium. A C

16 **Gll. olfactoriae**. Olfactory glands, tubular, branched seromucous glands in the Lamina propria of the Regio olfactoria. C

17 *Gll. nasales*. Nasal glands, tubuloalveolar, mixed, in the Regio respiratoria, few and small in Car. D

18 ***Gl. nasalis lateralis***. Lateral nasal gland, serous, in the maxillary sinus (recess, Car) or the nasomaxillary aperture. Absent in bo. B

19 ***Plexus cavernosi nasales***. Cavernous plexuses of the nose, dense venous networks in the submucosa. E

20 ***Meatus nasi dorsalis***. Dorsal nasal meatus, passage between dorsal concha and dorsal wall of the nasal cavity. E

21 ***Meatus nasi medius***. Middle nasal meatus, between dorsal and ventral conchae. B E

22 ***Meatus nasi ventralis****. Ventral nasal meatus, between ventral concha and floor of the nasal cavity. This is the only way to communicate with the nasopharynx for introducing an endoscope or a gastric tube. E

23 ***Meatus nasi communis***. Common nasal meatus, sagittal passage along the septum. E

24 ***Meatus ethmoidales***. Ethmoidal meatuses, passages between the ethmoidal conchae. A

25 **SINUS PARANASALES**. Paranasal sinuses.

26 ***Sinus conchae dorsalis***. Dorsal conchal sinus, cavity enclosed by the caudal part of concha. A

27 ***Bulla conchalis dorsalis***. Dorsal conchal bulla, enclosure formed by the rolled-up free border of the rostral part of the dorsal concha. A

28 *Cellulae*. Cells, compartments formed by transverse septa. A

29 ***Sinus conchae mediae***. Middle conchal sinus. A

30 ***Sinus conchae ventralis***. Ventral conchal sinus, cavity enclosed by the caudal part of the ventral concha. A

31 ***Bulla conchalis ventralis***. Ventral conchal bulla, enclosure formed by the rolled-up free border of the ventral concha. A E

32 *Cellulae*. Cells, compartments formed by transverse septa. E

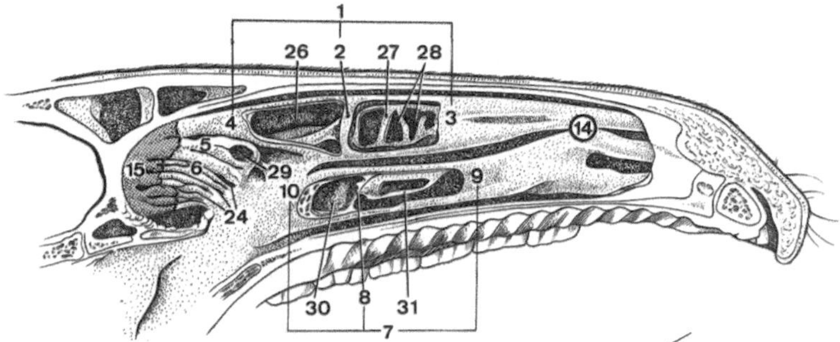

A Nasal cavity (septum removed), left medial aspect (eq)

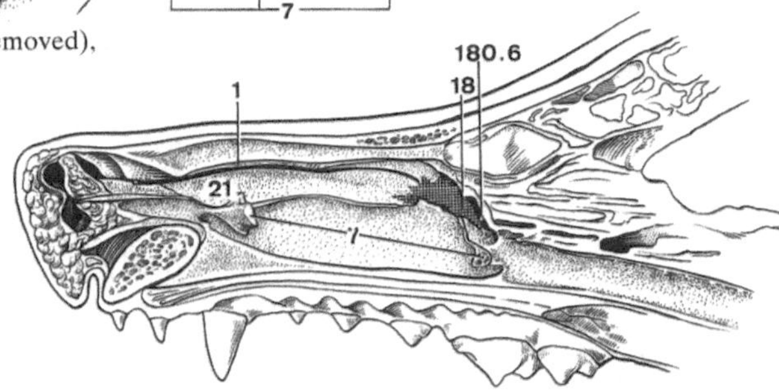

B Nasal cavity, medial aspect of right sagittal section (conchae largely removed) (ca)

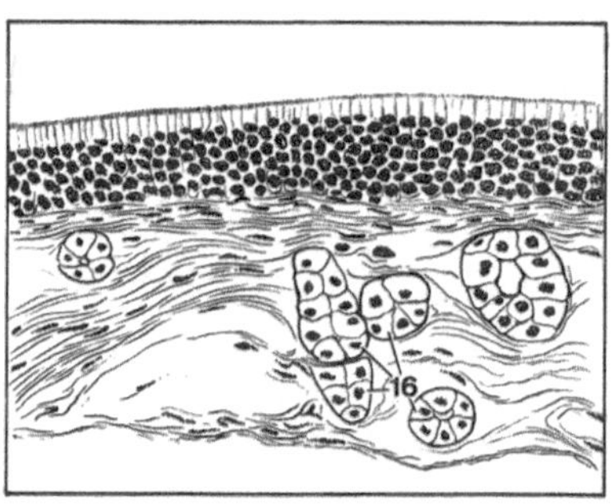

C Tunica mucosa of olfactory region, histological section (ca)

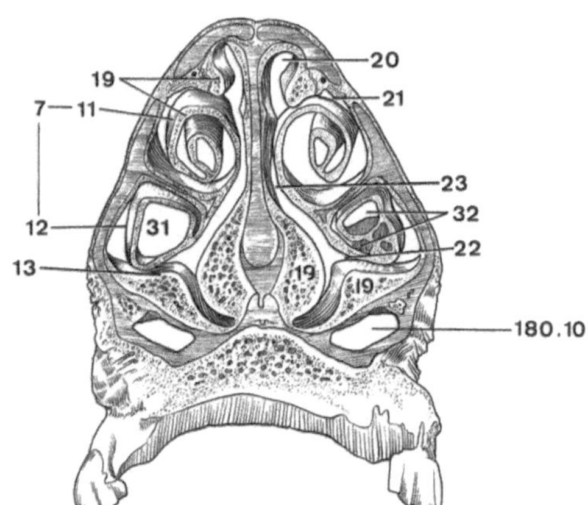

E Nasal cavity, transverse section rostral to 2nd premolar (bo)

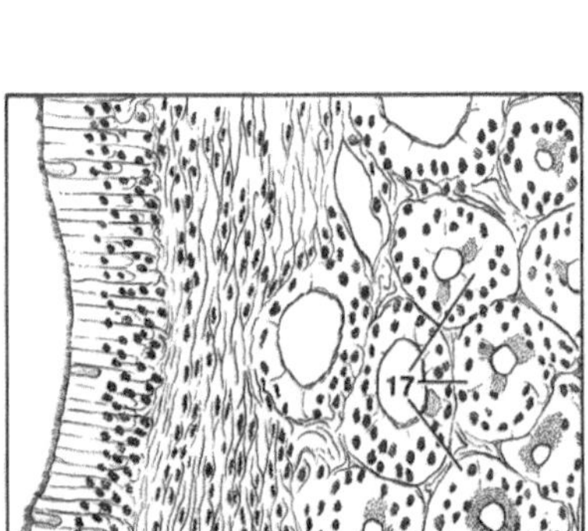

D Tunica mucosa of respiratory region, histological section (bo)

1 ***Sinus maxillaris.*** Maxillary sinus, between external and internal plates of facial bones. B

2 ***Sinus maxillaris rostralis.*** Rostral maxillary sinus in eq, separated by the maxillary septum from the caudal maxillary sinus. It opens freely into the ventral conchal sinus. A

3 ***Sinus maxillaris caudalis.*** Caudal maxillary sinus in eq, separated by the maxillary septum from the rostral maxillary sinus, communicates with the frontal and sphenopalatine sinuses, and opens in the middle nasal meatus. A

4 ***Septum sinuum maxillarium.*** Maxillary septum, between the rostral and caudal maxillary sinuses in eq. A

5 ***Recessus maxillaris*** (Car). Maxillary recess, between the ethmoid medially and the maxillary, palatine, and lacrimal bones laterally. C E

6 ***Apertura nasomaxillaris.*** Nasomaxillary opening, from the maxillary sinus or recess, to the middle nasal meatus. It is a common opening for both rostral and caudal maxillary sinuses in eq. A B C, 179 B

7 ***Apertura maxillopalatina*** (Ru). Maxillopalatine opening, wide passage over the infraorbital canal from the maxillary to the palatine sinus. B

8 ***Apertura conchomaxillaris*** (eq). Conchomaxillary opening, passage from the ventral conchal sinus to the rostral maxillary sinus. A

9 ***Sinus lacrimalis*** (su, Ru). Lacrimal sinus, in the lacrimal bone. B D

10 ***Sinus palatinus.*** Palatine sinus. In Ru in the hard palate, in eq in the Lamina perpendicularis of the palatine bone. 179 E

11 ***Sinus frontalis.*** Frontal sinus in fe and eq. Other species have more than one frontal sinus on each side. A E

12 ***Sinus frontalis rostralis*** (ca). Rostral frontal sinus. C

13 ***Sinus frontalis rostralis medialis*** (su, bo). Medial rostral frontal sinus. D

14 ***Sinus frontalis rostralis intermedius*** (bo). Middle rostral frontal sinus. D

15 ***Sinus frontalis rostralis lateralis*** (su, bo). Lateral rostral frontal sinus. D

16 ***Sinus frontalis medialis*** (ca, ov, cap). Medial frontal sinus. C

17 ***Sinus frontalis lateralis*** (ca, ov, cap). Lateral frontal sinus. C

18 ***Sinus frontalis caudalis*** (su, bo). Caudal frontal sinus. In the adult bo it has three diverticula: cornual, extended into the cornual process; nuchal, extended into the caudal wall of the skull, and postorbital, between the orbit and the cranial cavity. B D (The cornual diverticulum is opened in the dehorning of adult animals [large ruminants] [Nickel et al. 1979, p. 265].)

19 ***Aperturae sinuum frontalium.*** Openings of the frontal sinuses. D

20 ***Septa sinuum frontalium.*** Septa of the frontal sinuses, complete partitions between frontal sinuses. D

21 ***Lamellae intrasinuales.*** Intrasinusal lamellae, plates of bone that project into a sinus. D

22 ***Sinus conchofrontalis.*** Conchofrontal sinus is a compound term for the frontal sinus and the dorsal conchal sinus, which are continuous in eq. A

23 ***Apertura frontomaxillaris*** (eq). Frontomaxillary opening, between frontal sinus and caudal maxillary sinus. A

24 ***Sinus sphenoidalis.*** Sphenoidal sinus, cavity in the sphenoid bones. Absent in ca, ov, cap. E

25 *Septum sinuum sphenoidalium.* Septum between right and left sphenoidal sinuses. E

26 *Apertura sinus sphenoidalis.* Opening of the sphenoidal sinus. E

27 ***Sinus sphenopalatinus*** (eq). Sphenopalatine sinus. The sphenoid and palatine sinuses are continuous and open into the caudal maxillary sinus. A

28 ***Cellulae ethmoidales.*** Ethmoidal cells, enclosed by the ethmoidal conchae. A E

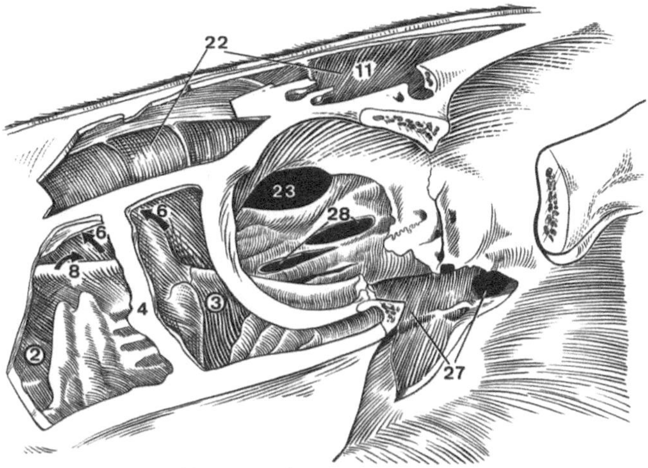

A Paranasal sinuses (medial wall of orbit removed), left lateral aspect (eq)

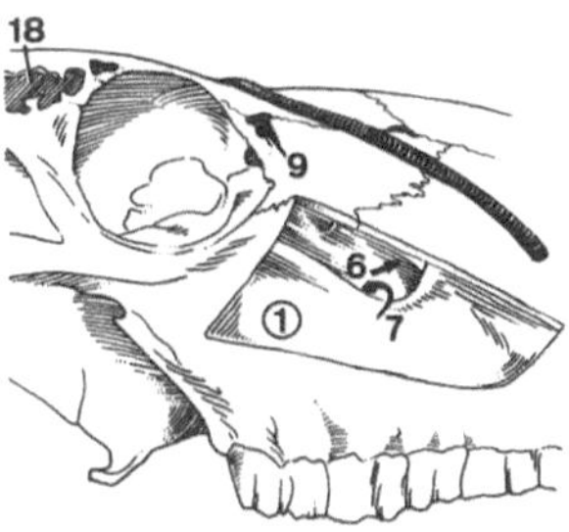

B Right maxillary sinus (bo)

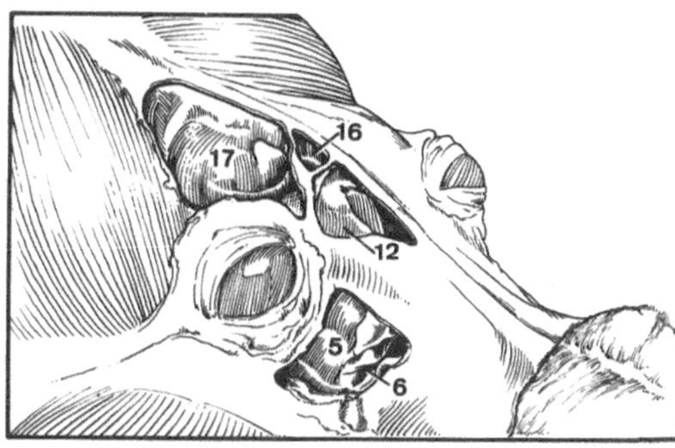

C Right frontal sinuses and maxillary recess (infraorbital canal removed) (ca)

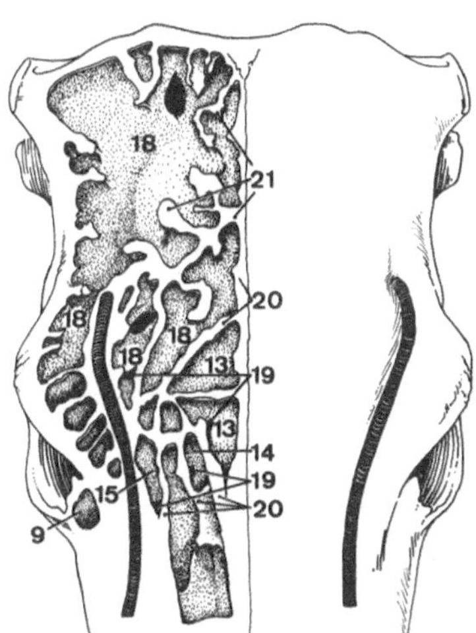

D Right frontal sinuses (bo)

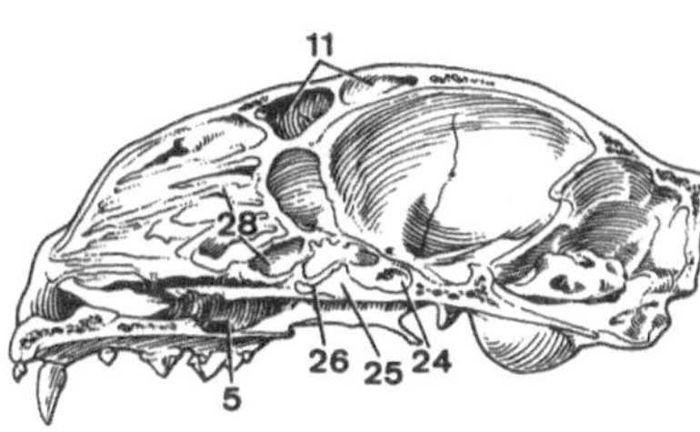

E Skull, medial aspect of right sagittal section (fe)

1 **LARYNX.** Organ of voice and transition between pharynx and trachea.

2 ***Prominentia laryngea.*** Ventral prominence of thyroid cartilage. A D

3 **Cartilagines laryngis.**

4 **Cartilago thyroidea [thyreoidea].** Thyroid cartilage. A D

5 ***Lamina [dextra et sinistra]**** . Right and left lamina, plates joined ventrally to form the thyroid cartilage. B D

6 ***Incisura thyroidea [thyreoidea] rostralis.*** Rostral thyroid notch in Ru. D

7 ***Incisura thyroidea [thyreoidea] caudalis**** . Caudal thyroid notch. B D

8 ***Linea obliqua.*** Oblique line on the lateral surface of the lamina for attachment of muscles. A

9 ***Cornu rostrale.*** Rostral horn, absent in su; articulates with the thyrohyoid bone. A D

10 ***Cornu caudale.*** Caudal horn, articulates with the cricoid cartilage. A D

11 ***Fissura thyroidea [thyreoidea].*** Thyroid fissure, between the rostral horn and the lamina. A

12 ***Foramen thyroideum [thyreoideum].*** Thyroid foramen, in the caudal end of the thyroid fissure, outlined by the cartilage and the perichondrium. A

13 ***Facies articularis cricoidea.*** Articular surface for cricoid cartilage on caudal horn. This is a syndesmosis in Ru. D

14 ***Facies articularis hyoidea.*** Articular surface for thyrohyoid bone on rostral horn. D

15 ***Articulatio thyrohyoidea [thyreo-].*** Thyrohyoid joint, between the thyroid cartilage and the thyrohyoid bone. A

16 ***Capsula articularis thyrohyoidea [thyreo-].*** Thyrohyoid joint capsule, absent in Car and su which is provided with a syndesmosis. A

17 ***Membrana thyrohyoidea [thyreo-].*** Thyrohyoid membrane, from the rostral border of the thyroid lamina to the basihyoid and thyrohyoid bones. A B

18 **Cartilago cricoidea.** Cricoid cartilage, the ring-shaped cartilage attached to the trachea. A C

19 ***Arcus cartilaginis cricoideae.*** Arch of the cricoid cartilage, the narrow ventral part. B C

20 ***Lamina cartilaginis cricoideae.*** Lamina of the cricoid cartilage, broad dorsal part. C

21 *Crista mediana.* Median crest on the lamina. C

22 *Facies articularis arytenoidea [arytaenoidea].* Articular surface for the arytenoid cartilage. C

23 *Facies articularis thyroidea [thyreoidea].* Articular surface for the thyroid cartilage. C

24 ***Articulatio cricothyroidea [-thyreoidea].*** Cricothyroid joint, between the cricoid and the thyroid cartilages. A

25 *Capsula articularis cricothyroidea [-thyreoidea].* Capsule of the cricothyroid joint. Absent in Ru, which have a syndesmosis here. A

26 *Lig. cricothyroideum [-thyreoideum]**. Cricothyroid ligament, from the cricoid cartilage to the thryoid laminae. B

27 ***Lig. cricotracheale.*** Cricotracheal ligament, the membrane between the cricoid cartilage and the first tracheal ring. B

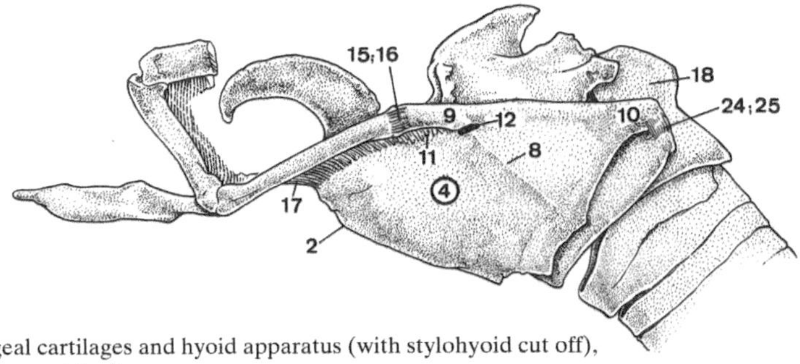

A Laryngeal cartilages and hyoid apparatus (with stylohyoid cut off), left lateral aspect (eq)

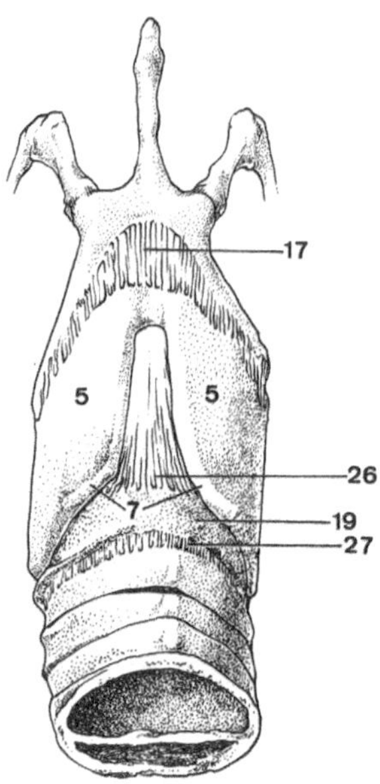

B Laryngeal cartilages and hyoid apparatus (with stylohyoid cut off), ventral aspect (eq)

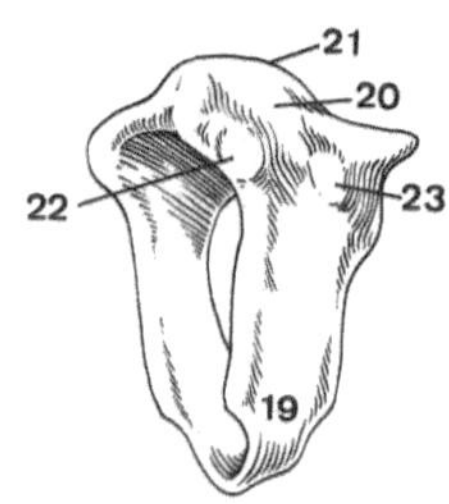

C Cricoid cartilage, rostrolateral left aspect (eq)

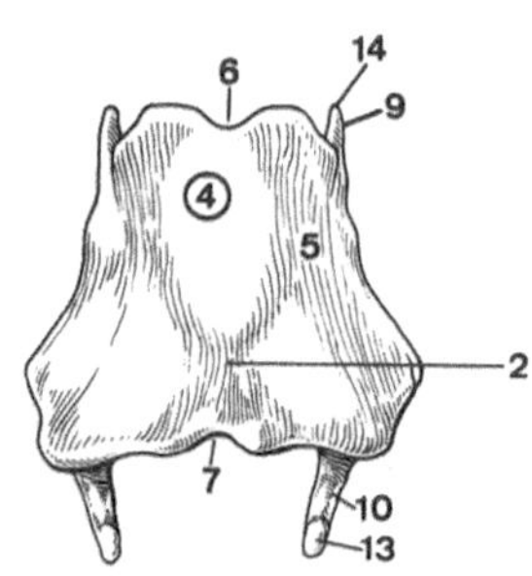

D Thyroid cartilage, ventral aspect (bo)

1 **Cartilago arytenoidea [arytaenoidea].** Arytenoid cartilage. Flattened pyramidal lever that widens and closes or narrows the glottis. A C D

2 ***Facies articularis.*** Articular surface for the cricoid cartilage. D

3 ***Basis cartilaginis arytenoideae [arytaenoideae].*** Base of the arytenoid cartilage, facing caudally toward the cricoid cartilage. C D

4 *Processus vocalis.* Vocal process, ventral projection for attachment of the vocal ligament. A C D

5 ***Facies lateralis.*** Lateral surface, separated from the dorsal surface by the Crista arcuata. C

6 *Processus muscularis.* Muscular process, at the caudal end of the Crista arcuata. B C

7 *Crista arcuata.* Arcuate crest, separates lateral and dorsal surfaces. C

8 ***Facies medialis.*** Medial surface, forms the dorsal part of the glottis. D

9 *Processus medialis.* Medial process, attachment of the Lig. arytenoideum transversum. B

10 ***Facies dorsalis.*** Dorsal surface. B C

11 *Apex cartilaginis arytenoideae [arytaenoideae].* Apex of the arytenoid cartilage, craniodorsal angle to which the corniculate process is attached. A C

12 **Processus corniculatus.** Corniculate process, may be independent, absent in fe. A B C

13 **Processus cuneiformis** (ca). Cuneiform process, rostrodorsal projection of the apex of the arytenoid, supports the Plica aryepiglottica and the Plica vestibuli. A B

14 ***Cartilago interarytenoidea [-arytaenoidea].*** Interarytenoid cartilage, dorsal to the Lig. arytenoideum transversum and just rostral to the cricoid cartilage in ca and su. A B

15 ***Cartilago sesamoidea.*** Symmetrical sesamoid cartilage, lies across the dorsal surface of the arytenoid cartilages caudal to the corniculate processes in Car. In ca it may be paired. A B

16 ***Lig. arytenoideum [arytaenoideum] transversum.*** Transverse arytenoid ligament, between the medial processes of the arytenoid cartilages. B

17 ***Lig. arycorniculatum.*** Arycorniculate ligament, from the Crista arcuata to the ventral half of the free border of the corniculate process. C (When the corniculate cartilage is independent, it is connected to the corresponding arytenoid cartilage by an amphiarthrosis including the arycorniculate ligament.)

18 ***Articulatio cricoarytenoidea [-arytaenoidea].*** Cricoarytenoid joint, between the cricoid cartilage and the arytenoid cartilages. B

19 *Capsula articularis cricoarytenoidea [-arytaenoidea].* Cricoarytenoid joint capsule. B D

20 *Lig. cricoarytenoideum [-arytaenoideum].* Cricoarytenoid ligament, from the cricoid lamina to the base of each arytenoid cartilage. A

21 **Epiglottis.** Most rostral component of the larynx. B E

22 ***Facies lingualis.*** Lingual surface. A

23 ***Facies laryngea.*** Laryngeal surface. E

24 ***Margines laterales.*** Lateral borders. E

25 ***Basis.*** Base, attached to the thyroid cartilage. E

26 ***Apex.*** Free rostral tip. A

27 ***Petiolus epiglotticus.*** Stem of the epiglottis, a median projection from the base. E

28 ***Cartilago epiglottica.*** Epiglottic cartilage. A

29 *Processus cuneiformis* (eq). Cuneiform process, projects in the vestibular fold. E

30 ***Lig. thyroepiglotticum [thyreo-].*** Thyroepiglottic ligament, attaches the base of the epiglottis to the thyroid cartilage. E

31 ***Lig. hyoepiglotticum.*** Hyoepiglottic ligament, from the basihyoid and keratohyoid bones, and, in su, also from the thyrohyoid bone, to the epiglottis. A 187 B

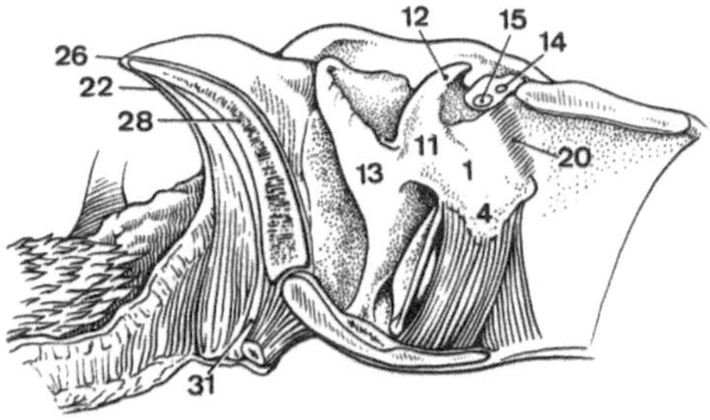

A Larynx, median section right medial aspect (mucosa partly removed) (ca)

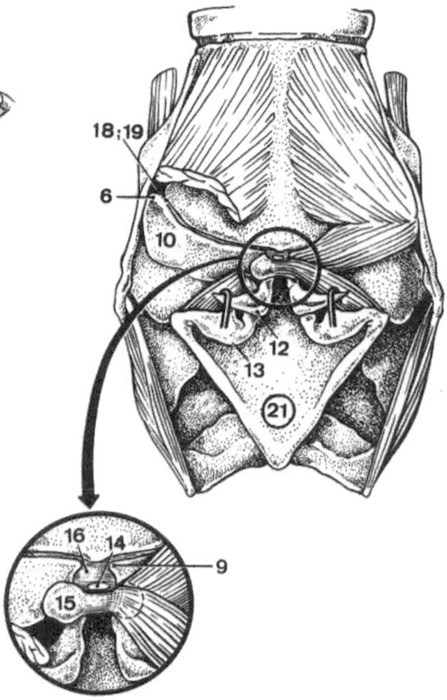

B Larynx (right M. arytenoideus transversus and terminations of M. cricoarytenoideus dorsalis and M. ventricularis removed), dorsal aspect (ca)

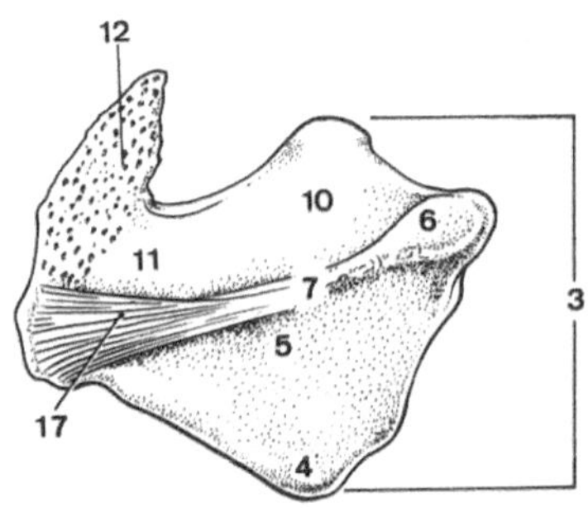

C Left arytenoid cartilage, lateral aspect (eq)

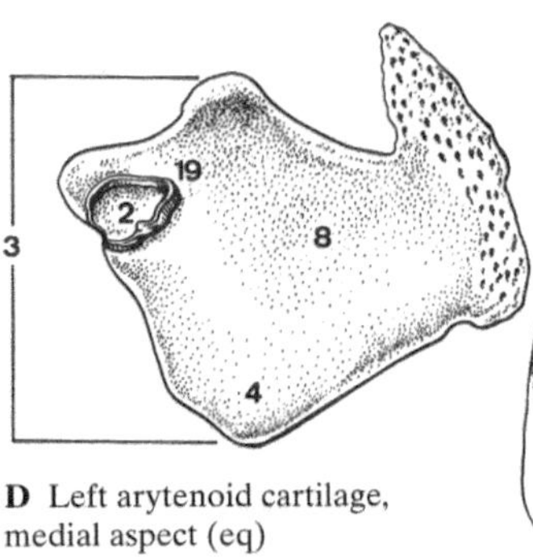

D Left arytenoid cartilage, medial aspect (eq)

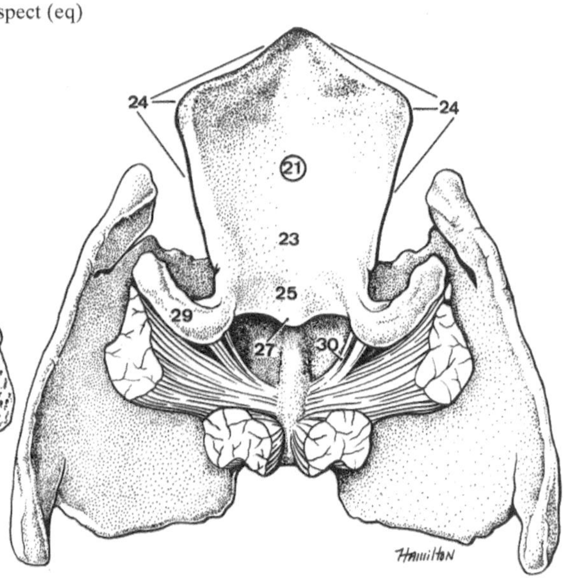

E Epiglottis and thyroid cartilage (the stumps of Mm. ventricularis and vocalis remain), caudodorsal aspect (eq)

1 **Musculi laryngis.**

2 ***M. cricothyroideus [-thyreoideus].*** O: cricoid arch. T: thyroid lamina. Tenses the vocal folds. A D

3 ***M. cricoarytenoideus [-arytaenoideus] dorsalis.*** O: cricoid lamina. T: Processus muscularis. Widens the glottis. A B

4 ***M. cricoarytenoideus [-arytaenoideus] lateralis.*** O: cricoid arch. T: Processus muscularis. Closes or narrows the glottis. A D

5 ***M. thyroarytenoideus [thyreoarytaenoideus].*** O: thyroid cartilage, epiglottis, Lig. cricothyroideum. T: Crista arcuata, muscular and vocal processes. A

6 *M. ventricularis.* Rostral part of M. thyroarytenoideus in ca and eq. A D

7 *M. vocalis.* In ca and eq, from thyroid cartilage and Lig. cricothyroideum to Crista arcuata and Processus vocalis. A D

8 ***M. thyroarytenoideus [thyreoarytaenoideus] accessorius*** (eq). O: thyroid cartilage. T: M. arytenoideus transversus. A

9 ***M. hyoepiglotticus.*** O: varies with species, basihyoid, keratohyoid, or both. T: epiglottic cartilage. B

10 ***M. tensor ventriculi laryngis*** (eq) O: Processus cuneiformis. T: ventral part of laryngeal ventricle.

11 ***M. arytenoideus [arytaenoideus] transversus.*** O: Crista arcuata of arytenoid cartilage. T: Contralateral muscle. A B

12 **Cavum laryngis.** Cavity of the larynx.

13 ***Aditus laryngis.*** Entrance to the larynx, bounded by the epiglottis, Plicae aryepiglotticae, and Tubercula corniculata (in fe arytenoid cartilages). C

14 *Tuberculum cuneiforme.* In the Plica aryepiglottica, formed by the Processus cuneiformis. C

15 *Tuberculum corniculatum.* Mucosal eminence formed by the Processus corniculatus, absent in fe. A B C

16 *Plica aryepiglottica.* From epiglottis to arytenoid cartilage in ca, eq, cricoid cartilage in fe, mucosa caudal to Tuberculum corniculatum in su, Ru. B C

17 *Incisura interarytenoidea [-arytaenoidea].* Interarytenoid notch, between the Processus corniculati. C

18 ***Vestibulum laryngis.*** Vestibule of the larynx, between the aditus and the vocal folds. B D

19 ***Plica vestibularis.*** Vestibular fold. In ca, eq supported by Lig. vestibulare and cuneiform process, in fe fold of mucosa; absent in su, Ru. B D

20 ***Rima vestibuli.*** Vestibular cleft, between right and left vestibular folds. D

21 ***Ventriculus laryngis.*** Laryngeal ventricle, between vestibular and vocal folds in ca, eq, between the two parts of the vocal fold in su. A B D (Called by veterinary clinicians "laryngeal saccule", which is a wrong term, not homologous to the human saccule, which is an appendix of the laryngeal ventricle.)

22 ***Recessus laryngis medianus.*** Median laryngeal recess, caudal to the epiglottis. B

23 ***Glottis.*** Vocal apparatus of the larynx, consists of vocal folds, arytenoid cartilages and Rima glottidis. B

24 ***Plica vocalis.*** Vocal fold, covers Lig. vocale and M. vocalis or the caudal part of M. thyroarytenoideus. B D

25 ***Rima glottidis.*** Cleft of the glottis, between vocal folds and arytenoid cartilages. D

26 *Pars intermembranacea.* Intermembranous part, between the vocal folds. B

27 *Pars intercartilaginea.* Intercartilaginous part, between the mucosa-covered arytenoid cartilages. B

28 ***Cavum infraglotticum.*** Infraglottic cavity, caudal to the glottis. B D

29 ***Tunica mucosa.*** Mucous membrane. Stratified squamous epithelium to the vocal folds, pseudostratified ciliated epithelium in the rest, including the Ventriculi laryngis in eq. D

30 ***Membrana fibroelastica laryngis.*** From the epiglottis to Lig. vestibulare and from Lig. vocale to the cricoid cartilage. D

31 *Lig. vestibulare.* Ca: thyroid cartilage to Processus cuneiformis; su: epiglottis to Processus corniculatus; eq; Processus cuneiformis to arytenoid cartilage. Absent in fe, Ru. D

32 *Lig. vocale.* From thyroid cartilage and Lig. cricothyroideum to Processus vocalis. D

33 ***Gll. laryngeae.*** Laryngeal glands. D

34 ***Lymphonoduli [Noduli lymphatici] laryngei.*** Lymph nodules of the larynx. D

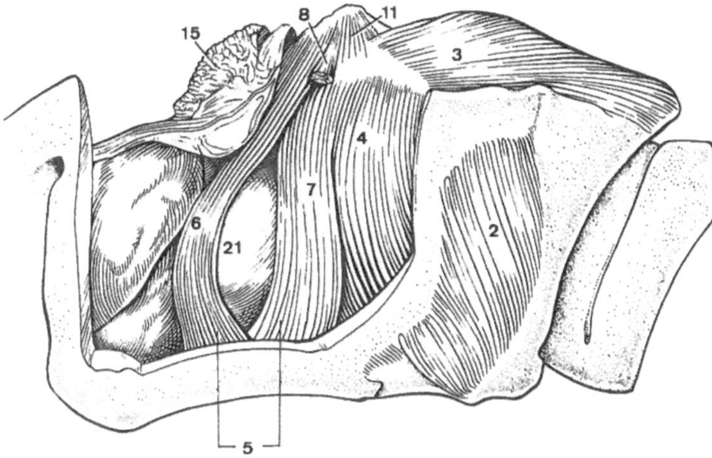

A Laryngeal muscles (most of the thyroid cartilage removed), left lateral aspect (eq)

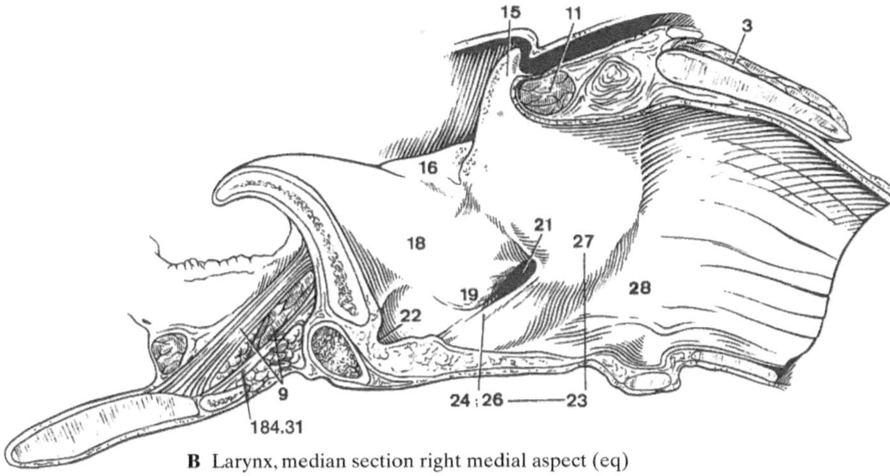

B Larynx, median section right medial aspect (eq)

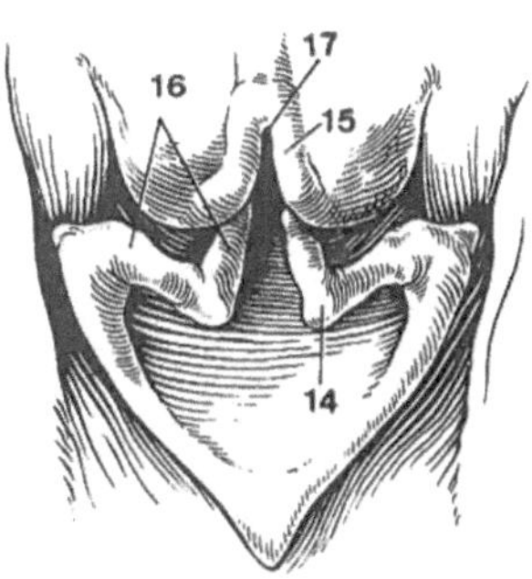

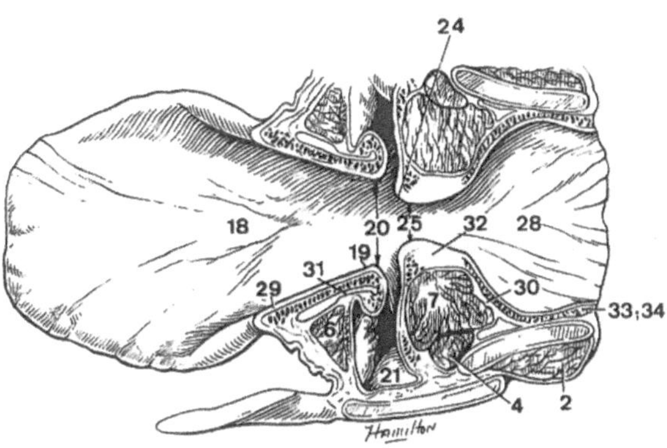

C Aditus laryngis dorsal aspect (ca) **D** Larynx, section perpendicular to vocal folds dorsal aspect (eq)

1 **TRACHEA***. Windpipe. A B

2 ***Pars cervicalis***. Cervical part.

3 ***Pars thoracica***. Thoracic part.

4 ***Cartilagines tracheales***. Tracheal cartilages, annular bands interrupted dorsally. A B C

5 ***Musculus trachealis***. Tracheal muscle, transverse bands of smooth muscle connecting the dorsal ends of the tracheal cartilages. The muscle is attached inside the cartilage except Car, where it is outside. B

6 ***Ligg. anularia [trachealia]***. Annular ligaments, the connective tissue between the tracheal cartilages. A C

7 ***Paries membranaceus***. Membranous wall continuation of perichondrium, when the dorsal ends of the tracheal cartilages do not meet. B

8 ***Tela submucosa***. Loose vascular connective tissue under the mucous membrane. C

9 *Gll. tracheales*. Tracheal glands, mixed glands in the submucosa. C

10 ***Tunica mucosa***. Mucous membrane, covered with pseudostratified ciliated epithelium. C

11 ***Bifurcatio trachea***. Tracheal bifurcation, where the right and left main bronchi arise. A D

12 *Carina tracheae*. Crest in the lumen on the caudal side of the bifurcation. D

13 **BRONCHI**. Branches of the trachea and their subdivisions.

14 ***Arbor bronchalis***. Bronchial tree. A

15 ***Bronchus principalis [dexter et sinister]***. Right and left main bronchus. A D

16 ***Bronchi lobares***. Lobar bronchi; each serves one whole lobe. A

17 *Bronchus trachealis* (su, Ru). Bronchus of the right cranial lobe, separate origin from the trachea. A

18 ***Bronchi segmentales***. Segmental bronchi; each serves one whole Segmentum bronchopulmonale. A

19 ***Cartilagines bronchales***. Bronchial ring-shaped cartilages, without interruption. D E

20 ***Tela submucosa***. Loose vascular connective tissue outside the mucosa. E

21 *Gll. bronchales*. Bronchial glands, mixed glands in the submucosa. E

22 ***Tunica mucosa***. Mucous membrane, covered by pseudostratified ciliated epithelium. E

23 *Lamina muscularis mucosae*. The bronchial musculature lies between the Lamina propria mucosae and the Tela submucosa. It is designated as the Musculus spiralis bronchalis in the Nomina Histologica Veterinaria. E

24 ***Lymphonoduli [Noduli lymphatici] bronchales***. Bronchial lymph nodules.

25 **PULMO [DEXTER ET SINISTER]**. Lung, right and left. F G

26 ***Basis pulmonis***. Base of the lung, caudal part. Its surface is in contact with the diaphragmatic pleura. G

27 ***Apex pulmonis***. Apex of the lung, the cranial extremity. F

28 ***Facies costalis***. Costal surface, in contact with the costal pleura. F

29 ***Facies medialis***. Medial surface. G

30 *Pars vertebralis*. Vertebral part, the dorsal zone along the vertebrae. G

31 *Pars mediastinalis*. Mediastinal part, in contact with the Mediastinum. G

32 *Impressio cardiaca*. Cardiac impression. G

33 *Impressio aortica*. Aortic impression. G

34 *Impressio esophagea [oesophagea]*. Esophageal impression. G

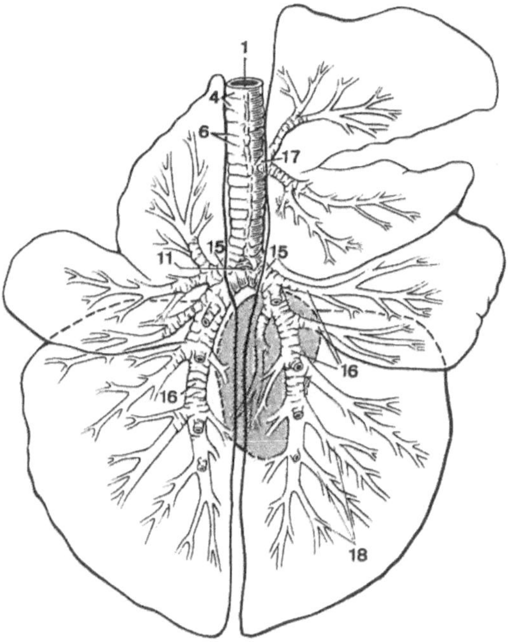

A Bronchial tree, dorsal aspect (bo) (Getty 1975)

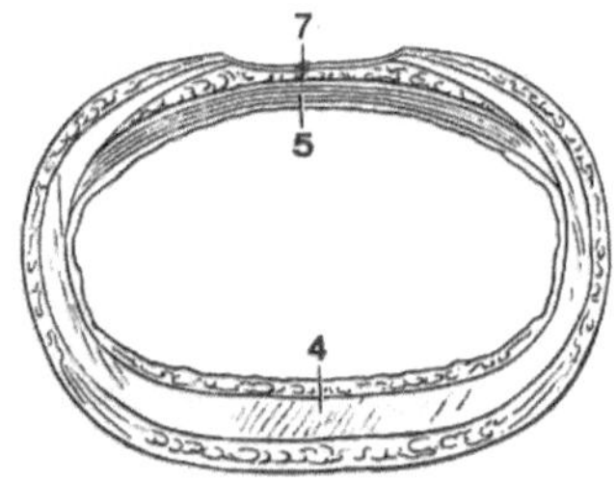

B Trachea, transverse section (eq)

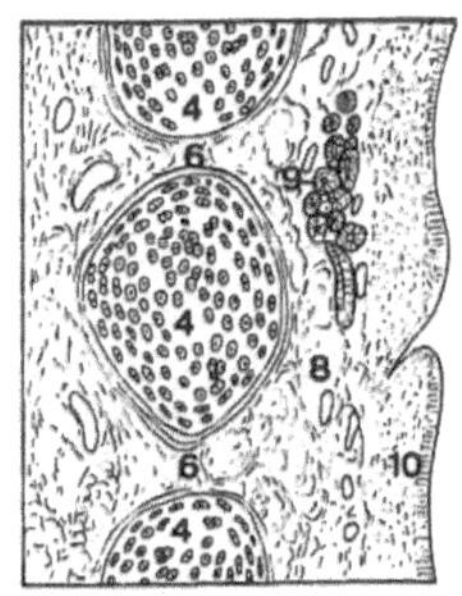

C Trachea, longitudinal section (su) (Trautmann and Fiebiger 1957)

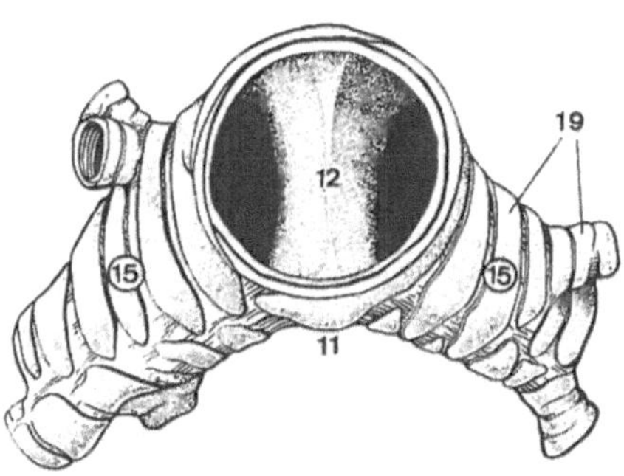

D Bifurcation of trachea, cranial aspect of section (eq)

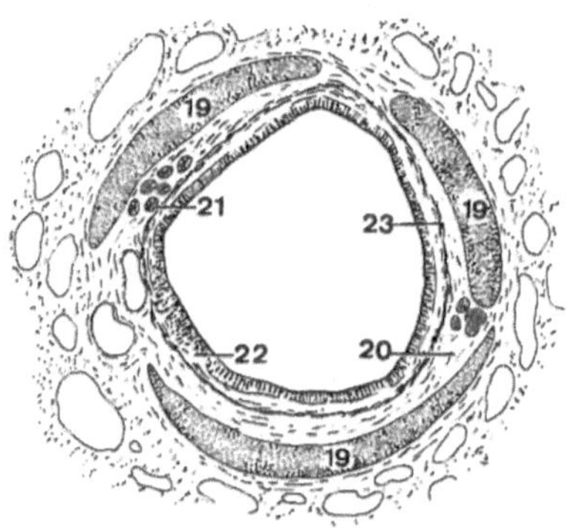

E Bronchus, transverse section (eq) (Trautmann and Fiebiger 1957)

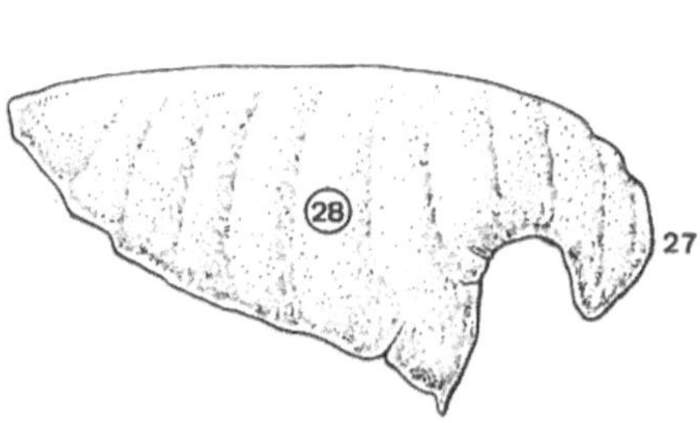

F Right lung, costal surface (eq) (Getty 1975)

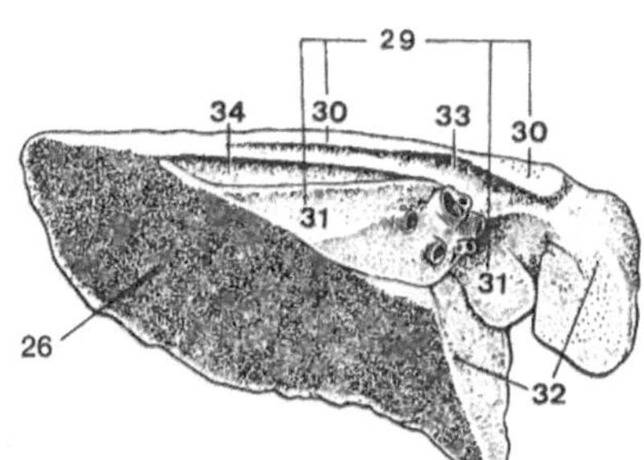

G Left lung, medial surface (eq) (Getty 1975)

1 *Sulcus venae cavae caudalis*. Groove for the caudal vena cava in the right lung between accessory lobe and middle and caudal lobes. A

2 ***Facies diaphragmatica***. Diaphragmatic surface. A

3 ***Facies interlobares***. Interlobar surfaces in the fissures between lobes.

4 ***Margo dorsalis [obtusus]***. Dorsal, thick, and rounded border. A B

5 ***Margo acutus***. Thin border. A

6 *Margo ventralis*. Ventral border, cranial to the tip of the middle lobe of the right lung or along the ventral border of the cranial lobe of the left lung. A B

7 *Margo basalis*. Basal border, cranioventrally oriented, where costal and diaphragmatic surfaces meet. A B

8 ***Hilus pulmonis***. Hilus of the lung, area where bronchus and vessels enter. A

9 ***Radix pulmonis***. Root of the lung, composed of the structures that enter the lung at the Hilus. A

10 ***Incisura cardiaca pulmonis dextri***. Cardiac notch of the right lung. A B C

11 ***Incisura cardiaca pulmonis sinistri***. Cardiac notch of the left lung. C

12 ***Lobus cranialis [pulm. dext.]***. Cranial lobe of the right lung. The scheme of lobation is determined by origin and division of the lobar bronchi. A B C (All species of domestic mammals have a cranial lobe and a caudal lobe on both lungs, and an accessory lobe on the right lung. All except eq have a middle lobe of the right lung. In all species except eq the cranial lobe of the left lung is divided into cranial and caudal parts. In Ru the right cranial lobe is also divided into cranial and caudal parts.)

13 *Pars cranialis*. Cranial part in Ru. B C

14 *Pars caudalis*. Caudal part in Ru. B C

15 ***Lobus cranialis [pulm. sin.]***. Cranial lobe of the left lung, divided into cranial and caudal parts (except eq). C

16 *Pars cranialis [Culmen]*. Cranial part. C

17 *Pars caudalis [Lingula]*. Caudal part. C

18 ***Lobus medius [pulm. dext.]***. Middle lobe of the right lung (except eq). A B

19 ***Lobus caudalis***. Caudal lobe. A B

20 ***Lobus accessorius [pulm. dext.]***. Accessory lobe (of the right lung). A

21 ***Fissura interlobaris cranialis [pulm. dext.]***. Cranial interlobar fissure of the right lung, between cranial and middle lobes, absent in eq. B

22 ***Fissura interlobaris caudalis***. Caudal interlobar fissure, between middle and caudal lobes of the right lung except eq (instead, in eq this fissure separates the cranial from the caudal lobes of the right lung), cranial and caudal lobes of the left lung. B

23 **Segmenta bronchopulmonalia***. Bronchopulmonary segments, segmentation based on the bronchi. They are accompanied by branches of A. bronchopulmonaris. C

24 ***Segmenta dorsalia lobi cranialis***. Dorsal segments of the cranial lobe. C

25 ***Segmenta ventralia lobi cranialis***. Ventral segments of the cranial lobe. C

26 ***Segmenta medialia lobi cranialis***. Medial segments of the cranial lobe.

27 ***Segmenta lateralia lobi cranialis***. Lateral segments of the cranial lobe.

28 ***Segmenta lobi medii***. Segments of the middle lobe, except eq. C

29 ***Segmenta dorsalia lobi caudalis***. Dorsal segments of the caudal lobe. C

30 ***Segmenta ventralia lobi caudalis***. Ventral segments of the caudal lobe. C

31 ***Segmenta medialia lobi caudalis***. Medial segments of the caudal lobe. C

32 ***Segmenta lateralia lobi caudalis***. Lateral segments of the caudal lobe.

33 ***Segmentum accessorium***. Accessory segment. C

34 ***Lobuli pulmonis***. Pulmonary lobules. A primary lobule is about 1 mm in diameter, a secondary lobule is a polyhedron with sides about 1 cm across. It contains about 50 primary lobules. B

35 ***Bronchuli***. Bronchioles, less than 1 mm in diameter, without cartilage. D

36 ***Bronchuli respiratorii***. Respiratory bronchioles, less than 0,5 mm in diameter, bear alveoli and branch. D

37 *Ductuli alveolares*. Alveolar ducts, walls riddled with the openings of alveoli. D

38 *Sacculi alveolares*. Alveolar sacs, bearing alveoli. D

39 *Alveoli pulmonis*. Pulmonary alveoli, the smallest respiratory chambers. D

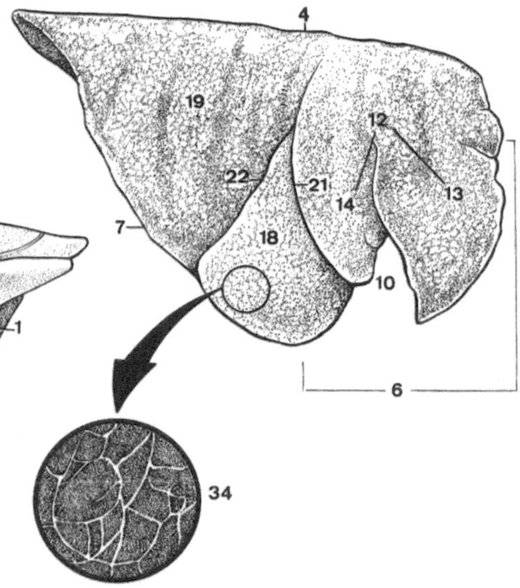

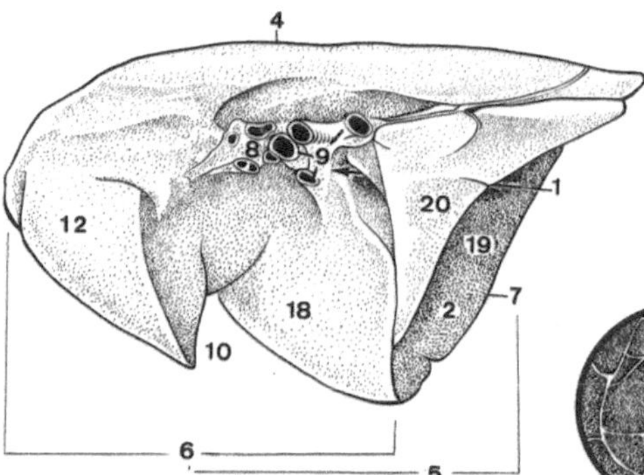

A Right lung, medial surface (ca) (Getty)

B Right lung, costal surface (bo) (Getty)

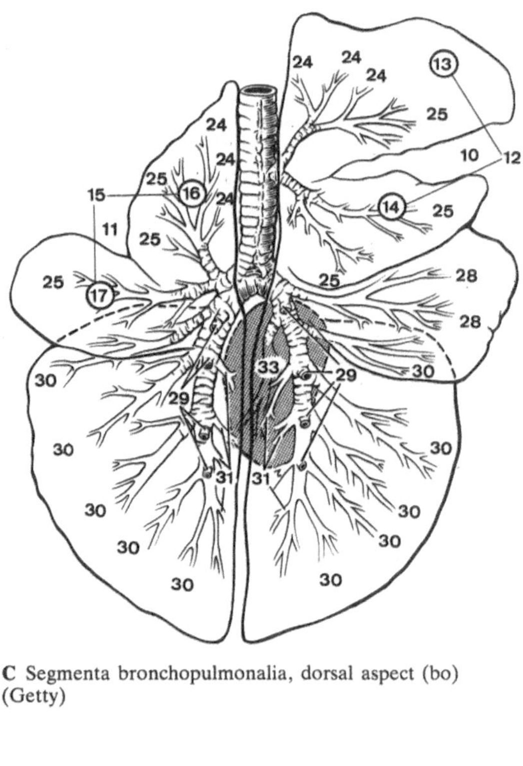

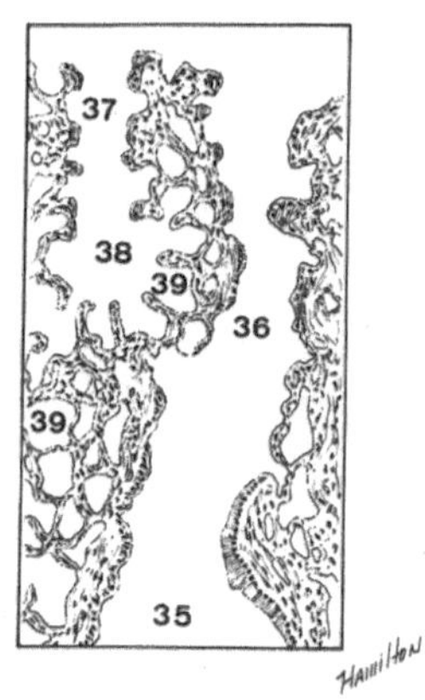

D Lung, histological section (ca)

C Segmenta bronchopulmonalia, dorsal aspect (bo) (Getty)

1 **CAVUM THORACIS**. Thoracic cavity. Its walls are formed by ribs, thoracic vertebrae, sternum, and associated muscles, including diaphragm. It is a truncated cone, flattened laterally in quadrupeds, with the apex between the first pair of ribs, and the concave oblique base at the diaphragm.

2 ***Fascia endothoracica***. Endothoracic fascia, connective tissue lining the thoracic walls outside of the Pleura parietalis. C

3 ***Cavum pleurae***. Pleural cavity, right and left, virtual and potential space between Pleura parietalis and pulmonalis and between the lobes of the lung. A C

4 ***Pleura***. Serous membrane that lines the thoracic cavity on either side of the mediastinum, medial side of ribs and, the diaphragm, and covers the lung. The Pleura parietalis is continuous with the Pleura pulmonalis at the root of the lung and the Lig. pulmonale. A

5 *Cupula pleurae*. Blind end of the pleural sacs at the thoracic inlet. A

6 *Pleura pulmonalis*. Pulmonary pleura, serous covering of the lung. C

7 *Pleura parietalis*. Parietal pleura, lining the walls of each pleural cavity.

8 **Pleura mediastinalis**. Mediastinal pleura. Part of the Pleura parietalis that covers the mediastinum on both sides. A C

9 **Pleura pericardiaca**. Pericardial pleura, Part of the Pleura mediastinalis that covers the Pericardium fibrosum. A C

10 **Pleura costalis**. Costal pleura, part of the Pleura parietalis that lines the ribs and intercostal muscles. C

11 **Pleura diaphragmatica**. Diaphragmatic pleura, part of the Pleura parietalis covering the diaphragm. D

12 ***Recessus pleurales***. Pleural recesses, clefts between reflected layers of Pleura parietalis allowing for movement of the walls and expansion of the lungs.

13 *Recessus costodiaphragmaticus**. Costodiaphragmatic recess, between Pleura costalis and diaphragmatica, caudoventral to the basal border of the lung. A D (The projection of this recess on the skin indicates the maximal ventral extent of the pleural cavity.)

14 *Recessus costomediastinalis*. Costomediastinal recess, between Pleura costalis and mediastinalis. C

15 *Recessus lumbodiaphragmaticus*. In Car, su, ov, cap the Pleura extends caudal to the vertebral end of the last rib to the first lumbar vertebra. B

16 *Recessus mediastinodiaphragmaticus sinister*. Left mediastinodiaphragmatic recess. Extension of the Recessus mediastini by leftward deviation of the attachment of mediastinum to the diaphragm. A D

17 ***Lig. pulmonale***. Pulmonary ligament, formed by the continuity of Pleura mediastinalis and pulmonalis caudal to the root of the lung. A C D

18 ***Mediastinum***. Deviant connective tissue septum and Pleurae mediastinales between the right and left pleural cavities. It contains most of the structures in the thoracic cavity except the lungs.

19 *Mediastinum craniale*. Cranial to the pericardium, contains great vessels, trachea, esophagus. A

20 *Mediastinum ventrale*. Between pericardium and sternum. A C

21 *Mediastinum medium*. Middle mediastinum, containing heart and pericardium. C

22 *Mediastinum dorsale*. Between pericardium and vertebrae. A

23 *Mediastinum caudale*. Caudal to the pericardium, the dorsal part contains aorta, esophagus; the ventral part is thin and attached to the left side of the diaphragm. A D

23a ***Fenestrae mediastini***. Small openings piercings the caudal mediastinum. Filled with fat in healthy animals. (Car, eq)

24 **Cavum mediastini serosum [Bursa infracardiaca]**. Serous cavity of the mediastinum on the right side of the esophagus in the Mediastinum caudale, extension of the Bursa omentalis. C D

25 **Plica venae cavae**. Fold for the caudal vena cava (and the right phrenic nerve), from the pericardium to the diaphragm, continuous ventrally with the Mediastinum caudale. D

26 **Recessus mediastini**. Mediastinal recess, evagination of the right pleural cavity between the Mediastinum caudale and the Plica venae cavae, contains the accessory lobe of the right lung. A D

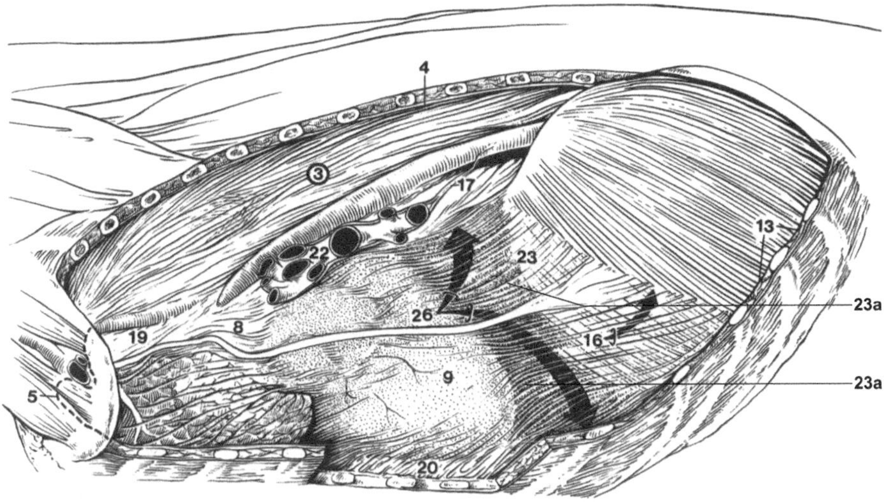

A Left pleural cavity (lung and ribs 2–12 removed) (ca)

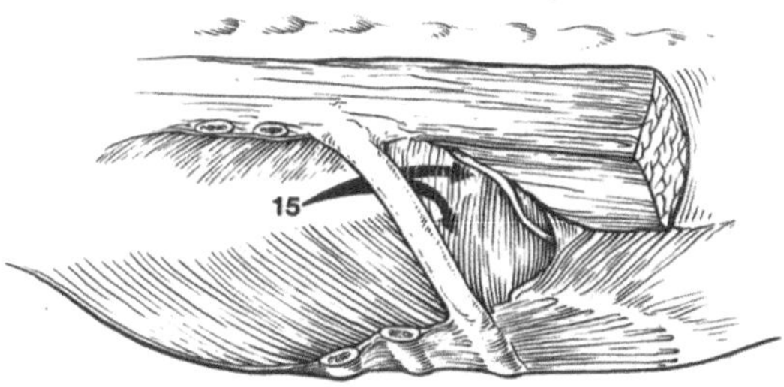

B Left thoracolumbar region, dorsolateral aspect (ca)

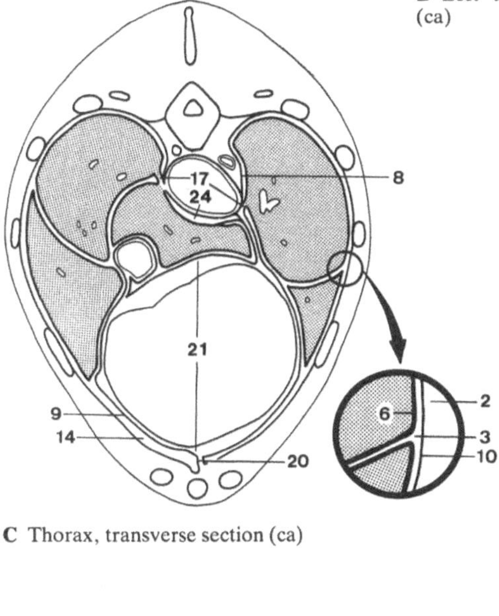

C Thorax, transverse section (ca)

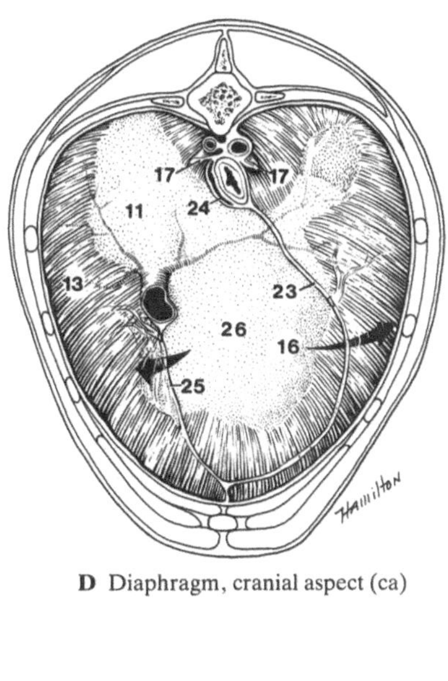

D Diaphragm, cranial aspect (ca)

1 **SYSTEMA UROGENITALE.**

2 **SYSTEMA URINARIUM.** Urinary organs.

3 **Ren [Nephros].** Kidney. A B 217 B

4 ***Margo lateralis.*** Lateral border. A B

5 ***Margo medialis.*** Medial border. A B

6 *Hilus renalis.* Renal hilus, the point on the medial border where the vessels and the ureter enter/exit the kidney. A B

7 *Sinus renalis.* Renal sinus, a cavity in the kidney at the hilus. It contains fat and connective tissue surrounding the renal pelvis and vessels. A

8 ***Facies ventralis.*** Ventral surface. C

9 ***Facies dorsalis.*** Dorsal surface. C

10 ***Extremitas cranialis.*** Cranial end. A B

11 ***Extremitas caudalis.*** Caudal end. A

12 ***Fascia renalis.*** Renal fascia, two layers enclose the kidney and the Capsula adiposa. C

13 ***Capsula adiposa.*** Fat capsule. It surrounds the kidney outside the Capsula fibrosa. C

14 ***Capsula fibrosa.*** Fibrous capsule on the surface of the kidney. D

15 ***Lobi renis.*** Renal lobes. Each consists of a renal pyramid and its cortical cap. Lobation is visible on the developing kidney of all species, but only in bo does it persist on the surface. It is indicated in other adult mammals by the renal pyramids and interlobar vessels seen in section. A B

16 ***Cortex renis.*** Renal cortex, outer layer of the kidney. It covers the bases of the pyramids and extends between them as Columnae renales. A B

17 *Lobuli corticales.* Cortical lobules. Each lobule consists of a medullary ray and the surrounding Pars convoluta. D

18 **Pars convoluta.** Consists of convoluted tubules and renal corpuscles. D

19 **Corpuscula renalia.** Renal corpuscles (former corpuscle of Malpighi). About 0.1–0.3 mm in diameter, consist of a glomerulum invaginated into a capsule (former capsule of Bowman). D

20 **Glomerula.** A glomerulum (former glomerulus of Malpighi) is a knot of capillaries in a Corpusculum renis. D

21 **Pars radiata.** Medullary rays, bundles of straight tubules extending from the medulla into the cortex. Each ray is the core of a cortical lobule. D

22 ***Medulla renis.*** Renal medulla, consists of the pyramids. A

23 *Pyramides renales.* Renal pyramids. The base of each is at the cortex and the apex is a renal papilla in the pelvis or calyx. A B

24 **Basis pyramidis.** Base of the pyramid, covered by the cortex. A B

25 **Papillae renales.** Apices of the pyramids. They are separate, each with its own calyx in su, bo, but fused to form a crest in Car, ov, cap, eq. B

26 **Ductus papillares.** Papillary ducts, large terminal ducts with columnar epithelium. B

27 **Crista renalis.** Renal crest. In Car, ov, cap, eq the Papillae renales are fused to form the Crista renalis. A C

28 **Area cribrosa.** Cribriform area of the papilla or of the crest perforated by the openings of the papillary ducts. B

29 **Foramina papillaria.** Openings of the papillary ducts. B

30 ***Columnae renales.*** Renal columns, sections of crests of cortical tissue extending into the medulla around and between the pyramids. A

31 ***Tubuli renales.*** Renal tubules. D

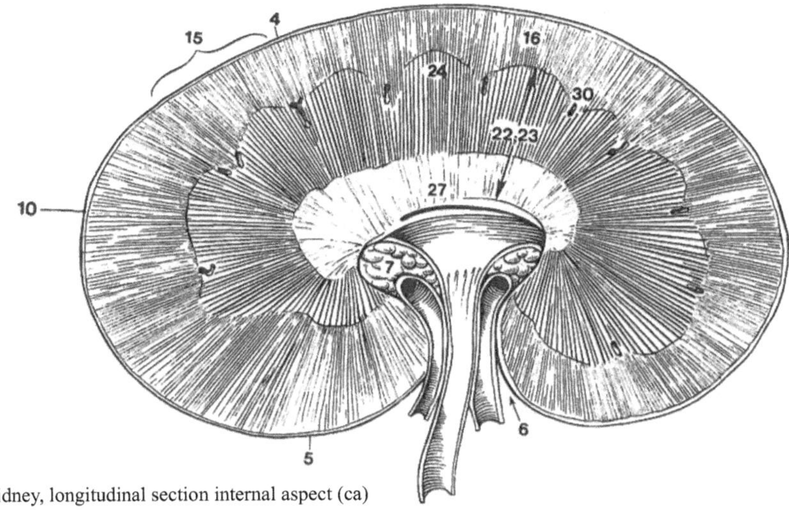

A Kidney, longitudinal section internal aspect (ca)

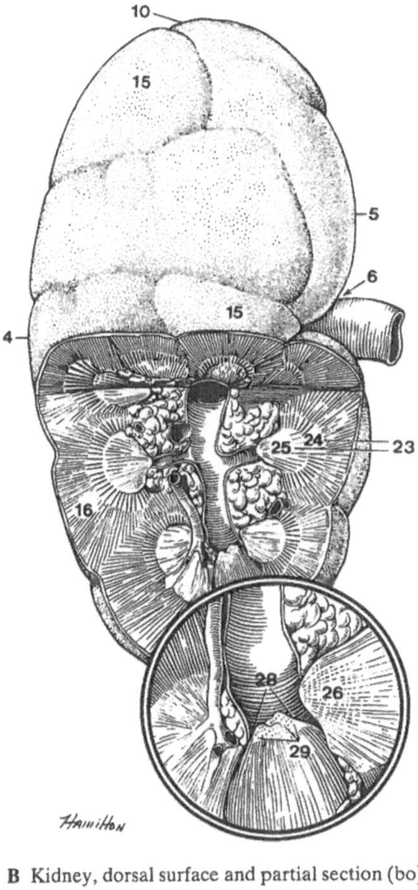

B Kidney, dorsal surface and partial section (bo)

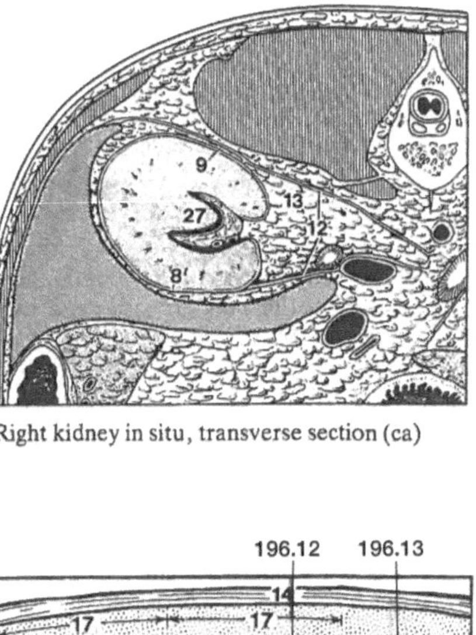

C Right kidney in situ, transverse section (ca)

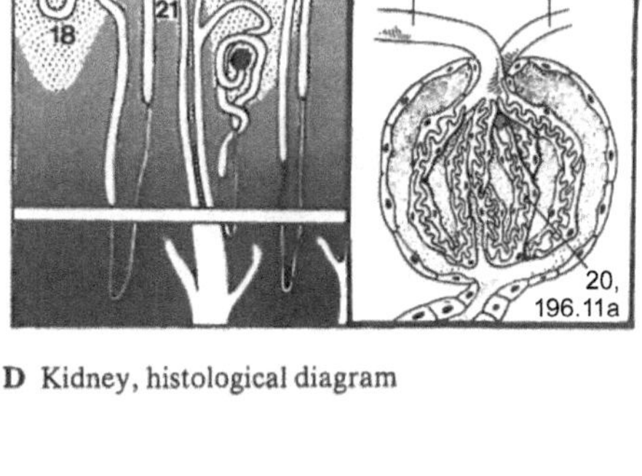

D Kidney, histological diagram

1 ***Pelvis renalis***. Renal pelvis, the space which collects urine, situated within Sinus renalis at the beginning of the ureter. It is not enlarged in some pigs and most oxen. A B D

2 ***Recessus pelvis***. Recess of the pelvis, one of several expansions of the pelvis, sac-like diverticula between the Pyramides renales. They occur in Car, ov, cap, or. Each recess embraces a ridge formed by a pyramid leading to the renal crest. The interlobar vessels run in grooves between the recesses. B

3 ***Gll. pelvis renalis*** (eq). Mucous glands of renal pelvis. D

4 ***Calices renales***. Renal calices. They are now included in the Pelvis renalis.

5 *Calices renales majores*. Major enlarged renal calices, the primary branches of the pelvis (su, bo). A

6 *Calices renales minores*. Minor renal calices, those receiving papillae (in some pigs and most oxen). A

7 ***Recessus terminales***. Terminal recesses, tubular diverticula of the equine renal pelvis which extend into the cranial and caudal ends of the kidney. They are not part of the renal pelvis, as they are not located within the renal sinus and are lined by the same two-layered epithelium that covers the renal crest. D

8 **Vasa sanguinea renis**. Vessels of the kidney. C

8a ***Arteria renalis***. The artery sending branches into the kidney. C

9 *Arteriae interlobares*. The interlobar arteries run from the sinus toward the cortex between the pyramids. C D

10 **Arteriae arcuatae**. Arched arteries, branches arising from the Aa. interlobares. C

11 *Arteriae interlobulares*. Interlobular arteries arise from the Aa. arcuatae and penetrate the Pars convoluta of the cortex. C

11a *Arteriae intralobulares*. Intralobular arteries. 195 D

12 *Arteriola glomerularis afferens*. Afferent vessel to the glomerulum from a A. interlobularis. C 195 D

12a *Rete capillare glomerulare*. Capillary network of the glomerulum. 195 D.20

13 *Arteriola glomerularis efferens*. Efferent vessel from the glomerulum to capillaries between tubules. C 195 D

14 *Rami capsulares*. Capsular branches from Aa. interlobulares to the fibrous capsule of the kidney. C

15 *Arteriolae rectae*. Straight arterioles, descend from the Arteriolae glomerulares efferentes or Aa. arcuatae into the medulla. (The new edition of the N.A.V. listed Arteriolae recte below Arteriae arcuatae). C

16 ***Vena renalis***. Venous branches inside of the kidney. C

17 *Venae interlobares*. Interlobar veins, between the renal pyramids. C D

18 **Venae arcuatae**. Arched veins. They form arches between Vv. interlobares at the corticomedullary junction. C

19 *Venae interlobulares*. In the Pars convoluta of the cortex. C

19a *Venae intralobulares*. Intralobular veins. C

20 *Venulae stellatae*. Stellate venules, capsular branches of Vv. interlobulares, visible in ca, ov, cap, eq. C

21 *Venulae rectae*. Straight venules drain the medulla to the Vv. arcuatae. C

22 ***Venae capsulares*** (fe). Capsular veins that branch off the V. renalis at the hilus and form a characteristic tree-like network. E

23 **Ureter**. Duct from kidney to urinary bladder. A D E 217 B

24 ***Pars abdominalis***. Abdominal part.

25 ***Pars pelvina***. Pelvic part.

26 ***Tunica adventitia***. External coat of connective tissue. F

27 ***Tunica muscularis***. Muscular coat. F

28 ***Tunica mucosa***. Mucous membrane, lined by transitional epithelium. F

29 *Gll. uretericae* (eq). Ureteral glands, mucous glands in the renal end of the ureter. F

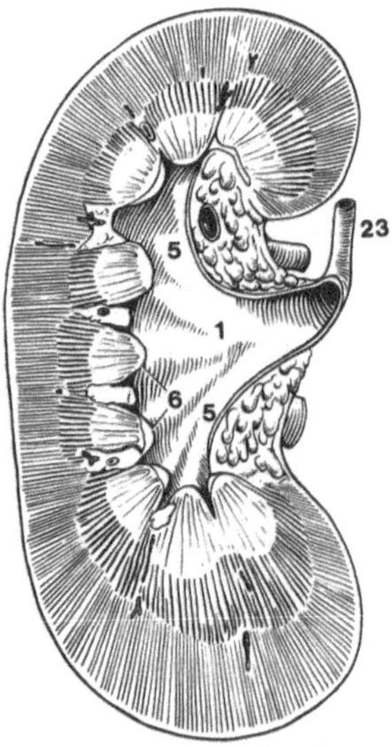

A Kidney, longitudinal section through hilus internal aspect (su)

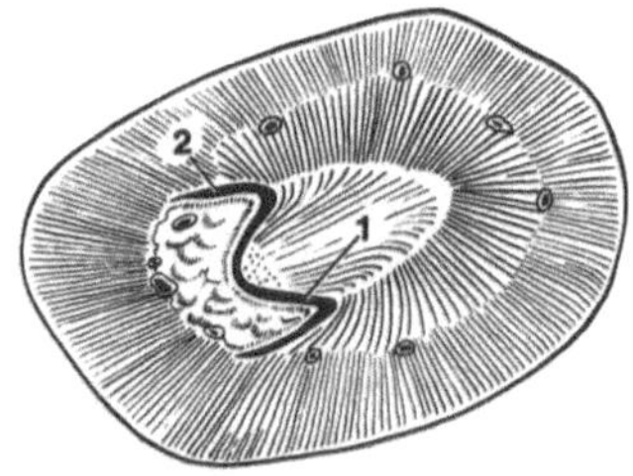

B Kidney, transverse section (ca)

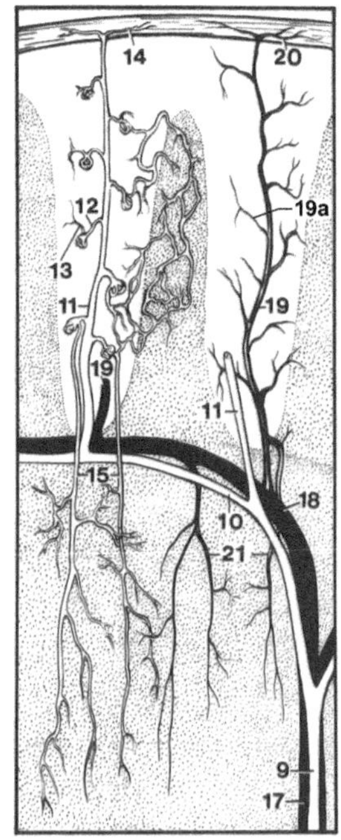

C Diagram of renal vessels (in the cortex, Pars radiata stippled, convoluta white)

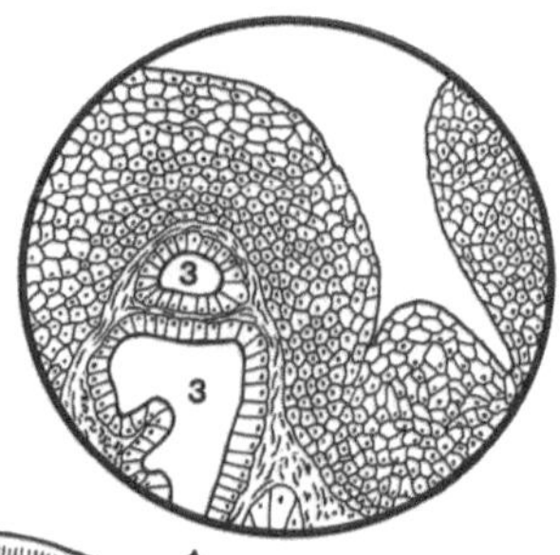

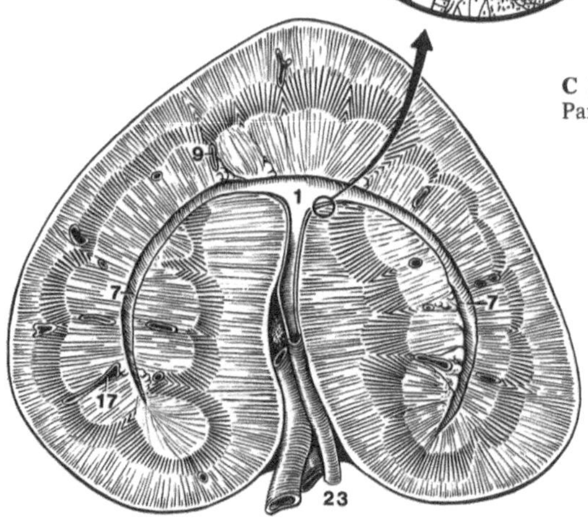

D Right kidney, longitudinal section through hilus internal aspect (eq)

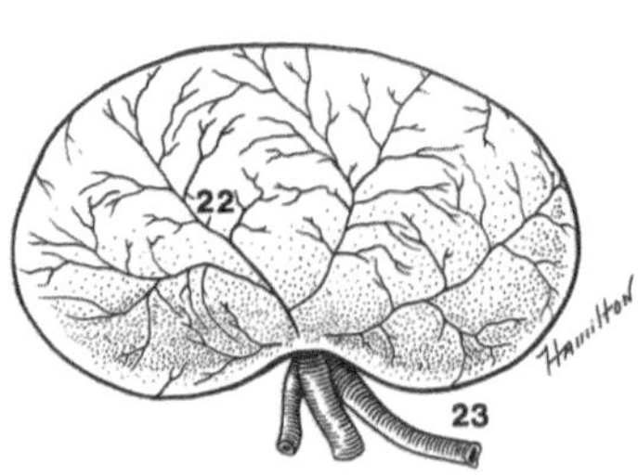

E Left kidney, ventral surface (fe)

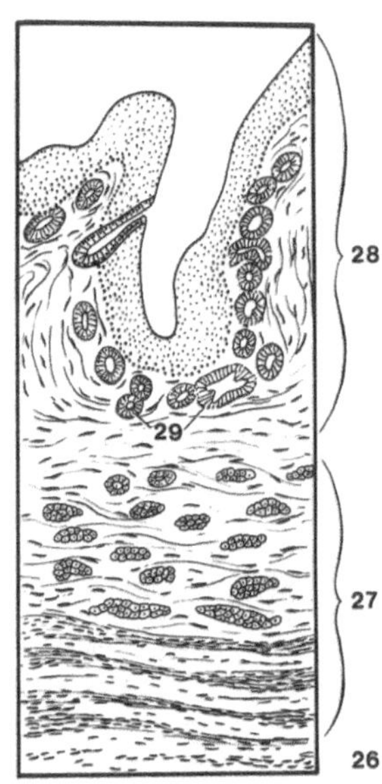

F Ureter, histological section (eq)

1 **Vesica urinaria**. Urinary bladder. A C 217 B

2 ***Apex vesicae [Vertex vesicae]***. Apex of the urinary bladder, the blind cranial end. A C (There are many "bladders" in the body, and this should be called "urinary bladder", similar to the "gall bladder", for example.)

3 ***Corpus vesicae***. Body of the urinary bladder. The dorsal wall of the urinary bladder does not form a Fundus vesicae in domestic mammals. A C

4 ***Cervix vesicae***. Neck of the urinary bladder. A

5 ***Facies dorsalis***. Dorsal surface. A

6 ***Facies ventralis***. Ventral surface. A

7 ***Lig. vesicae medianum***. Middle ligament of the urinary bladder, a peritoneal fold attaching the ventral surface of the urinary bladder to the Symphysis pelvina and the Linea alba. In the fetus it contains the Urachus (C.8) in its free border. A C

8 ***Urachus*** (ont). Fetal duct from the bladder through the umbilical cord to the allantoic cavity. It is enclosed in the Lig. vesicae medianum. C (This structure was omitted from the 5th edition of the N. A. V., because it is an ontogenetic term.)

9 ***Lig. vesicae laterale***. Lateral ligament of the urinary bladder, a peritoneal fold attached to the dorsolateral pelvic wall in the male and to the broad ligament in the female. It contains the Lig. teres vesicae. A C

10 *Lig. teres vesicae*. Round ligament of the urinary bladder, symmetrical, vestige of the A. umbilicalis in the Lig. vesicae laterale. A C

11 ***Tunica serosa***. Serous coat, the visceral peritoneum of the urinary bladder. B

12 ***Tela subserosa***. Subserous tissue, the connective tissue between serous and muscular layers. B

13 ***Tunica muscularis (M. detrussor vesicae)***. Muscular coat, smooth muscle of the wall of the urinary bladder. The term M. sphincter vesicae was omitted because there is no evidence of such a sphincter apart from the striated M. urethralis. B (The term detrussor vesicae was introduced as alternative name for the whole Tunica muscularis, which acts to expel urine.)

14 ***M. pubovesicalis***. Smooth muscle in the Lig. pubovesicale from the Symphysis pubica to the Cervix vesicae. A

15 ***M. rectourethralis***. O: ventral longitudinal muscle of the rectum. T: in the male, on the urethra; in the female, in the smooth muscle of the vestibule and labia. In the bull it is variable in occurrence and position. C

16 ***Tela submucosa***. Loose vascular connective tissue under the Tunica mucosa. B

17 ***Tunica mucosa***. Mucous membrane, covered by transitional epithelium. B

18 ***Trigonum vesicae***. Triangle of the urinary bladder, smooth area of mucous membrane between the ureteral and urethral orifices. D

19 ***Columna ureterica***. Ureteral column, the elevation of the mucosa produced by the ureter in its course within the wall of the urinary bladder. D

20 ***Ostium ureteris***. Opening of the ureter. D

21 ***Plica ureterica***. Ureteral fold, the lateral boundary of the Trigonum vesicae. D

22 ***Ostium urethrae internum***. Internal urethral orifice. D

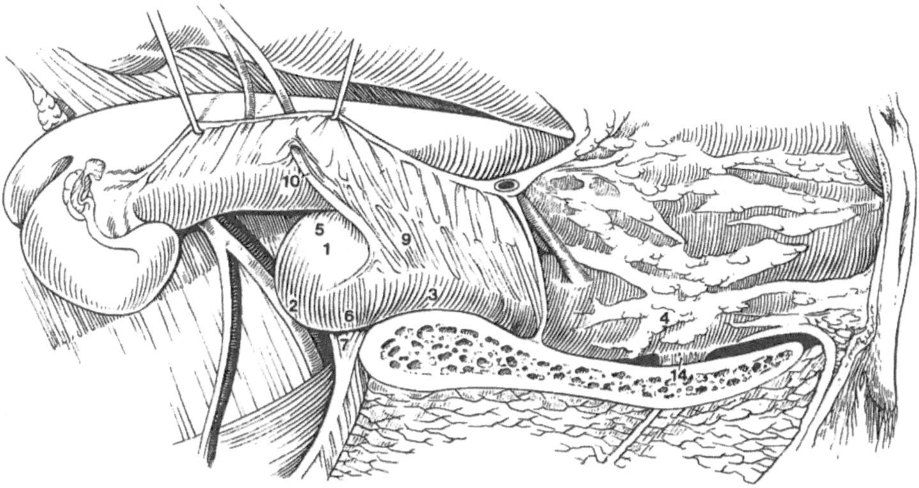

A Genital organs and bladder in situ (the cut edge of the broad ligament is held by hooks), left lateral aspect (bo fem)

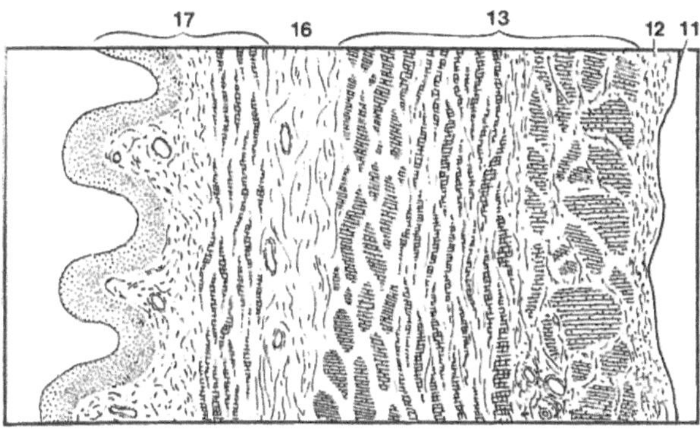

B Wall of urinary bladder, histological section (bo) (Trautmann and Fiebiger)

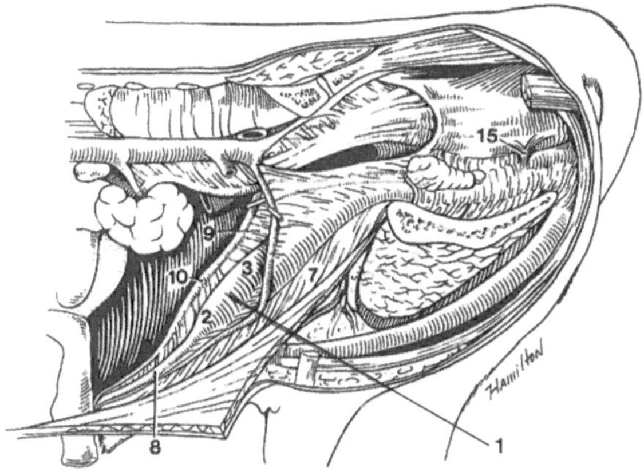

C Urogenital organs in situ, left lateral aspect (bo masc, newborn) (Popesko)

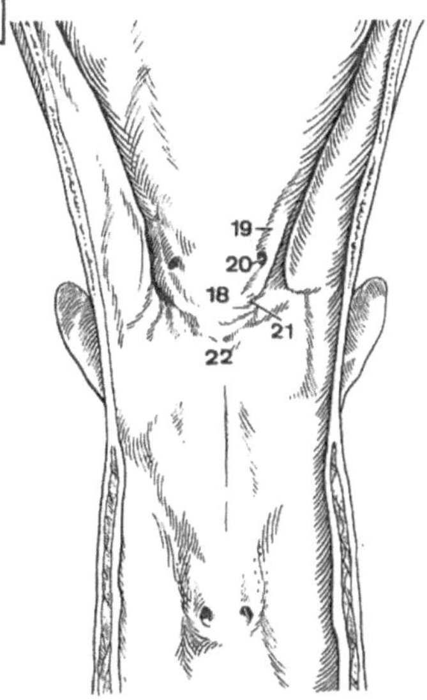

D Dorsal wall of urinary bladder and male urethra, seen from inside (eq)

1 **ORGANA GENITALIA MASCULINA**. Male genital organs.

2 **Testis [Orchis]***. Testicle. The different position of testicles in the scrotum, from horizontal to oblique and to vertical makes the names of the borders species specific. To avoid confusion, the medial border in Ru, cranial in su and dorsal in most of species, corresponding to the Corpus epididymidis is called Margo epididymalis, and the opposite Margo liber. A C 203 E

3 ***Extremitas capitata***. Head end, related to the Caput epididymidis, cranial in most species, but dorsal in Ru. A

4 ***Extremitas caudata***. Tail end, related to the Cauda epididymidis, caudal in most species, but ventral in Ru. A

5 ***Facies lateralis***. Lateral surface. The corresponding surface is caudal in Ru. A Cc

6 ***Facies medialis***. Medial surface. The corresponding surface is cranial in Ru.

7 ***Margo liber***. Free border, ventral in most species, but caudal in su, lateral in Ru. A Ca

8 ***Margo epididymalis***. Epididymal border, dorsal in most species, but cranial in su medial in Ru. A Cb

9 ***Tunica albuginea***. Dense white capsule of the testis. B

10 ***Mediastinum testis***. Axial strand of connective tissue from which the septula radiate. It is absent in eq. B

11 ***Septula testis***. Minute interlobular connective tissue partitions extending from the Mediastinum testis to the Tunica albuginea. B

12 ***Lobuli testis***. Lobules of the testis. B

13 ***Parenchyma testis***. Consists of the seminiferous tubules. B

14 ***Tubuli seminiferi contorti***. Convoluted seminiferous tubules. B

15 ***Tubuli seminiferi recti***. Straight seminiferous tubules, from the convoluted tubules to the Rete testis. B

16 ***Rete testis***. Network of ducts in the Mediastinum testis connecting the Tubuli seminiferi recti to the Ductuli efferentes. It is absent in eq. B

16a ***(Appendix testis)***. Appendage of the testicle, a wrinkled wart-like process on the testis near the Caput epididymidis. It is a vestige of the cranial end of the paramesonephric duct and occurs always in eq, and occasionally in the ca, su, ov, cap. A

17 **Epididymis***. Organ attached to the testis, covered by Tunica albuginea originating from the Testis and enclosing the Ductuli efferentes testis and the coiled Ductus epididymidis. A B 203 E

18 ***Caput epididymidis***. Head of the epididymis, contains the Lobuli epididymidis. In Ru it has descending and ascending limbs. A B C

19 *Ductuli efferentes testis*. Efferent ductules, lead from the Rete testis to the Ductus epididymidis. They are coiled to form the Lobuli epididymidis. B

20 ***Corpus epididymidis***. Body of the epididymis, consists of the coiled duct. A B C

21 ***Cauda epididymidis***. Tail of the epididymis, where the Ductus epididymidis continues with the Ductus deferens. A B C

22 ***Lobuli epididymidis [Coni epididymidis]***. Lobules of the epididymis, containing the coiled Ductuli efferentes testis in the Caput epididymidis. B

23 ***Ductus epididymidis***. Convoluted duct of the epididymis, 70–80 m long in eq. B

24 ***(Ductuli aberrantes)***. Aberrant ductules, blind branches of the Ductus epididymidis or of Ductuli efferentes testis. They are rare vestiges of the mesonephric tubules, appearing as cysts on the epididymis. B C

24a ***(Appendix epididymidis)***. Appendage of the head of epididymis, vestige of the mesonephros. Always present in eq, and occasionally in ca, su, ov, and cap.

25 ***(Paradidymis)***. Detached mesonephric tubules in the spermatic cord just proximal to the head of the epididymis. B C

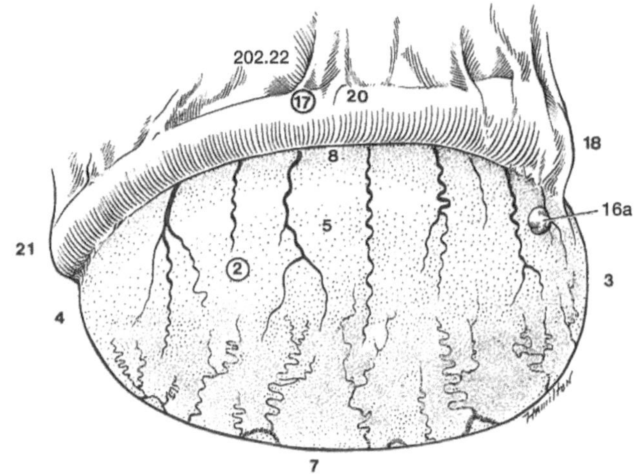

A Right testis and epididymis, lateral surface (eq)

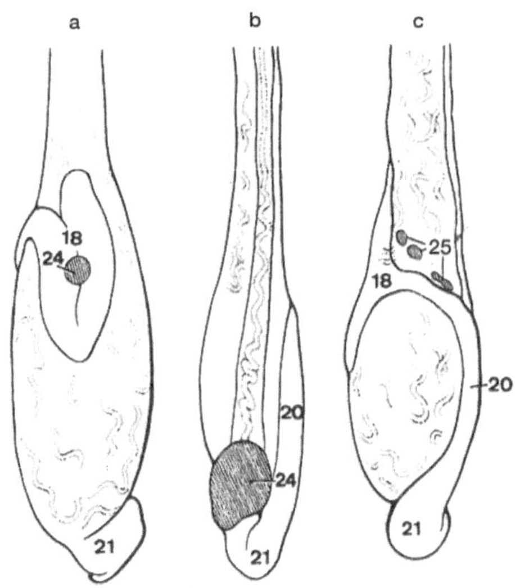

C Testis and epididymis. a: free border, right testis; b: epididymal border, right testis; c: caudal surface, left testis (bo, young) (Blom and Christensen 1958)

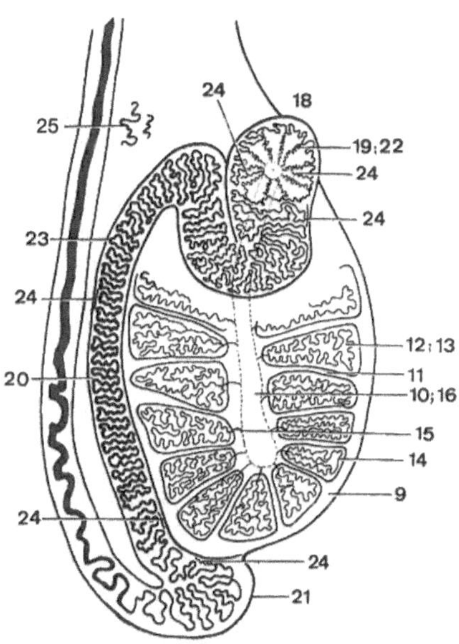

B Diagram of testis and epididymis (bo) (Blom and Christensen 1960)

1 **Ductus deferens***. Deferent duct. Extends from the Ductus epididymidis through the Funiculus spermaticus to the Colliculus seminalis in the urethra. A D

2 ***Ampulla ductus deferentis***. Enlargement of the terminal part of the Ductus deferens, produced by a glandular thickening of its wall, absent in fe, su. A B

3 *Gll. ampullae.* Glands of the ampulla. In domestic mammals they are branched tubular glands. B

4 ***Tunica adventitia***. Outer connective tissue coat of the Ductus deferens in its retroperitoneal course.

5 ***Tunica serosa***. Serous coat of the Ductus deferens, present in quadrupeds. B

6 ***Tunica muscularis***. Smooth muscle of the Ductus deferens. B

7 ***Tunica mucosa***. Mucous membrane. B

8 ***Ductus ejaculatorius*** (Ru, eq). Ejaculatory duct, short, inconstant common excretory passage in the Colliculus seminalis for the Ductus deferens and the duct of the Glandula vesicularis. A

9 **Funiculus spermaticus***. Spermatic cord, including the blood vessels, lymphatics, and nerves of the testis and epididymis, together with the Ductus deferens and the Lamina visceralis tunicae vaginalis. C D

10 **Tunicae funiculi spermatici et testis***. Coverings of the spermatic cord and testicle. (As far as origin, the testicular tunics consist of two groups of structures: intraabdominal, brought by the testicle during its descent [the internal spermatic fascia and the vaginal tunic with the parietal and visceral laminae], and extraabdominal, those preexistent to the testicular descent [the external spermatic fascia and the scrotum with the scrotal skin and the tunica dartos].)

11 ***Fascia spermatica externa***. External spermatic fascia, continuation of Fascia m. obliqui externi abdominis. It continues in the perineal region as the Fascia perinealis profunda C D

12 ***M. cremaster***. Strand of muscle fibers from M. obliquus internus abdominis on Tunica vaginalis. O: Fascia iliaca. T: Tunica vaginalis near the testis. It lies between the internal and external spermatic fasciae and draws the testis toward the inguinal canal. C D

13 ***Fascia cremasterica***. Cremasteric fascia on the M. cremaster. D

14 ***Fascia spermatica interna***. Internal spermatic fascia, continuation of Fascia transversalis. C D

15 ***Tunica vaginalis***. Vaginal tunic, the serous membranes covering the spermatic cord and testis, and lining the Tunica spermatica interna. It is a fetal evagination of the peritoneum into the inguinal canal. In males it becomes the Tunica vaginalis after the descent of the Testis. In females the Processus vaginalis is often present in ca and is absent in fe. D (Watson 2009)

16 *Lamina parietalis*. Parietal layer, continuation of the parietal peritoneum. C D

17 *Lamina visceralis*. Visceral layer, adherent to the testis, epididymis and spermatic cord. C D

18 *Anulus vaginalis*. Vaginal ring, where the parietal peritoneum is evaginated to form the Lamina parietalis of the Tunica vaginalis. It seats inside of the deep inguinal ring, lining it. A

19 *Canalis vaginalis*. Vaginal canal, potential space between Lamina parietalis and visceralis around the spermatic cord. C D

20 *Cavum vaginale*. Vaginal cavity, between Lamina parietalis and visceralis around the testis. C

21 **Mesorchium**. Peritoneal fold containing vessels and nerves of testis. D E (In domestic mammals following the descent of the testis, the Ductus deferens, Mesoductus deferens and Mesorchium retain their identity in the spermatic cord.)

22 *Mesorchium proximale [Plica vasculosa]*. Proximal mesorchium (vascular fold). It extends from the origin of the testicular vessels to the mesepididymis. C E 201 A

23 **Mesofuniculus**. Strip of Mesorchium between origin of Mesoductus deferens and Lamina parietalis. D

24 *Mesorchium distale*. Extends from Mesepididymis to the testis, forming part of the wall of Bursa testicularis. C E

25 ***Mesoductus deferens [Plica ductus deferentis]***. Attaches the Ductus deferens to the mesorchium and to the abdominal and pelvic walls. D

26 ***Mesepididymis***. Attaches the epididymis between Mesorchium proximale et distale. E

27 ***Lig. testis proprium***[1]. Proper ligament of the testis, from the testis to the tail of the epididymis. C

28 ***Lig. caudae epididymidis***[1]. Between the tail of the epididymis and the Lamina parietalis (Un). In Car the tail of the epididymis is adherent to the Fascia spermatica interna, therefore there is no ligament of the tail of epididymis in Car. However, the scrotal ligament is present in Car. C

cont. p. 204 ►

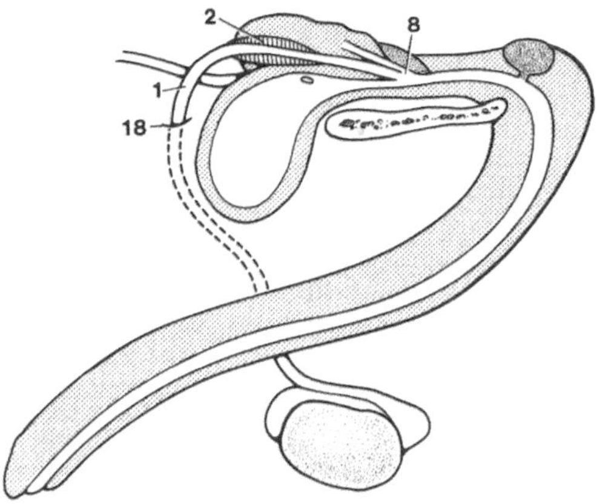

A Diagram of male genital organs, showing right testis (eq) (Nickel et al. 1979)

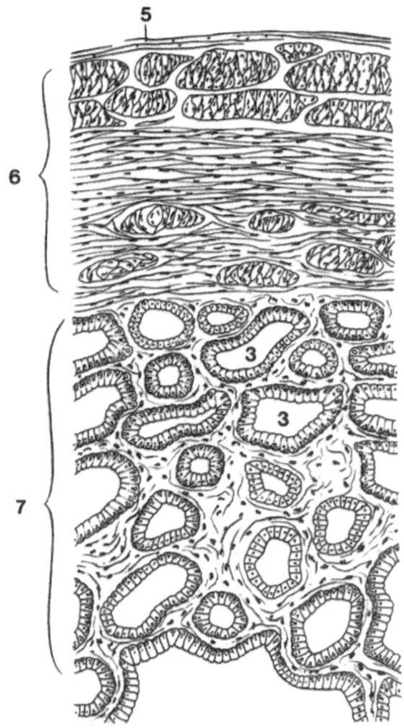

B Ampulla of Ductus deferens, histological section (bo)

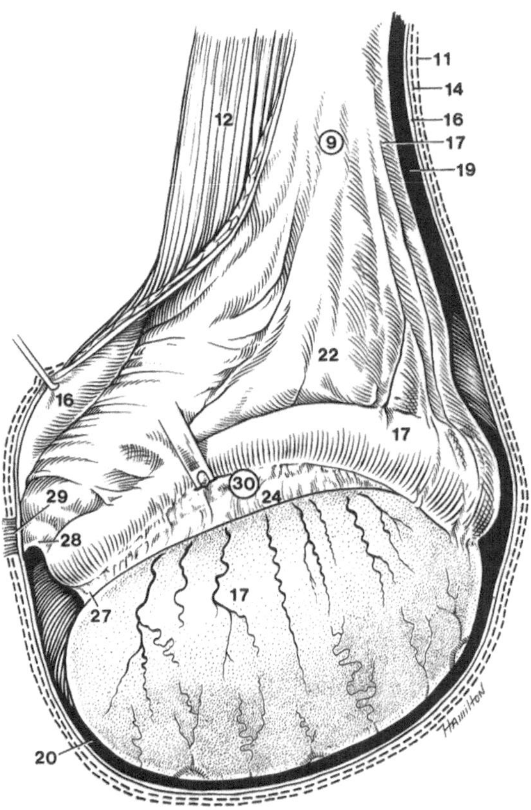

C Right testis and spermatic cord, lateral surface (fasciae, M. cremaster and parietal tunic opened) (eq)

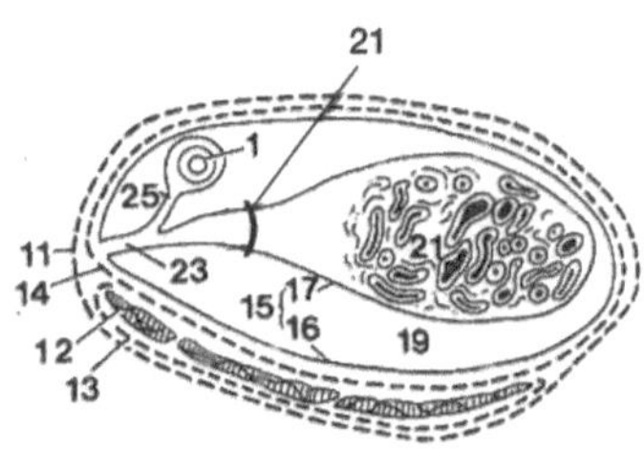

D Right spermatic cord, transsected, distal surface (eq)

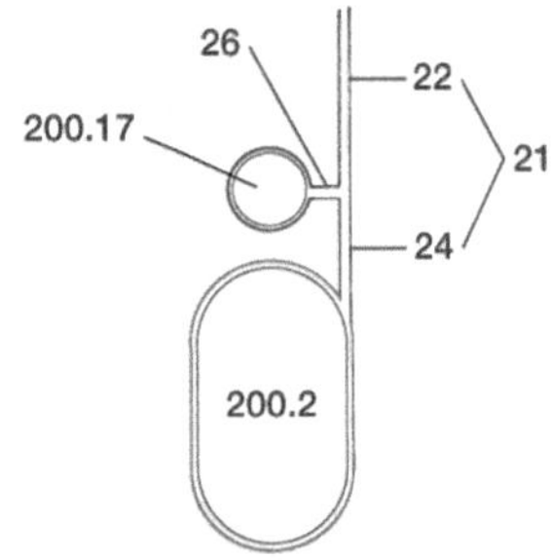

E Mesorchium and mesepididymis (schematic)

29 ***Lig. scroti***[1]. Scrotal ligament, strand of connective tissue between Tunica dartos and Lig. caudae epididymidis (Un) or the tail of the epididymis (Car). C

30 ***Bursa testicularis [Sinus epididymalis]***. Testicular bursa [epididymal sinus], formed by Mesorchium distale, testis, and epididymis. C

1) They are vestiges of Gubernaculum testis.

---

1 ***Processus vaginalis peritonei [peritonaei]***. Vaginal process, fetal cylindrical evagination of peritoneum into the inguinal canal before the descent of the testis; thereafter in males it becomes the Tunica vaginalis. In adult females the Processus vaginalis is often present in ca and is absent in fe. A (Watson 2009)

2 ***Descensus testis*** (ont) [1]. Descent of the testicle from its original position to the scrotum. A

3 ***Gubernaculum testis*** (ont)[1]. Guide of the testicle, a mesenchymal tract from the testis to the tail of the epididymis and thence to the deep inguinal ring and through the inguinal canal. The vestiges of the gubernaculum are the Lig. proprium testis, the Lig. caudae epididymidis, and the Lig. scroti. A

4 **Glandulae genitales accessoriae**. Accessory genital glands. C

5 **Ampulla ductus deferentis**. See 202.2. C

6 **Glandula vesicularis** (Un). Vesicular gland. In su, Ru, a compound tubular lobulated gland on the neck of the bladder; in eq, a flask-shaped organ with a muscular wall and a central collecting space, folds of the Tunica mucosa form a complex system of glandular recesses. It is absent in Car. B C (The vesicular gland in eq is sometimes called Vesicula seminalis, due to its appearance and structure.)

7 ***Tunica adventitia***. Outer connective tissue coat of the gland. B

8 ***Tunica muscularis***. A continous muscular coat is present only in eq. B

9 ***Tunica mucosa***. Mucous membrane (eq).

10 ***Ductus excretorius***. Excretory duct, opens on the Colliculus seminalis, sometimes via a Ductus ejaculatorius. D

11 **Prostata***. Prostate, gland secreting into the pelvic part of the male urethra. C

12 ***Facies ventralis***. Ventral surface.

13 ***Facies dorsalis***. Dorsal surface. C

14 ***Corpus prostatae***. Body of the prostate, at the beginning of the pelvic urethra in Car, su, bo and eq. D

15 ***Pars disseminata prostatae***. Disseminate part of the prostate. It forms a glandular layer in the wall of the pelvic urethra in su, bo, cap, but is deficient ventrally in ov, and is represented only by a few lobules in Car. E

16 ***Lobus [dexter et sinister]***. Right and left lobes. In eq, right and left lobes are connected by an isthmus (C); in Car they are partially divided by a groove.

17 ***Isthmus prostatae***. Isthmus of the prostate. In eq, it lies between the lobes, across the dorsal surface of the neck of the urinary bladder. C

18 ***Parenchyma***. Glandular substance. D E

19 ***Ductuli prostatici***. Prostatic ductules. Numerous excretory ductules open into the urethra. D

20 ***Substantia muscularis***. Muscular substance. The septa that radiate through the gland to the capsule contain much smooth muscle. D E

21 ***Capsula prostatae***. Capsule of the prostate, containing smooth muscle. D E

22 **Glandula bulbourethralis***. Bulbourethral gland. Secreting into the caudal end of the pelvic urethra, it bulges dorsolaterally between M. urethralis and M. bulbospongiosus. In su it extends cranially the full length of the pelvic urethra. It is absent in ca. C

23 ***Ductus gl. bulbourethralis***. Duct of the bulbourethral gland. 211 D

1) These terms were omitted from the 5th edition of the N. A. V., because they are ontogenetic terms. However, we keep them for better understanding the transition between the structures during the developmental life, and those after birth.

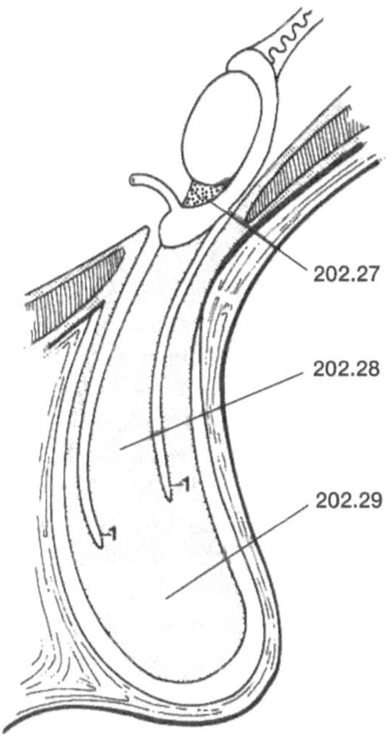

A Processus vaginalis peritonei and Gubernaculum testis within the inguinal canal (su) (Backhouse and Butler)

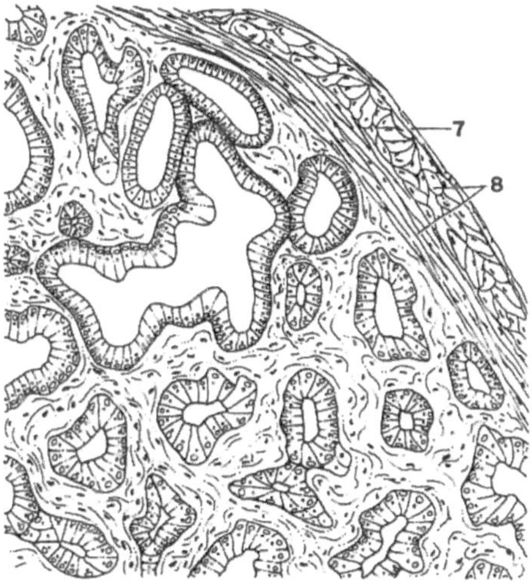

B Vesicular gland, histological section (bo)

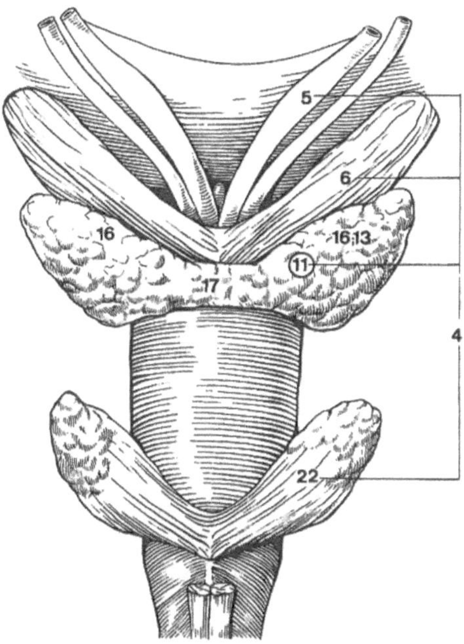

C Glandulae genitales accessoriae, dorsal aspect (eq) (Nickel et al., 1979)

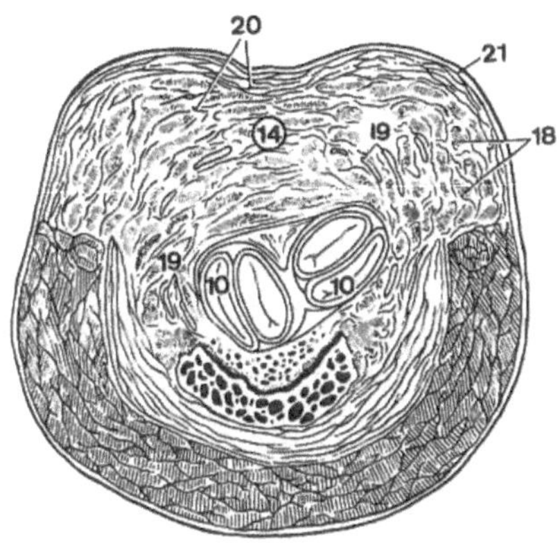

D Body of the prostate, transverse section of pelvic part of urethra and Stratum spongiosum (deferent ducts medial and dorsal to 10) (bo)

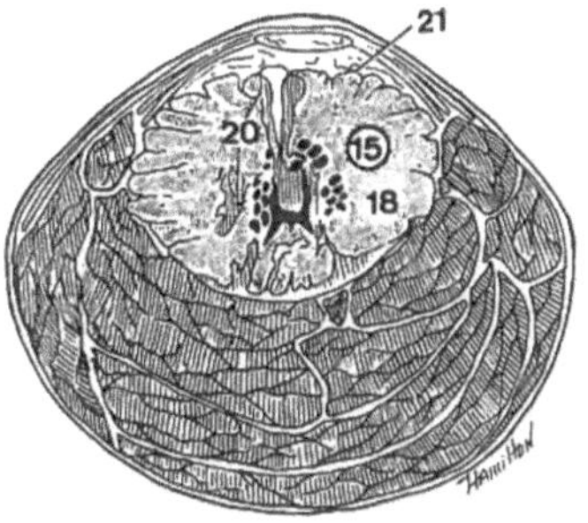

E Disseminate prostate (ventral and lateral parts of the section consist of M. urethralis) (bo)

1 **PARTES GENITALES MASCULINAE EXTERNAE.** External male genitalia: penis, prepuce, and scrotum.

2 **Penis***. Male organ of copulation. A

3 ***Radix penis***. Root of the penis, composed of the two Crura and the Bulbus penis. A

4 ***Crus penis***. Proximal end of each Corpus cavernosum penis attached to the Arcus ischiadicus and covered by M. ischiocavernosus. A

5 ***Corpus penis***. Body of the penis, the shaft from the root to the glans. A

6 ***Dorsum penis***. Back of the penis when erect, the surface opposite the urethral surface. A

7 *Sulcus dorsalis penis*. Dorsal groove of the penis (eq). B

8 ***Facies urethralis***. Urethral surface. A

9 *Sulcus urethralis*. Urethral groove in the body of the penis, containing Corpus spongiosum and urethra. B

10 ***Flexura sigmoidea penis*** (su, Ru). S-shaped bend in the flaccid penis between the thighs. E H

11 ***Pars libera penis***. Free part of the penis, distal to the attachment of the prepuce. E F H

12 ***Glans penis***. Head of the penis, containing the Corpus spongiosum glandis. The glans of Ru was formerly called the Galea glandis in the belief that the whole Pars libera penis was the glans. A glans is a cushion outside the Tunica albuginea corporum cavernosorum. It is very different among species as far as texture and extent. It may be predominantly vascular (Car, eq), predominantly fibrous (Ru), or practically absent (su). It may involve most of the Pars libera (eq), more than the Pars libera (ca), all of the Pars libera (fe), or only a small part of Pars libera (Ru). A C D E F G

13 *Processus dorsalis glandis* (eq). Dorsal process of the glans. It extends caudally about 10 cm. A D

14 *Pars longa glandis* (ca). Long part of the glans, the distal, cylindrical part. G

15 *Bulbus glandis* (ca). Bulb of the glans, the proximal part. G

16 *Corona glandis*. Crown of the glans. A D G

17 *Septum glandis*. Septum of the glans, incomplete median ventral septum. C

18 *Collum glandis*. Neck of the glans, constriction proximal to the Corona glandis. A D

19 *Fossa glandis* (eq). Fossa of the glans, circular excavation around the Processus urethralis. C D

20 **Sinus urethralis** (eq). Urethral sinus, a dorsal diverticulum of the Fossa glandis. C D

21 ***Preputium [Praeputium]***. Sheath, foreskin, surrounding the Pars libera penis when not erect. It is a fold consisting of a Lamina externa and a Lamina interna, continuous at Ostium preputiale. Tha Lamina interna terminates at its attachment to the penis. H

22 *Lamina externa*. External layer of the fold of skin forming the prepuce. D

23 *Raphe preputii [Rhaphe praeputii]*. Median ventral seam of the prepuce, continuous with the Raphe scroti. F

24 *Ostium preputiale [prae-]*. Preputial orifice where the Lamina externa is reflected as the Lamina interna. D E

25 *Cavum preputiale [prae-]*. Preputial cavity, between the Lamina interna and the Pars libera penis. In eq the cavity is divided by the Plica preputialis into two concentric recesses. D E H

26 *Lamina interna*. Internal layer of the fold of skin forming the prepuce. It is attached to the penis at the proximal end of the Pars libera, where it is continuous with the skin of the free end of penis and glans. D F G

27 **Plica preputialis [prae-]** (eq). Preputial fold, a cylindrical fold of the Lamina interna, reflected at the Anulus preputialis. D

28 **Anulus preputialis [prae-]** (eq). Preputial ring, a thickened band of skin at the reflection of the preputial fold. D

29 *Diverticulum preputiale [prae-]* (su). Bilobed large dorsal sac connected with the cranial end of the preputial cavity. H

30 *Frenulum preputii [prae-]*. Rudimentary fold of skin connecting the Raphe preputii to Raphe penis in fe, Ru. F

C Glans penis, cut caudal to opening between 19 and 20 (eq)

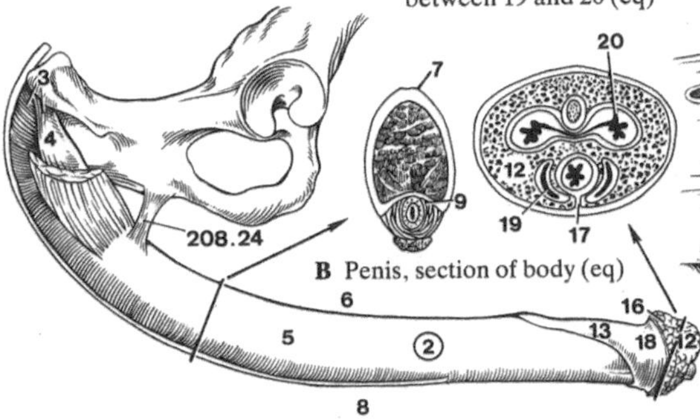

B Penis, section of body (eq)

A Penis, dissection lateral aspect (right M. ischiocavernosus partly removed) (eq)

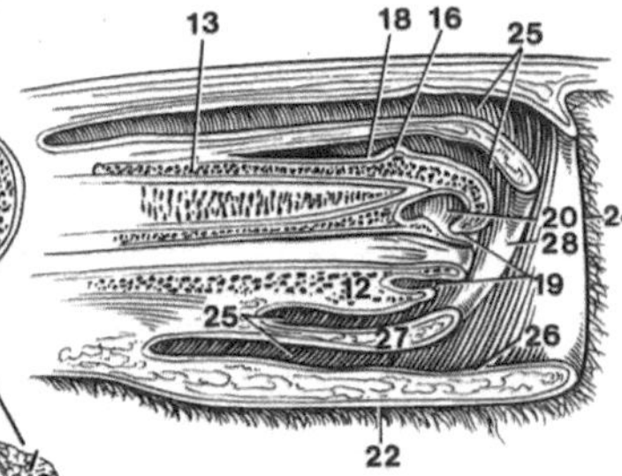

D Penis, prepuce and abdominal wall, longitudinal section internal aspect (eq)

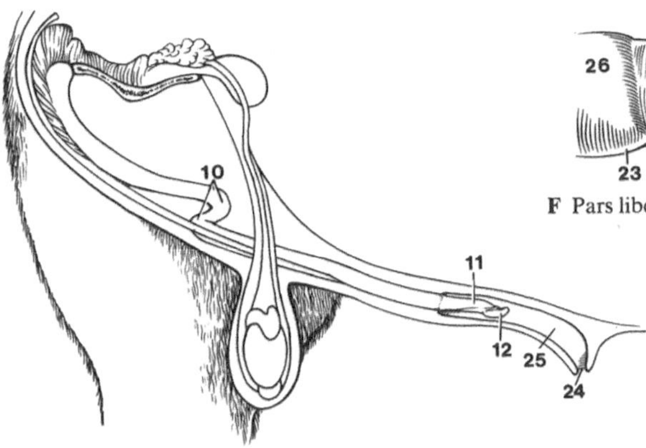

E Penis and prepuce (right wall of prepuce removed) lateral aspect (bo)

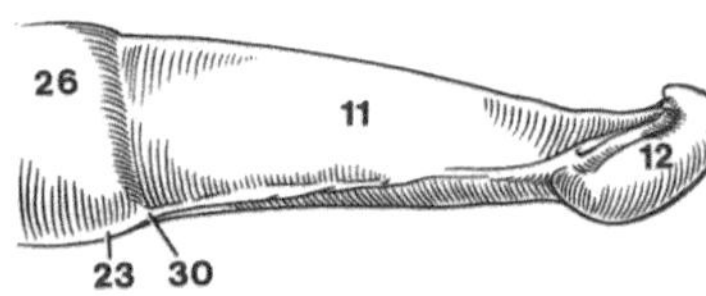

F Pars libera penis, right lateral surface (bo)

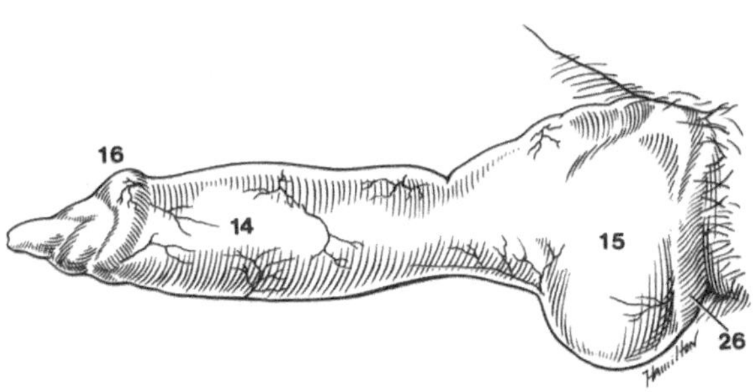

G Glans penis, erect, left craniolateral aspect (ca) (Hart and Kitchell)

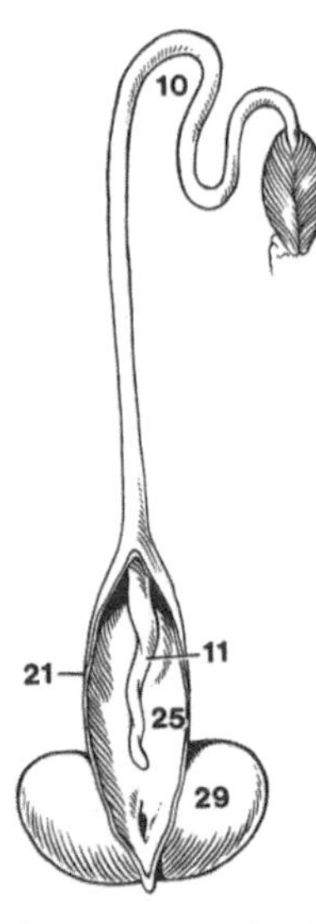

H Prepuce and penis (prepuce opened and portion with orifice removed), ventral aspect (su) Ellenberger and Baum)

1 *Gll. preputiales [prae-].* Preputial glands, modified sebaceous and sudoriferous glands in the Lamina interna near the preputial orifice, in eq they extend to the preputial ring. A

2 *Lymphonoduli [Noduli lymphatici] preputiales [prae-].* Preputial lymph nodules.

3 ***M. preputialis [prae-] cranialis.*** Cutaneous muscle, absent in eq. O: Superficial fascia in the xiphoid region; in bo, also transverse from M. cutaneus trunci to Ostium preputiale T: prepuce; right and left muscles form a loop around the orifice. B

4 ***M. preputialis [prae-] caudalis.*** Cutaneus muscle in fe, Ru; rudimentary in ca, su; absent in eq. O: in fe, on M. sphincter ani externus; in Ru, inguinal fascia lateral and medial to Tunica vaginalis. T: prepuce. B

5 ***Raphe [Rhaphe] penis.*** Seam on the free part of the penis from the Fenulum preputii to the glans in su and Ru. The former term Raphe glandis (Ru) is omitted because the greater part of this raphe is not on the glans. C

6 ***Corpus cavernosum penis.*** Cavernous body of the penis. Right and left Corpora cavernosa are fused in the body of the penis. D G

7 ***Os penis.*** Bone of the penis (Car), ossified distal part of the fused Corpora cavernosa in the Glans penis. In fe it is mostly cartilaginous. D

8 ***Corpus spongiosum penis.*** Spongy body of the penis, erectile tissue surrounding the urethra, formely Corpus cavernosum urethrae. D

9 ***Corpus spongiosum glandis.*** Spongy body of the glans, continous with the Corpus spongiosum penis. D

10 ***Bulbus penis.*** Bulb of the penis, caudal expansion of the Corpus spongiosum penis, formely Bulbus urethrae. D

11 ***Tuberculum spongiosum.*** Spongy tubercle (ov), rounded process of the Corpus spongiosum on the left ventral side of the Pars libera penis. C

12 ***Tunica albuginea corporum cavernosorum.*** Dense white fibrous coat around the Corpora cavernosa. D F G

13 *Lig. apicale penis* (Ru). Apical lig. of the penis, a thick longitudinal band arising from the dorsal surface of the Tunica albuginea distal to the sigmoid flexure and inserted into the Tunica albuginea near the apex. E

14 ***Tunica albuginea corporis spongiosi.*** Fibrous coat of the spongy body. F

15 ***Septum penis.*** Median septum between the Corpora cavernosa penis. F

16 ***Trabeculae corporum cavernosorum.*** Fibromuscular partitions between the Cavernae corporum cavernosorum. F

17 ***Trabeculae corporis spongiosi.*** Fibromuscular partitions between the Cavernae corporis spongiosi. F

18 ***Cavernae corporum cavernosorum.*** Vascular spaces within the cavernous bodies. F

19 ***Cavernae corporis spongiosi.*** Vascular spaces within the spongy body. F

20 ***Arteriae helicinae.*** Helicine arteries, terminal branches of the A. profunda penis, coiled and closed in the flaccid state, open to the cavernae in erection. F

21 ***Venae cavernosae.*** Veins draining the cavernous spaces of the erectile tissue. F

22 ***Fascia penis superficialis.*** Superficial fascia of the penis. It extends to the glans and into the prepuce and is continuous with the superficial perineal fascia, the Septum scroti, and the external spermatic fascia. B G

23 ***Fascia penis profunda.*** Deep fascia of the penis. Closely surrounds Corpora cavernosa and Corpus spongiosum, blends with the suspensory ligament of the penis, and is continuous with the deep perineal fascia. B G

24 ***Lig. suspensorium penis.*** Suspensory lig. of the penis, bilateral collagenous laminae that extend from the caudal part of the Symphysis pelvina to the Corpora cavernosa, enclosing the dorsal vessels and nerves of the penis. 207 A

25 ***Lig. fundiforme penis.*** Sling-shaped ligament of the penis, bilateral elastic bands from the median ventral surface of the Tendo prepubicus. They pass around the sides of the penis and blend with the Septum scroti. G

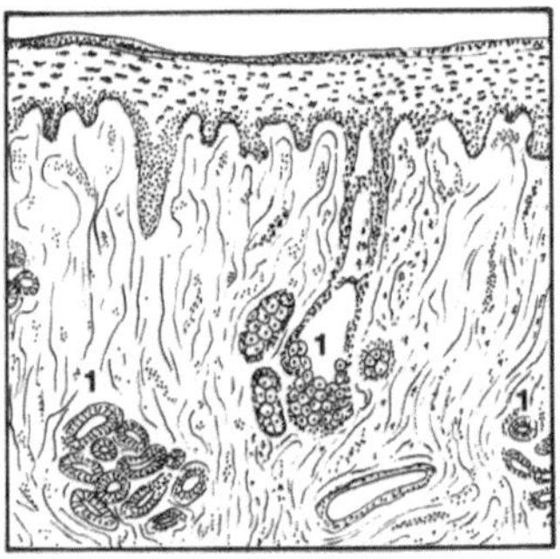

A Lamina interna of prepuce, histological section (eq) (Krage)

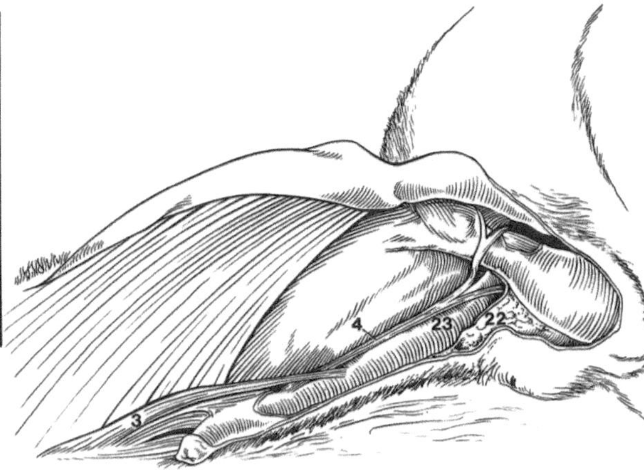

B Preputial muscles (external spermatic fascia fenestrated over M. cremaster), left ventral aspect (cap)

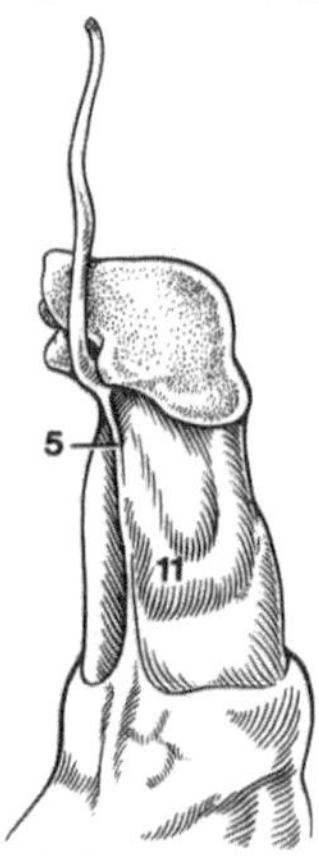

C Penis, left ventral aspect (ov) (Nickel et al. 1979)

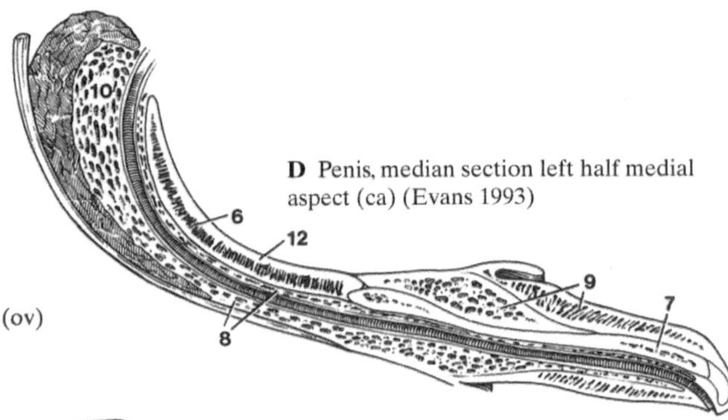

D Penis, median section left half medial aspect (ca) (Evans 1993)

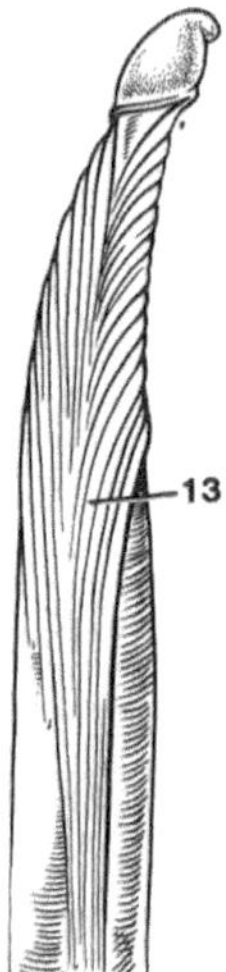

E Penis (skin and superficial fascia removed, except from the glans), dorsal aspect (bo)

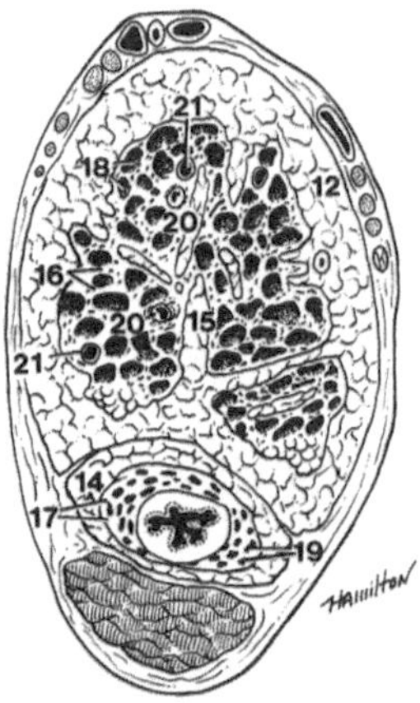

F Penis, histological section (fe)

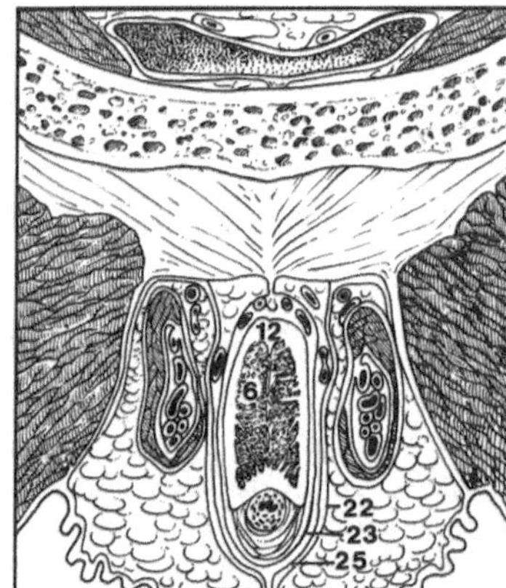

G Penis, transverse section through prepubic tendon, cranial to scrotum (spermatic cords cut obliquely) (eq)

1 **Urethra masculina***. Male urethra, excretory passage for urine and semen.

2 ***Pars pelvina***. Pelvic part. A D

3 *Pars preprostatica [prae-]*. Part between the urinary bladder and the Prostata, longest in fe. A

4 *Pars prostatica*. Part associated with the Prostata. A C

4a *Pars postprostatica*. Part between the Prostata and the Isthmus urethreae. In the NAV 2017 it is listed after "sinus prostaticus". A

5 **Crista urethralis**. Urethral crest, dorsal longitudinal mucosal ridge from the junction of the Plicae uretericae to the Colliculus seminalis. It extends farther caudally in some species. C

6 **Colliculus seminalis**. Seminal hillock, an eminence on the Crista urethralis, bearing on each side the Ostium ejaculatorium or separate openings of the Ductus deferens and the excretory duct of the Glandula vesicularis. A

7 **Ostium ejaculatorium**. Ejaculatory orifice, the opening of the Ductus ejaculatorius on the Colliculus seminalis. A

8 **Uterus masculinus**. Rudimentary male uterus, largest and most constant in eq. The cranial part is often bifurcated and lies in the genital fold between the ampullae. The caudal end may open on the Colliculus seminalis. B

9 **Sinus prostaticus**. Recess between the Colliculus seminalis and the lateral urethral wall. A C

10 *Stratum spongiosum*. Spongy layer, cavernous tissue surrounding the pelvic urethra. C F

11 *Isthmus urethrae*. Narrow segment of the urethra where it turns around the ischial arch. D

12 ***Pars penina***. Penile part of urethra. It is surrounded by the Corpus spongiosum. D E

13 *Recessus urethralis* (su, Ru). Caudodorsal to the urethra at the Arcus ischiadicus. Opens ventrally into the urethra. D

14 *Fossa navicularis urethrae* (su, eq). Navicular fossa of the urethra, a slight dilatation near the distal end in eq. E

15 *Processus urethrae*. Urethral process, free distal part of the urethra. It is longest in ov, cap; absent in fe, su. E

16 ***Ostium urethrae externum***. External urethral orifice. E

17 ***Tunica muscularis***. Smooth muscle of the pelvic urethra. It surrounds the Pars disseminata prostatae where that is present, or the Stratum spongiosum. It is not to be confused with the thick, striated M. urethralis, external to it. C F

18 ***Tunica mucosa***. Mucous membrane, covered by transitional epithelium, except near the external orifice, where it becomes stratified squamous. F

19 ***Lacunae urethrales***. Pockets formed by the surface epithelium. F

20 ***Gll. urethrales***. Urethral glands, isolated small branched glands in the Pars pelvina in ca, eq, and also in the Pars penina of su, eq. F

21 **Scrotum**. Cutaneous pouch containing the testes. G (The scrotal skin, the tunica dartos and the external spermatic fascia are considered as the extraabdominal testicular tunics. As far as origin, the testicular tunics consist of two groups of structures: intraabdominal, brought by the testicle during its descent [the internal spermatic fascia and the vaginal tunic with the parietal and visceral laminae], and extraabdominal, those preexistent to the testicular descent [the external spermatic fascia and the scrotum consisting of the scrotal skin and the tunica dartos].)

22 ***Cutis scroti***. Skin of the scrotum. G

23 *Raphe [Rhaphe] scroti*. Median seam of the Cutis scroti. G

24 ***Tunica dartos***. Layer of smooth muscle in the subcutaneous tissue. It wrinkles the skin, and continues as the Fascia perinealis superficialis. G

25 *Septum scroti*. Scrotal septum. Median partition formed by the Tunica dartos. G

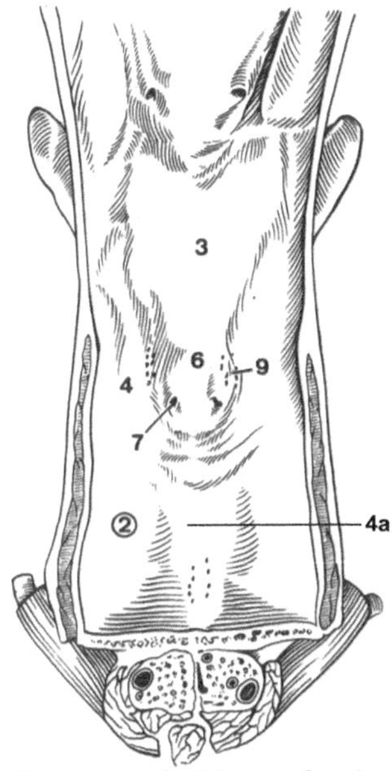

A Dorsal wall of pelvic part of urethra, seen from inside (the bulb of the penis is shown in section at the bottom, and the Trigonum vesicae above) (eq)

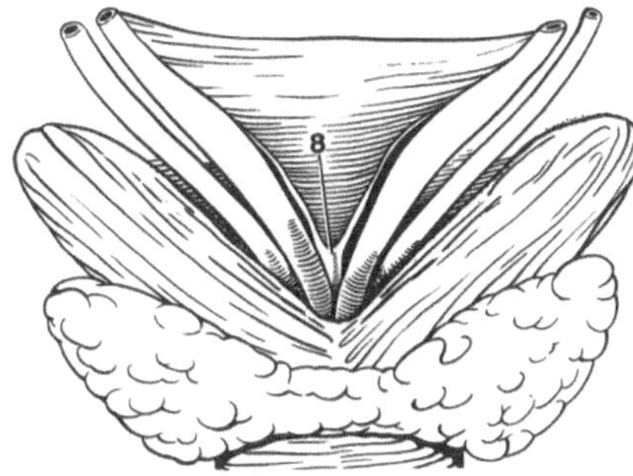

B Uterus masculinus, dorsal aspect (eq)

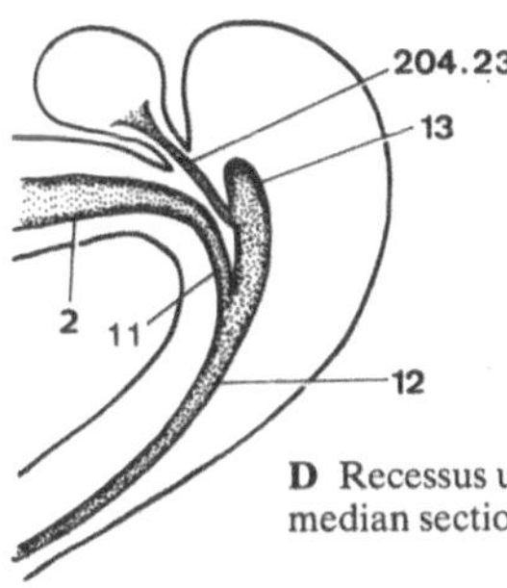

D Recessus urethralis median section (bo) (Garrett)

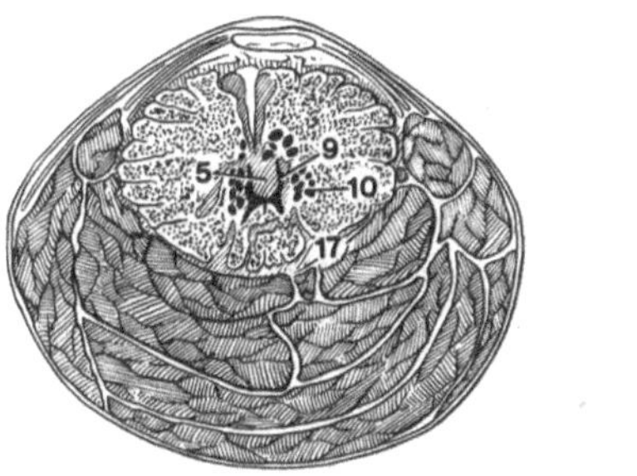

C Prostatic part of urethra, transverse section (M. urethralis is shown on the ventral and lateral surfaces) (bo)

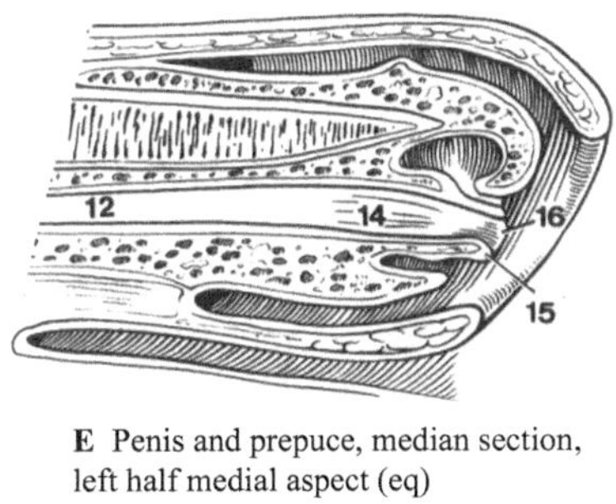

E Penis and prepuce, median section, left half medial aspect (eq)

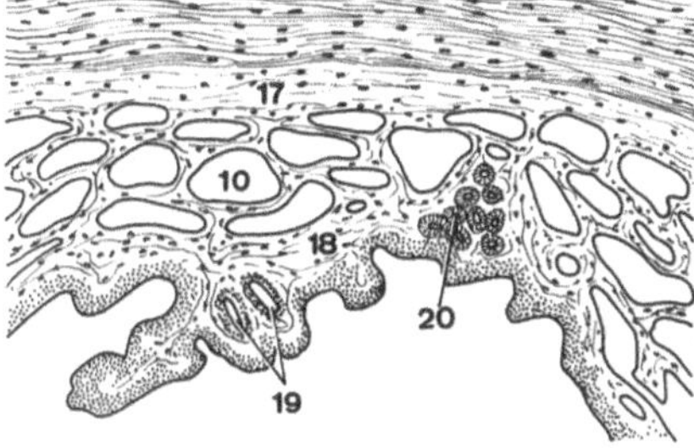

F Pelvic part of urethra, histological section (ca)

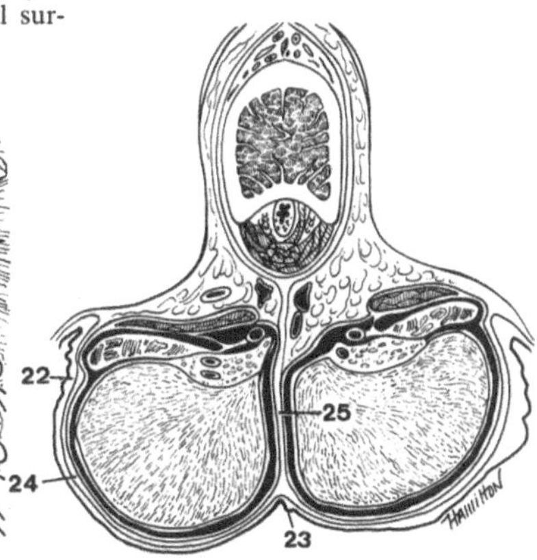

G Scrotum and penis, transverse section, caudal aspect (eq)

1 **ORGANA GENITALIA FEMININA**. Female genital organs.

2 ***Ovarium***. Ovary. A B C

3 ***Hilus ovarii***. Hilus of ovary, area of attachment of mesovarium and entrance of ovarian vessels. B

4 ***Facies medialis***. Medial surface. A

5 ***Facies lateralis***. Lateral surface.

6 ***Margo liber***. Free border. A

7 *Fossa ovarii* (eq). Ovarian fossa, depression on the free border where ovulation occurs. A

8 ***Margo mesovaricus***. Mesovarian border, where the Mesovarium is attached. A

9 ***Extremitas tubaria***. Tubal end, the end nearer to the Infundibulum tubae, opposite to the Extremitas uterina. A

10 ***Extremitas uterina***. Uterine end, the end attached to the uterus by the proper ligament. A

11 ***Margo limitans peritonei [peritonaei]***. Terminal border of the peritoneum, the line of attachment of the mesovarium to the ovary, also the transition from squamous mesothelium to cuboidal superficial epithelium; in eq, the termination of the Zona vasculosa around the Fossa ovarii. A B

12 ***Epithelium superficiale***. The superficial epithelium of the ovary in the young animal is cuboidal, and is restricted to the Fossa ovarii in eq. A B C

13 ***Tunica albuginea***. In the Cortex ovarii the amount of collagen fibers is very small, and therefore the term Tunica albuginea does not apply and was deleted from the 6th edition of the N.A.V.

14 ***Cortex ovarii [Zona parenchymatosa]***. Although in most species the tissue containing the follicles is peripheral and may be called a cortex, in eq it is central and requires a non-topographic name, the parenchymatous zone. B

15 ***Medulla ovarii [Zona vasculosa]***. In the Cortex ovarii the amount of collagen fibers is very small, and therefore the term Tunica albuginea does not apply and was deleted. In eq the vascular zone is peripheral and cannot be called a medulla, as it is in other species. B

16 ***Stroma ovarii***. Connective tissue of the ovary. B C

17 ***Folliculi ovarici primarii***. Primary ovarian follicles, consist of an ovocyte surrounded by one or more layers of follicular cells before the appearance of an antrum filled with Liquor folliculi. C

18 ***Folliculi ovarici vesiculosi***. Vesicular follicles have a fluid-filled cavity that enlarges with maturation. B C

19 ***Corpus luteum****. Yellow body, developed from cells of the Stratum granulosum and Theca interna after ovulation. B

20 ***Corpus albicans***. White body remaining after degeneration of a Corpus luteum. The color varies with species. It is red in bo. B

21 ***Lig. ovarii proprium***. Proper ligament of the ovary, band of connective tissue covered with peritoneum between Extremitas uterina ovarii and the apex of the uterine horn or nearby mesometrium. A

22 **Epoophoron**. Complex of vestigial tubules occasionally giving rise to cysts in the mesovarium and mesosalpinx. D

23 ***Ductus epoophori longitudinalis****. Duct of the epoöphoron, the vestige of the cranial part of the mesonephric duct, former the duct of Gärtner (see 216.23). D

24 *Ductuli transversi*. Transverse ductules, remnants of mesonephric tubules which run from the hilus of the ovary through the mesovarium and mesosalpinx to the Ductus epoöphori. D

25 ***Appendices vesiculosae***. Vesicular appendages, pedunculated cysts near the Infundibulum tubae. D

26 **Paroophoron**. Group of caudal mesonephric tubules in the Mesosalpinx near the Extremitas uterina ovarii. D

27 **Tuba uterina [Salpinx]**. Uterine tube, the conduit for ova from the ovary to the uterus. A

28 ***Ostium abdominale tubae uterinae***. Abdominal opening of the uterine tube in the infundibulum. A

29 ***Infundibulum tubae uterinae***. Funnel-shaped ovarian end of the tube. A

30 ***Fimbriae tubae***. Fringe of processes around the opening of the infundibulum. A

31 *Fimbria ovarica*. Ovarian fimbria, attached to the ovary. A

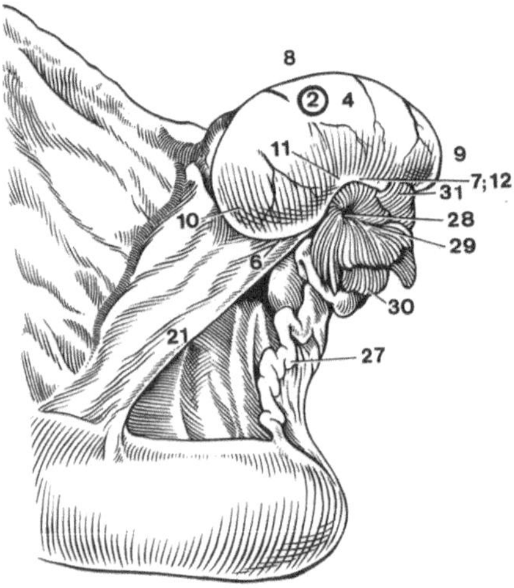

A Left ovary and ovarian bursa, medial aspect (eq)

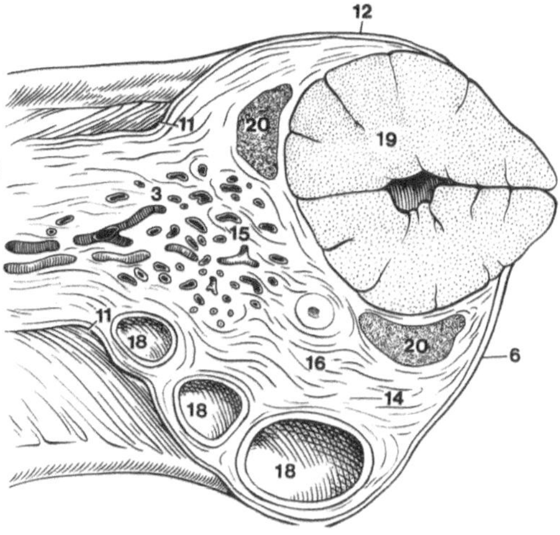

B Ovary and mesovarium, gross section (bo)

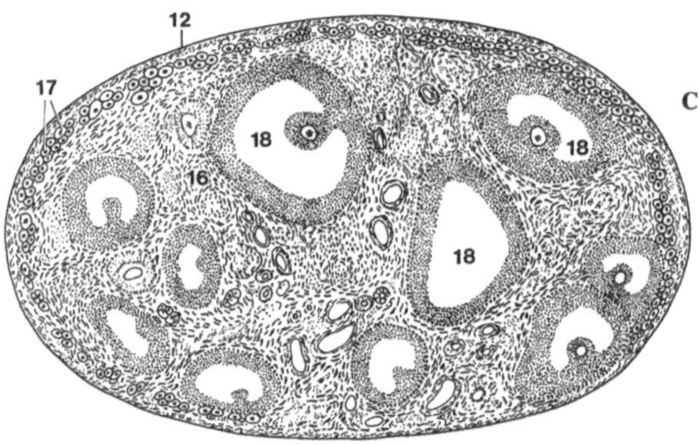

C Ovary, histological section (fe)

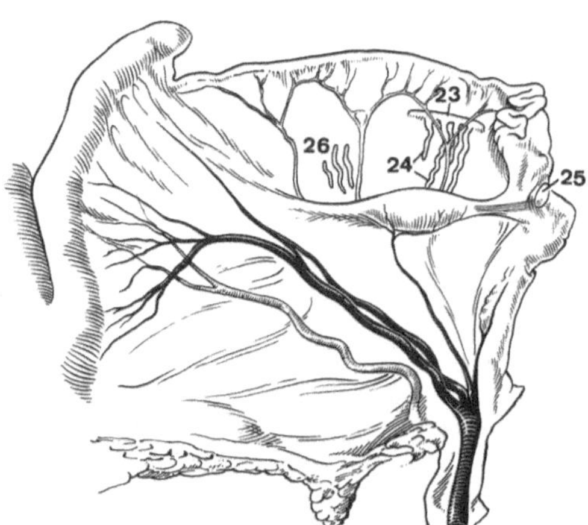

D Right ovary and uterine horn, epoöphoron and paroöphoron, dorsal aspect (ov)

1 ***Ampulla tubae uterinae***. Relatively wide part from the abdominal opening to the isthmus. A B

2 ***Isthmus tubae uterinae***. Narrow portion leading to the uterus. A

3 ***Pars uterina***. Uterine part. In Car, eq, the part of the tube in the wall of the uterus is distinct and ends on a papilla. In su, Ru, the tube is gradually continuous with the uterine horn. A

4 ***Ostium uterinum tubae***. Uterine orifice of the tube. A

5 ***Tunica serosa***. Serous coat. B

6 ***Tela subserosa***. Layer of loose connective tissue under the Tunica serosa. B

7 ***Tunica muscularis***. Smooth muscle coat. It is thickest in the Pars uterina. B

8 ***Tunica mucosa***. Mucous membrane lining the tube. B

9 *Plicae tubariae*. Tubal folds of mucous membrane. B

10 **Uterus**. Womb, organ of gestation. C D

11 ***Uterus bicornis***. Uterus with two horns and a single body and cervix, as in domestic mammals. C D

12 ***Cornu uteri [dextrum et sinistrum]****. Right and left horns of the uterus. D

13 *Margo mesometricus*. Mesometrial border, the side of the uterine horn attached to the mesometrium. D

14 *Margo liber*. Free border, the side of the uterine horn opposite to the mesometrium. D

15 ***Lig. intercornuale***. Intercornual lig. in ov, cap. Fold of serosa containing smooth muscle, crosses the acute angle between the cornua.

16 *Lig. intercornuale dorsale* (bo)*. Dorsal intercornual ligament. D

17 *Lig. intercornuale ventrale* (bo)*. Ventral intercornual ligament. D

18 ***Corpus uteri****. Body of the uterus, undivided part between the cornua and the cervix. D

19 ***Margo uteri [dexter et sinister]***. Right and left borders of the corpus and cervix to which the mesometrium is attached. D

20 ***Facies dorsalis***. Dorsal surface. C

21 ***Cavum uteri***. Cavity of the uterus. D

22 ***Facies ventralis***. Ventral surface.

23 ***Velum uteri***. Median partition formed by the fusion of the medial walls of the uterine horns in Car, su, Ru, absent in eq. D

24 ***Fundus uteri***. Cranial end of the body of the uterus in eq. C

25 ***Cervix uteri****. Neck of the uterus, thick-walled vaginal end which effects the closure of the uterus. D

26 *Portio prevaginalis [prae-] [cervicis]*. Part of the cervix cranial to the vagina. D

27 *Portio vaginalis [cervicis]**. Part of the cervix that projects into the vagina. In the female dog, the very prominent dorsal median mucosal fold of the vagina extends cranially to a cervical tubercle, which is the vaginal portion of the cervix. D (McCarthy 2005)

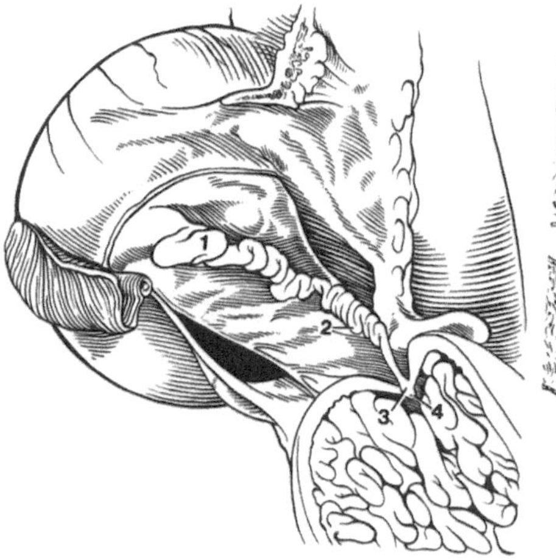

A Ovary, uterine tube, and mesosalpinx, lateral surface (uterine horn, lower right, has ben opened) (eq)

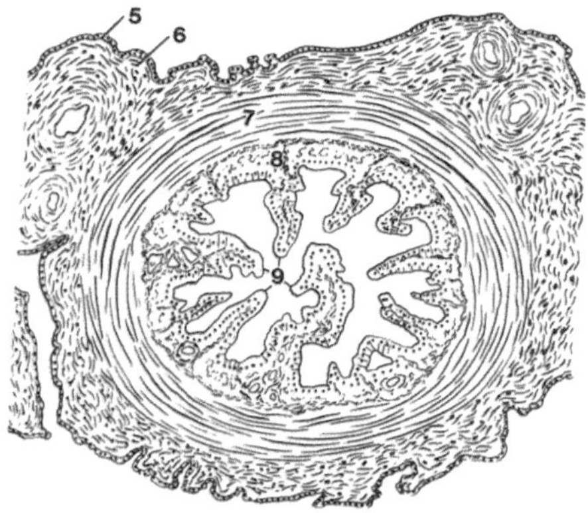

B Ampulla of uterine tube, histological section (bo)

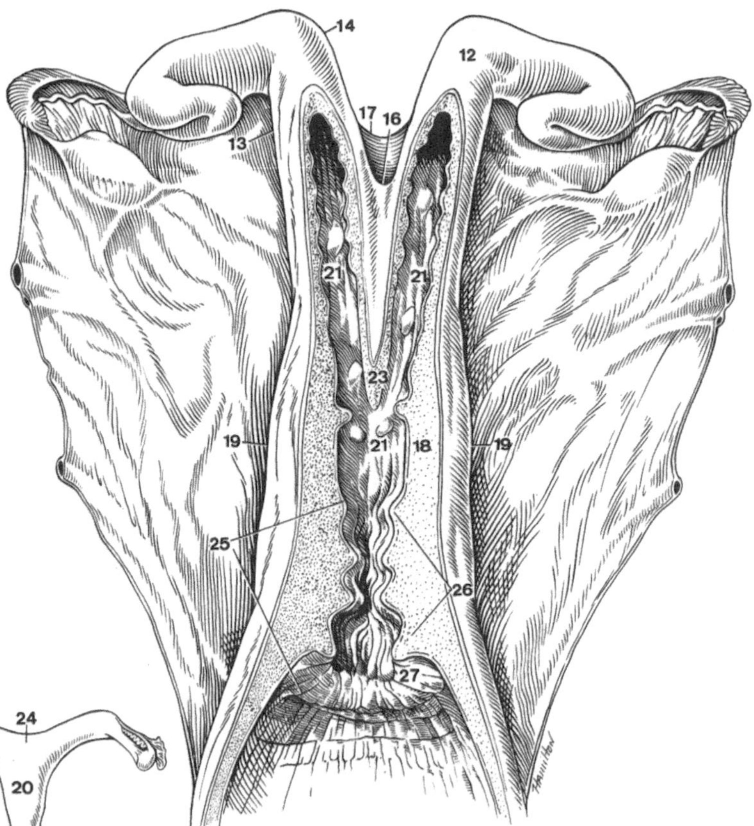

D Uterus, opened dorsally (bo)

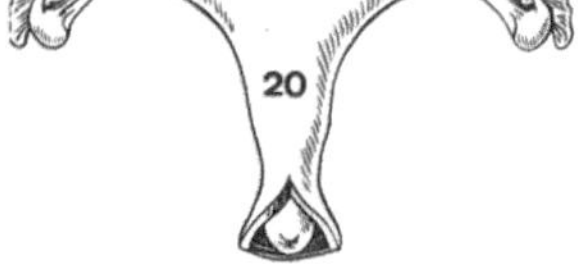

C Uterus, dorsal surface (ovaries displaced laterally) (eq)

1 ***Ostium uteri internum***. Internal orifice of the uterus, between the body of the uterus and the cervix. A

2 ***Ostium uteri externum****. External orifice of the uterus, between the cervix and the vagina. A E

3 ***Canalis cervicis uteri***. Cervical canal. A C

4 *Plicae longitudinales*. Longitudinal folds of cervical mucosa. A

5 *Plicae circulares* (Ru)*. Circular or crescentic folds of cervical mucosa which close the canal. A

6 *Pulvini cervicales* (su)*. Cervical cushions, interdigitating processes which close the canal. C

7 *Gll. cervicales*. Cervical glands. Simple tubular glands in Car, su, ov, cap, but the cervical mucus is secreted primarily by the epithelium.

8 ***Parametrium***. Connective tissue, smooth muscle, vessels, and nerves between the peritoneal laminae of the mesometrium. D

9 ***Tunica serosa [Perimetrium]***. Visceral peritoneum on the uterus. D

10 ***Tela subserosa***. Layer of loose connective tissue under the Tunica serosa. D

11 ***Tunica muscularis [Myometrium]***. Smooth muscle of the uterus. The inner, circular and oblique layer is thick, the outer longitudinal is associated with the perimetrium. A vascular layer separates circular and longitudinal layers. D

12 ***Tunica mucosa [Endometrium]***. Mucous membrane. It has a thick glandular Lamina propria and is covered by columnar epithelium. D

13 *Carunculae**. Caruncles, eminences of the endometrium in Ru, the term for the maternal parts of the placentomes. They enlarge in pregnancy and receive the chorionic villi of the cotyledons (the fetal part of the placentomes – listed in the Nomina Embryologica Veterinaria) to form placentomes. A

14 *Gll. uterini*. Uterine glands. Branched tubular glands extend through the endometrium. D

15 ***Lig. teres uteri***. Round ligament of the uterus. It extends from the tip of the uterine horn to the deep inguinal ring, enclosed in a lateral fold of the Lig. latum. The longest ligament is found in the dog, in which it passes through the inguinal canal concealed within the vaginal process. It is palpable under the skin from the inguinal region to the labia of the vulva. In the cat it passes through the inguinal canal without the vaginal process around[1]. B

16 ***Processus vaginalis peritonei [peritonaei]***. Vaginal process of the peritoneum in the inguinal canal. In males it becomes the Tunica vaginalis after the descent of the testis. In females it often persists in ca, absent in fe [1]. B

17 **Vagina**. Canal from the cervix to the hymen or vestibule. A E

18 ***Fornix vaginae****. Fornix of the vagina, the cranial blind pouch of the vagina surrounding the Portio vaginalis cervicis. A E

19 ***Paries ventralis***. Ventral wall of the vagina. A

20 ***Paries dorsalis***. Dorsal wall of the vagina. A

21 ***Hymen***. Fold of mucosa just cranial to the transverse plane of the urethral orifice, marking the Ostium vaginae in virgins. It is poorly developed in domestic mammals. E

22 ***Ostium vaginae***. Opening of the vagina into the vestibule. It is marked by the hymen or a transverse plane just cranial to the urethral orifice. A

23 ***(Ductus deferens vestigialis)***. Remnant of the caudal part of the mesonephric duct, formerly called Gärtner's duct (see 212.23). It is often present in the floor of the bovine vagina, opening craniolateral to the urethral orifice. A

24 ***Tunica serosa***. Peritoneal covering of the cranial end of the vagina. A

25 ***Tela subserosa***. Loose connective tissue under the serosa. A

26 ***Tunica adventitia***. Connective tissue covering the retroperitoneal part of the vagina. A

27 ***Tunica muscularis***. Smooth muscle of the vaginal wall. A

28 ***Tunica mucosa***. Mucous membrane. The lining epithelium varies from secretory columnar to stratified squamous according to species and stage of the estrus cycle. In addition to the dorsal mucosal fold of the vagina (see 214.27), in anestrus prominent longitudinal mucosal folds can be seen in the dog. A (McCarthy 2005)

29 *Rugae vaginales*. Vaginal ridges, around the cervix in the Fornix vaginae of bo. A

30 *Lymphonoduli [Noduli lymphatici] vaginales*. In the Lamina propria.

1) Watson 2009

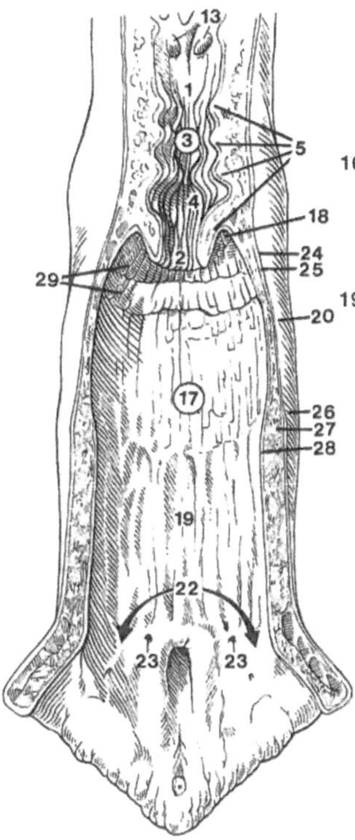

A Cervix and vagina, opened dorsally (bo)

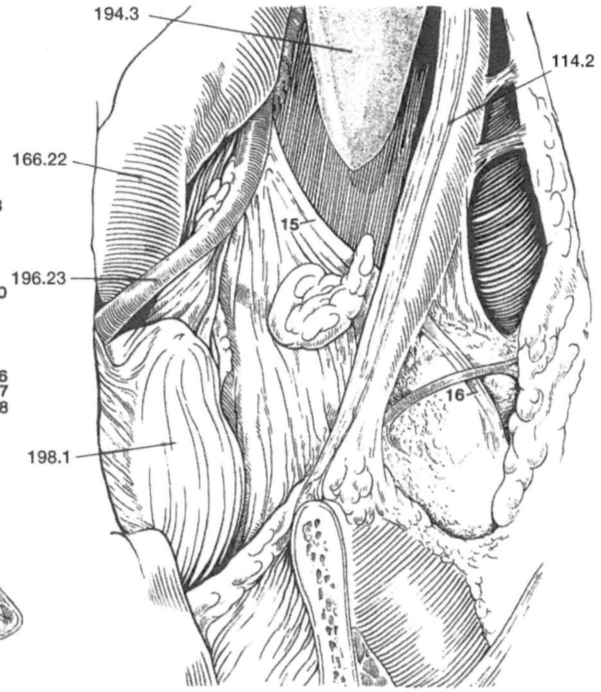

B Left inguinal region (abdomen opened midventrally, mammae and fat separated from the abdominal wall) (ca fem)

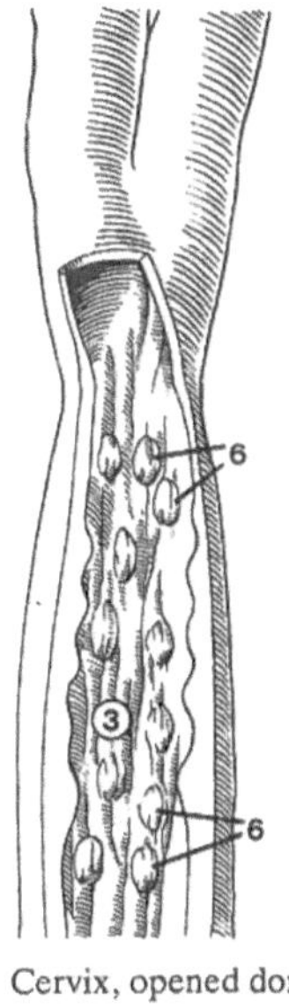

C Cervix, opened dorsally (su)

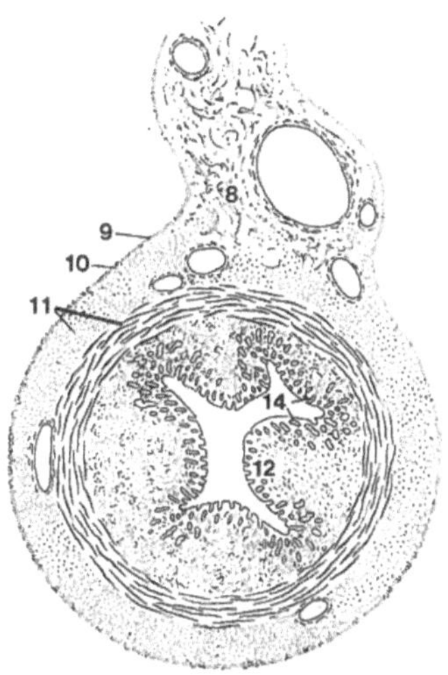

D Uterine horn with mesometrium, histological section (fe)

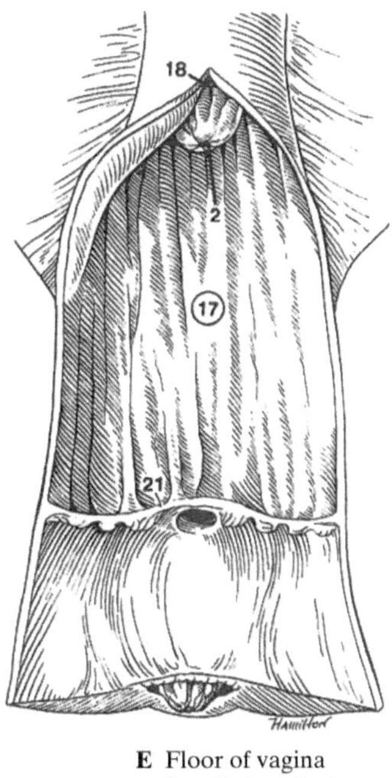

E Floor of vagina and vesibulum (eq)

1 **Vestibulum vaginae**. Vestibule, the part of the female genital canal from the hymen to the labia. The human vestibule is so shallow that it is included with the external genitalia. In quadrupeds, where it is much deeper (in fe it is about the same length as the vagina) it is not included in the Pudendum femininum (the external part of female genitalia). A B E

2 ***Bulbus vestibuli***. Vestibular bulb, cavernous tissue in the lateral wall of the vestibule in ca, eq. C

3 ***Pars intermedia bulborum***. Commissure of bulbi. B

4 ***Gll. vestibulares minores***. Minor vestibular gll., microscopic branched tubular glands in the ventral and lateral walls.

5 ***Gl. vestibularis major***. Major vestibular gland (fe, bo, ov), a lobulated gland cranial to Membrana perinei and M. constrictor vestibuli. The duct opens on the lateral wall of the vestibule. A

6 ***Diverticulum suburethrale*** (su, Ru)*. Suburethral diverticulum, a blind sac ventral to the urethra and opening into the urethral orifice. A

7 ***Tuberculum urethrale*** (ca)*. Urethral tubercle, an elevation bearing the urethral orifice at the vestibulovaginal junction. On both sides of the tubercle two curved mucosal folds run cranially in a divergent direction in the dog. An annular, narrow, bandlike constriction unofficially called “cingulum” acts as a functional sphincter at the vestibulovaginal junction. B (McCarthy 2005)

8 **PARTES GENITALES FEMININAE EXTERNAE**. External female genitalia, the vulva and clitoris. The vestibule in domestic mammals is not considered an external organ.

9 **Vulva [Pudendum femininum]**. Labia and their commissures.

10 ***Labium vulvae [pudendi]****. Labium of the vulva. Major and minor labia are not distinguishable in domestic mammals, with the possible exception of or and Car. The outer surface of the labium is covered with sparsely haired skin, and the inner surface with Tunica mucosa bearing stratified squamous epithelium. A B C D

11 *Commissura labiorum ventralis**. Ventral commissure of the labia. A B C D

12 *Commissura labiorum dorsalis**. Dorsal commissure of the labia. B C

13 *Rima pudendi [vulvae]*. Pudendal fissure between right and left labia, the external urogenital opening. B

14 **Clitoris**. Rudimentary partial homologue of the penis in the ventral wall of the vestibule. C

15 ***Crus clitoridis***. Crus of the clitoris. Right and left crura are attached to the ischial arch and join the body of the clitoris. A C

16 ***Corpus clitoridis***. Body of the clitoris, composed of the fused Corpora cavernosa. It is tortuous in bo. A B C

17 ***Glans clitoridis***. Glans of the clitoris, best developed in ca and eq. B C D

18 *Sinus clitoridis**. In eq three clitoral sinuses open on dorsal surface of glans, near frenulum; the median sinus occupies the central part of glans, and the lateral sinuses are shallow and inconstant. Other sinuses may occur ventral to the glans. D

19 *Frenulum clitoridis*. Median dorsal attachment of glans to vestibular wall of Preputium in ca, eq. In other species the separation of Preputium from glans is insufficient to isolate a Frenulum. B C D

20 ***Preputium [Praeputium] clitoridis***. Prepuce of the clitoris. In domestic mammals the prepuce is formed by the ventral commissure of the labia and by a transverse fold of vestibular mucosa to which the frenulum is attached. B C D

21 *Fossa clitoridis*. Fossa of the clitoris, the preputial cavity, it is almost obliterated by adhesion of the prepuce to the glans in fe, su, Ru. In ca, eq it surrounds the glans except at the Frenulum. B C D

22 ***Corpus cavernosum clitoridis***. Cavernous body of the clitoris. Right and left cavernous bodies are fused to form the body of the clitoris. In ca most of the erectile tissue is replaced by fat. In fe it contains a cartilage corresponding to the Os penis. In Un it is mostly fibrous. E

23 ***Septum corporum cavernosorum***. Partial septum between the cavernous bodies. E

24 ***Corpus spongiosum glandis*** (ca, eq). Spongy body of the glans, continuous with the Pars intermedia bulborum. B

25 ***Fascia clitoridis***. Fascia of the clitoris. E

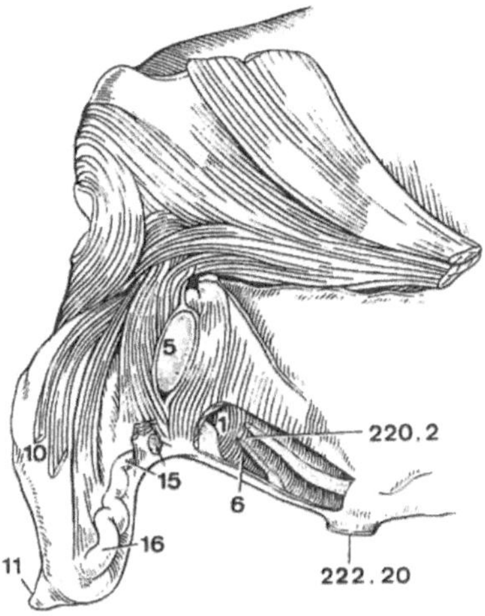

A Female genital organs (left lateral wall fenestrated) (bo)

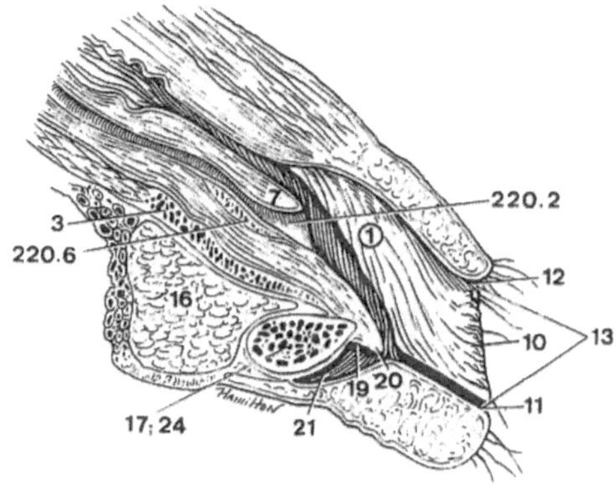

B Female genital organs, median section (ca)

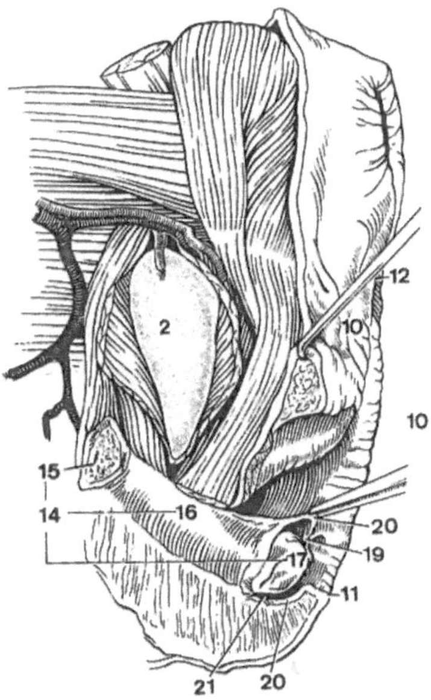

C Female genital organs, left lateral aspect (ventral part of left labium removed and M. constrictor vestibuli cut to expose bulbus vestibuli) (eq)

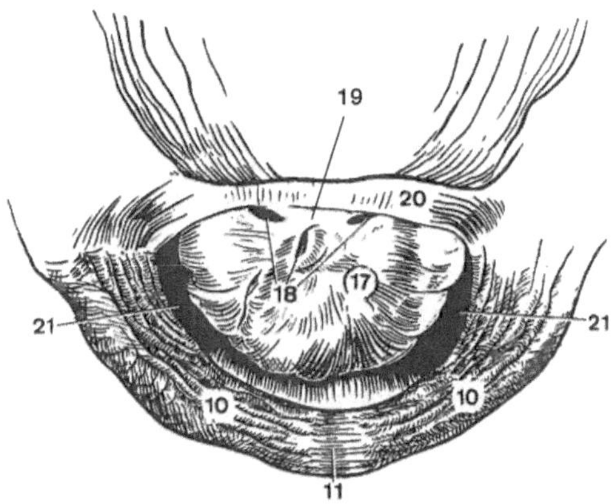

D Glans clitoridis (eq) (De Schaepdrijver et al. 1988)

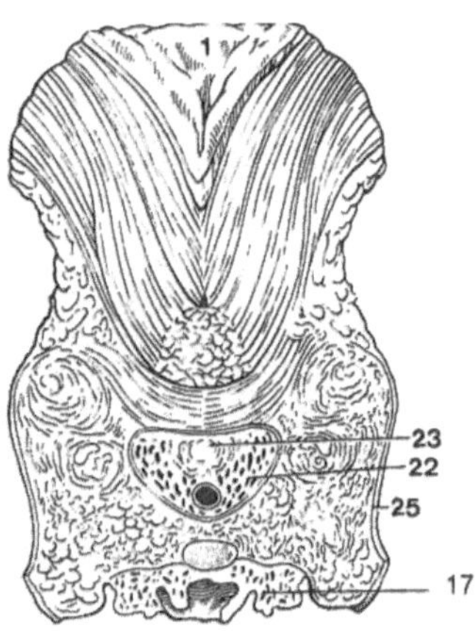

E Corpus clitoridis, transverse section ventral to vestibule (17 is the ventral process of the glans) (eq)

1 **Urethra Feminina.** Female urethra, corresponds to the male preprostatic part. A B

2 ***Ostium urethrae externum.*** External urethral orifice. 219 A

3 ***Tunica adventitia.*** Loose connective tissue covering the urethra. A

4 ***Tunica muscularis.*** Muscular coat, smooth muscle of the wall. A

5 ***Tunica mucosa.*** Mucous membrane, lined by stratified epithelium, squamous at the end, cubiodal to columnar in the middle, transitional near the urinary bladder. A

6 *Stratum spongiosum.* Spongy layer, cavernous tissue around the urethra. 219 B

7 *Gll. urethrales.* Urethral glands in bo, may open either on the surface or into a lacuna. A

8 *Lacunae urethrales.* Tubular evaginations of the surface epithelium in su, bo, eq. A

9 *(Ductus paraurethrales).* Paraurethral ducts in fe, su, ov, blind epithelial tubules, 1–2 cm long, in the angle between the urethra and the vagina. In fe, su, they are the ducts of small paraurethral glands, which are absent in ov. They open near the urethral orifice. B

10 *(Gll. paraurethrales).* Paraurethral glands, appended to the paraurethral ducts in fe, su. B

11 ***Crista urethralis.*** Urethral crest, dorsal longitudinal mucosal ridge extending from the junction of the Plicae uretericae caudally to the middle of the urethra. A

12 **TERMINI ONTOGENETICI.** Developmental terms. (All of the ontogenetic terms were omitted from the 5th edition of the N. A. V. They are listed in Nomina Embryologica Veterinaria.)

Membranae fetales.

Amnion.

Allantois.

Chorion.

Villi chorii.

Placenta.

Pars uterina.

Pars fetalis.

Placenta diffusa.

Placenta multiplex.

Placentomus.

Caruncula.

Cotyledon.

Placenta zonaria.

Funiculus umbilicalis.

Mesonephros.

Ductus mesonephricus.

Ductus paramesonephricus.

Sinus urogenitalis.

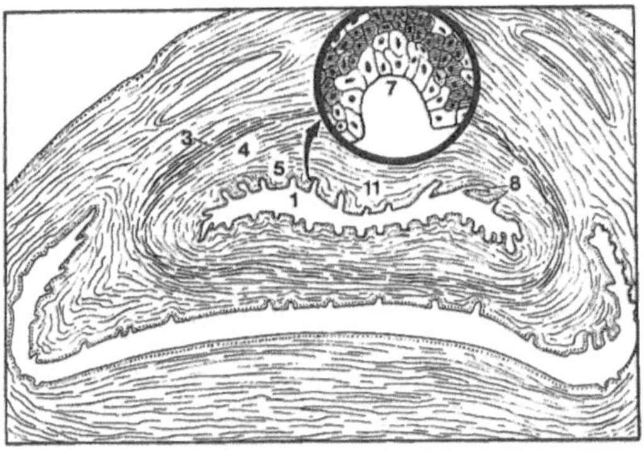

A Female urethra, transverse section (above the urethra the vestigial deferent ducts, and below the suburethral diverticulum (bo) (Schmaltz)

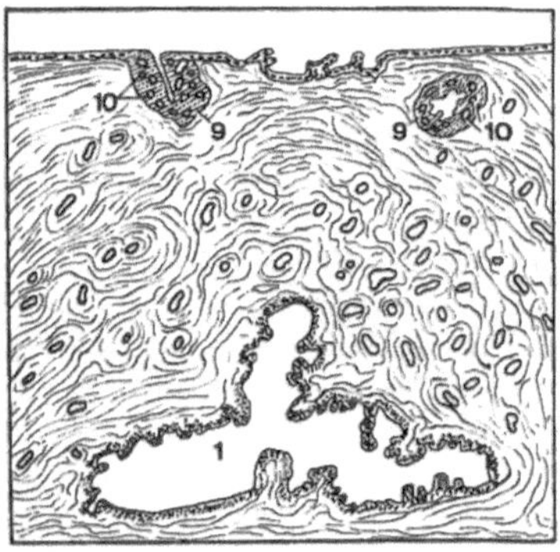

B Female urethra, transverse section (vaginal mucosa above) (su)

1 **PERINEUM**. Part of the body wall that closes the Apertura pelvis caudalis and surrounds the anal and urogenital canals. A

2 ***Raphe [Rhaphe]***. Median cutaneous seam prolonging the Raphe scroti on the perineum in eq. B

3 ***Musculi perinei***. Muscles of the perineum.

4 ***Diaphragma pelvis***. Pelvic diaphragm, composed of M. levator ani and M. coccygeus and the internal and external fasciae. C

5 *M. levator ani**. Lateral to the rectum, medial to M. coccygeus. Car: divided into Mm. iliocaudalis and pubocaudalis. Un: O: Spina ischiadica or Lig. sacrotuberale latum. T: M. sphincter ani externus, in su also caudal vertebrae 2–5. There are three fascicles in Un: coccygeal (Ca Fa), anal (Cb Fb), and perineal (Cc Fc). C E F

6 **M. iliocaudalis [-coccygeus]** (Car). O: Corpus ossis ilii. T: caudal vertebrae 1–3 in fe, 3–7 in ca; also M. sphincter ani externus by means of the pelvic fasciae. D

7 **M. pubocaudalis [-coccygeus]** (Car). O: Ramus cranialis ossis pubis, Symphysis pelvina. T: caudal vertebrae 1–3 in fe, 3–7 in ca; also M. sphincter ani externus by means of the pelvic fasciae. D

8 **(Arcus tendineus m. levatoris ani)**. Tendinous arch of M. levator ani, reinforcement of the Fascia obturatoria extending from the caudal end of the Symphysis pelvina to the Spina ischiadica at the origin of M. levator ani in Ru, eq. E

9 *M. Coccygeus**. O: Spina ischiadica. T: caudal vertebrae 1–4. C E

10 *Fascia diaphragmatis pelvis interna*. Medial to Mm. coccygeus and levator, at their borders joining the external fascia, caudally reflected on the rectum. E

11 *Fascia diaphragmatis pelvis externa*. Lateral to Mm. coccygeus and levator, at their borders joining the internal fascia, dorsally continuous with the deep caudal fascia. C

12 ***M. sphincter ani externus****. External anal sphincter, striated muscle surrounding the M. sphincter ani internus. C

13 *Pars cutanea*. Cutaneous part, thin fiberbundles passing dorsoventrally around the anus or radially. C

14 *Pars superficialis*. Superficial part, main part in Un, with the most circular fibers. Many fiber bundles pass through a ventral decussation into M. constrictor vulvae, or end on M. bulbospongiosus in the male. In eq divided into a large circular caudal portion and a small, paired cranial portion. C F

15 *Pars profunda*. Deep part, intimately associated or continuous with the M. levator ani. C

16 ***Fascia pelvis***. Pelvic fascia, in the pelvic cavity. E

17 *F. pelvis parietalis*. Parietal pelvic fascia, lining the walls of the pelvic cavity, includes Fascia diaphragmatis pelvis interna and Fascia obturatoria. E

18 **Fascia obturatoria**. On the dorsal surface of M. obturatorius internus in Car and eq, Pars pelvina of M. obturatorius externus in su and Ru. E

19 *Arcus tendineus fasciae pelvis*. Tendinous arch of the pelvic fascia, indistinct zone on the Fascia diaphragmatis pelvis interna along the ventral border of M. levator ani where the Septum rectovaginale is attached in Ru, eq. E

20 *Lig. pubovesicale*. From Symphysis pelvina to Cervix vesicae. 219 A

21 *F. pelvis visceralis*. Covering the pelvic organs. E

22 **Fascia prostatae**. Prostatic fascia, covering the prostate.

23 **Septum rectovaginale**. Attached laterally to the Arcus tendineus fasciae pelvis extending in a dorsal plane between rectum and vagina. E

24 ***Septum perineale***. Quadrilateral sheet of fascia in eq. From the dorsal surface of the vestibule deep to the M. constrictor vulvae, it extends dorsocranially to the Pars rectalis m. retractoris clitoridis and the rectum. The ventral part of the M. levator ani is attached to its craniolateral angle, the M. constrictor vestibuli originates from its lateral border. F

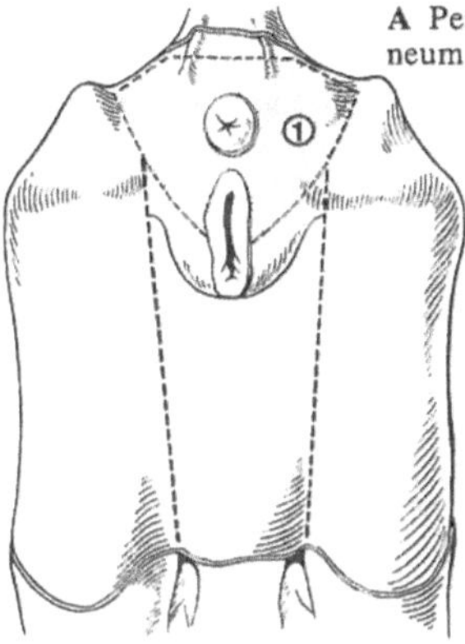

A Perineum (gray; perineal region includes the perineum and extends to the udder) (bo)

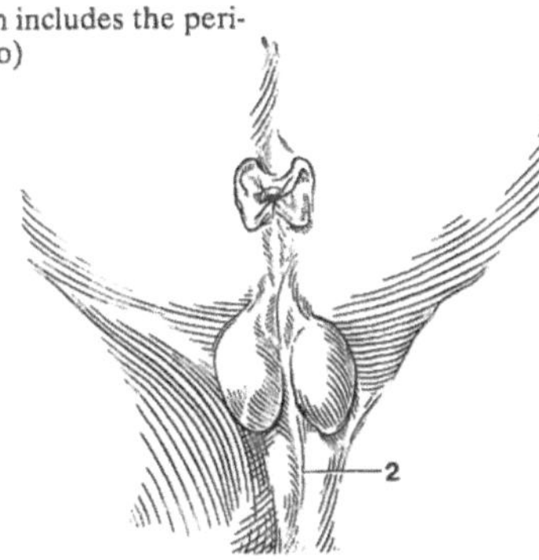

B Male genitalia, ventral surface (eq)

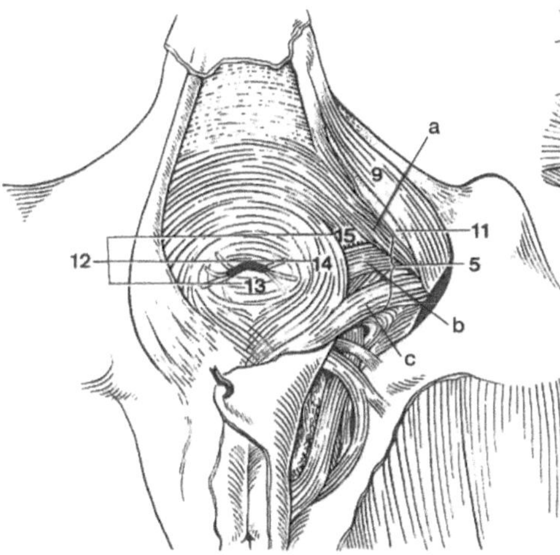

C Pelvic diaphragm (bo)

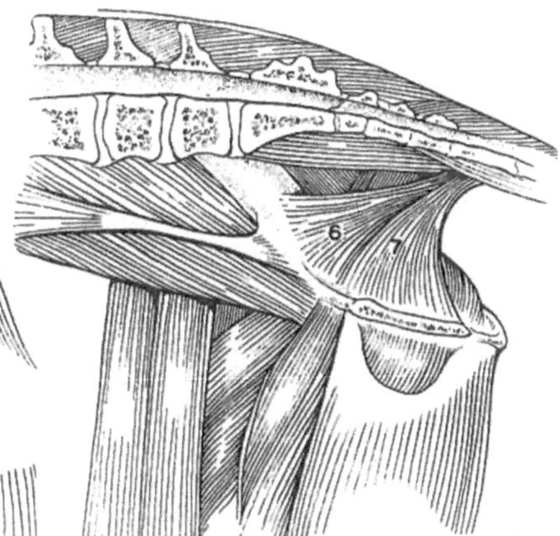

D Pelvic wall, right medial aspect (ca) (Nickel et al. 1954)

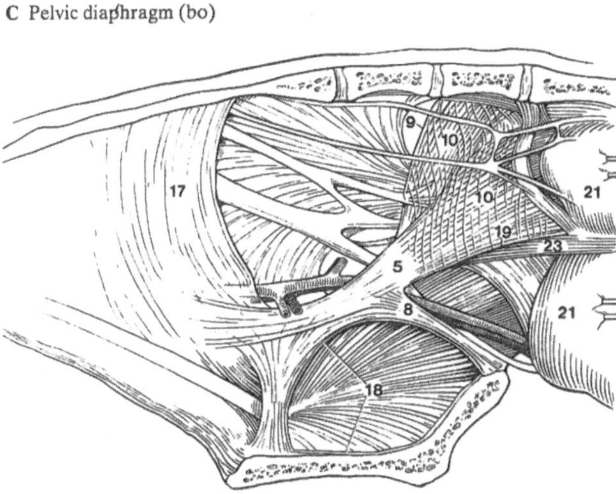

E Fascia pelvis, medial aspect (rectum and vagina reflected caudally, 17 and 18 partly removed) (bo)

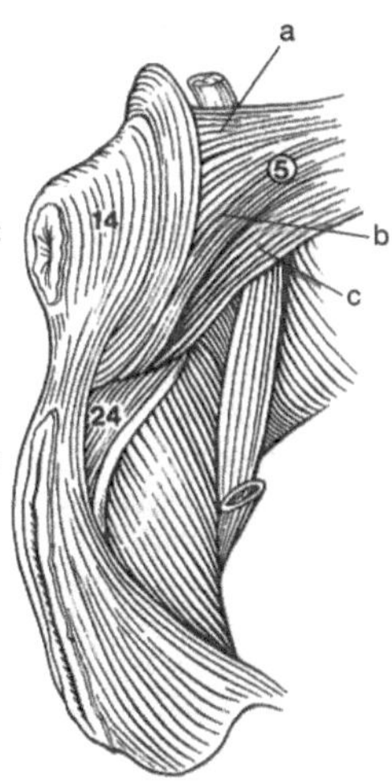

F Perineal muscles, caudolateral aspect (eq)

1 ***Centrum tendineum perinei [Corpus perineale].*** Tendinous center of the perineum [perineal body]. Fibromuscular node between anus und vulva or the Bulbus penis, where are attached: Mm. sphincter ani externus, bulbospongiosus, levator ani, and transversus perinei superficialis. A D

2 ***M. urethralis.*** Striated muscle of pelvic urethra, which it surrounds in male. In female originates from sides of vagina and forms a sling ventral to urethra. B E

3 ***M. ischiourethralis.*** O: Arcus ischiadicus. T: in ca, on Lig. transversum perinei. Compresses V. dorsalis penis. In the mare it terminates on dorsolateral wall of vagina; in other Un, on M. urethralis. Lies between Fascia pelvis parietalis and Membrana perinei. C

4 ***M. bulboglandularis.*** Striated muscle on Gl. bulbourethralis (male) or Gl. vestibularis major (female). B

5 ***Membrana perinei.*** Perineal membrane. Deep perineal fascia that closes the urogenital triangle between Arcus ischiadicus and Diaphragma pelvis. Attached to male urethra or Vestibulum vaginae between M. urethralis and M. bulbospongiosus. C D

6 *Lig. transversum perinei.* Transverse perineal ligament. Ventral band of Membrana perinei attached to Ossa ischii across Symphysis ischiadica.

7 ***M. transversus perinei superficialis.*** Rudimentary band of muscle in Ru, eq. O: fascia in the region of the Tuber ischiadicum. T: Centrum tendineum perinei. D

8 ***M. ischiocavernosus.*** O: Tuber ischiadicum in male, Arcus ischiadicus in female. T: Corpus penis at junction of crura, encloses Crus penis. It is rudimentary in female. B C

9 ***M. bulbospongiosus.*** Formerly M. bulbocavernosus. O: Tunica albuginea lateral to Corpus spongiosum penis, which is compressed by the muscle. T: median septum. B F. In female domestic mammals, because of the elongated vestibule, M. bulbospongiosus is divided into the following two muscles.

10 *M. constrictor vestibuli.* O: in Car, ov, cap, from M. sphincter ani externus; in bo, eq, from ventral border of M. levator ani; in eq, also from Septum perineale and M. retractor clitoridis. T: an aponeurosis joins right and left muscles ventral to the vestibule. Other attachments are vestibule, clitoris, and urogenital diaphragm, depending on species. D

11 *M. constrictor vulvae.* Striated muscle in the labium. O: superficial part of M. sphincter ani externus. T: labium and, in Ru, eq, perineal fascia ventrolateral to vulva. A C D

12 ***M. retractor penis.*** Predominantly smooth. O: caudal vertebrae 1–4, depending on species; sacrum in su. Passes ventrally between rectum and M. levator ani. F

13 ***M. retractor clitoridis.*** See 12. In su the vertebral origin is absent, Pars clitoridea originates from the rectum. D

14 *Pars analis.* Anal part, caudal portion inserted dorsolaterally on and under anal sphincters in Car. F

15 *Pars rectalis.* Rectal part, cranial portion inserted on lateral wall of rectum. Absent in sow, and sometimes in ca, in eq it joins contralateral muscle ventral to rectum, and was formerly known as suspensory lig. of the anus. A F

16 *Pars penina.* Penile part, runs on urethral surface of the penis, except across Flexura sigmoidea in su, Ru. B F

17 *Pars clitoridea.* Clitoridean part, absent in ca. Passes deep to M. constrictor vestibuli to reach the labium and (exc. eq) the clitoris. A C D

18 ***Fascia perinei superficialis.*** Superficial fascia of the perineal region. C

19 ***M. longitudinalis perinei cutaneus.*** Fine fiber bundles that extend from anus to vulva just under the skin. Demonstrated in the female cat and dog.

20 ***M. sphincter labiorum cutaneus.*** Cutaneous sphincter of the labia. It lies between M. constrictor vulvae and skin. Demonstrated in the female cat and dog.

21 ***Fossa ischiorectalis.*** Ischiorectal fossa, fat-filled space between Diaphragma pelvis medially, Lig. sacrotuberale laterally, Fascia obturatoria ventrally. D E

22 *Corpus adiposum fossae ischiorectalis.* Fat pad of ischiorectal fossa. E

23 *Canalis pudendalis.* Pudendal canal, fascial conduit in Fossa ischiorectalis for internal pudendal vessels and the pudendal nerve. E

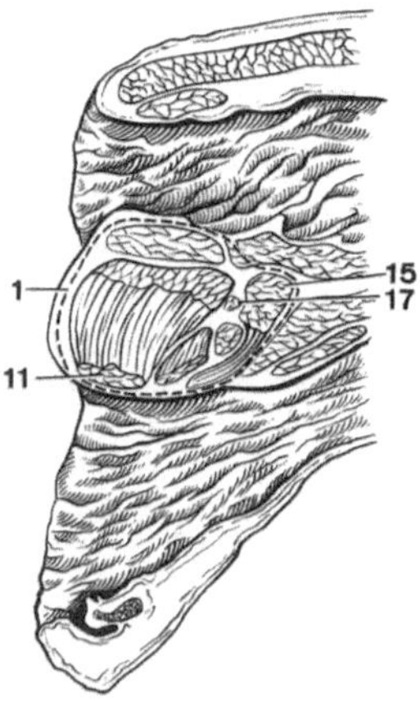

A Anus, perineal body, and vulva, median section left side (eq)

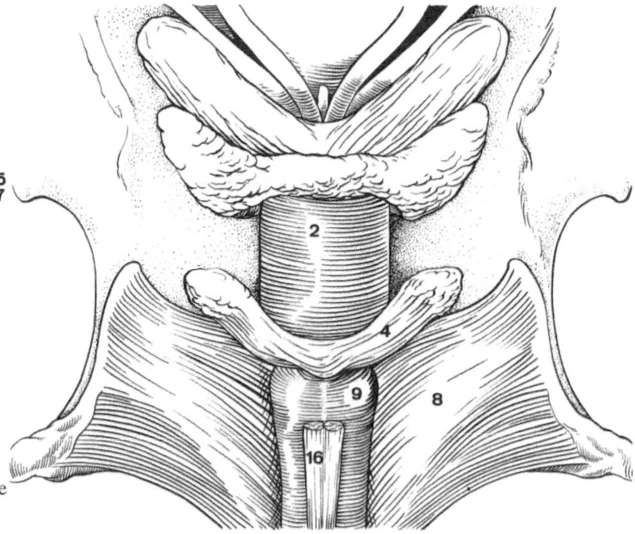

B Pelvic part of urethra and root of the penis, dorsal surface (eq) (Nickel et al. 1979)

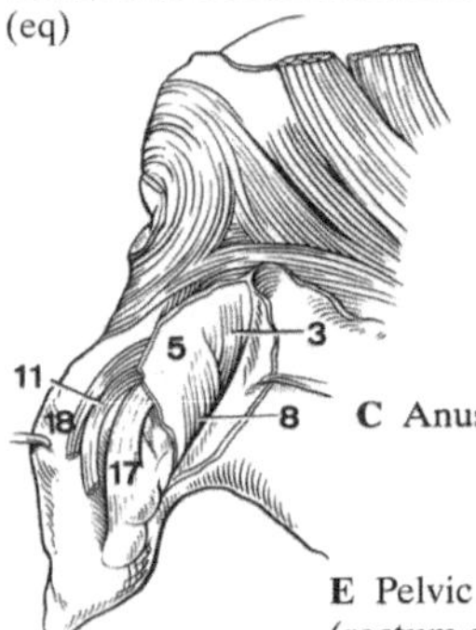

C Anus and vulva, right side (bo)

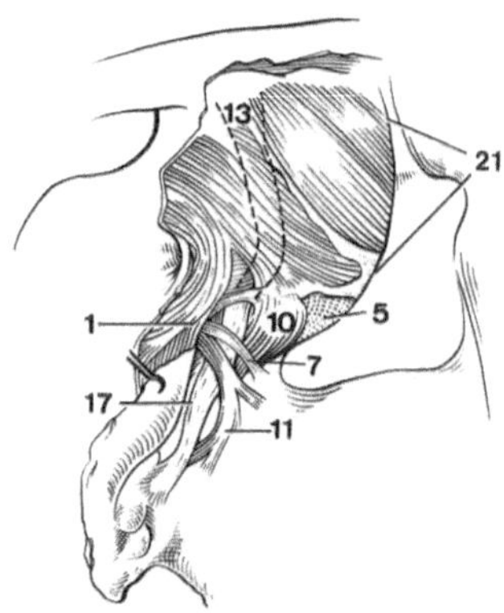

D Perineum, right caudolateral aspect (bo fem)

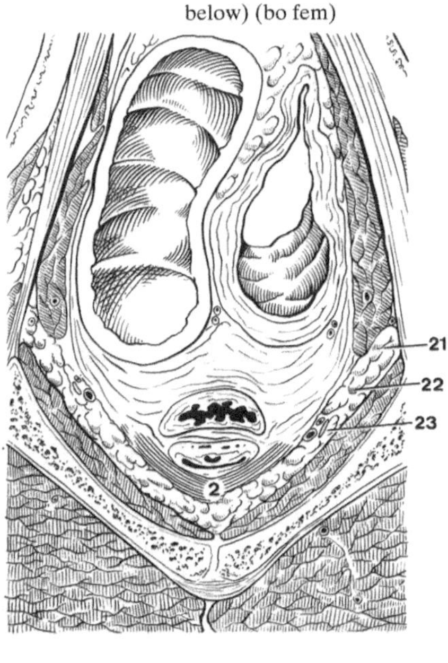

E Pelvic cavity transverse section (rectum and cecum above; vagina, urethra, and suburethral diverticulum below) (bo fem)

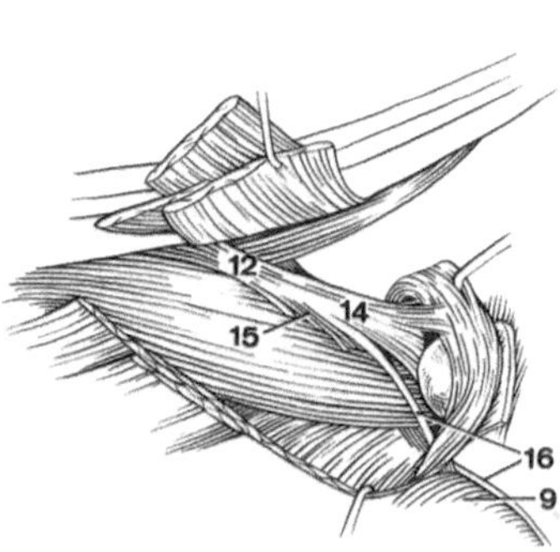

F Perineal muscles, left lateral aspect (muscles of pelvic diaphragm transected and retracted) (ca) (Miller et al.)

1 **PERITONEUM [PERITONAEUM].** Serous membrane lining the abdominal, pelvic, and scrotal cavities, and covering the organs contained therein. A

2 ***Peritoneum [Peritonaeum] parietale.*** Serous membrane on the walls of the above cavities. A

3 *Tunica serosa.* Serous membrane, composed of a layer of mesothelium and a layer of connective tissue.

4 *Tela subserosa.* Layer of loose connective tissue and fat present under the serosa in certain areas.

5 ***Peritoneum [Peritonaeum] viscerale.*** Serous membrane covering the organs. The transition between the parietal peritoneum and the visceral peritoneum is made by folds, omenta, mesos, mesentery, and ligaments with specific names. A

6 *Tunica serosa.* See 3.

7 *Tela subserosa.* See 4.

8 ***Cavum peritonei [peritonaei].*** Peritoneal cavity, the potential space containing peritoneal fluid between the parietal and visceral peritoneum. A

9 ***Foramen omentale [epiploicum]*.*** Omental [epiploic] foramen, opening from the greater peritoneal sac to the Vestibulum bursae omentalis. It passes between V. cava caudalis dorsally, V. portae included into the hepatoduodenal ligament ventrally, the caudate lobe of liver cranially, and the pancreas caudally. B C (formerly called "Hiatus of Winslow")

10 ***Bursa omentalis.*** Omental bursa, lesser peritoneal sac, the potential space enclosed by the two omenta, the stomach and the liver. It communicates with the greater peritoneal sac through the omental foramen. B D

11 *Vestibulum bursae omentalis.* Vestibule of the omental bursa, enclosed by Omentum minus, stomach and liver. B C D

12 *Recessus dorsalis omentalis.* Dorsal omental recess. A minor diverticulum of the vestibule between right crus of the diaphragm and liver, and between esophagus and Vena cava caudalis. C

13 *Aditus ad recessum caudalem.* Opening to caudal recess from vestibule. It is bounded by Plica gastropancreatica, Plica hepatopancreatica, Curvatura ventriculi minor, and duodenum. B C D

14 *Recessus caudalis omentalis.* Caudal omental recess, cavity enclosed by the Omentum majus. B D

15 *Recessus lienalis.* Splenic recess, the left extremity of the Bursa omentalis, enclosed by the Ligg. gastrophrenicum, gastrolienale, and phrenicolienale, and in eq lienorenale. B

16 *Plica gastropancreatica.* Fold of the wall of the bursa containing left gastric vessels. B C

17 *Plica hepatopancreatica*.* Fold of the wall of the bursa containing A. hepatica. B C

18 ***Recessus supraomentalis*** (Ru)*. Supraomental recess, the part of the peritoneal cavity dorsal to the Omentum majus. It contains the intestinal mass. D

19 ***Mesenterium dorsale primitivum*** (ont)[1)]. Primitive dorsal mesentery, double peritoneal sheet connecting dorsal body wall to the intestine. A B

20 *Mesogastrium dorsale* (ont)[1)]. Dorsal mesogastrium, the primordium of the Omentum majus.

21 ***Omentum majus [Epiploon].*** Greater omentum, peritoneal sac between intestines and ventral abdominal wall, encloses the Recessus caudalis omentalis. B D

22 *Paries superficialis*.* Superficial wall, from Curvatura ventriculi major to the caudal reflection in species with a simple stomach, or from the left longitudinal groove of rumen to descending and cranial duodenum, and greater curvature of abomasum in Ru. B D

23 *Paries profundus*.* Deep wall, from the caudal reflection to its dorsal attachment in species with a simple stomach. In Ru from the right longitudinal groove of rumen to descending and cranial duodenum, and greater curvature of abomasum. B D

24 *Ligamentum gastrophrenicum.* Gastrophrenic ligament, extends from the diaphragm to the fundus of the stomach. C

25 *Ligamentum gastrolienale.* Gastrosplenic ligament, between stomach and spleen. B C

26 *Ligamentum phrenicolienale.* Phrenicosplenic ligament, from the diaphragm to the spleen. C

26a *Ligamentum lienorenale.* The left portion of Ligamentum phrenicolienale to the left kidney in eq. C

27 *Velum omentale* (ca). This sagittal membrane connects Paries profundus of Omentum majus with the left surface of Mesocolon descendens. It has a free caudal border. C (ca was omitted from the 5th edition of the N. A. V. by a typo mistake.)

1) These structures were omitted from the 5th edition of the N. A. V. because they are ontogenetic terms. However, we keep them for understanding the origin of some structures after birth.

A Schematic representation of embryonic peritoneum

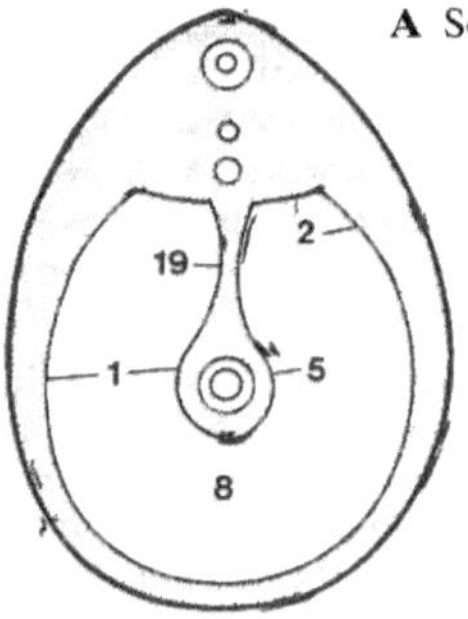

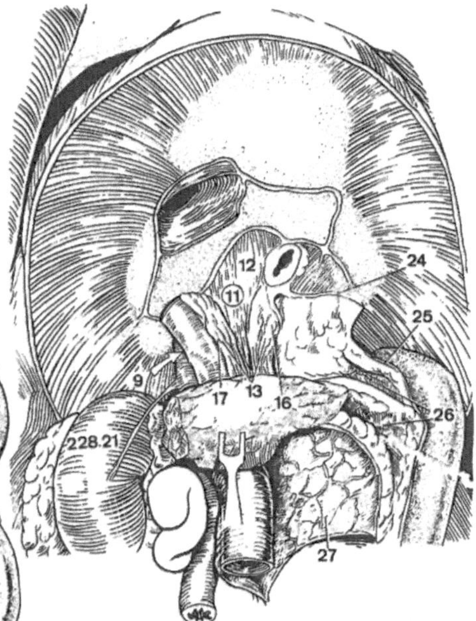

C Dorsal abdominal wall (stomach, liver, and right lobe of pancreas removed), caudoventral aspect (ca)

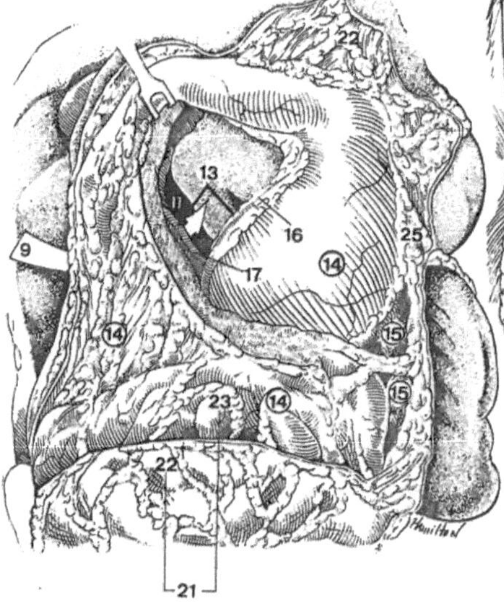

B Bursa omentalis (superficial wall reflected cranially with stomach; 13 is on papillary process of liver) (ca)

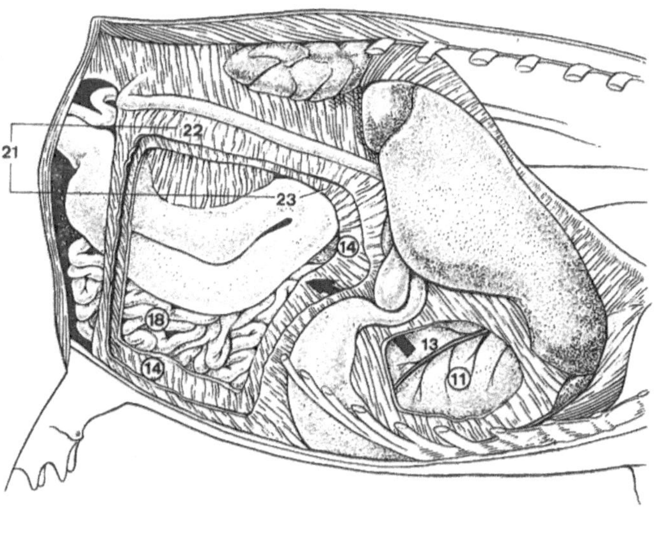

D Bursa omentalis (greater omentum fenestrated to show jejunum, cecum, and ascending colon on the left, lesser omentum fenestrated to show omasum on the right) (bo)

1 ***Mesoduodenum***. Mesentery of the duodenum. A B

2 ***Mesenterium****. Mesentery in the specific sense, attached to Jejunum and Ileum.

3 *Radix mesenterii**. Root of the mesentery, dorsal attachment containing A. mesenterica cranialis. A

4 *Mesojejunum*. Mesentery of the jejunum. A

5 *Mesoileum*. Mesentery of the ileum. A

6 ***Mesocolon****. Mesentery of the colon.

7 *Mesocolon ascendens*. Ascending mesocolon, attached to Colon ascendens. A

8 *Mesocolon transversum*. Transverse mesocolon, attached to Colon transversum. A

9 *Mesocolon descendens*. Descending mesocolon, attached to Colon descendens. A B

10 *Mesocolon sigmoideum*. Sigmoid mesocolon, attached to Colon sigmoideum (in bo).

11 ***Mesorectum***. Attached to rectum. A

12 ***Mesenterium ventrale primitivum*** (ont)[1)].

13 *Mesogastrium ventrale* (ont.) [1)].

14 ***Omentum minus****. Lesser omentum, connects Curvatura ventriculi minor and Pars cranialis duodeni to the visceral surface of the liver. C E

15 *Ligamentum hepatogastricum*. Hepatogastric ligament, the greater part of the Omentum minus, from liver to stomach. C

16 *Ligamentum hepatoduodenale*. Hepatoduodenal ligament, the free right border of the Omentum minus. It connects liver to Pars cranialis duodeni, contains V. portae, A. hepatica, and Ductus choledochus, and forms the ventral boundary of the Foramen omentale. C

17 ***Ligamentum falciforme hepatis****. Falciform ligament of the liver, a derivative of the primitive ventral mesentery between parietal surface of the liver, and diaphragm and ventral abdominal wall. In ca, the caudal portion, extending to the umbilicus, is usually filled with fat. C D E

18 ***Ligamentum coronarium hepatis***. Coronary ligament, attaches liver to diaphragm, surrounding Area nuda and Sulcus venae cavae, and connecting Ligg. triangularia and falciforme. E

19 ***Ligamentum triangulare dextrum***. Right triangular ligament, right free fold of the Lig. coronarium between right lobe of the liver and diaphragm. E

20 ***Ligamentum triangulare sinistrum***. Left triangular ligament, left free fold of the Lig. coronarium between left lobe of the liver and diaphragm. D E

21 ***Ligamentum hepatorenale***. Hepatorenal ligament, between Processus caudatus and right kidney. 227 C

22 ***Plica duodenocolica***. Duodenocolic fold, a fold of peritoneum between Duodenum ascendens and Colon descendens (Mesocolon descendens in ca). A

23 ***Recessus duodenalis caudalis***. Caudal duodenal recess (ca), small blind sac in the peritoneum on the attached surface of the end of the Duodenum ascendens. It opens cranially. B

1) These structures were omitted from the 5th edition of the N. A. V. because they are ontogenetic terms.

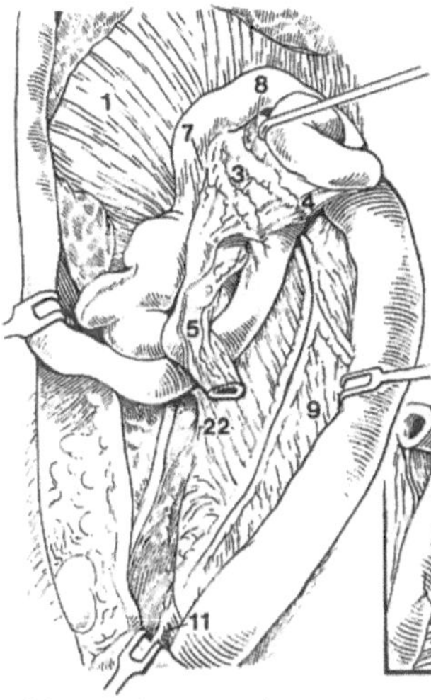

A Mesenteries, ventral aspect most of jejunum removed) (ca)

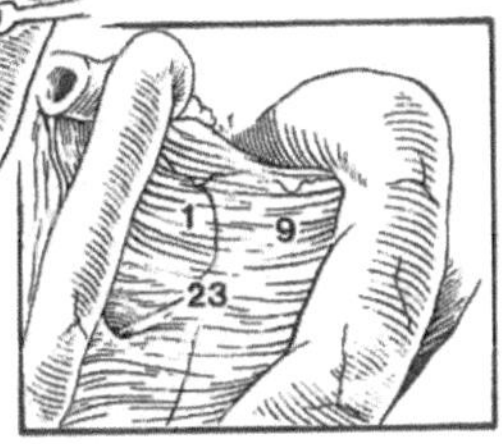

B Caudal duodenal recess, left ventrolateral aspect (duodenojejunal flexure and descending colon shown) (ca)

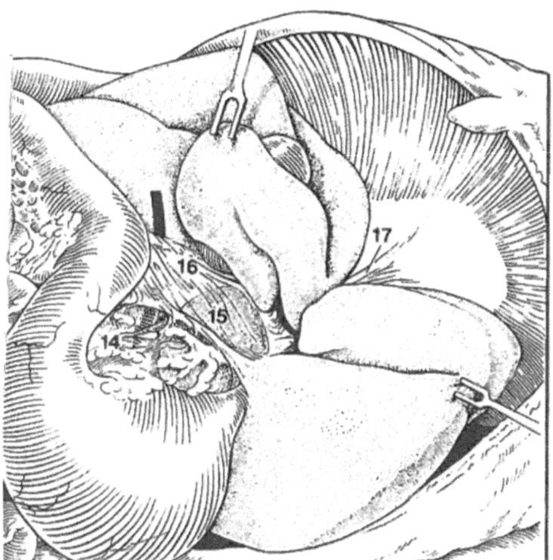

C Lesser omentum, left caudoventral aspect (left ribs 7–13 removed. Arrow indicates omental foramen) (ca)

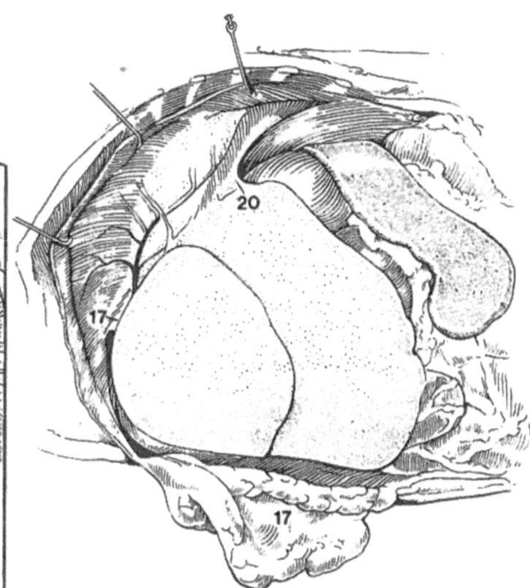

D Liver in situ, left lateral aspect (diaphragm retained by hooks) (ca)

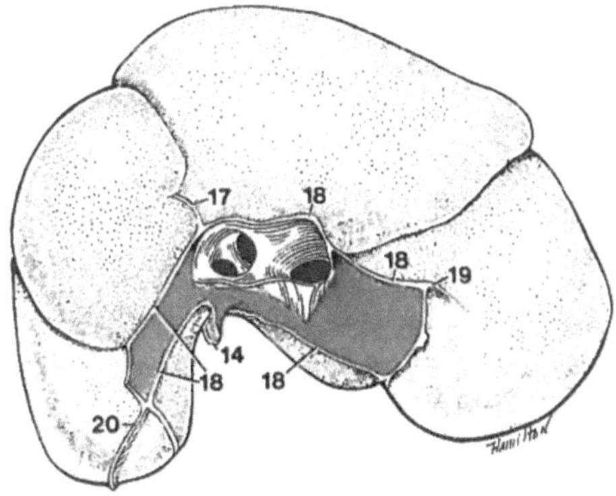

E Liver, diaphragmatic surface (dorsal aspect, fixed in situ) (ca)

1 ***Plica ileocecalis [-caecalis]****. Ileocecal fold, between the antimesenteric curvature of ileum and cecum. In eq it is attached to the Tenia dorsalis ceci. B

2 ***Plica cecocolica [caeco-]*** (eq)*. Cecocolic fold between Tenia libera lateralis of the right ventral colon and Tenia lateralis ceci. A

3 ***Lig. vesicae medianum***. (See 198.7)

4 ***Lig. vesicae laterale***. (See 198.9)

5 ***Trigonum inguinale***. Inguinal triangle, bounded by Arcus inguinalis, lateral border of M. rectus abdominis, and the line formed by Truncus pudendoepigastricus and A. epigastrica caudalis. C

6 ***Fossa inguinalis lateralis***. Lateral inguinal fossa, depression over the Anulus inguinalis profundus lateral to the A. epigastrica caudalis. C

7 ***Mesorchium***. (See 202.21)

8 ***Mesoductus deferens***. (See 202.25)

9 ***Mesepididymis***. (See 202.26)

10 ***Bursa testicularis [Sinus epididymalis]***. (See 202.30)

11 ***Processus vaginalis peritonei [peritonaei]***. (See 204.1)

12 ***Plica genitalis***. Genital fold, separates Excavatio rectogenitalis from Excavatio vesicogenitalis in the male, contains the Ductus deferens and the Uterus masculinus. C

13 ***Lig. latum uteri****. Broad ligament of the uterus, fold of peritoneum attaching the intraperitoneal female genital organs to the dorsolateral body wall. D

14 *Mesometrium*. Part of the broad ligament attached to the uterus. D

15 *Mesosalpinx*. Fold laterally detached from broad ligament, contains uterine tube, forms lateral wall of ovarian bursa, completely surrounds ovary in Car and su. It separates the Mesovarium proximale from the Mesovarium distale. D

16 *Mesovarium*. Part of the broad ligament attached to the ovary, contains the ovarian vessels and is homologous to the mesorchium. D

17 **Mesovarium proximale**. From the abdominal wall to the origin of mesosalpinx. D

18 **Mesovarium distale**. From the origin of Mesosalpinx to the ovary. D

19 *Bursa ovarica*. Ovarian bursa, cavity enclosed by mesosalpinx, distal mesovarium, and ovary. D

20 ***Lig. suspensorium ovarii****. Free border of the mesovarium. D

21 ***Excavatio rectogenitalis***. Rectogenital pouch, recess of the peritoneal cavity between rectum and Plica genitalis (male), uterus and Ligg. lata (female). C

22 *Fossa pararectalis*. Symmetrical extension of Excavatio rectogenitalis lateral to rectum and mesorectum. C

23 ***Excavatio vesicogenitalis***. Vesicogenital pouch, recess of the peritoneal cavity between the urinary bladder and Plica genitalis (male), uterus and Ligg. lata (female). C

24 ***Excavatio pubovesicalis***. Pubovesical pouch, peritoneal recess ventral to the urinary bladder and Ligg. vesicae lateralia. C

25 ***Spatium retroperitoneale [-peritonaeale]***. Space filled with connective tissue and fat between peritoneum and body wall. C

26 **SYSTEMA ENDOCRINUM**. Endocrine glands, ductless glands that secrete hormones into the bloodstream.

27 **Glandula thyroidea [thyreoidea]**. Thyroid gland, on the cranial end of the trachea. E F

28 ***Lobus [dexter et sinister]***. Lobe, right and left. E

29 ***Isthmus glandularis*** (Car, bo). Glandular band connecting the caudal ends of the lobes, may be absent in Car. E

30 ***Isthmus fibrosus*** (ov, cap, eq). Connecting fibrous band between the caudal ends of the lobes, sometimes absent.

31 ***Lobus pyramidalis***. Pyramidal lobe, variable median ventral lobe projecting cranially, occurs in su. F

32 ***Capsula fibrosa***. Capsule. G

33 ***Stroma***. Connective tissue framework. G

34 ***Parenchyma***. Glandular substance, composed of follicles. G

35 *Lobuli*. Lobules. E

36 *Folliculi*. Follicles, epithelial sacs containing colloid. G

37 ***(Gll. thyroideae [thyreoideae] accessoriae)***. Small nodules of thyroid tissue anywhere between tongue and heart.

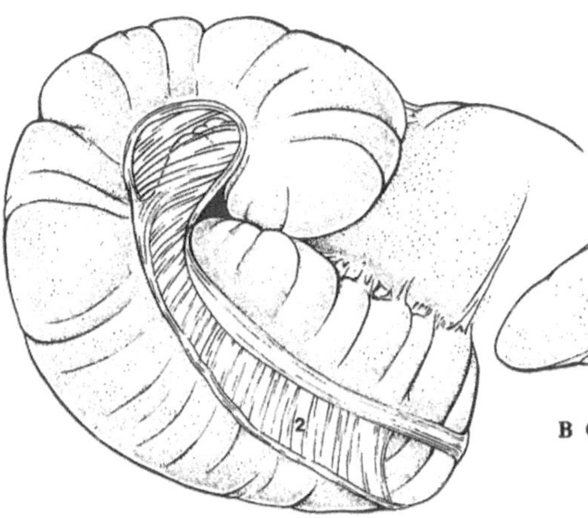

A Cecum and right dorsal and ventral colon, right lateral aspect (eq)

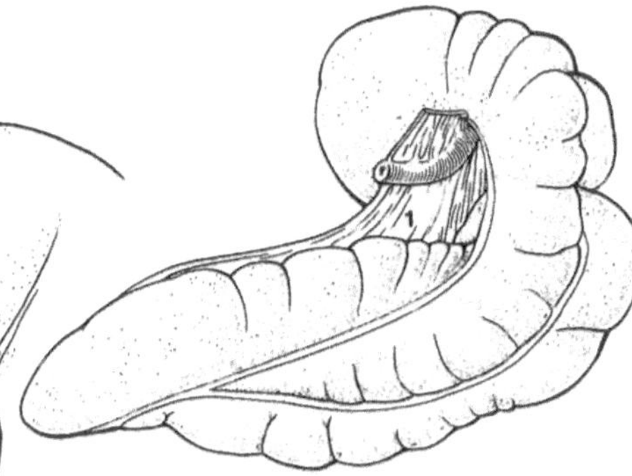

B Cecum and ileum, medial aspect (eq) (Getty)

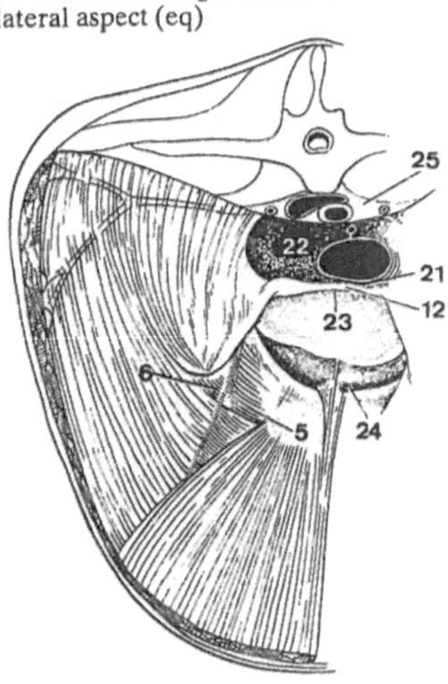

C Abdominal and pelvic cavities, cranial aspect (eq) (Getty)

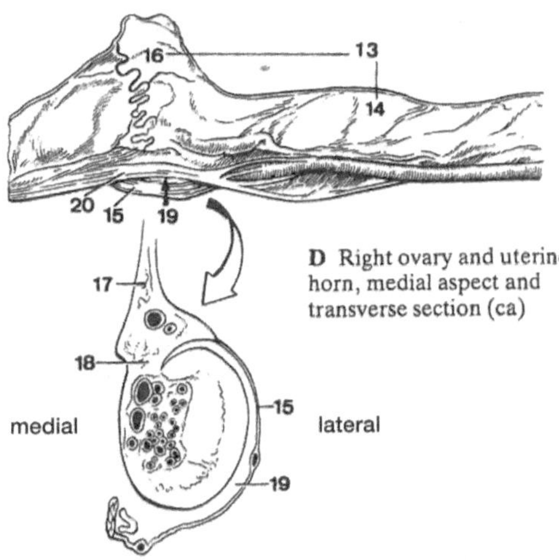

D Right ovary and uterine horn, medial aspect and transverse section (ca)

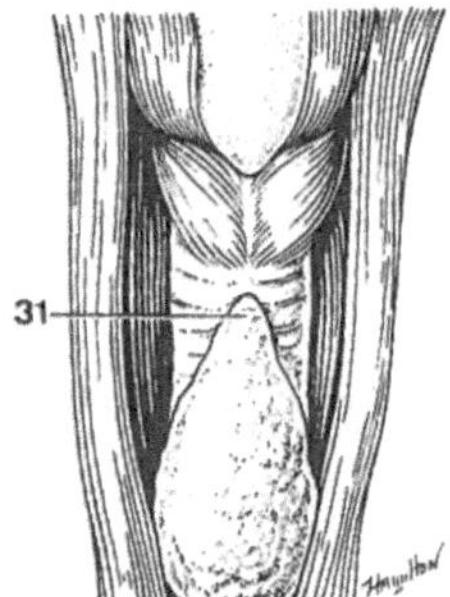

F Thyroid gland, ventral aspect (su)

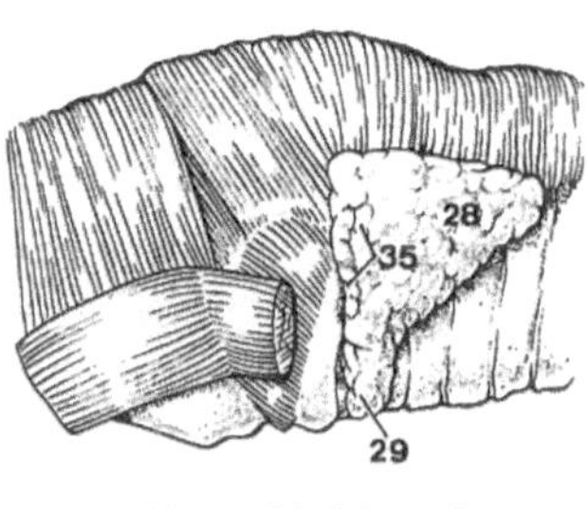

E Thyroid gland, left lateral aspect (bo)

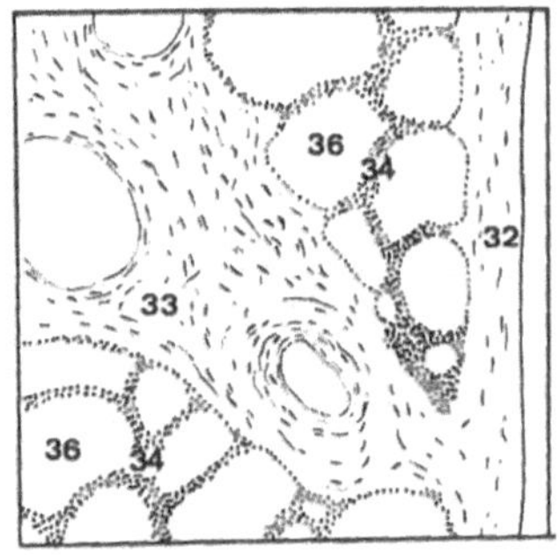

G Thyroid gland, histological section (ca)

1 **Glandula parathyroidea [-thyreoidea] interna [IV]** [1]. Internal parathyroid gland, from the fourth pharyngeal pouch. In the thyroid lobe in Car, absent in su, embedded in the medial surface of the thyroid lobe in Ru, on the surface of the cranial half of the thyroid lobe in eq. A

2 **Glandula parathyroidea [-thyreoidea] externa [III]** [1]. External parathyroid gland, from the third pharyngeal pouch. On the lateral surface of the thyroid lobe in Car, near the end of the A. carotis communis in su and Ru, near the thoracic inlet in eq. A

3 **Hypophysis [Glandula pituitaria].** Hypophysis or pituitary gland, in the Fossa hypophysialis on the basisphenoid. Neural and glandular components provide link between hypothalamus and endocrine glands. B

4 ***Adenohypophysis.*** Glandular lobe, derived from the stomodeal epithelium. The term anterior lobe is not applicable to domestic mammals. B

5 *Pars tuberalis.* Tuberal part, covers the infundibulum up to the Tuber cinereum. B

6 *Pars intermedia.* Intermediate part, lies between Pars distalis and Neurohypophysis, surrounds the Neurohypophysis in Car and eq. B

7 *Pars distalis.* Distal part, largest part of the Adenohypophysis. B

8 *(Pars pharyngea).* Pharyngeal part, a remnant of the Saccus hypophysialis (Rathke's pouch) in the dorsal mucosa of the nasopharynx (Car, eq).

9 ***Neurohypophysis.*** Ventral outgrowth of the hypothalamus, composed of infundibulum and neural lobe. In a caudodorsal groove of the Adenohypophysis in su, Ru, surrounded by it in Car, eq. Therefore the term posterior lobe is not suitable for domestic mammals. B

10 *Infundibulum.* Funnel-shaped stalk of the Neurohypophysis. B

11 **Radix.** Root, the histological zone where the nerve fibers of the infundibulum join the Tuber cinereum.

12 **Pars cava.** Hollow part, containing a recessof the third ventricle. B

13 **Pars compacta.** Solid part. B

14 *Pars distalis neurohypophysis.* Neural lobe, part of the Neurohypophysis distal to the Diaphragma sellae. B

15 ***Cavum hypophysis.*** Cavity of the hypophysis, a remnant of the cavity of the Saccus hypophysialis (Rathke's pouch) between Pars intermedia and Pars distalis, absent in eq. B

16 **Glandula pinealis** (vide Epithalamus). Epiphysis cerebri or pineal gland.

17 **Glandula adrenalis.** Adrenal gland, medial to the cranial half of the kidney, but the left gland in bo is cranial to the kidney near the A. mesenterica cranialis. C D

18 ***Facies ventralis.*** Ventral surface. D

19 ***Facies dorsalis.*** Dorsal surface.

20 ***Margo lateralis.*** Lateral border. C

21 ***Margo medialis.*** Medial border. C

22 ***Hilus.*** Depression on the medial border where the vein joins the gland. D

23 ***Capsula.*** Capsule, connective tissue covering. C

24 ***Cortex.*** Outer yellowish portion consisting of cords and clusters of epithelial cells. C

25 ***Medulla.*** Central brown zone of chromaffin (adrenalin secreting) cells and sympathetic ganglion cells. C

26 ***(Gll. adrenales [suprarenales] accessoriae).*** Accessory adrenal glands, may contain cortical and medullary tissue, retroperitoneally in the lumbar region.

27 **Insulae pancreaticae.** Pancreatic islets, small (.04–.2 mm) groups of endocrine cells which secrete insulin and glucagon. E

28 **Thymus** (vide Systema lymphaticum).

[1] The variation in number and position of the parathyroid glands in domestic mammals makes it necessary to add the numbers IV and III to indicate their origin from the epithelium of the fourth and third pharyngeal pouch, respectively.

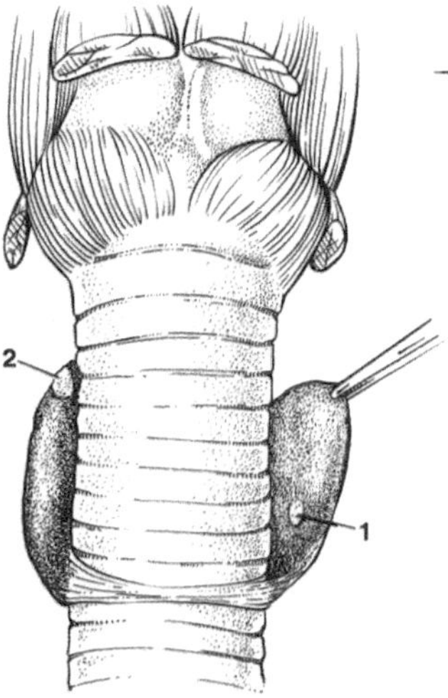

A Larynx and trachea, thyroid and parathyroid glands, ventral aspect (ca)

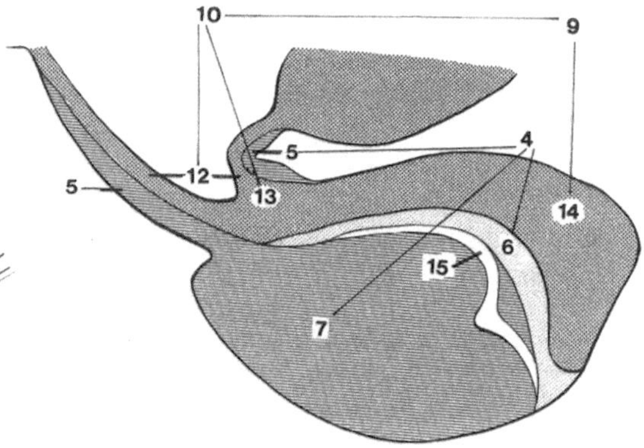

B Hypophysis, median section (bo)

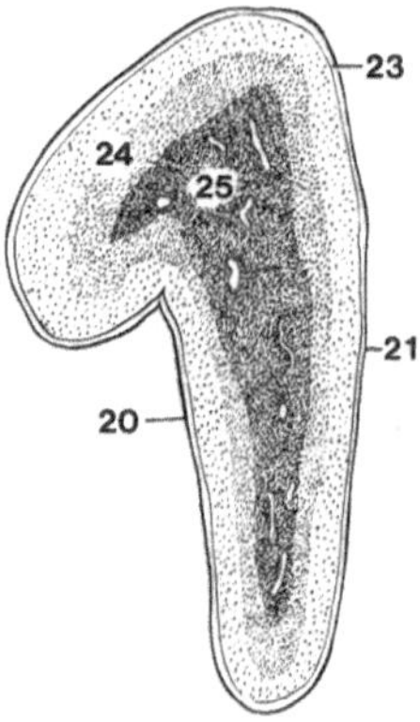

C Right adrenal gland, sectioned longitudinally, ventral aspect (ca)

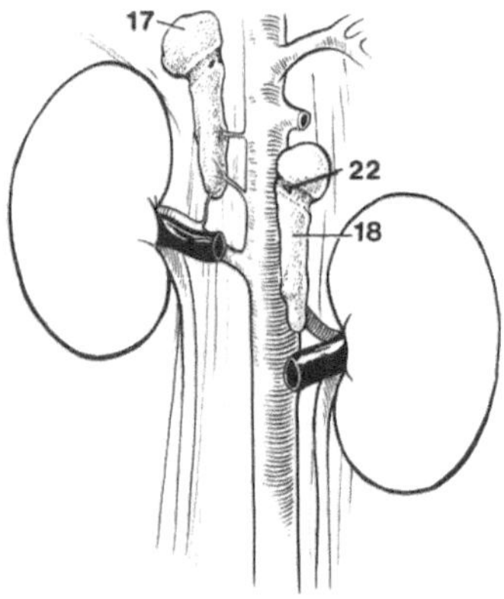

D Adrenal glands and kidneys, ventral aspect (Vv. cava caudalis and phrenicoabdominalis removed) (ca)

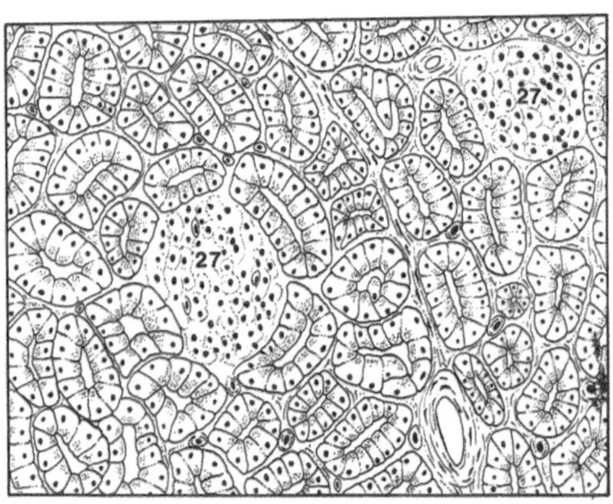

E Pancreatic islets, histological section (su)

1 **PERICARDIUM**. Conical sack-like structure enclosing the heart and the roots of the largest vessels. Covered by Pleura pericardiaca. Consists of an outer fibrous and an inner bilaminar serous portion. B C D E

2 ***Pericardium fibrosum***. Outer fibrous part of pericardium. C D E

3 *Ligg. sternopericardiaca*. Bilateral connective band between Pericardium fibrosum and sternum (Ru). C

4 *Lig. sternopericardiacum*. Singular connective band between Pericardium fibrosum and sternum (eq). E

5 *Lig. phrenicopericardiacum*. Band between Pericardium fibrosum and Diaphragma (Car, su). B

6 ***Pericardium serosum***. Closed sac surrounded by Pericardium fibrosum. Encloses a cavity into which about one-half of its wall is invaginated by the heart to form the Lamina visceralis, while its uninvaginated Lamina parietalis is firmly fused with Pericardium fibrosum. C D E

7 *Lamina parietalis*. Serous internal covering of Pericardium fibrosum. C D E

8 *Lamina visceralis [Epicardium]*. Serous covering of the surface of the heart and the roots of the great vessels. C D E

9 ***Cavum pericardii***. Body cavity between Lamina parietalis and Lamina visceralis of Pericardium serosum. Contains a small amount of serous fluid. C D E

10 *Sinus transversus pericardii*. Tunnel-shaped extension of Cavum pericardii between the united Aorta and Truncus pulmonalis, and the concave wall-parts of the adjacent atria. D E

10a *Sinus obliquus pericardii*. Recess in Cavum pericardii between the right pulmonary veins and V. cava caudalis, and between the right and left Vv. pulmonales. (according to the N. A.)

11 **COR**. Heart. Cone-shaped (Un) to ovoid (Car) hollow muscular organ enclosed by pericardium. Center of the vascular system. A C E

12 ***Basis cordis***. Dorsocranially (Car, su) to dorsally (Ru, eq) directed upper surface of the heart, ventrally marked out by Sulcus coronarius. A E

13 ***Facies auricularis***. Heart surface marked by the tips of Auriculae atriorum, facing the left thoracic wall. A E

14 ***Facies atrialis***. Heart surface on the side of the atrial mass. Opposite Facies auricularis, it faces the right thoracic wall. A C

15 ***Margo ventricularis dexter***. Part of the cranially situated convex border of the heart, which belongs to Ventriculus dexter. A C E

16 ***Margo ventricularis sinister***. Side of Ventriculus sinister turned to Diaphragma, forming the caudal border of the heart. C E

17 ***Apex cordis***. By Ventriculus sinister formed tip, opposite to Basis cordis. C E

18 *Incisura apicis cordis*. Notch underneath Margo ventricularis dexter near Apex cordis. Formed by the continuation of Sulcus interventricularis paraconalis. C E

19 ***Sulcus interventricularis paraconalis***. Longitudinal groove on Facies auricularis. Descends from Sulcus coronarius along Conus arteriosus, outside of Septum interventriculare. A E

20 ***Sulcus interventricularis subsinuosus***. Longitudinal groove on Facies atrialis outside of Septum interventriculare. Begins at Sulcus coronarius, ventral to Sinus venarum cavarum and Sinus coronarius. A C

21 ***Sulcus coronarius***. Groove that encircles the heart completely, except at Conus arteriosus. Indicates externally the limit between Atria and Ventriculi cordis. A C

* Reminder: the structures followed by an asterisk are landmarks for physical examination and/or clinical approach.

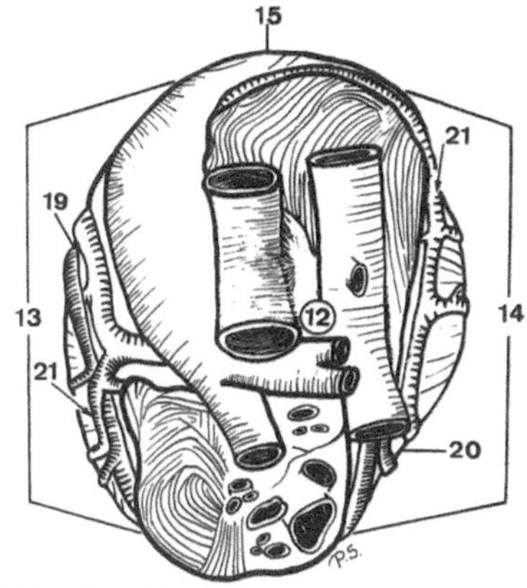

A Basis cordis, dorsal aspect (eq)

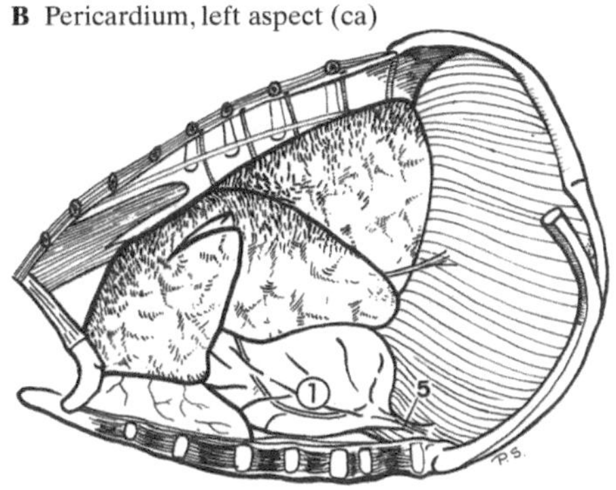

B Pericardium, left aspect (ca)

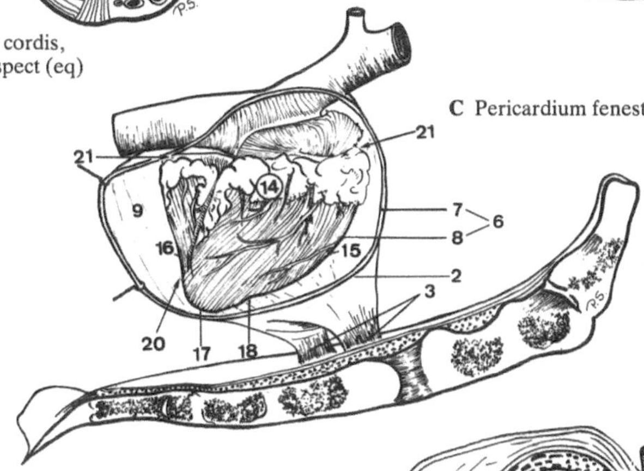

C Pericardium fenestrated, heart (bo, young)

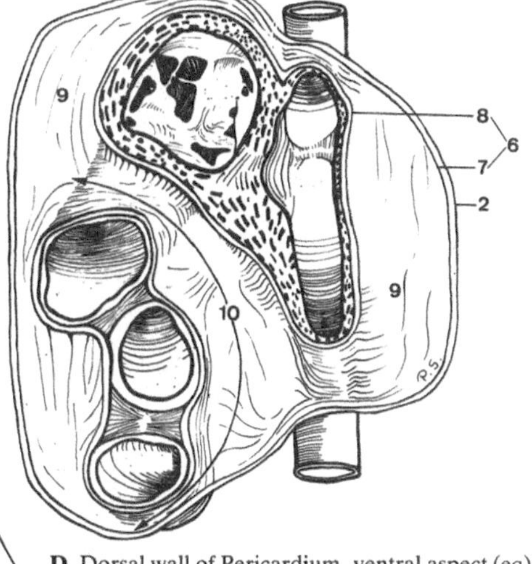

D Dorsal wall of Pericardium, ventral aspect (eq)

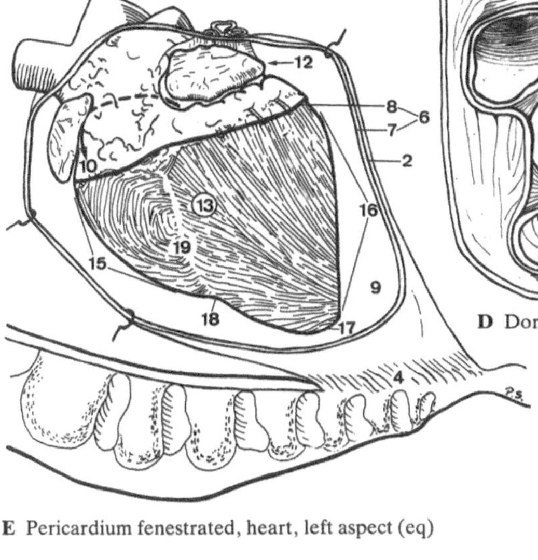

E Pericardium fenestrated, heart, left aspect (eq)

1 ***Ventriculus cordis***. Each of both heart chambers ventral to the level of Sulcus coronarius. A B D

2 ***Septum interventriculare***. Longitudinal partition-wall between both Ventriculi cordis, externally indicated by Sulci interventriculares. D E

3 *Pars muscularis*. Larger and thicker portion of Septum interventriculare, formed by myocardium of the two contiguous ventricular septal walls. D

4 *Pars membranacea*. Very small dorsal membranous portion of Septum interventriculare. Most distinct in the cat, absent in adult oxen. D

5 ***Septum atrioventriculare***. Small membranous contact-wall between Atrium dextrum and Ventriculus sinister. Situated dorsal to the base of Cuspis septalis of Valva atrioventricularis dextra. D

6 ***Atrium cordis***. Each of both chambers at Basis cordis. At the level of Sulcus coronarius separated from the corresponding Ventriculus cordis by an Anulus fibrosus. D E

7 *Auricula atrii*. Blind, ear-shaped diverticulum of the left and right Atrium cordis. D

8 ***Septum interatriale***. Muscular partition between both Atria cordis. D

9 ***Ostium atrioventriculare [dext. et sin.]***. By Anuli fibrosi surrounded large openings of the left and right Atrium cordis into the corresponding Ventriculus cordis. A

10 ***Ostium trunci pulmonalis***. Opening of Ventriculus dexter into Truncus pulmonalis. Surrounded by an Anulus fibrosus to which a valve system is attached. A

11 ***Ostium aortae***. Opening of Ventriculus sinister into Aorta ascendens. Surrounded by an Anulus fibrosus to which a valve system is attached. A D

12 ***Trabeculae carneae***. Subendocardial myocardial ridges of the ventriclewall, projecting into the lumen of the heart. D

13 ***Foramina venarum minimarum***. Openings of Vv. cordis minimae. D (The Vv. cordis minimae empty into all four chambers of the heart.)

14 ***Vortex cordis***. Swirl of myocardial fibers at Apex cordis. B

15 ***Musculi papillares***. Conical myocardial projections into the ventricular lumen. Connected with the atrioventricular cusps by Chordae tendineae. D E

16 ***Chordae tendineae***. Fibromuscular cords between Valvae atrioventriculares and the apices of Mm. papillares. A D

17 ***Trigona fibrosa***. Pair of adjacent triangular areas of dense connective tissue, located between both Ostia atrioventricularia and Ostium aortae. A

18 ***Anuli fibrosi***. Connective tissue rings surrounding Ostia atrioventricularia, Ostium aortae, and Ostium trunci pulmonalis. Give rise to the corresponding valve systems. A

19 ***Cartilago cordis***. Amount of cartilage in or near the aortic Anulus fibrosus (Car, su, eq). Sometimes absent (Car), frequently senilely calcified (su, eq) or plural (eq). A

20 ***Ossa cordis***. Pair of bones in the aortic Anulus fibrosus. Usually single in ov. C

21 **Myocardium**. Striated cardiac musculature including the internal conducting system listed thereunder. D E (In the last decades of the 20th Century the following structures of the excitation and conducting system of the heart were found: left AV Kent fibers, James atrio-His pathway, James internodal tract, James intranodal tract, Mahaim nodoventricular fibers, Mahaim nodofascicular fibers, and Mahaim fasciculoventricular fibers [Constantinescu 2002, p. 195].)

22 ***Nodus sinuatrialis***. Keith-Flack node, a small complex of special cardiac muscle tissue located at Sulcus terminalis near Ostium venae cavae cranialis. This is the pacemaker of the heart. E

23 ***Nodus atrioventricularis***. Aschoff-Tawara node a small complex of special cardiac muscle tissue located in the base of the septal wall of Atrium dextrum, close to the opening of Sinus coronarius. E

24 ***Fasciculus atrioventricularis***. His fascicle, a bundle of modified cardiac muscle fibers. Contains Nodus atrioventricularis in its first section, and conducts from the atrial to the ventricular, esp. papillary musculature. E

25 *Truncus fasciculi atrioventricularis*. Section of the Fasciculus atrioventricularis before its division at Septum interventriculare. D

26 **Crus fasciculi atrioventricularis dextrum**. Right limb of the atrioventricular conducting system that finally ramifies inside Mm. papillares of the right ventricle as Purkinje fibers. E

26a **Crus fasciculi atrioventricularis sinistrum**. Left limb of the atrioventricular conducting system that finally ramifies inside Mm. papillares of the left ventricle as Purkinje fibers. E

27 **Endocardium**. Glistening membrane lining the internal surface of the heart chambers. D E

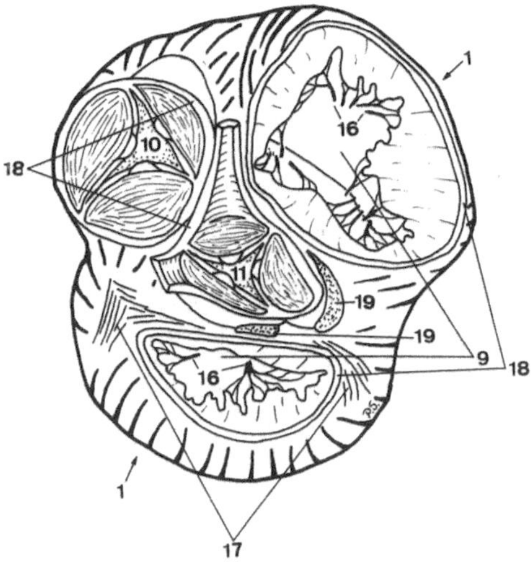

A Ventriculi cordis (atria removed), dorsal aspect (eq)

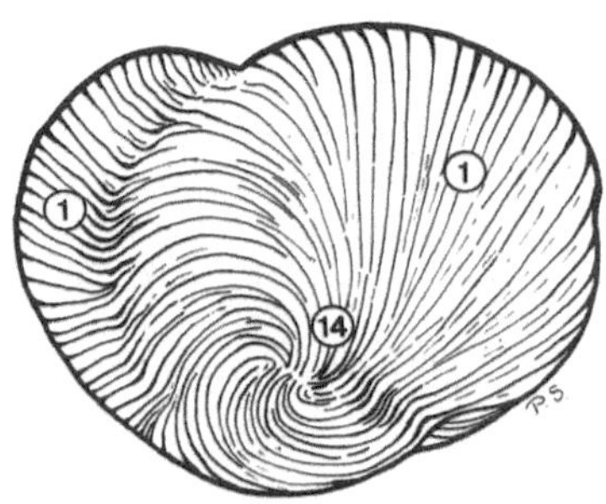

B Apex cordis, ventral aspect (eq)

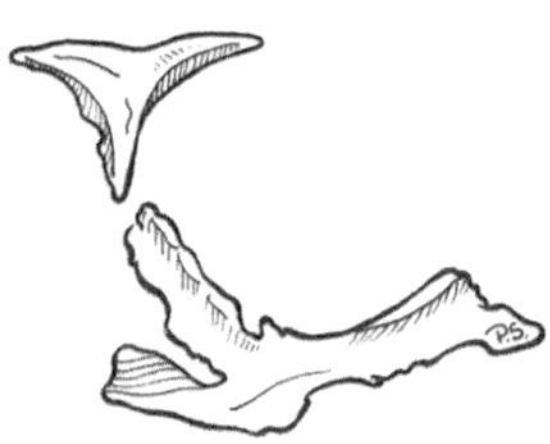

C Ossa cordis, right caudodorsal aspect (bo)

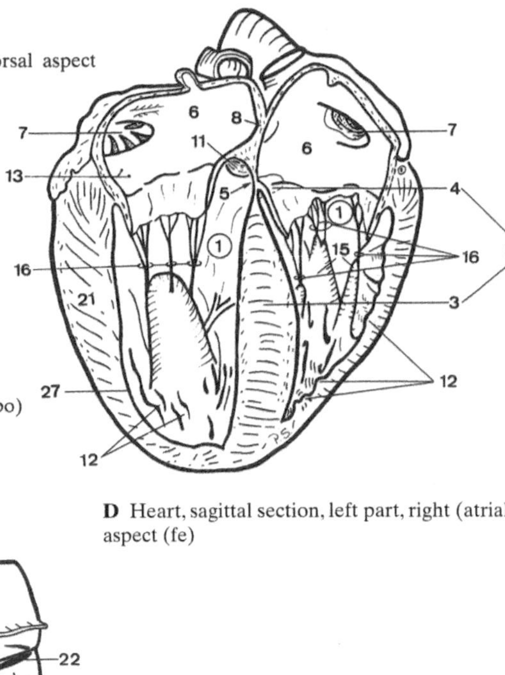

D Heart, sagittal section, left part, right (atrial) aspect (fe)

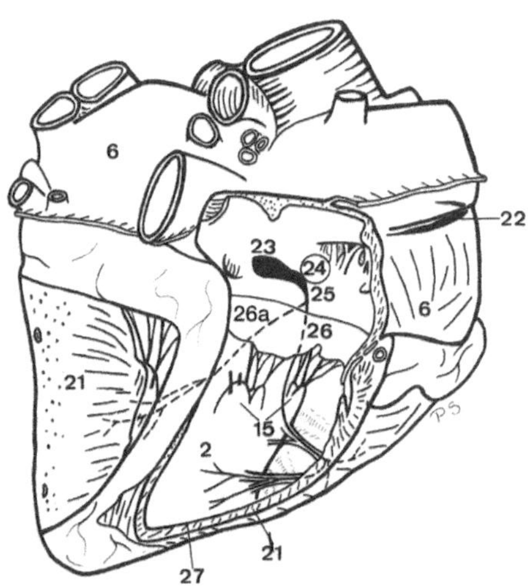

E Facies atrialis of the heart (ventricular walls partly removed) (eq)

1 **Atrium dextrum**. Atrium on the right cranial part of Basis cordis, situated dorsal (Un) or dorsocranial (Car) to Ventriculus dexter. It consists of three compartments: Auricula dextra, Sinus venarum cavarum, and Atrium dextrum proper in between. A B

2 ***Mm. pectinati***. Muscular ridges on the wall of Auricula dextra and Atrium dextrum proper. Most of them radiate from Crista terminalis. A B

3 ***Sulcus terminalis***. Often poorly defined (esp. Car) external groove opposite Crista terminalis. A

4 ***Crista terminalis***. Internal muscular ridge on the wall of Atrium dextrum between Sinus venarum cavarum and Auricula dextra . A B

5 ***Sinus venarum cavarum***. Smooth-walled part of Atrium dextrum between the wide openings of both Vv. cavae and Ostium atrioventriculare dextrum, bounded by Septum interatriale and Crista terminalis. A B

6 ***Fossa ovalis***. Depression in the septal wall of Atrium dextrum at Ostium venae cavae caudalis, caudal to Tuberculum intervenosum. Remnant of the fetal Foramen ovale (Botali). A

7 ***Limbus fossae ovalis***. Elevated rim of Fossa ovalis. A

8 ***Foramen ovale*** (ont). Orifice in Septum interatriale, sometimes persisting in adults. B (The Foramen ovale was omitted from the 5th edition of the N. A. V. because it is an ontogenetic term. However, in some individuals it can be identified after birth. The condition is called Atrial Septal Defect [ASD].)

9 ***Auricula dextra***. Blind diverticulum of Atrium dextrum. Curves around the right and cranial surfaces of Aorta ascendens. B

10 ***Ostium venae cavae cranialis***. Craniodorsally situated opening of V. cava cranialis into Sinus venarum cavarum. A B

11 ***Ostium venae cavae caudalis***. Caudally situated opening of V. cava caudalis into Sinus venarum cavarum. A B

12 ***Tuberculum intervenosum***. Internal transverse ridge on the dorsal wall of Atrium dextrum, placed between the openings of both Vv. cavae. A B

13 ***Valvula venae cavae caudalis***. Valve-like fold near Ostium venae cavae caudalis, frequently disappeared (adults) or absent (foal). B

13a ***Ostium sinus coronarii***. The opening of the Sinus coronarius that contains the small Valvula sinus coronarii. A

14 ***Valvula sinus coronarii***. Semilunar fold at the orifice of Sinus coronarius. May be indistinct or even absent, esp. in eq. A B

15 **Ventriculus dexter**. Heart chamber that constitutes the right cranial part of the ventricular mass. A C D

16 ***Ostium atrioventriculare dextrum***. Opening between Atrium dextrum and Ventriculus dexter. A C D

17 ***Valva atrioventricularis dextra [Valva tricuspidalis]***. The entire valve system of Ostium atrioventriculare dextrum, basically composed of three large cusps, possibly accompanied by small intermediate cusps. C D

18 *Cuspis angularis*. Cusp in the cranial corner of Ostium atrioventiculare dextrum. Arises from the septal and parietal walls of Ventriculus dexter. A C D (Cuspis anterior in the N.A.)

19 *Cuspis parietalis*. Cusp arising from the parietal margin of Ostium atrioventriculare dextrum. C D (Cuspis posterior in the N.A.)

20 *Cuspis septalis*. Cusp arising from the septal margin of Ostium atrioventriculare dextrum. C D

21 ***Crista supraventricularis***. Muscular ridge which separates Ostium atrioventriculare dextrum from Conus arteriosus. C

22 ***Conus arteriosus***. Dilatation at the left craniodorsal angle of Ventriculus dexter from which Truncus pulmonalis arises. C D

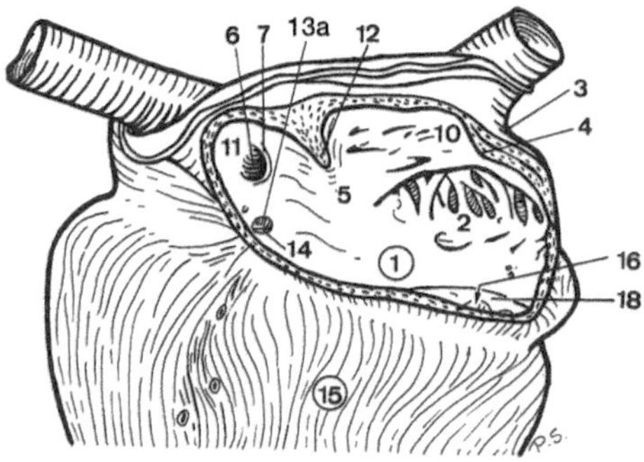

A Heart, Atrium dextrum opened (eq)

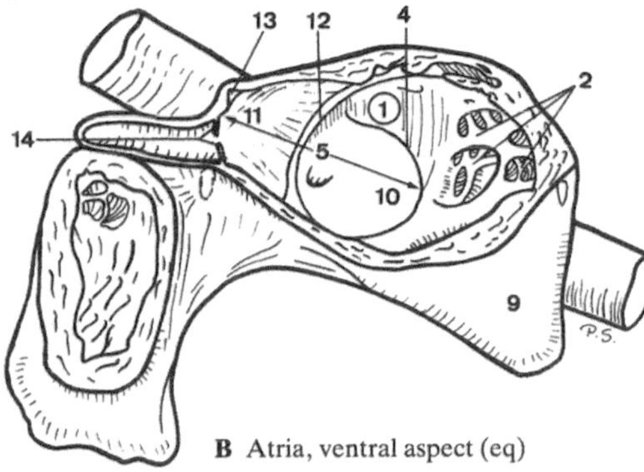

B Atria, ventral aspect (eq)

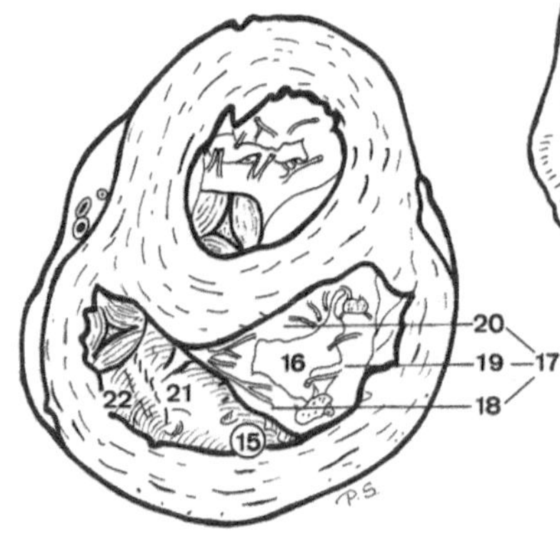

C Ventriculi, horizontal section, ventral aspect (cap)

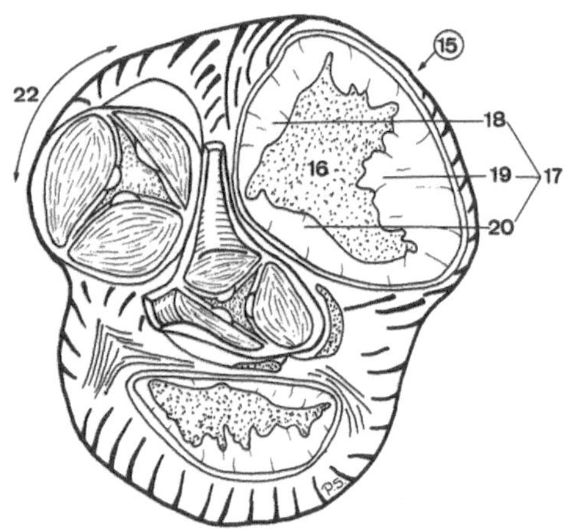

D Heart (atria removed), dorsal aspect (eq)

1 ***Ostium trunci pulmonalis***. Opening between Conus arteriosus and Truncus pulmonalis. A

2 ***Valva trunci pulmonalis***. Valve apparatus composed of three crescent-shaped leaflets, attached to the Anulus fibrosus of Ostium trunci pulmonalis. A

3 *Valvula semilunaris intermedia*. Left-cranially situated semilunar leaflet (valvule). A B (Valvula semilunaris anterior in the N.A.)

4 *Valvula semilunaris dextra*. Right-cranially situated semilunar leaflet (valvule). A B

5 *Valvula semilunaris sinistra*. Caudally situated semilunar leaflet (valvule). A B

6 *Noduli valvularum semilunarium*. Small elevations near the middle of the free concave margins of Valvulae semilunares. B

7 *Lunulae valvularum semilunarium*. Crescentic ridges on the free valvular rims, extending on both sides of each Nodulus valvulae semilunaris. B

8 ***Musculus papillaris magnus***. Eminent and usually largest M. papillaris of Ventriculus dexter, situated on the parietal wall (Un) or related to the septal wall (Car) of that heart chamber. B (M. papillaris anterior in the N.A.)

9 ***Musculi papillares parvi***. Generally grouped, medium-sized Mm. papillares. Mostly caudally situated on the septal wall. B (M. papillaris posterior in the N.A. [there is only one muscle in humans, not several as in the domestic mammals])

10 ***Musculus papillaris subarteriosus***. Situated on the septal wall, ventral to Ostium trunci pulmonalis. B (Mm. papillares septales in the N.A. [there are several muscles in humans, only one in the domestic mammals])

11 ***Trabecula septomarginalis dextra***. Myocardial strand extending from Septum interventriculare to the opposite parietal wall. Frequently plural and branched. This is a shortcut for the Crus fasciculi atrioventricularis dexter. B

12 **Atrium sinistrum**. Atrium on the left caudal half of Basis cordis, dorsal to Ventriculus sinister. C

13 ***Mm. pectinati***. Muscular ridges on wall of Auricula sinistra. C

14 ***Auricula sinistra***. Blind diverticulum of Atrium sinistrum. Extends around the caudal surface of Truncus pulmonalis, pointing to the left thoracic wall. C

15 ***Valvula foraminis ovalis***. Floor of Fossa ovalis located on Septum interatriale. C

16 ***Ostia venarum pulmonalium***. Entrances of Vv. pulmonales into the left atrium. C

17 **Ventriculus sinister**. Heart chamber that constitutes the left caudal portion of the ventricular mass. C

18 ***Ostium atrioventriculare sinistrum***. Opening between Atrium sinistrum and Ventriculus sinister. A

19 ***Valva atrioventricularis sinistra [Valva bicuspidalis, mitralis]***. Entire valve system of Ostium atrioventriculare sinistrum, basically composed of two large cusps, usually attended by accessory intermediate cusps. A

20 *Cuspis septalis*. Cusp arising from the septal margin of Ostium atrioventriculare sinistrum, separating the latter from Ostium aortae. A C (Cuspis anterior in the N.A.)

21 *Cuspis parietalis*. Cusp arising from the parietal margin of Ostium atrioventriculare sinistrum. A C (Cuspis posterior in the N.A.)

22 ***Ostium aortae***. Opening of Ventriculus sinister into Aorta ascendens. A

23 ***Valva aortae***. Valve apparatus composed of three crescent-shaped leaflets, attached on the Anulus fibrosus of Ostium aortae. A

24 *Valvula semilunaris septalis*. Right-caudally situated semilunar leaflet (valvule) facing Septum interatriale. A C (Valvula septalis posterior in the N.A.)

25 *Valvula semilunaris dextra*. Cranially situated semilunar leaflet (valvule) facing Ventriculus dexter. A C

26 *Valvula semilunaris sinistra*. Left caudally situated semilunar leaflet (valvule) facing the center of Ventriculus sinister. A C

27 *Noduli valvularum semilunarium*. Small elevations near the middle of the free concave margins of Valvulae semilunares. C

28 *Lunulae valvularum semilunarium*. Crescentic ridges on the free valvular rims extending on both sides of each Nodulus valvulae semilunaris. C

29 ***Musculus papillaris subauricularis***. Located on the parietal wall, ventral to Auricula sinistra. C (M. papillaris anterior in the N.A.)

30 ***Musculus papillaris subatrialis***. Located on the parietal wall, ventral to Atrium sinistrum. C (M. papillaris posterior in the N.A.)

31 ***Trabeculae septomarginales sinistrae***. Extend from Septum interventriculare through ventricular lumen into Mm. papillares. They are shortcuts for the Crus fasciculi atrioventricularis sinister. C

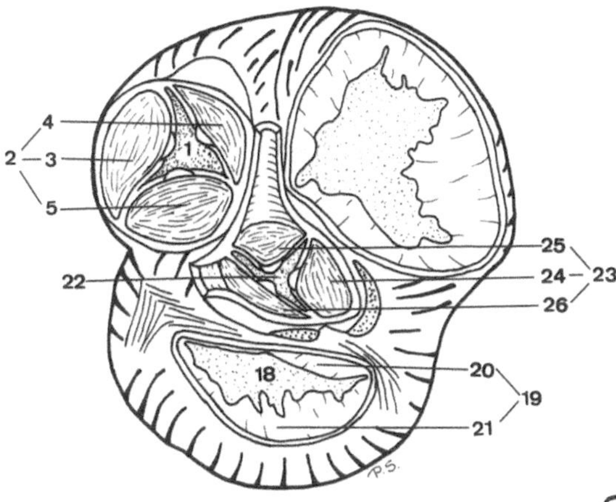

A Ventriculi cordis (atria removed), dorsal aspect (eq)

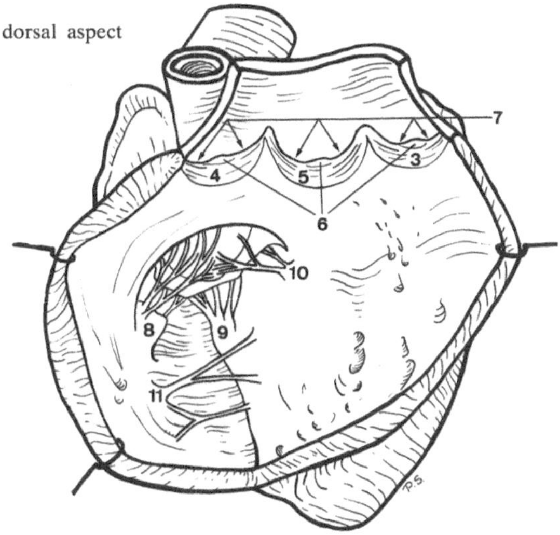

B Ventriculus dexter, opened, cranial aspect (eq)

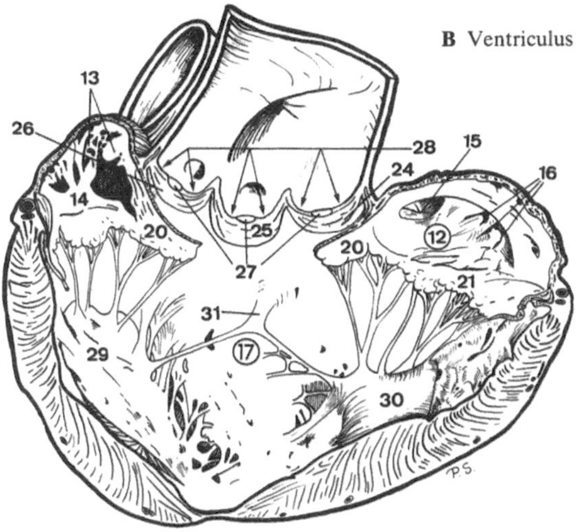

C Atrium sinistrum and Ventriculus sinister, opened, caudal aspect (eq)

1 **ARTERIAE**. Arteries, conveying the blood from the heart to the lungs and the periphery.

2 **TRUNCUS PULMONALIS**. Arterial trunk between Conus arteriosus and the beginning of Aa. pulmonales. A E

3 ***Sinus trunci pulmonalis***. Three dilatations of Truncus pulmonalis, dorsal to the roots of Valvulae semilunares. B D

4 **A. pulmonalis dextra**. Passes on the caudal side of Aorta ascendens into the hilus of the right lung, crossing the ventral aspect of trachea. A C

5 ***Ramus lobi cranialis***. Branch to Lobus cranialis of the right lung. A

6 *Ramus ascendens*. To the cranial part of the divided Lobus cranialis. (Ru). A

7 *Ramus descendens*. To the caudal part of the divided Lobus cranialis. (Ru). A

8 ***Ramus lobi medii***. Branch to Lobus medius of the right lung (absent in eq). A

9 ***Ramus lobi caudalis***. Branch to Lobus caudalis of the right lung. A

10 *Ramus lobi accessorii*. Enters Lobus accessorius (of the right lung). A

11 **A. pulmonalis sinistra**. Enters the hilus of the left lung. A C E

12 ***Ramus lobi cranialis***. Branch to Lobus cranialis of the left lung. A

13 *Ramus ascendens*. To the cranial part of the divided Lobus cranialis (absent in eq). A

14 *Ramus descendens*. To the caudal part of the divided Lobus cranialis (absent in eq). A

15 ***Ramus lobi caudalis***. Branch to Lobus caudalis of the left lung. A

16 ***Ductus arteriosus*** (ont). Patent duct between Truncus pulmonalis and Arcus aortae. E (The Ductus arteriosus was omitted from the 5th edition of the N. A. V. because it is an ontogenetic term. If persists after birth it causes a condition called Patent Ductus Arteriosus [PDA].)

17 ***Ligamentum arteriosum****. Fibrous remnant of the fetal Ductus arteriosus. A

18 **AORTA**. Main artery of the body. Arises from Ventriculus sinister. A B C E

19 **AORTA ASCENDENS**. Craniodorsally directed initial part of aorta. Located within pericardium and continues with Arcus aortae. B

20 ***Bulbus aortae***. Bulb of the aorta, internally occupied by Sinus aortae. D

21 *Sinus aortae*. Three dilatations of the aortic wall, each of them located dorsal to the corresponding Valvula semilunaris. D

22 ***A. coronaria dextra***. Arises from the Sinus aortae above Valvula semilunaris dextra and follows, subepicardially, the right part of Sulcus coronarius. B C D

23 *Ramus interventricularis subsinuosus*. Branch of A. coronaria dextra that descends in Sulcus interventricularis subsinuosus (su, eq, sometimes fe). In fe this branch is very variable and may arise from both coronary arteries. C (Posterior interventricular branch in the N.A.)

24 **Rami septales**. Run into Septum interventriculare. C

25 ***A. coronaria sinistra***. Arises from the Sinus aortae above Valvula semilunaris sinistra. B D E

26 *Ramus interventricularis paraconalis*. Descends in Sulcus interventricularis paraconalis. B D E (Anterior interventricular branch in the N.A. – L.A.D. [Left Anterior Descending])

27 **Rami septales**. Run into Septum interventriculare. B D

28 *Ramus circumflexus*. Continuation of A. coronaria sinistra into the left and caudal parts of Sulcus coronarius, also reaching the right caudal part of it. B D E

29 **Ramus intermedius [marginis ventricularis sinistri]**. Branch that descends in the longitudinal groove on Margo ventricularis sinister (Car, su, Ru). D E

30 **Ramus interventricularis subsinuosus**. Branch of Ramus circumflexus that descends in Sulcus interventricularis subsinuosus (Car, Ru, exceptionally eq). D

31 **Rami septales**. Arise from the preceding mentioned Ramus interventricularis subsinuosus and run into Septum interventriculare. D

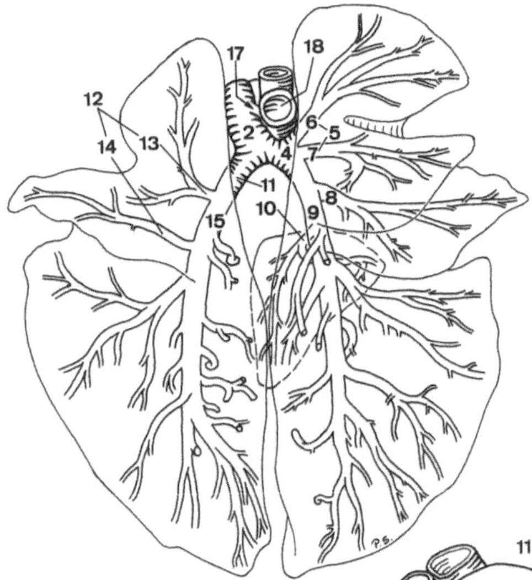

A Truncus pulmonalis, dorsal aspect of horizontally spread lungs (cap)

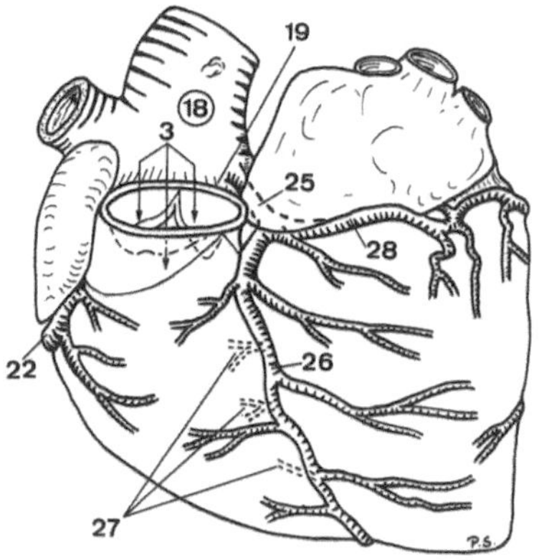

B A. coronaria sinistra (eq)

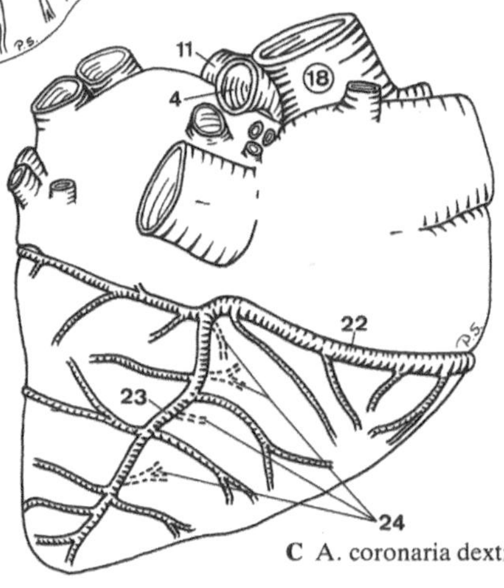

C A. coronaria dextra (eq)

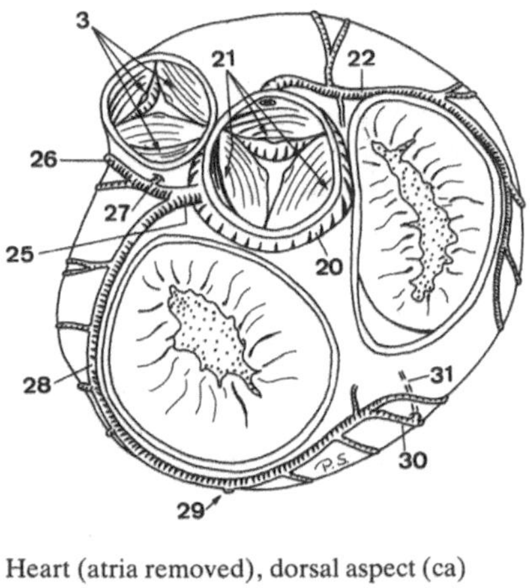

D Heart (atria removed), dorsal aspect (ca)

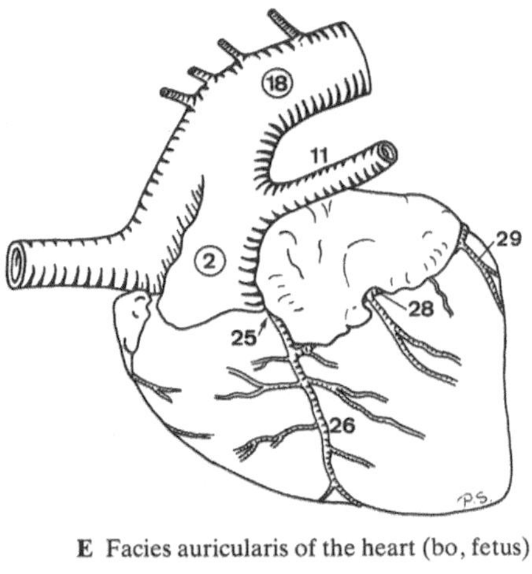

E Facies auricularis of the heart (bo, fetus)

1 **ARCUS AORTAE**. Caudodorsally curved segment between Aorta ascendens and Aorta descendens, begins intrapericardially. It continues into Aorta descendens after attachment of Ligamentum arteriosum. A

2 ***Corpora paraaortica***. Paraganglia, scattered along Arcus aortae and the roots of its great vessels. A

3 **TRUNCUS BRACHIOCEPHALICUS**. Craniodorsally directed large trunk arising from Arcus aortae. Extends to the bifurcation into A. subclavia dextra and Truncus bicaroticus or, the latter being absent, A. carotis communis dextra. A

4 **TRUNCUS BICAROTICUS**. Common trunk for the left and right A. carotis communis. Arises from Truncus brachiocephalicus and is usually (Car) or exceptionally (su, Ru, eq) absent. A

5 **ARTERIA CAROTIS COMMUNIS**. Cranially directed bilateral stem for A. carotis externa and A. carotis interna. Arises from Truncus brachiocephalicus via the occasional Truncus bicaroticus. A B C D E

CARNIVORA

6 **A. thyroidea [thyreoidea] caudalis**. Rarely present and variably arising artery that runs cranially towards the caudal part of Gl. thyroidea. B

7 **A. thyroidea [thyreoidea] cranialis**. Curves ventrally and branches into the cranial pole of Gl. thyroidea. B

8 ***Ramus sternocleidomastoideus***. To M. sternocephalicus and M. cleidomastoideus. B

9 ***Ramus pharyngeus***. Courses craniodorsally and supplies Mm. constrictores pharyngis. B

10 ***Ramus cricothyroideus [-thyreoideus]***. Runs cranioventrally, branches enter the M. cricothyroideus. B

11 ***Ramus laryngeus caudalis***. Runs parallel to N. laryngeus caudalis and enters larynx from caudally. B

SUS

12 **A. thyroidea [thyreoidea] caudalis**. Penetrates into the caudal pole of Gl. thyroidea. Inconstant. C

13 **A. thyroidea [thyreoidea] cranialis**. Branches and enters into the cranial pole of Gl. thyroidea. Inconstant. C

14 ***Ramus pharyngeus***. Cranially directed supply for Mm. constrictores pharyngis caudales. C

15 ***Ramus cricothyroideus [-thyreoideus]***. To M. cricothyroideus. C

16 ***Ramus laryngeus caudalis***. Passes caudally, accompanying N. laryngeus caudalis. C

17 **A. laryngea cranialis**. Arises close to the terminal division of A. carotis communis and accompanies N. laryngeus cranialis to larynx. C

18 ***Ramus pharyngeus***. To Mm. constrictores pharyngis caudales. C

19 ***Ramus laryngeus***. Continuation of A. laryngea cranialis that enters larynx cranially and reaches the medial aspect of Cartilago thyroidea. C

RUMINANTIA

20 **Rami sternocleidomastoidei**. Variably originated branches for M. sternomastoideus and M. cleidomastoideus. D E

21 **A. thyroidea [thyreoidea] caudalis**. Enters the caudal pole of Gl. thyroidea. Present in ov, inconstant in bo, cap. D E

22 **A. thyroidea [thyreoidea] cranialis**. Curves to, and supplies, the cranial pole of Gl. thyroidea. D E

23 ***Ramus pharyngeus***. To the pharyngeal wall. D E

24 ***Ramus cricothyroideus [-thyreoideus]*** (bo, ov). Supplies M. cricothyroideus and may be plural in ov. D E

25 ***Ramus laryngeus caudalis***. Runs parallel to N. laryngeus caudalis and enters larynx between Cartilago thyroidea and Cartilago cricoidea. D E

26 **A. laryngea cranialis**. Runs cranioventrally to larynx. Has variable origin within species. D E

27 ***Ramus pharyngeus***. For the pharyngeal wall and its constrictor musculature. D E

28 ***Ramus laryngeus***. Continuation of the parent stem that enters larynx. D E

29 **A. pharyngea ascendens**. Runs craniomedially to the dorsal wall of pharynx. D E

30 ***Rami palatini*** (bo). To Palatum molle. D

31 ***Rami tonsillares*** (bo). Pass to Tonsillae. D

32 ***Rami pharyngei***. Small branches supplying the pharyngeal wall and its musculature. D E

33 **A. palatina ascendens** (ov, cap). Courses craniomedially to Palatum molle. E

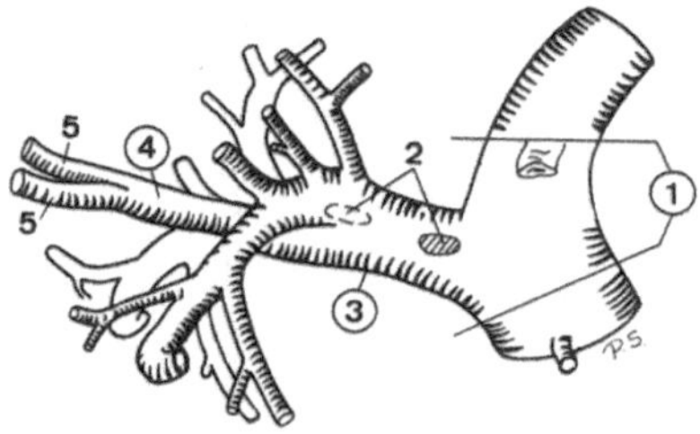

A Arcus aortae, left lateral aspect (eq)

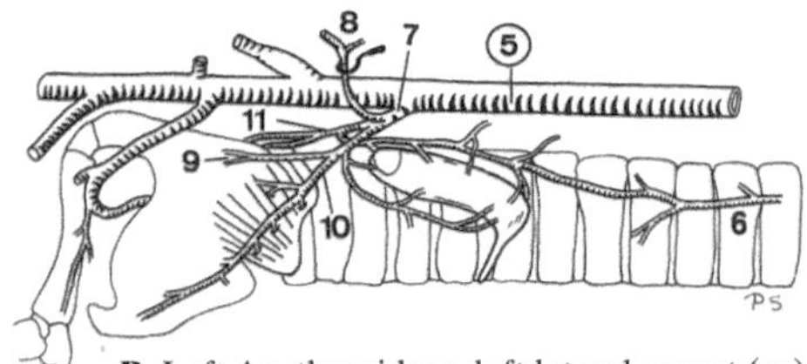

B Left Aa. thyroideae, left lateral aspect (ca)

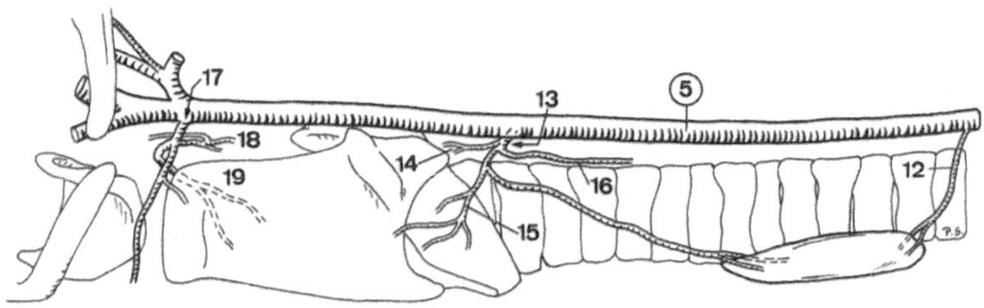

C Left A. carotis communis, lateral aspect (su)

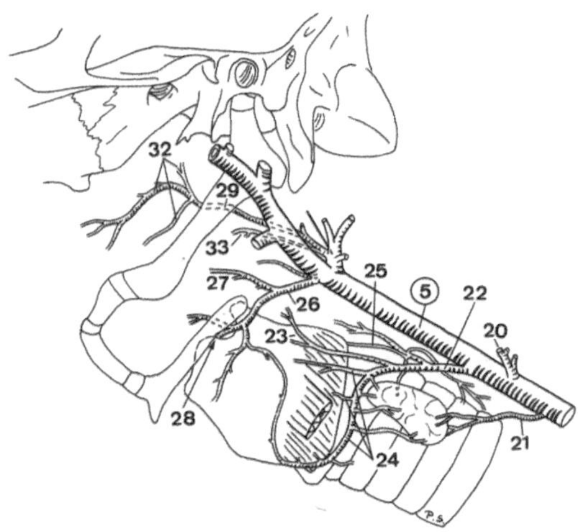

E Left A. carotis communis, lateral aspect (ov)

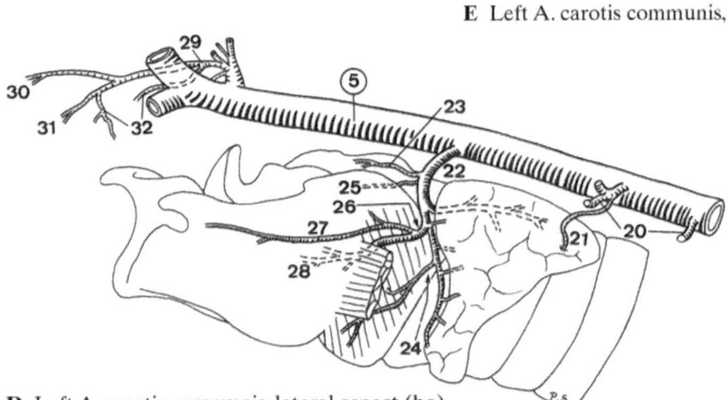

D Left A. carotis communis, lateral aspect (bo)

EQUUS

1 **(A. thyroidea [thyreoidea] caudalis).** Inconstant vessel which sends branches into the caudal pole of Gl. thyroidea. A

2 **A. thyroidea [thyreoidea] cranialis.** Curves around and supplies the cranial pole of Gl. thyroidea. A

3 ***Ramus pharyngeus.*** Courses cranially into the caudal part of the pharyngeal wall. A

4 ***Ramus cricothyroideus [-thyreoideus].*** To M. cricothyroideus. A

5 ***Ramus laryngeus caudalis.*** Runs parallel to N. laryngeus caudalis to the larynx. A

6 ***A. pharyngea ascendens.*** Passes dorsocranially into the pharyngeal musculature. A

7 *Rami palatini.* To Palatum molle. A

8 *Rami pharyngei.* Enter the caudal half of pharyngeal wall. A

9 ***A. laryngea cranialis.*** Courses cranioventrally to larynx. A

10 *Ramus pharyngeus.* To Mm. constrictores pharyngis. A

11 *Ramus laryngeus.* Enters larynx between Cartilagines thyroidea and cricoidea. A

TERMINUS COMMUNIS

12 **A. CAROTIS EXTERNA.** Continuation of A. carotis communis beyond the origin of A. carotis interna (Car, su, eq) or A. occipitalis (adult Ru). A B D

CARNIVORA

13 **A. occipitalis.** Extends dorsally to the neck and the occipital region of the skull. B D

14 ***A. condylaris.*** Courses in Fossa condylaris ventralis and reaches Cavum cranii through Canalis n. hypoglossi and Foramen jugulare. B

15 ***Ramus occipitalis.*** Branched continuation of A. occipitalis beyond the connection with Ramus anastomoticus cum a. occipitali from A. vertebralis. B

16 *A. meningea caudalis* (ca). Enters Meatus temporalis via Foramen mastoideum and reaches Cavum cranii where it ramifies in Dura mater encephali. B

17 **A. tympanica caudalis.** Supplies Auris media and Auris interna. B

18 **A. laryngea cranialis.** Courses ventrally towards larynx. B D

19 ***Ramus pharyngeus.*** Dorsally directed supply for Mm. hyo-, thyro-, and cricopharyngei. B

20 ***Ramus laryngeus.*** Enters larynx through Fissura thyroidea. B

21 **A. pharyngea ascendens.** Runs dorsorostrally to the medial aspect of Bulla tympanica and anastomoses with A. carotis interna. B D

22 ***Rami palatini.*** To Palatum molle. May be singular in fe. D

23 ***Rami pharyngei.*** Primarily to the cranial part of pharynx. D

24 **A. lingualis.** Courses rostroventrally and enters the tongue between Os hyoideum and M. hyoglossus. B D

25 ***A. palatina ascendens.*** Usually represented by two small vessels, supplies Radix linguae, Palatum molle and the adjacent part of pharynx. B D

26 ***Rami perihyoidei.*** Arise at various levels and supply the structures around Os hyoideum and Tonsilla palatina. B D

27 ***A. profunda linguae.*** Rostral continuation of A. lingualis, coursing on the lateral aspect of M. genioglossus towards Apex linguae. D

28 *Rami dorsales linguae.* Run flexuously to Dorsum linguae. D

29 **A. facialis.** Courses cranioventrally, crosses Margo ventralis of Mandibula and ascends along the rostral border of M. masseter. B C

30 ***Ramus glandularis.*** To Gl. mandibularis and Gll. sublinguales. B

31 ***A. sublingualis.*** Courses rostrally along the medial aspect of Margo ventralis of Mandibula and ramifies on the floor of the mouth after piercing M. mylohyoideus. B C D

32 *A. submentalis.* Follows Margo ventralis of Mandibula ventral to M. mylohyoideus to the chin. C D

33 ***A. labialis inferior.*** Passes rostrally to the lower lip. B C

34 ***Aa. angulares oris.*** Run to Angulus oris. C

35 ***A. labialis superior.*** Courses rostrally to the upper lip. C

36 ***Ramus anastomoticus cum a. infraorbitali.*** Connection to A. infraorbitalis. C

37 ***A. angularis oculi*** (fe). Curves caudodorsally towards Angulus oculi medialis. Also reported in the dog. C

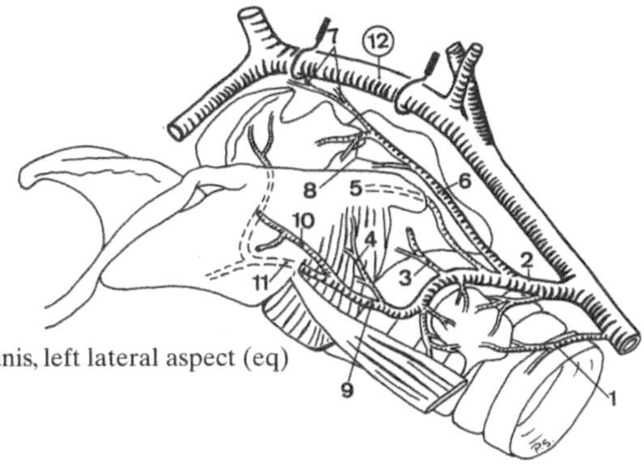

A A. carotis communis, left lateral aspect (eq)

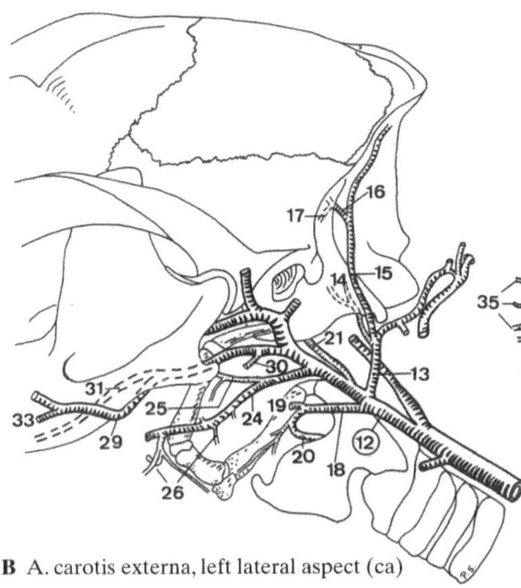

B A. carotis externa, left lateral aspect (ca)

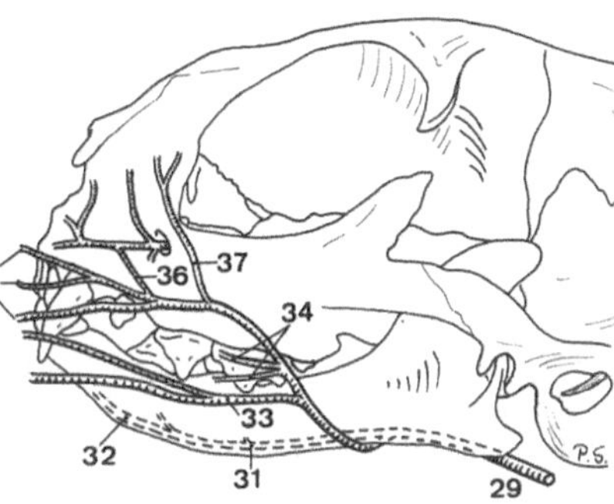

C A. Facialis, left lateral aspect (fe)

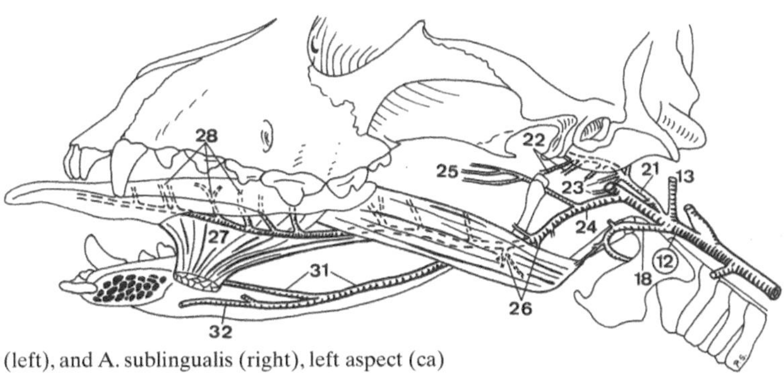

D A. lingualis (left), and A. sublingualis (right), left aspect (ca)

1 **A. auricularis caudalis**. Circles around the caudal part of the base of the ear. A B C

2 ***A. stylomastoidea***. Enters Foramen stylomastoideum, passes to Auris media. A B C

3 ***Ramus parotideus***. Variable branch for Gl. parotis. A B C

4 ***Ramus sternocleidomastoideus*** (ca). Occasionally double branch to the conjoined tendons of M. sternomastoideus and M. cleidomastoideus. A C

5 *Ramus glandularis*. To Gl. mandibularis. C

6 ***Ramus auricularis lateralis***. On Dorsum auriculae along Margo antitragicus. Frequently double (esp. fe). A B C

7 ***Ramus auricularis intermedius***. Runs in the middle of Dorsum auriculae. A B C

8 ***Ramus auricularis medialis***. On Dorsum auriculae along Margo tragicus. A B C

9 ***Ramus occipitalis***. Enters the caudal border of M. temporalis. A B C

10 ***A. auricularis profunda***. Sends branches to the internal surface of Auris externa and ramifies in Mm. auriculares and M. temporalis. A B C

11 **A. parotidea**. Main vessel to Gl. parotis. A B C

12 **A. temporalis superficialis**. Courses dorsally, bends rostrally. A B C

13 ***A. transversa faciei***. Emerges from the medial aspect of Gl. parotis, continues rostrally. C

14 ***A. auricularis rostralis***. Courses between Gl. parotis and M. temporalis to Auricula. C

15 ***A. palbebralis inferior lateralis***. Enters Palpebra inferior from lateral. C

16 ***A. palpebralis superior lateralis***. Enters Palpebra superior from lateral. C

17 *A. dorsalis nasi caudalis* (ca). Runs rostrally to Regio dorsalis nasi. C

18 **A. maxillaris**. Traverses Canalis alaris (ca) to Fossa pterygopalatina. A B C

19 ***Ramus articularis temporomandibularis***. Sometimes plural. A C

20 ***A. alveolaris interior***. Courses between Ramus mandibulae and M. pterygoideus medialis, enters Canalis mandibulae. A B C

21 *Ramus mylohyoideus*. To M. mylohyoideus. B C

22 *Rami dentales*. Branches for teeth. C

23 *Rami mentales*. Emerge through Foramina mentalia. C

24 ***A. temporalis profunda caudalis***. To M. temporalis. A B

25 *A. masseterica*. Passes through Incisura mandibulae to M. masseter. A B

26 ***A. tympanica rostralis***. Passes to Auris media through Fissura petrotympanica. A B

27 ***A. meningea media***. Passes through Foramen ovale, Incisura spinosa, or Foramen spinosum to Dura mater. A B

28 *Ramus anastomoticus cum a. carotide interna*. Joins the homonymous branch of A. ophthalmica externa (ca) or Rami retis (fe), to reach A. carotis interna. A

29 ***Rete mirabile a. maxillaris*** (fe). Extracranial network formed by A. maxillaris. B

30 *Rami retis*. Pierce through Fissura orbitalis to Circulus arteriosus cerebri directly, or by joining A. carotis interna. B

31 *A. temporalis profunda rostralis*. Ramifies in M. temporalis. B

32 *Ramus anastomoticus cum a. ophthalmica interna*. Joins A. ophthalmica interna medial to N. opticus. 251 A

33 **A. centralis retinae**. Collective term for the extrabulbar stem vessels of Arteriolae retinae.

34 **Aa. ciliares posteriores longae**. Lateral and medial, perforate anterior part of sclera, supply Tunica vasculosa bulbi. 251 A

35 **Aa. ciliares posteriores breves**. Penetrate sclera near Area cribrosa, supply Choroidea. 251 A

36 **Aa. episclerales**. On the external surface of sclera.

37 *Rami musculares*. Primarily for Mm. bulbi. 251 A

38 **Aa. ciliares anteriores**. Penetrate sclera near Sulcus sclerae, supply Tunicae fibrosa and vasculosa bulbi.

39 **Aa. episclerales**. Course on the outer surface of scleara.

40 **Aa. conjunctivales posteriores**. To Tunica conjunctiva.

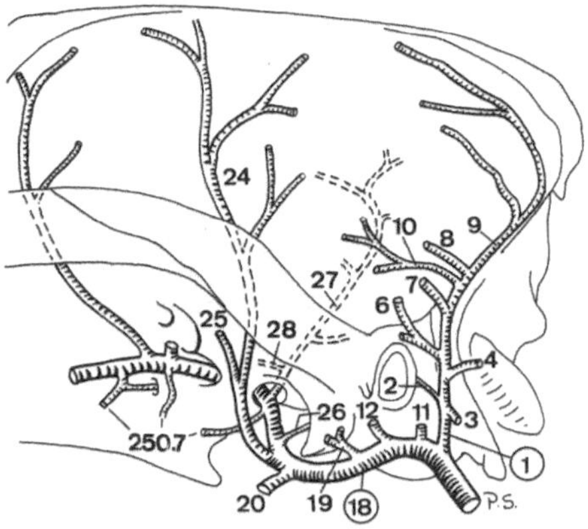

A A. maxillaris, left lateral aspect (ca)

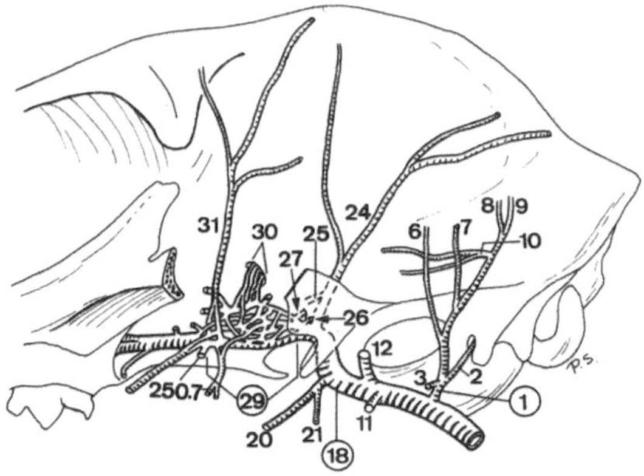

B A. maxillaris (semischematic), left lateral aspect (fe)

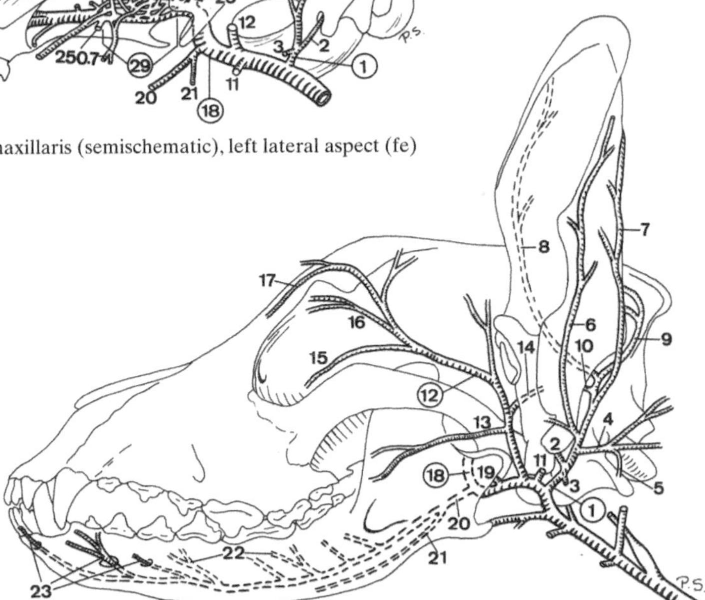

C Branches of A. carotis externa, left lateral aspect (ca)

1 *A. lacrimalis*. Accompanies N. lacrimalis to Gl. lacrimalis. A

2 *A. ethmoidalis externa*. Courses into Cavum cranii via Foramen ethmoidale. A

3 **Aa. nasales septales caudales.** Pass through Lamina cribrosa into Cavum nasi.

4 *A. supraorbitalis*. Perforates periorbita and crosses the dorsomedial border of Orbita. A

5 *A. buccalis*. Courses ventrorostrally to the cheek. A

6 **Rami glandulares zygomatici.** To Gl. zygomatica.

7 ***Rami pterygoidei.*** Variable branches to Mm. pterygoidei. 249 A B

8 ***A. ophthalmica externa*** (ca). Leaves A. maxillaris rostral to Canalis alaris, enters periorbita and runs rostrodorsally. B C

9 *Ramus anastomoticus cum a. carotide interna*. Pierces through Fissura orbitalis into Cavum cranii, anastomoses with A. carotis interna. B C

10 **Ramus anastomoticus cum a. meningea media.** Intracranially arisen branch to Ramus anastomoticus cum a. carotide interna of A. meningea media. B

11 *Ramus anastomoticus cum a. ophthalmica interna*. See 248.32. B C

12 **A. centralis retinae.** See 248.33. B

13 **Aa. ciliares posteriores longae.** See 248.34. B

14 **Aa. ciliares posteriores breves.** See 248.35. B

15 **Aa. episclerales.** See 248.36. B

16 *Rami musculares*. See 248.37. B C

17 **Aa. ciliares anteriores.** See 248.38

18 **Aa. episclerales.** See 248.39

19 **Aa. conjunctivales posteriores.** See 248.40 C

20 *A. lacrimalis*. See 1. B C

21 *A. ethmoidalis externa*. See 2. B C

22 **A. meningea rostralis.** Ramifies in dura at the caudal margin of Lamina cribrosa. B

23 **Aa. nasales septales caudales.** See 3. B

24 ***A. temporalis profunda rostralis*** (ca). Enters M. temporalis near the middle of its rostral border. B

25 ***A. buccalis*** (ca). See 5. B

26 *Rami glandulares zygomatici*. See 6. B

27 ***A. infraorbitalis.*** Enters Canalis infraorbitalis via Foramen maxillare and emerges through Foramen infraorbitale. A B D

28 *A. malaris*. Passes dorsorostrally to Angulus oculi medialis. A B D

29 **A. palpebralis inferior medialis.** Enters the medial part of Palpebra inferior. B D

30 **A. palpebralis superior medialis.** Supplies the medial part of Palpebra superior. B D

31 **A. palpebrae tertiae.** To Plica semilunaris conjunctivae. B D

32 *Rami dentales*. To the superior teeth. A D

32a *A. dorsalis nasi* (fe). Supplies Regio dorsalis nasi in the cat, because unlike in the dog, there is no A. dorsalis nasi caudalis in the cat. A

33 *A. dorsalis nasi rostralis* (ca). Passes through Canalis infraorbitalis (fe) and runs rostrodorsally to Regio dorsalis nasi. A D

34 *A. lateralis nasi*. To Regio lateralis nasi and Labium superius. A D

35 *A. palatina minor*. Courses to Palatum durum and Palatum molle. A B D

36 ***A. palatina descendens.*** Rostroventral continuation of A. maxillaris at the rostral end of Fossa pterygopalatina. A B D

37 *A. palatina major*. Traverses Canalis palatinus major and continues rostrally inside Sulcus palatinus. A B D

38 *A. sphenopalatina*. Courses towards Cavum nasi via Foramen sphenopalatinum. B D

39 **Aa. nasales caudales, laterales et septales.** To Cavum nasi. D

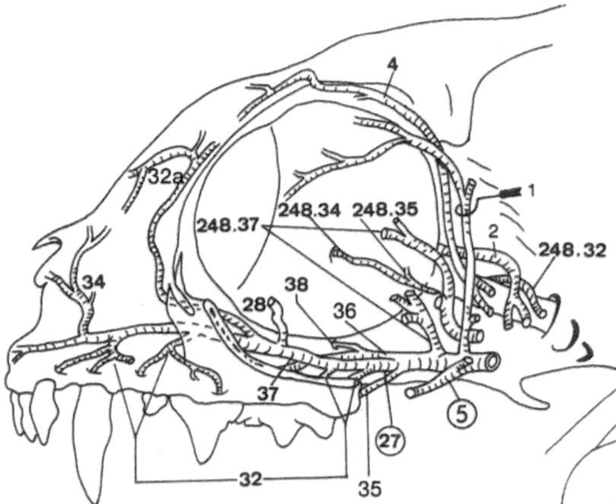

A Branches of left A. carotis externa, lateral aspect (fe)

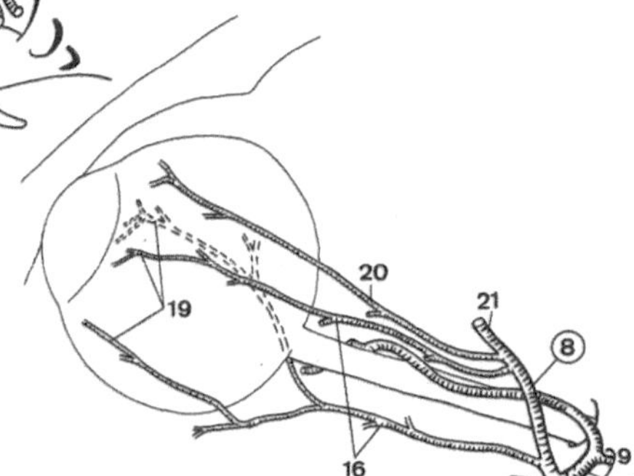

C Left A. ophthalmica externa, lateral aspect (ca)

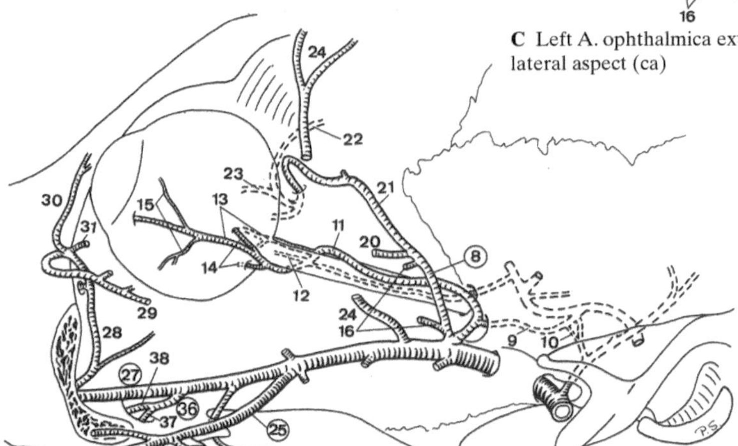

B Branches of left A. maxillaris, lateral aspect (ca)

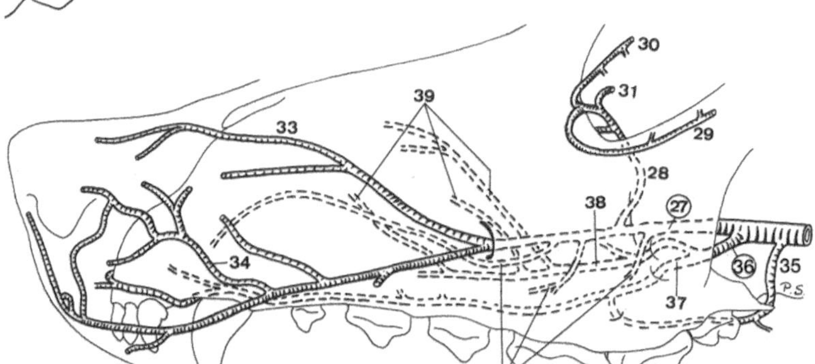

D Terminal branches of left A. maxillaris, lateral aspect (ca)

SUS

1 **A. lingualis**. Enters the tongue between Os hyoideum and M. hyoglossus. B C

2 ***Rami perihyoidei***. Branching vessels around Os hyoideum. Mainly tend to the median plane. B

3 ***A. palatina ascendens***. Courses at the medial aspect of Stylohyoideum into Palatum molle and its musculature. B

4 ***A. pharyngea ascendens***. Dorsally directed vessel which may be double. B

5 *Rami palatini*. Supply Mm. palati. B

6 *Rami pharyngei*. Ramify in the pharyngeal wall. B

7 ***A. sublingualis***. Runs rostrally over the lateral aspect of M. genioglossus at the dorsal border of M. geniohyoideus and supplies the floor of the mouth and Gl. sublingualis polystomatica. A B

8 ***A. profunda linguae***. Flexuous rostral continuation of A. lingualis along the lateral aspect of M. genioglossus. B

9 *Rami dorsales linguae*. Course on the medial aspect of M. hyoglossus and M. styloglossus towards Dorsum linguae. B

10 **A. facialis**. Runs rostroventrally and enters with plural branches the ventral part of M. masseter after crossing Margo ventralis of Mandibula. A B C

11 ***Ramus pharyngeus***. To the lateral pharyngeal wall. A C

12 ***Rami glandulares***. To Gl. mandibularis, Gl. parotis and Gl. sublingualis monostomatica. A C

13 ***A. submentalis***. Courses rostrally on the ventrolateral aspect of M. mylohyoideus. A

14 **A. auricularis caudalis**. Runs dorsally to the caudal aspect of the ear and ramifies variably. A C

15 ***Ramus parotideus***. To Gl. parotis. C

16 ***Ramus sternocleidomastoideus***. To M. cleidocephalicus and M. sternomastoideus. C

17 ***Ramus auricularis lateralis***. Courses apically on Dorsum auriculae, following Margo antitragicus. C

18 ***Ramus auricularis intermedius***. Runs towards Apex auriculae on the middle of Dorsum auriculae. C

19 ***Ramus auricularis medialis***. Courses apically on Dorsum auriculae along Margo tragicus. C

20 ***A. auricularis profunda***. Ramifies in Mm. auriculares and M. temporalis and also supplies the surface of Auris externa. C

21 **Rami parotidei**. To Gl. parotis. A C

22 **A. temporalis superficialis**. Courses dorsally across the lateral aspect of Arcus zygomaticus. A C

23 ***A. transversa faciei***. Surrounds Collum mandibulae laterally and continues rostrally over the M. masseter. C

24 *Ramus articularis temporomandibularis*. Courses dorsally to Articulatio temporomandibularis. C

25 ***Aa. auriculares rostrales***. Run caudally to Meatus acusticus externus and supply Mm. auriculares and the internal surface of Auris externa. C

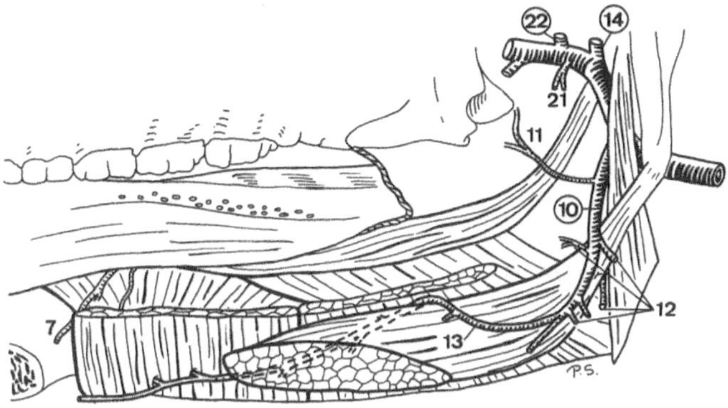

A Left A. facialis, lateral aspect (su)

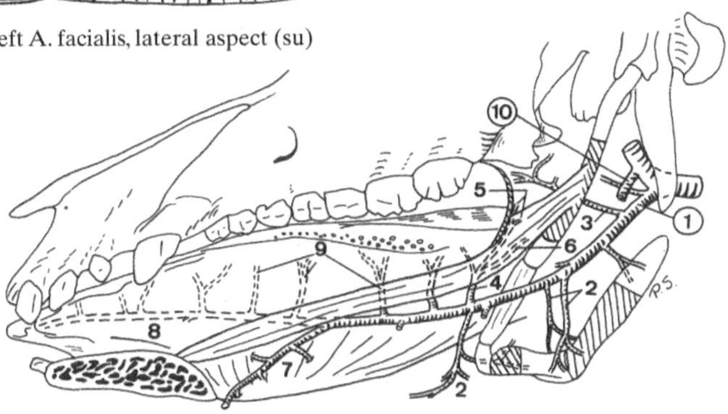

B Left A. lingualis, lateral aspect (su)

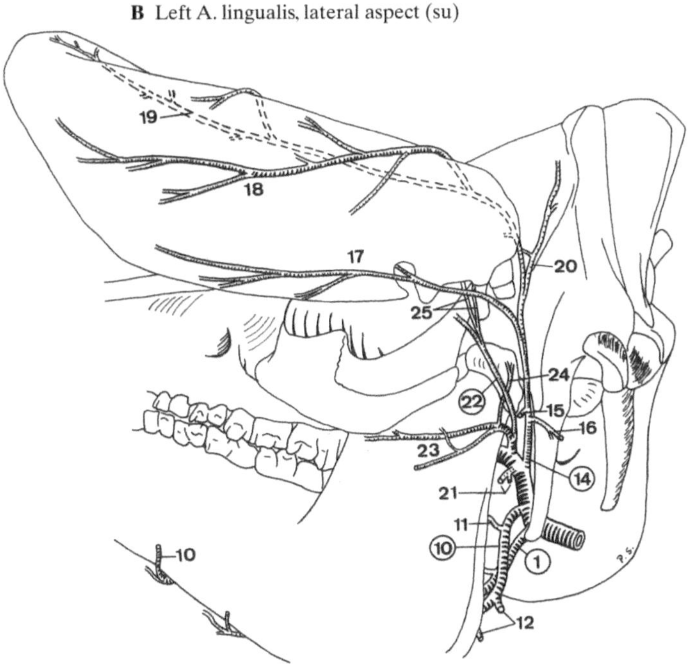

C Branches of left A. carotis externa, caudolateral aspect (su)

1 **A. maxillaris**. Pursues a flexuous course to Fossa pterygopalatina. A

2 ***A. meningea media***. Passes caudomedially through Incisura spinosa into dura. A

3 *Ramus ad rete mirabile epidurale rostrale*. Concurs to the formation of Rete mirabile epidurale rostrale. A

4 ***A. temporalis profunda caudalis***. Crosses the medial aspect of Arcus zygomaticus and enters M. temporalis. A

5 *A. masseterica*. Passes via Incisura mandibulae into M. masseter. A

6 ***Rami pterygoidei***. Branches for the homonymous muscles. A

7 ***A. alveolaris inferior***. Runs rostroventrally and enters through Foramen mandibulae in Canalis mandibulae. A

8 *Ramus mylohyoideus*. Branch for M. mylohyoideus. A

9 *Rami dentales*. To the mandibular teeth. A

10 *Rami mentales*. Emerge via Foramina mentalia lateralia and ramify in Regio mentalis and Labium inferius. A

11 ***A. buccalis***. Courses between Tuber maxillae and Ramus mandibulae to the cheek and ramifies at the rostral border of M. masseter. A

12 *A. temporalis profunda rostralis*. Passes dorsally into M. temporalis. A

13 *A. angularis oculi*. Runs rostrodorsally and then curves caudodorsally to Angulus oculi medialis. A

14 **A. palpebralis inferior medialis**. Runs to the medial part of Palpebra inferior and supplies it. A

15 *A. angularis oris*. Passes rostroventrally to Angulus oris. A

16 *A. labialis inferior*. Runs rostroventrally to supply Labium inferius and Gll. buccales ventrales. A

17 *A. labialis superior*. Supplies Labium superius and Gll. buccales dorsales. A

18 ***A. ophthalmica externa***. Pierces through periorbita and passes between Mm. recti dorsalis and lateralis to the dorsal aspect of M. retractor bulbi. A B

19 *A. meningea rostralis*. Enters Foramen orbitorotundum to supply dura. A

20 **Ramus ad rete mirabile epidurale rostrale**. Intracranially arisen branch that concurs in the formation of Rete mirabile epidurale rostrale. A

21 *A. supratrochlearis*. Pierces through periorbita, curves upon Mm. bulbi and perforates the periorbita again to reach Processus zygomaticus of Os frontale. A B

22 **A. palpebralis superior medialis**. Courses medially along the rostral aspect of Processus zygomaticus and supplies the medial part of Palpebra superior. A

23 *A. supraorbitalis*. Penetrates through periorbita into Canalis supraorbitalis and may emerge through Foramen supraorbitale. A B

24 *Aa. ciliares anteriores*. Perforate sclera near Sulcus sclerae and supply Tunica vasculosa bulbi. B

25 *A. ethmoidalis externa*. Perforates periorbita, enters Cavum cranii via Foramen ethmoidale and comes through Lamina cribrosa towards Cavum nasi. A B

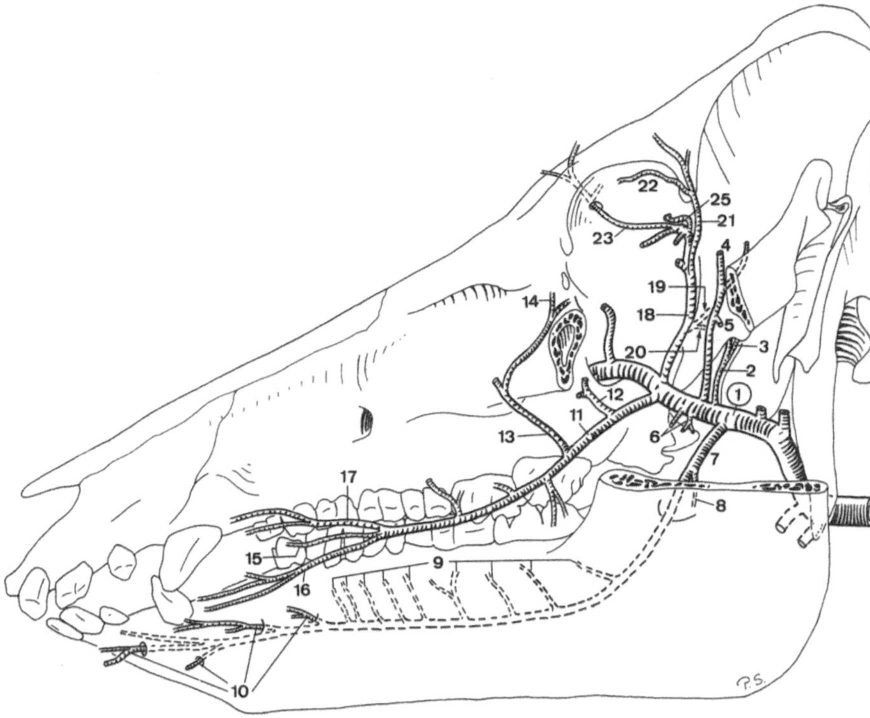

A Left A. maxillaris, lateral aspect (su)

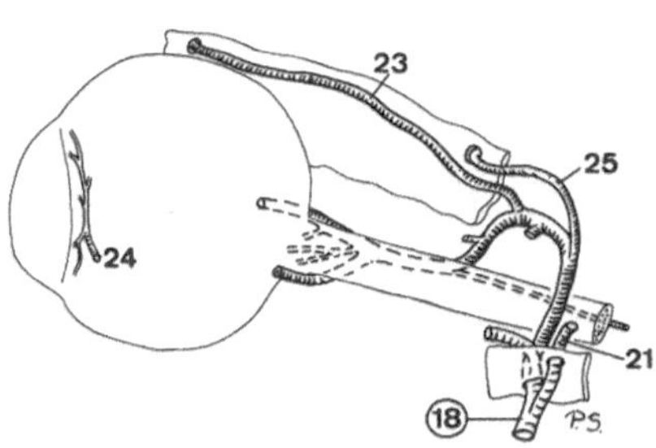

B Left A. ophthalmica externa (periorbita partly represented), lateral aspect (su)

1 *A. lacrimalis*. Courses rostrodorsally within periorbita to Gl. lacrimalis. C

2 **A. palpebralis inferior lateralis.** Enters Palpebra inferior from lateral. C

3 **A. palpebralis superior lateralis.** Courses to the lateral aspect of Palpebra superior. C

4 *Rami musculares*. Variable branches for Mm. bulbi. A

5 *Ramus anastomoticus cum a. ophthalmica interna*. Connects with A. ophthalmica interna on the medial aspect of Nervus opticus and continues rostrally. A

6 **A. centralis retinae.** Collective term for the extrabulbar stem vessels of the Arteriolae retinae. A

7 **Aa. ciliares posteriores longae.** Pair of vessels which perforate the anteriolateral and anteriomedial aspect of sclera to supply Tunica vasculosa bulbi. A

8 **Aa. ciliares posteriores breves.** Branches of Aa. ciliares posteriores longae which perforate sclera near N. opticus, and ramify in choroidea. A

9 **Aa. episclerales.** Branches of Aa. ciliares posteriores longae which run on the outer surface of sclera and supply it. A

10 **Aa. conjunctivales posteriores.** Extend along sclera into Tunica conjunctiva. A

11 ***A. malaris.*** Crosses the medial aspect of Processus temporalis of Os zygomaticum, pierces through periorbita and courses towards Angulus oculi medialis. B

12 *A. palpebrae tertiae*. Supplies Palpebra tertia. B

13 *Ramus frontalis*. Arises outside periorbita and continues upon the ventromedial part of Orbita to Angulus oculi medialis. B [1)]

14 **A. palpebralis inferior medialis.** Enters Palpebra inferior from medial. B [1)]

15 *Aa. conjunctivales anteriores*. Supply Tunica conjunctiva. B [1)]

16 *A. dorsalis nasi*. Emerges from Orbita and courses to Regio dorsalis nasi, as a branch of Ramus frontalis. B[1)]

17 ***A. infraorbitalis.*** Enters Canalis infraorbitalis through Foramen maxillare and emerges through Foramen infraorbitale. B

18 *Rami dentales*. To the superior teeth. B

19 *Aa. laterales nasi*. Run rostrally and dorsally in Regio lateralis nasi. B

20 ***A. palatina descendens.*** Courses rostroventrally at the rostral end of Fossa pterygopalatina. B C

21 *A. sphenopalatina*. Courses towards Cavum nasi through Foramen sphenopalatinum. C

22 **Aa. nasales caudales, laterales et septales.** Ramify in Tunica mucosa nasi. C

23 **A. palatina minor.** Courses between Processus pyramidalis of Os palatinum and Tuber maxillae to Palatum molle. Inconstant. C

24 **A. palatina major.** Courses rostrally through Canalis palatinus major and continues rostrally in Sulcus palatinus. Sends branches to Palatum durum, to its heterolateral counterpart, to the snout and, via Fissura palatina to Tunica mucosa nasi. C

1) A change of order from 13–14–15–16 to 15–13–14–16 and other changes are suggested by Prof. Dr. Paul Simoens albeit they are not (yet) implemented in the N. A. V., as follows:

13 **Aa. conjunctivales anteriores.**

14 *Ramus frontalis.*

15 **A. palpebralis inferior medialis.**

16 **A. dorsalis nasi.**

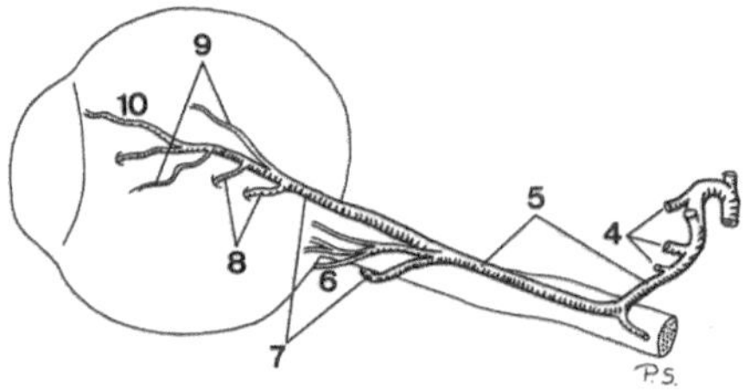

A Arteries of the right eye, medial aspect (su)

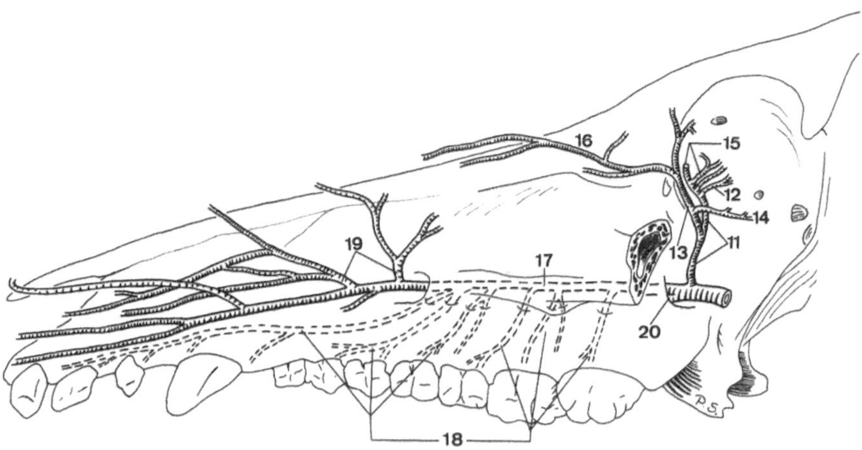

B Left A. infraorbitalis and A. malaris, lateral aspect (su)

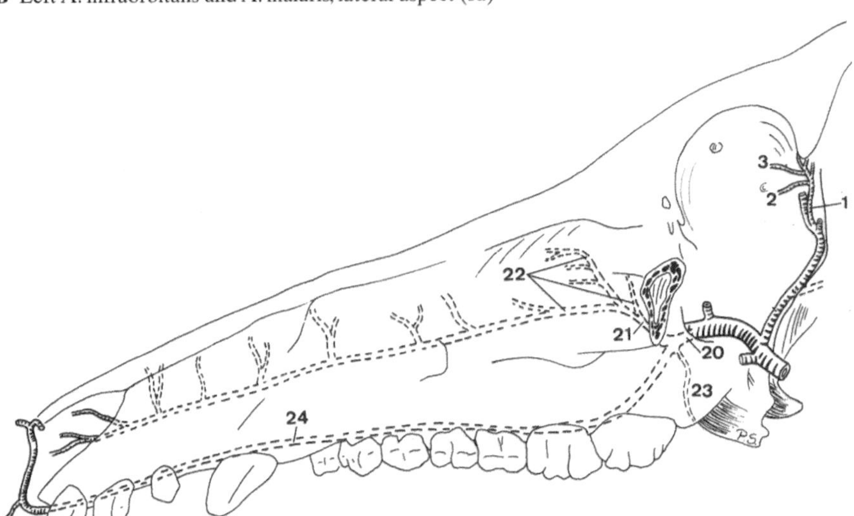

C Left A. maxillaris, lateral aspect (su)

RUMINANTIA

1 **Truncus linguofacialis**. Common trunk for A. lingualis and A. facialis. Usually present in bo; A. facialis is absent in ov and cap. B

2 **A. lingualis.** Courses rostroventrally and enters the tongue at the medial aspect of M. hyoglossus. A B C

3 ***Rami glandulares***. Variable branches to Gl. mandibularis. A

4 ***Rami perihyoidei***. Surround Os hyoideum and usually anastomose by a distinct branch with their heterolateral counterparts. A

5 ***A. sublingualis***. Courses rostrally on the medial aspect of M. hyoglossus. May be unilaterally regressed (ov, cap). A

6 *A. submentalis* (ov, cap). Occasionally present, perforates M. mylohyoideus and continues superficially to the chin. A

7 ***A. profunda linguae***. Passes rostrally along the lateral aspect of M. genioglossus. A

8 *Rami dorsales linguae*. Arise inside the tongue and course towards Dorsum linguae. A

9 **A. facialis** (bo)*. Courses rostroventrally, crosses Margo ventralis of Mandibula at Incisura vasorum facialium* and ascends along the rostral border of M. masseter. B

10 ***Ramus glandularis***. Occasionally plural branch to Gl. mandibularis. B

11 ***A. submentalis***. Runs rostrally on the ventrolateral aspect of M. mylohyoideus. B

12 ***Aa. labiales inferiores***. Rostrally directed pair of vessels for Labium inferius. B

13 ***A. labialis superior***. Passes rostrally into Labium superius and Planum nasolabiale. B

14 ***A. angularis oris***. Supplies Angulus oris. Very small or absent. B

15 ***Ramus lateralis nasi rostralis***. Runs on the lateral aspect of the nose. Frequently represented by several branches. B

16 *Ramus anastomoticus cum a. infraorbitali*. Connection with branches of A. infraorbitalis. B

17 ***Ramus angularis oculi***. Variable and inconstant branch towards Angulus oculi medialis.

18 **A. auricularis caudalis.** Courses caudodorsally towards the base of the ear. B C

19 ***Rami parotidei***. To Gl. parotis. B C

20 ***A. stylomastoidea***. Passes through Foramen stylomastoideum into Canalis facialis and ramifies in Auris media. B C

21 ***Ramus meningeus*** (ov, cap). Enters Os temporale near Porus acusticus externus and traverses Meatus temporalis into Cavum cranii where it supplies meninges. C

22 ***Ramus sternocleidomastoideus*** (cap). To M. sternomastoideus and M. cleidocephalicus. C

23 ***Ramus auricularis lateralis***. Runs on Dorsum auriculae along Margo antitragicus towards the Apex auriculae. B C

24 ***Ramus auricularis intermedius*** (ov, cap). Runs apically on the middle of Dorsum auriculae. Occurs exceptionally in bo. C

25 ***Ramus auricularis intermedius lateralis*** (bo). Lateral intermediate branch that runs apically on Dorsum auriculae. B

26 ***Ramus auricularis intermedius medialis*** (bo). Medial intermediate branch that runs apically on Dorsum auriculae. B

27 ***Ramus occipitalis***. Runs towards Regio occipitalis. B C

28 ***A. auricularis profunda***. Sends a branch to the internal surface of Auris externa and also supplies Mm. auriculares and M. temporalis. B C

29 **Ramus massetericus** (bo). Runs rostroventrally into the caudal part of M. masseter. B

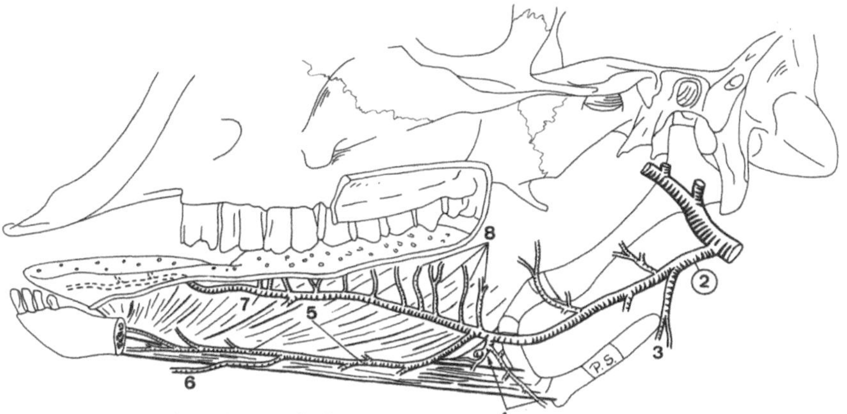

A Left A. lingualis, lateral aspect (ov)

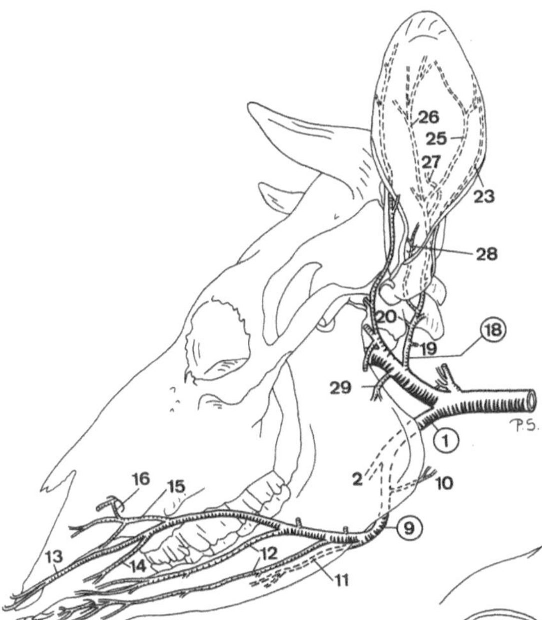

B Arteries of the head, left lateral aspect (bo)

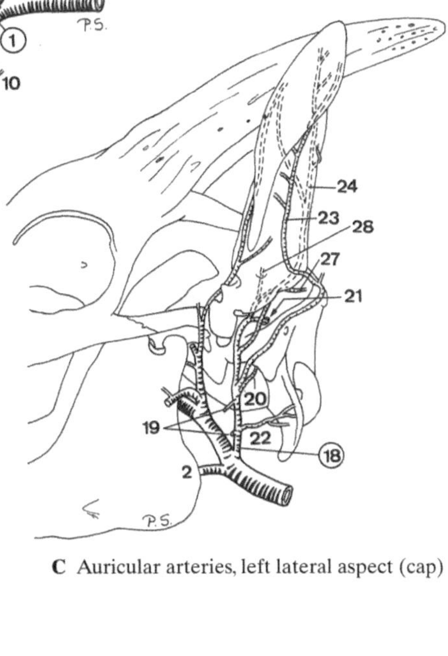

C Auricular arteries, left lateral aspect (cap)

1 **A. temporalis superficialis.** Courses dorsally across the lateral aspect of Arcus zygomaticus and ramifies in Regio frontalis. A B

2 ***A. auricularis rostralis*** (ov, cap). Crosses the lateral aspect of Arcus zygomaticus and reaches the cranial part of the base of the ear. A

3 *Ramus auricularis medialis.* Runs on Dorsum auriculae along Margo tragicus towards the apex of the ear. A

4 ***A. transversa faciei.*** Crosses Ramus mandibulae and courses rostroventrally on the lateral surface of M. masseter. A B

5 *Ramus articularis temporomandibularis* (bo). To the homonymous joint, from variable origins. B

6 *Ramus massetericus* (ov, cap). To M. masseter. A

7 *A. labialis inferior* (ov, cap). Runs in Labium inferius. A

8 *A. labialis superior* (ov, cap). Courses in Labium superius. A

9 **A. angularis oris.** Tends to Angulus oris. A

10 **Ramus anastomoticus cum a. infraorbitali.** Usually plural connection with A. infraorbitalis. A

11 ***A. auricularis rostralis*** (bo). Runs towards the rostral aspect of the base of the ear. B

12 *Ramus meningeus.* Courses through Meatus temporalis into Cavum cranii where it ramifies in meninges. B

13 *Ramus auricularis medialis.* Courses towards the Apex auriculae on Dorsum auriculae, parallel to Margo tragicus. B

14 ***A. cornualis****. Courses caudomedially to Basis cornus. Developed to variable size, dependent on the development of the horn, often represented by several vessels. A B

15 ***Ramus lacrimalis*** (bo, ov). Branch which arises at variable level and, after piercing through periorbita, courses into Gl. lacrimalis. B

16 ***A. palpebralis superior lateralis.*** Courses rostromedially into Palpebra superior. A B

17 ***A. palpebralis inferior lateralis.*** Runs rostromedially into Palpebra inferior. Often absent in ov. A B

18 ***A. dorsalis nasi*** (cap). Courses rostrally on Dorsum nasi. A

19 **A. maxillaris.** Passes rostrodorsally to Fossa pterygopalatina. A B

20 ***Ramus pterygoideus.*** Variable branch for Mm. pterygoidei. A B

21 ***A. alveolaris inferior.*** Pierces through Foramen mandibulae and courses within Canalis mandibulae. A B

22 *Ramus mylohyoideus.* To M. mylohyoideus. Arises before its parent vessel entered Canalis mandibulae. A

23 *Rami dentales.* To the mandibular teeth. A

24 *A. mentalis.* Continuation of A. alveolaris inferior which emerges from Foramen mentale. A

25 ***A. temporalis profunda*** (ov, cap). Pursues a short rostral course, bends dorsally, and ramifies in M. temporalis. A

26 *Ramus articularis temporomandibularis.* To the homonymous joint. A

27 ***A. temporalis profunda caudalis*** (bo). Supplies M. temporalis. B

28 *A. masseterica.* Passes through Incisura mandibulae into M. masseter. B

29 ***A. buccalis.*** Courses over Tuber maxillae into the caudal part of the cheek. A B

30 *A. temporalis profunda rostralis* (bo). Runs into M. temporalis. B

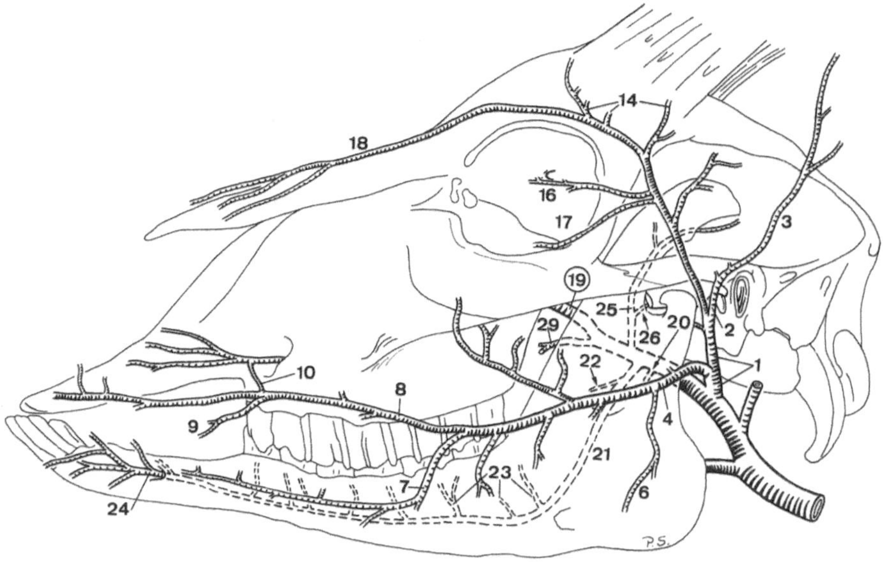

A Arteries of the head, left aspect (cap)

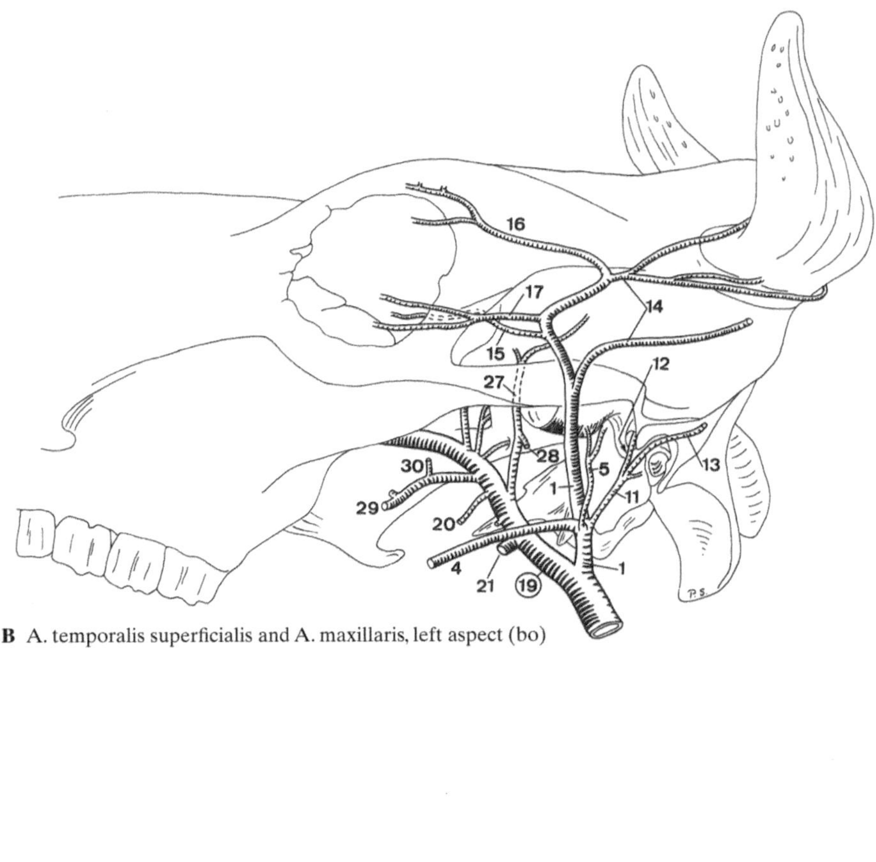

B A. temporalis superficialis and A. maxillaris, left aspect (bo)

1 ***Ramus caudalis ad rete mirabile epidurale rostrale.*** Passes through Foramen ovale to rete, may also pierce the skull near Foramen ovale. A C

2 ***Rami rostrales ad rete mirabile epidurale rostrale.*** Course through Foramen orbitorotundum to Rete mirabile epidurale rostrale. A C

3 ***A. ophthalmica externa.*** Perforates periorbita, passes between Mm. recti dorsalis and lateralis upon M. retractor bulbi, and continues rostrally upon N. opticus. A B C

4 *Rete mirabile ophthalmicum.* Arterial network in the course of A. ophthalmica externa. A B

5 *A. supraorbitalis.* Passes through Canalis supraorbitalis to Regio frontalis (bo, sometimes ov). A B

6 **A. ethmoidalis externa.** Enters through Foramen ethmoidale in Cavum cranii and continues through Lamina cribrosa towards Cavum nasi. A

7 **Aa. conjunctivales anteriores.** Variably originating vessels to Tunica conjunctiva. A B

8 *A. lacrimalis.* Courses along M. rectus dorsalis into Gl. lacrimalis. Absent in ov. A

9 *Ramus anastomoticus cum a. ophthalmica interna.* Short branch which joins A. ophthalmica interna at the rostromedial aspect of N. opticus. B

10 *Rami musculares.* Mainly to Mm. bulbi. Mostly arisen from Rete mirabile ophthalmicum. B

11 **Aa. ciliares anteriores.** Perforate the anterior aspect of sclera and ramify in choroidea.

12 **Aa. episclerales.** Course on sclera and supply it.

13 **Aa. conjunctivales posteriores.** Run along sclera to Tunica conjunctiva.

14 *Aa. ciliares posteriores longae.* Pair of vessels which run anteriorly on the lateral and medial aspects of Bulbus oculi and penetrate sclera to Tunica vasculosa. B

15 **A. centralis retinae.** Usually double parent trunk for the Arteriolae retinae. B

16 **Aa. ciliares posteriores breves.** Perforate sclera near Area cribrosa and ramify in choroidea. B

17 **Aa. episclerales.** Supply sclera from the outside. B

18 ***A. malaris.*** Passes dorsorostrally in Orbita to Angulus oculi medialis and continues onto the lateral aspect of the face. A C

19 *A. palpebrae tertiae.* Supplies Palpebra tertia. A C

20 *A. palpebralis inferior medialis.* Courses laterally, supplying Palpebra inferior. A C

21 *A. palpebralis superior medialis* (ov, cap). Courses laterally in Palpebra superior. Inconstant (esp. ov). A

22 *A. angularis oculi* (bo). Passes caudally to Angulus oculi medialis. C

23 *A. lateralis nasi caudalis.* Courses rostrally on Regio nasalis. A C

24 *A. dorsalis nasi* (bo, ov). Courses rostrally on the dorsal surface of the nose. A C

25 ***A. infraorbitalis.*** Pierces through Foramen maxillare in Canalis infraorbitalis and, after emerging from Foramen infraorbitale, ramifies on the lateral aspect of the face. A C

26 *Rami dentales.* To the superior teeth. A C

27 *A. lateralis nasi rostralis.* To Regio nasalis. A

28 ***A. palatina descendens.*** Rostroventrally directed continuation of A. maxillaris. A C

29 *A. sphenopalatina.* Courses through Foramen sphenopalatinum towards Cavum nasi. A C

30 **Aa. nasales caudales, laterales et septales.** Supply the caudoventral parts of Tunica mucosa nasi. A C

31 **A. palatina minor.** Supplies Palatum molle and the adjacent structures. A C

32 **A. palatina major.** Traverses Canalis palatinus major, continues rostrally in Sulcus palatinus, supplies Palatum durum, and, anastomosing with its heterolateral counterpart, also Tunica mucosa nasi. A C

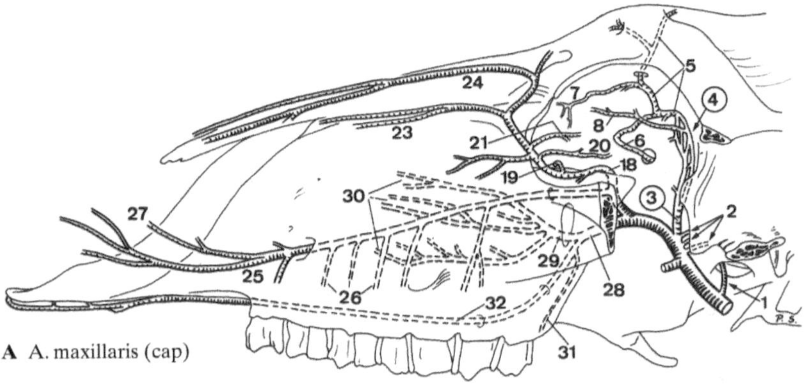

A A. maxillaris (cap)

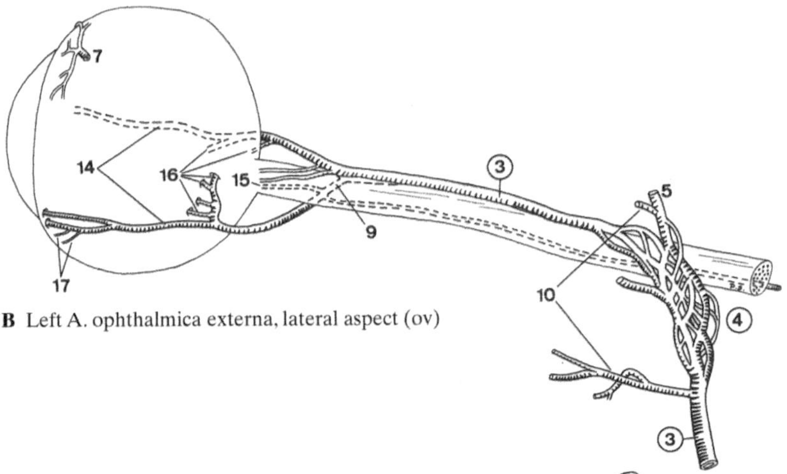

B Left A. ophthalmica externa, lateral aspect (ov)

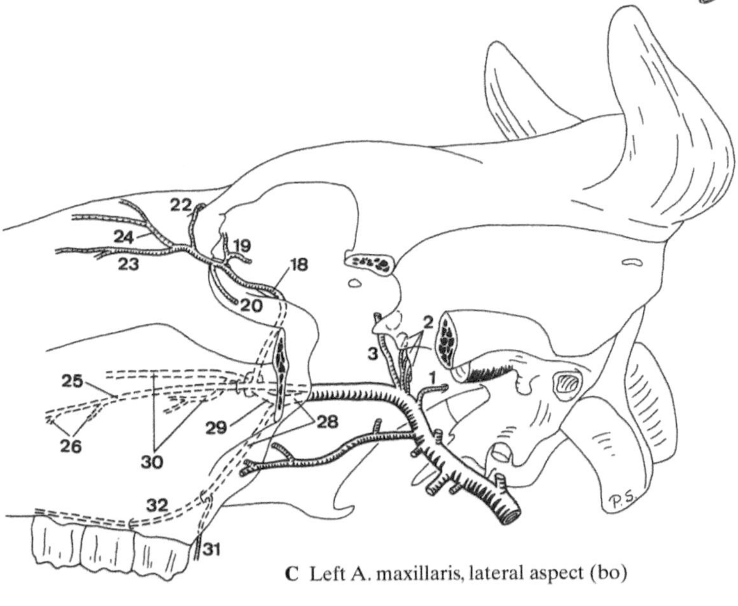

C Left A. maxillaris, lateral aspect (bo)

EQUUS

1 **A. occipitalis**. Arises in common with, or immediately rostral to A. carotis interna and pursues a somewhat flexuous course to Fossa atlantis. A B

2 ***Ramus glandularis***. To Gl. mandibularis. A B

3 ***A. condylaris***. Passes rostrodorsally and divides in muscular and meningeal branches. The latter enter cranium via Foramen jugulare and Canalis n. hypoglossi. A B

4 ***Ramus occipitalis***. Continuation of the parent stem beyond its connection with Ramus anastomoticus cum a. occipitali from A. vertebralis. Extends towards Crista nuchae. A B

5 *A. meningea caudalis*. Runs rostrodorsally, comes through Foramen mastoideum into Meatus temporalis and reaches Cavum cranii to supply dura. A B

6 **Truncus linguofacialis**. Exceptionally absent common trunk for A. lingualis and A. facialis, from which also A. palatina ascendens arises. Runs rostroventrally along Stylohyoideum on the medial aspect of M. stylohyoideus. A B C

7 **A. palatina ascendens**. Runs rostrally between Stylohyoideum and M. stylopharyngeus and chiefly supplies Palatum molle. C

8 **A. lingualis**. Usually enters the tongue between M. hyoglossus and M. ceratohyoideus. C

9 ***Rami perihyoidei***. Branching vessels which arise near Os hyoideum and supply the latter, pharynx, and epiglottis. C

10 ***A. profunda linguae***. Runs rostrally in the tongue along the lateral aspect of M. genioglossus. C

11 *Rami dorsales linguae*. Course to Dorsum linguae. C

12 **A. facialis***. Courses rostroventrally on the medial surface of M. pterygoideus medialis, turns around Incisura vasorum facialium* and ascends on the face at the rostral border of M. masseter. A C

13 ***Ramus pharyngeus***. Inconstant branch to the pharyngeal wall. (The Ramus pharyngeus was omitted from the 5th edition of the N.A.V.)

14 ***A. sublingualis***. Courses rostroventrally between Mandibula and M. mylohyoideus and, after perforating the latter, runs along the ventral border of Gl. sublingualis polystomatica to the floor of the mouth. C

15 *A. submentalis*. Runs rostrally on the ventrolateral aspect of M. mylohyoideus. C

16 ***A. labialis inferior***. Passes rostrally to Labium inferius. A

17 *A. angularis oris*. To Angulus oris. A

18 ***A. labialis superior***. Courses rostrally to Labium superius. A

19 ***A. lateralis nasi***. Often double supply for Regio lateralis nasi. A

20 *Ramus anastomoticus cum a. infraorbitali*. Communication with branches of A. infraorbitalis. A

21 ***A. dorsalis nasi***. Passes rostrodorsally to Regio dorsalis nasi. A

22 ***A. angularis oculi***. Curves towards Angulus oculi medialis. A

23 **Ramus massetericus**. Courses cranioventrally across Ramus mandibulae and continues on the ventral aspect of M. masseter. A B

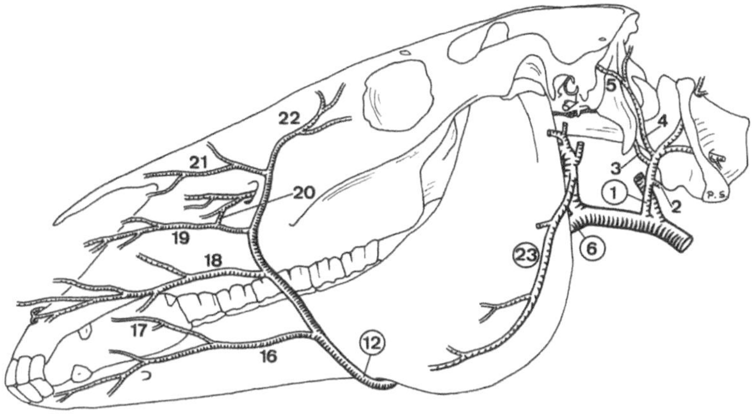

A Left A. facialis, lateral aspect (eq)

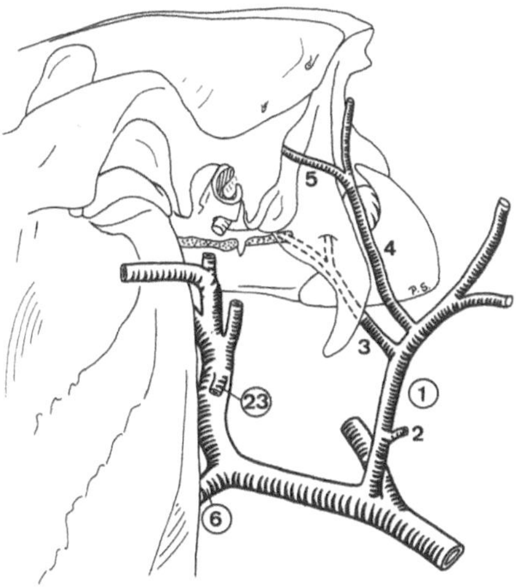

B Left A. occipitalis, lateral aspect (eq)

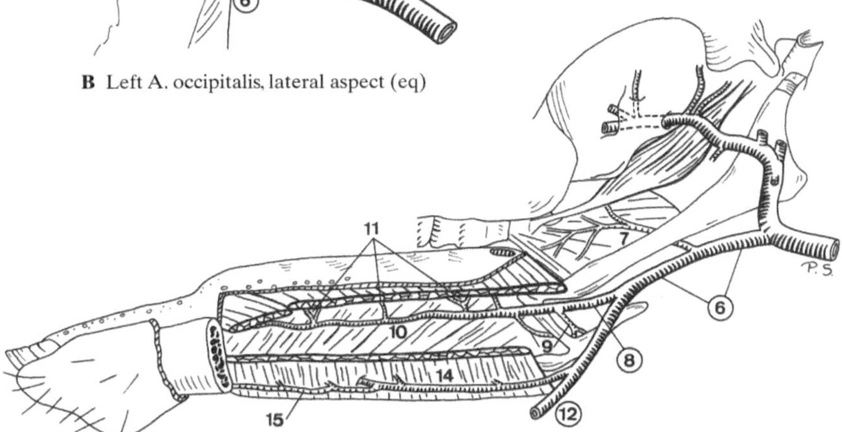

C Left Truncus linguofacialis, lateral aspect (eq)

1 **A. auricularis caudalis**. Passes dorsally to the base of the ear. A D

2 ***Rami parotidei***. Several branches to Gl. parotis. A

3 ***Ramus auricularis lateralis***. Runs towards the Apex auriculae on Dorsum auriculae, following Margo antitragicus. A

4 ***Ramus auricularis intermedius***. Passes apically in the middle of Dorsum auriculae. A

5 ***Ramus auricularis medialis***. Runs apically along Margo tragicus on Dorsum auriculae. A

6 ***Ramus occipitalis***. Courses towards Regio occipitalis and Regio temporalis. A

7 ***A. auricularis profunda***. Courses between Meatus acusticus externus and Processus mastoideus and gives off muscular branches and one or more branches to the interior of Auris externa. A B C

8 *A. stylomastoidea*. Passes through or near Foramen stylomastoideum into Cavum tympani. C

9 *A. tympanica caudalis*. Supplies Auris media and its muscles. C

10 **A. temporalis superficialis**. Passes dorsally between Auris externa and Articulatio temporomandibularis and finally divides in muscular branches at the level of M. temporalis. A D

11 ***A. transversa faciei***. Courses rostrally upon M. masseter and supplies it. A D

12 ***Ramus articularis temporomandibularis***. To the homonymous joint. A

13 ***A. auricularis rostralis***. Courses to the rostral part of the base of the ear. A

14 **A. maxillaris**. Curves to Basis cranii externa and passes through Canalis alaris to Fossa pterygopalatina. A B D

15 ***A. alveolaris inferior****. Passes ventrorostrally and pierces through Foramen mandibulae* into Canalis mandibulae. A B D

16 *Rami dentales*. To the mandibular teeth. D

17 *A. mentalis**. Emerges through Foramen mentale*. D

18 ***Rami pterygoidei***. To Mm. pterygoidei. A B

19 ***A. tympanica rostralis***. Courses along Tuba auditiva and pierces through Fissura petrotympanica into Auris media. B C

20 ***A. meningea media***. Runs caudally, enters Cavum cranii through Incisura spinosa and supplies dura. B C

21 ***A. temporalis profunda caudalis***. Passes caudodorsally into M. temporalis. A B

22 ***A. temporalis profunda rostralis***. Emerges from Canalis alaris through Foramen alare parvum and chiefly supplies M. temporalis. A B

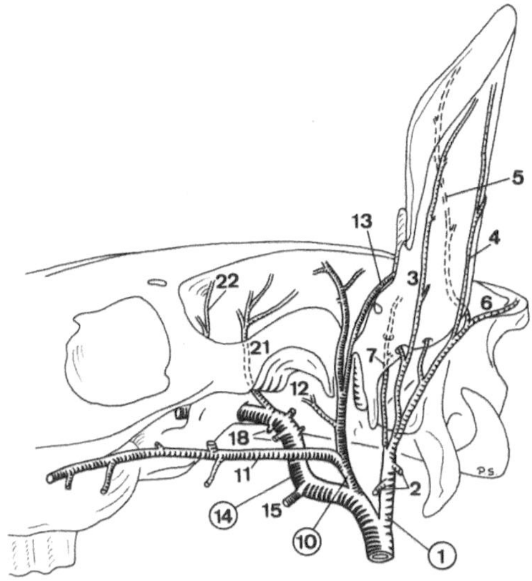

A Auricular arteries, left lateral aspect (eq)

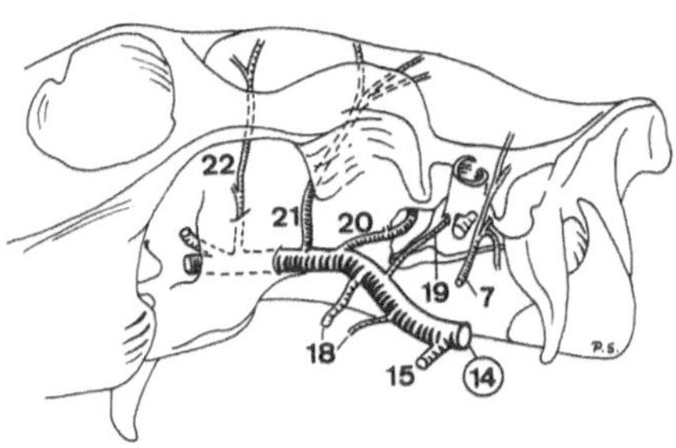

B Left A. maxillaris, ventrolateral aspect (eq)

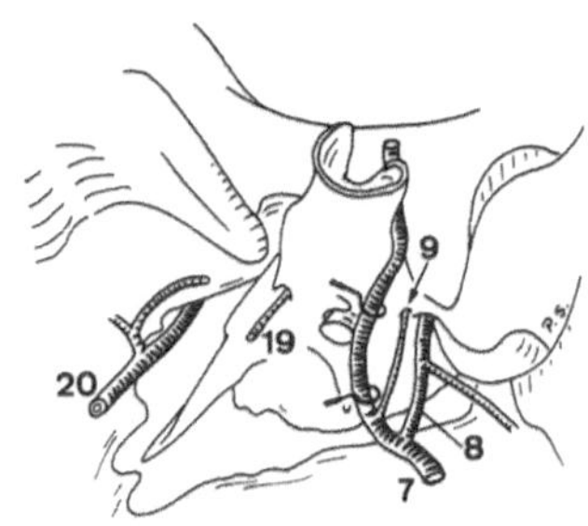

C Arteries in relation to left temporal bone, ventrolateral aspect (eq)

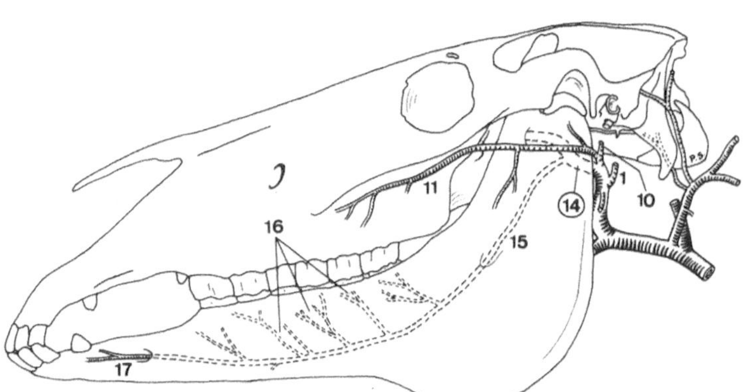

D Arteries of the head, left lateral aspect (eq)

1 **A. ophthalmica externa**. Leaves Canalis alaris through Foramen alare rostrale, enters periorbita, courses between Mm. recti dorsalis and lateralis, to the dorsal aspect of M. retractor bulbi. A B C

2 *Ramus anastomoticus cum a. ophthalmica interna*. Courses to the medial aspect of N. opticus where it joins A. ophthalmica interna. A B

3 **A. centralis retinae**. Collective term for the extrabulbar stem vessels for the Arteriolae retinae. A

4 **Aa. ciliares posteriores longae**. Lateral and medial arteries that pierce the posterior part of sclera and run anteriorly in Lamina suprachoroidea to Corpus ciliare and iris. A B

5 **Aa. ciliares posteriores breves**. Short branches of Aa. ciliares posteriores longae that perforate sclera near Area cribrosa and ramify in choroidea. A B

6 **Aa. episclerales**. Supply sclera from outside. A B

7 *Rami musculares*. Variably arising branches for Mm. bulbi. A B

8 **Aa. ciliares anteriores**. Pierce through sclera near Sulcus sclerae and ramify in Tunica vasculosa. A

9 **Aa. episclerales**. Course on sclera and supply it. A

10 *Aa. conjunctivales posteriores*. To Tunica conjunctiva. A

11 *A. supraorbitalis*. Pierces through Foramen supraorbitale accompanied by N. frontalis. A B C

12 *A. lacrimalis*. Runs rostrodorsally within periorbita into Gl. lacrimalis. A B

13 **A. palpebralis superior lateralis**. Courses from lateral in Palpebra superior. B

14 **A. palpebralis inferior lateralis**. Enters Palpebra inferior from lateral. B

15 *A. ethmoidalis externa*. Enters Cavum cranii via Foramen ethmoidale accompanied by N. ethmoidalis and passes through Lamina cribrosa towards Cavum nasi. A B C

16 **A. meningea rostralis**. Arises at Fossa ethmoidalis and ramifies in the rostral part of dura. A B C

17 *A. palpebrae tertiae*. To Palpebra tertia. A B

18 ***A. buccalis***. Courses between Tuber maxillae and Ramus mandibulae, ramifies in the cheek structures. A B C

19 ***A. infraorbitalis***. Passes through Foramen maxillare in Canalis infraorbitalis and emerges from Foramen infraorbitale with variable size accompanied by N. infraorbitalis. A B C

20 *A. malaris*. Passes between periorbita and the rostromedial wall of Orbita into structures at Angulus oculi medialis. C

21 **A. palpebralis superior medialis**. Pursues a lateral course in Palpebra superior. C

22 **A. palpebralis inferior medialis**. Supplies the medial part of Palpebra inferior. C

23 Rami dentales. To the superior teeth. C

24 ***A. palatina descendens***. Variably dividing rostroventral continuation of A. maxillaris accompanied by N. pterygopalatinus. A B C

25 *A. palatina minor*. Runs rostroventrally at the medial side of Tuber maxillae to Palatum molle accompanied by N. palatinus minor. May be absent. C

26 *A. palatina major*. Enters Foramen palatinum majus, traverses Canalis palatinus major and continues rostrally in Sulcus palatinus accompanied by N. palatinus major. Anastomoses with its heterolateral counterpart and then enters as a single vessel in Canalis interincisivus. C

27 *A. sphenopalatina*. Passes through Foramen sphenopalatinum into Cavum nasi accompanied by N. nasalis caudalis. C

28 **Aa. nasales caudales, laterales et septales**. Supply the caudoventral parts of Tunica mucosa nasi. C

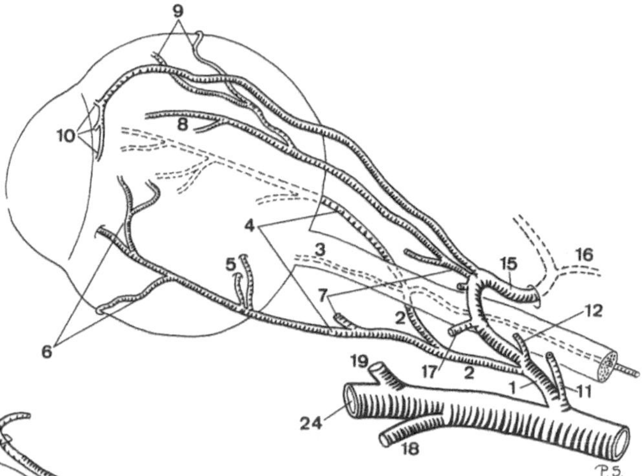

A Left A. ophthalmica externa, lateral aspect (eq)

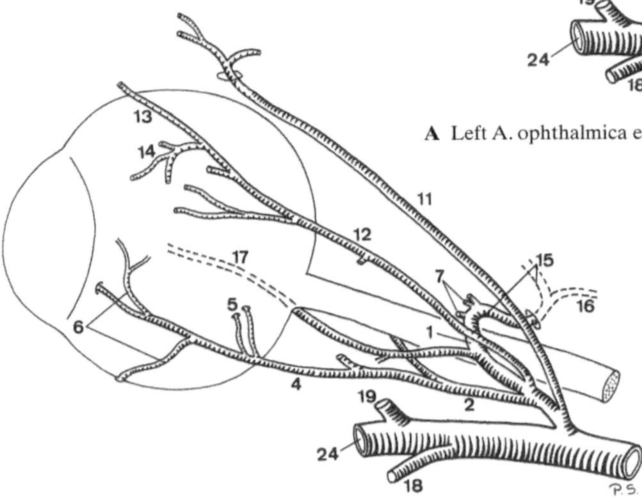

B Left A. ophthalmica externa, lateral aspect (eq)

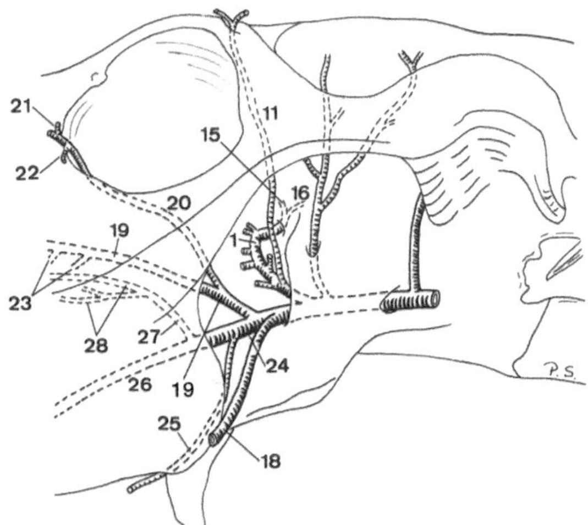

C Left A. maxillaris, ventrolateral aspect (eq)

TERMINI COMMUNES

1 **ARTERIA CAROTIS INTERNA**. Arises from A. carotis communis, often together with A. occipitalis (esp. su, Ru). Enters Cavum cranii through Canalis caroticus (Car), Foramen jugulare (su), Fissura petrooccipitalis (Ru), or Incisura carotica (eq). The extracranial segment is regressed in the adult fe, su, Ru. A B C D E F

2 ***Glomus caroticum***. Small nodule containing epitheloid chemoreceptor cells, located at the division of A. carotis communis. B

3 ***Sinus caroticus***. Variably distinct enlargement at the origin of A. carotis interna. D E

4 ***A. caroticobasilaris*** (eq). Inconstant caudomedially directed connection between A. carotis interna and A. basilaris. A

5 ***A. intercarotica caudalis*** (Car, eq). Connects both Aa. carotides internae at the caudal aspect of hypophysis. May be slightly reticulated (esp. Car). A C

6 ***A. intercarotica rostralis*** (Car). Connection between left and right A. carotis interna or A. cerebri rostralis (fe), located at the rostral aspect of hypophysis. C

SUS

7 **A. occipitalis**. Dorsal branch of A. carotis interna. B F

8 ***Ramus occipitalis***. Continuation of A. occipitalis beyond the connection with Ramus communicans cum a. occipitali from A. vertebralis. Runs towards Crista nuchae. B F

9 *A. meningea caudalis*. Enters Cavum cranii via Meatus temporalis and ramifies in dura. B

10 **A. condylaris**. Reaches Fossa condylaris ventralis and enters Cavum cranii through Canalis n. hypoglossi and Foramen jugulare. B F

11 ***A. stylomastoidea***. Pierces through Foramen stylomastoideum and traverses Canalis facialis in order to reach Auris media. B

12 ***Rete mirabile epidurale caudale***. Epidurally located arterial network at the level of atlas. Formed by the terminal segment of A. vertebralis, its Ramus spinalis that enters between atlas and axis, and A. condylaris. F

13 **Ramus ad rete mirabile epidurale rostrale**. Large branch that courses to Foramen lacerum where it joins Rete mirabile epidurale rostrale. B F

14 **Rete mirabile epidurale rostrale**. Network of small arteries formed by branches of A. carotis interna, A. meningea media, A. meningea rostralis, and A. maxillaris. Consists of an extracranial and an intracranial part. F

RUMINANTIA

15 **A. occipitalis**. Arises with the vestigial A. carotis interna at the level of transition between A. carotis communis and A. carotis externa. D E

16 ***A. palatina ascendens*** (bo). Crosses the pharyngeal wall and supplies Palatum molle. D E

17 ***A. stylomastoidea profunda*** (bo). Passes through Foramen stylomastoideum into Auris media. D E

18 ***A. meningea media***. Enters Cavum cranii via Foramen jugulare. D E

19 ***A. condylaris***. Runs into Fossa condylaris ventralis and, frequently double, enters Cavum cranii through the likewise double Canalis n. hypoglossi. Joins A. vertebralis and Rete mirabile epidurale caudale (bo). D E

20 ***Ramus occipitalis***. Continuation of A. occipitalis beyond the contact with Ramus anastomoticus cum a. occipitali from A. vertebralis or A. condylaris. Ramifies on the nuchal aspect of Os occipitale. D E

21 *A. meningea caudalis*. Reaches meninges via the openings near Margo mastoideus of Squama occipitalis. May be absent (bo). D

22 **Rete mirabile epidurale rostrale**. Anastomotic arterial network located in Sinus cavernosus. Developed in the intracranial course of A. carotis interna, supplied by branches of A. maxillaris. Continuous with Rete mirabile epidurale caudale (bo). E

23 ***Rete chiasmaticum*** (bo). Reticular extension of Rete mirabile epidurale rostrale to Chiasma opticum. E

24 *A. ophthalmica interna*. Accompanies N. opticus through Canalis opticus to the Orbita, where it anastomoses with A. ophthalmica externa. E

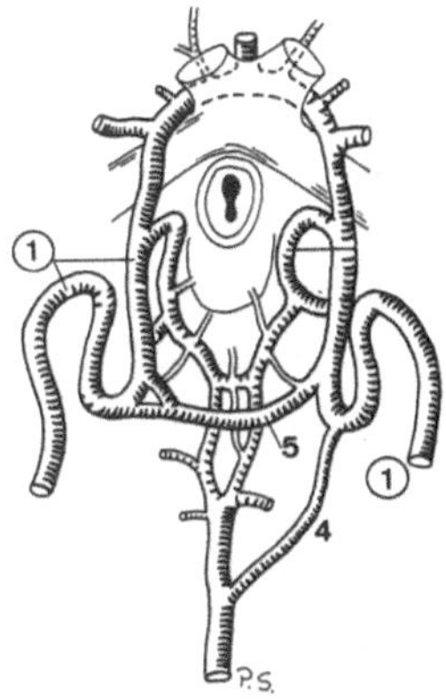

A Aa. carotides internae, ventral aspect (eq)

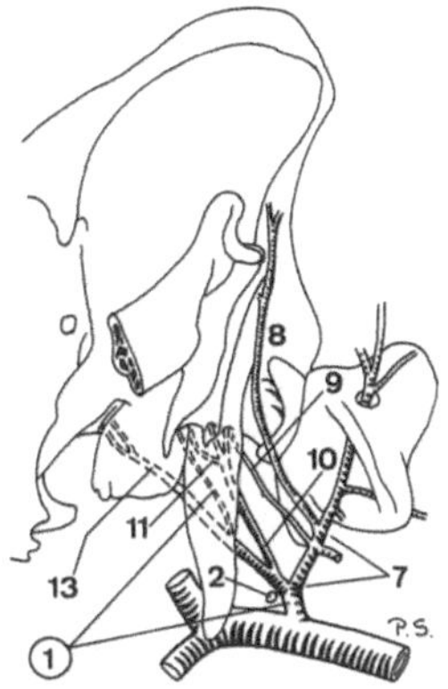

B Left A. carotis interna, lateral aspect (su)

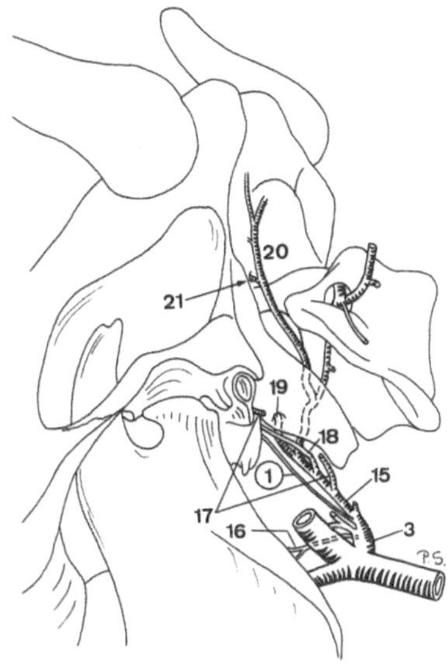

D Left A. carotis interna, lateral aspect (bo)

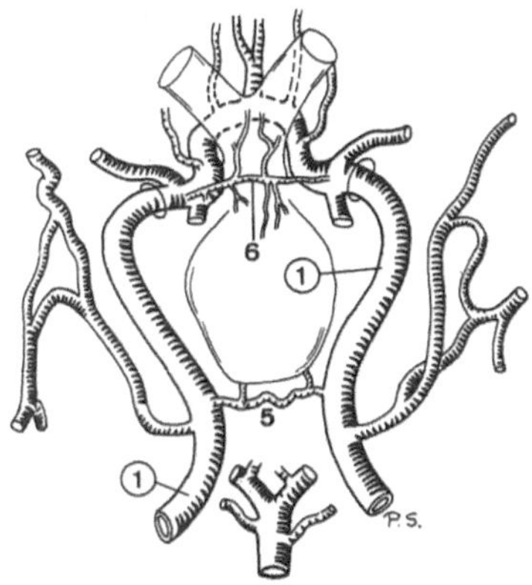

C Aa. carotides internae, ventral aspect (ca)

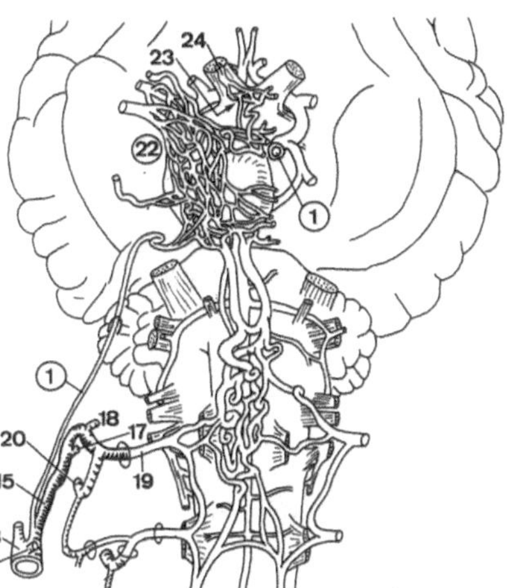

E Aa. carotides internae, ventral aspect (bo)

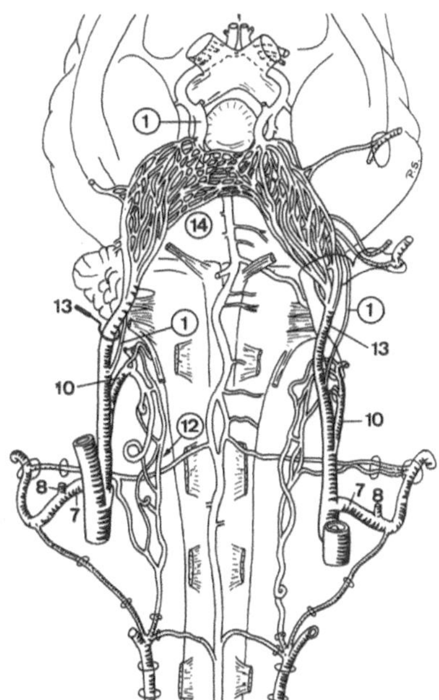

F Aa. carotides internae, ventral aspect (su)

TERMINI COMMUNES

1 **ARTERIAE CEREBRI**. Supply the brain.

2 ***Circulus arteriosus cerebri***. Willis' arterial circle, surounds Hypophysis and Chiasma opticum. Formed by A. communicans rostralis, Aa. cerebri rostrales, and Aa. communicantes caudales. A B

3 ***A. choroidea [chorioidea] rostralis***. Mainly contributes to Plexus choroideus ventriculi lateralis. A B

4 **A. cerebri rostralis**. Originates directly from A. carotis interna, forms the rostrolateral quadrant of Circulus arteriosus cerebri and continues curving on Facies medialis of Hemispherium. A B C (Three segments are considered as parts of this artery: the initial part is situated between the terminal division of A. carotis interna and the origin of A. cerebri media; the second segment extends between the origin of A. cerebri media and the Chiasma opticum, where the symmetrical arteries join with each other and form the A. communicans rostralis; the third segment runs rostrally in the Fissura longitudinalis cerebri and curves caudally at the Genu corporis callosi to continue caudally on Facies medialis of Hemispherium [Simoens et al. 1978].)

5 ***A. ophthalmica interna***. Accompanies N. opticus through Canalis opticus, anastomoses with A. ophthalmica externa. Given off by Rete mirabile epidurale rostrale through Rete chiasmaticum in bo. A B C

6 *A. meningea rostralis* (fe). Rostrally directed single branch to Dura mater encephali. Arises from the intracranial connection between both Aa. ophthalmicae internae. B

7 ***A. ethmoidalis interna***. Courses rostrally to Fossa ethmoidalis where it ramifies. A C

8 ***A. communicans rostralis***. Connection between right and left A. cerebri rostralis just rostral to Chiasma opticum. Constant in su, inconstant in Car and Ru, absent in eq. Occasionally plural in su and Ru. C

9 ***Rami corticales***. Supply Cortex cerebri. A C

10 ***Rami centrales***. Penetrate deeply into the brain. A

11 **A. cerebri media**. Arises from Circulus arteriosus cerebri, passes laterally to Lobus piriformis. Represented by two or three branches in su. A B C

12 ***Rami corticales***. To Cortex cerebri. A C

13 ***Rami centrales***. Penetrate into the brain. A

14 *Rami striati*. Supply Corpus striatum and associated structures. A

15 **A. communicans caudalis**. Connects A. carotis interna with A. basilaris and forms the caudolateral quadrant of Circulus arteriosus cerebri. A B C

16 ***A. cerebri caudalis***. Originating from the caudolateral part of Circulus arteriosus cerebri, courses dorsolaterally around Crus cerebri. Often double in eq, plural in ca. A B C

17 *Rami choroidei [choriodei] caudales*. Reach Plexus choroideus ventriculi tertii. A

18 *Rami corticales*. To the cortex. A C

19 *Rami centrales*. Penetrate into the brain. A

20 ***A. cerebelli rostralis***. Arises from A. communicans caudalis, occasionally (su, ov, eq) from A. basilaris. Crosses Crus cerebri and courses dorsocaudally to the lateral aspect of cerebellum. May be plural (fe, su, ov, eq). A B C

21 **ARTERIA SUBCLAVIA**. Intrathoracic portion of the parent artery to Membrum thoracicum. The left arises from Arcus aortae (Car, su) or Truncus brachiocephalicus (Ru, eq), the right is usually given off by Truncus brachiocephalicus. D

CARNIVORA

22 **A. vertebralis**. Passes cranially inside Foramina transversaria of Vertebrae cervicales VI–I, turns dorsally through Incisura alaris and enters Canalis vertebralis via Foramen vertebrale laterale of atlas. Then the right and left join to form A. basilaris. A B C D

23 ***Rami spinales***. Enter Canalis vertebralis through the cervical Foramina intervertebralia. A D

24 *A. spinalis ventralis*. Unpaired vessel at Fissura mediana. A B C

25 ***Ramus anastomoticus cum a. occipitali***. Joins A. occipitalis. May be partially absent in fe. A

26 ***Ramus descendens***. Muscular branch, emerges dorsally through Incisura alaris. A

27 A. basilaris. Unpaired vessel on the ventral surface of rhombencephalon, formed by the union of both Aa. vertebrales. A B C

28 *A. cerebelli caudalis*. To the caudal aspect of cerebellum. May be plural or has a different origin. A B C

29 *A. labyrinthi*. Enters Meatus acusticus internus and supplies Auris interna. May have a different origin. A B C

30 *Rami ad pontem*. Branches for pons. May be absent in ca. A B C

B Circulus arteriosus cerebri, ventral aspect (fe)

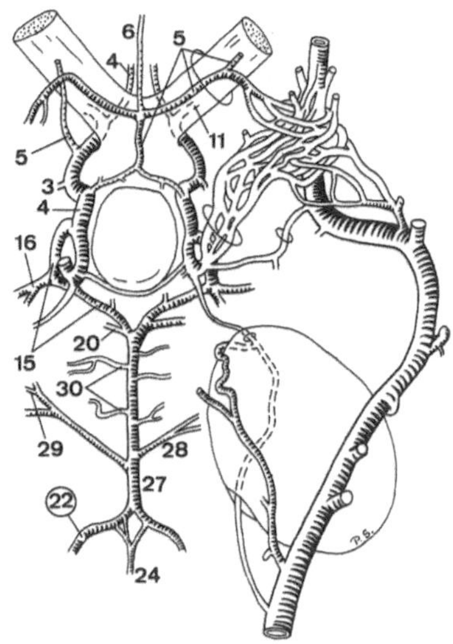

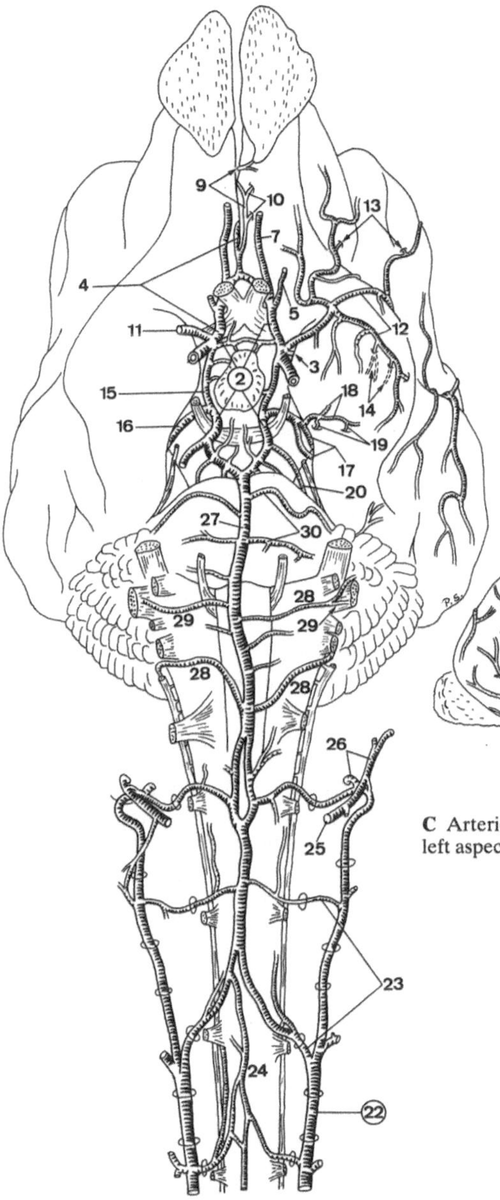

A Aa. cerebri and A. vertebralis, ventral aspect (ca)

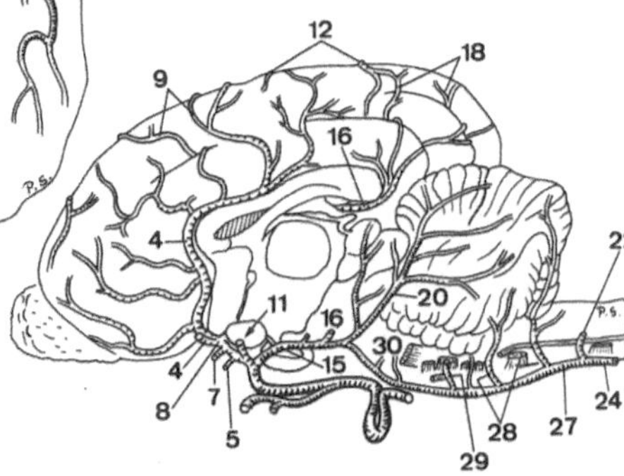

C Arteries of the brain (left hemisphere removed), left aspect (ca)

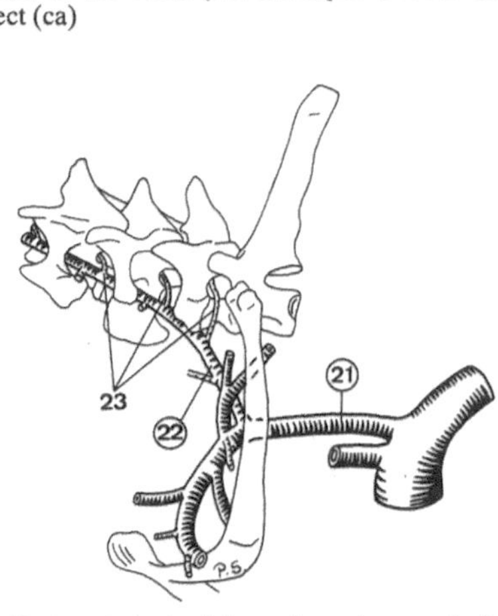

D A. subclavia sinistra, lateral aspect (ca)

1 **Truncus costocervicalis**. Dorsally directed arterial trunk. Inconstant in fe. A

2 ***A. intercostalis dorsalis*** I. Supplies the first Spatium intercostale. May even extend into the second and the third in Car. A

3 ***A. scapularis dorsalis***. Courses dorsally through the first Spatium intercostale or at the cranial aspect of Costa I. A

4 ***A. cervicalis profunda***. Leaves Cavum thoracis through the first Spatium intercostale and curves dorsocranially into the cervical musculature. A

5 ***A. vertebralis thoracica*** (ca). Courses caudally on the dorsal aspect of the necks of 2nd and 3rd ribs, therefore this artery of the dog is not homologous to A. intercostalis suprema of the other domestic mammals (which runs on the ventral aspects of the neck of the ribs). A (In the 5th edition of the N. A. V. [ca] is not mentioned. Maybe a typo mistake, since this artery is found only in the dog.)

6 *Aa. intercostales dorsales II et III*. Course ventrally in the corresponding Spatium intercostale. A

7 *Rami dorsales*. Course dorsally to Mm. dorsi. A

8 **Ramus spinalis**. Enters Canalis vertebralis via the corresponding Foramen intervertebrale. A

9 ***A. intercostalis suprema*** (fe). Courses caudally on the ventral aspects of the necks of the 2nd and 3rd ribs. May be absent. B

10 *Aa. intercostales dorsales II et III*. Course ventrally in the respective Spatium intercostale. B

11 **Ramus dorsalis**. Courses dorsally to Mm. dorsi. B

12 **Ramus spinalis**. Enters Canalis vertebralis via the corresponding Foramen intervertebrale. B

13 **A. thoracica interna**. Curves caudoventrally and passes between sternum and M. transversus thoracis. A

14 ***A. pericardiacophrenica***. Runs caudally with N. phrenicus to pericardium, and reaches Diaphragma occasionally. A

15 ***Rami thymici***. Supply thymus. May be single (esp. fe). A

16 ***Rami mediastinales***. Essentially to Mediastinum craniale. A

17 ***Rami perforantes***. Leave Cavum thoracis via the ventral parts of Spatia intercostalia. A

18 *Rami sternales*. To the sternebrae. A

19 *Rami mammarii*. Supply the medial portions of the Mammae thoracicae. A

20 ***Rami intercostales ventrales***. Frequently double segmental branches which supply the ventral parts of Spatia intercostalia II–VIII, usually absent in the second in fe. A

21 ***A. musculophrenica***. Courses caudodorsolaterally, perforates Diaphragma and continues subperitoneally. A

22 *Rami intercostales ventrales*. Often double segmental branches supplying the ventral parts of Spatia intercostalia VIII–X (XI). A

23 ***A. epigastrica cranialis***. Leaves thorax caudally and continues on the dorsal aspect of M. rectus abdominis. A

24 *A. epigastrica cranialis superficialis*. Perforates M. rectus abdominis and continues subcutaneously. A

25 **Rami mammarii**. To the caudal thoracic and cranial abdominal mammae. A

26 **A. cervicalis superficialis**. Dorsocranially directed arterial stem leaving Apertura thoracis cranialis. A C

27 ***Ramus deltoideus***. May have different origins. It accompanies V. cephalica in Sulcus pectoralis lateralis. A C

28 ***Ramus ascendens***. Cranially directed muscular branch at the medial aspect of M. cleidocephalicus. Frequently double. C

29 ***Ramus prescapularis [prae-]***. Continuation of A. cervicalis superficialis beyond the origin of A. suprascapularis. Runs parallel to Margo cranialis of scapula. C

30 ***A. suprascapularis***. Accompanies N. suprascapularis and divides at the cranial aspect of Collum scapulae. C

31 *Ramus acromialis*. Courses on the lateral aspect of scapula and crosses Collum scapulae. C

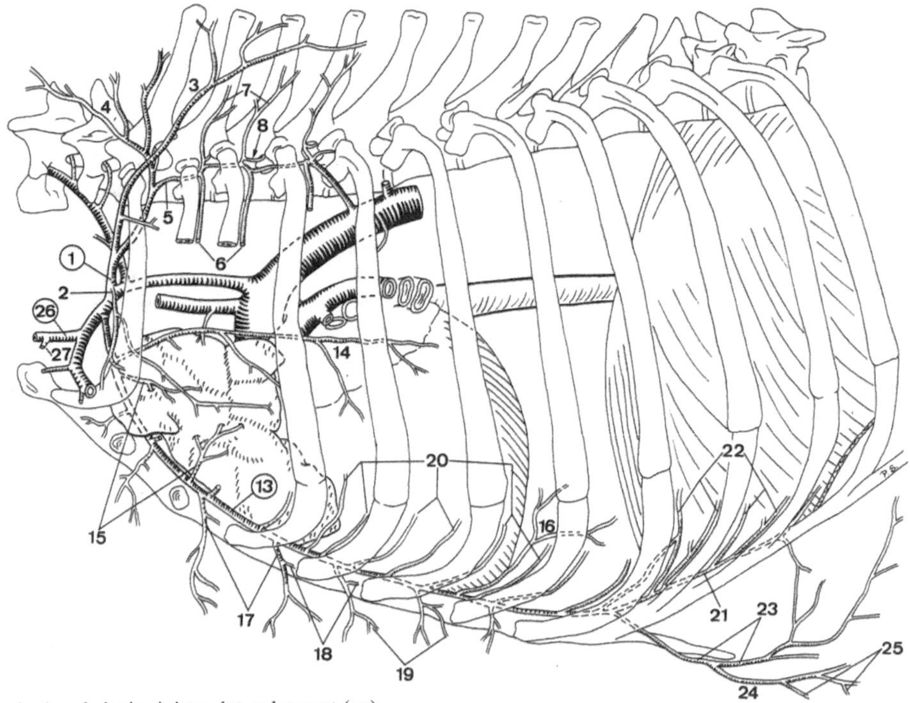

A A. subclavia sinistra, lateral aspect (ca)

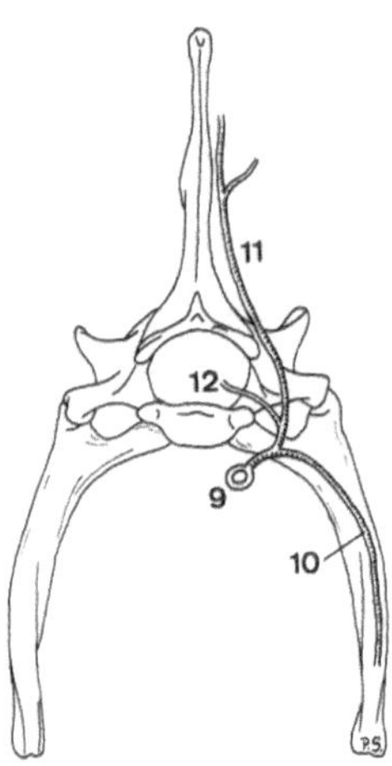

B Branches of right A. intercostalis suprema, caudal aspect (fe)

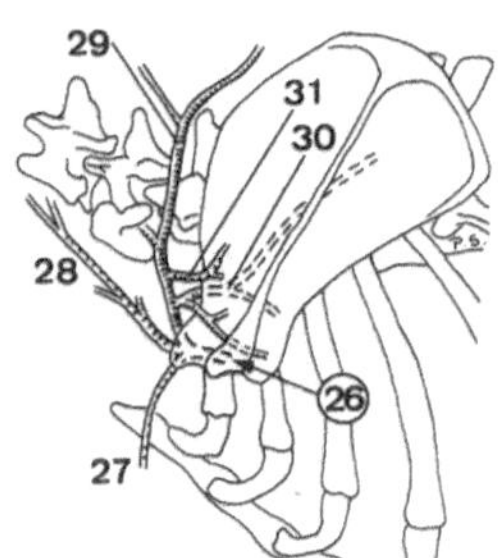

C Left A. cervicalis superficialis, lateral aspect (ca)

SUS

1 **A. vertebralis.** Courses cranially inside Foramina transversaria of Vertebrae cervicales (VI) V–I, continues through Fossa atlantis, Foramen alare, and Foramen vertebrale laterale of atlas. Then the right and left arteries connect with A. basilaris. A B C

2 ***A. intercostalis dorsalis I dextra.*** May have different origins. It courses ventrally in the first Spatium intercostale. C

3 ***Rami spinales.*** Enter Canalis vertebralis through the cervical Foramina intervertebralia (VIII) VII–III and Foramen vertebrale laterale of axis. A B C

4 *A. spinalis dorsalis.* Small, near Radices dorsales of Nervi spinales. B

5 *A. spinalis ventralis.* Unpaired at Fissura mediana. B

6 ***Ramus anastomoticus cum a. occipitali.*** Arises in Fossa atlantis and joins A. occipitalis. A B

7 ***Ramus descendens.*** Muscular branch, emerges dorsally trough Foramen alare. A B

8 ***Rete mirabile epidurale caudale.*** Arterial network near the beginning of canalis vertebralis. Supplied by A. vertebralis and A. condylaris. B (This term was omitted from the 5th edition of the N. A. V. It is already listed at page 270.12.)

9 A. basilaris. Unpaired vessel on the ventral surface of rhombencephalon. Formed by the union of both Aa. vertebrales. B

10 *A. cerebelli caudalis.* Courses dorsolaterally to the caudal aspect of cerebellum. Exceptionally double. B

11 *A. labyrinthi.* Enters Meatus acusticus internus and supplies Auris interna. B

12 *Rami ad pontem.* Branches for pons. B

13 **A. scapularis dorsalis.** Leaves Cavum thoracis via the first Spatium intercostale and/or pierces through Foramen vertebrale laterale of Vertebra thoracica I. A C

14 ***A. intercostalis dorsalis II.*** Courses ventrally in the second Spatium intercostale. A

15 **Truncus costocervicalis.** Common stem for A. cervicalis profunda and A. intercostalis suprema. Occasionally absent. A C

16 ***A. cervicalis profunda.*** Passes through Foramen vertebrale laterale of Vertebra thoracica II. A C

17 *A. intercostalis dorsalis I sinistra.* Courses ventrally in the first Spatium intercostale. A

18 ***A. intercostalis suprema.*** Runs on the dorsolateral aspect of M. longus colli. A C

19 *Aa. intercostales dorsales III–V.* Course ventrally in the corresponding Spatium intercostale. A C

20 **Ramus dorsalis.** Courses dorsally and passes through Foramen vertebrale laterale of the corresponding vertebra. Frequently double. A C

21 **Ramus spinalis.** Passes through Foramen intervertebrale or Foramen vertebrale laterale. A C

22 **Truncus thyrocervicalis [thyreo-].** Trunk for A. cervicalis superficialis and A. thyroidea caudalis, usually only on the right side. C

23 ***A. thyroidea [thyreoidea] caudalis dextra.*** Courses cranially to Gl. thyroidea. C

24 **A. cervicalis superficialis.** Courses in a craniodorsal direction. C

25 *Ramus ascendens.* Craniodorsally directed muscular branch. C

26 *Ramus prescapularis [prae-].* Continuation of A. cervicalis superficialis along the cranial border of M. subclavius. C

27 *Ramus acromialis.* Enters the lateral aspect of M. supraspinatus, crosses Collum scapulae laterally. C

28 **A. cervicalis superficialis sinistra.** Courses cranioventrally and continues craniodorsally. A

29 ***Ramus ascendens.*** Craniodorsally directed muscular branch along the medial aspect of M. cleidocephalicus. A

30 ***Ramus prescapularis [prae-].*** Courses along the cranial border of M. subclavius. A

31 ***Ramus acromialis.*** Enters the lateral aspect of M. supraspinatus and crosses Collum scapulae laterally. A

Note: The labels 22 and 23 are omitted from the 5th edition of the N.A.V. The labels 24 to 27 indicate branches of the A. cervicalis superficialis dextra, whereas the labels 28 to 31 indicate branches of the A. cervicalis superficialis sinistra, as it shows on the next page. None of the terms “dextra” or “sinistra” are listed in the 5th edition of the N.A.V. The 5th edition is listing only the A. cervicalis superficialis with its three branches.

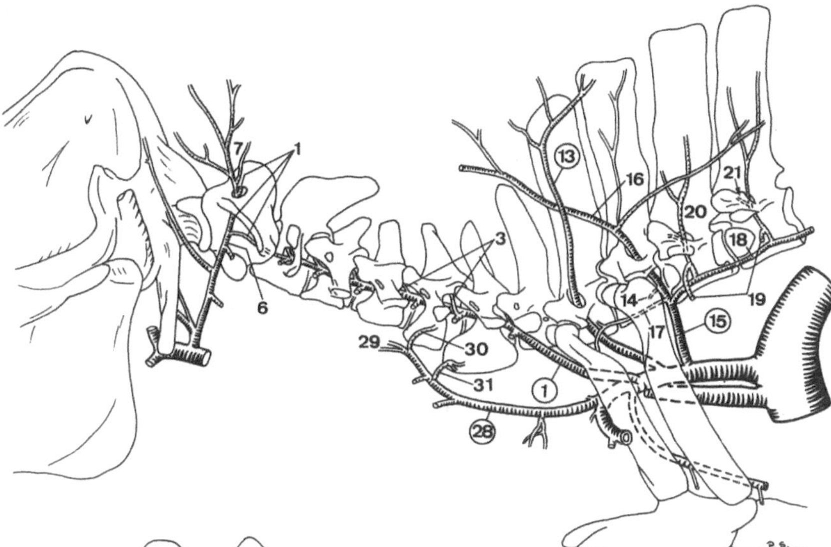

A A. subclavia sinistra, lateral aspect (su)

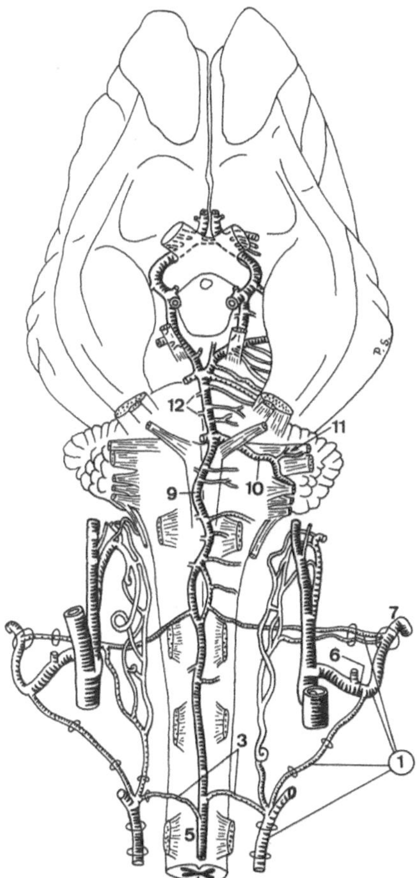

B A. vertebralis, ventral aspect (su)

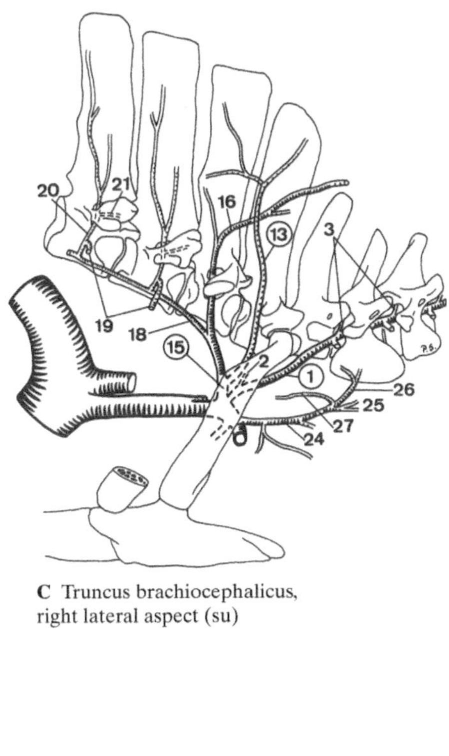

C Truncus brachiocephalicus, right lateral aspect (su)

1 **A. thoracica interna**. Courses caudoventrally and continues caudally on the ventral aspect of M. transversus thoracis. A

2 ***A. pericardiacophrenica***. Courses caudally to pericardium and may reach Diaphragma. Occasionally absent. A

3 ***Rami thymici***. To Thymus. A

4 ***Rami mediastinales***. Lie in Mediastinum craniale. A

5 ***Rami perforantes***. Perforate Mm. intercostales near sternum. A

6 *Rami sternales*. To sternum. A

7 *Rami mammarii*. Supply the Mammae thoracicae. A

8 ***Rami intercostales ventrales***. Supply the ventral parts of the first 6 or 7 Spatia intercostalia. May be absent or indistinct in some segments. A

9 ***A. musculophrenica***. Pierces through Diaphragma after coursing caudodorsally along the medial aspect of Arcus costalis. A

10 *Rami intercostales ventrales*. Supply the ventral parts of Spatia intercostalia (VI) VII and VIII. A

11 ***A. epigastrica cranialis***. Courses caudally on the dorsal aspect of M. rectus abdominis. A

12 *Rami intercostales ventrales*. Run dorsally to Spatia intercostalia IX–XII (XIII). May be absent in the caudal segments. A

13 *Ramus costoabdominalis ventralis*. Courses dorsally on the caudal aspect of last rib. A

14 *Rami mammarii*. To the first two Mammae abdominales. A

RUMINANTIA

15 **Truncus costocervicalis**. Craniodorsally directed, variably branching arterial trunk, given off by A. subclavia. B

16 ***A. scapularis dorsalis***. Crosses the vertebral end of the first rib cranially, and continues caudodorsally. B

17 ***A. intercostalis suprema***. Courses caudally on the ventral aspect of the necks of 1st, 2nd (3rd) rib, exceptionally on their dorsal aspect (cap, ov). B

18 *Aa. intercostales dorsales I et II (III)*. Course ventrally at the caudal margin of the corresponding rib. B

19 **Ramus dorsalis**. Runs dorsally to Mm. dorsi. B

20 **Ramus spinalis**. Given off by Ramus dorsalis, occasionally by A. intercostalis dorsalis (bo). Enters Canalis vertebralis via the corresponding Foramen vertebrale laterale (bo) or Foramen intervertebrale (ov, cap). B

21 ***A. cervicalis profunda***. Passes dorsally at the caudal (exceptionally cranial) aspect of Processus transversus of the seventh Vertebra cervicalis. Continues far cranially in the neck (bo). B

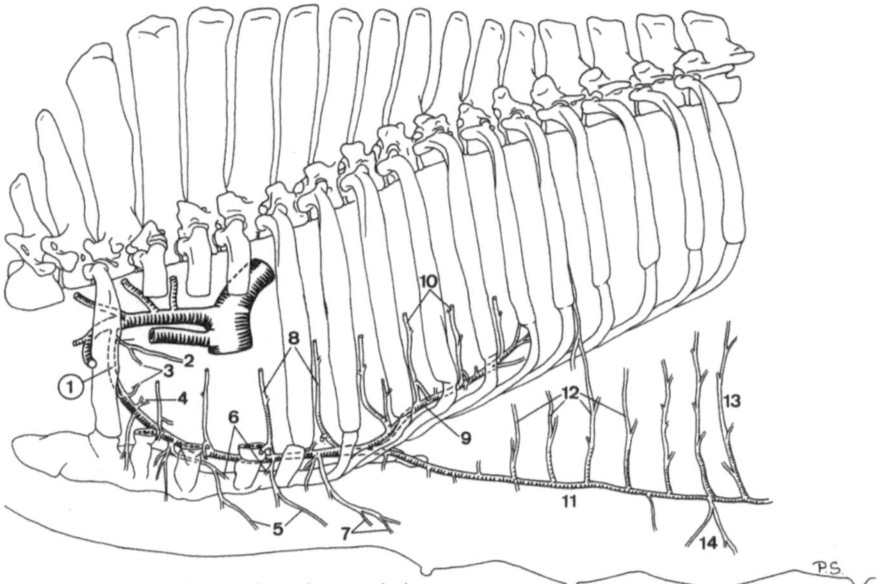

A Left A. thoracica interna, lateral aspect (su)

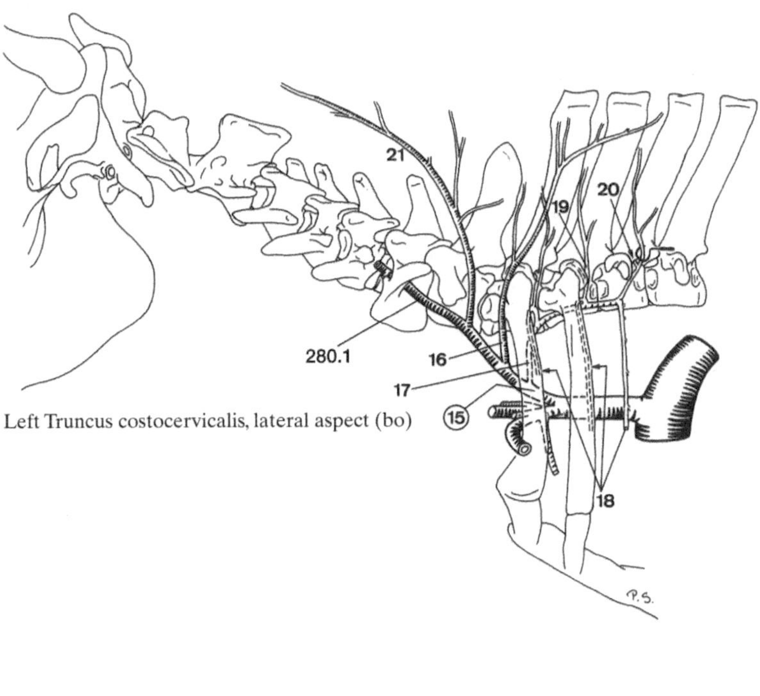

B Left Truncus costocervicalis, lateral aspect (bo)

1 **A. vertebralis**. Continuation of Truncus costocervicalis that courses craniodorsally through Foramina transversaria of Vertebrae cervicales VI–III. Then most blood is conducted in Canalis vertebralis by the Ramus spinalis between Vertebrae cervicales II and III (exc. III and IV). The course along the lateral aspect of atlas and axis is represented by a branch which usually traverses the Foramen transversarium of axis and gives rise to small branches which join Ramus descendens and Ramus anastomoticus cum a occipitali. A B 279 B

2 ***Rami spinales***. Enter the Foramina intervertebralia VII (except some ov), VI–III and Foramen vertebrale laterale of axis. A B

3 *A. spinalis dorsalis*. Irregular vessel along Radices dorsales of Nervi spinales. Absent at some levels. B

4 *A. spinalis ventralis*. Unpaired vessel at Fissura mediana. B

5 A. basilaris. Large unpaired vessel between the union of both Aa. communicantes caudales and A. spinalis ventralis. B

6 **A. cerebelli caudalis**. Courses dorsolaterally to the caudal aspect of cerebellum. B

7 **A. labyrinthi**. Enters Meatus acusticus internus and supplies Auris interna. B

8 **Rami ad pontem**. Branches for pons. B

9 ***Ramus descendens***. Large muscular branch which emerges through Foramen vertebrale laterale of atlas. A B

10 *Ramus anastomoticus cum a. occipitali*. Passes through Foramen alare to join A. occipitalis. Sometimes absent in bo and ov. A B

11 ***Rete mirabile epidurale caudale***. Epidural arterial network at Os occipitale. Formed in the ox by A. vertebralis and A. condylaris. Continuous with the Rete mirabile epidurale rostrale. It is absent in the sheep and goat. B

12 **A. cervicalis superficialis**. Cranially directed branch of A. subclavia. A C D

13 ***Ramus deltoideus***. Accompanies V. cephalica in Sulcus pectoralis lateralis. Inconstant. A

14 ***Ramus ascendens***. Courses craniodorsally at the medial face of M. brachiocephalicus. A C

15 ***Ramus prescapularis [prae-]****. Courses at the cranial margin of M. supraspinatus. It supplies the enormous Ln. cervicalis superficiualis. A C

16 ***A. suprascapularis*** (ov, cap). Accompanies N. suprascapularis and extends across the craniomedial face of M. supraspinatus. C

17 *Ramus acromialis*. Courses laterally to the craniolateral aspect of M. supraspinatus. C

18 ***Ramus suprascapularis*** (bo). Small vessel accompanying N. suprascapularis. A

19 *Ramus acromialis*. Crosses M. supraspinatus cranially. A

20 **A. thoracica interna**. Curves caudoventrally and continues caudally on the ventral aspect of M. transversus thoracis. A D

21 ***A. pericardiacophrenica***. Courses caudally to pericardium and may reach Diaphragma. Occasionally absent. D

22 ***Rami thymici***. To thymus. Usually singular or even absent. D

23 ***Rami mediastinales***. To mediastinum. D

24 ***Rami perforantes***. Pass through the ventral parts of Spatia intercostalia I–VI. D

25 *Rami sternales*. To the adjacent Sternebrae. D

26 ***Rami intercostales ventrales***. Course dorsally at the caudal margin of Costae I–VI. D

27 ***A. musculophrenica***. Courses caudodorsally, perforates Diaphragma and continues parallel to Arcus costalis. D

28 *Rami intercostales ventrales*. Course dorsally along the caudal margin of Costae VII–VIII (IX, X). D

29 ***Ramus phrenicus***. Enters Pars sternalis of Diaphragma. D

30 ***A. epigastrica cranialis***. Pierces between Arcus costalis and Processus xiphoideus (bo, ov) or passes through Spatium intercostale VII (cap). Continues caudally to the dorsal aspect of M. rectus abdominis and finally enters it. D

31 *A. epigastrica cranialis superficialis*. Becomes subcutaneous. D

32 *Rami intercostales ventrales*. Course dorsally to Costae (IX, X) XI–XII. D

33 *Ramus costoabdominalis ventralis*. Runs dorsally towards the caudal aspect of the last rib. D

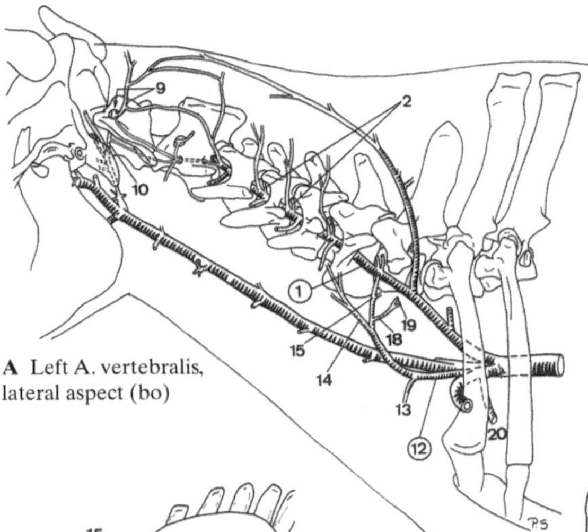

A Left A. vertebralis, lateral aspect (bo)

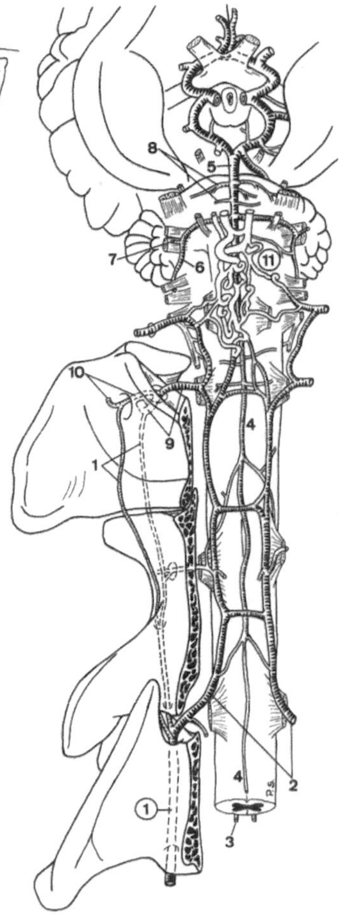

B A. vertebralis, ventral aspect (bo)

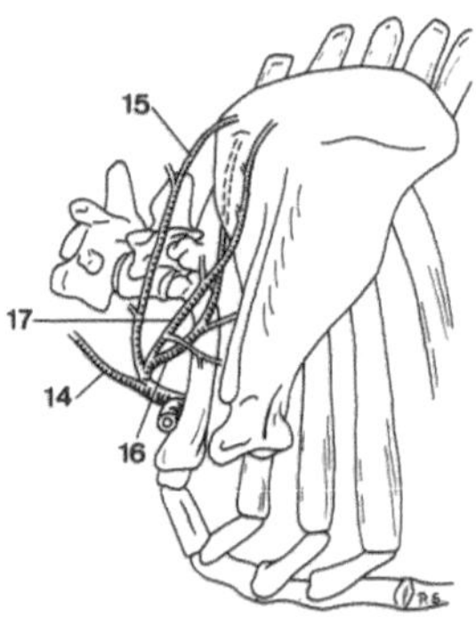

C Branches of left A. cervicalis superficialis, lateral aspect (ov)

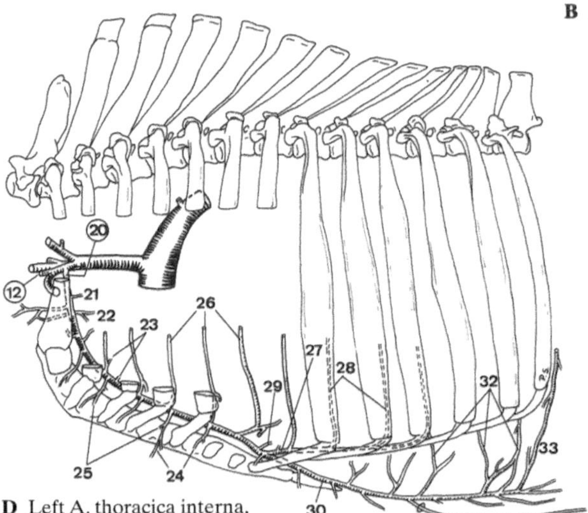

D Left A. thoracica interna, lateral aspect (bo)

EQUUS

1 **Truncus costocervicalis**. Dorsally directed arterial trunk. May arise from Truncus brachiocephalicus (esp. on the right), exceptionally from aorta. A C

2 ***A. intercostalis suprema***. Courses caudally on the lateral aspect of M. longus colli. A C

3 *Aa. intercostales dorsales II–V.* Course ventrally along the caudal margin of the corresponding rib. A

4 **Ramus dorsalis**. Courses dorsally to Mm. dorsi. A

5 **Ramus spinalis**. Through the corresponding Foramen intervertebrale in Canalis vertebralis. A

6 ***A. scapularis dorsalis***. Emerges through Spatium intercostale II (exc. III). A C

7 **A. cervicalis profunda**. Passes through Spatium intercostale I or II. May arise from Truncus costocervicalis. A C

8 ***A. intercostalis dorsalis I***. Runs ventrally in Spatium intercostale I. A

9 **A. vertebralis**. Courses through Foramina transversaria of Vertebrae cervicales (VII, VI), V–I, continues through Fossa atlantis, Foramen alare, and enters Canalis vertebralis via Foramen vertebrale laterale of atlas. Then both Aa. vertebrales join to form A. basilaris. Given off from Truncus brachiocephalicus on the right. A B C

10 ***Rami spinales***. Enter Canalis vertebralis via cervical Foramina intervertebralia VIII–III and Foramen vertebrale laterale of axis. A

11 *A. spinalis dorsalis*. On the dorsolateral aspect of Medulla spinalis. B

12 *A. spinalis ventralis*. Unpaired at Fissura mediana. B

13 ***Ramus anastomoticus cum a. occipitali***. Anastomosis with A. occipitalis. A B

14 ***Ramus descendens***. Muscular branch, emerges dorsally through Foramen alare. A B

15 A. basilaris. Unpaired, formed by the union of both Aa. vertebrales. Runs rostrally on the ventral surface of rhombencephalon. B

16 **Aa. cerebelli caudales**. Course laterally to the caudal aspect of cerebellum. Frequently singular. B

17 **A. labyrinthi**. Passes to Auris interna via Meatus acusticus internus. Usually given off by one of the Aa. cerebelli caudales. B

18 **Rami ad pontem**. Branches for pons. B

19 **A. thoracica interna**. Curves ventrocaudally and passes on the ventral aspect of M. transversus thoracis. A C

20 ***A. pericardiacophrenica***. Supplies pericardium and accompanies N. phrenicus to Diaphragma. C

21 ***Rami thymici***. To thymus. C

22 ***Rami mediastinales***. Supply Mediastinum craniale. C

23 ***Rami perforantes***. Perforate Mm. intercostales near sternum. C

24 *Rami sternales*. To sternum. C

25 ***Rami intercostales ventrales***. Course dorsally at the caudal margin of the first (6) 7 ribs. C

26 ***A. musculophrenica***. Runs caudodorsally, perforates Diaphragma and continues parallel to the costal arch. C

27 *Rami intercostales ventrales*. Course dorsally in Spatia intercostalia (VII) VIII–XI (–XVI). C

28 ***A. epigastrica cranialis***. Emerges between Cartilago costalis IX and Cartilago xiphoidea and passes into the abdominal wall. C

29 **A. cervicalis superficialis**. Cranioventrally directed. A C

30 ***Ramus deltoideus****. Accompanies V. cephalica in Sulcus pectoralis lateralis*. A

31 ***Ramus prescapularis [prae-]***. Runs parallel to the cranial border of M. subclavius. A

32 ***Ramus ascendens***. Courses craniodorsally at the medial side of M. brachiocephalicus. A

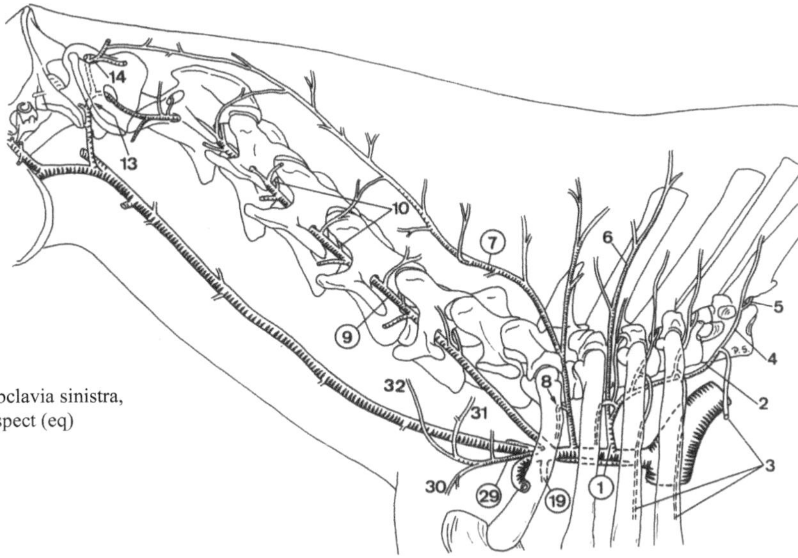

A A. subclavia sinistra, lateral aspect (eq)

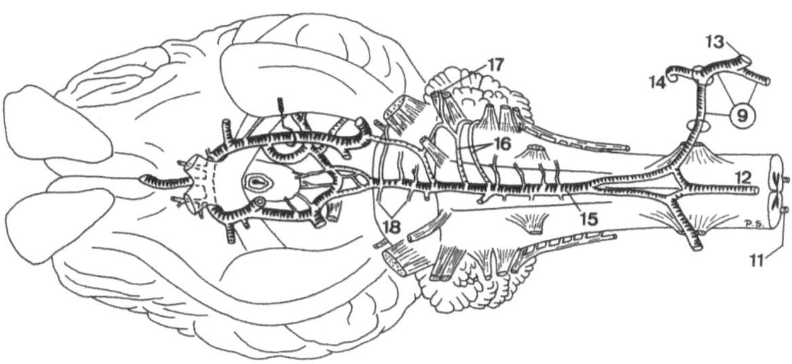

B Right A. thoracica interna, lateral aspect (eq)

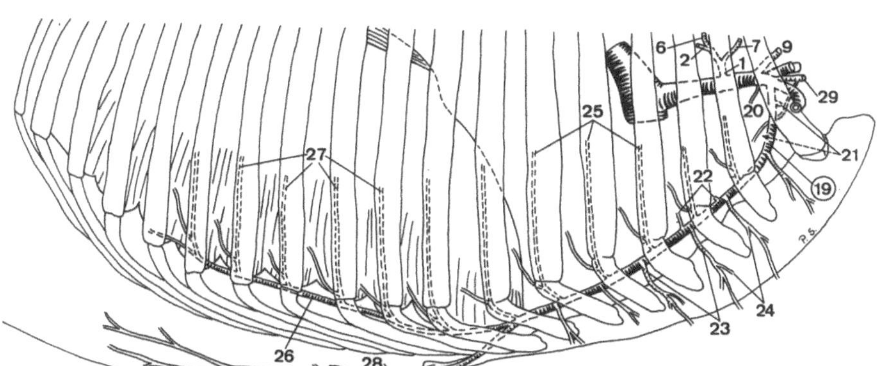

C A. basilaris, ventral aspect (eq)

TERMINUS COMMUNIS

1 **ARTERIA AXILLARIS.** Continuation of A. subclavia beyond the origin of A. cervicalis superficialis. A B (Some of the arteries nourishing the bones of the thoracic limb are not listed in the 5th edition of the N. A. V.)

CARNIVORA

2 ***Ramus deltoideus*** (ca). Accompanies V. cephalica in Sulcus pectoralis lateralis. B

3 ***A. thoracica externa.*** Courses across the cranial border of M. pectoralis profundus, supplies the pectoral muscles. B

4 ***A. thoracica lateralis.*** Runs caudally toward the ventral thoracic wall. B

5 *Rami mammarii laterales.* Supply the Mammae thoracicae. B

6 ***A. subscapularis.*** Courses along the caudal border of scapula. A B

7 *A. circumflexa humeri caudalis.* Courses across the caudal aspect of Articulatio humeri. A B

8 **A. collateralis radialis.** Accompanies N. radialis onto the surface of M. brachialis. A B

9 **A. nutricia humeri** (ca). Variable origin. See 17a. A B

10 **A. collateralis media.** Branch of A. collateralis radialis to Rete articulare cubiti. May be absent (ca). A B

11 *A. thoracodorsalis.* Passes across the medial surface of M. teres major to M. latissimus dorsi. A B

12 *A. circumflexa scapulae.* Passes craniodorsally across the lateral and medial aspects of scapula. A B

13 ***A. circumflexa humeri cranialis.*** Curves cranially along the medial aspect of humerus. A B

FELIS

14 **A. brachialis***. Runs distally with N. medianus, traverses Foramen supracondylare. A

15 ***A. profunda brachii.*** To the muscles of the caudal side of brachium. A

16 ***A. brachialis superficialis.*** Courses along M. biceps brachii to the cranial aspect to Articulatio cubiti. A

17 *A. bicipitalis.* Supplies M. biceps brachii. A

17a *A. nutricia humeri.* Spplies the humerus. A

18 *A. collateralis ulnaris.* Ramifies at olecranon. A

19 **Rete articulare cubiti.** Network at the caudal aspect of Articulatio cubiti supplied by many arteries, including A. collateralis media and A. recurrens interossea. A

20 *Aa. radiales superficiales.* Accompany N. cutaneus antebrachii medialis. A

21 *A. antebrachialis superficialis cranialis.* Courses along the craniomedial aspect of antebrachium. A C

21a A. digitalis dorsalis I abaxialis. Runs along the abaxial side of Digitus I.

22 **Arcus dorsalis superficialis.** Subcutaneous communication to Ramus dorsalis of A. ulnaris in Regio metacarpi dorsalis. C

23 **Aa. digitales dorsales communes I–IV.** Superficial branches of Arcus dorsalis superficialis. C

24 **Aa. digitales dorsales propriae.** Arise from the bifurcation of Aa. digitales dorsales communes. C

25 ***A. transversa cubiti.*** Curves laterally across the cranial surface of Articulatio cubiti. A

26 ***A. profunda antebrachii.*** Plural and variable, to caudal muscles of antebrachium. A (A. profunda antebrachii supplies in all species the muscles of the caudal side of the forearm. This term is a generic name for all major branches which supply those muscles, and arise with a species specific origin either from A. brachialis, or from A. mediana [Simoens et al. 1980].)

27 ***A. interossea cranialis.*** Pierces the Spatium interosseum antebrachii, continues on the cranial aspect of Membrana interossea antebrachii. A C

28 *A. recurrens interossea.* Passes proximally to the lateral aspect of Articulatio cubiti. A

29 *Ramus carpeus dorsalis.* Often double contribution to Rete carpi dorsale. C

30 ***A. interossea caudalis.*** Courses between Membrana interossea antebrachii and M. pronator quadratus. A

31 *A. ulnaris.* Accompanies N. ulnaris along the caudal border of Antebrachium. A

32 **A. recurrens ulnaris.** Courses proximally as an ascending (recurrent) artery at the medial aspect of olecranon, anastomoses with A. collateralis ulnaris. A (The A. recurrens ulnaris is described in various books either as a caudodistal [descending] branch of A. brachialis, or as a caudodorsal [ascending – read recurrent] branch of A. ulnaris. Therefore the "ascending" branch is better compatible with the meaning of the term "recurrent ulnar" [Simoens et al. 1980].)

33 **Ramus dorsalis.** To Arcus dorsalis superficialis. A C

34 **Ramus carpeus dorsalis.** Branch of Ramus dorsalis to Rete carpi dorsale. C

35 **A. digitalis dorsalis V. abaxialis.** Arises from Arcus dorsalis superficialis. C

B Arteries of left axilla, medial aspect (ca)

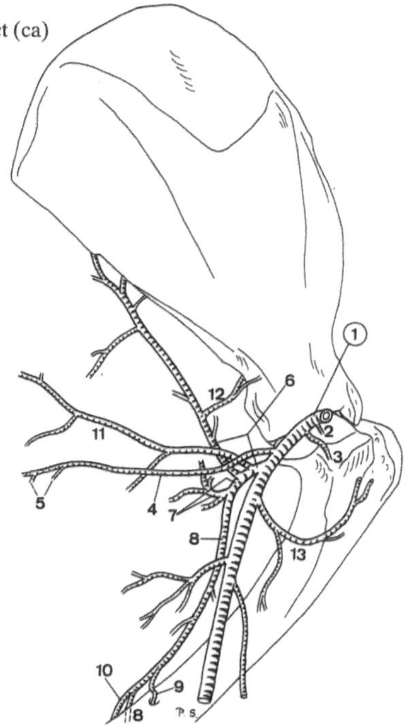

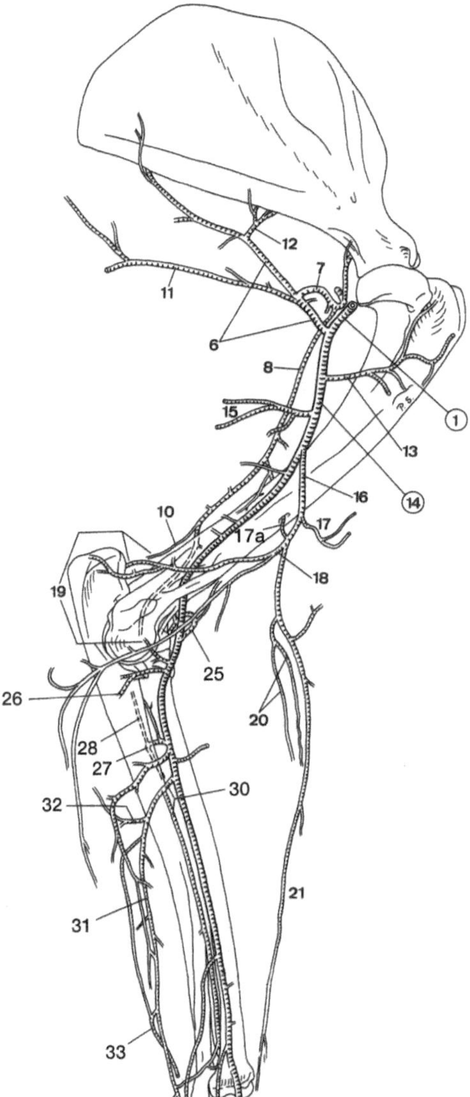

A Arteries of left thoracic limb, medial aspect (fe)

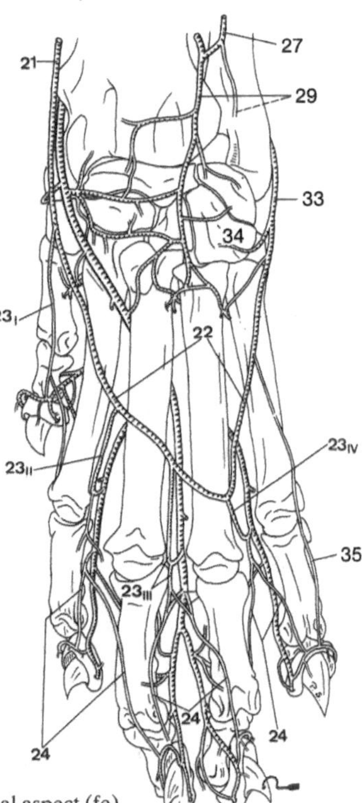

C Arteries of left manus, dorsal aspect (fe)

1 **Ramus interosseus.** Branch of A. interossea caudalis, passes through the distal part of Spatium interosseum antebrachii, joins A. interossea cranialis. A

2 **Ramus carpeus dorsalis.** Branch to the dorsal aspect of carpus. C

2a **Ramus carpeus palmaris.** Small branch, runs on the palmr aspect of carpus. A

3 Ramus palmaris. Continuation of A. interossea caudalis beyond the origin of Ramus carpeus palmaris. Joins A. ulnaris. A

4 **Ramus superficialis.** Courses at the lateropalmar aspect of metacarpus. Joins Arcus palmaris superficialis and/or continues as A. digitalis palmaris communis IV and A. digitalis palmaris V abaxialis. A

5 **Ramus profundus.** Passes to Mm. interossei, forming the lateral contribution to Arcus palmaris profundus. A

CANIS

6 **A. brachialis.** Continuation of A. axillaris. Runs distally across the medial aspect of humerus. B

7 ***A. profunda brachii.*** To the caudal musculature of brachium. B

8 ***A. bicipitalis.*** Supply for M. biceps brachii. B

9 ***A. collateralis ulnaris.*** Courses caudally and, near N. ulnaris, ramifies at olecranon. B

10 *Rete articulare cubiti.* Arterial network at the caudal aspect of Articulatio cubiti. B

11 ***A. brachialis superficialis.*** Courses craniodistally across the distal part of M. biceps brachii. B

12 *Aa. radiales superficiales.* Pair of small superficial vessels that accompany N. cutaneus antebrachii medialis. B

13 *A. antebrachialis superficialis cranialis.* Continuation of A. brachialis superficialis in the antebrachium. Immediately bifurcated. B

14 **Ramus medialis.** Runs along the craniomedial border of M. extensor carpi radialis and on the dorsomedial aspect of carpus. B C

15 **A. digitalis dorsalis communis I.** Continuation of Ramus medialis of A. antebrachialis superficialis cranialis. C

16 **Ramus lateralis.** Runs on the cranial aspect of antebrachium and the dorsal aspect of carpus. B C

17 **Aa. digitales dorsales communes II–IV.** Run on the superficial surface of the extensor tendons. C

18 **Aa. digitales dorsales propriae.** Three pairs of vessels, arisen from the bifurcation of Aa. digitales dorsales communes II–IV. Run along the dorsal parts of the adjacent surface of digits. C

19 ***A. transversa cubiti.*** Curves laterally across Articulatio cubiti. B

20 ***A. profunda antebrachii.*** Variable supply for the muscles on the caudal side of antebrachium. B (See the text within parenthesis on page 284.26.)

21 ***A. interossea communis.*** Proceeds to the Spatium interosseum antebrachii. B

22 *A. ulnaris.* Runs caudally across the medial aspect of ulna, where it joins N. ulnaris. Continues along the lateral surface of M. flexor carpi ulnaris. B

23 **A. recurrens ulnaris.** Courses proximally along the medial aspect of olecranon and joins Rete articulare cubiti. B (The A. recurrens ulnaris is described in various books either as a caudodistal [descending] branch of A. brachialis, or as a caudodorsal [ascending – read recurrent] branch of A. ulnaris. Therefore the "ascending" branch is better compatible with the meaning of the term "recurrent ulnar" [Simoens et al. 1980].)

24 **Ramus dorsalis.** Courses along the lateral border of M. flexor carpi ulnaris to Regio carpi lateralis. B C

25 **Ramus carpeus dorsalis.** To Rete carpi dorsale. C

26 **A. digitalis dorsalis V abaxialis.** Runs along the dorsolateral surface of metacarpus and digit V. C

27 **Ramus carpeus palmaris.** (This artery was omitted from the 5th edition of the N. A. V.)

28 *A. interossea cranialis.* Passes cranially through the proximal part of Spatium interosseum antebrachii and continues distally along the cranial aspect of Membrana interossea antebrachii. B C

29 **A. recurrens interossea.** Courses proximally to the lateral aspect of Articulatio cubiti and contributes to Rete articulare cubiti. B

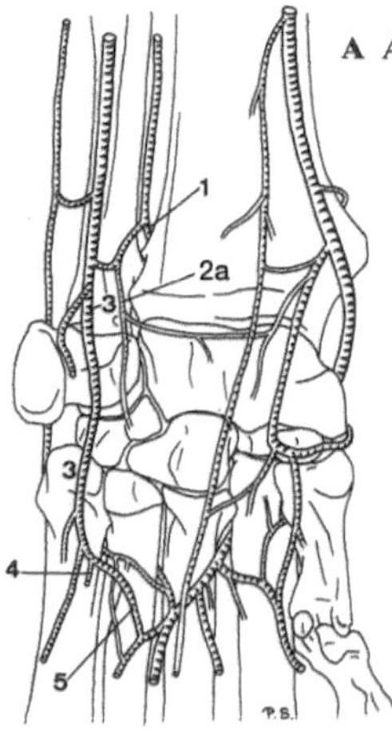

A Arteries of left carpus, palmar aspect (fe)

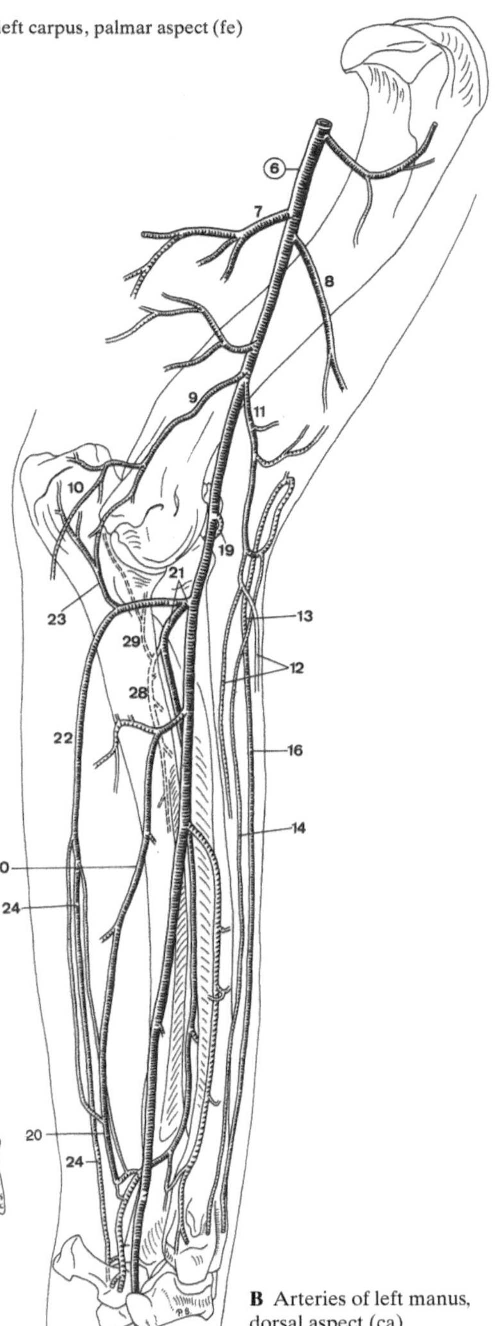

B Arteries of left manus, dorsal aspect (ca)

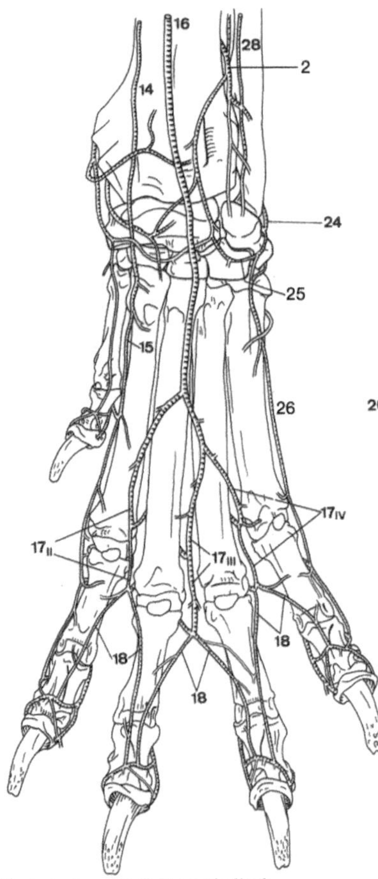

C Arteries of left thoracic limb, medial aspect (ca)

1 *A. interossea caudalis*. Courses between Membrana interossea antebrachii and M. pronator quadratus. B

2 **Ramus interosseus.** Passes cranially through the distal part of Spatium interosseum antebrachii. A

3 **Ramus carpeus dorsalis.** Branch of Ramus interosseus to Rete carpi dorsale. A

4 **Ramus carpeus palmaris.** Small branch to the palmar aspect of carpus. B

5 **Ramus palmaris.** Continuation of A. interossea caudalis. Joins A. ulnaris and/or A. profunda antebrachii. B

6 **Ramus superficialis.** Lateral contribution to Arcus palmaris superficialis. B

7 **Ramus profundus.** Lateral contribution to Arcus palmaris profundus. B

CARNIVORA

8 **A. mediana.** Continuation of A. brachialis beyond the origin of A. interossea communis (ca) s. caudalis (fe). Courses along the caudomedial aspect of antebrachium, passes through Canalis carpi to Regio metacarpi palmaris. Distal to the origin of A. radialis it is much diminished in size in fe. B

9 ***A. radialis.*** Courses along the caudomedial border of radius and in Retinaculum flexorum to the mediopalmar aspect of carpus. Most of the blood of the feline A. mediana is conducted in A. radialis, and continues through Ramus carpeus dorsalis. B

10 *Ramus carpeus palmaris*. Courses to the palmar aspect of carpus. B

11 *Ramus carpeus dorsalis*. Runs dorsodistally across the medial aspect of carpus. Usually plural. A B

11a **A. digitalis dorsalis I abaxialis.** The continuation of the previous branch on the dorsal aspect of the digit I.

12 **Rete carpi dorsale.** Network on the dorsal aspect of carpus. A

13 **Aa. metacarpeae dorsales I–IV.** Small branches of Rete carpi dorsale which join A. interdigitalis (I) s. Ramus perforans distalis (II–IV). A

14 *Ramus palmaris superficialis*. Joins Arcus palmaris superficialis, or may continue as A. digitalis palmaris communis II (most fe). B

15 *Arcus palmaris profundus*. Lies across the palmar aspect of Mm. interossei. May be incomplete, or be complemented by a supplementary arch on the dorsal aspect of Mm. interossei (ca). In fe mainly supplied via Ramus carpeus dorsalis of A. radialis. B

16 **Aa. metacarpeae palmares I–IV.** In fe they are the largest arteries of the metapodium. B

17 **Ramus perforans proximalis.** Connects each of the Aa. metacarpeae palmares with its dorsal counterpart by piercing through the proximal part of the corresponding Spatium interosseum metacarpi. In fe the A. radialis mainly contributes to the Ramus perforans proximalis II, which joins the Arcus palmaris profundus. A B

18 **Ramus perforans distalis.** Connects each of the Aa. metacarpeae palmares II–IV with its dorsal counterpart by traversing the distal part of the corresponding Spatium interosseum metacarpi. Also connected with Aa. digitales dorsales et palmares communes II–IV. Many variations may be seen in the dog. A B

19 ***Arcus palmaris superficialis.*** Situated between M. flexor digitorum profundus and M. flexor digitorum superficialis. Usually absent in fe. B

20 *Aa. digitales palmares communes I–IV.* In fe, most of the blood is furnished by the Aa. metacarpeae palmares via the Rami perforantes distales. B

21 **Ramus tori metacarpei.** Usually double branch, supplies Torus metacarpeus. B

22 **A. interdigitalis.** Connects each of the Aa. digitales palmares communes with the corresponding A. digitalis dorsalis communis (Car) or Aa. digitales dorsales propriae (fe). A B

23 **Aa. digitales palmares propriae.** Pairs of arteries which course distally along the adjacent palmar aspects of digits. Finally enter Foramen soleare axiale s. abaxiale of Phalanx distalis. They display a constant branching pattern, as in the other domestic mammals, which is listed below. B

23a **Ramus palmaris phalangis proximalis.** Supplies palmar structures of Phalanx proximalis.

23b **(Ramus dorsalis phalangis proximalis).** Supplies dorsal structures of Phalanx proximalis. A

24 **Ramus tori digitalis.** Usually double branch, supplies the Torus digitalis. B

25 *A. digitalis palmaris V abaxialis*. Finally enters Foramen soleare abaxiale of Phalanx distalis V. B (This artery was omitted from the 5th edition of the N. A. V.)

26 **Ramus palmaris phalangis mediae.** For the palmar structures of Phalanx media. B

27 **(Ramus dorsalis phalangis mediae).** For the dorsal structures of Phalanx media. B

28 **A. coronalis.** Supplies structures of Regio coronalis.

29 **Ramus palmaris phalangis distalis.** For the palmar structures of Phalanx distalis. B

30 **Arcus terminalis.** Arch inside Phalanx distalis, formed by the axial and abaxial Aa. digitales palmares propriae.

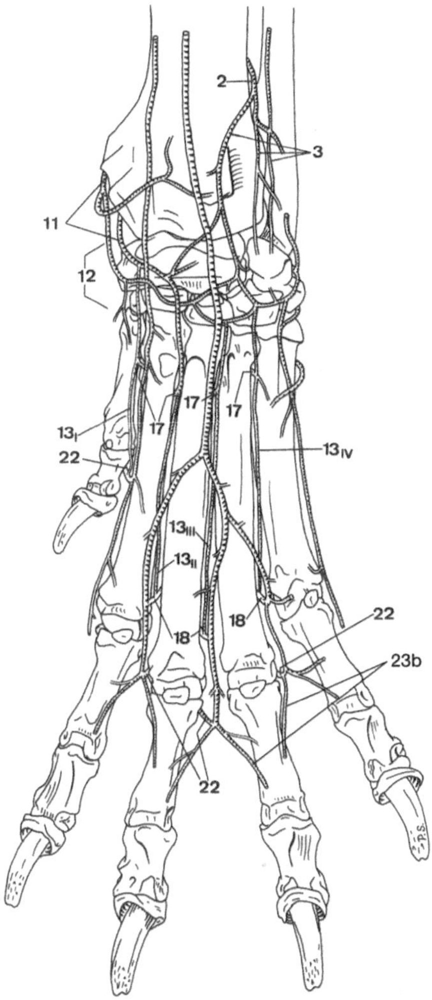

A Arteries of left manus, dorsal aspect (ca)

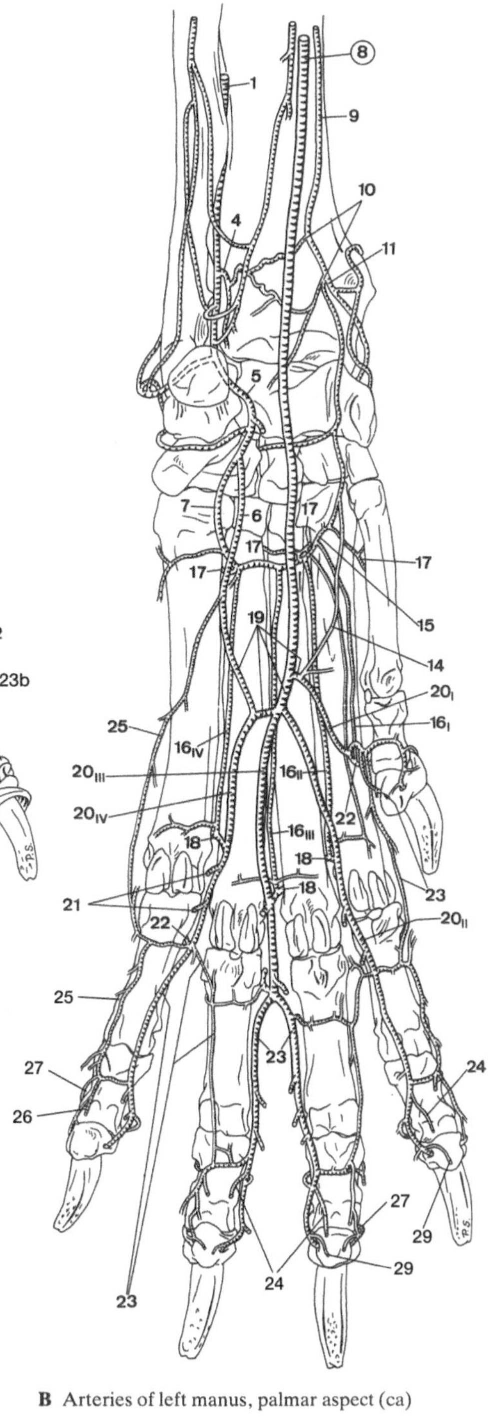

B Arteries of left manus, palmar aspect (ca)

SUS

1 ***Ramus deltoideus.*** Accompanies V. cephalica in Sulcus pectoralis lateralis. A

2 ***A. thoracica externa.*** Arises at the medial aspect of the first rib, emerges from Apertura thoracis cranialis and supplies the pectoral muscles. A

3 *A. thoracica lateralis.* Accompanies N. thoracicus lateralis, coursing caudally along the medial aspect of M. pectoralis profundus. A

4 **Rami mammarii.** Supply the first (and occasionally also second) Mamma thoracica. A

5 ***A. subscapularis.*** Courses dorsocaudally along Margo caudalis of scapula. A B

6 *A. thoracodorsalis.* Runs across the medial surface of M. teres major and M. latissimus dorsi. A B

7 *A. circumflexa humeri caudalis.* Courses along the caudal aspect of Articulatio humeri. A B

8 **A. suprascapularis.** Runs dorsocranially across the medial aspect of Collum scapulae and continues along Margo cranialis of scapula. A B

9 **A. circumflexa humeri cranialis.** Courses craniodistally through, or lateral to, M. coracobrachialis. May arise directly form the A. axillaris (the origin of this artery indicates the transition between A. axillaris and A. brachialis). A

10 **A. collateralis radialis.** Accompanies N. radialis upon M. brachialis. A B

11 **A. nutricia humeri.** Branch of A. collateralis radialis to Foramen nutricium. A B

12 **A. collateralis media.** Caudodistal branch of A. collateralis radialis towards Rete articulare cubiti. A B

13 **A. antebrachialis superficialis cranialis.** Continuation of A. collateralis radialis along M. extensor carpi radialis. A B

14 **A. digitalis dorsalis communis III.** Superficial continuation of A. antebrachialis superficialis cranialis. A B

15 **Aa. digitales dorsales propriae.** Continuations of A. digitalis dorsalis communis III. A

16 *A. circumflexa scapulae.* Courses toward Margo caudalis and mainly Facies lateralis scapulae. A B

17 **A. brachialis.** Continuation of A. axillaris, runs across the medial aspect of brachium. A B

18 ***A. profunda brachii.*** To M. triceps brachii. A B

19 ***A. bicipitalis.*** To M. biceps brachii. A

20 ***A. collateralis ulnaris.*** Accompanies N. ulnaris. Usually reinforced by branches of A. profunda antebrachii. A

21 *Rete articulare cubiti.* Network supplying the elbow joint. A

22 *Ramus carpeus palmaris.* (This artery was omitted from the 5th edition of the N. A. V.)

23 ***A. transversa cubiti.*** Courses laterally across the cranial aspect of humerus. A B

24 ***A. profunda antebrachii.*** Usually plural, to the caudal musculature of antebrachium. A (See the text within parenthesis on page 284.26.)

25 ***A. interossea communis.*** Runs laterally to the proximal part of Spatium interosseum antebrachii. A

26 *A. interossea cranialis.* Passes laterally through the proximal part of Spatium interosseum antebrachii and continues distally. B

27 **A. recurrens interossea.** Runs proximally to Rete articulare cubiti. B

28 *A. interossea caudalis.* Courses between radius und ulna. Enveloped in a fine arterial network. A

29 **Ramus interosseus.** Passes through the distal part of Spatium interosseum antebrachii and joins A. interossea cranialis. B

30 **Ramus carpeus dorsalis.** Branch of Ramus interosseus to Rete carpi dorsale. B

31 **Ramus carpeus palmaris.** Deep branch to the palmar aspect of carpus. A

32 **Ramus palmaris.** Continuation of A. interossea caudalis. Receives A. collateralis ulnaris, continues distally along the medial aspect of Os accessorium. A

32a *Ramus carpeus dorsalis.* To the dorsal aspect of carpus. A (This artery was moved as 32a according to the 5th edition of the N. A. V., because it is not a branch of A. collateralis ulnaris, but of A. interossea caudalis.)

33 **Ramus superficialis.** Branch of Ramus palmaris, courses distally along the lateropalmar border of metacarpus, joins Arcus palmaris superficialis. A

34 **Ramus profundus.** Inconstant deep branch of Ramus palmaris to Arcus palmaris profundus. A

A Arteries of left thoracic limb, medial aspect (su)

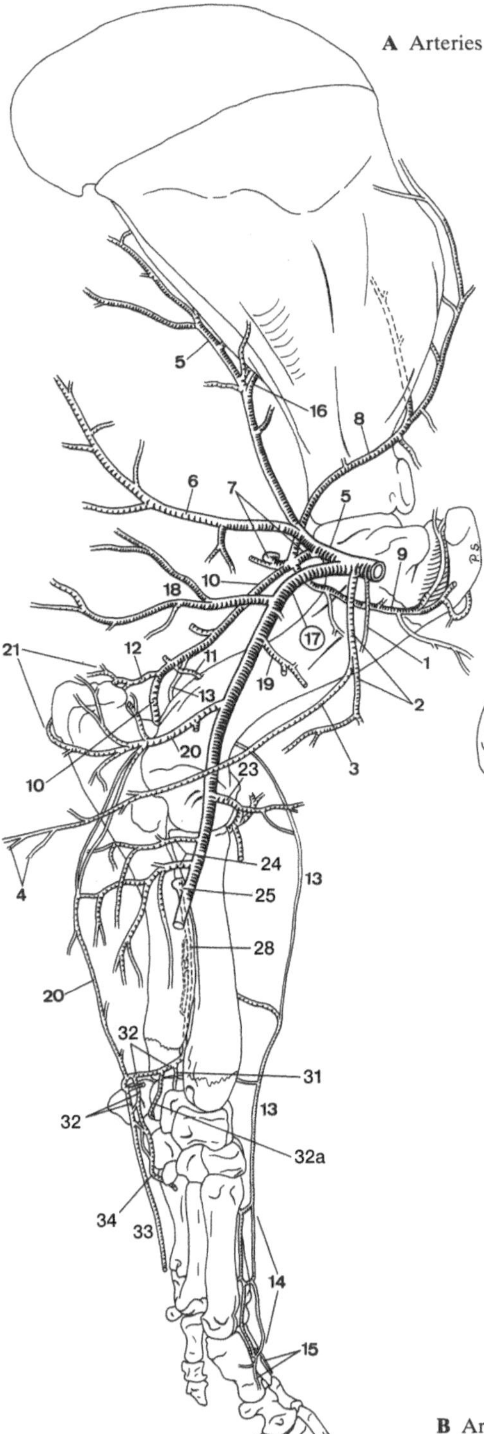

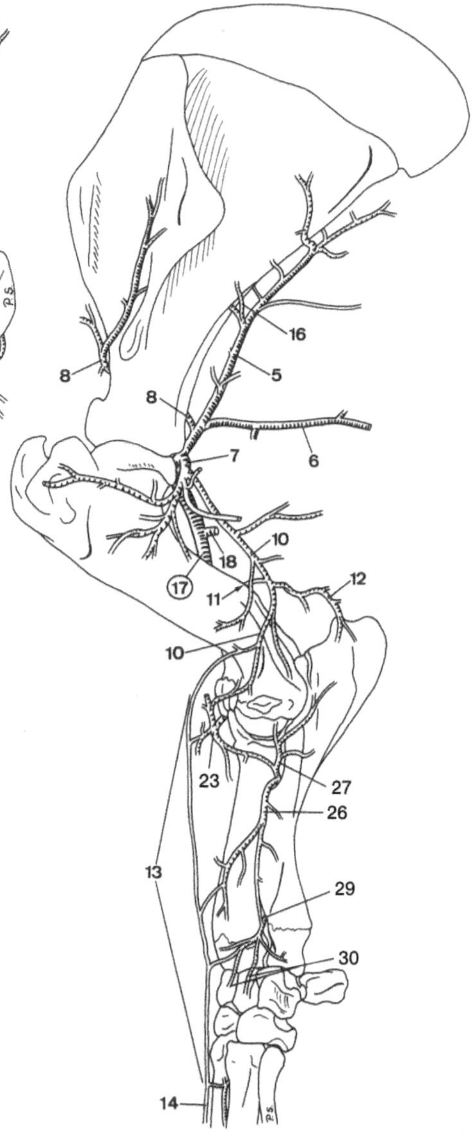

B Arteries of left thoracic limb, lateral aspect (su)

1 **A. mediana**. Continuation of A. brachialis distal to the origin of A. interossea communis. Runs distally, medial to the digital flexor tendons surrounded by a fine arterial network, and continues through Canalis carpi. A

2 ***A. radialis***. Courses along the caudomedial aspect of radius, surrounded by a fine arterial network, continues superficially on the mediopalmar aspect of carpus. A

3 *Ramus carpeus palmaris*. Small branch to the palmar aspect of carpus. A

4 *Ramus carpeus dorsalis*. Courses dorsally across the medial aspect of carpus. A B

5 **Rete carpi dorsale**. Arterial network on the dorsal aspect of carpus. B

6 **Aa. metacarpeae dorsales II et IV**. Small branches of Rete carpi dorsale which are reinforced by Rami perforantes proximales IV. B

7 **Aa. digitales dorsales propriae**. Slender superficial terminal branches of A. metacarpea dorsalis II s. IV along the adjacent sides of Digiti II and III s. IV and V. B

8 **A. metacarpea dorsalis III**. Arises from Rete carpi dorsale, reinforced by Ramus perforans proximalis. B C

9 *Ramus palmaris superficialis*. Courses distally along the medial aspect of the flexor tendons of the third digit and joins Arcus palmaris superficialis. A

10 *Arcus palmaris profundus*. Transverse connection between A. radialis and Ramus profundus of Ramus palmaris of A. interossea caudalis across the dorsal aspect of Mm. interossei, often complemented by an arch on the palmar aspect. A

11 **Aa. metacarpeae palmares II–IV**. Join Ramus perforans distalis after running axially across the heads of Os metacarpale III et IV. A

12 **Ramus perforans proximalis**. Connects each of Aa. metacarpeae palmares II–IV with its dorsal counterpart through the proximal part of Spatium interosseum metacarpi. A B

13 **Ramus perforans distalis III**. Connects A. metacarpea palmaris III with its dorsal counterpart, by traversing the distal part of the space between Ossa metacarpalia III et IV. A B

14 ***Ramus ulnaris***. Transverse connection between A. mediana and Ramus palmaris of A. interossea caudalis. A

15 ***Arcus palmaris superficialis***. Variable, subfascial connection between Ramus palmaris superficialis of A. radialis, A. mediana, and Ramus superficialis of Ramus palmaris of A. interossea caudalis. A

16 *Aa. digitales palmares communes II–IV*. The arteries II and IV run toward the interdigital spaces II-III and III-IV to divide into the corresponding palmar proper digital arteries, whereas the artery III runs in the interdigital space III-IV and bifurcates into the (axial) palmar proper digital arteries III and IV. A C

17 **Aa. digitales palmares propriae**. Enter Foramen axiale of the corresponding Phalanx distalis. A B C

18 **A. interdigitalis**. Each of the four arteries which traverse Spatia interdigitalia, connecting the axial and abaxial Aa. digitales palmares propriae III et IV with their dorsal analogues. A B C

19 **Ramus dorsalis phalangis proximalis**. Each of the six vessels which arise usually from A. interdigitalis (Digiti III et IV) or Ramus palmaris phalangis proximalis (Digiti II et V) and ramify on the dorsal side of the corresponding Phalanx proximalis. B

20 **Ramus palmaris phalangis proximalis**. Transverse branch of each A. digitalis palmaris propria which courses across the palmar surface of the corresponding Phalanx proximalis. A B C

21 **Ramus tori digitalis**. Branch of Aa. digitales palmares propriae III et IV and Rami palmares phalangis proximalis II et V, supplying the corresponding Torus ungulae. A C

22 **Ramus dorsalis phalangis mediae**. Transverse branch of each A. digitalis palmaris propria across the dorsal aspect of the corresponding Phalanx media. A B C

23 **A. coronalis**. Superficial branch of each axial Ramus dorsalis phalangis mediae (II–V), which courses abaxially towards the corresponding Corona ungulae. B

24 **Ramus palmaris phalangis mediae**. Transverse branch of each A. digitalis palmaris propria which runs across the palmar aspect of the corresponding Phalanx media. A C

24a Ramus palmaris phalangis distalis. Runs on the palmar side of Phalanx distalis. A

25 **Ramus dorsalis phalangis distalis**. Slender branch of each axial A. digitalis palmaris propria which courses dorsally along Facies axialis of the corresponding Phalanx distalis. B C

26 **Arcus terminalis**. Arterial arch inside Phalanx distalis. A

A Arteries of left manus, palmar aspect (su)

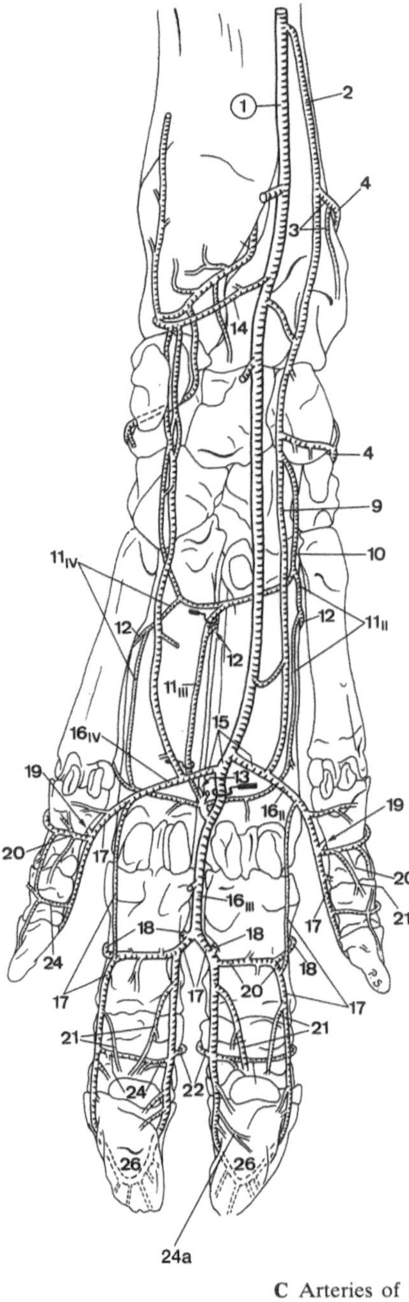

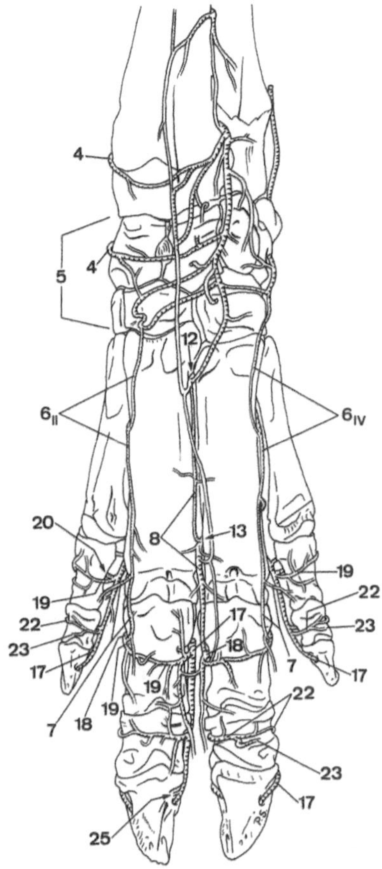

B Arteries of left manus, dorsal aspect (su)

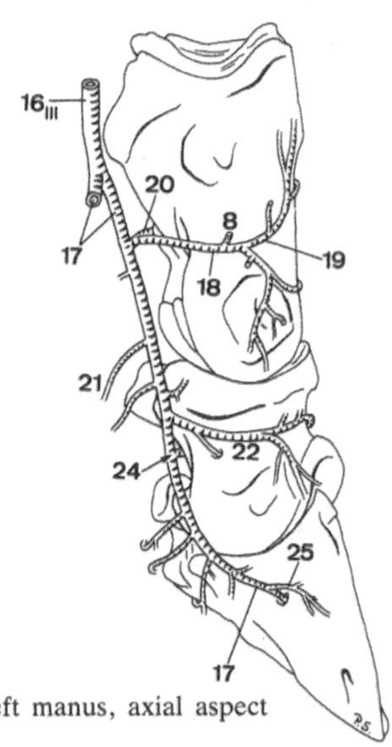

C Arteries of fourth digit, left manus, axial aspect (su)

RUMINANTIA

1 ***A. thoracica externa***. Suplies mainly Mm. pectorales. A

2 *Ramus deltoideus* (bo). Accompanies V. cephalica in Sulcus pectoralis lateralis. A

3 ***A. suprascapularis*** (bo). Principal vessel accompanying N. suprascapularis. A B

4 ***A. subscapularis***. Passes dorsocaudally along Margo caudalis of scapula. A B

5 *A. thoracodorsalis*. Caudodorsally directed muscular vessel. A B

6 *A. circumflexa humeri caudalis*. Runs laterally passing the flexor angle of Articulatio humeri. A B

7 **A. collateralis radialis**. Runs distocaudally, accompanying N. radialis. A B

8 **A. antebrachialis superficialis cranialis**. Small branch of A. collateralis radialis, accompanies Ramus superficialis of N. radialis. Reinforced by A. transversa cubiti and A. interossea cranialis. B D

9 **Aa. digitales dorsales communes II et III**. Very small branches given off by A. antebrachialis superficialis cranialis. D

10 **Aa. digitales dorsales propriae**. The medial one forms the continuation of A. digitalis dorsalis communis II, both axial originate from the bifurcation of A. digitalis dorsalis communis III. D

11 **A. nutricia humeri**. Branch of A. collateralis radialis. A B

12 **A. collateralis media**. Arises from A. collateralis radialis and proceeds caudally towards Articulatio cubiti. A B

13 **A. circumflexa scapulae**. Courses dorsocranially to the caudal border of scapula and continues across its lateral and medial aspects. A B

14 *A. circumflexa humeri cranialis*. Courses cranially across the medial aspect of humerus. May arise variably from A. axillaris, A. subscapularis, A. circumflexa humeri caudalis, or A. thoracodorsalis (the origin of this artery indicates the transition between A. axillaris and A. brachialis). A

15 **A. brachialis**. Continuation of A. axillaris. Courses across the medial aspect of brachium. A B

16 ***A. profunda brachii***. Caudally directed trunk which soon divides in muscular branches. A

17 ***A. collateralis ulnaris***. Courses caudally, and usually gives off a distal continuation between Mm. extensor and flexor carpi ulnaris. A B C

18 *Rete articulare cubiti*. Arterial network which supplies the elbow joint. A

19 *Ramus carpeus palmaris*. (This artery was omitted from the 5th edition of the N. A. V.) C

19a *Ramus carpeus dorsalis*. Courses to Regio carpi dorsalis. B C D

20 **A. digitalis dorsalis communis IV**. Runs superficially on the dorsal aspect of metacarpus. D

21 ***A. bicipitalis***. Short muscular branch, mainly for M. biceps brachii. A

22 ***A. transversa cubiti***. Cranially directed trunk which ramifies into muscular branches on the flexor aspect of Articulatio cubiti. A B

23 ***A. interossea communis***. Passes caudolaterally along the caudomedial aspect of radius, may enter Spatium interosseum antebrachii proximale (bo, cap). A

24 *A. interossea cranialis*. Continuation of A. interossea communis. Traverses Spatium interosseum antebrachii proximale with some exceptions, courses distally in the craniolateral groove between radius and ulna. B D

25 **A. recurrens interossea**. Courses proximally to the lateral aspect of olecranon. B

26 **Ramus carpeus dorsalis**. Courses distodorsally and ramifies on the dorsolateral aspect of carpus. B D

27 **Ramus interosseus**. Caudal continuation of A. interossea cranialis through Spatium interosseum antebrachii distale. B C 297 A

28 **Ramus carpeus palmaris**. Deep branch of Ramus interosseus to the palmar aspect of carpus. B C 297 A

29 **Ramus palmaris**. Continuation of Ramus interosseus. Receives A. collateralis ulnaris, and, usually split, continues along the lateropalmar aspect of carpus. B C 297 A

30 **Ramus superficialis**. Branch of Ramus palmaris which courses along the lateral aspect of the flexor tendons of the digits and usually joins Arcus palmaris superficialis. C 297 A

31 **Ramus profundus**. Deep branch of Ramus palmaris which pierces between metacarpus and M. interosseus into Arcus palmaris profundus. C 297 A

32 *A. interossea caudalis*. Courses along the medial groove between radius and ulna. A

B Arteries of left thoracic limb, lateral aspect (bo)

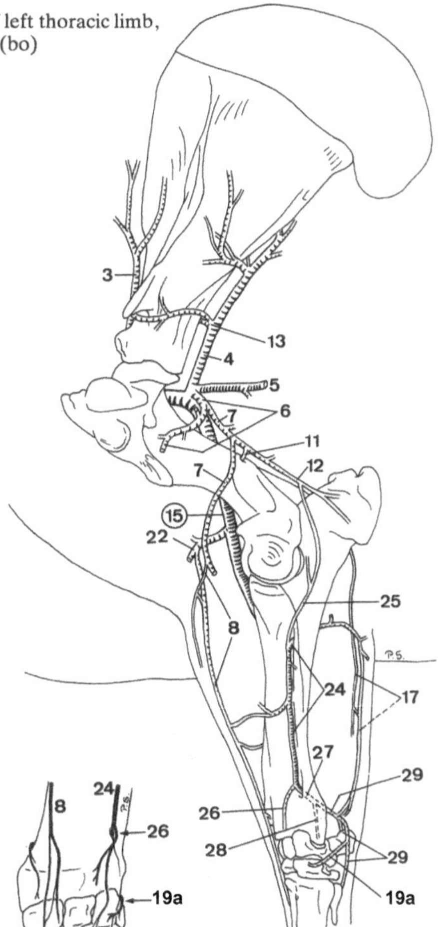

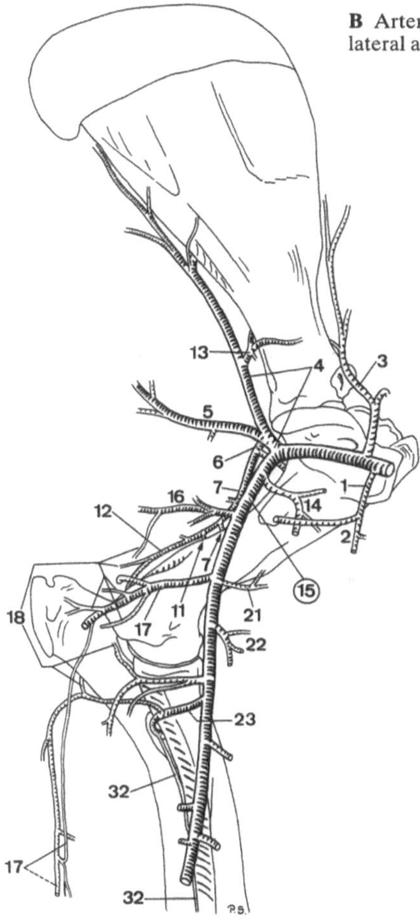

A Arteries of left thoracic limb, medial aspect (bo)

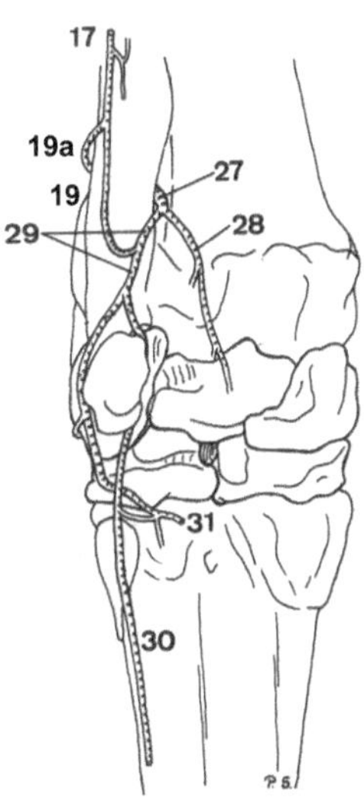

C Arteries of left carpus, palmar aspect (bo)

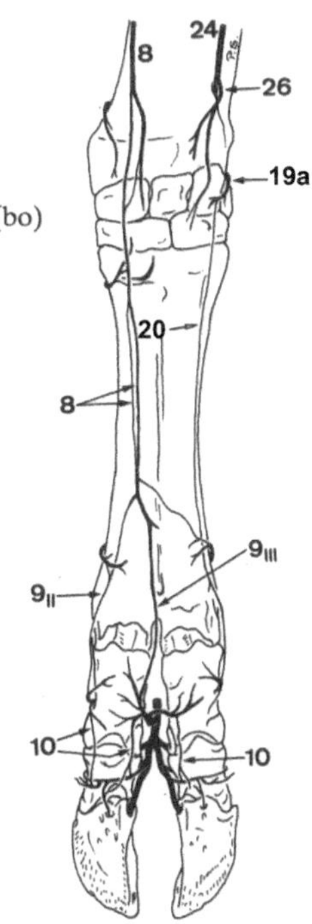

D Arteries of left manus, dorsal aspect (bo)

1 **A. mediana.** Continuation of A. brachialis distal to the origin of A. interossea communis. Passes through Sulcus carpi. A C D

2 ***A. profunda antebrachii.*** To the muscles on the caudal side of the forearm. A (See the text within parentheses on page 284.26.)

3 ***A. radialis.*** Continues superficially on the mediopalmar aspect of carpus. A

4 *Ramus carpeus palmaris.* Slender artery in bo. A

5 *Ramus carpeus dorsalis.* Usually double branch to the dorsal aspect of carpus. A B

6 **Rete carpi dorsale.** Network on the dorsal aspect of carpus. B

7 **A. metacarpea dorsalis III.** Proceeds from Rete carpi dorsale in Sulcus longitudinalis dorsalis of Os metacarpale III et IV, joins A. interdigitalis. B D

8 *Ramus palmaris superficialis.* Courses underneath Fascia palmaris, joins Arcus palmaris superficialis, or continues in A. digitalis palmaris communis II. A C D

9 *Arcus palmaris profundus.* Connection between A. radialis and Ramus interosseus between Os metacarpale III et IV and M. interosseus. A

10 **Aa. metacarpeae palmares II–IV.** Interanastomosing arteries between Os metacarpale III et IV and M. interosseus. A C D

11 **Ramus perforans proximalis III.** Connects A. metacarpea palmaris III or Arcus palmaris profundus through Canalis metacarpi proximalis with A. metacarpea dorsalis III. A B

12 **Ramus perforans distalis III.** Connects A. metacarpea palmaris III with A. metacarpea dorsalis III through Canalis metacarpi distalis. A B D

13 ***Arcus palmaris superficialis.*** Variably developed subfascial arch connecting Ramus interosseus via A. mediana, with Ramus palmaris superficialis of A. radialis. A C D

14 *A. digitalis palmaris communis II.* A C D

15 **A. digitalis palmaris propria II axialis.** Courses subfascially to the medial dew claw. A C

16 **A. digitalis palmaris propria III abaxialis.** Runs along the mediopalmar side of the flexor tendons of the third digit and finally enters the mediopalmar aspect of Phalanx distalis III. A C

17 **Ramus dorsalis phalangis proximalis.** Branch of A. digitalis palmaris propria III abaxialis to the dorsal aspect of Phalanx proximalis. A B C

18 **Ramus tori digitalis.** Branch of A. digitalis palmaris propria III abaxialis to Torus ungulae. A C

19 **Ramus dorsalis phalangis mediae.** Branch of A. digitalis palmaris propria III abaxialis to the dorsal aspect of Phalanx media. A B C

20 **Ramus palmaris phalangis distalis.** Runs on the palmar aspect of Phalanx distalis. A C

21 **Ramus dorsalis phalangis distalis.** Runs on the dorsal aspect of Phalanx distalis.

22 *A. digitalis palmaris communis III.* Continuation of A. mediana beyond Arcus palmaris superficialis. A B C D

23 **Rami palmares phalangium proximalium.** Course across the palmar surface of Phalanx proximalis, join A. digitalis palmaris propria abaxialis. A D

24 **A. interdigitalis.** Communication with A. metacarpea dorsalis III through Spatium interdigitale. A B D

25 **Rami dorsales phalangium proximalium.** Branches of A. interdigitalis to the dorsal aspect of Phalanx proximalis. D

26 *Aa. digitales palmares propriae III et IV axiales.* Course to the corresponding Foramen axiale, through which they enter Phalanx distalis. A B D

27 **Ramus tori digitalis.** Branch of A. digitalis palmaris propria axialis to Torus ungulae. A C D

28 **Ramus palmaris phalangis mediae.** Branch of A. digitalis palmaris propria III s. IV axialis which courses transversely across the palmar aspect of Phalanx media III s. IV. A D

29 **Ramus dorsalis phalangis mediae.** Branch of A. digitalis palmaris propria axialis to the dorsal aspect of Phalanx media. A branch of it (arrows in figures C and D) enters the Foramen axiale phalangis distalis and joins the Arcus terminalis. B C D

30 **A. coronalis.** Arises from the axial Ramus dorsalis phalangis mediae (bo) or A. digitalis palmaris propria axialis, courses into the abaxial part of Corona ungulae. B C D

31 **Ramus palmaris phalangis distalis.** Continuation of A. digitalis palmaris propria III s. IV axialis. A D

32 **Ramus dorsalis phalangis distalis.** Branch of Ramus palmaris phalangis distalis, courses dorsally along Facies axialis of Phalanx distalis. D

33 **Arcus terminalis.** Arterial arch inside Phalanx distalis. A D

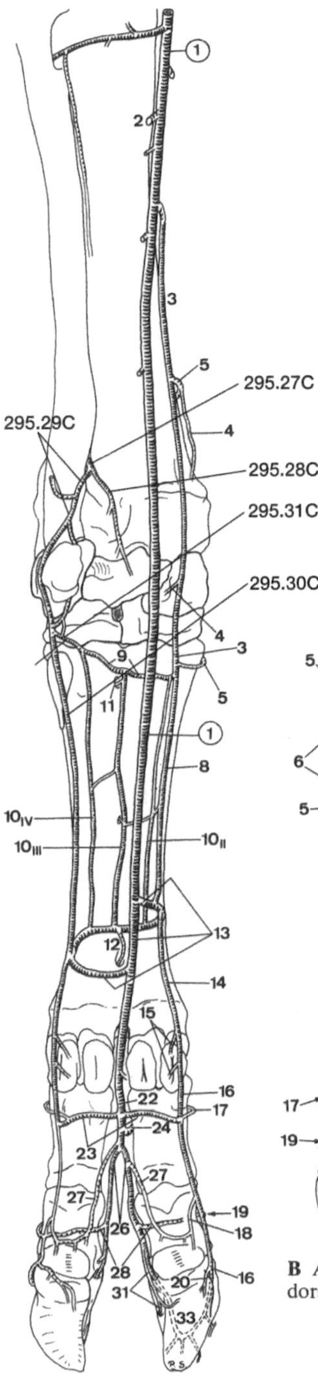

A Arteries of left thoracic limb, palmar aspect (bo)

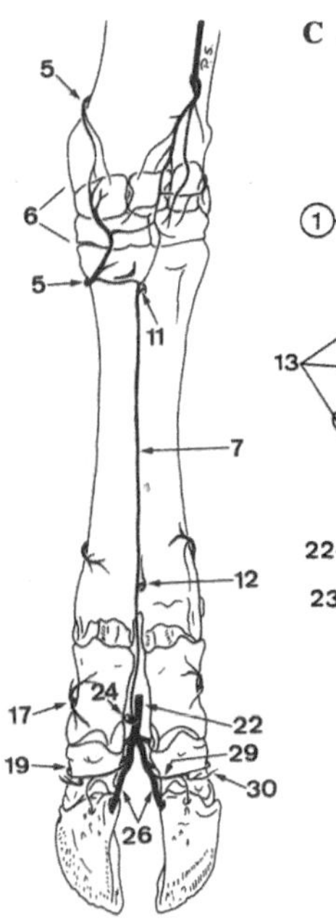

B Arteries of left manus, dorsal aspect (bo)

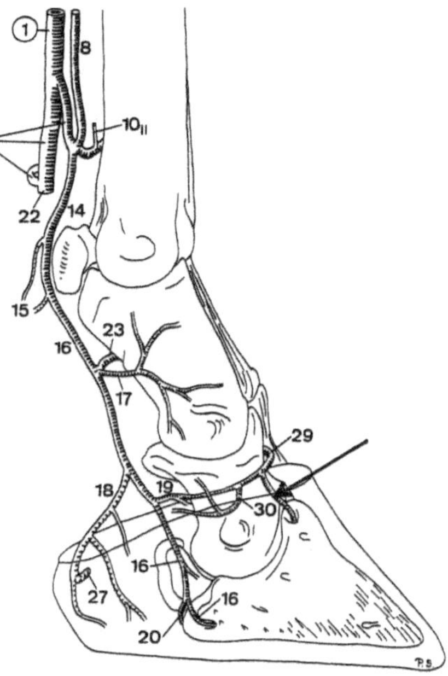

C Arteries of left manus, medial aspect (bo)

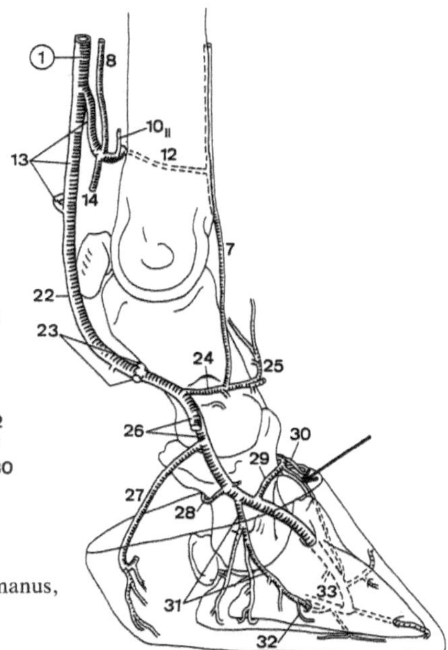

D Arteries of left manus (third digit removed), medial aspect (bo)

1 ***A. digitalis palmaris communis IV.*** Palmar common digital A. IV. A

2 *A. digitalis palmaris propria IV abaxialis*. Runs along the lateropalmar side of the flexor tendons of the fourth digit. A

3 **Ramus dorsalis phalangis proximalis.** Branch of A. digitalis palmaris propria IV abaxialis, to the dorsal aspect of Phalanx proximalis IV. A

4 **Ramus tori digitalis.** Branch of A. digitalis palmaris propria IV abaxialis, enters Torus ungulae IV laterally. A

5 **Ramus dorsalis phalangis mediae.** Branch of A. digitalis palmaris propria IV abaxialis, to the dorsal aspect of Phalanx media IV. A

6 **Ramus palmaris phalangis distalis.** Branch of A. digitalis palmaris propria IV abaxialis, courses axially across the palmar aspect of Phalanx distalis IV. A

7 **Ramus dorsalis phalangis distalis.** Dorsal branch for the distal phalanx.

8 **A. digitalis palmaris propria V axialis.** Courses subfascially to the lateral dew claw. A

EQUUS

9 ***A. thoracica externa.*** Courses caudoventrally to Mm. pectorales. Variable and inconstant. B

10 ***A. suprascapularis.*** Runs dorsally to the furrow between M. subscapularis and M. supraspinatus, accompanying N. suprascapularis. Often double. B C

11 ***A. subscapularis.*** Courses caudodorsally between M. subscapularis and M. teres major towards Angulus caudalis of scapula. B C

12 *A. thoracodorsalis.* Crosses the medial face of M. teres major and continues caudodorsally on M. latissimus dorsi. B C

13 *A. circumflexa humeri caudalis.* Passes laterally with N. axillaris, caudal to Articulatio humeri. B C

14 *A. circumflexa scapulae.* Runs between M. subscapularis and Caput longum of M. triceps brachii and gives off cranial branches at each side of scapula. B C (The A. nutricia scapulae is missing from the 5th edition of the N. A. V., albeit it is shown in the figure C, as a branch of 14.)

15 ***A. circumflexa humeri cranialis.*** Courses distocranially across the medial aspect of humerus. B C

16 **A. brachialis.** Continuation of A. axillaris distal to the place where A. circumflexa humeri cranialis arises. Courses across the medial surface of humerus to the craniomedial aspect of Articulatio cubiti. B C

17 ***A. profunda brachii.*** Caudally directed trunk which primarily supplies the musculature of the caudal side of brachium. B C

18 *A. collateralis radialis.* Courses to the cranial aspect of Articulatio cubiti, accompanying N. radialis in Sulcus m. brachialis. B C

19 **A. collateralis media.** Runs towards Fossa olecrani and contributes to Rete articulare cubiti. C

20 ***A. bicipitalis.*** Cranially and slightly distally directed muscular trunk, mainly for M. biceps brachii. B

21 ***A. nutricia humeri.*** Enters Foramen nutricium of humerus. B

22 ***A. collateralis ulnaris.*** Passes caudodistally across the medial surface of humerus and continues distally between Mm. extensor and flexor carpi ulnaris. Joins Ramus palmaris of A. mediana just proximal to carpus. B C

23 *Rete articulare cubiti.* Network around Articulatio cubiti. B C

23a *Ramus dorsalis.* Dorsal branch.

24 ***A. transversa cubiti.*** Passes distolaterally over the cranial aspect of Articulatio cubiti and continues on the cranial surface of radius towards carpus. B C 301 B

25 ***A. interossea communis.*** Courses caudolaterally towards Spatium interosseum antebrachii. B

26 *A. interossea cranialis.* Traverses Spatium interosseum antebrachii and courses distally on the lateral border of radius. B C 301 B

27 **A. recurrens interossea.** Courses proximally along the lateral aspect of ulna. C

28 **Rami carpei dorsales.** Concur to form the Rete carpi dorsale. C

29 *A. interossea caudalis.* Very slender and inconstant, runs along the caudal surface of radius. B

A Arteries of left manus, abaxial aspect (bo)

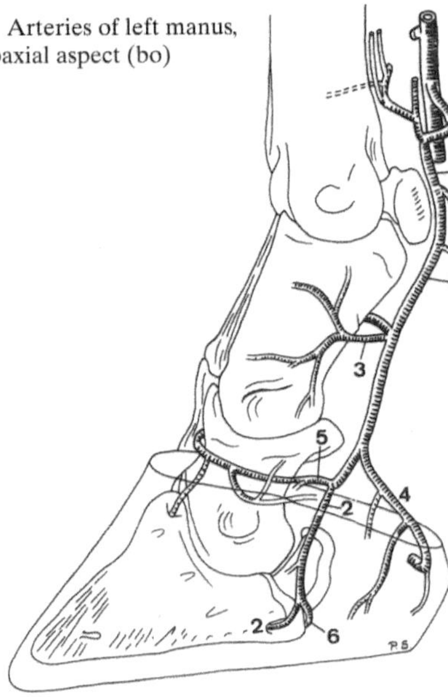

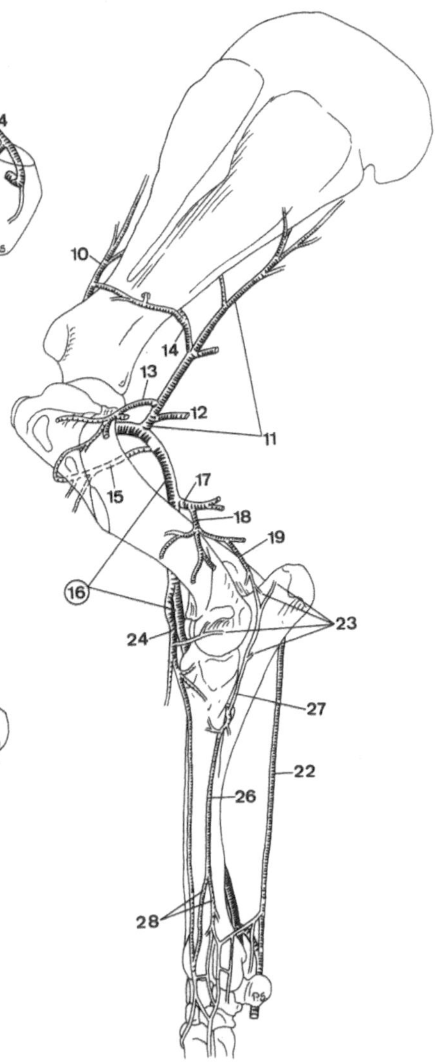

C Arteries of left thoracic limb, lateral aspect (eq)

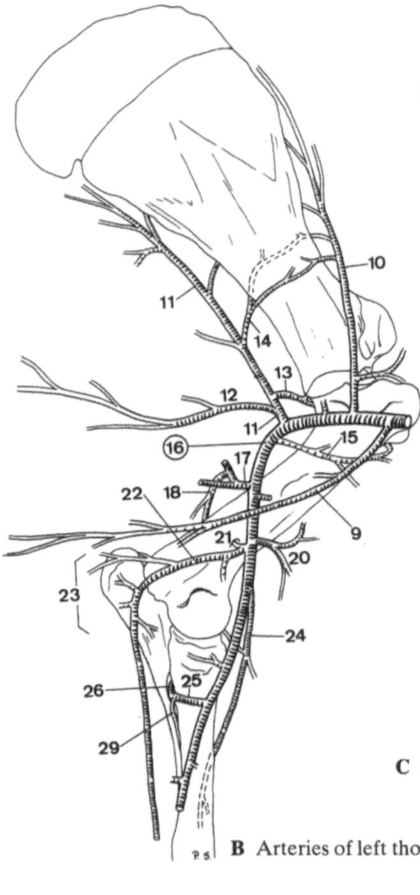

B Arteries of left thoracic limb, medial aspect (eq)

1 **A. mediana**. Continuation of A. brachialis distal to the origin of A. interossea communis. Passes through Canalis carpi and continues along the medial aspect of the digital flexor tendons. A

2 ***A. profunda antebrachii***. Supplies the caudal muscles on antebrachium. A (See the text within parentheses on page 284.26.)

3 ***A. radialis proximalis***. Small artery which courses on the caudal surface of radius. A

4 *Ramus carpeus dorsalis*. Branch to Rete carpi dorsale. A B

5 **Rete carpi dorsale**. Network on the dorsal surface of carpus. B

6 **Aa. metacarpeae dorsales II et III**. Run in the dorsal grooves between Ossa metacarpalia II–III s. III–IV. B C D

7 *Ramus carpeus palmaris**. Supplies the palmar aspect of carpus. A (This small branch is highly significant in the Proximal check ligament desmotomy.)

8 ***A. radialis***. Courses on the palmar surface of carpus. A

8a *Ramus carpeus dorsalis*. Surrounds the medial border of Regio carpi (at the level of Os carpi radiale) and becomes a dorsal branch. A

9 *Ramus anastomoticus cum a. metacarpea dorsali II*. Courses around the Basis of Os metacarpale II. A B

10 *Arcus palmaris profundus*. Connection between A. radialis and Ramus palmaris of A. mediana. Usually represented on both surfaces of M. interosseus. A

11 **Aa. metacarpeae palmares II et III**. Run along the palmar groove between Ossa metacarpalia II–III s. III–IV. A C D

12 **Ramus perforans distalis**. Branch of A. metacarpea palmaris, penetrates between Ossa metacarpalia, joins A. metacarpea dorsalis. A C D

13 ***Ramus palmaris***. Courses laterodistally, joins A. collateralis ulnaris and continues distally. A

14 *Ramus superficialis*. Concurs to Arcus palmaris superficialis. A

15 **A. digitalis palmaris communis III**. Continuation of Ramus superficialis distal to the point where it joins Arcus palmaris superficialis. A D

16 *Ramus profundus*. Concurs to Arcus palmaris profundus. A

17 *Ramus anastomoticus cum a. metacarpea dorsali III*. Courses around the lateral surface of Basis of Os metacarpale IV, joins A. metacarpea dorsalis III. A B

18 *(Arcus palmaris superficialis)*. Subfascial connection of A. mediana and Ramus superficialis of Ramus palmaris. A

19 ***A. digitalis palmaris communis II***. Continuation of A. mediana distal to the point where Arcus palmaris superficialis normally arises. A C D

20 *A. digitalis [palmaris propria III] medialis*. Passes on the abaxial side of the medial Os sesamoideum proximale, reaches Sulcus solearis, enters Foramen soleare. A C D

21 **Ramus palmaris phalangis proximalis**. Courses laterally across the palmar aspect of Phalanx proximalis. A C

22 **Ramus dorsalis phalangis proximalis**. Dorsally directed branch, given off by Ramus palmaris phalangis proximalis. A C

23 **Ramus palmaris phalangis mediae**. Courses laterally across the palmar aspect of Phalanx media. A

24 **Ramus dorsalis phalangis mediae**. Passes on the lateral aspect of Cartilago ungularis medialis to the dorsal surface of Phalanx media. C

25 **Ramus tori digitalis**. Runs in a distopalmar direction and ramifies chiefly in Torus ungulae. A C

26 **A. coronalis**. Arises from Ramus tori digitalis, courses dorsally along the proximal border of Cartilago ungularis medialis and Capsula ungulae. A C

27 **Ramus dorsalis phalangis distalis**. Passes through Foramen or Incisura processus palmaris and continues dorsally in Sulcus parietalis medialis. A C

28 **Arcus terminalis**. Arch inside Canalis solearis, formed by the union of Aa. digitales medialis and lateralis. A

28a **A. marginis solearis**. Surrounds the Margo solearis phalangis distalis. C D

29 *A. digitalis [palmaris propria III] lateralis*. Courses laterally between M. interosseus medius and M. flexor digitalis profundus, takes up Aa. metacarpeae palmares and A. digitalis palmaris communis III. Continues on the abaxial side of the lateral Os sesamoideum proximale. Reaches Sulcus solearis, enters Foramen soleare. A C D

30 **Ramus palmaris phalangis proximalis**. See 21. A D

31 **Ramus dorsalis phalangis proximallis**. See 22. A D

32 **Ramus palmaris phalangis mediae**. See 23. A

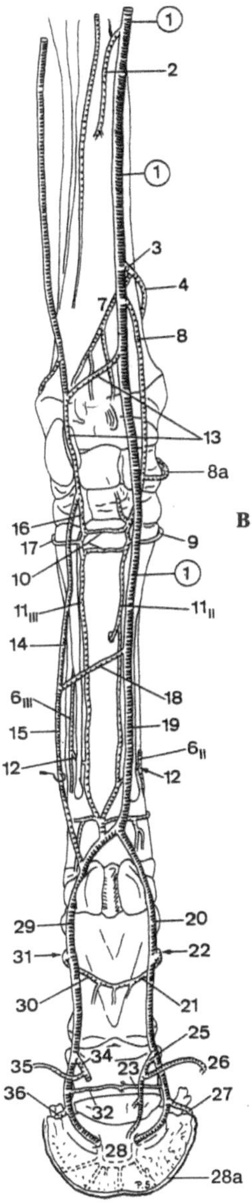

A Arteries of left thoracic limb, palmar aspect (eq)

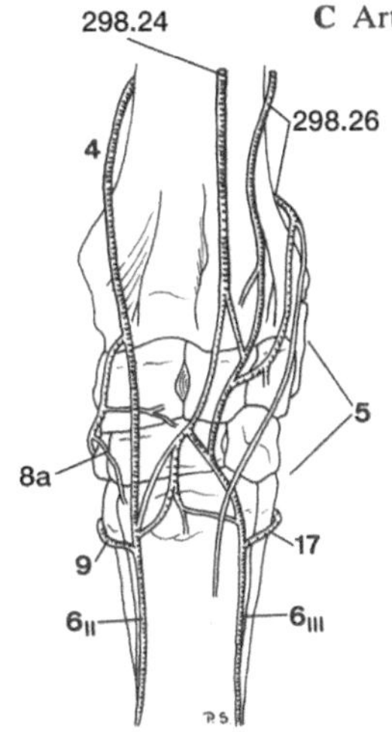

B Arteries of left carpus, dorsal aspect (eq)

C Arteries of left manus, medial aspect (eq)

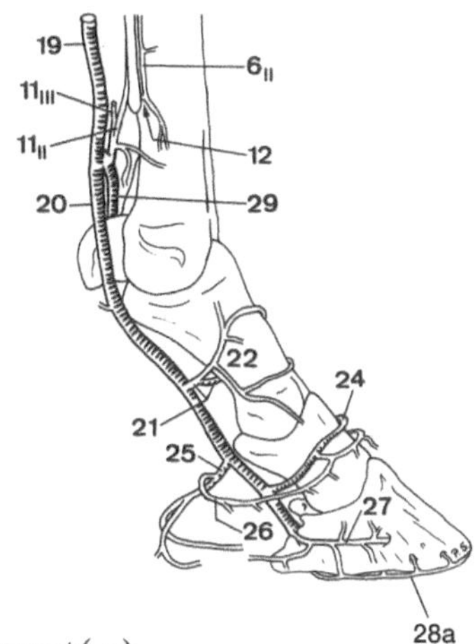

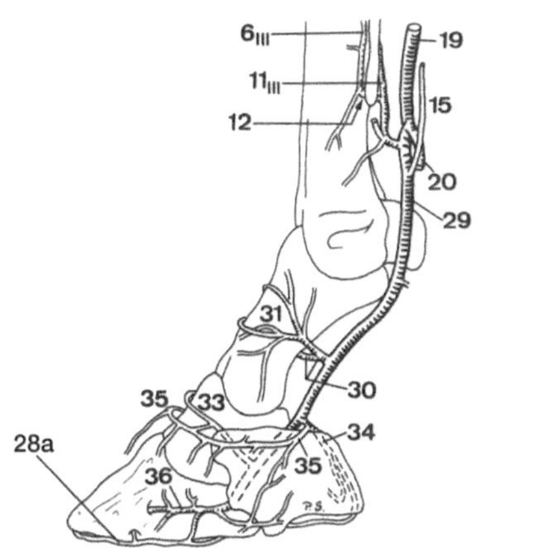

D Arteries of left manus, lateral aspect (eq)

33 **Ramus dorsalis phalangis mediae.** Counterpart of 24. D

34 **Ramus tori digitalis.** See 25. A D

35 **A. coronalis.** See 26. A D

36 **Ramus dorsalis phalangis distalis.** Counterpart of 27. A D

TERMINI COMMUNES

1 **AORTA DESCENDENS.** Caudal continuation of aorta beyond Arcus aortae. A C

2 **AORTA THORACIA.** Intrathoracic segment of Aorta descendens. Extends to Hiatus aorticus of the Diaphragma. A B C

3 ***A. broncho-esophagea [-oesophagea].*** Variable trunk for the supply of lungs and esophagus. A

4 *Ramus bronchalis.* Variably developed vessel which divides at Bifurcatio tracheae in left and right branches which enter the hilus of the corresponding lung along the bronchi. A

5 *Ramus esophageus [oesophageus].* Passes caudally along esophagus. A

6 ***Rami esophagei [oesophagei].*** Small branches to esophagus, in su and ov.

7 ***Rami pericardiaci.*** Variably arising branches to pericardium in ca. A

8 ***Rami mediastinales.*** Small branches to Mediastinum dorsale in ca. A

9 ***A. phrenica cranialis*** (eq). Intrathoracic branch to Pars lumbalis of the Diaphragma. Also described in su, ov, bo. C

10 ***Aa. intercostales dorsales.*** Symmetrical vessels which pass across the Corpus vertebrae to the Spatium intercostale and continue along Sulcus costae. Often fuse with the initial segments of adjacent fellow vessels. A B C

11 *Ramus dorsalis.* Courses dorsally to Mm. dorsi. Passes through Foramen vertebrale laterale in su. B C

12 **Ramus spinalis.** Enters Canalis vertebralis via Foramen intervertebrale, Foramen vertebrale laterale or both openings (su). Contributes to A. spinalis ventralis. B C

13 **Ramus cutaneus medialis.** Superficial continuation of Ramus dorsalis. Absent in su. B

14 **Ramus cutaneus lateralis.**[1)]

15 *Ramus collateralis* (Car, su). Courses across the medial aspect of the corresponding rib to the preceding Spatium intercostale. An analogous branch, but towards the cranial border of the following rib, is described in eq. B

16 *Rami cutanei laterales.* Perforating branches to the skin of the lateral thoracic wall. B

17 **Rami mammarii.** To the Mammae thoracicae (Car, su). B

18 *Rami phrenici.* Arise from the caudal Aa. intercostales dorsales and supply Pars costalis of Diaphragma.

19 ***A. costoabdominalis dorsalis.*** Courses along the caudal aspect of the last rib. Given off by Aorta abdominalis in eq. C

20 *Ramus dorsalis.* Runs dorsally to Mm. dorsi. Passes through Foramen vertebrale laterale of the last Vertebra thoracica in su. C

21 **Ramus spinalis.** Enters Canalis vertebralis via the thoracolumbar Foramen intervertebrale and (su)/or Foramen vertebrale laterale and joins A. spinalis ventralis. C

22 **Ramus cutaneus medialis.** Superficial continuation of Ramus dorsalis. C

23 **Ramus cutaneus lateralis.**[1)]

24 *Rami cutanei laterales.* Pass laterally to the adjacent skin segments. C

1) These arteries were omitted from the 5th edition of the N. A. V.

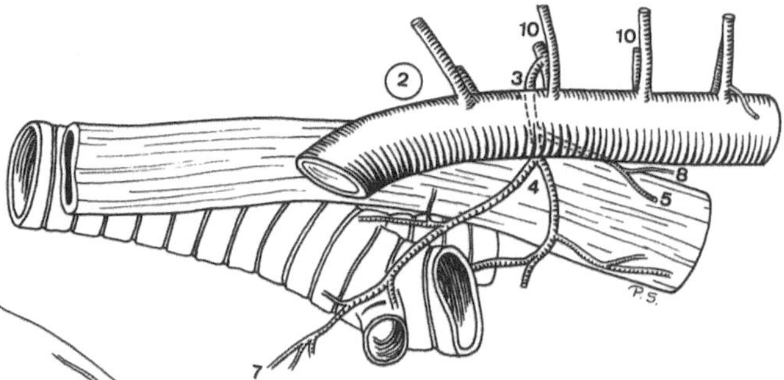

A Aorta descendens, left lateral aspect (ca)

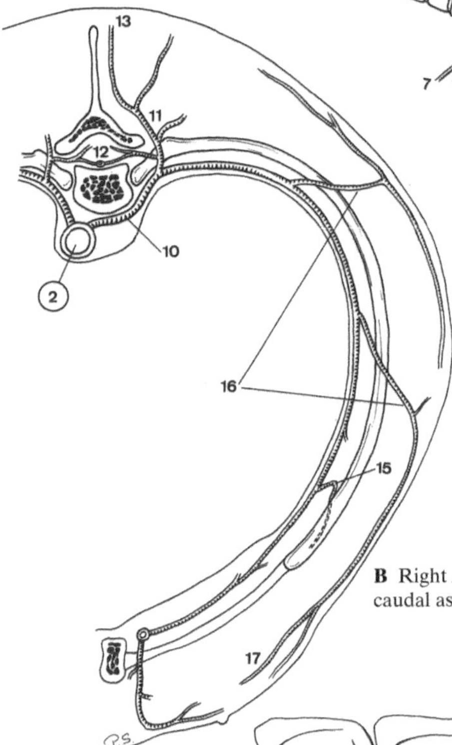

B Right A. intercostalis dorsalis V, caudal aspect (ca)

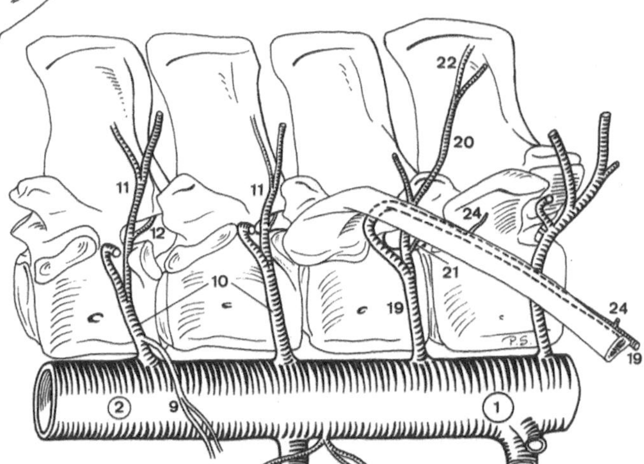

C Thoracolumbar segment of Aorta descendens, left lateral aspect (eq)

1 **AORTA ABDOMINALIS**. Intra-abdominal segment of Aorta descendens. A B

2 **A. phrenica caudalis**. Courses cranially into Pars lumbalis of Diaphragma. Originates by a common trunk with the A. abdominalis cranialis in Car, from A. celiaca in su and Ru, and is absent in eq. A

3 ***Rami adrenales [supra-] craniales***. Run caudally to Gl. adrenalis. Arise variably. A

4 **A. abdominalis cranialis**. Passes to the lateral abdominal wall. It occurs in Car and su, in Car arises by a common trunk with the A. phrenica caudalis. A

5 **Aa. lumbales**. Often initially fused segmental vessels, pass across Corpus of the corresponding Vertebra lumbalis to the caudal border of its Processus costalis. The first 2 or 3 arise from Aorta thoracica in Car, the last arises variably. A B C

6 ***Rami phrenici*** (su, Ru). Arise from the cranial Aa. lumbales and course cranially to Pars lumbalis of Diaphragma. May be absent (esp. su).

7 ***Rami adrenales [supra-]*** (ca, Ru). Arise from the cranial Aa. lumbales and supply Gl. adrenalis.

8 ***Ramus spinalis***. Enters Canalis vertebralis through the corresponding Foramen intervertebrale or Foramen vertebrale laterale and joins A. spinalis ventralis. B C

9 ***Ramus dorsalis***. Courses dorsally to the epaxial muscles. Passes through Foramen vertebrale laterale of the corresponding Vertebra lumbalis in su. B C

10 *Ramus cutaneus medialis*. Runs to the medial region of the skin of the dorsum. B

11 ***Ramus cutaneus lateralis***. Superficial continuation of Ramus dorsalis into the skin of the Dorsum.

12 **A. circumflexa ilium profunda**. Arises from the Aorta in Carnivora, and from A. iliaca externa in the other domestic mammals. The branching is also different in Carnivora . A (A. circumflexa ilium profunda arises from A. iliaca communis in rabbits. The term "A. iliaca communis" is not yet officially introduced nor listed in the N. A. V.)

13 ***Rami craniales***. Course cranioventrally in the flank. A

14 ***Rami caudales***. Ventrally or ventrocaudally directed branches to the flank and the thigh. A

15 **(A. sacralis mediana)** (eq). Continuation of the aorta along Facies pelvina of Os sacrum. Slender or absent. (Should be listed as 22a according to the 5th edition of the N. A. V.)

16 **A. sacralis mediana** (Car, su, Ru). Continuation of aorta along Facies pelvina of Os sacrum. May be paired (ca, ov). A B C

17 ***A. lumbalis VI (VII)*** (su, ov, cap). Often initially fused, passes across the corpus of the corresponding Vertebra lumbalis to the caudal border of its Processus costalis. B

18 ***Rami sacrales***. Often initially fused segmental arteries, course dorsally into the corresponding Foramen sacrale ventrale. The last pair pierces between Os sacrum and Vertebra caudalis I. A B C

19 *Ramus spinalis*. Joins A. spinalis ventralis. B C

20 *Ramus dorsalis*. Emerges through Foramen sacrale dorsale or between the last sacral and first caudal vertebrae respectively, and supplies the epaxial musculature. B C

21 ***A. sacralis lateralis*** (fe). Anastomosis between Rami sacrales along the ventral aspect of Os sacrum. C

22 ***(A. sacralis lateralis)*** (ca). Anastomosis between Rami sacrales along the ventral aspect of Os sacrum.

23 **A. caudalis [coccygea] mediana**. Continuation of A. sacralis mediana (except eq) along the ventral surface of Vertebrae caudales. Locally enclosed by Processus hemales or Arcus hemales. In eq it usually arises from the left or right A. glutea caudalis. A B C

24 ***Rami caudales [coccygei]***. Sometimes initially fused (ca, su) segmental branches, course dorsally across the corpus of the corresponding Vertebra caudalis. A B C

25 *A. caudalis [coccygea] ventrolateralis*. Chain of anastomoses bwtween the Rami caudales, located along the ventrolateral aspect of Vertebrae caudales. A B C

26 *A. caudalis [coccygea] dorsolateralis*. Chain of anastomoses between the Rami caudales, located along the dorsolateral aspect of Vertebrae caudales. B C

27 ***Corpora caudalia [coccygea]***. Small nodules of arteriovenous anastomoses, located in the tail.

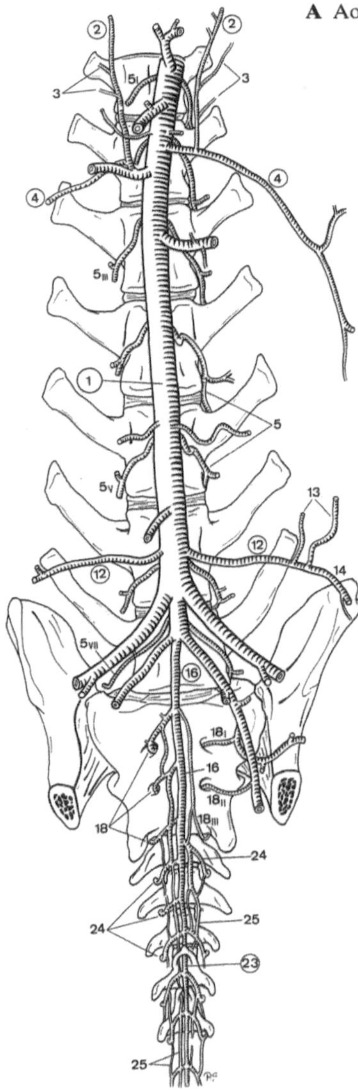

A Aorta abdominalis, ventral aspect (ca)

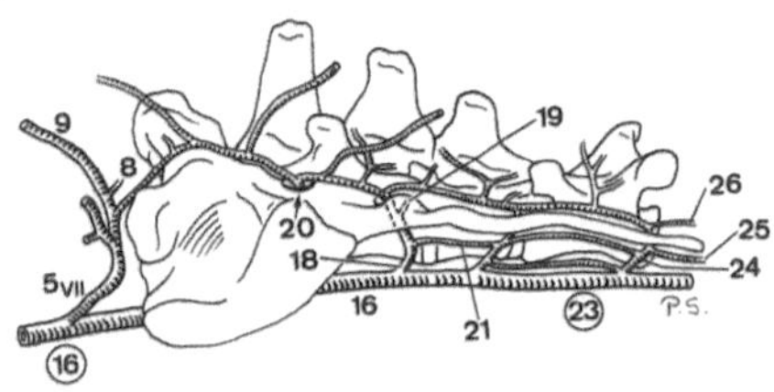

C Branches of A. sacralis mediana and A. caudalis mediana, left lateral aspect (fe)

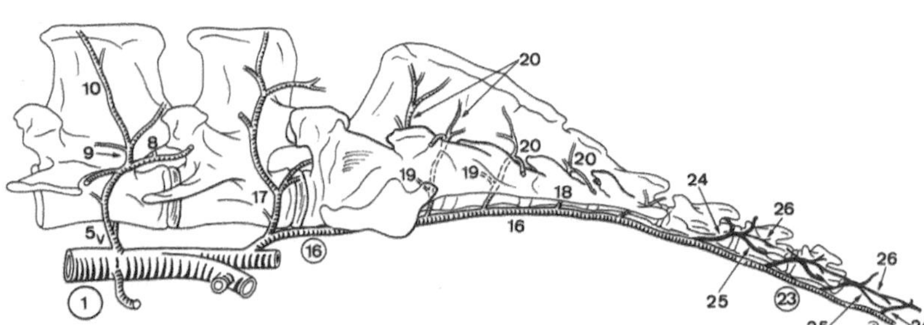

B Segmental branches of Aorta abdominalis, A. sacralis mediana, and A. caudalis mediana, left lateral aspect (cap)

1 **A. celiaca [coeliaca]**. Unpaired, leaves the initial part of Aorta abdominalis. A B C

CARNIVORA

2 *(**A. phrenica caudalis**)* (fe). Courses cranially to Pars lumbalis of Diaphragma.

3 ***A. gastrica sinistra***. Runs to Pars cardiaca of the stomach, continues to the right along Curvatura ventriculi minor. A B

4 *Rami esophagei [oesophagei]*. Run through Hiatus esophageus. A

5 ***A. hepatica***. Courses cranioventrally and to the right toward the liver. A B

6 *Ramus dexter lateralis*. To Lobus hepatis dexter lateralis. B

7 **A. lobi caudati**. Supplies Lobus caudatus of the liver. B

8 *Ramus dexter medialis*. Supplies Lobus hepatis dexter medialis. May be plural. B

9 *Ramus sinister*. Trunk of branches to the left portion of the liver. B

10 **Rami sinistri mediales**. Branches for Lobus hepatis sinister medialis and Lobus quadratus. B

11 **A. cystica**. Arises from one of the Rami sinistri mediales or Ramus dexter medialis, to Vesica fellea. B

12 **Rami sinistri laterales**. Branches to Lobus hepatis sinister lateralis. B

13 *A. gastrica dextra*. Runs to the left along Curvatura ventriculi minor. A B

14 *A. gastroduodenalis*. Short arterial stem, located between pancreas and Pars cranialis of the duodenum. A B

15 **A. pancreaticoduodenalis cranialis**. In mesoduodenum, branches to pancreas and Pars descendens duodeni. It anastomoses by inosculation with the A. pancreaticoduodenalis caudalis. A (The term "inosculation" is given to two arteries which anastomose with one another in a straight line, therefore it is impossible to know where is the origin and/or termination of either of them; it applies mainly to the arteries of the abdominopelvic viscera.)

16 **A. gastroepiploica dextra**. Curves to the left in Omentum majus along Curvatura ventriculi major. It anastomoses by inosculation with the A. gastroepiploica sinistra. A

17 ***A. lienalis***. Runs to the left along Lobus pancreatis sinister, to the spleen. A B

18 *Rami pancreatici*. Enter Lobus pancreatis sinister. A

19 *Aa. gastricae breves*. To Curvatura ventriculi major via Lig. gastrolienale. A

20 *A. gastroepiploica sinistra*. Courses along Curvatura ventriculi major to the right, anastomoses by inosculation with A. gastroepiploica dextra. A

SUS

21 ***A. phrenica caudalis***. Courses cranially to Pars lumbalis of Diaphragma. C

22 ***A. hepatica***. Courses cranioventrally and to the right toward the liver. C D

23 *Rami pancreatici*. Pass caudoventrally to the pancreas. C

24 *Ramus dexter lateralis*. Slender branch, essentially supplying Lobus hepatis dexter lateralis. C D

25 **A. lobi caudati**. Supplies Lobus caudatus of the liver. D

26 *A. gastroduodenalis*. Courses ventrally through the pancreas to the duodenum. C D

27 **A. pancreaticoduodenalis cranialis**. Runs caudodorsally between Lobus pancreatis dexter and the duodenum. It anastomoses by inosculation with the A. pancreaticoduodenalis caudalis. C

28 **A. gastroepiploica dextra**. Passes along Curvatura ventriculi major. It anastomoses by inosculation with the A. gastroepiploica sinistra. C

29 *Ramus dexter medialis*. Supplies chiefly Lobus hepatis dexter medialis. C

30 **A. cystica**. Courses ventrally along Ductus cysticus to Vesica fellea. D

31 *Ramus sinister*. Large branch to the left half of the liver. C D

32 **Rami sinistri laterales**. Supply Lobus hepatis sinister lateralis. D

33 **Rami sinistri mediales**. Supply Lobus hepatis sinister medialis. D

34 *A. gastrica dextra*. Courses ventrally in Omentum minus and ramifies on Facies parietalis of the stomach. D

35 ***A. lienalis***. Runs to the left, reaches Extremitas dorsalis of the spleen, and courses ventrally along Hilus lienis. C

36 *A. gastrica sinistra*. Courses ventrally to Curvatura ventriculi minor and ramifies on Facies visceralis of the stomach. C

37 **Rami esophagei [oesophagei]**. Run cranially across Curvatura ventriculi minor to the caudal portion of the esophagus. C

38 *A. diverticuli*. Reaches the medial aspect of Diverticulum ventriculi. C

39 *Ramus pancreaticus*. To Lobus pancreatis sinister. C

40 *Ramus gastrolienalis*. Short trunk which supplies small dorsal parts of stomach and spleen. C

41 *A. gastroepiploica sinistra*. Courses in Lig. gastrolienale to Curvatura ventriculi major. Anastomoses by inosculation with A. gastroepiploica dextra. C

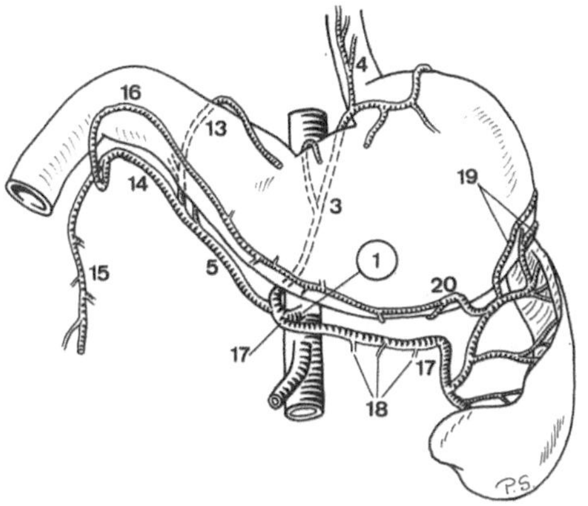

A Arteries of stomach and spleen, ventral aspect (ca)

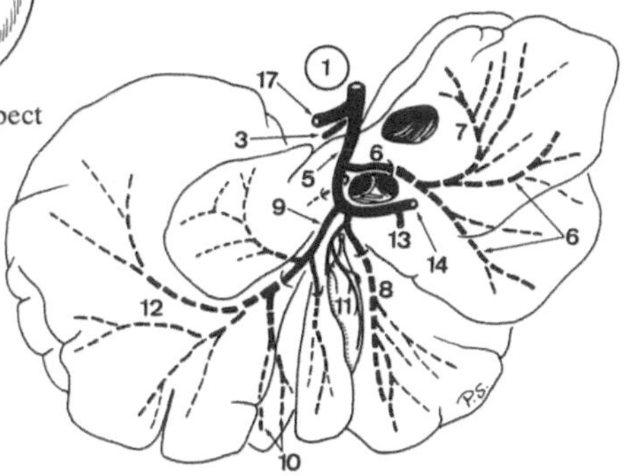

B A. hepatica, caudal aspect (ca)

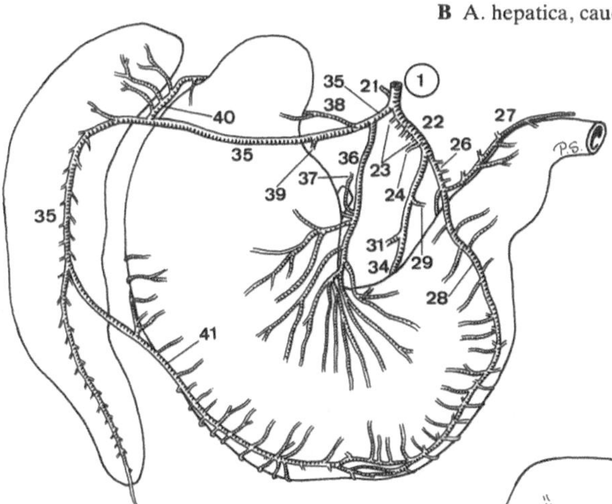

C Arteries of stomach and spleen, caudal aspect (su)

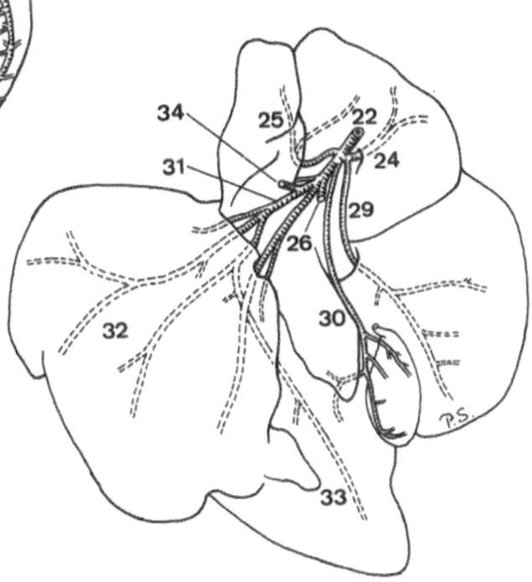

D A. hepatica, caudal aspect (su)

RUMINANTIA

1 **Aa. phrenicae caudales.** Course cranioventrally to Pars lumbalis of Diaphragma. A

2 ***Rami adrenales [supra-] craniales.*** Inconstant branches to Gl. adrenalis. A

3 ***A. gastrica sinistra.*** Courses on the right side of Atrium ruminis and Basis omasi to Curvatura minor of abomasum. Arises often from A. hepatica in ov, cap. It anastomoses by inosculation with the A. gastrica dextra. A (see 306.15)

4 *A. gastroepiploica sinistra.* Runs across the left caudal aspect of Collum omasi to Curvatura major of abomasum. A

5 *A. reticularis accessoria.* Courses to reticulum. May be absent (bo). A

6 ***A. hepatica.*** Passes to the right and cranioventrally towards the liver. A B

7 *Rami pancreatici.* Run caudodorsally towards pancreas. B

8 *Ramus dexter.* Often double branch to Lobus hepatis dexter. B

9 **A. lobi caudati.** To Lobus caudatus of the liver. B

10 **A. cystica.** Courses along Ductus cysticus to Vesica fellea, originates from A. gastroduodenalis in bo. B

11 *Ramus sinister.* Supplies Lobi hepatis sinister, caudatus, and quadratus. B

12 *A. gastrica dextra.* Courses in Omentum minus along duodenum to Curvatura minor of abomasum. It anastomoses by inosculation with A. gastrica sinistra. A B

13 *A. gastroduodenalis.* Courses towards the duodenum. A B

14 **A. pancreaticoduodenalis cranialis.** Courses along Pars descendens of duodenum. It anastomoses by inosculation with A. pancreaticoduodenalis caudalis. A B

15 **A. gastroepiploica dextra.** Courses along Curvatura major of abomasum. It anastomoses by inosculation with A. gastroepiploica sinistra. A B

16 ***A. lienalis.*** Passes to the left across the rumen, enters Hilus lienis. A

17 *Rami pancreatici.* Into Lobus pancreatis sinister. A

18 *A. ruminalis sinistra.* Curves across Atrium ruminis and through Sulcus cranialis to Facies parietalis. Arises often from A. gastrica sinistra in ov. A

19 **A. reticularis.** Passes to the left across the rumen into Sulcus ruminoreticularis. Arises often from A. lienalis or gastrica sinistra in ov, cap. A

20 **Rami phrenici.** Branches of A. reticularis to Pars lumbalis of Diaphragma. A

21 **Rami esophagei [oesophagei].** Branches of A. reticularis to esophagus. A

22 *Ramus epiploicus.* Runs caudally in Paries profundus of Omentum majus, continues through Sulcus caudalis of the rumen. Absent in bo. A

23 *A. ruminalis dextra.* Courses in Sulcus longitudinalis dexter, in Sulcus accessorius dexter (cap) and passes via Sulcus caudalis to Facies parietalis (ov, cap), or continues cranially in Sulcus longitudinalis sinister (bo) of the rumen. A

EQUUS

24 ***A. gastrica sinistra.*** Passes in Lig. gastrophrenicum towards Curvatura ventriculi minor. It anastomoses by inosculation with the A. gastrica dextra. In 15% of individuals it originates from A. lienalis. Exceptionally, it is a double artery, originating one from the A. lienalis and the other from A. hepatica. C

25 *Ramus visceralis.* Ramifies on Facies visceralis of the stomach. C

26 *Ramus parietalis.* Ramifies on Facies parietalis of the stomach. C

27 *Ramus esophageus [oesophageus].* Passes through Hiatus esophageus along the dorsal aspect of the esophagus. C

28 ***A. hepatica.*** Passes cranioventrally and to the right into Porta hepatis. C

29 *Rami pancreatici.* Enter Facies dorsalis of the pancreas. C

30 *A. gastrica dextra.* Runs to Ampulla duodeni, curves along Curvatura ventriculi minor. It anastomoses by inosculation with the A. gastrica sinistra. C

31 *A. gastroduodenalis.* Common trunk for A. pancreaticoduodenalis cranialis and A. gastroepiploica dextra. C

32 **A. pancreaticoduodenalis cranialis.** Supplies Corpus pancreatis and continues along Ansa sigmoidea of the duodenum. It anastomoses by inosculation with A. pancreaticoduodenalis caudalis. C

33 **A. gastroepiploica dextra.** Crosses Ampulla duodeni caudally, courses along Curvatura ventriculi major. It anastomoses by inosculation with A. gastroepiploica sinistra. C

34 *Ramus dexter.* Variably branching supply for the right half of the liver. C

35 *Ramus sinister.* Supplies Lobi hepatis sinistri and Lobus quadratus. C

36 ***A. lienalis.*** Passes to the left via Lig. gastrolienale, continues along Hilus lienis to Extremitas ventralis of the spleen. C

37 *Rami pancreatici.* Supply Lobus pancreatis sinister. C

38 *Aa. gastricae breves.* Pass in Ligamentum gastrolienale to Curvatura ventriculi major. C

39 *A. gastroepiploica sinistra.* Passes to the right along Curvatura ventriculi major and anastomoses by inosculation with A. gastroepiploica dextra (306.15). C

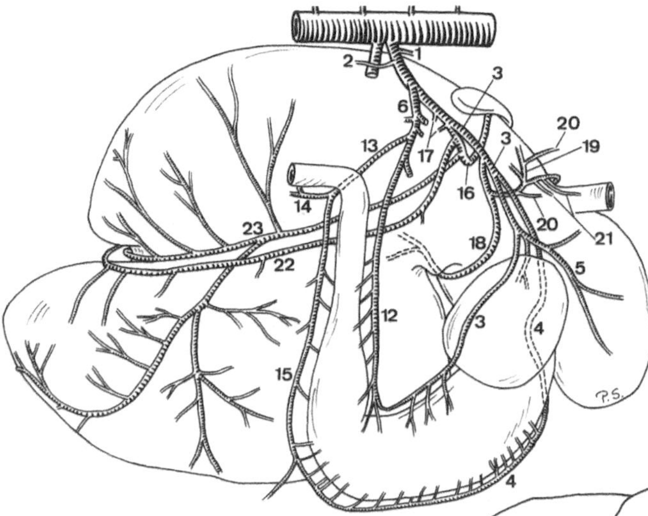

A Arteries of the stomach, right aspect (cap)

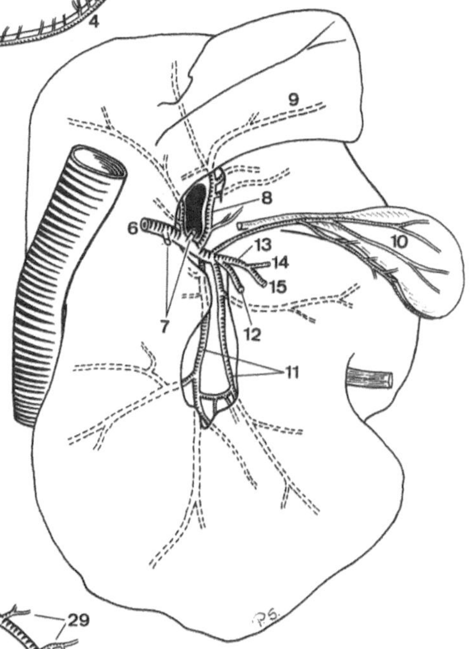

B Arteries of the liver, caudal aspect (bo)

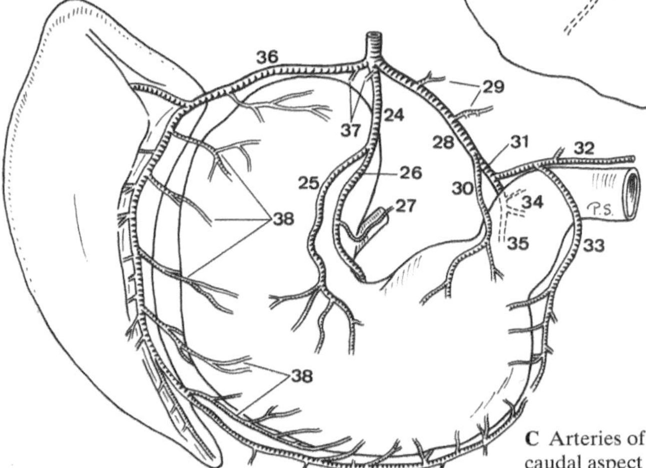

C Arteries of stomach and spleen, caudal aspect (eq)

TERMINI COMMUNES

1 **A. mesenterica cranialis.** Unpaired visceral branch of aorta in Radix mesenterii. The branches are listed in the order of the segments of the intestine supplied. A B C (This is a substantial difference from the 4th edition of the N. A. V., and much easier to follow.)

2 ***Rami pancreatici*** (Ru). To Lobus pancreatis dexter. A

3 ***A. pancreaticoduodenalis caudalis.*** Supplies parts of pancreas and duodenum. It anastomoses by inosculation with A. pancreaticoduodenalis cranialis. A (see 306.15)

4 ***Aa. jejunales.*** Course radially in mesojejunum and, interconnected by arches, supply jejunum. A B

4a *Rami colici dextri* (ov, cap). Supply the last Gyrus centrifugalis, which is closely related to the jejunum.

5 ***Ramus collateralis*** (bo). Curves caudoventrally in mesojejunum, rejoins A. mesenterica cranialis. A

6 ***Aa. ilei.*** Variably arising branches of A. mesenterica cranialis and A. ileocolica located in mesoileum, supply ileum. A

7 ***A. ileocolica.*** Variably composed trunk, branches to ileum, cecum, and colon. A B

8 *Ramus ilei mesenterialis.* Runs inside mesoileum along the lesser curvature of ileum and anastomoses with the ileal arteries. A B

9 *A. cecalis [caecalis]* (Car, su, Ru). Passes along the dorsal border of cecum (fe), in the axis of the cecal loops (ca), in Plica ileocecalis (su, Ru) towards the apex. A

10 ***Ramus ilei antimesenterialis*** (Car, Ru). Courses in Plica ileocecalis along the major curvature of ileum towards jejunum. A

11 *A. cecalis [caecalis] medialis* (eq). Passes along Tenia medialis towards Apex ceci. B

12 *A. cecalis [caecalis] lateralis* (eq). Courses along Tenia lateralis towards Apex ceci. B

13 *Ramus colicus.* Supplies the initial segment of Colon ascendens, i. e. Gyri centripetales (su), Colon ventrale (eq). Anastomoses by inosculation with A. colica dextra. Surrounded by an arterial network in su. B

14 *Rami colici.* Occur in Ru, course at the right aspect of Colon ascendens, supply Ansa proximalis and Gyri centripetales, and are homologous to Ramus colicus of the other domestic mammals and to A. ascendens of the N.A. They arise from the distal part of A. ileocolica and may originate by a common trunk with Aa. colicae dextrae. A

15 *Aa. colicae dextrae* (Ru). Supply Gyri centrifugales and Ansa distalis, and are homologous to A. colica dextra of the other domestic mammals. They arise from the proximal part of A. ileocolica and may originate by a common trunk with Rami colici. A

16 ***A. colica dextra.*** Arises by a common trunk with A. ileocolica and A. colica media in Car, together with A. colica media from A. mesenterica cranialis (su, eq). Supplies the terminal segment of Colon ascendens, i. e. Gyri centrifugales (su), or Colon dorsale (eq). Anastomoses by inosculation with Ramus colicus and with A. colica media. B

17 ***A. colica media.*** Arises directly (fe, Ru) or together with A. colica dextra (su, eq), or originates from A. ileocolica (Car, exceptionally ov). Supplies Colon transversum and, in Car and Ru, the initial segment of Colon descendens. It anastomoses by inosculation with A. colica dextra and with A. colica sinistra. A B

18 **A. mesenterica caudalis.** Unpaired visceral branch of the aorta. Supplies the terminal portion of intestine. A B

19 ***A. colica sinistra.*** In Mesocolon descendens, supplies Colon descendens. It anastomoses by inosculation with A. colica media. A B

20 ***Aa. sigmoideae.*** Branches of A. colica sinistra and A. rectalis cranialis to Colon sigmoideum. A B

21 ***A. rectalis cranialis.*** Courses in mesorectum along the dorsal border of rectum. A B

22 **A. adrenalis [supra-] media** (Car). Branch to Gl. adrenalis. C

23 **Aa. adrenales [supra-] mediae** (su). To the middle segment of Gl. adrenalis.

24 **A. renalis.** To the Hilus renalis, ramifies usually before entering the kidney. The intrarenal blood vessels are listed in the chapter Splanchnologia (vide Vasa sanguinea renis). C

25 ***Rami adrenales [supra-] caudales.*** Run cranially towards Gl. adrenalis. C

26 ***Ramus uretericus.*** To Pars abdominalis of the ureter. C

27 **A. testicularis.** Passes in Mesorchium proximale through Canalis inguinalis to testis. D

28 ***Rami epididymales.*** To Epididymis. D

29 *Rami ductus deferentis.* Branch to the initial segment of Ductus deferens in cap.

30 **A. ovarica.** Passes coiled via mesovarium to Ovarium. C

31 ***Ramus tubarius.*** Courses in Mesosalpinx, supplies Tuba uterina. C

32 ***Ramus uterinus.*** Runs in mesometrium, supplies the cranial part of Cornu uteri. C

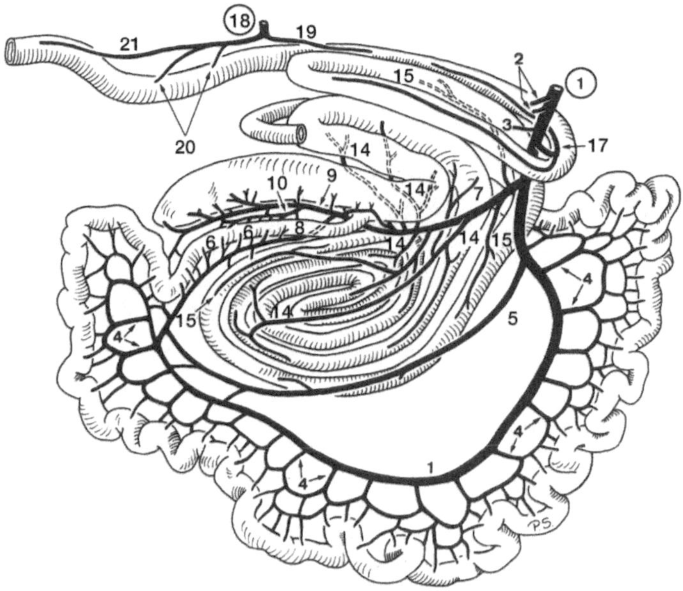

A Arteries of the intestinal tract, right aspect (bo)

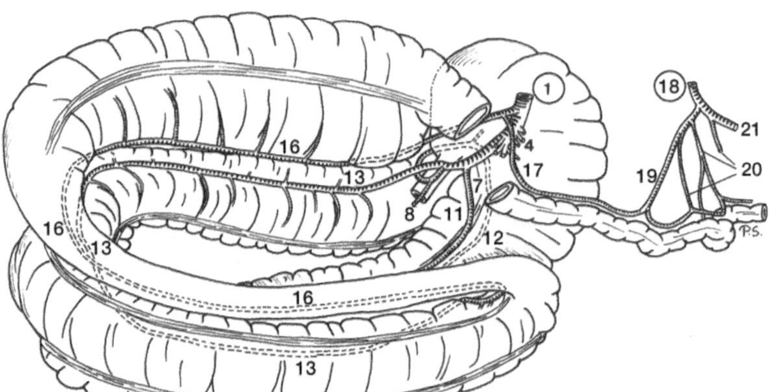

B Arteries of the large intestine, left aspect (eq)

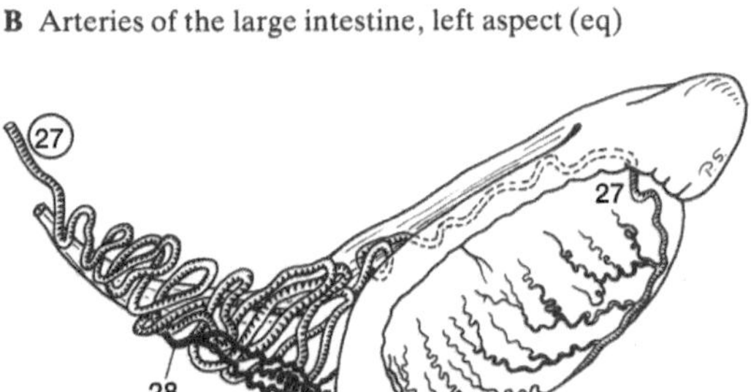

D Left A. testicularis, lateral aspect (su)

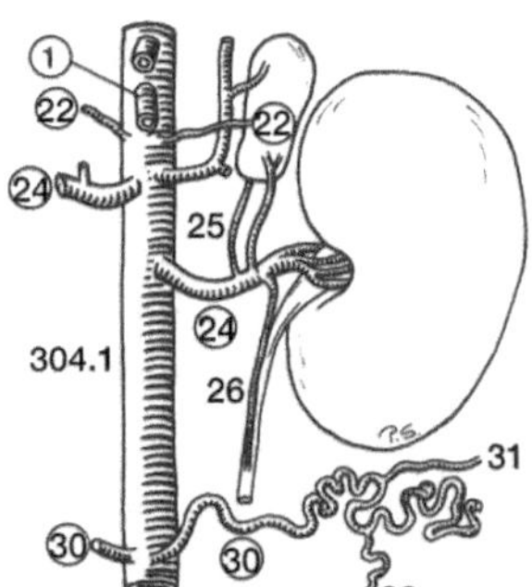

C Aorta abdominalis and left kidney, ventral aspect (ca)

1 **A. ILIACA INTERNA**. Bilateral large branch of Aorta abdominalis, which extends in Cavum pelvis and, after a short (Car, eq) or long (su, Ru) course, ends by dividing into A. glutea caudalis and A. pudenda interna. Leaves Cavum pelvis via Foramen ischiadicum majus and courses on the lateral aspect of Lig. sacrotuberale latum in su. A B (A. iliaca interna arises from A. iliaca communis in the rabbit, but this term is not yet officially discussed, approved, nor listed in the N. A. V., as stated before.)

CARNIVORA

2 **A. umbilicalis**. Enters Lig. vesicae laterale. In the fetus it continues through the umbilicus to the placenta. Becomes postnatally vestigial in its distal segment. A B

3 ***A. vesicalis cranialis*** (fe). Supplies the craniodorsal segment of Vesica urinaria. Normally plural. A

4 ***(A. vesicalis cranialis)*** (ca). Supplies the craniodorsal aspect of Vesica urinaria. B

5 ***Ligamentum teres vesicae***. Vestige of A. umbilicalis located near the cranial border of Lig. vesicae laterale. A B

6 **A. glutea [glutaea] cranialis** (fe). Courses across Incisura ischiadica major. A

7 ***A. obturatoria***. Acompanies N. obturatorius towards Foramen obturatum. Inconstant. A

8 ***A. iliolumbalis***. Passes between Os ilium and M. iliopsoas. A

9 **A. glutea [glutaea] caudalis**. Runs along the dorsal border of Spina ischiadica and courses laterally over Incisura ischiadica minor. A B

10 ***A. iliolumbalis*** (ca). Runs between M. iliopsoas and Os ilium. B

11 ***A. glutea [glutaea] cranialis*** (ca). Runs across the cranial part of Incisura ischiadica major. B

12 ***A. comitans n. ischiadici***. Accompanies N. ischiadicus. A B

13 ***A. caudalis [coccygea] lateralis***. Courses along the lateral aspect of the tail. A B

14 ***A. perinealis dorsalis***. Supplies the dorsal part of perineum. A B

15 **A. pudenda interna**. Courses along Spina ischiadica. A B

16 ***A. prostatica***. To Prostata. The main supplier of pelvic viscera in male. A

17 *A. ductus deferentis*. Courses along Ductus deferens. A

18 **A. vesicalis caudalis**. Reaches Cervix vesicae and ramifies on Vesica urinaria. A

19 **Ramus uretericus**. Branch of A. vesicalis caudalis, to the terminal segment of ureter. In fe it may arise from A. pudenda interna. A

20 **Ramus urethralis**. Branch of A. vesicalis caudalis (ca) or A. ductus deferentis (fe) to the initial portion of urethra. A

21 *A. rectalis media*. To rectum. A

22 ***A. vaginalis***. Ramifies in the lateral wall of vagina. The main supplier of pelvic viscera in female. B

23 *A. uterina*. Main artery of the uterus, coursing along Cervix, Corpus, and Cornu uteri in mesometrium. B

24 **A. vesicalis caudalis**. To Cervix vesicae. B

25 **Ramus uretericus**. Branch of A. vesicalis caudalis to the terminal portion of ureter. B

26 **Ramus urethralis**. Branch of A. vesicalis caudalis to the initial segment of urethra. B

27 *A. rectalis media*. Courses dorsally to rectum. B

28 ***A. urethralis***. Supplies the caudal pelvic part of urethra. Inconstant origin. A B

29 ***A. perinealis ventralis***. Courses along rectum to perineum. A B

30 *A. rectalis caudalis*. To Rectum and Canalis analis. A B

31 *Ramus scrotalis dorsalis*. To the caudodorsal segment of scrotum. A

32 *Ramus labialis dorsalis*. To Labium pudendi. B

33 ***A. penis***. Stem for the supply of the penis. A

34 *A. bulbi penis*. Into Bulbus penis, continues in Corpus spongiosum penis. A

35 *A. profunda penis*. Enters Crus penis and continues in Corpus cavernosum penis. A

36 *A. dorsalis penis*. Courses on Dorsum penis toward glans. A

37 ***A. clitoridis***. Curves across the lateral aspect of Vestibulum vaginae to the clitoris. B

38 *A. bulbi vestibuli*. Enters Bulbus vestibuli. B

39 *A. profunda clitoridis*. Supplies Corpus cavernosum clitoridis. B

40 *A. dorsalis clitoridis*. Courses along the cranioventral border of Corpus clitoridis towards glans. B

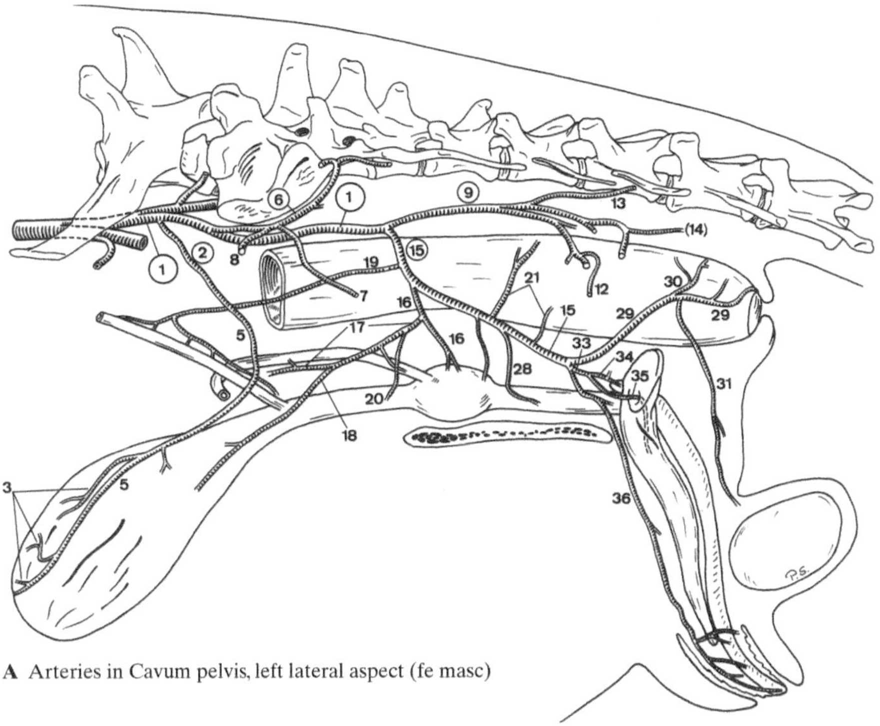

A Arteries in Cavum pelvis, left lateral aspect (fe masc)

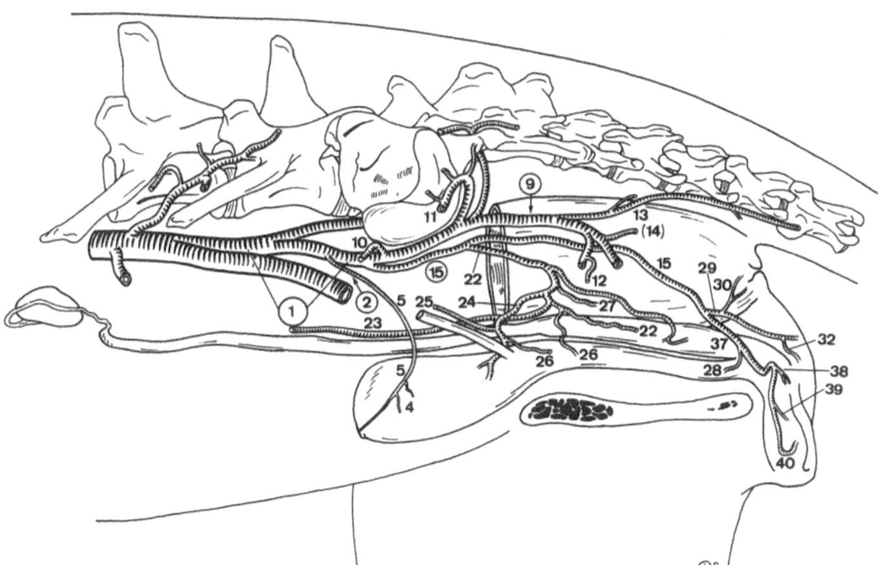

B Arteries in Cavum pelvis, left lateral aspect (ca fem)

SUS

1 **A. umbilicalis**. Enters Lig. vesicae laterale. In the fetus it continues in Funiculus umbilicalis to the placenta. A B

2 ***A. ductus deferentis***. Courses along Ductus deferens. A

3 *Ramus uretericus*. Ramifies along ureter. A

4 ***A. uterina***. Courses in Lig. latum uteri, supplies Cervix, Corpus, and Cornu uteri. B

5 *Ramus uretericus*. Ramifies along ureter. B

6 ***Aa. vesicales craniales***. Supply the cranial portion of Vesica urinaria. A B

7 ***Ligamentum teres vesicae***. Vestige of A. umbilicalis near the cranial border of Lig. vesicae laterale. A B

8 **A. iliolumbalis**. To the lumbar musculature. A B

9 ***A. obturatoria***. Passes with N. obturatorius towards Foramen obturatum. A B

10 **A. glutea [glutaea] cranialis**. Courses over Incisura ischiadica major. A B

11 **A. prostatica**. Runs over the lateral aspect of the rectum and Glandula vesicularis to prostata. It is the main supplier of pelvic viscera in male. A

12 ***Ramus ductus deferentis***. Supplies the terminal segment of Ductus deferens. A

13 *A. vesicalis caudalis*. To the caudal part of Vesica urinaria. A

14 **Ramus uretericus**. Supplies the terminal segment of ureter. A

15 ***Ramus urethralis***. Supplies the cranial segment of Pars pelvina of urethra. A

16 **A. vaginalis**. Courses along the lateral wall of the rectum to the vagina. It is the main supplier of pelvic viscera in female. B

17 ***Ramus uterinus***. Runs along Cervix and Corpus uteri. B

18 *A. vesicalis caudalis*. Passes to the caudal part of Vesica urinaria. B

19 **Ramus uretericus**. Supplies the terminal segment of ureter. B

20 **Ramus urethralis**. Supplies the cranial segment of urethra. B

21 ***A. rectalis media***. Inconstant, to rectum. B

22 ***A. perinealis dorsalis***. Runs to perineum. Also described in male su as branch of A. prostatica or A. glutea caudalis. A B

23 *A. rectalis caudalis*. Supplies Canalis analis. B

24 **A. glutea [glutaea] caudalis**. Courses laterally at Incisura ischiadica minor to the musculature at Regio clunis. A B

25 **A. pudenda interna**. Enters Cavum pelvis by piercing medially through Foramen ischiadicum minus and passes caudoventrally towards Arcus ischiadicus. A B

26 ***A. urethralis***. Runs to the caudal portion of Urethra feminina s. Pars pelvina of Urethra masculina. May form a common initial trunk with its counterpart. A B

27 ***A. perinealis ventralis***. Passes to perineum. A B

28 *A. rectalis caudalis*. Supplies Canalis analis. A

29 *Rami scrotales dorsales*. Ramify in the dorsal aspect of scrotum. A

30 *Rami labiales dorsales*. Ramify in Labium pudendi. B

31 ***A. penis***. Courses towards Radix penis. A

32 *A. bulbi penis*. Enters Bulbus penis and ramifies in Corpus spongiosum penis. A

33 *A. profunda penis*. Enters Corpus cavernosum penis. A

34 *A. dorsalis penis*. Courses along Dorsum penis. Fuses with its counterpart or continues unilaterally at Flexura sigmoidea penis. A

35 ***A. clitoridis***. Courses to Crus clitoridis. B

36 *A. bulbi vestibuli*. Courses to Bulbus vestibuli. B

37 *A. profunda clitoridis*. Enters Corpus cavernosum clitoridis. B

38 *A. dorsalis clitoridis*. Courses along the ventral aspect of Corpus clitoridis. The right may arise from its left counterpart. B

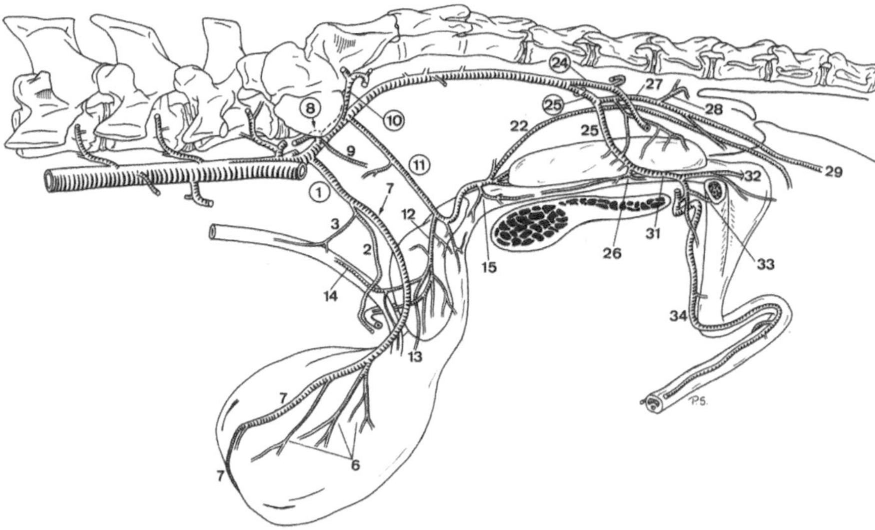

A Arteries in Cavum pelvis, left lateral aspect (su masc)

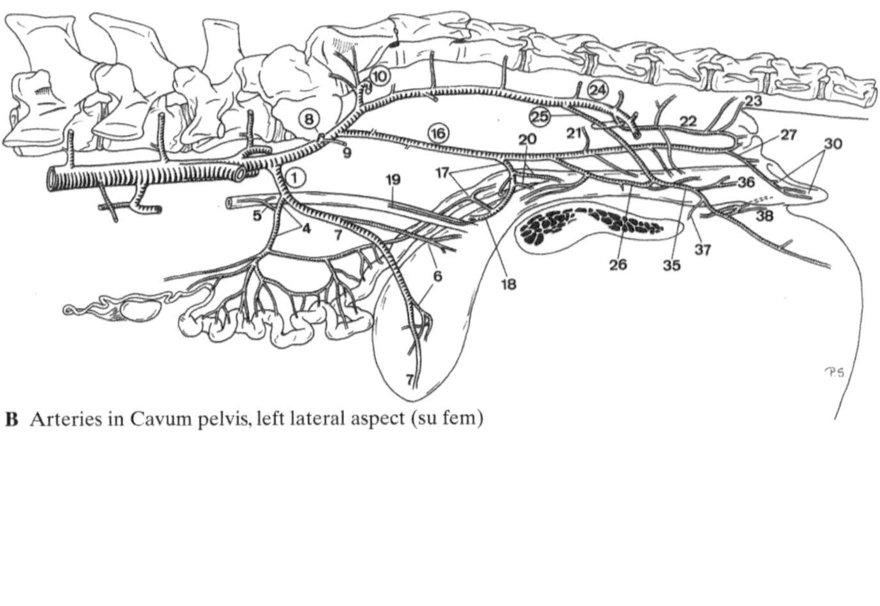

B Arteries in Cavum pelvis, left lateral aspect (su fem)

RUMINANTIA

1 **A. umbilicalis**. Curves in Lig. vesicae laterale. In the fetus it continues via Funiculus umbilicalis to the placenta. A B

2 ***A. ductus deferentis***. Courses along Ductus deferens. A

3 ***A. uterina***. Courses in Lig. latum uteri, supplies Cervix, Corpus, and Cornu uteri. B

4 ***Ramus uretericus***. To the caudal segment of ureter. A B

5 ***Aa. vesicales craniales***. Supply the cranial part of Vesica urinaria. A B

6 ***Ligamentum teres vesicae***. Vestige of A. umbilicalis near cranial border of Lig. vesicae laterale. A B

7 **A. iliolumbalis**. Courses laterally between Os ilium and M. iliopsoas. A B

8 ***A. lumbalis VI*** (bo). Runs towards the last Vertebra lumbalis. A

9 **A. glutea [glutaea] cranialis**. Courses laterally through Foramen ischiadicum majus. Often plural. A B

10 ***Rami sacrales I et II*** (bo). Course dorsally into the corresponding Foramen sacrale ventrale, leave the corresponding Foramen sacrale dorsale as Ramus dorsalis. A

11 **A. prostatica**. To Glandula vesicularis and prostata. It is the main supplier of pelvic viscera in male. A

12 ***Ramus ductus deferentis***. Supplies the terminal segment of Ductus deferens. A

13 *A. vesicalis caudalis*. Supplies the caudal part of Vesica urinaria. A

14 **Ramus uretericus**. To the terminal segment of ureter. A

15 ***Ramus urethralis***. Supplies the initial segment of Urethra masculina. A

16 **A. vaginalis**. Courses to the vagina. It is the main supplier of pelvic viscera in female. B

17 ***Ramus uterinus***. Courses along vagina and Cervix uteri. B

18 *A. vesicalis caudalis*. Supplies the caudal part of Vesica urinaria. B

19 **Ramus uretericus**. To the terminal segment of ureter. B

20 **Ramus urethralis**. Passes to the initial segment of urethra. B

21 ***A. rectalis media***. To the rectum. Also described in the male, as branch of A. prostatica. B

22 ***A. perinealis dorsalis***. Runs toward anus. Also described in the male, as branch of A. prostatica. B

23 *A. rectalis caudalis*. Supplies the caudal segment of rectum and the Canalis analis. B

24 *Ramus labialis dorsalis*. Enters the dorsal aspect of Labium pudendi. B

25 **A. glutea [glutaea] caudalis**. Leaves Cavum pelvis thorugh Foramen ischiadicum minus. A B

26 **A. pudenda interna**. Runs toward Arcus ischiadicus. A B

27 ***A. urethralis*** (bo). Supplies the caudal segment of Urethra feminina s. Pars pelvina of Urethra masculina. A

28 ***A. vestibularis*** (bo). Courses ventrally to the lateral wall of Vestibulum vaginae.

29 ***A. perinealis ventralis***. Courses to perineum. A B

30 *A. rectalis caudalis*. Supplies the caudal segment of rectum and the Canalis analis of the male. A

31 *Ramus labialis dorsalis et mammarius*. Ramifies in Labium pudendi and continues at Regio supramammaria. B

32 ***A. urethralis*** (ov, cap). Supplies the caudal segment of Urethra feminina s. Pars pelvina of Urethra masculina. B

33 ***A. penis***. Courses to Radix penis. A

34 *A. bulbi penis*. Enters Bulbus penis and continues in Corpus spongiosum penis. A

35 *A. profunda penis*. Enters Crus penis and runs in Corpus cavernosum penis. A

36 *A dorsalis penis*. Courses along Dorsum penis towards glans and Preputium. Usually asymmetrical. A

37 ***A. clitoridis***. To Crus clitoridis. B

38 *A. bulbi vestibuli* (ov, cap). Ramifies in Bulbus vestibuli. B

39 *A. profunda clitoridis*. Enters Corpus cavernosum clitoridis. B

40 *A. dorsalis clitoridis*. Courses along the ventral aspect of Corpus clitoridis. B

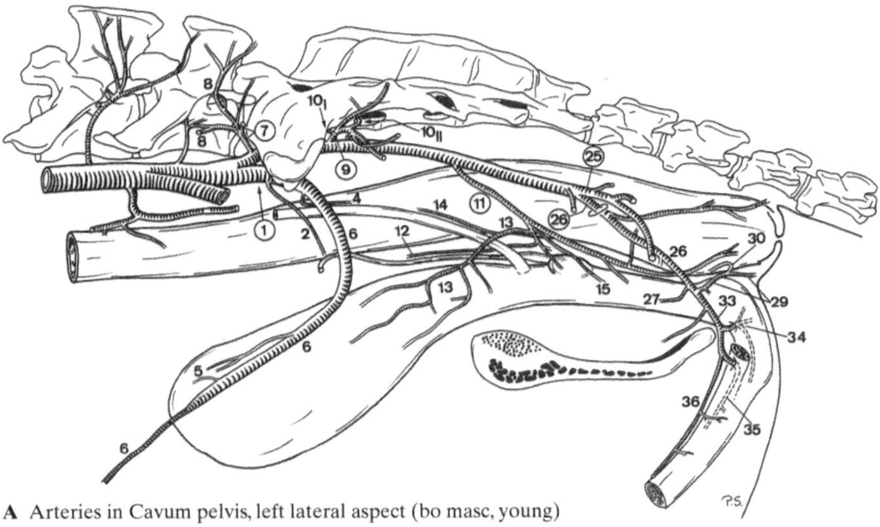

A Arteries in Cavum pelvis, left lateral aspect (bo masc, young)

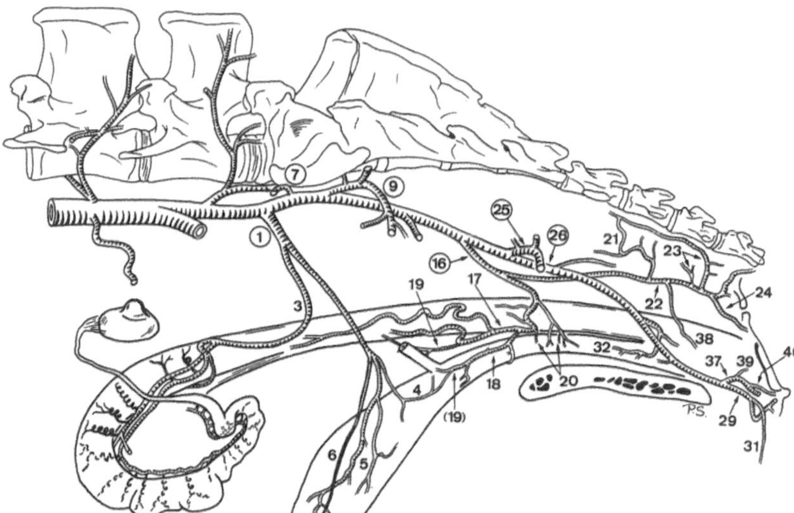

B Arteries in Cavum pelvis, left lateral aspect (cap fem)

EQUUS

1 **Aa. lumbales V et VI**. Supply structures dorsal to Processus costalis of vertebra lumbalis V et VI. A B

2 **A. glutea [glutaea] caudalis**. Passes through the dorsal part of Lig. sacrotuberale latum. A B

3 ***A. glutea [glutaea] cranialis***. Curves caudoventrally at the medial aspect of Os ilium. Passes through Foramen ischiadicum majus. A B

4 *A. iliolumbalis*. Runs across the ventromedial aspect of Ala ossis ilium and continues craniodorsally between Ala ossis ilium and Vertebra lumbalis VI. May arise from A. glutea caudalis. A B

5 *A. obturatoria*. Leaves Cavum pelvis through Foramen obturatum. A B

6 **A. iliacofemoralis**. Curves across the craniomedial aspect of Corpus ossis ilium. A B

7 **Ramus ascendens**. Courses along M. tensor fasciae latae. A B

8 **A. penis media**. To Dorsum penis, joins A. dorsalis penis. A

9 **A. clitoridis media**. To Crus clitoridis, branches into the following two arteries. B

10 **A. profunda clitoridis**. Supplies Corpus cavernosum clitoridis. B

11 **A. dorsalis clitoridis**. Courses along the ventral border of Corpus clitoridis towards glans. B

12 ***Rami sacrales***. Course into the corresponding Foramen sacrale pelvinum. A B

13 *Ramus spinalis*. To A. spinalis ventralis. A

14 *Ramus dorsalis*. Emerges through Foramen sacrale dorsale. A

15 ***A. caudalis [coccygea] mediana***. Arises from the left or right A. glutea caudalis or A. caudalis ventrolateralis, exceptionally from A. sacralis mediana. A B

16 ***A. caudalis [coccygea] ventrolateralis***. Continues along the ventrolateral aspect of Vertebrae caudales. A B

17 *Rami caudales [coccygei]*. Course dorsally to the caudal aspect of the corresponding Vertebra caudalis. A B

18 *A. caudalis [coccygea] dorsolateralis*. Chain of anastomoses between the Rami caudales at the dorsolateral aspect of Vertebrae caudales. A

19 ***Corpora caudalia [coccygea]***. Nodules of arteriovenous anastomoses in the tail.

20 **A. pudenda interna**. Continues along the Spina ischiadica. A B

21 ***A. umbilicalis***. Curves in Lig. vesicae laterale. In the fetus it continues to the placenta. A B

22 *A. ductus deferentis*. Courses along Ductus deferens. A

23 **Ramus uretericus**. Supplies ureter. A

24 *Aa. vesicales craniales*. Supply Vesica urinaria. A B

25 *Ligamentum teres vesicae*. Vestige of A. umbilicalis near the cranial border of Lig. vesicae laterale. A B

26 ***A. prostatica***. To Prostata. It is the main supplier of pelvic viscera in male. A

27 *Ramus ductus deferentis*. Supplies the terminal segment of Ductus deferens. A

28 **A. vesicalis caudalis**. To Vesica urinaria. A

29 **Ramus uretericus**. Supplies the terminal segment of ureter. A

30 **Ramus urethralis**. Supplies the cranial segment of Urethra masculina. A

31 *A. rectalis media*. Ramifies in the wall of rectum. A

32 ***A. vaginalis***. Supply for the pelvic viscera, esp. vagina. It is the main supplier of pelvic viscera in female. B

33 *Ramus uterinus*. To Cervix and Corpus uteri. B

34 **A. vesicalis caudalis**. To the caudal segment of Vesica urinaria. B

35 **Ramus uretericus**. Supplies the terminal segment of ureter. B

36 **Ramus urethralis**. Supplies the cranial segment of Urethra feminina. B

37 *A. rectalis media*. To the rectum. B

38 ***Ramus vestibularis***. Passes around the Vestibulum vaginae. B

39 ***A. perinealis ventralis***. To perineum. A B

40 *A. rectalis caudalis*. To the caudal segment of rectum and Canalis analis. A B

41 *Ramus labialis dorsalis*. To Labium pudendi. B

42 ***A. penis***. To Radix penis. A

43 *A. bulbi penis*. Enters Bulbus penis and continues in Corpus spongiosum penis. A

44 *A. profunda penis*. Enters Corpus cavernosum penis. A

45 *A. dorsalis penis*. Courses along Dorsum penis, is reinforced by A. penis media. A

46 ***A. bulbi vestibuli***. To Bulbus vestibuli. B

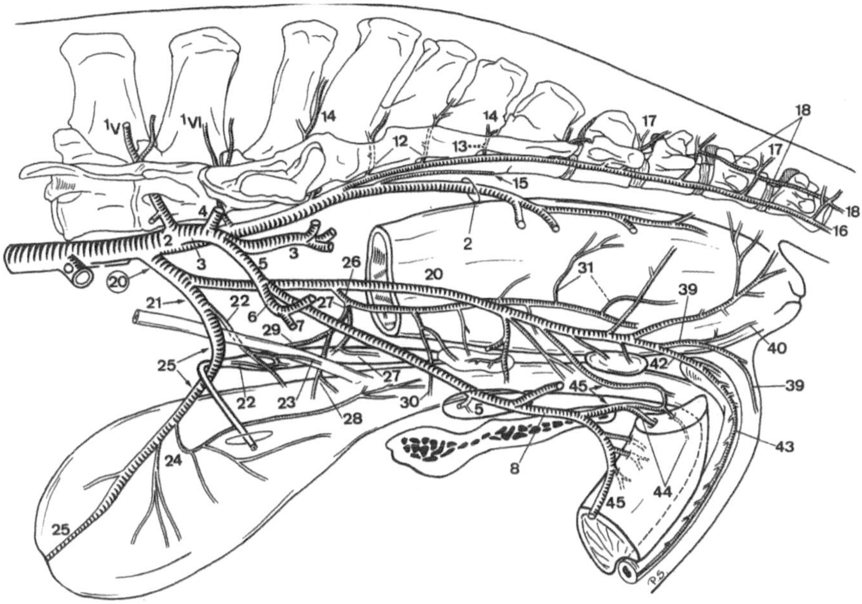

A Arteries in Cavum pelvis, left lateral aspect (eq masc)

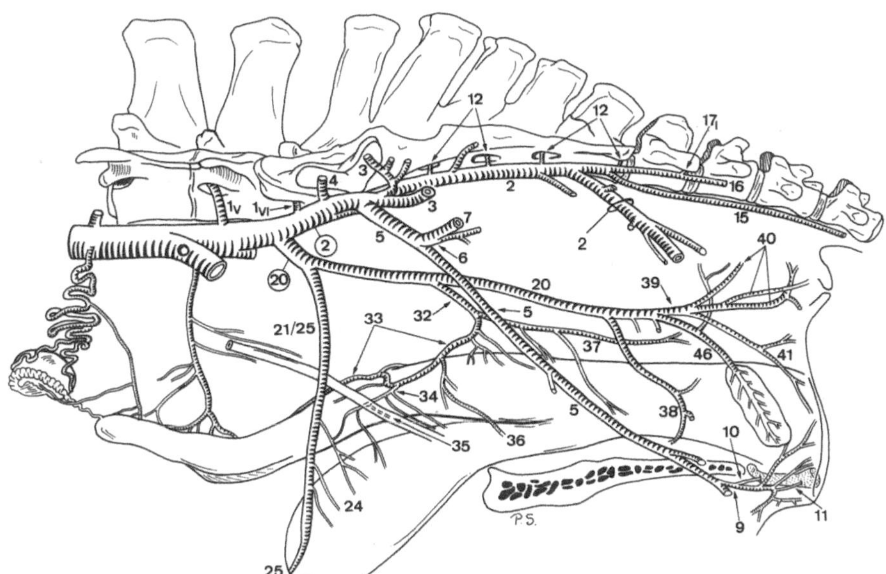

B Arteries in Cavum pelvis, left lateral aspect (eq fem)

TERMINI COMMUNES

1 **A. ILIACA EXTERNA**. Branch of aorta, courses to Lacuna vasorum. A B C (Some of the arteries nourishing the bones of the pelvic limb are not listed in the 5th edition of the N. A. V. In the rabbit the A. iliaca externa branches from A. iliaca communis. As stated before, the term "A. iliaca communis" is not yet officially introduced nor listed in the N. A. V., because rabbit features are incompletely introduced up to now.)

2 **A. circumflexa ilium profunda**. Branch of Aorta in Car, of A. iliaca communis in or, and of A. iliaca externa in the other domestic mammals. The branching is also different in Car. Courses to the cranial aspect of Tuber coxae. A

3 ***Ramus cranialis***. Runs in the lateral abdominal wall. A

4 ***Ramus caudalis***. Runs in the caudolateral abdominal wall. A

5 **A. cremasterica** (eq). Courses through Canalis inguinalis to M. cremaster. C

6 **A. uterina** (eq). Courses in Lig. latum uteri to Corpus and Cornu uteri.

7 **A. profunda femoris**. Stem for Truncus pudendoepigastricus and A. circumflexa femoris medialis. A B C

8 ***Truncus pudendoepigastricus***. Trunk for A. epigastrica caudalis and A. pudenda externa. Inconstant in fe. A B C

9 *A. abdominalis caudalis* (bo, ov). Courses into M. obliquus internus abdominis.

10 *A. cremasterica* (bo, cap). Courses through Canalis inguinalis to M. cremaster.

11 *A. epigastrica caudalis*. Runs along M. rectus abdominis. A B C

12 **A. vesicalis media** (su). Supplies Vesica urinaria. Also described in ov. A

13 **A. cremasterica** (ov). Courses through Canalis inguinalis to M. cremaster.

14 *A. vesicalis media* (Car). To Vesica urinaria. B

15 *A. cremasterica* (Car, su). Runs through Canalis inguinalis to M. cremaster. A

16 *A. lig. teretis uteri* (Car). To Ligamentum teres uteri. B

17 *A. pudenda externa*. Through Canalis inguinalis to Regio inguinalis. A B C

18 **Ramus scrotalis ventralis**. To scrotum. A C

19 **Ramus labialis ventralis [A. mammaria caudalis (Ru, eq)]**. To Labium pudendi, branches to the inguinal mamma. B

20 **A. penis cranialis** (eq.) Joins A. dorsalis penis. C

21 **A. epigastrica caudalis superficialis [A. mammaria cranialis (Ru, eq)]**. Courses superficially in the ventral abdominal wall. A B C

22 **Rami preputiales [prae-]**. Branches of A. epigastrica caudalis superficialis to preputium. A C

23 **Rami mammarii**. Branches of A. epigastrica caudalis superficialis to the abdominal and inguinal mammae. B

24 ***A. circumflexa femoris medialis***. Continuation of A. profunda femoris to the medial surface of Os femoris. A B C

25 *Ramus obturatorius*. Enters Cavum pelvis through Foramen obturatum. A B

26 *Ramus profundus*. Courses distally along the caudal aspect of Os femoris. A B

27 *Ramus ascendens*. Courses across the medial aspect of Os femoris. A B

28 *Ramus transversus*. Curves across the medial aspect of Os femoris. A B

29 *Ramus acetabularis*. Enters Articulatio coxae through Incisura acetabuli. A B

30 **A. abdominalis caudalis** (Car). Courses at the inner surface of M. obliquus internus abdominis. B

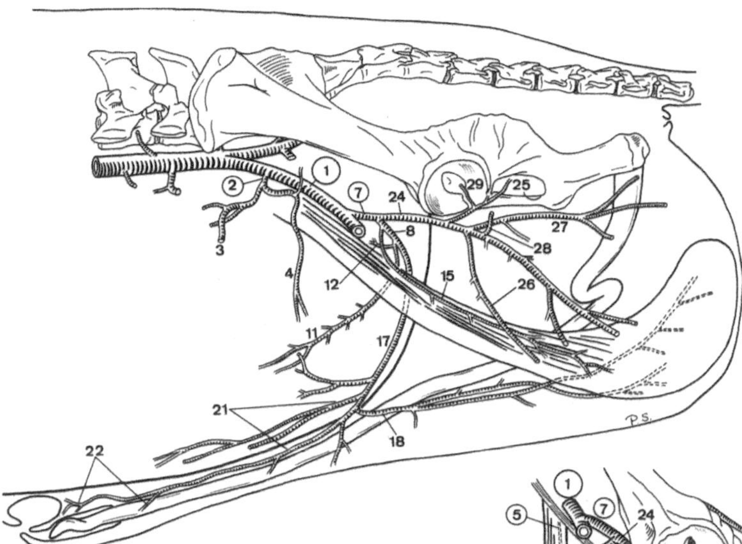

A A. iliaca externa, left lateral aspect (su masc)

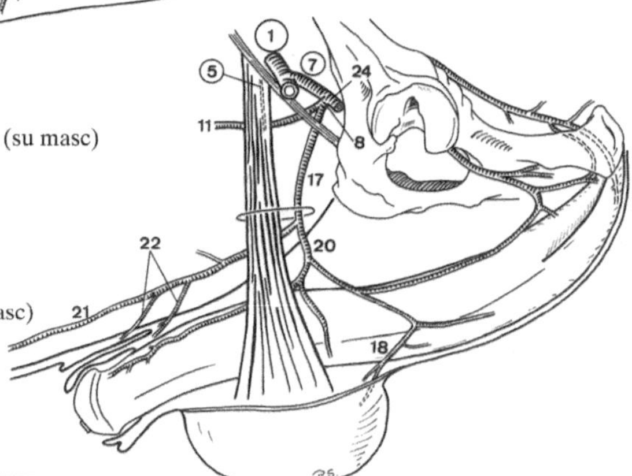

C A. iliaca externa, left lateral aspect (eq masc)

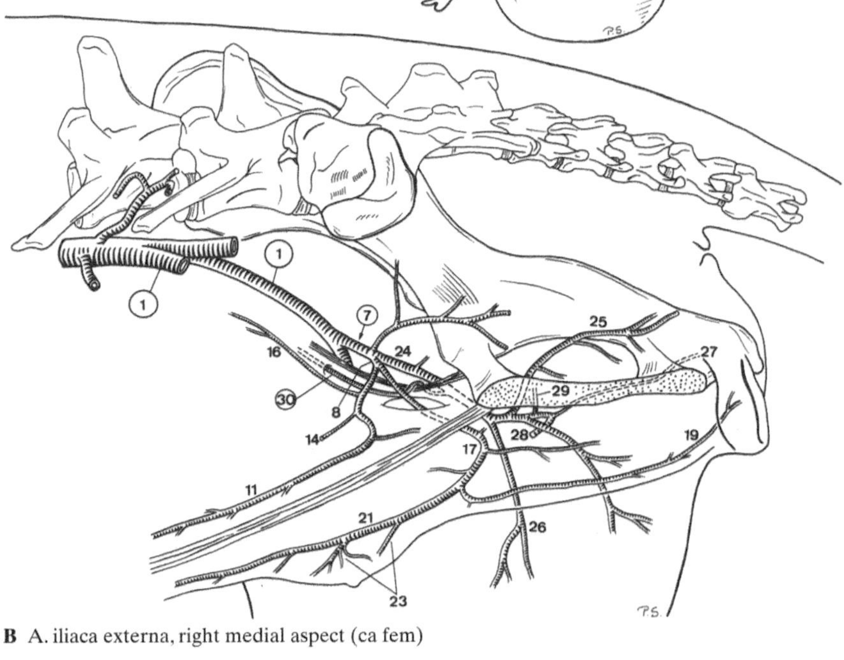

B A. iliaca externa, right medial aspect (ca fem)

CARNIVORA

1 **A. femoralis**. Continuation of A. iliaca externa, courses through Canalis femoralis. A

2 ***A. circumflexa ilium superficialis*** (ca). Also described in fe as branch of A. circumflexa femoris lateralis. A

3 ***A. circumflexa femoris lateralis***. Courses laterally between M. vastus medialis and M. rectus femoris. A

4 *Ramus ascendens*. Courses proximally. A

5 *Ramus descendens*. Courses distolaterally inside of M. quadriceps femoris. A

6 *Ramus transversus*. A

7 ***A. caudalis femoris proximalis***. Muscular branch, usually coursing across the lateral surface of M. gracilis. A

8 ***A. genus descendens***. To the medial aspect of Articulatio genus. A

8a ***A. nutricia ossis femoris****. A constant artery which arises variably from A. femoralis in Car.

9 ***A. saphena***. Courses superficially to Condylus medialis tibiae. A

10 *Ramus articularis genus*. Courses over M. sartorius to Articulatio genus. A

11 *Ramus cranialis*. Runs over Facies medialis of Corpus tibiae, continues onto Dorsum pedis. A B

12 **A. digitalis dorsalis II abaxialis** (fe). Turns dosomedially to the abaxial side of Digitus I. B

13 **Aa. digitales dorsales communes II–IV** (fe), **I–IV** (ca). Subcutaneous arteries, run to the Articulationes metatarsophalangeae where they bifurcate. B

14 **Aa. digitales dorsales propriae**. Arise from the bifurcation of Aa. digitales dorsales communes, run along the dorsal parts of the adjacent surfaces of the digits. B

15 **A. digitalis dorsalis V abaxialis** (fe). Passes along the dorsolateral aspect of Digitus V. B

16 *Ramus caudalis*. Courses superficially along the medial border of Corpus tibiae to the medioplantar aspect of tarsus. A C

17 **Rami calcanei**. To calcaneus. C

18 **Rete calcaneum**. Network at Tuber calcanei. C

19 **A. plantaris medialis**. Larger terminal branch at the medial aspect of the tarsus. C

20 **Ramus profundus** (ca). Passes along the medial border of the tendon of M. flexor digitorum profundus, lateral contribution to Arcus plantaris profundus. Also described in fe. C

21 **Ramus superficialis**. Runs along the medial border of the tendon of M. flexor digitorum superficialis. C

22 **Aa. digitales plantares communes II–IV**. Superficial branches of Ramus superficialis of A. plantaris medialis. C

23 **Ramus tori metatarsei**. Branch for Torus metatarseus, given off by each A. digitalis plantaris communis. C

24 **A. interdigitalis**. Connects each A. digitalis plantaris communis with the corresponding A. digitalis dorsalis communis or Aa. digitales dorsales propriae (ca). B C

25 **Aa. digitales plantares propriae**. Arise from the bifurcation of Aa. digitales plantares communes, course along the plantar aspects of adjacent digits, enter Foramen soleare axiale s. abaxiale of Phalanx distalis. C

26 **Ramus plantaris phalangis proximalis**.[1)]

27 **(Ramus dorsalis phalangis proximalis)**.[1)]

28 **Ramus tori digitalis**. Supplies the Torus digitalis.[1)] C

29 **Ramus plantaris phalangis mediae**.[1)]

30 **(Ramus dorsalis phalangis mediae)**.[1)]

31 **A. coronalis**. Supplies structures of Regio coronalis. [1)]

32 **Ramus plantaris phalangis distalis**.[1)]

33 **Arcus terminalis**. Arch inside Phalanx distalis, formed by the axial and abaxial Aa. digitales plantares propriae.[1)]

34 **A. plantaris lateralis**. Runs between Mm. flexores digitorum superficialis and profundus, continues along the lateral aspect of the tendon of M. flexor digitorum profundus. C

35 **Arcus plantaris profundus**. Courses transversely across the plantar aspect of Mm. interossei, joins Ramus profundus of A. plantaris medialis. Receives most of its blood via Ramus perforans proximalis II. C

36 **Aa. metatarseae plantares II–IV**. Branches of Arcus plantaris profundus along the lateroplantar aspect of the corresponding Os metatarsale. C

37 **Ramus perforans distalis**. Connects each A. metatarsea plantaris with its dorsal counterpart by traversing the Spatium interosseum metatarsi. Also connected with A. digitals dorsalis and plantaris communis. C

38 ***A. caudalis femoris media***. Muscular branch for M. adductor and M. semimembranosus. A

39 ***A. caudalis femoris distalis***. Large muscular branch in the poples. A

1) See details on 288.23–30 of the thoracic limb and replace “palmar” with “plantar”.

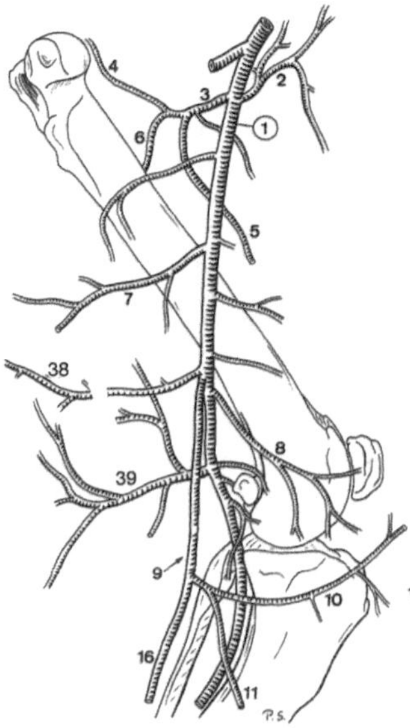

A Arteries of left femur, medial aspect (ca)

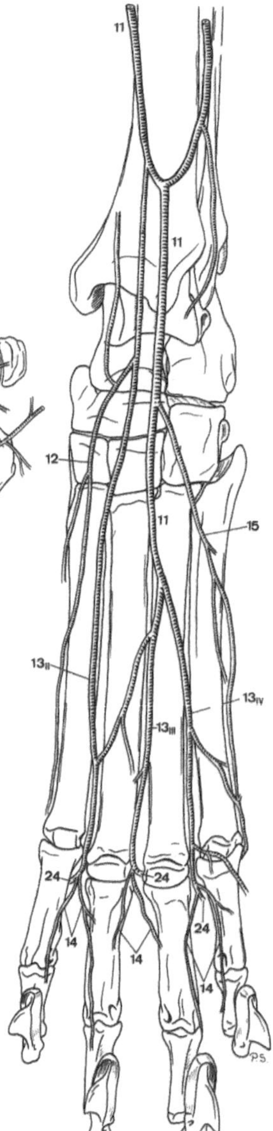

B Arteries of left pes, dorsal aspect (fe)

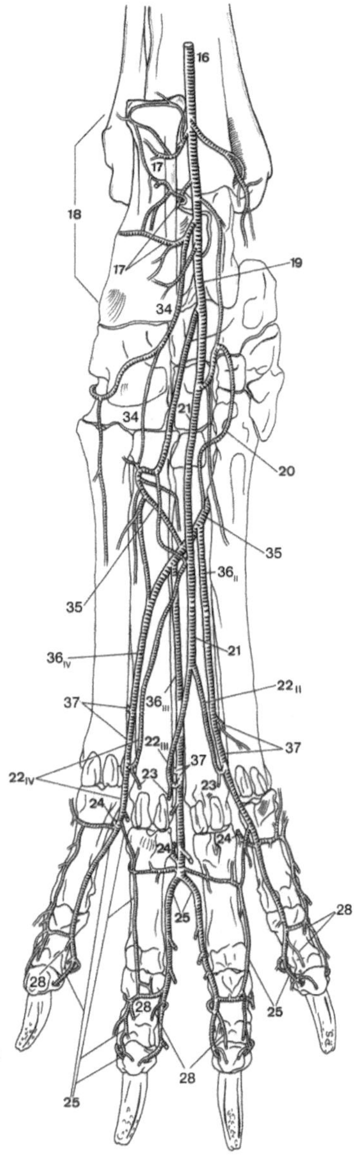

C Arteries of left pes, plantar aspect (ca)

1 **A. poplitea**. Continuation of A. femoralis beyond the origin of A. caudalis femoris distalis. Passes over the flexor surface of Articulatio femorotibialis. A B

2 ***A. genus proximalis lateralis***. Ramifies in joint capsule along Condylus lateralis of Os femoris. B

3 ***A. genus proximalis medialis***. Ramifies in joint capsule along Condylus medialis of Os femoris. A

4 ***A. genus media****. Passes cranially to Fossa intercondylaris of Os femoris. A B

5 ***Aa. surales***. Course to the muscles along the caudal aspect of crus. A B

6 ***A. genus distalis lateralis***. Courses over the medial surface of Ligamentum collaterale laterale of Articulatio femorotibialis to the lateral aspect of Articulatio genus. B

7 ***A. genus distalis medialis***. Passes over the lateral surface of Ligamentum collaterale mediale of Articulatio femorotibialis to the medial aspect of Articulatio genus. A

8 ***Rete articulare genus***. Network around Articulatio genus. A B

9 ***Rete patellae***. Network at the patella. A B

10 ***A. recurrens tibialis caudalis***. Courses proximally along the caudal aspect of tibia to Articulatio femorotibialis. Also in fe is described as a branch of A. tibialis cranialis. A

11 **A. tibialis cranialis**. Larger terminal branch of A. poplitea, courses craniodistally through the proximal part of Membrana interossea cruris and continues along the craniolateral aspect of tibia. A B C

12 ***A. recurrens tibialis cranialis***. Courses proximally over Facies lateralis of tibia toward Articulatio genus. A B

13 ***A. nutricia tibiae et fibulae****. Stem for the nutrient arteries for tibia and fibula. In many cases these two branches arise separately. A B

14 ***Ramus superficialis***. Courses along Facies lateralis of Corpus tibiae and usually joins Ramus cranialis of A. saphena at the tarsus. B C

15 *A. digitalis dorsalis V abaxialis* (ca). Runs along the dorsolateral aspect of tarsus, metatarsus and Digitus V. B

16 ***Ramus interosseus***. Occurs in fe, courses caudally through the distal part of Membrana interossea cruris, and connects A. tibialis cranialis with A. femoralis by branches of A. caudalis femoris distalis. Also connected with Ramus cranialis (and Ramus caudalis) of A. saphena. C

17 ***Rami malleolares***. Course to Malleolus medialis and Malleolus lateralis. C

18 **A. dorsalis pedis**. Extension of A. tibialis cranialis distal to Articulatio tarsocruralis on the dorsal and axial aspect of the tarsus. C

19 ***A. tarsea lateralis***. Courses to the lateral aspect of tarsus. C

20 ***A. tarsea medialis***. Courses to the medial aspect of tarsus. C

21 ***A. arcuata***. Courses laterally across the dorsal and lateral aspect of tarsus. C

22 *Aa. metatarseae dorsales II–IV.* Run along the dorsolateral aspects of Ossa metatarsalia II–IV and join the corresponding Ramus perforans distalis. C

23 **Ramus perforans proximalis II**. Large branch of A. metatarsea dorsalis II which courses to the plantar aspect of Metatarsus by passing between the proximal ends of Ossa metatarsalia II and III. Joins Arcus plantaris profundus. C

24 **A. tibialis caudalis**. Small terminal branch of A. poplitea at the caudal aspect of Skeleton cruris. A B

A Arteries of left stifle, medial aspect (ca)

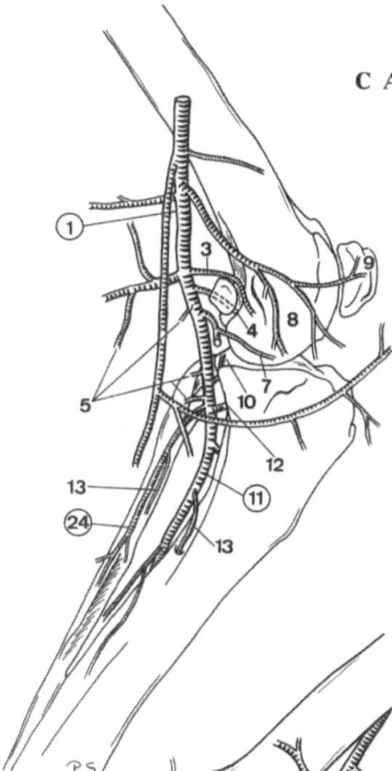

C Arteries of left pes, dorsal aspect (fe)

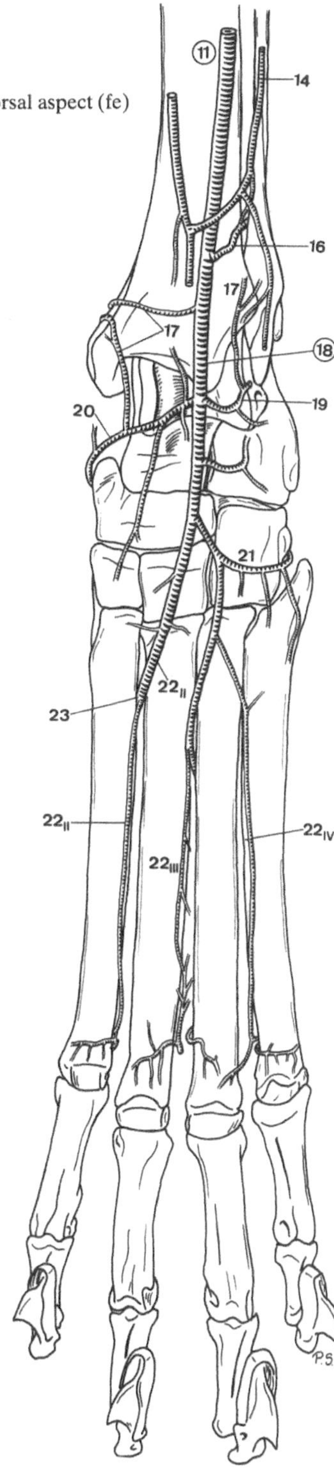

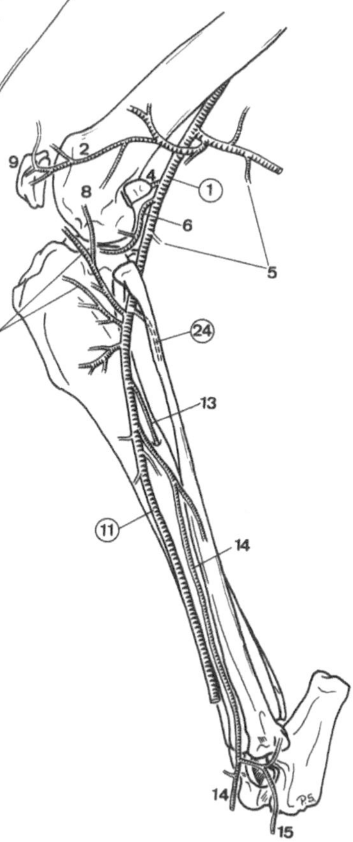

B Arteries of left stifle, lateral aspect (ca)

SUS

1 **A. femoralis**. Continuation of A. iliaca externa through Canalis femoralis. A

2 ***A. circumflexa femoris lateralis***. Courses laterally inside of M. quadriceps femoris. A

3 *Ramus ascendens*. Runs proximally. A

4 *Ramus descendens*. Courses craniodistally inside of M. quadriceps femoris. A

5 *Ramus transversus*. Crosses the lateral aspect of proximal femur. A

6 ***A. saphena***. Curves craniodistally to the medial aspect of Articulatio genus, continues subcutaneously and caudodistally to the medioplantar aspect of tarsus. A

7 *Ramus caudalis*. Superficial continuation to the medioplantar aspect of tarsus. A C

8 **Rami malleolares mediales**. Ramify at Malleolus medialis. C

9 **Rami calcanei**. To Tuber calcanei. C

10 **Rete calcaneum**. Network around Tuber calcanei. C

11 **A. plantaris medialis**. Larger terminal branch of Ramus caudalis of A. saphena at the medioplantar aspect of tarsus. C

12 **Ramus profundus**. Receives A. tarsea perforans distalis, joins Arcus plantaris profundus. C

13 **Ramus superficialis**. Courses along the medial aspect of the digital flexor tendons. C

14 **Aa. digitales plantares communes II–IV**. Superficial branches of Ramus superficialis of A. plantaris medialis. C

15 **Aa. digitales plantares propriae**. Arise from the bifurcation of Aa. digitales plantares communes, course along the plantar aspects of adjacent digits, enter Foramen axiale s. Facies parietalis of Phalanx distalis. C

16 **A. interdigitalis**. Connects each A. digitalis plantaris propria with its dorsal counterpart through Spatium interdigitale. B C

17 **Ramus dorsalis phalangis proximalis**. Ramifies on the dorsal aspect of Phalanx proximalis. Arises from A. interdigitalis or Ramus plantaris phalangis proximalis (digit II and V). B C

18 **Ramus plantaris phalangis proximalis**. Transverse branch across the plantar surface of Phalanx proximalis. C

19 **Ramus tori digitalis**. Supplies the Torus ungulae. C

20 **Ramus dorsalis phalangis mediae**. Runs across the dorsal aspect of Phalanx media. B C

21 **A. coronalis**. Superficial branch of the axial Ramus dorsalis phalangis mediae, courses abaxially along the Corona ungulae. B

22 **Ramus plantaris phalangis mediae**. Runs across the plantar aspect of Phalanx media. C

22a **Ramus plantaris phalangis distalis**. Runs across the plantar surface of Phalanx distalis.

23 **Ramus dorsalis phalangis distalis**. Courses dorsally along Facies axialis of Phalanx distalis. B C

24 **Arcus terminalis**. Arch inside Phalanx distalis, formed by the axial and abaxial Aa. digitales plantares propriae. C

25 **A. plantaris lateralis**. Smaller terminal branch of Ramus caudalis of A. saphena. Courses across the plantar aspect of tarsus, receives A. tarsea perforans proximalis, continues along the lateroplantar aspect of metatarsus, anastomoses with A. digitalis plantaris communis IV. C

26 **Arcus plantaris profundus**. Connection of A. plantaris lateralis and Ramus profundus of A. plantaris medialis across the dorsal (usually also the plantar) side of Mm. interossei. C

27 **Aa. metatarseae plantares II–IV**. Branches of Arcus plantaris profundus at the lateroplantar aspect of the corresponding Os metatarsale, join Ramus perforans distalis III. C

28 **Rami perforantes proximales II–IV**. Branches of Aa. metatarseae plantares II–IV through Spatium interosseum metatarsi. B C

29 **Aa. metatarseae dorsales II et IV**. Continuations of Rami perforantes proximales II and IV on the dorsoabaxial aspect of Ossa metatarsalia III s. IV. B

30 **Aa. digitales dorsales propriae**. Continuations of Aa. metatarseae dorsales II and IV along the adjacent sides of Digiti II–III s. IV–V. B

31 **Ramus perforans distalis III**. Connects A. metatarsea plantaris III with its dorsal counterpart. Connected also with Aa. metatarseae plantares II and IV and A. digitalis plantaris communis III. B C

31a **Ramus superficialis**. Continuation of A. plantaris lateralis which joins A. digitalis plantaris communis IV.

32 ***Aa. caudales femoris***. Muscular branches in the poples. A

33 ***A. genus descendens***. To the medial aspect of Articulatio genus. A

34 *A. genus proximalis medialis*. Inconstant, to the medial aspect of Articulatio genus. A

35 ***A. nutricia ossis femoris***. A constant artery, which arises variably from A. femoralis.

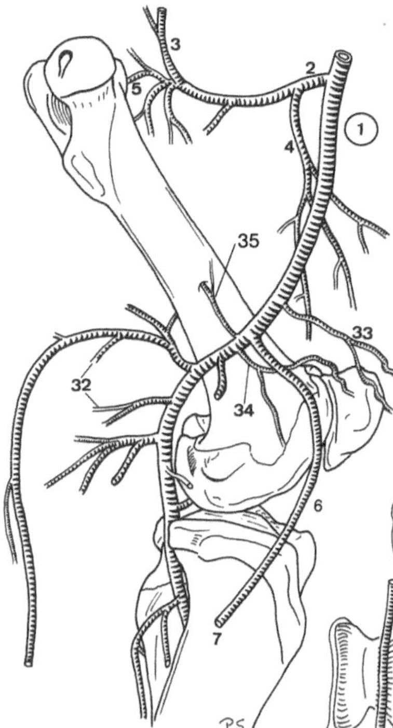

A Arteries of left femur, medial aspect (su)

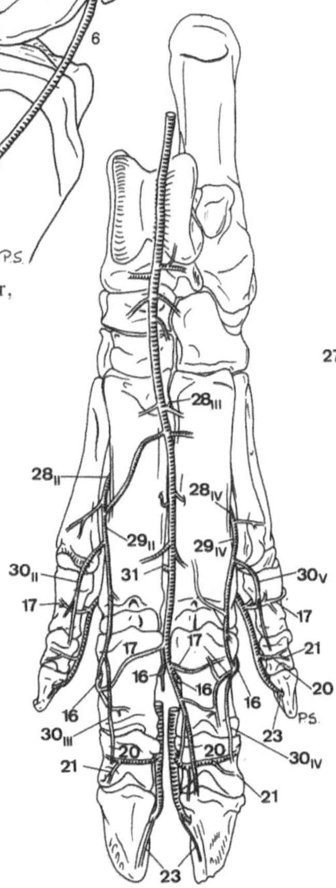

B Arteries of left pes, dorsal aspect (su)

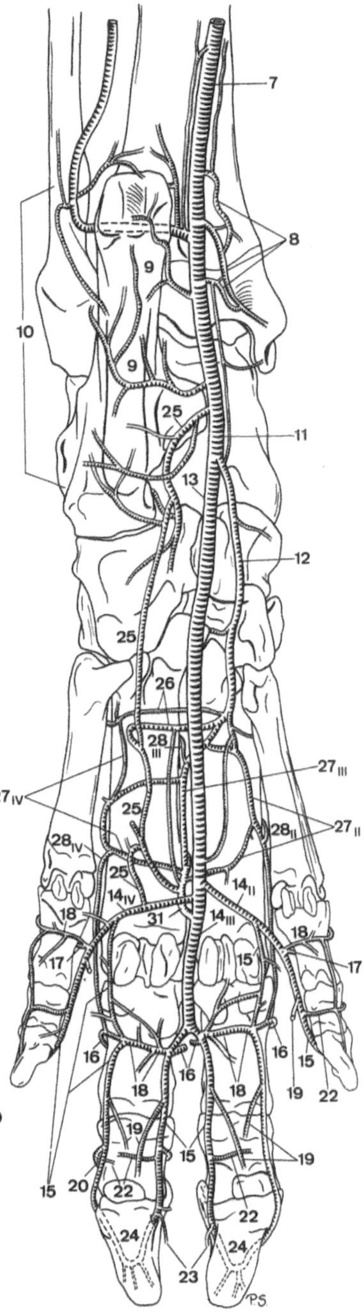

C Arteries of left pes, plantar aspect (su)

1 **A. poplitea.** Continuation of A. femoralis in poples, runs over the flexor surface of Articulatio femorotibialis. A

2 ***A. genus proximalis lateralis.*** Courses to the lateral aspect of Articulatio genus. A

3 ***Aa. surales.*** Caudodistal branches for the musculature at the caudal aspect of crus. A

4 ***A. genus distalis lateralis.*** Courses to the lateral aspect of Articulatio genus. A

5 ***A. genus distalis medialis.*** Courses to the medial aspect of Articulatio genus. A

6 ***A. genus media.*** Runs cranially between Condylus lateralis and Condylus medialis of Os femoris to the cranial aspect of Articulatio genus. A

7 ***Rete articulare genus.*** Arterial network surrounding Articulatio genus. A

8 ***Rete patellae.*** Network at the patella. A

9 **A. tibialis cranialis.** Larger terminal branch of A. poplitea which courses through the proximal part of Membrana interossea cruris and continues along the lateral border of tibia. A B

10 ***A. recurrens tibialis cranialis.*** Courses proximally over Condylus lateralis of tibia towards Articulatio genus. A

11 ***A. interossea cruris.*** Runs along the caudal surface of Membrana interossea cruris. A B

12 *A. nutricia tibiae.* Enters Foramen nutricium of tibia. A

13 *A. nutricia fibulae.* Enters Foramen nutricium of fibula. A

14 *Ramus perforans.* Passes cranially through the distal part of Membrana interossea cruris and joins A. tibialis cranialis. May be represented by two branches. A B

15 *Ramus anastomoticus cum a. tibiali caudali.* Passes caudomedially over the distal aspect of tibia, anastomoses with A. tibialis caudalis. A B

16 **Rami malleolares mediales.** Reach Malleolus medialis. A

17 *Rami malleolares laterales.* To Malleolus lateralis. A

18 ***A. malleolaris cranialis lateralis.*** Passes caudolaterally to Malleolus lateralis. Inconstant. A B

19 ***A. malleolaris cranialis medialis.*** Passes to Malleolus medialis. B

20 **A. dorsalis pedis.** Continuation of A. tibialis cranialis, distal to Articulatio tarsocruralis. Lies on the dorsal aspect of tarsus. A B

21 ***A. tarsea lateralis.*** Courses laterally to the lateral aspect of tarsus, divides in proximal and distal branches. B

22 *A. tarsea perforans proximalis.* Pierces between talus and calcaneus, joins A. plantaris lateralis. B

23 ***A. tarsea medialis.*** Courses to the medial aspect of tarsus. B

24 ***A. tarsea perforans distalis.*** Pierces between Os tarsale III and IV, joins Ramus profundus of A. plantaris medialis. B

25 ***A. metatarsea dorsalis III.*** Continuation of A. dorsalis pedis, courses at the dorsal aspect of metatarsus. Joined by Ramus perforans distalis, finally reaches the paired A. interdigitalis III. B

26 *Aa. digitales dorsales propriae.* Dorsal vessels which course along the axial aspects of Digiti III et IV. B

27 **A. tibialis caudalis.** Smaller terminal branch of A. poplitea, coursing distally along the caudal aspect of crus. A

28 ***Ramus circumflexus fibulae.*** Passes laterally around fibula. A

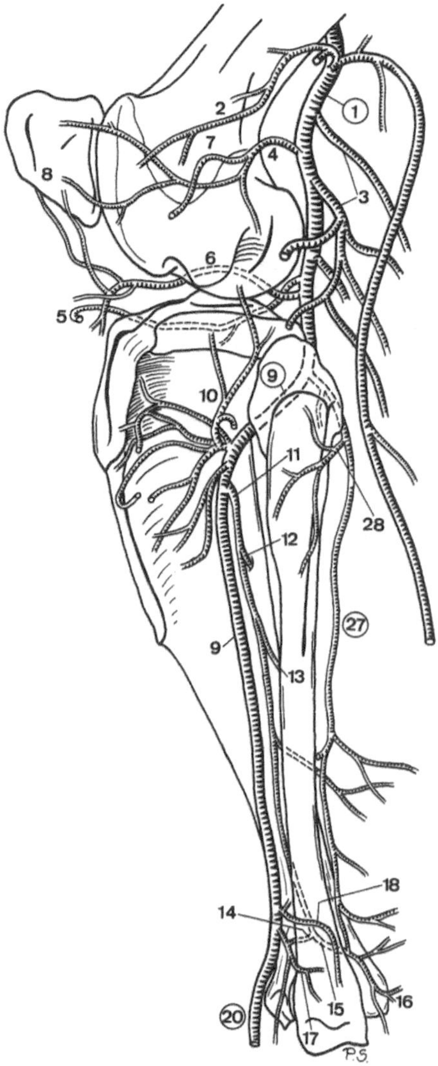

A Arteries of left stifle, lateral aspect (su)

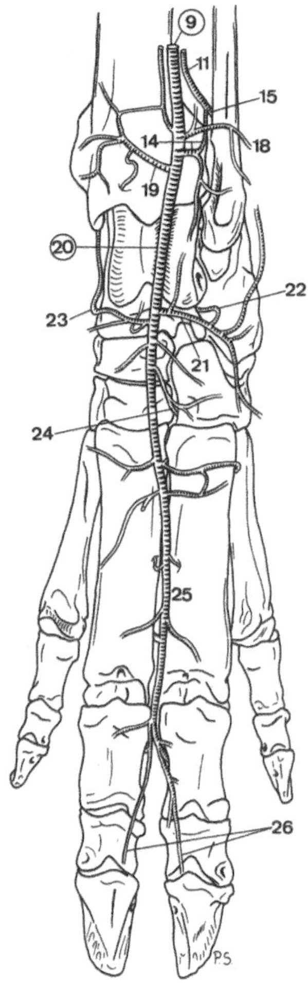

B Arteries of left pes, dorsal aspect (su)

RUMINANTIA

1 **A. femoralis**. Continuation of A. iliaca externa, passes in Canalis femoralis. A

2 ***A. circumflexa femoris lateralis.*** Courses laterally inside of M. quadriceps femoris. A

3 *Ramus ascendens*. Courses proximally. A

4 *Ramus descendens*. Passes craniodistally in M. quadriceps femoris. A

5 *Ramus transversus*. Anastomoses with A. circumflexa femoris medialis. A

6 ***A. saphena.*** Leaves the distal end of Trigonum femorale on the medial surface of the thigh. A

7 *Ramus caudalis*. Continuation to the medioplantar side of crus. A B

8 **Rami malleolares mediales**. Ramify at Malleolus medialis. B

9 **Rami calcanei**. To Tuber calcanei. B

10 **Rete calcaneum**. Network around Tuber calcanei. B

11 **A. plantaris medialis**. Larger terminal branch of Ramus caudalis of A. saphena at the medioplantar aspect of tarsus. B

12 **Ramus profundus**. Joins Arcus plantaris profundus. B

13 **Ramus superficialis**. Courses along the medial border of the tendon of M. flexor digitorum profundus. B

14 **A. digitalis plantaris communis II.** Medial continuation of Ramus superficialis of A. plantaris medialis. B C

15 **A. digitalis plantaris propria II axialis**. Enters the base of the medial dew claw. C

16 **A. digitalis plantaris propria III abaxialis**. Continuation of A. digitalis plantaris communis II along the abaxial side of the flexor tendons of Digitus III. C

17 **Ramus dorsalis phalangis proximalis**. Branch of to the dorsal aspect of Phalanx proximalis. C

18 **Ramus tori digitalis**. Enters Torus ungulae. C

19 **Ramus dorsalis phalangis mediae.** To the dorsal aspect of Phalanx media. C

20 **Ramus plantaris phalangis distalis.** Courses around the plantar aspect of Phalanx distalis. C

21 **Ramus dorsalis phalangis distalis.** Runs dorsally along Facies parietalis of Phalanx distalis. C

22 **A. digitalis plantaris communis III.** Lateral continuation of Ramus superficialis of A. plantaris medialis. B D

23 **Rami plantares phalangium proximalium**. Branches of A. digitalis plantaris communis III, course across the plantar surface of Phalanx proximalis III s. IV and join the corresponding A. digitalis plantaris propria abaxialis. C D

24 **A. interdigitalis**. Communication between A. digitalis plantaris communis III and A. metatarsea dorsalis III through Spatium interdigitale. D

25 **Rami dorsales phalangium proximalium**. Branches of A. interdigitalis to the dorsal aspect of Phalanx proximalis III s. IV. D

26 **Aa. digitales plantares propriae III et IV axiales**. Terminal branches of A. digitalis plantaris communis III which course distally to the corresponding Foramen axiale. D

27 **Ramus tori digitalis**. To Torus ungulae. D

28 **Ramus plantaris phalangis mediae.** Courses across the plantar aspect of Phalanx media. C D

29 **Ramus dorsalis phalangis mediae.** To the dorsal aspect of Phalanx media. C D

30 **A. coronalis.** Arises from the corresponding axial Ramus dorsalis phalangis mediae and courses superficially along Corona ungulae. C D

31 **Ramus plantaris phalangis distalis.** Supplies Facies solearis of Phalanx distalis, enters Facies axialis to join Arcus terminalis. D

32 **Ramus dorsalis phalangis distalis.** Courses dorsally along Facies axialis of Phalanx distalis. D

33 **Arcus terminalis**. Arch inside Phalanx distalis, formed by the union of axial and abaxial Aa. digitales plantares propriae III. s. IV. D

34 **A. plantaris lateralis**. Smaller terminal branch of Ramus caudalis of A. saphena, at the plantar aspect of tarsus. B

35 **Arcus plantaris profundus.** Connection between A. plantaris lateralis and Ramus profundus of A. plantaris medialis between Os metatarsale III et IV and M. interosseus. B

36 **Aa. metatarseae plantares II–IV.** Branches of Arcus plantaris profundus between Os metatarsale III et IV and M. interosseus. B D

37 **Ramus perforans proximalis III** (bo). Small connection with A. metatarsea dorsalis III, which enters the dorsoproximal aspect of Os metatarsale III et IV. D

38 **Ramus perforans distalis III**. Connects A. metatarsea plantaris III with its dorsal counterpart. B

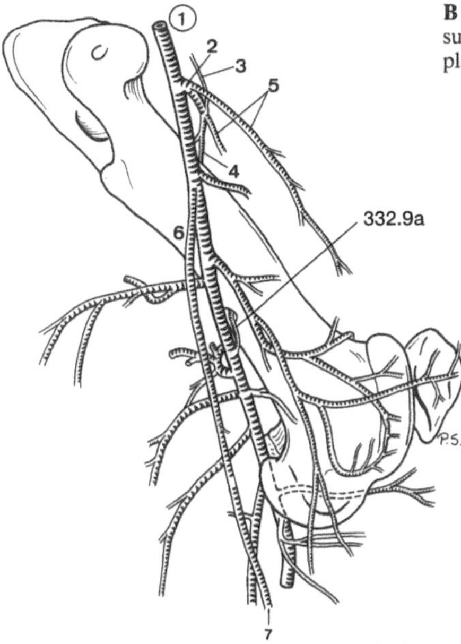

A Arteries of left femur, medial aspect (bo)

B Arteries of left tarsus and metatarsus, plantar aspect (bo)

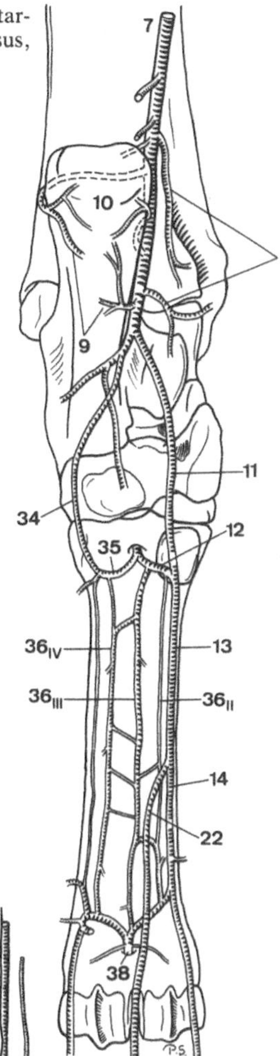

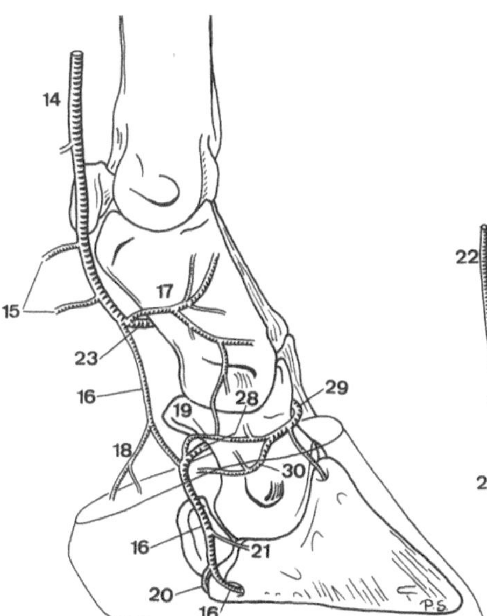

C Arteries of left pes, abaxial aspect (bo)

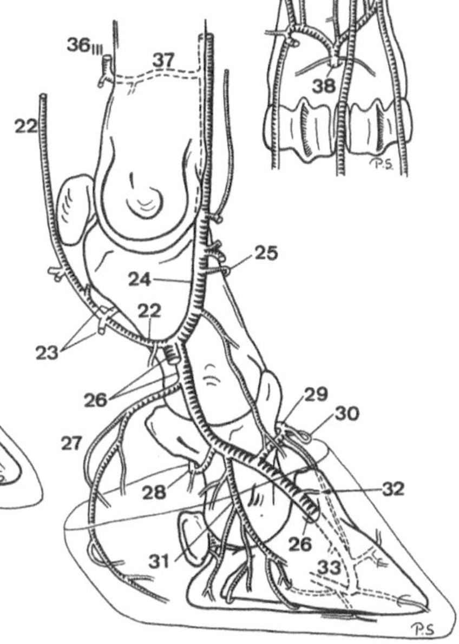

D Arteries of left pes (third digit removed), axial aspect (bo)

1 **Ramus superficialis [A. digitalis plantaris communis IV].** Continuation of A. plantaris lateralis along the lateral border of the tendon of M. flexor digitorum profundus. A

2 **A. digitalis plantaris propria IV abaxialis.** Continuation of Ramus superficialis of A. plantaris lateralis. A

3 **Ramus dorsalis phalangis proximalis.** To the dorsal aspect of Phalanx proximalis IV. A

4 **Ramus tori digitalis.** Enters Torus ungulae. A

5 **Ramus dorsalis phalangis mediae.** To the dorsal aspect of Phalanx media. A

6 **Ramus plantaris phalangis distalis.** Courses axially across the plantar aspect of Phalanx distalis. A

7 **Ramus dorsalis phalangis distalis.** Courses dorsally along Facies parietalis of Phalanx distalis. A

8 **A. digitalis plantaris propria V axialis.** Branch of Ramus superficialis of A. plantaris lateralis which enters the base of the lateral dew claw. A

9 ***A. genus descendens.*** To the medial aspect of Articulatio genus. B

9a ***A. nutricia ossis femoris.*** A constant artery, which arises variably from A. femoralis. 331 A

10 ***A. caudalis femoris.*** Supplies the musculature in the poples with proximal and distal branches. B

11 *A. genus proximalis lateralis.* Ramifies at the lateral aspect of Articulatio genus. B

12 **A. poplitea.** Continuation of A. femoralis. Runs over the flexor surface of Articulatio femorotibialis. B

13 ***A. genus media.*** Courses between Ligamenta cruciata genus to the cranial aspect of Articulatio genus. B

14 ***Aa. surales.*** Branches for the musculature at the caudal aspect of crus. B

15 ***A. genus distalis lateralis.*** To the lateral side of Articulatio genus. B

16 ***A. genus distalis medialis.*** To the medial side of Articulatio genus. B

17 ***Rete articulare genus.*** Network surrounding Articulatio genus. B

18 ***Rete patellae.*** Network around patella. B

19 **A. tibialis cranialis.** Larger terminal branch of A. poplitea along the craniolateral aspect of tibia. B C

20 ***A. recurrens tibialis cranialis*** (bo). Runs over Condylus lateralis tibiae towards Articulatio genus. B

21 ***A. interossea cruris.*** Runs along Margo lateralis of Corpus tibiae. B

22 *Ramus perforans.* Passes cranially over Margo lateralis ossis tibiae and joins A. tibialis cranialis or A. malleolaris cranialis lateralis. B

23 *Ramus anastomoticus cum a tibiali caudali.* Joins A. tibialis caudalis on the distal part of tibia. B

24 *Rami malleolares mediales.* To Malleolus medialis. B

25 *Rami malleolares laterales.* To Malleolus lateralis. B

26 ***A. nutricia tibiae.*** Enters Foramen nutricium of tibia. B

27 ***A. malleolaris cranialis lateralis.*** To Malleolus lateralis. B

28 ***A. malleolaris cranialis medialis.*** To Malleolus medialis. B C

29 ***Ramus superficialis.*** Superficial branch at the dorsal aspect of tarsus, together with N. fibularis superficialis. B C

30 *A. digitalis dorsalis communis III (ov, cap), II–IV (bo).* Continuation of Ramus superficialis of A. tibialis cranialis, III joins A. interdigitalis. C

31 **Aa. digitales dorsales propriae.** Superficial digital arteries on the dorsoaxial and dorsoabaxial (bo) aspect of digits. C

32 **A. dorsalis pedis.** Continuation of A. tibialis cranialis distal to Articulatio tarsocruralis. B C

33 ***A. tarsea lateralis.*** Ramifies at the dorsolateral aspect of tarsus. B C

34 ***A. tarsea medialis.*** Ramifies at the dorsomedial aspect of tarsus. B C

35 ***A. tarsea perforans.*** Pierces between Os centroquartale and Os tarsale II et III and continues in Canalis metatarsi proximalis. Joins A. plantaris medialis (ov, cap), A. metatarsea plantaris III (bo), or Arcus plantaris profundus (bo). May be absent (bo). B C

36 ***A. metatarsea dorsalis III.*** Continuation of A. dorsalis pedis in Sulcus longitudinalis dorsalis of Os metatarsale III et IV. Joins A. interdigitalis III. B C

37 **A. tibialis caudalis.** Smaller terminal branch of A. poplitea, at the caudal aspect of tibia. B

38 ***Rami malleolares mediales*** (bo). To Malleolus medialis. B

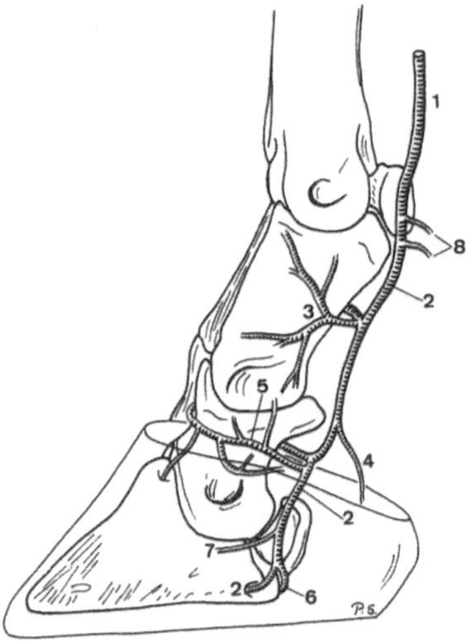

A Arteries of left pes, abaxial aspect (bo)

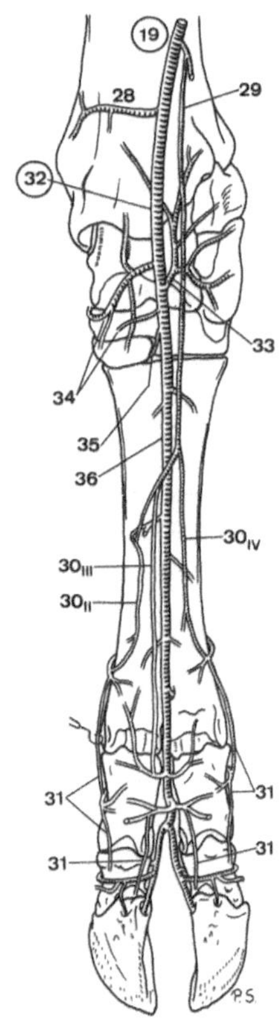

C Arteries of left pes, dorsal aspect (bo)

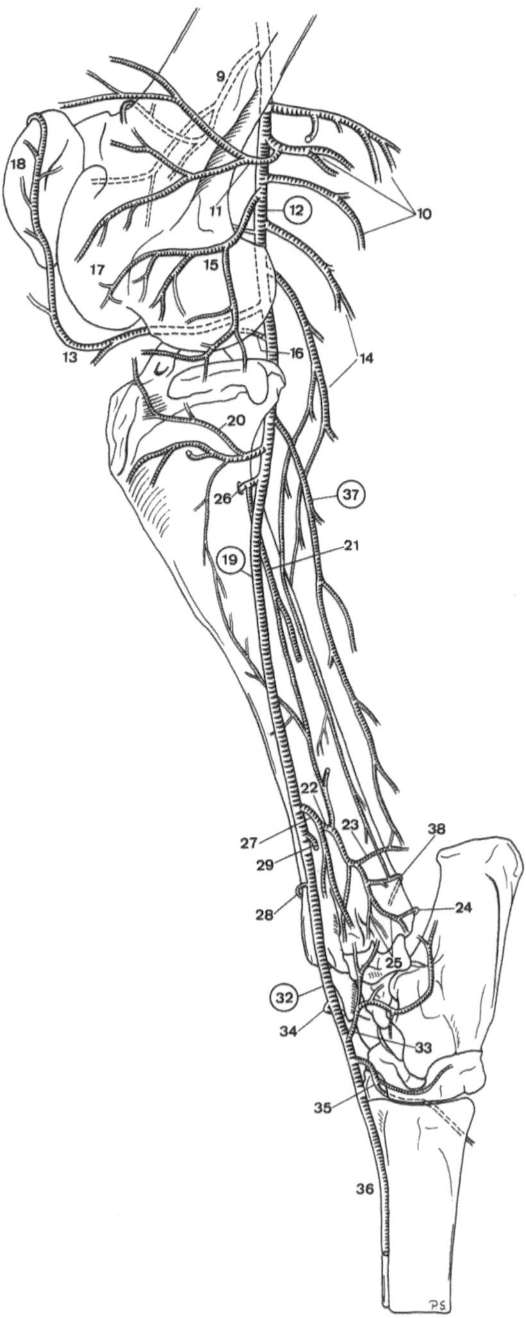

B Arteries of left crus, lateral aspect (bo)

EQUUS

1 **A. femoralis**. Continuation of A. iliaca externa in Canalis femoralis. A

2 ***A. circumflexa femoris lateralis***. Runs craniolaterally between M. rectus femoris and M. vastus medialis. A

3 *Ramus descendens*. Passes distally in M. quadriceps femoris. A

4 ***A. saphena***. Leaves the distal end of Canalis femoralis medially, and pursues a caudodistally curved superficial course over the medial surface of the thigh. A

5 *Ramus cranialis*. Slender craniodistal branch, courses over Facies medialis of tibia. A

6 *Ramus caudalis*. Caudodistal continuation of A. saphena. Reinforced by a branch of A. caudalis femoris (usually), A. malleolaris caudalis lateralis (occasionally), and Ramus anastomoticus cum A. saphena of A. tibialis caudalis (usually). Continues distally over the medioplantar aspect of the tarsus. A B

7 **A. plantaris medialis**. Courses distally along the medioplantar aspect of tarsus. A B

8 **Ramus profundus**. Deep branch of A. plantaris medialis, pierces dorsolaterally into Arcus plantaris profundus. A B

9 **Ramus superficialis [A. digitalis plantaris communis II]**. Superficial continuation of A. plantaris medialis, courses along the medial border of the tendon of M. flexor digitalis profundus. Joins A. digitalis medialis, Ramus perforans distalis III or Ramus superficialis of A. plantaris lateralis. A B

10 **A. plantaris lateralis**. Passes laterodistally to the lateral aspect of the tendon of M. flexor digitalis profundus. A B

11 **Arcus plantaris profundus**. Connection between A. plantaris lateralis and Ramus profundus of A. plantaris medialis. Usually double, upon the dorsal and plantar surfaces of M. interosseus medius in the proximal part of metatarsus. B

12 **Aa. metatarseae plantares II et III**. Branches of Arcus plantaris profundus which run along the medial s. lateral border of the M. interosseus medius. Usually they join Ramus perforans distalis III. B

13 **Ramus perforans distalis II**. Slender branch of A. metatarsea plantaris II which courses dorsally between Ossa metatarsalia II et III, and joins the slender dorsomedial metatarsal artery. B

14 **Ramus superficialis [A. digitalis plantaris communis III]**. Superficial continuation of A. plantaris lateralis which courses along the lateral border of the tendon of M. flexor digitalis profundus. Joins A. digitalis lateralis, Ramus perforans distalis III, or Ramus superficialis of A. plantaris medialis. B

15 ***A. genus descendens***. Courses craniodistally along the medial border of M. vastus medialis to the medial aspect of Articulatio genus. A

15a ***A. nutricia ossis femoris***. A constant artery, which arises variably from A. femoralis. A

16 ***A. caudalis femoris***. Large artery which supplies the musculature in the poples. A

17 **A. poplitea**. Continuation of A. femoralis beyond the origin of A. caudalis femoris. Runs over the flexor surface of Articulatio femorotibialis. A

18 ***A. genus proximalis lateralis***. Runs craniolaterally to the lateral aspect of Articulatio genus. A

19 ***A. genus proximalis medialis***. Runs craniomedially to the medial aspect of Articulatio genus. A

20 ***A. genus media***. Runs cranially between Ligamenta cruciata genus to the cranial aspect of Articulatio genus. A

21 ***A. genus distalis lateralis***. Courses over the medial surface of Ligamentum collaterale laterale of Articulatio femorotibialis to the lateral side of Articulatio genus. A

22 ***A. genus distalis medialis***. Passes over the lateral surface of Ligamentum collaterale mediale of Articulatio femorotibialis to the medial side of Articulatio genus. A

23 ***Rete articulare genus***. Network surrounding Articulatio genus. A

24 ***Rete patellae***. Network around patella. A

B Arteries of left tarsus and metatarsus, plantar aspect (eq)

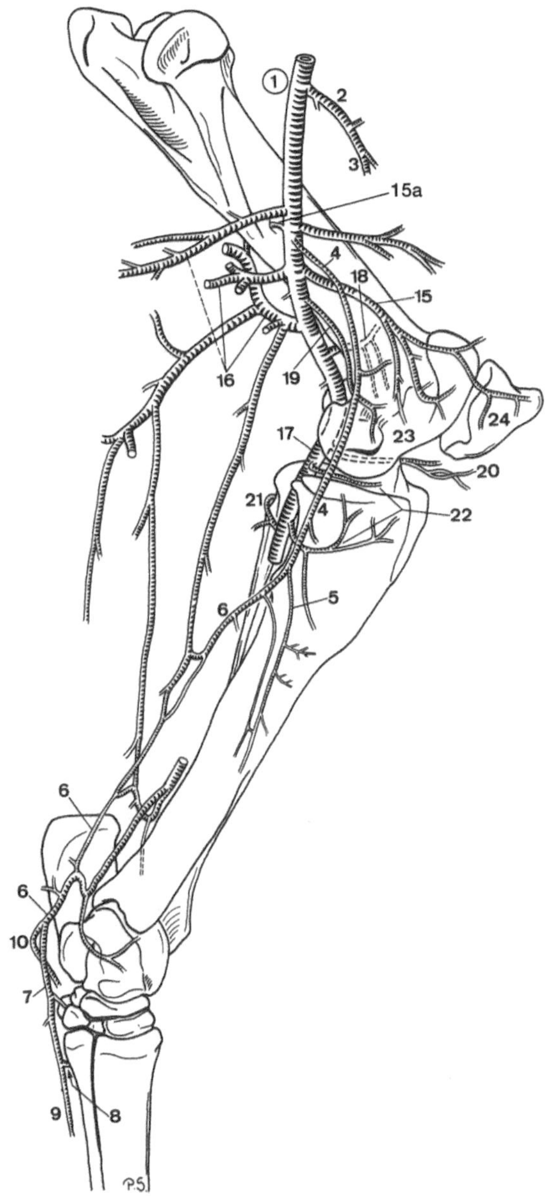

A Arteries of left pelvic limb, medial aspect (eq)

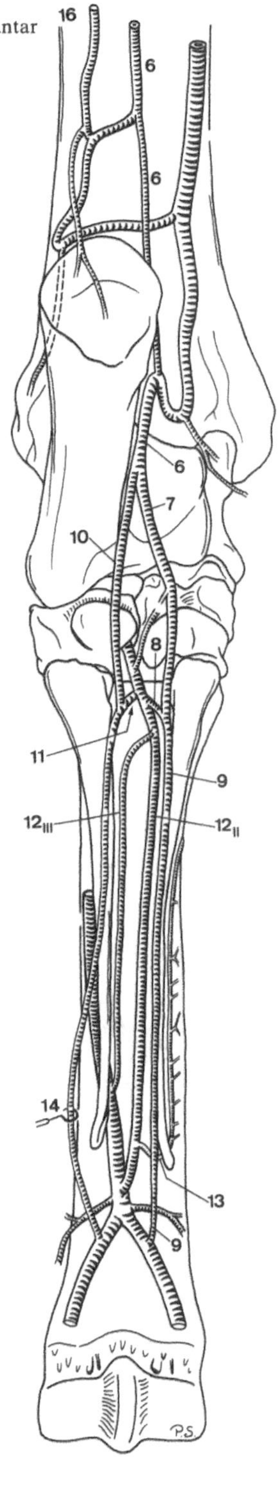

1 **A. tibialis cranialis.** Larger terminal branch of A. poplitea along the craniolateral aspect of tibia. A B

2 ***Ramus superficialis.*** Superficial branch, courses on the craniolateral aspect of the crus along N. fibularis superficialis. A

3 **A. dorsalis pedis.** Continuation of A. tibialis cranialis distally, on the dorsal aspect of tarsus. A B

4 ***A. tarsea perforans.*** Courses through Canalis tarsi, joins Arcus plantaris profundus, A. plantaris lateralis, or A. metatarsea plantaris II. A B

5 ***A. metatarsea dorsalis III.*** Continuation of A. dorsalis pedis, curves over the dorsolateral surface of Os metatarsale III, continues in the dorsal groove between Ossa metatarsalia III and IV. A

6 *Ramus perforans distalis.* Continuation of A. metatarsea dorsalis III, passes along the plantar surface of metatarsus by piercing between Ossa metatarsalia III and IV. A C D

7 **A. digitalis [plantaris propria III] medialis.** Medial terminal branch of Ramus perforans distalis III. Enters Foramen soleare mediale. A C D

8 **Ramus plantaris phalangis proximalis.** To the plantar aspect of Phalanx proximalis. C

9 **Ramus dorsalis phalangis proximalis.** To the dorsomedial surface of Phalanx proximalis. C D

10 **Ramus plantaris phalangis mediae.** To the plantar aspect of Phalanx media. C

11 **Ramus dorsalis phalangis mediae.** Branch of A. digitalis medialis which passes at the lateral aspect of Cartilago ungularis medialis to the dorsal surface of Phalanx media. D

12 **Ramus tori digitalis.** Ramifies in Torus ungulae. C D

13 **A. coronalis.** Arises from Ramus tori digitalis or A. digitalis medialis, courses dorsally along the proximal border of Cartilago ungularis medialis. C D

14 **Ramus dorsalis phalangis distalis.** Passes through Foramen or Incisura of Processus plantaris medialis and continues dorsally in Sulcus parietalis medialis. C D

15 **Arcus terminalis.** Arch inside Canalis solearis, formed by the anastomosis of Aa. digitales medialis and lateralis. C

15a **A. marginis solearis.** Around the Margo solearis phalangis distalis. C

16 **A. digitalis [plantaris propria III] lateralis.** Lateral terminal branch of Ramus perforans distalis III. Enters Foramen soleare laterale. A C D

17 **Ramus plantaris phalangis proximalis.** To the plantar aspect of Phalanx proximalis. A C

18 **Ramus dorsalis phalangis proximalis.** Ramifies on the dorsolateral surface of Phalanx proximalis. A C

19 **Ramus plantaris phalangis mediae.** To the plantar aspect of Phalanx media. C

20 **Ramus dorsalis phalangis mediae.** Passes along the medial aspect of Cartilago ungularis lateralis to the dorsal surface of Phalanx media. A

21 **Ramus tori digitalis.** Ramifies in Torus ungulae. A C

22 **A. coronalis.** Arises from Ramus tori digitalis or A. digitalis lateralis, courses along the proximal border of Cartilago ungularis lateralis. A C

23 **Ramus dorsalis phalangis distalis.** Passes through Foramen or Incisura of Processus plantaris lateralis, and continues in Sulcus parietalis lateralis. A C

24 **A. tibialis caudalis.** Smaller terminal branch of A. poplitea, courses at the caudal aspect of tibia. A B

25 ***A. nutricia tibiae.*** Enters Foramen nutricium of tibia. A

26 ***A. malleolaris caudalis lateralis.*** Passes laterally between tibia and M. flexor digitalis profundus, branches to Malleolus lateralis. A B

27 *Rami calcanei.* To Tuber calcanei. A B

28 **Rete calcaneum.** Network surrounding Tuber calcanei. A B

29 ***Ramus anastomoticus cum a saphena.*** Curved continuation of A. tibialis caudalis beyond the origin of A. malleolaris caudalis lateralis. Joins and reinforces Ramus caudalis of A. saphena. Exceptionally absent. A B

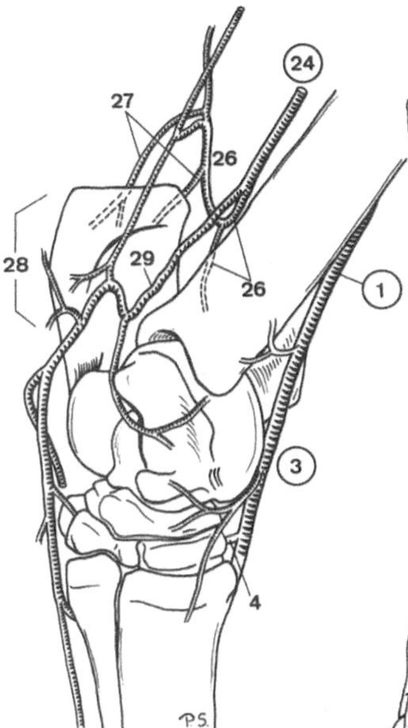

B Arteries of left tarsus, medial aspect (eq)

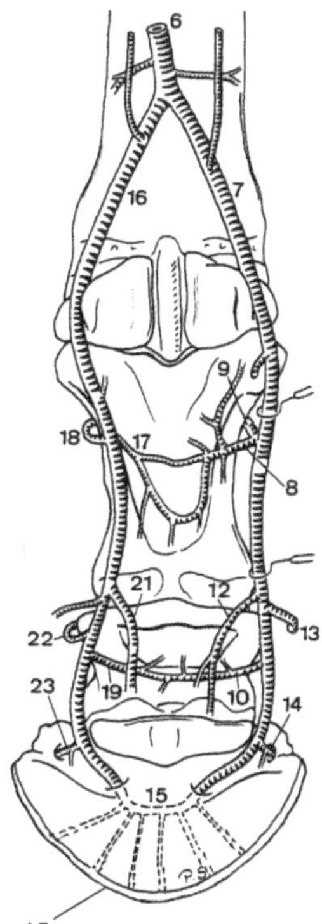

C Arteries of left pes, plantar aspect (eq)

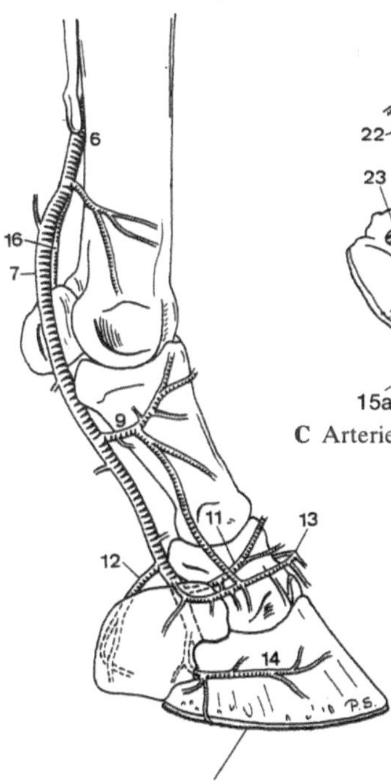

D Arteries of left pes, medial aspect (eq)

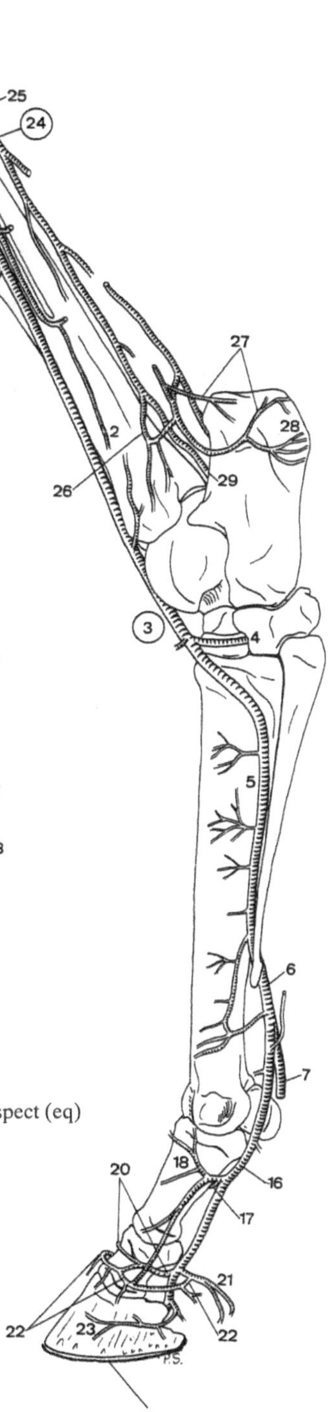

A Arteries of left pelvic limb, lateral aspect (eq)

TERMINI COMMUNES

1 **VENAE**[1]. Veins, conveying the blood from the lungs and the periphery, to the heart.

2 **VENAE PULMONALES**. Pulmonary veins, collect the oxygenated blood from the lungs and discharge it in Atrium sinistrum. May be fused with each other or plural. A B

3 ***V. pulmonalis lobi cranialis dextri.*** Collects the blood from Lobus cranialis of the right lung. A B

4 ***V. pulmonalis lobi medii.*** Collects the blood from Lobus medius of the right lung, absent in eq. A B

5 ***V. pulmonalis lobi caudalis dextri.*** Collects the blood from Lobus caudalis of the right lung. A B

6 *Ramus lobi accessorii*. Collects the blood from Lobus accessorius. A B

7 ***V. pulmonalis lobi cranialis sinistri.*** Collects the blood from Lobus cranialis of the left lung. A B

8 ***V. pulmonalis lobi caudalis sinistri.*** Collects the blood from Lobus caudalis of the left lung. A B

9 **VENAE CORDIS**. Veins of heart. B C

10 ***Sinus coronarius.*** Venous enlargement in Sulcus coronarius at the opening into the Atrium dextrum. Receives blood from Vv. cordis media et magna, obliqua atrii sinistri, and Vena azygos sinistra. B C

11 *V. cordis media*. In Sulcus interventricularis subsinousus, discharges into Sinus coronarius or Atrium dextrum (eq). It may join the Atrium dextrum at some distance from the coronary sinus[1]. B

12 *V. cordis magna*. Continuation of Sinus coronarius in Sulcus interventricularis paraconalis. B C

13 **Ramus intermedius [V. marginis ventricularis sinistri]**. On Margo ventricularis sinister. C

14 *V. obliqua atrii sinistri* (Car, eq). Conducts blood from the wall of Atrium sinistrum into Sinus coronarius. Remnant of the left V. cardinalis communis. B

15 ***Vv. cordis dextrae.*** Collect blood from Ventriculus dexter, discharge into Atrium dextrum. B

16 ***Vv. cordis minimae.*** Slender veins, discharge into all heart chambers, esp. atria.

17 ***Plica v. cavae sinistrae*** (Car). Remnant of the V. cava cranialis sinistra. (This structure was omitted from the 5th edition of the N. A. V.)

18 **V. AZYGOS SINISTRA**. Arises from Sinus coronarius in su and Ru, curves caudodorsally, continues along the left-dorsal surface of aorta. C

19 ***Vv. esophageae [oesophageae].*** To the thoracic part of esophagus. C

20 ***Vv. bronchales.*** Course along trachea and Bronchi principales, continue in su and bo along the intrapulmonary bronchi. C

21 ***(V. hemiazygos dextra)*** (su, Ru). Caudal complement of V. azygos sinistra along the right surface of aorta.

22 ***Vv. intercostales dorsales.*** Segmental, pass dorsally across Corpus vertebrae to Spatium intercostale, continue along Sulcus costae. D

23 *Ramus dorsalis*. Courses dorsally into Plexus vertebralis externus dorsalis. D

24 **V. intervertebralis.** Passes through the Foramen intervertebrale, connects Plexus vertebrales externi and internus. D

25 **Plexus vertebralis externus ventralis.** Network at the ventral aspect of Columna vertebralis. E

26 **Plexus vertebralis externus dorsalis.** Network at the dorsal aspect of Columna vertebralis. D E

27 **Plexus vertebralis internus ventralis.** Network on the floor of Canalis vertebralis. D E

28 **Rami interarcuales.** Bilateral branches which penetrate Ligamenta flava and join Plexus vertebralis externus dorsalis. E

29 **Rami spinales.** Connect Plexus vertebralis internus ventralis with Vv. spinales by piercing through dura. D E

30 **Vv. spinales.** Longitudinal veins along Medulla spinalis. D E

31 **Vv. basivertebrales.** Perforate the Corpus vertebrae and usually join Plexus vertebralis externus ventralis. E

32 ***V. costoabdominalis dorsalis.*** Accompanies corresponding artery. D

33 *Ramus dorsalis*. To Plexus vertebralis externus dorsalis. D

34 **V. intervertebralis.** Passes through the thoracolumbar Foramen intervertebrale. D

35 ***Vv. lumbales I et II.*** Pass across the body of vertebra to the caudal border of Processus costalis. D

36 *Ramus dorsalis*. To Plexus vertebralis externus dorsalis. D

37 **V. intervertebralis.** Passes through the Foramen intervertebrale to Plexus vertebralis internus. D

[1] According to the definition of the veins "conveying the blood from the lungs and the periphery to the heart", the veins should be

cont. p. 339 ►

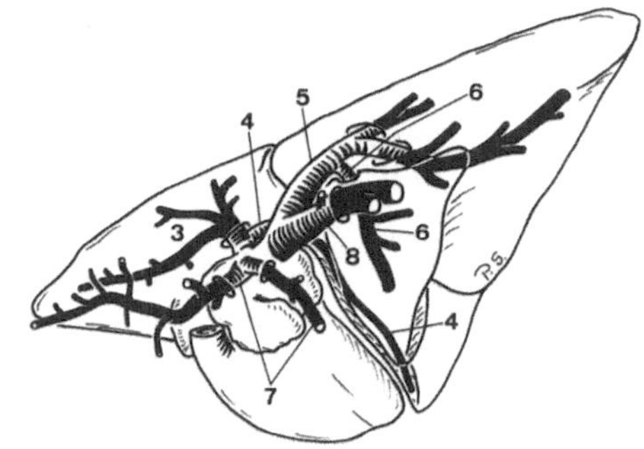

A Venae pulmonales (left lung removed) (fe)

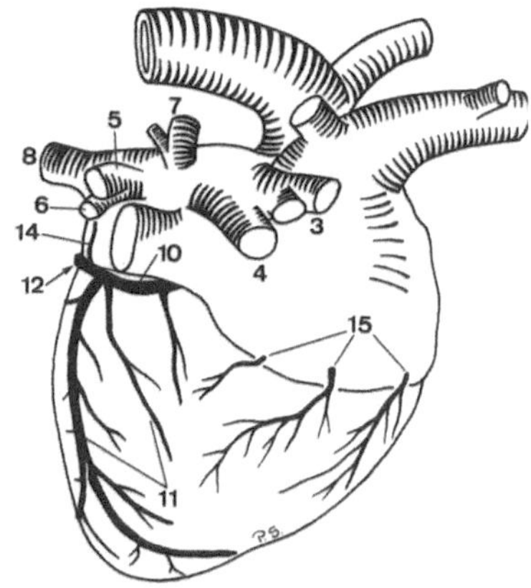

B Veins on Facies atrialis of the heart (ca)

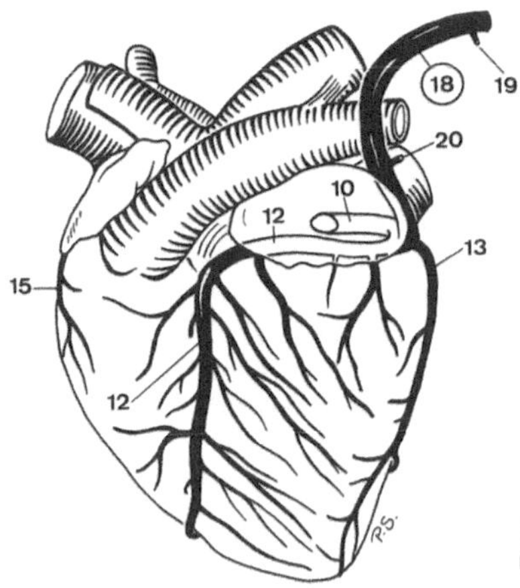

C Veins on Facies auricularis of the heart (bo)

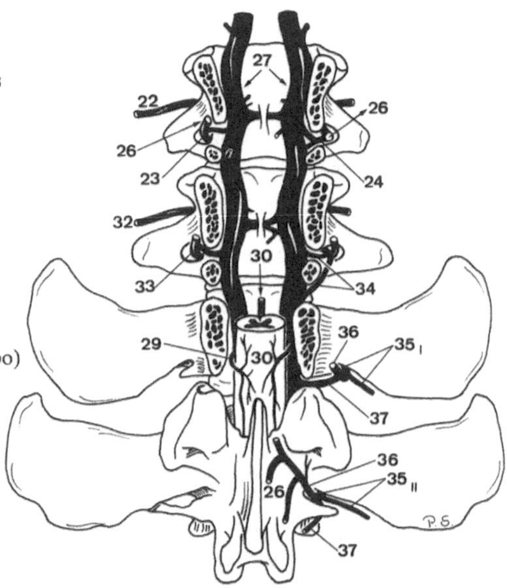

D Veins in relation to Vertebrae thoracicae and lumbales (Arcus partly removed) (su)

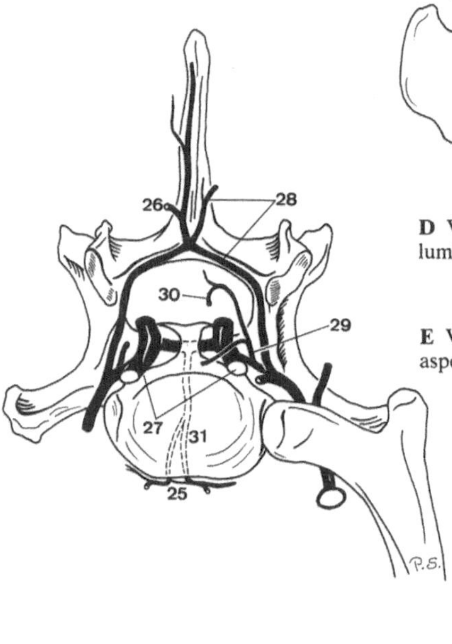

E Veins in relation to Vertebra cervicalis VII, caudal aspect (ca)

listed as such. Instead, the N. A. V. adopted the proposal that the origin of veins should be considered similar to that of the arteries and not following the blood flow, the larger veins being listed before their tributaries, except for the Vv. pulmonales. In anatomical texts the endings of the affluents/tributaries are designated as the origin of the venous branches, following the blood flow.

1 **VENA CAVA CRANIALIS.** Large unpaired vein which leaves Sinus venarum cavarum, courses cranially in Mediastinum craniale towards Apertura thoracis cranialis. Bifurcates in the left and right Vv. brachiocephalicae (Car, su, sometime cap) or gives rise to the left and right Vv. subclaviae (Ru, eq). A

2 **V. azygos dextra.** Occurs in Car, Ru, eq, and sometimes su. Unpaired vein, curves across the right aspect of trachea and esophagus, continues along the right-dorsal surface of Aorta thoracica. A B

3 ***V. broncho-esophagea [-oesophagea]*** (ca, eq). Bilateral (ca) s. unpaired (eq) vein which gives rise to bronchal and esophageal branches. A

4 ***(V. hemiazygos sinistra)*** (ca, eq). Inconstant and variably developed. Unpaired complement or replacement of the caudal portion of V. azygos dextra. Arises from the latter vein in the caudal half on the thorax, crosses Columna vertebralis ventrally and continues caudally along the left surface of Aorta descendens. B

5 ***Vv. intercostales dorsales.*** Accompany corresponding arteries. A B

6 *Ramus dorsalis.* To Plexus vertebralis externus dorsalis. A B

7 **V. intervertebralis.** Passes through the Foramen intervertebrale, connects Plexus vertebrales externi and internus. A B

8 ***V. costoabdominalis dorsalis.*** Accompanies corresponding artery. B

9 *Ramus dorsalis.* To Plexus vertebralis externus dorsalis. B

10 **V. intervertebralis.** Passes through Foramen intervertebrale, connects Plexus vertebrales externi and internus. B

11 ***Vv. lumbales I et II (III).*** Bilateral, but often initially fused, accompany corresponding arteries. B

12 *Ramus dorsalis.* To Plexus vertebralis externus dorsalis. B

13 **V. intervertebralis.** Passes through Foramen intervertebrale, connects Plexus vertebrales externi and internus. B

14 **V. broncho-esophagea [-oesophagea]** (fe). Gives rise to bronchal and esophageal branches.

15 **V. costocervicalis.** V. costocervicalis sinistra originates from V. brachiocephalica sinistra in Car. A

CARNIVORA

16 ***V. vertebralis.*** Accompanies corresponding artery. A C

17 *Vv. intervertebrales.* Pass through the Foramen intervertebrale s. Foramen vertebrale laterale of atlas and connect Plexus vertebrales externi and internus. A C

18 *Ramus anastomoticus cum v. jugulari interna.* Originates in Fossa atlantis, courses across the ventrolateral surface of Articulatio atlanto-occipitalis to V. jugularis interna. C

19 ***V. scapularis dorsalis.*** Accompanies corresponding artery. A

20 ***V. intercostalis dorsalis I.*** Accompanies corresponding artery. A

21 ***V. cervicalis profunda.*** Accompanies corresponding artery. A

22 *V. vertebralis thoracica.* Accompanies corresponding artery in ca. A

23 **Vv. intercostales dorsales III et IV.** Accompany corresponding arteries. A

24 **Rami dorsales.** To Plexus vertebralis externus dorsalis. A

25 **V. intervertebralis.** Branch of Ramus dorsalis, passes through the Foramen intervertebrale, connects Plexus vertebrales externi and internus. A

26 ***V. intercostalis suprema.*** Accompanies corresponding artery. May be absent in ca. A

27 *V. intercostalis dorsalis II.* Accompanies corresponding artery. A

28 **Ramus dorsalis.** To Plexus vertebralis externus dorsalis. A

29 **V. intervertebralis.** Branch of Ramus dorsalis, passes through Foramen intervertebrale, connects Plexus vertebrales externi and internus. A

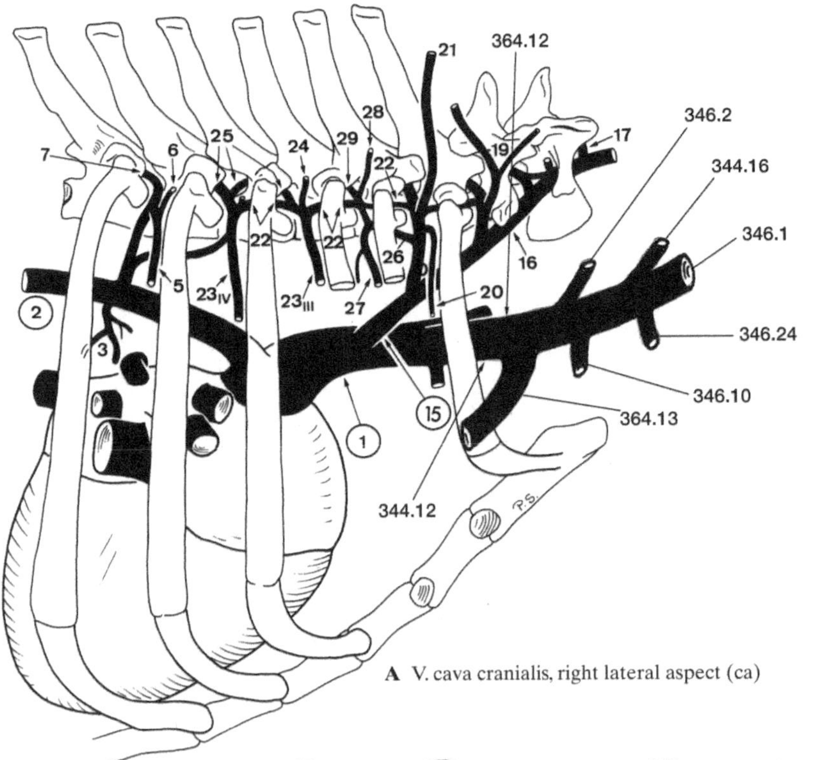

A V. cava cranialis, right lateral aspect (ca)

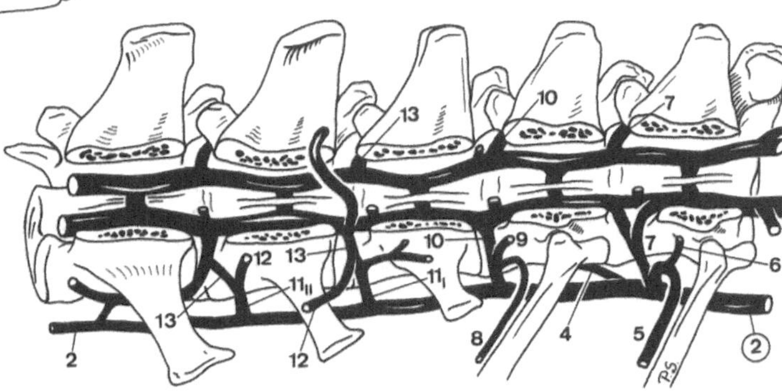

B Veins in relation to Vertebrae thoracicae and lumbales (Arcus removed), dorsal (and right) aspect (ca)

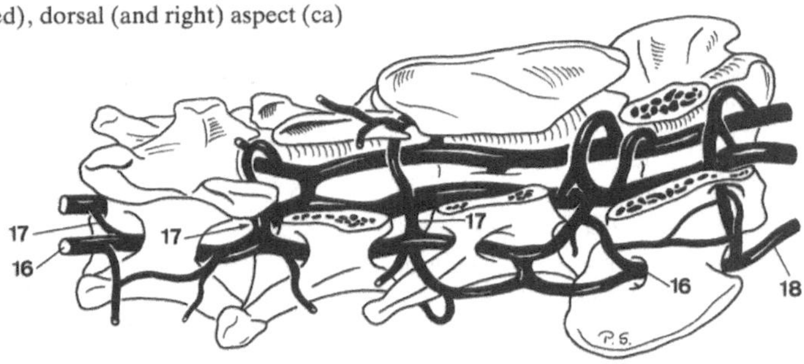

C Veins in relation to Vertebrae cervicales I–IV, (Arcus partly removed), right dorsal aspect (ca)

SUS

1 ***V. vertebralis***. Accompanies corresponding artery. A B

2 *Vv. intervertebrales*. Pass through Foramen intervertebrale s. Foramen vertebrale laterale of axis or atlas, connect Plexus vertebrales externi and internus. B

3 *Ramus anastomoticus cum v. occipitali*. Connection to V. occipitalis in Fossa atlantis. Accompanied by a similar branch at the level of axis. B

4 *Ramus descendens*. Emerges dorsally from Foramen alare and joins Plexus vertebralis externus dorsalis. B

5 ***V. intercostalis suprema***. Accompanies corresponding artery. A

6 *Vv. intercostales dorsales III et IV (V)*. Accompany corresponding arteries. A

7 **Ramus dorsalis**. Courses dorsally through Foramen vertebrale laterale, joins Plexus vertebralis externus dorsalis. A

8 **V. intervertebralis**. Enter Foramen intervertebrale, connects Plexus vertebrales externi and internus. A

9 ***V. intercostalis dorsalis II***. Accompanies corresponding artery. A

10 ***V. scapularis dorsalis***. Courses through Foramen vertebrale laterale of Vertebra thoracica I and contributes to Plexus vertebralis externus dorsalis. A

11 ***V. cervicalis profunda***. Courses through Foramen vertebrale laterale of Vertebra thoracica II (seldom I) and ramifies in branches which contribute to Plexus vertebralis externus dorsalis. A

12 *V. vertebralis thoracica*. Runs caudally upon the dorsal aspect of Colla costarum. A

13 *V. intercostalis dorsalis* I. Accompanies corresponding artery. A

RUMINANTIA

14 ***V. intercostalis suprema***. Accompanies corresponding artery. C

15 *Vv. intercostales dorsales*. Course distally in Spatium intercostale I–III (IV) at the left side and, inconstantly present, in the right Spatium intercostale I. C

16 **Ramus dorsalis**. Contributes to Plexus vertebralis externus dorsalis. C

17 **V. intervertebralis**. Branch of Ramus dorsalis, passes through Foramen intervertebrale, connects Plexus vertebrales externi and internus. C

18 ***V. scapularis dorsalis***. Accompanies corresponding artery. C

19 ***V. cervicalis profunda***. Accompanies corresponding artery. C

20 *V. vertebralis thoracica*. Courses caudally over the dorsal surface of Colla costarum. Inconstant in ov and cap. C

21 ***V. vertebralis***. Accompanies corresponding artery. C D

22 *Vv. intervertebrales*. Enter Foramen intervertebrale s. Foramen vertebrale laterale of axis, connect Plexus vertebrales externi and internus. C D

23 *Ramus descendens*. Branch of the intravertebral segment of V. vertebralis, leaves Canalis vertebralis through Foramen vertebrale laterale of atlas, and joins Plexus vertebralis externus dorsalis. D

24 **Ramus anastomoticus cum v. occipitali**. Passes through Foramen alare of atlas, joins V. occipitalis. D

EQUUS

25 ***V. cervicalis profunda***. Accompanies corresponding artery. E

26 *V. intercostalis dorsalis I. Accompanies corresponding artery. E*

27 ***V. intercostalis suprema***. Accompanies corresponding artery. E

28 *Vv. intercostales dorsales II–VI (sin), II–IV (dext)*. Accompany corresponding arteries. E

29 **Ramus dorsalis**. Contributes to Plexus vertebralis externus dorsalis. E

30 **V. intervertebralis**. Branch of Ramus dorsalis, enters Foramen intervertebrale, connects Plexus vertebrales externi and internus. E

31 ***V. scapularis dorsalis***. Contributes to Plexus vertebralis externus dorsalis. E

32 ***V. vertebralis***. Accompanies corresponding artery. E F

33 *Vv. intervertebrales*. Pass through Foramen intervertebrale s. Foramen vertebrale laterale of axis s. atlas, connect Plexus vertebrales externi and internus. F

34 *Ramus anastomoticus cum v. occipitali*. Connection to V. occipitalis in Fossa atlantis. A similar anastomosis may arise at the level of axis. F

35 *Ramus descendens*. Emerges dorsally from Foramen alare and ramifies. F

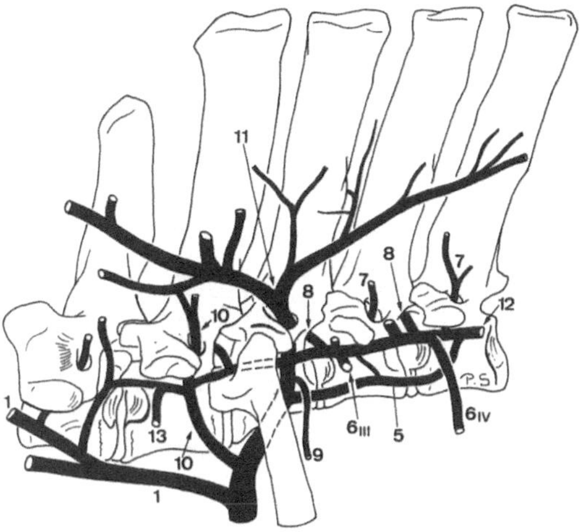

A Veins in relation to Vertebrae cervicalis VII–thoracica IV, left lateral aspect (su)

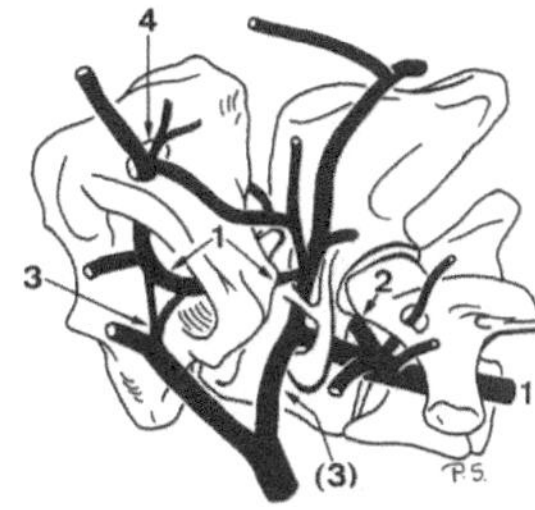

B Veins in relation to Vertebrae cervicales I–III, left lateral aspect (su)

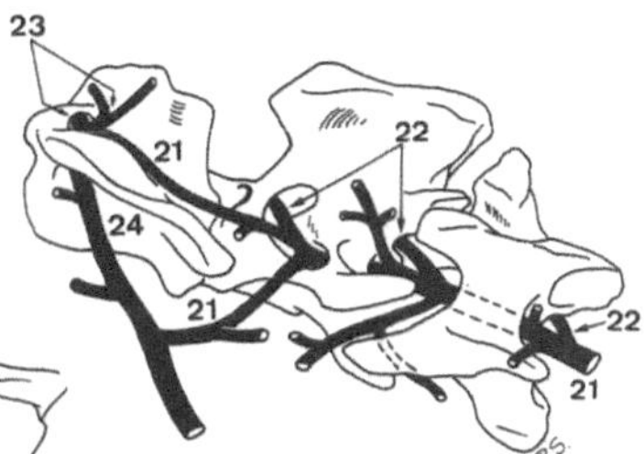

D Veins in relation to Vertebrae cervicales I–III, left lateral aspect (bo)

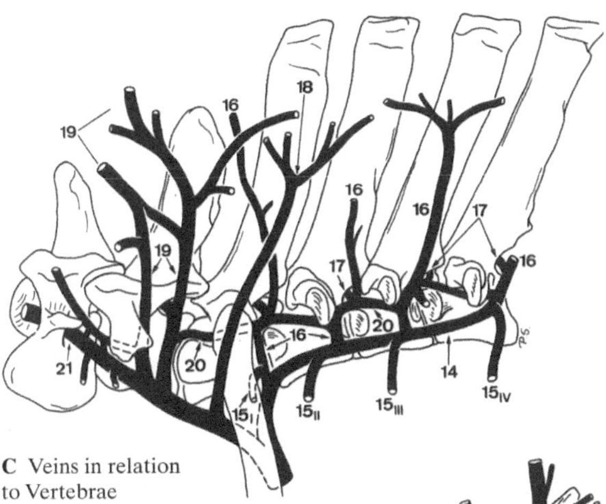

C Veins in relation to Vertebrae cervicalis VI–thoracica IV, left lateral aspect (bo)

E Veins in relation to Vertebrae thoracicae I–V, left lateral aspect (eq)

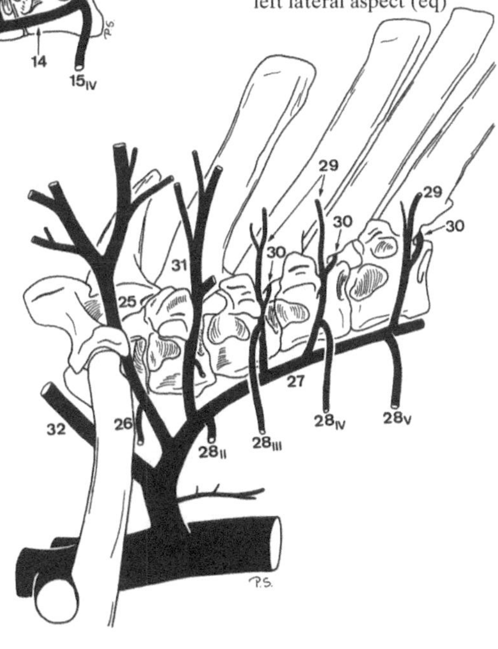

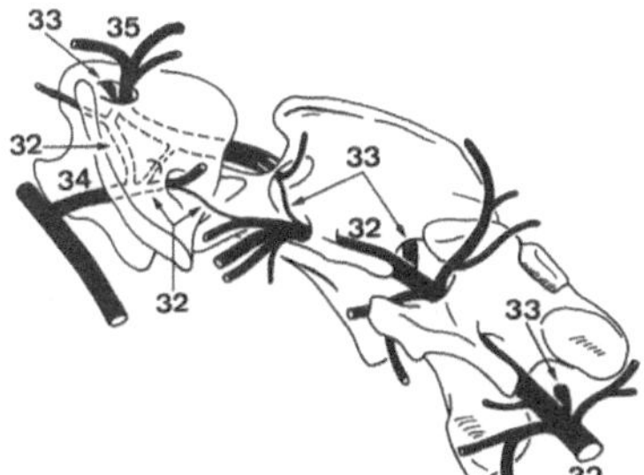

F Veins in relation to Vertebrae cervicales I–III, left lateral aspect (eq)

TERMINI COMMUNES

1 **V. thoracica interna**. Arises by a common trunk with its counterpart in fe and often ca. The left vein may arise from V. brachiocephalica sinistra (ca). Accompanies corresponding artery. A B

2 ***V. pericardiacophrenica***. Indistinct vein to pericardium and Diaphragma.

3 ***Vv. thymicae***. To Lobus thoracicus of thymus. Variable in origin and development.

4 ***Vv. mediastinales***. To mediastinum. A

5 ***Vv. perforantes***. Perforate Mm. intercostales. A

6 ***Vv. intercostales ventrales***. Variably arising veins which course dorsally in the first 6 (bo), 7 (fe, eq) or 8 (ca, su, ov, cap) Spatia intercostalia. Absent in Spatium intercostale I in su. Sometimes present in Spatium intercostale IX (su, ov, cap). A

7 ***V. musculophrenica***. Caudodorsal vein which enters Pars sternalis of Diaphragma (su, ov, cap) or perforates Diaphragma and continues along the abdominal surface of Pars costalis of Diaphragma (Car, bo, eq). A

8 *Vv. intercostales ventrales*. Course dorsally in the middle Spatia intercostalia. A

9 ***V. epigastrica cranialis***. Accompanies corresponding artery. A

10 *V. epigastrica cranialis superficialis [V. subcutanea abdominis]* (Car, su, Ru). Courses subcutaneously in the ventral abdominal wall and anastomoses by inosculation with V. epigastrica caudalis superficialis. Arises from V. thoracica superficialis in eq. A (see 306.15)

11 *Rami phrenici* (Ru). To Pars costalis of Diaphragma. A

12 **V. BRACHIOCEPHALICA**. Paired branch of V. cava cranialis in Car, su (in most pigs it is double), sometimes cap, gives rise to V. subclavia and V. jugularis externa. B 341A

13 ***V. thyroidea [thyreoidea] caudalis***. Unpaired vein in Car, courses along the ventral surface of trachea to Gl. thyroidea. B

14 ***V. costocervicalis sinistra*** (Car). Trunk collecting most left major veins in the cranial part of Cavum thoracis. B

15 **TRUNCUS BIJUGULARIS**. Unpaired continuation of V. cava cranialis, cranial to Vv. subclaviae, in Ru, eq, sometimes su. A (The Truncus bijugularis was omitted from the 5th edition of the N. A. V. The venous trunk which was previously indicated by this term is actually the cranialmost segment of V. cava cranialis.)

16 **V. JUGULARIS INTERNA.** This vein is present in Car, su, bo, and most eq. It arises from the ipsilateral V. jugularis externa in Car, su, some bo, and most eq, or from the cranial end of V. Cava cranialis in most bo and some eq. It is absent in ov and cap, and the veins listed hereunder are branches of V. jugularis externa. When V. jugularis interna occurs in eq, it does not have the branches listed here. A B C 341 A

17 ***V. thyroidea [thyreoidea] media***. Inconstant, enters the caudal pole of Gl. thyroidea. B

18 ***V. thyroidea [thyreoidea] cranialis***. Arises variably, enters the cranial pole of Gl. thyroidea. B

19 *V. cricothyroidea [-thyreoidea]*. To M. cricothyroideus. B

20 *Ramus laryngeus caudalis*. Supplies the caudal part of larynx. B

21 **Arcus laryngeus caudalis** (Car). Transverse connection between left and right Ramus laryngeus caudalis at the ventral aspect of larynx. B

22 *V. laryngea cranialis* (bo). Enters larynx between Cartilago thyroidea and Cartilago cricoidea.

23 ***V. occipitalis*** (fe, su, Ru). Runs towards Fossa atlantis, arises from V. jugularis externa in ov, cap, sometimes bo. C

24 *V. pharyngea ascendens* (bo). To the dorsal pharyngeal wall.

25 *V. stylomastoidea* (su). Enters Foramen stylomastoideum.

26 *Ramus occipitalis*. To Regio occipitalis. C

27 ***V. comitans a. carotidis externae*** (Car, su). Runs along A. carotis externa. C

28 *V. laryngea cranialis* (su). Enters larynx.

29 *V. pharyngea*. To Plexus pharyngeus. C

30 *V. comitans a lingualis*. Accompanies A. lingualis, joins V. lingualis. C

31 *V. palatina* (fe, su). Courses along the medial surface of M. pterygoideus medialis to supply Palatum durum. C

32 **Plexus palatinus**. Network within Palatum durum. C

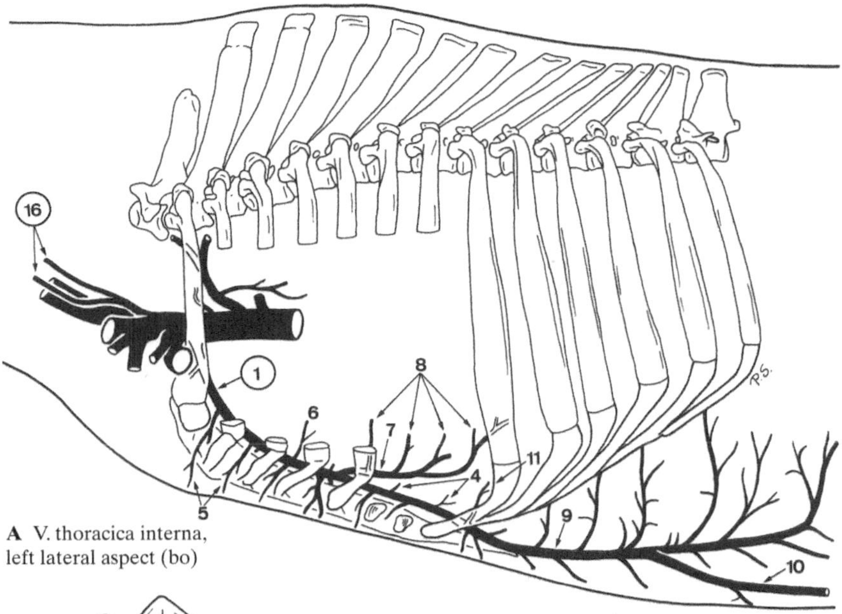

A V. thoracica interna, left lateral aspect (bo)

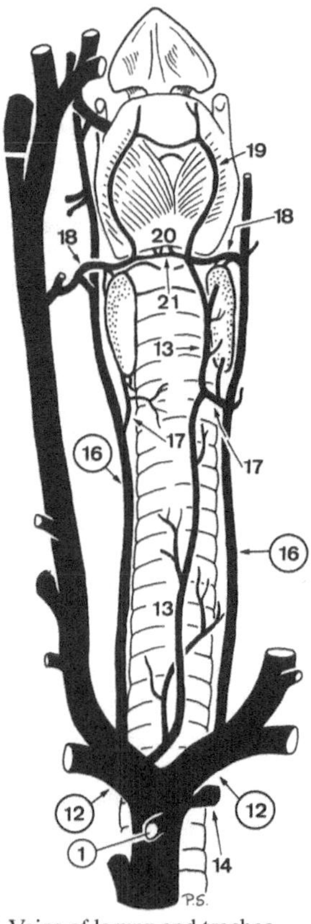

B Veins of larynx and trachea, ventral aspect (ca)

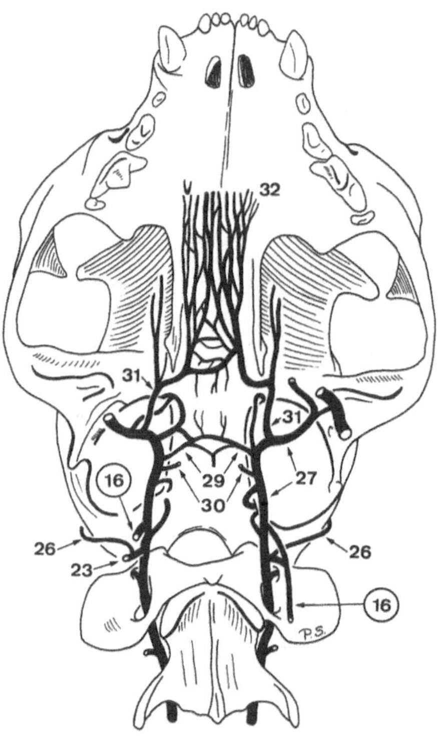

C V. jugularis interna (Mandibula removed), ventral aspect (fe)

1 **V. JUGULARIS EXTERNA**. Superficial and principal vein of the neck, arises from V. brachiocephalica in Car (su, cap), V. cava cranialis (ov), or Truncus bijugularis in Un (except sometimes su, ov, cap), courses in Sulcus jugularis and bifurcates into V. linguofacialis and V. maxillaris. A B 341 A

2 **V. cervicalis superficialis**. Accompanies corresponding artery. A B 341 A

3 ***Ramus ascendens***. Accompanies corresponding artery. A B

4 *Ramus auricularis* (su). Anastomoses with V. auricularis caudalis.

5 ***V. suprascapularis*** (Car). Accompanies N. suprascapularis. A

6 ***Ramus suprascapularis*** (Ru). Accompanies corresponding artery. B

7 *Ramus acromialis*. Accompanies corresponding artery. B

8 ***Ramus acromialis*** (Car, su). Accompanies corresponding artery. A

9 ***Ramus prescapularis [prae-]***. Accompanies corresponding artery. A B

10 **V. cephalica**. Branch of V. jugularis externa (ca, Un), or V. cervicalis superficialis (fe), courses in Sulcus pectoralis lateralis (and caudomedial to M. brachiocephalicus in ca). Continues superficially along the medial border of M. extensor carpi radialis. Ends at the mediopalmar aspect of carpus by joining V. radialis. B D 341 A 365 E (For practical purposes, some anatomists and clinicians divide this vein unofficially into an antebrachial segment and a brachial segment, similar to the continuation of A. brachialis superficialis with the A. antebrachialis superficialis.)

11 ***V. mediana cubiti***. Caudodistal (Car, su, Ru) or caudoproximal (eq) connection to V. brachialis, V. mediana (bo, cap) and/ or V. brachialis superficialis (Car) at the cranial aspect of Regio cubiti. D

12 ***V. cephalica accessoria***. Subcutaneous branch, arising halfway Regio brachialis (su: first root), in the proximal (eq), lower middle (Car) or distal (su: second root, Ru) segment of antebrachium. Courses over the dorsomedial aspect of carpus and metacarpus. C D

CARNIVORA, SUS

13 *Ramus carpeus dorsalis* (Car.) Branch to the Rete carpi dorsale, often plural. D

14 *Vv. digitales dorsales communes I–IV (Car), II–IV (su)*. Run over the superficial surface of the digital extensor tendons towards the lateral aspect of the corresponding Articulatio metacarpophalangea, where they bifurcate. D

15 **Vv. digitales dorsales propriae**. Three (su) s. four (Car) pairs of dorsal veins, arising from the bifurcation of Vv. digitales dorsales communes. D

16 *V. digitalis dorsalis V abaxialis* (ca). Accompanies corresponding artery. D

RUMINANTIA

17 *V. digitalis dorsalis communis II*. Courses mediodistally across the middle segment of metacarpus and joins Arcus palmaris profundus distalis or V. digitalis palmaris communis II (bo). C

18 *V. digitalis dorsalis communis III*. Continuation of V. cephalica accessoria. C

19 **Vv. digitales dorsales propriae**. Pair of superficial dorsal axial veins, course along tendons of M. extensor digitorum communis. C

20 **Ramus dorsalis phalangis proximalis**. Branch of V. digitalis dorsalis communis III (bo), courses abaxially across the dorsal surface of Phalanx proximalis. C

21 **Ramus dorsalis phalangis mediae**. Branch of V. digitalis dorsalis propria, courses abaxially across the dorsal surface of Phalanx media. C

22 **V. coronalis**. Superficial branch of V. digitalis dorsalis propria, courses abaxially in Sulcus coronalis of Ungula. C

22a **Plexus ungularis**. Surrounds the Facies parietalis phalangis distalis. This network extends also on the solear surface. Therefore, it is suggested to define the plexus as the dense venous network in Dermis ungulae.

23 *V. digitalis dorsalis communis IV*. Inconstant, courses laterodistally across the middle segment of metacarpus, joins Arcus palmaris profundus distalis or V. digitalis palmaris communis IV (bo). C

TERMINI COMMUNES

24 **V. omobrachialis** (ca). Courses caudodistally across the lateral surface of M. brachiocephalicus and M. deltoideus, joins V. axillobrachialis. A 341A 365 E

25 **V. thyroidea [thyreoidea] media** (ov, cap). Courses cranially to the caudal pole of Gl. thyroidea where it ramifies. B

26 **V. thyroidea [thyreoidea] cranialis** (ov, cap). Ramifies at the rostral pole of Gl. thyroidea. B

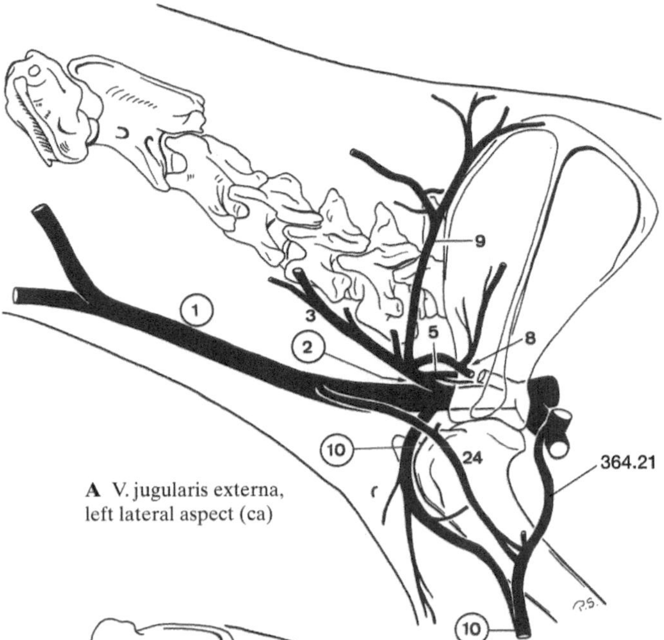

A V. jugularis externa, left lateral aspect (ca)

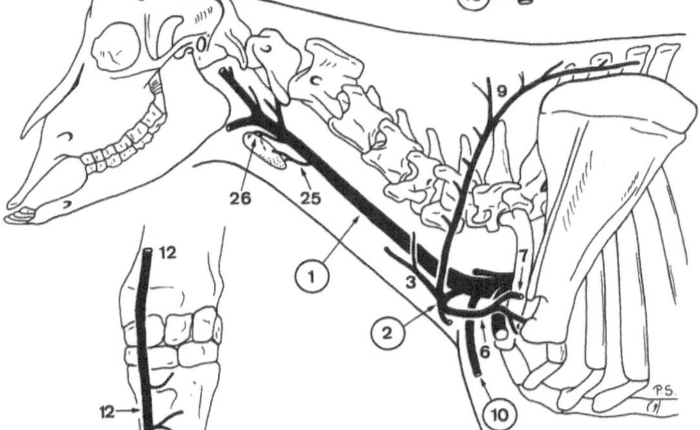

B V. jugularis externa, left lateral aspect (cap)

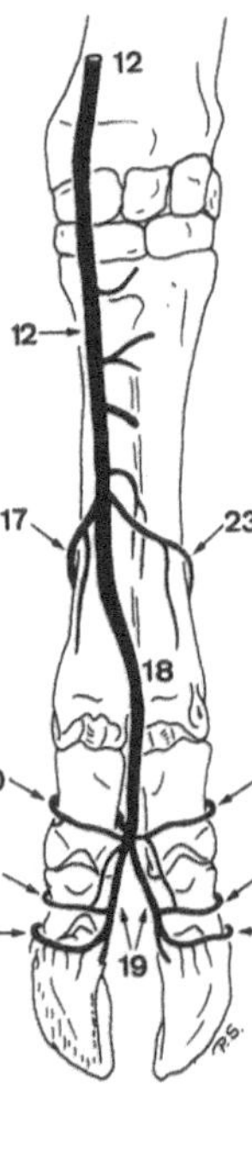

C Left V. cephalica accessoria, dorsal aspect (bo)

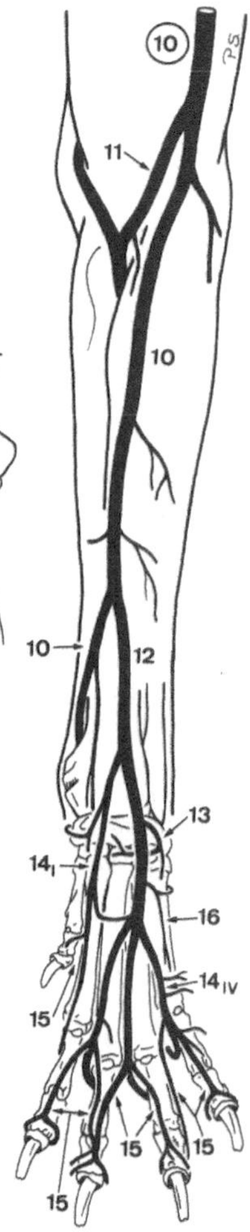

D Left V. cephalica, cranial aspect (ca)

1 **V. linguofacialis**. Rostrodorsally (Car) or rostroventrally (Un) directed terminal branch of V. jugularis externa. Common stem for V. lingualis and V. facialis. A B

FELIS

2 ***V. glandularis***. To Gl. mandibularis. A C

3 ***Arcus hyoideus***. Connection of both Vv. linguofaciales. A B C

4 *V. laryngea impar*. Unpaired vein supplying the larynx. A B

5 *V. lingualis impar*. Unpaired, into the tongue. A B C

6 **V. pharyngea ascendens**. To the pharyngeal wall. B C

7 **Plexus pharyngeus**. Network in the pharyngeal wall. B C

8 **V. laryngea cranialis**. Enters larynx through Fissura thyroidea. B C

9 **V. palatina ascendens**. To Palatum molle, supplies Tonsilla palatina. B C

10 **Ramus lingualis**. To the tongue. B C

11 **Vv. dorsales linguae**. Course dorsally in the tongue. B C

12 ***V. lingualis***. Into the tongue. A B C

13 *V. submentalis*. Courses along the ventromedial border of Corpus mandibulae. B C

14 *V. sublingualis*. To the floor of the mouth. B C

15 *V. profunda linguae*. Accompanies corresponding artery. B C

16 **Vv. dorsales linguae**. Ramify at Dorsum linguae. B C

17 ***V. facialis***. Courses over the lateral surface of Mandibula and over Facies towards Angulus oculi medialis. A B C

18 *V. labialis inferior*. Passes into Labium inferius. Usually represented by a superficial and a deep branch. A B

19 *V. angularis oris*. Runs to Angulus oris. A

20 *V. profunda faciei*. Courses dorsomedially to the medial aspect of Processus temporalis of Os zygomaticum. A B

21 **Ramus anastomoticus cum v. temporali superficiali**. To V. temporalis superficialis. A

22 **Ramus anastomoticus cum v. ophthalmica externa ventrali**. Perforates periorbita, joins V. ophthalmica externa ventralis. A

23 **Ramus infraorbitalis**. Courses through Canalis infraorbitalis. A

24 **V. palatina descendens**. Ramifies in Fossa pterygopalatina. A B

25 **V. palatina minor**. To Palatum molle. B

26 **V. palatina major**. Contributes to Plexus palatinus. B

27 **V. sphenopalatina**. Accompanies corresponding artery. B

28 *V. labialis superior*. Accompanies corresponding artery. A

29 *V. palpebralis inferior*. To Palpebra inferior. A

30 *V. lateralis nasi*. To Regio lateralis nasi. A

31 *V. dorsalis nasi*. To Regio dorsalis nasi. A

32 *V. angularis oculi*. Continuation of V. facialis across the mediodorsal border of Orbita. A

33 **V. frontalis [supratrochlearis]**. Courses along Margo supraorbitalis, anastomoses with V. auricularis rostralis. A

33a **V. palpebralis superior lateralis**. To the lateral portion of palpebra superior. A

34 **V. palpebralis superior medialis**. To the medial portion of Palpebra superior. A

35 **V. palpebralis inferior medialis**. To the medial portion of Palpebra inferior. A (This vein was omitted from the 5th edition of the N. A. V.)

36 **Ramus anastomoticus cum v. ophthalmica externa dorsali**. Intraorbital continuation of V. angularis oculi, joins V. ophthalmica externa dorsalis. A

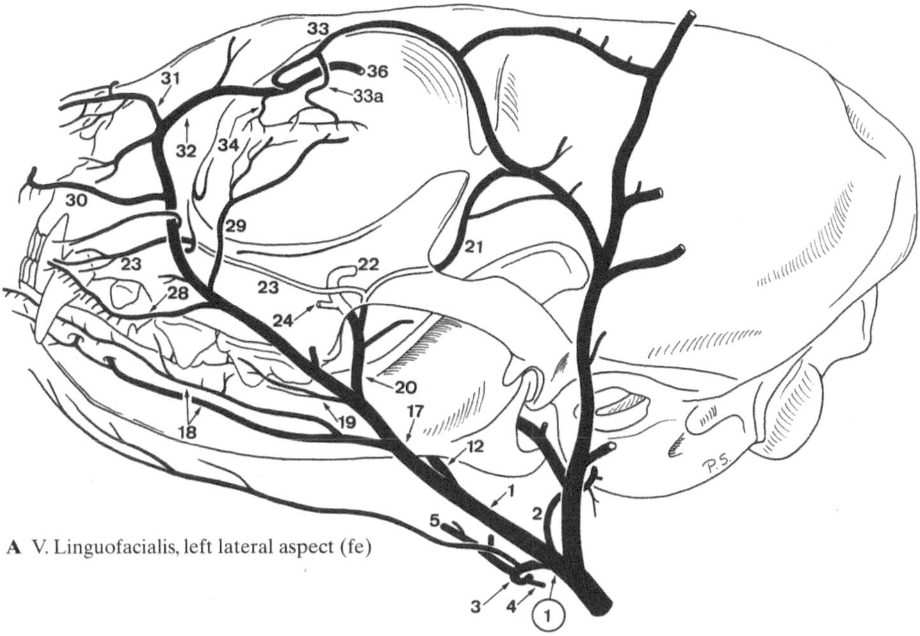

A V. Linguofacialis, left lateral aspect (fe)

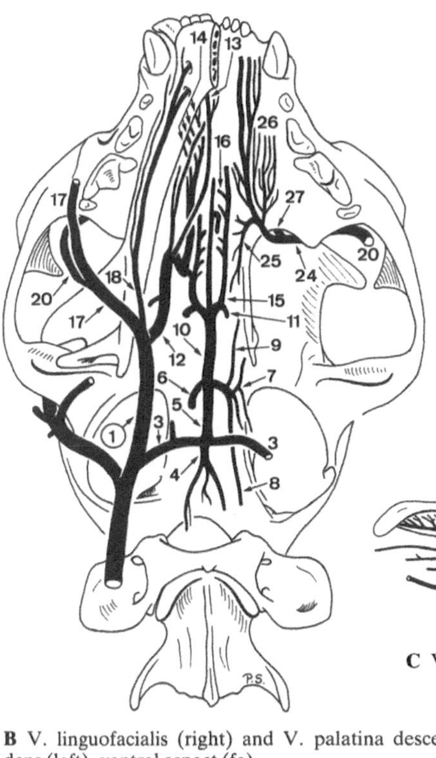

B V. linguofacialis (right) and V. palatina descendens (left), ventral aspect (fe)

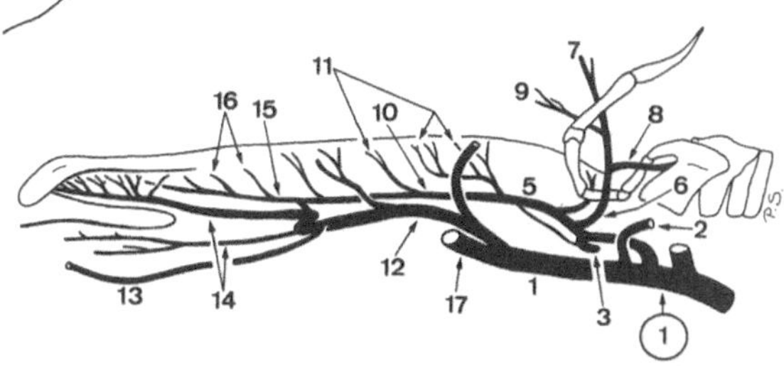

C V. lingualis, lateral aspect, left lateral aspect (fe)

CANIS

1 ***V. lingualis***. Into the tongue. A B C D

2 *V. glandularis*. To Gl. mandibularis. A

3 *V. pharyngea ascendens*. To the pharyngeal wall. A B C

4 **Plexus pharyngeus**. Network in the pharyngeal wall. A B

5 **V. laryngea cranialis**. Enters larynx through Fissura thyroidea. A B C

6 **V. palatina ascendens**. Joins Plexus palatinus. A B C

7 *Arcus hyoideus*. Connection between both Vv. linguales. Often (partly) double or plural. A B C

8 **V. laryngea impar**. Unpaired. B C

9 **Ramus submentalis**. Variably developed unpaired branch, courses over the ventral aspect of Mm. mylohyoidei. A B C

10 *V. sublingualis*. To the floor of the mouth. A B C

11 **V. superficialis ventralis linguae**. Ramifies in the ventral mucosa of Apex linguae. B

12 *V. profunda linguae*. Accompanies corresponding artery. B C

13 **Arcus hyoideus profundus**. Arch between the initial segments of the Vv. profundae linguae, deep into the tongue. B C

14 **Vv. dorsales linguae**. Ramify at Dorsum linguae. B C

15 ***V. facialis***. Runs over the lateral surface of Mandibula and over Facies towards Angulus oculi medialis. A C D

16 *V. submentalis*. Courses along the ventromedial border of Corpus mandibulae. A C

17 *V. labialis inferior*. Passes into Labium inferius. A C

18 *V. angularis oris*. Runs to Angulus oris. A

19 *V. profunda faciei*. Courses dorsomedially to the medial aspect of Processus temporalis of Os zygomaticum. A D

20 **Ramus anastomoticus cum v. temporali superficiali**. To V. temporalis superficialis. A D

21 **Rami glandulares zygomatici**. Branches of Ramus anastomoticus cum v. temporali superficiali or V. profunda faciei, supply Gl. zygomatica. A

22 **Rami dentales**. Arise from Ramus anastomoticus cum v. temporali superficiali, usually by one common trunk. Pierce through small openings in Tuber maxillae to the upper Dentes molares. A D

23 **Ramus anastomoticus cum v. ophthalmica externa ventrali**. Courses dorsomedially and pierces periorbita, joins V. ophthalmica externa ventralis. A D

24 **V. infraorbitalis**. Accompanies corresponding artery. A D

25 **V. malaris**. Branch of V. infraorbitalis or Ramus anastomoticus cum v. ophthalmica externa ventrali to the ventromedial border of Orbita. A

26 **V. palatina descendens**. Ramifies in Fossa pterygopalatina. A D

27 **V. palatina minor**. To Palatum molle. A D

28 **V. palatina major**. Joins Plexus palatinus. A D

29 **V. sphenopalatina**. Accompanies corresponding artery. A D

30 *V. labialis superior*. Accompanies corresponding artery. A D

31 *V. palpebralis inferior*. To Palpebra inferior. A D

32 *V. lateralis nasi*. To Regio lateralis nasi. A D

33 *V. dorsalis nasi*. To Dorsum nasi. A D

34 *V. angularis oculi*. Continuation of V. facialis across the dorsomedial border of Orbita. A D

35 **Ramus anastomoticus cum v. ophthalmica externa dorsali**. Pierces periorbita, continues as V. ophthalmica externa dorsalis. A D

36 **V. palpebralis superior medialis**. Ramifies in Palpebra superior. A

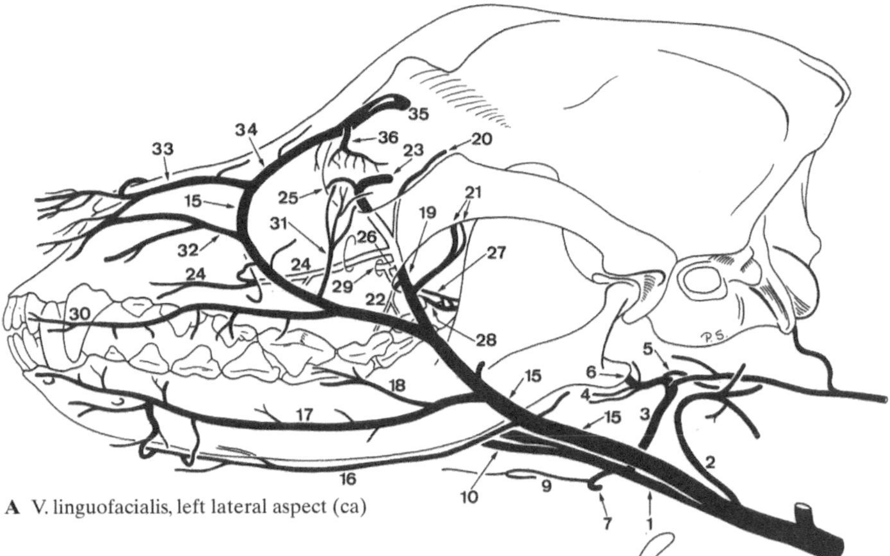

A V. linguofacialis, left lateral aspect (ca)

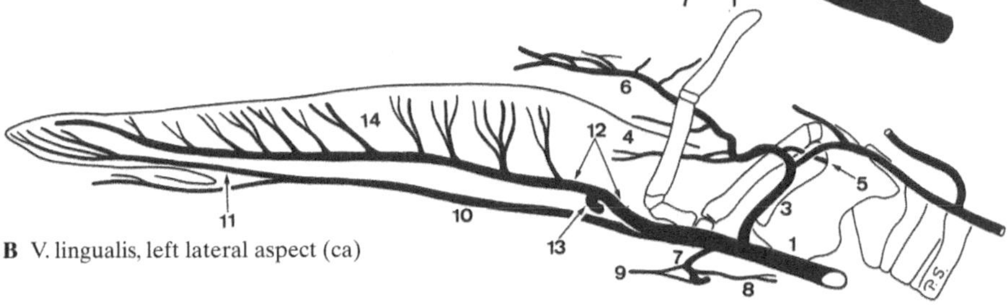

B V. lingualis, left lateral aspect (ca)

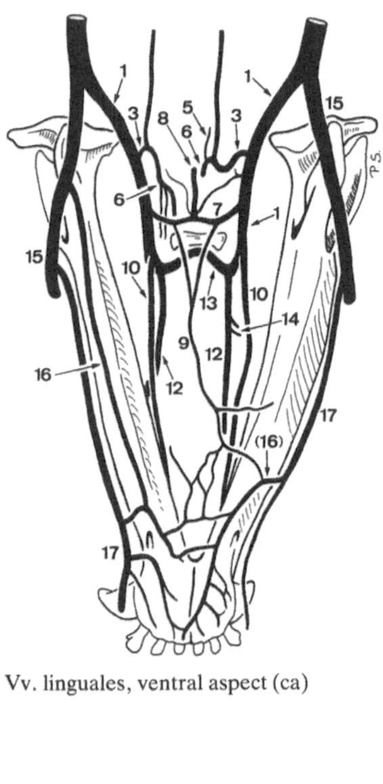

C Vv. linguales, ventral aspect (ca)

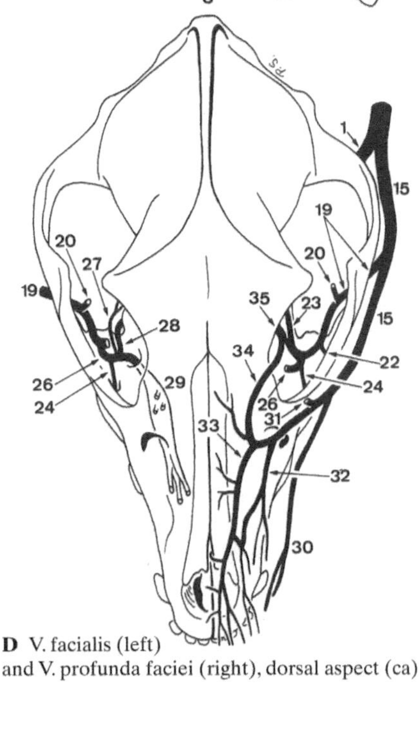

D V. facialis (left)
and V. profunda faciei (right), dorsal aspect (ca)

SUS, RUMINANTIA, EQUUS

1 ***Vv. glandulares***. To Gl. mandibularis. A B

2 ***V. laryngea cranialis*** (ov). Enters larynx through Foramen thyroideum.

3 ***V. lingualis***. To the tongue. Joins V. comitans a. lingualis (su), courses along the medial surface of M. styloglossus or perforates M. mylohyoideus (cap, eq). A B C

4 *Arcus hyoideus* (su, Ru). Transverse anastomosis between the symmetrical Vv. linguales, at the caudoventral aspect of Mm. geniohyoidei (su) or deep into the tongue (Ru). B

5 *V. sublingualis*. Courses along the medial aspect of M. mylohyoideus to the floor of the mouth. B

6 **V. pharyngea ascendens** (su). To the pharyngeal wall. B

7 **Plexus pharyngeus**. Network in the pharyngeal wall. Drains into V. pharyngea ascendens and V. pharyngea. B

8 **V. submentalis** (su, ov, cap, eq). Runs along the ventrolateral aspect of M. mylohyoideus towards the chin. Represented by a vein which courses at the lateral aspect of M. geniohyoideus into Foramen mentale mediale in su. B

9 *V. profunda linguae*. Runs along the medial aspect of M. hyoglossus towards Apex linguae. B

10 **Vv. dorsales linguae**. Ramify at Dorsum linguae. B

11 ***V. facialis***. Courses across Incisura vasorum facialium, continues along the rostral border of M. masseter. A B C

12 *V. submentalis* (bo). Runs along the ventrolateral aspect of M. mylohyoideus towards the chin. A

13 *V. labialis inferior* (su, eq). Into Labium inferius. C (These veins are species specific, and even though they are not listed as such in the 5th edition of the N. A. V., it is important to know that they are found only in su and eq.)

14 *Vv. labiales inferiores* (Ru). Single (ov, cap) or superficial and deep veins (bo) into Labium inferius. A

15 **V. angularis oris**. Inconstant, to Angulus oris. A

16 *V. angularis oris* (eq). Variably arising branch to Angulus oris. C

17 *V. labialis superior* (eq). Into Labium superius. C

18 *V. profunda faciei*. Courses at the medial surface of M. masseter and curves at the caudal aspect of Tuber maxillae towards Fossa pterygopalatina. A B C

19 **Plexus v. profundae faciei** (Ru). Anastomosing branches of V. faciei profunda, at the medial aspect of M. masseter. A

20 **Sinus v. profundae faciei** (eq). Long spindle-shaped enlargement of V. profunda faciei. C

21 **V. ophthalmica externa ventralis**. Continuation of V. profunda faciei into Sinus (su) or Plexus (eq) ophthalmicus. B

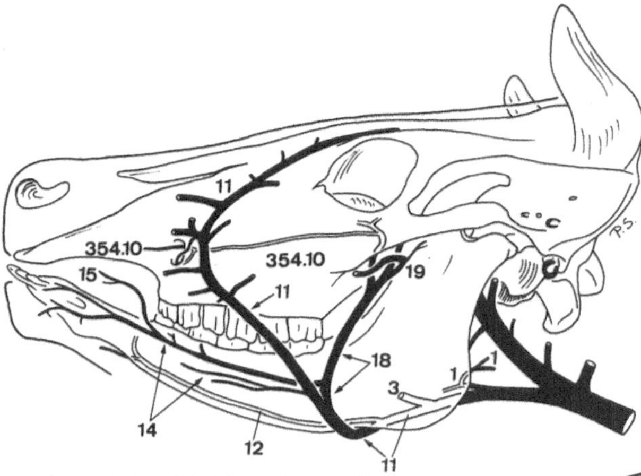

A Veins of the head, left lateral aspect (bo)

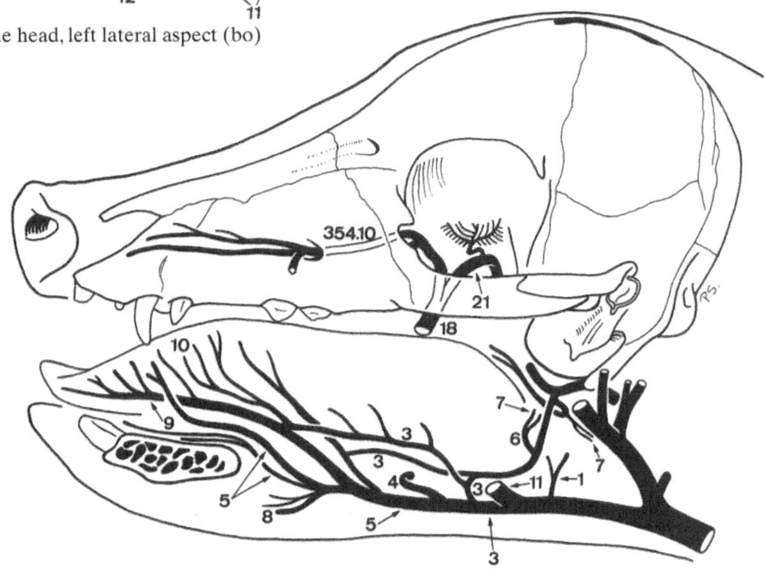

B Veins of the head, left lateral aspect (su, neonate)

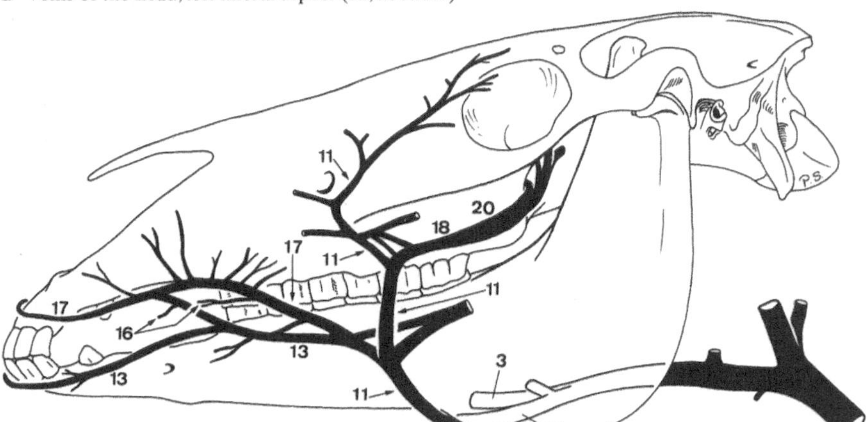

C V. facialis, left lateral aspect (eq)

1 **Sinus ophthalmicus** (su), Plexus ophthalmicus (eq). Venous enlargement, and network in Orbita, respectively. A.

2 **Vv. vorticosae.** Four veins which ramify in choroidea. A B

3 **Vv. ciliares.** Anterior branches of Vv. vorticosae to Corpus ciliare. B

4 **Vv. conjunctivales.** To Tunica conjunctiva. A

5 **V. lacrimalis.** To Gl. lacrimalis. A

6 **V. ethmoidalis externa.** Enters Foramen ethmoidale. A

7 **V. malaris.** Arises from Plexus ophthalmicus (eq), V. ophthalmica externa ventralis (su), courses to Angulus oculi medialis. A

8 **V. ophthalmica externa dorsalis.** Courses between M. obliquus dorsalis and M. levator palpebrae superioris. A

9 **V. supraorbitalis.** Lies dorsomedially in the Orbita, leaves through Foramen supraorbitale. Anastomoses with V. facialis in su. A

10 **V. infraorbitalis.** Passes through Canalis infraorbitalis. Originates from V. palatina descendens in Ru. 353 A B

11 **V. palatina descendens.** Continuation of V. profunda faciei in Fossa pterygopalatina. D

12 **V. palatina minor.** Inconstant branch to Palatum molle.

13 **V. palatina major.** Branch of V. palatina descendens, curves over Facies pterygopalatina of Corpus maxillae (su, bo, eq) or through Canalis palatinus major (ov, cap) to Palatum durum. A

14 **V. sphenopalatina.** Branch of V. palatina descendens, enters Cavum nasi through Foramen sphenopalatinum. A

15 *V. labialis superior* (su). Into Labium superius. C

16 **V. angularis oris.** To Angulus oris. Complemented by one or two branches of V. labialis inferior. C

17 *Vv. labiales superiores* (Ru). Superficial and deep veins into Labium superius. D

18 *V. lateralis nasi.* Variably developed vein in Regio lateralis nasi. C D

19 *Vv. dorsales nasi* (Ru). Variable branches in Regio dorsalis nasi. D

20 *V. palpebralis inferior medialis* (su, Ru). Enters the medial part of Palpebra inferior. Arises usually from V. angularis oculi in bo. C D

21 *V. dorsalis nasi* (su, eq). Ramifies in Regio dorsalis nasi. C

22 *V. angularis oculi.* Continuation of V. facialis along Angulus oculi medialis. C D

23 **V. palpebralis superior medialis.** To the medial part of Palpebra superior. C D

24 **Ramus anastomoticus cum v. ophthalmica externa dorsali** (su). Anastomoses with V. ophthalmica externa dorsalis. C

25 **V. frontalis [supratrochlearis]** (Ru). Courses along Margo supraorbitalis, ramifies in Regio frontalis. D

26 **V. palpebralis inferior medialis** (eq). To the medial part of Palpebra inferior. A

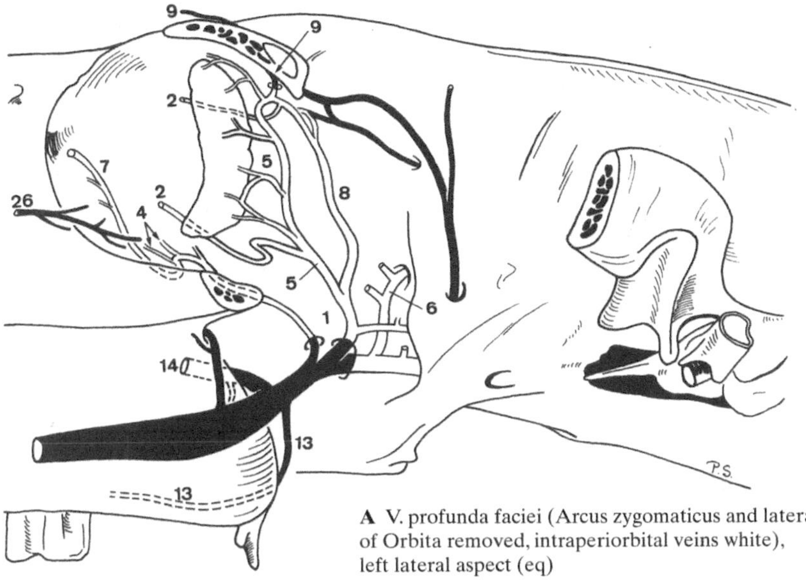

A V. profunda faciei (Arcus zygomaticus and lateral wall of Orbita removed, intraperiorbital veins white), left lateral aspect (eq)

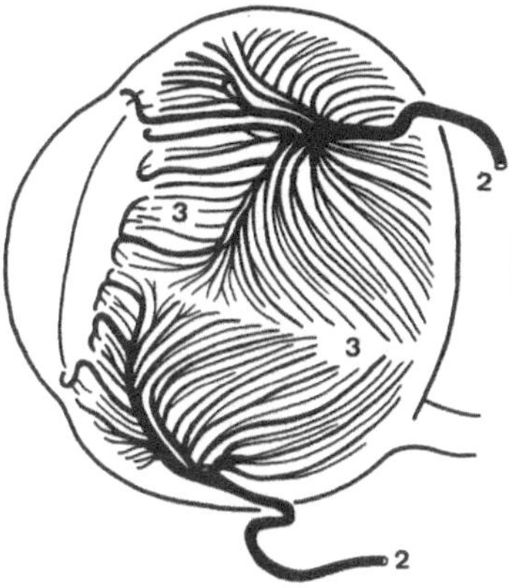

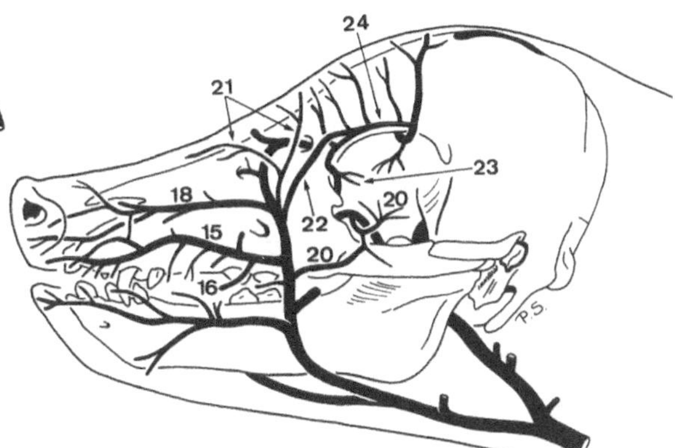

B Veins of the left eyeball, lateral aspect (eq) **C** Veins of the head, left lateral aspect (su, neonate)

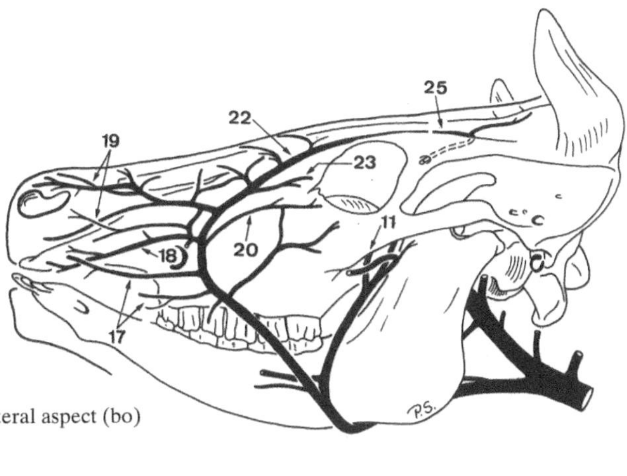

D V. facialis, left lateral aspect (bo)

TERMINUS COMMUNIS

1 **V. maxillaris.** Terminal branch of V. jugularis externa, courses towards the ventral aspect of Articulatio temporomandibularis, continues rostrally along the dorsolateral aspect of Mm. pterygoidei. A B D (The ventral [initial] segment of V. maxillaris is often designated as "V. retromandibularis". This viewpoint of Prof. Barone has frequently been discussed by the Subcommittee of Angiologia, but was never accepted. However, somehow it was apparently approved by W.A.V.A. in Rio de Janeiro, but still it never made it into our list.)

CARNIVORA, SUS

2 ***V. sternocleidomastoidea.*** To Mm. sterno- and cleidocephalicus. May be double in su. B D

3 ***V. glandularis*** (Car). To Gl. mandibularis (ca). B

4 ***V. auricularis caudalis.*** Accompanies corresponding artery. A B D

5 *Rami parotidei.* To Gl. parotis. A B D

6 *V. auricularis lateralis* (ca, su). On Dorsum auriculae along Margo antitragicus. May arise from V. maxillaris or V. temporalis superficialis in su. B D

7 *V. auricularis intermedia.* On the middle of Dorsum auriculae. A B D

8 *V. auricularis profunda* (ca, su). Courses along the surface of M. temporalis. B D

9 **V. stylomastoidea** (ca). Enters Foramen stylomastoideum. B

10 ***V. temporalis superficialis.*** Accompanies corresponding artery. A B D

11 *V. transversa faciei* (ca, su). Courses along the ventral aspect of Arcus zygomaticus. B D

12 **V. palpebralis inferior lateralis** (su). To the lateral part of Palpebra inferior. D

13 *V. auricularis lateralis* (fe). On Dorsum auriculae along Margo antitragicus. A

14 *V. auricularis rostralis.* Courses at the rostral aspect of Auris externa. A B D

15 **V. auricularis medialis.** Along Margo tragicus on Dorsum auriculae. A B D

16 *Ramus anastomoticus cum plexu ophthalmico* (fe). Perforates periorbita, joins Plexus ophthalmicus. A

17 *V. palpebralis superior lateralis* (su). To the lateral segment of Palpebra superior. D

18 ***V. auricularis profunda*** (fe). Runs across the medial aspect of V. temporalis superficialis, turns around the caudal aspect of the base of the ear and ramifies in Mm. auriculares and M. temporalis. A

19 *V. stylomastoidea.* Enters Foramen stylomastoideum. A

20 ***Plexus pterygoideus.*** Confluence of veins at the caudal aspect of Mm. pterygoidei, in continuation of V. maxillaris. A B

21 *V. masseterica.* Reaches M. masseter through Incisura mandibulae. B

22 *Vv. articulares temporomandibulares.* Form a network around Articulatio temporomandibularis. B D

23 *V. palatina* (ca). Into Palatum molle. B

24 **Plexus palatinus.** Network in Palatum molle. B

25 *V. alveolaris inferior.* Courses between M. pterygoideus medialis and Ramus mandibulae, enters Canalis mandibulae. A B

26 *V. buccalis* (Car). To the cheek. Usually given off by V. facialis or V. labialis inferior.

27 *Vv. temporales profundae.* Run at the rostral aspect of Articulatio temporomandibularis into M. temporalis. A

28 *Vv. pterygoideae.* Into Mm. pterygoidei. A B

29 *V. buccalis* (su). Large cheek vein, anastomoses with V. facialis. D

30 *V. infraorbitalis* (fe). Through canalis infraorbitalis. A

31 *Plexus ophthalmicus* (Car). Network in the caudoventral segment of the Orbita. A B

32 **Vv. vorticosae.** Perforate sclera and ramify in the anterior area of choroidea. A C

33 **Vv. ciliares.** Branches of Vv. vorticosae to Corpus ciliare C

34 **Vv. conjuctivales.** To Tunica conjunctiva. C

35 **V. lacrimalis.** To Gl. lacrimalis. A

36 **V. ethmoidalis externa.** Enters Cavum cranii through Foramen ethmoidale. May be double and join V. ophthalmica externa dorsalis in ca. B

37 **V. ophthalmica externa ventralis.** Courses within the ventromedial aspect of Orbita. Double in fe. Connected with V. profunda faciei by a large Ramus anastomoticus. A B C

38 **V. ophthalmica externa dorsalis.** Courses within the dorsomedial aspect of Orbita. Anastomoses with V. angularis oculi and V. ophthalmica externa ventralis. A B C

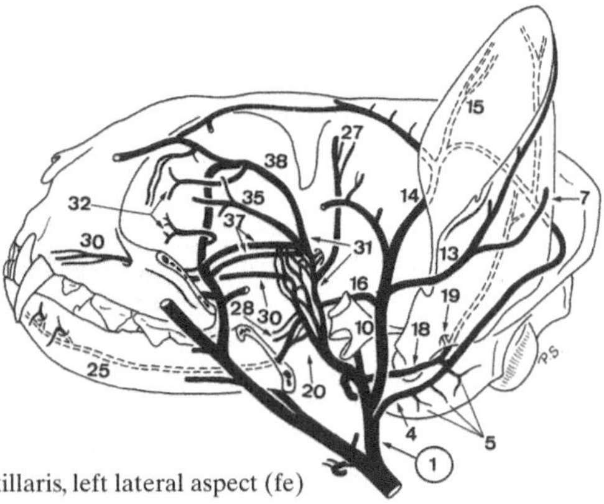

A V. maxillaris, left lateral aspect (fe)

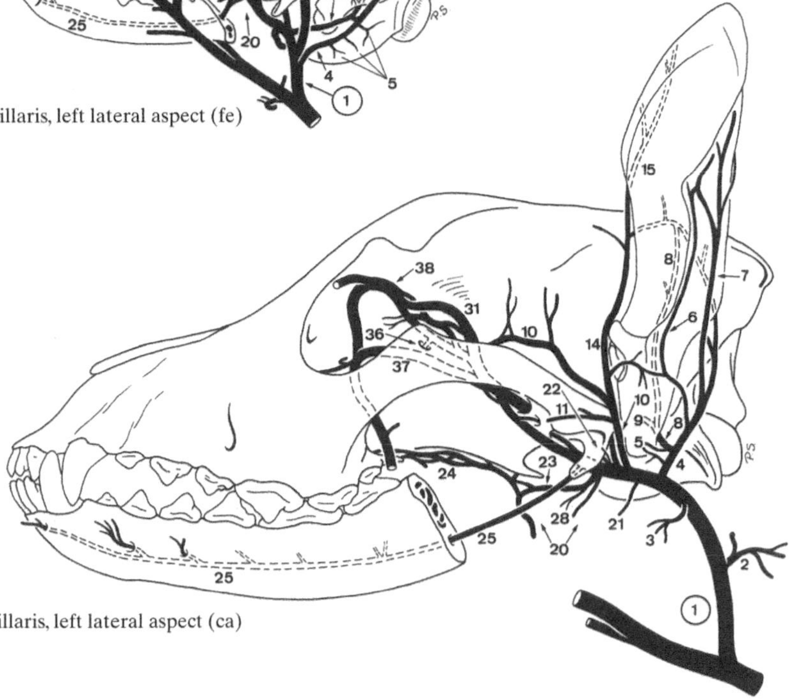

B V. maxillaris, left lateral aspect (ca)

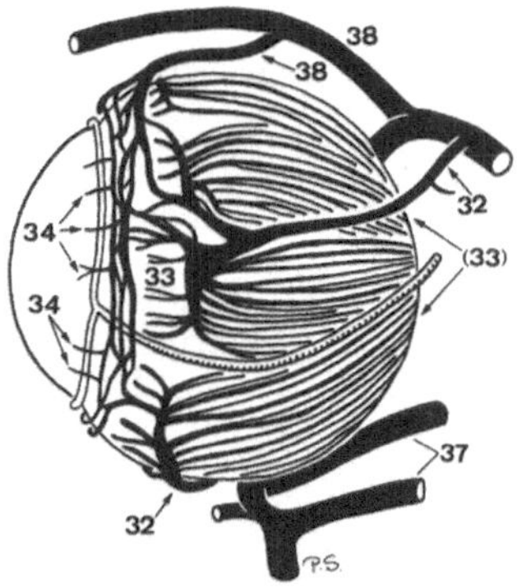

C Veins of the left eyeball, lateral aspect (fe)

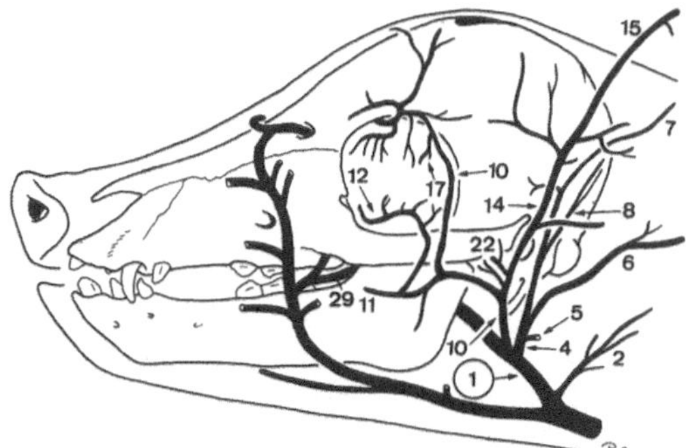

D V. maxillaris, left lateral aspect (su, neonate)

RUMINANTIA

1 *V. auricularis caudalis*. Passes towards the base of the ear. A

2 *Vv. glandulares*. To Gl. parotis (Ru) and Gl. mandibularis (bo). A

3 *V. stylomastoidea*. Enters Foramen stylomastoideum. A

4 *V. auricularis lateralis*. On Dorsum auriculae along Margo antitragicus. A

5 *V. auricularis intermedia*. In the middle of Dorsum auriculae. A

6 *V. auricularis profunda*. Ramifies in muscular branches. A

7 ***V. masseterica ventralis***. Into M. masseter. A B

8 ***V. temporalis superficialis***. Runs across Arcus zygomaticus into M. temporalis. A B

9 *V. auricularis rostralis*. Runs over Cartilago scutiformis to Regio occipitalis. A

10 **V. auricularis medialis**. On Dorsum auriculae along Margo tragicus. A

11 *V. transversa faciei*. Accompanies corresponding artery. A

12 **V. palpebralis inferior lateralis**. To the lateral part of Palpebra inferior. Replaced or accompanied by a branch of V. masseterica (bo). A

13 *V. palpebralis superior lateralis*. Enters Palpebra superior laterally. A

14 *V. cornualis**. Along Linea temporalis to Basis cornus. A

15 *V. ophthalmica externa dorsalis*. Perforates periorbita, continues along the dorsal border of M. rectus lateralis. A B

16 **Plexus ophthalmicus**. Network inside periorbita. B

17 **Vv. vorticosae**. Four veins which arise from Plexus ophthalmicus, perforate sclera, ramify in Choroidea. B C

18 **Vv. ciliares**. Anterior branches of Vv. vorticosae to Corpus ciliare. C

19 **Vv. conjunctivales**. Branches of Plexus ophthalmicus to Tunica conjunctiva.

20 **V. lacrimalis**. Branch of Plexus ophthalmicus to Gl. lacrimalis. B

21 **V. ethmoidalis externa**. Through Foramen ethmoidale, continues through Lamina cribrosa into Cavum nasi. B

22 **V. supraorbitalis**. Branch of Plexus ophthalmicus, traverses Canalis supraorbitalis, anastomoses with V. frontalis. B

23 **V. malaris**. Branch of Plexus ophthalmicus to Angulus oculi medialis. B

24 **V. palpebrae tertiae**. Branch of V. malaris into Palpebra III. Usually plural. B

25 ***Plexus pterygoideus***. Network at the caudolateral aspect of Mm. pterygoidei. B

26 *Vv. palatinae*. To Palatum molle. B

27 **Plexus palatinus**. Network around Tonsilla palatina and in Palatum molle. B

28 *Vv. pharyngeae*. Ramify in the pharyngeal wall. B

29 *V. alveolaris inferior*. Enters Canalis mandibulae. B

30 **V. mentalis**. Emerges from Foramen mentale, ramifies in the chin. A

31 *V. temporalis profunda*. Courses across the rostral aspect of Articulatio temporomandibularis into M. temporalis. B

32 *V. masseterica*. Through Incisura mandibulae into M. masseter. A B

33 *Vv. articulares temporomandibulares*. To Articulatio temporomandibularis. A B

34 *V. buccalis*. Vein to the cheek. B

35 *Vv. pterygoideae*. To Mm. pterygoidei. B

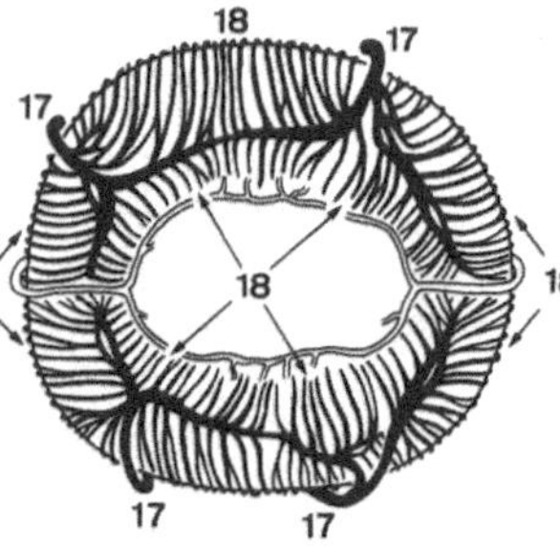

C Veins of the left eyeball, anterior aspect (ov)

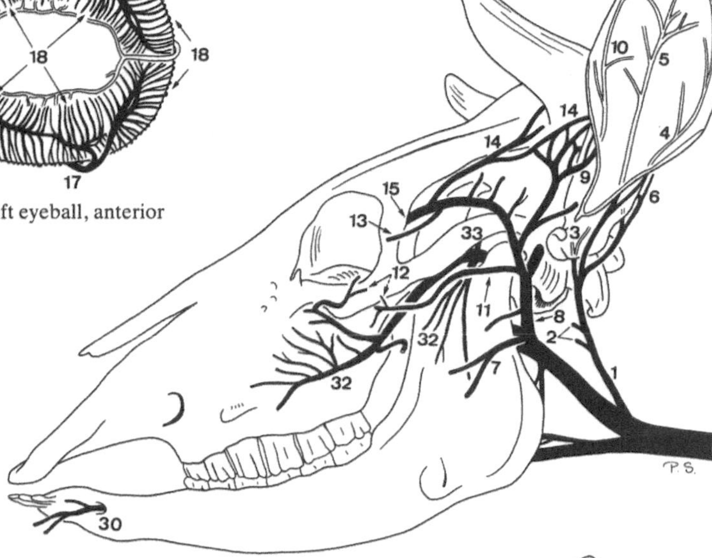

A Veins of the head, left lateral aspect (bo)

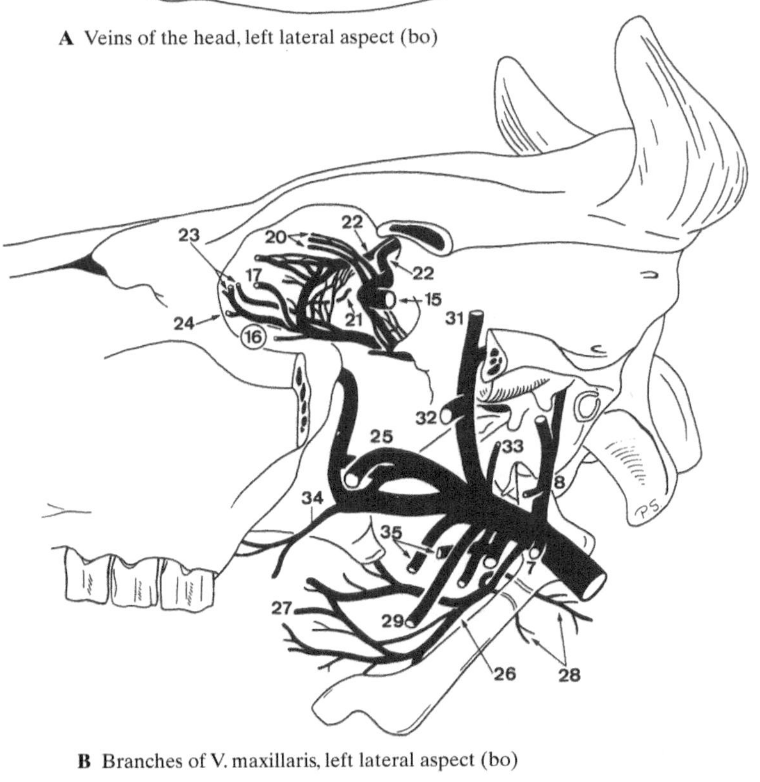

B Branches of V. maxillaris, left lateral aspect (bo)

EQUUS

1 ***V. thyroidea [thyreoidea] cranialis.*** Curves around the cranial pole of Gl. thyroidea. B

2 *(V. thyroidea [thyreoidea] media).* Inconstant, enters the middle segment of Gl. thyroidea. B

3 *V. pharyngea ascendens.* Into the pharyngeal musculature. B

4 **Plexus pharyngeus.** Network around Pharynx. B

5 *V. cricothyroidea [-thyreoidea].* To M. cricothyroideus. B

6 *Ramus laryngeus caudalis.* Enters larynx between Cartilago thyroidea and Cartilago cricoidea and parallels N. laryngeus caudalis. B

7 ***V. occipitalis.*** To Fossa atlantis, receives a Ramus anastomoticus from V. vertebralis, continues along the medial aspect of Processus paracondylaris, joins the extracranial segment of Sinus petrosus ventralis. A

8 *V. stylomastoidea.* To Foramen stylomastoideum.

9 *Ramus occipitalis.* Extends towards Crista nuchae. Usually replaced by a slender branch of V. vertebralis. A

10 ***V. auricularis caudalis.*** To the base of the ear. A B

11 *Rami parotidei.* To Gl. parotis. B

12 *V. auricularis lateralis.* On Dorsum auriculae along Margo antitragicus. B

13 *V. auricularis intermedia.* In the middle of Dorsum auriculae. B

14 *V. auricularis medialis.* On Dorsum auriculae along Margo tragicus. B

15 ***V. masseterica ventralis.*** Into M. masseter. A B

16 ***V. temporalis superficialis.*** Passes between Auris externa and Articulatio temporomandibularis, ramifies in M. temporalis. A B

17 *V. transversa faciei.* Courses along the ventral border of Crista facialis, joins V. facialis. A B

18 **Sinus v. transversae faciei.** Long enlargement of V. transversa faciei. A

19 *V. auricularis rostralis.* To the rostral part of the base of the ear. A B

20 **V. auricularis profunda.** Ramifies into muscular branches. B

21 ***Plexus pterygoideus.*** Network at the caudolateral aspect of Mm. pterygoidei. B

22 *Vv. pharyngeae.* Form a network in the pharyngeal wall. B

23 *Vv. palatinae.* Into Palatum molle. B

24 **Plexus palatinus.** Network in Palatum molle and Palatum durum. B

25 *V. alveolaris inferior.* Into Canalis mandibulae. A B

26 **V. mentalis.** Emerges from Foramen mentale. A

27 *Ramus sublingualis.* Into the tongue. A B

28 *V. temporalis profunda.* Into M. temporalis. B

29 *Vv. articulares temporomandibulares.* To Articulatio temporomandibularis. B

30 *Vv. pterygoideae.* Ramify in Mm. pterygoidei. A B

31 *V. buccalis.* Courses along the medial surface of M. masseter, joins V. facialis. A B

32 **Sinus v. buccalis.** Large spindle-shaped dilatation of V. buccalis. A

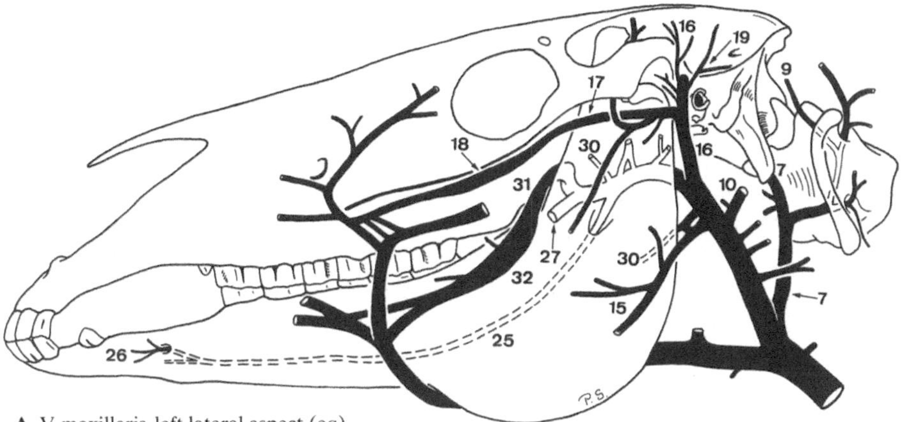

A V. maxillaris, left lateral aspect (eq)

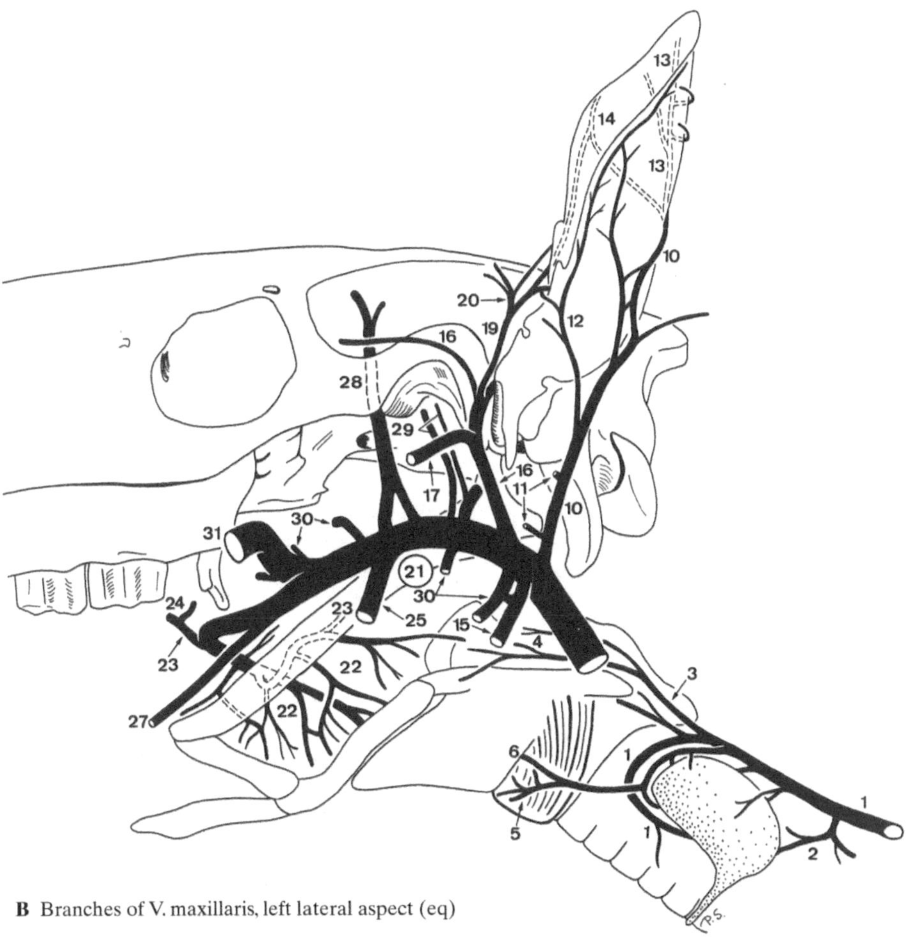

B Branches of V. maxillaris, left lateral aspect (eq)

TERMINI COMMUNES

1 **SINUS DURAE MATRIS.** Channels within dura. Receive blood from Encephalon and Calvaria, drain into Vv. emissariae and Plexus vertebralis internus ventralis.

2 ***Sinus transversus.*** Located within Tentorium cerebelli osseum (Car, eq) s. membranaceum (su, Ru). A B C D

2a ***Sinus communicans.*** Connects the right and left Sinus transversus.

3 ***Sinus temporalis.*** Continuation of Sinus transversus with V. emissaria foraminis retroarticularis in Car, Ru, eq through Meatus temporalis. A B C D

4 ***Sinus sigmoideus.*** Continuation of Sinus transversus with V. emissaria foraminis jugularis in Car, su, Ru along the caudal aspect of Pars petrosa. A B D E

5 ***Confluens sinuum.*** Triangular (eq, often fe), plexiform (su, Ru), or asymmetrical (Car) confluence of sinus. A B C D

6 ***Sinus basilaris.*** Continuation of Plexus vertebralis internus ventralis upon clivus. Contains in bo the Rete mirabile epidurale caudale. A B C D E

7 *Sinus interbasilaris.* Ventral connection of left and right Sinus basilaris. May be complemented dorsally (Car). A B E

8 ***Sinus sagittalis dorsalis.*** In the rim of Falx cerebri along Crista sagittalis interna. A B C D

9 *Lacunae laterales.* Enlargements into which the Vv. cerebri dorsales discharge. A C

10 ***Sinus sagittalis ventralis*** (eq). In the free margin of Falx cerebri. C

11 ***(Sinus sagittalis ventralis)*** (Car). Ventral sagittal sinus.

12 ***Sinus rectus.*** Unpaired continuation of V. cerebri magna inside Falx cerebri. A C

13 ***Sinus petrosus ventralis.*** Caudal extension of Sinus cavernosus, intracranial in Car, leaves Cavum cranii through Foramen lacerum in eq, Fissura petrooccipitalis in Ru. A B C E

14 *Vv. labyrinthi.* Enter Meatus acusticus internus.

15 ***Sinus petrosus dorsalis*** (Car, eq). Courses in Tentorium cerebelli membranaceum along Pars petrosa to Sinus transversus. Described also in Ru. A B C D

16 ***Sinus cavernosus.*** Located at the lateral aspect of hypophysis. Encloses A. carotis interna (Car, eq) or Rete mirabile epidurale rostrale (su, Ru). A B E

17 *Sinus intercavernosi.* Connections between left and right Sinus cavernosi, rostral and caudal to hypophysis. A B E

18 **Vv. diploicae.** Conduct blood from Diploë of Calvaria into Sinus durae matris.

19 ***V. diploica frontalis.*** Ramifies in Diploë of Os frontale, discharges into Sinus sagittalis dorsalis. A

20 ***V. diploica parietalis.*** Ramifies in Os parietale, discharges into Sinus transversus (Ru) or Sinus sagittalis dorsalis. A

21 ***V. diploica occipitalis.*** Ramifies in Os occipitale, discharges in Confluens sinuum or Sinus transversus (ca). A B

22 **Vv. emissariae.** Connections between Sinus durae matris and veins of skull.

23 ***V. emissaria mastoidea*** (ca, bo). Leaves Sinus sigmoideus, perforates through Foramen mastoideum. Joins V. emissaria occipitalis in ca. A B

24 ***V. emissaria occipitalis.*** Leaves Sinus transversus, perforates Os occipitale near Crista nuchae, joins V. emissaria mastoidea in ca. A

25 ***V. emissaria canalis n. hypoglossi.*** Connects Sinus basilaris via Canalis n. hypoglossi with various veins. A C E

26 ***V. emissaria foraminis jugularis.*** Connects Sinus sigmoideus (Car, su, cap) s. Sinus basilaris (ca, su, Ru) through Foramen jugulare with various veins. A E

27 ***V. emissaria foraminis retroarticularis*** (ca, Ru, eq). Connects Sinus temporalis with V. maxillaris (ca, Ru) or V. temporalis superficialis (eq). A C D

28 ***V. emissaria canalis carotici.*** Leaves Sinus petrosus ventralis, emerges at the rostral aspect of Bulla tympanica, joins V. maxillaris in Car. A

29 ***V. emissaria foraminis ovalis.*** Connects Sinus cavernosus through Foramen ovale with V. maxillaris in Car, Ru. B E

30 ***V. emissaria foraminis laceri.*** Connects Sinus cavernosus with V. jugularis interna (su) or extracranial segments of Sinus petrosus ventralis (eq). C

31 ***V. emissaria foraminis rotundi.*** Connects Sinus cavernosus with V. maxillaris or Plexus ophthalmicus in Car. B

32 ***V. emissaria fissurae orbitalis.*** Connects Sinus cavernosus via Fissura orbitalis with Plexus ophthalmicus, in Car, eq. A B C

33 ***V. emissaria foraminis orbitorotundi.*** Connects Sinus cavernosus with Sinus s. Plexus ophthalmicus in su, Ru. E

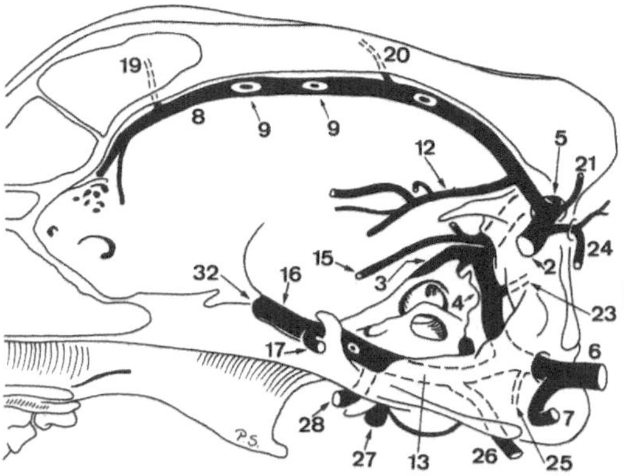

A Sinus durae matris, right medial aspect (ca)

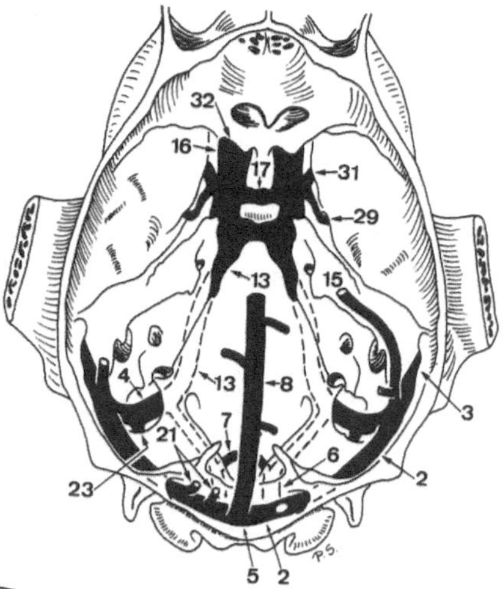

B Sinus durae matris, dorsal aspect (ca)

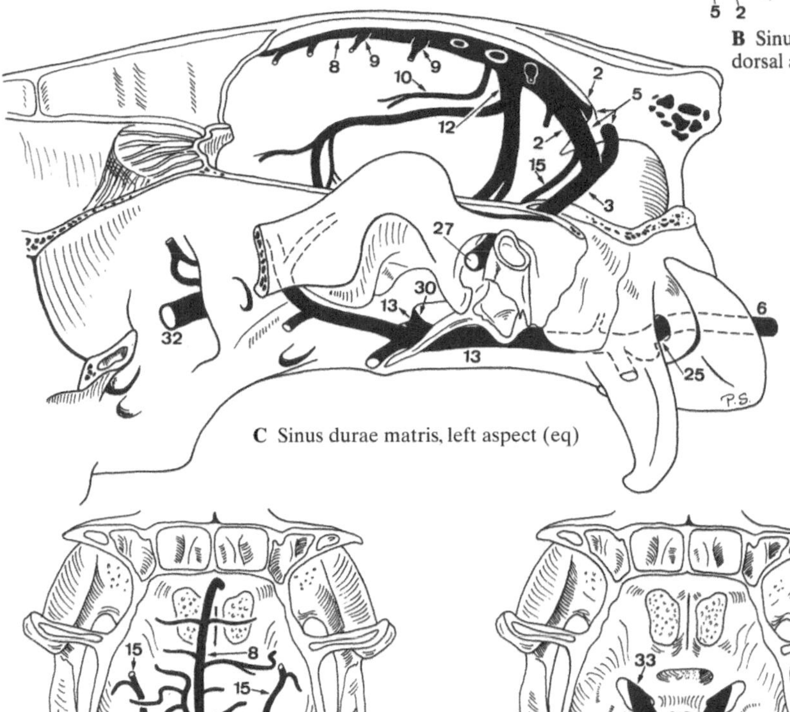

C Sinus durae matris, left aspect (eq)

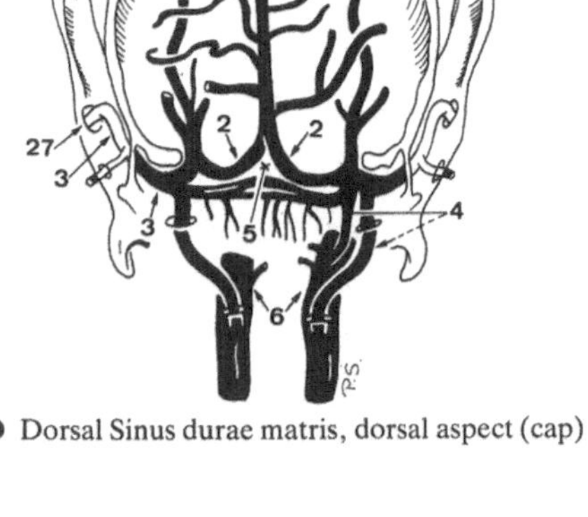

D Dorsal Sinus durae matris, dorsal aspect (cap)

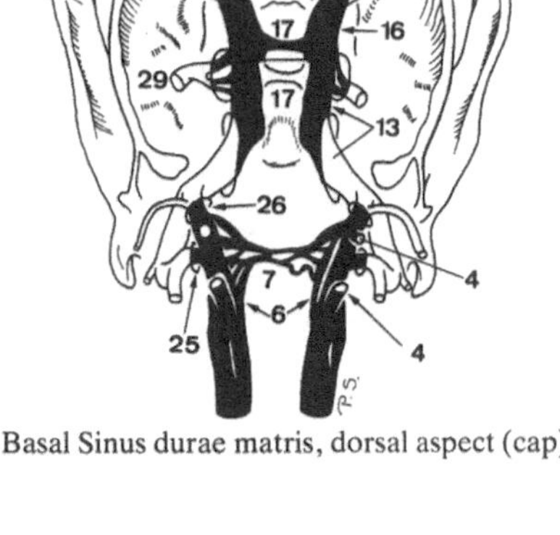

E Basal Sinus durae matris, dorsal aspect (cap)

1 **Vv. cerebri**. Valveless veins of cerebrum. Discharge into Sinus durae matris.

2 ***Vv. cerebri dorsales***. Ramify on Facies convexa and medialis of Hemispheria cerebri. A B C

3 ***Vv. cerebri ventrales***. Ramify on Facies basilaris of Hemispheria cerebri, and Pars basalis rhinencephali. A B C

4 ***V. cerebri magna***. Unpaired trunk formed by left and right Vv. cerebri internae in Tela choroidea ventriculi tertii, continues inside Falx cerebri as Sinus rectus. B D

5 *(V. corporis callosi)*. Unpaired, courses caudally along the dorsal surface of Corpus callosum. B

6 *Vv. cerebri internae*. Bilateral venous trunks in Tela choroidea ventriculi tertii, collect blood from V. choroidea and V. thalamostriata. B D

7 ***V. choroidea [chorioidea]***. Collects blood from Plexus choroideus ventriculi lateralis (et tertii). D

8 **V. thalamostriata**. Curves along the medial border of Nucleus caudatus, drains Corpus striatum and thalamus. D

9 ***Vv. cerebelli dorsales***. Ramify on the dorsal surface of Vermis and Hemispheria cerebelli. A

10 ***Vv. cerebelli ventrales***. Collect blood from the ventral surface of cerebellum and adjacent segments of Rhombencephalon including Plexus choroideus ventriculi quarti. C

11 **V. ophthalmica interna**. Branch of Plexus s. Sinus ophthalmicus along N. opticus, receives Venulae retinae and Vv. ciliares.

12 **V. SUBCLAVIA**. Arises from V. brachiocephalica (Car, su, sometimes cap) or V. cava cranialis (Ru, eq), curves laterally to the cranial border of the first rib. Very short and double in su. G 341A

13 **V. axillaris**. Continuation of V. subclavia beyond the cranial border of Costa I. Courses into axilla. Double in su. E F G 341A

14 ***V. thoracica externa***. Double (bo, sometimes eq) or plural (Car, su) vein, courses into Mm. pectorales. G

15 ***V. thoracica superficialis*** (Ru). Courses over M. serratus ventralis thoracis, continues subcutaneously.

16 ***V. thoracica lateralis*** (Car, su). Courses along the dorsal border of M. pectoralis profundus.

17 ***V. suprascapularis*** (Un). Accompanies corresponding artery. F G

18 ***V. subscapularis***. Accompanies corresponding artery. E F G

19 *V. circumflexa humeri cranialis* (Ru). Accompanies corresponding artery.

20 *V. circumflexa humeri caudalis*. Accompanies corresponding artery. E F G

21 **V. axillobrachialis** (ca). Anastomotic branch between V. circumflexa humeri caudalis (where it originates from), and V. cephalica. Receives V. omobrachialis. E 347 A (V. axillobrachialis is listed in the 5th edition of the N. A. V. under the V. circumflexa humeri caudalis, because of its role to connect the V. cephalica to the V. circumflexa humeri caudalis in the dog only. Therefore, the species designation is necessary, albeit [ca] is not listed in the 5th edition of the N. A. V.)

22 **V. collateralis radialis** (Car, su, cap). Accompanies corresponding artery. Arises from V. circumflexa humeri cranialis, or V. brachialis in su. E F

23 **V. collateralis media**. Accompanies corresponding artery. E F

24 *Ramus suprascapularis* (su). Courses craniodorsally between scapula and M. subscapularis, joins V. suprascapularis. F

25 *V. circumflexa scapulae*. Accompanies corresponding artery. E F G

26 ***V. circumflexa humeri cranialis*** (su). Accompanies corresponding artery. F

27 ***V. thoracodorsalis***. Accompanies corresponding artery. E F G

28 *V. thoracica superficialis* (eq). Courses over M. serratus ventralis thoracis, drains the lateral thoracic wall. G

29 **V. epigastrica cranialis superficialis [V. subcutanea abdominis]**. Subcutaneous continuation of V. thoracica superficialis, towards Regio inguinalis. It anastomoses by inosculation (see 306.15) with the V. epigastrica caudalis superficialis. G

30 ***V. circumflexa humeri cranialis*** (Car, eq). Accompanies corresponding artery. G

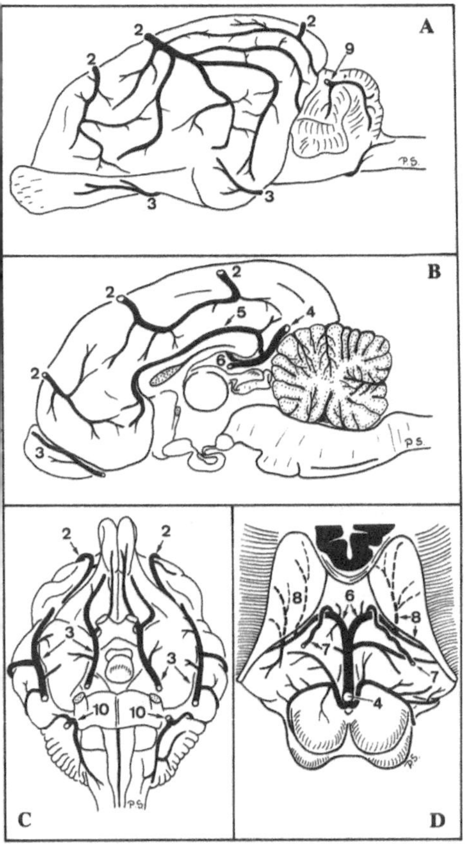

A Veins of the brain, left lateral aspect (ca)
B Veins of the brain (median section), right lateral aspect (ca)
C Veins of the brain, ventral aspect (fe)
D Veins of Nucleus caudatus, Thalamus, and Tectum mesencephali, dorsal aspect (bo)

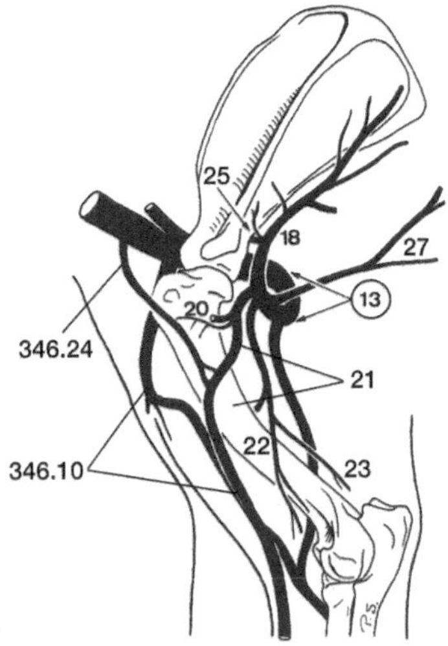

E Veins of left thoracic limb, lateral aspect (ca)

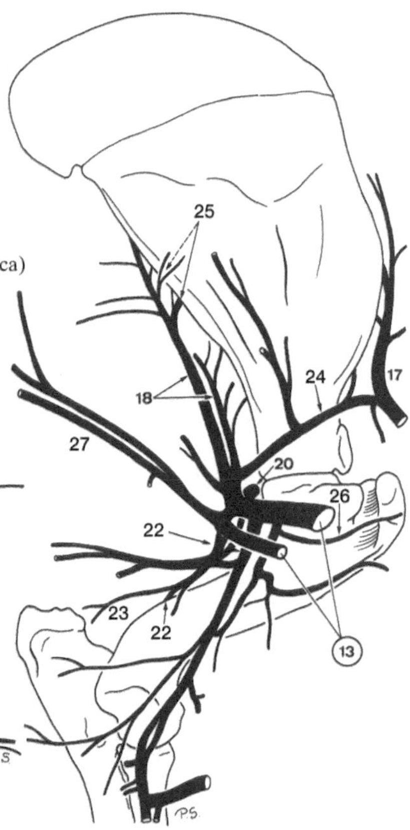

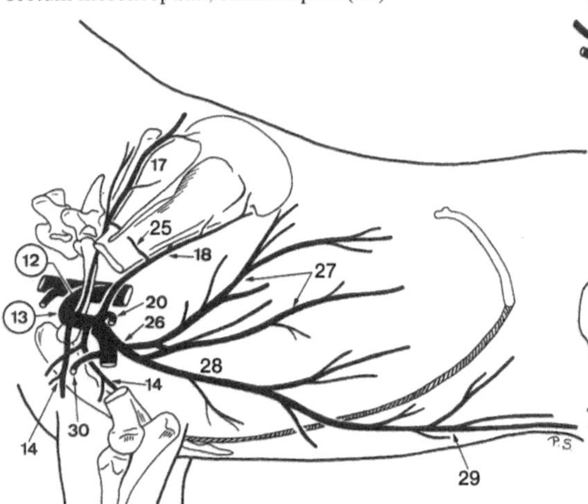

G V. subclavia, left lateral aspect (eq)

F Veins of left thoracic limb, medial aspect (su)

1 **V. brachialis.** Continuation of V. axillaris. Accompanies corresponding artery. Double in su. A C E

CARNIVORA, SUS

2 ***V. profunda brachii.*** Accompanies corresponding artery. A

3 ***V. bicipitalis*** (ca, su). Accompanies corresponding artery. A

4 ***V. collateralis ulnaris.*** Ramifies at olecranon, sends a branch distally anastomosing with V. ulnaris (ca) or V. interossea caudalis (su). Double in su. A C

5 ***V. brachialis superficialis*** (Car). Accompanies corresponding artery. A

6 *V. bicipitalis* (fe). Enters M. biceps brachii. C

7 *Vv. radiales superficiales.* Accompany corresponding arteries. A

8 ***V. transversa cubiti.*** Accompanies corresponding artery. A C

9 ***V. interossea communis*** (ca, su). Accompanies corresponding artery. A

10 *V. ulnaris* (ca). Accompanies corresponding artery. Joins the palmar branch of V. interossea caudalis. A

11 **V. recurrens ulnaris.** Accompanies corresponding artery. Joins V. collateralis ulnaris. A

12 *V. interossea cranialis.* Accompanies corresponding artery. B

13 **V. recurrens interossea.** Accompanies corresponding artery. B

14 *V. interossea caudalis.* Accompanies corresponding artery. Double in su. A

15 **Ramus interosseus.** Accompanies corresponding artery. A

16 **Ramus palmaris.** Accompanies corresponding artery. A

17 **Ramus superficialis.** Accompanies corresponding artery. A

18 **Ramus profundus.** Accompanies corresponding artery. A

19 ***V. interossea cranialis*** (fe). Accompanies corresponding artery. C

20 *V. recurrens interossea.* Accompanies corresponding artery.

21 ***V. interossea caudalis*** (fe). Accompanies corresponding artery. C D

22 *V. ulnaris.* Accompanies corresponding artery. Joins Ramus palmaris of V. interossea caudalis. C D

23 **Ramus dorsalis.** Courses to the dorsolateral side of carpus. D

24 *Ramus interosseus.* Accompanies corresponding artery. D

25 *Ramus palmaris.* Accompanies corresponding artery. D

26 **Ramus superficialis.** Courses at the lateropalmar aspect of metacarpus, joins Arcus palmaris superficialis. D

27 **V. digitalis palmaris V abaxialis.** Continuation of Ramus superficialis of Ramus palmaris of V. interossea caudalis. D

28 **Ramus profundus.** Accompanies corresponding artery. D

RUMINANTIA, EQUUS

29 ***V. profunda brachii.*** Accompanies corresponding artery. E

30 *V. collateralis radialis* (bo, ov, eq). Accompanies corresponding artery. E

31 **V. collateralis media.** Courses caudodistally towards Articulatio cubiti. E

32 ***V. bicipitalis*** (eq). To M. biceps brachii.

33 ***V. collateralis ulnaris.*** Accompanies corresponding artery. A small branch joins the palmar continuation of V. interossea cranialis (Ru) s. Ramus palmaris of V. mediana (eq). E

34 ***V. transversa cubiti.*** Accompanies corresponding artery. E

35 *V. bicipitalis* (Ru). Accompanies corresponding artery. E

36 ***V. interossea communis.*** Accompanies corresponding artery. Double in bo, ov, and sometimes cap. E

37 *V. recurrens ulnaris* (bo). Courses proximally along the medial surface of olecranon, joins V. collateralis ulnaris. E

38 *V. interossea caudalis.* Very slender or absent. E

39 *V. interossea cranialis.* Accompanies corresponding artery. E

40 **V. recurrens interossea.** Accompanies corresponding artery.

41 **Ramus interosseus** (Ru). Accompanies corresponding artery. E

42 **Ramus palmaris.** Accompanies corresponding artery. 371 A

43 **Ramus superficialis.** Inconstant. 371 A

44 **Ramus profundus.** To Arcus palmaris profundus. 371 A

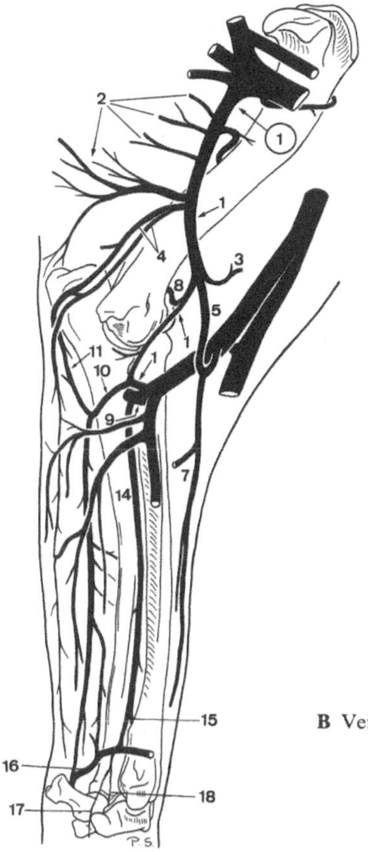

A Veins of left thoracic limb, medial aspect (ca)

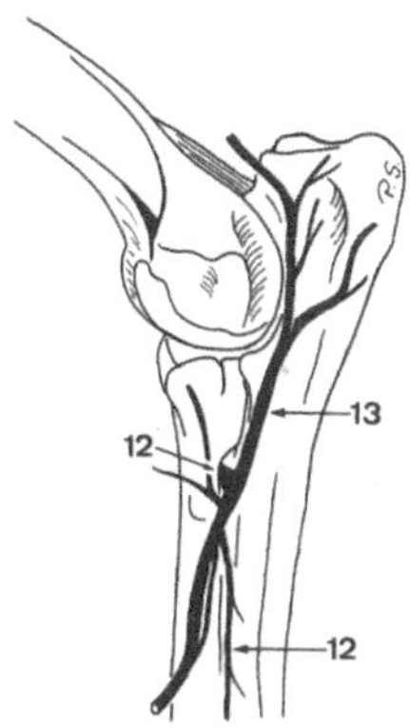

B Veins of left elbow, lateral aspect (ca)

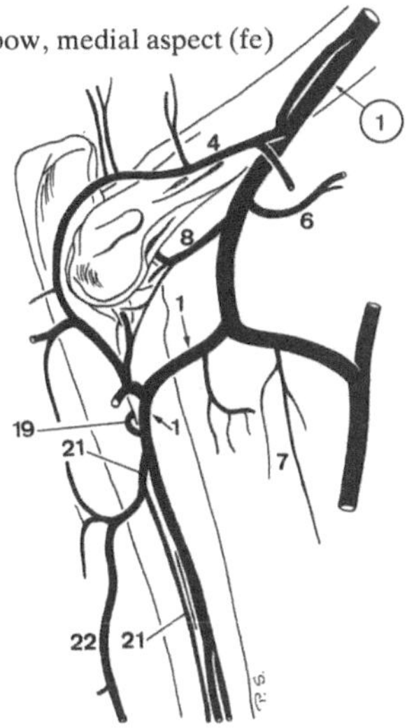

C Veins of left elbow, medial aspect (fe)

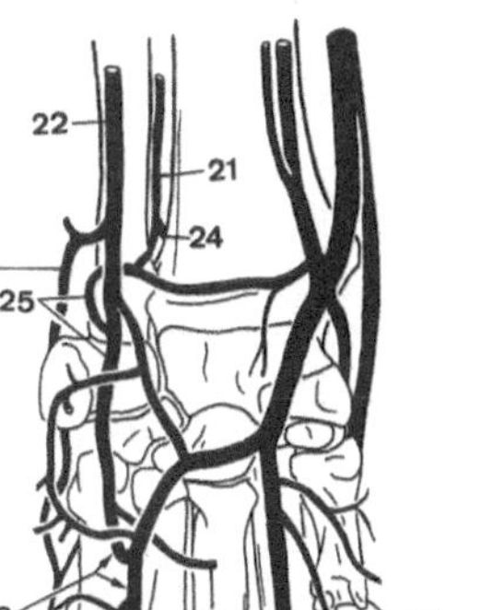

D Veins of left manus, palmar aspect (fe)

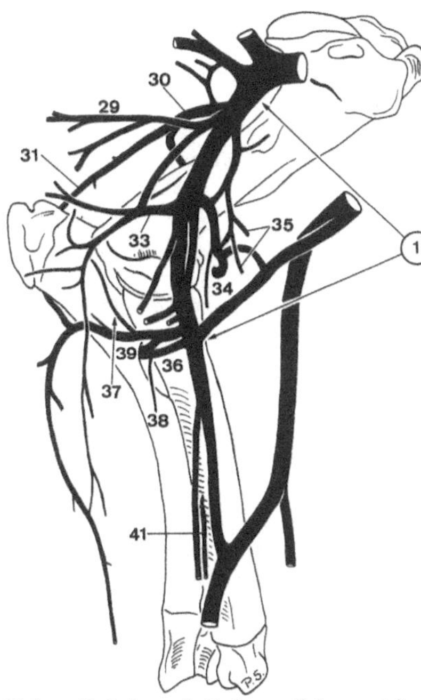

E Veins of left thoracic limb, medial aspect (bo)

TERMINUS COMMUNIS

1 **V. mediana**. Accompanies corresponding artery. A C

CARNIVORA

2 ***V. profunda antebrachii***. Accompanies corresponding artery.

3 ***V. radialis***. Courses along the caudomedial border of radius, receives V. cephalica, continues superficially over the mediopalmar surface of carpus. Double in fe. Forms the major continuation of V. mediana in fe. A

4 *Ramus carpeus dorsalis*. Accompanies corresponding artery. Plural in ca. A B

5 **Rete carpi dorsale**. Network on the dorsal aspect of carpus. Mainly supplied by branches of V. radialis, Vv. interosseae cranialis and caudalis, and V. cephalica accessoria. B

6 **Vv. metacarpeae dorsales I–IV**. Accompany corresponding arteries. Join V. digitalis propria I axialis s. V. digitalis dorsalis communis (II – IV) (ca). B

7 *Arcus palmaris profundus*. Lies across the palmar aspect of Ossa metacarpalia. Reinforced by Ramus carpeus dorsalis of V. radialis in fe. A

8 **Vv. metacarpeae palmares I–IV**. Accompany corresponding arteries. A

9 *Arcus palmaris superficialis*. Usually double, across the palmar aspect of the flexor tendons at Torus metacarpeus. A complementary superficial (fe) s. intermediate (ca) arch in the proximal half of metacarpus, receives V. mediana in ca. A

10 **Vv. digitales palmares communes I–IV**. May be absent, as their Vv. digitales palmares propriae may arise directly from Arcus palmaris superficialis. A

11 **V. interdigitalis**. Accompanies corresponding artery. A

12 **Vv. digitales palmares propriae**. Accompany corresponding arteries. A

SUS

13 ***V. radialis***. Accompanies corresponding artery. C D

14 *Arcus palmaris profundus*. Lies between Ossa metacarpalia and Mm. interossei. C

15 **Vv. metacarpeae palmares II–IV**. Accompany corresponding arteries. End in the distal half of metacarpus by a transverse anastomosis which joins Arcus palmaris superficialis. C

16 **Ramus perforans proximalis**. Branch of V. metacarpea palmaris, pierces through the proximal half of the Spatium interosseum metacarpi. C D

17 **V. metacarpea dorsalis**. Slender continuation of Ramus perforans proximalis. Joins V. digitalis dorsalis communis. D

18 *Arcus palmaris superficialis*. Connection between V. radialis and Ramus superficialis of Ramus palmaris of V. interossea caudalis across the palmar aspect of the flexor tendons. C D

19 **Vv. digitales palmares communes II–IV**. Accompany corresponding arteries. C

20 **Rami palmares phalangium proximalium**. Transverse branches of each V. digitalis palmaris communis and/or propria across the palmar surface of the corresponding Phalanx proximalis. C D

21 **V. interdigitalis**. Branch of V. digitalis palmaris communis to the corresponding V. digitalis dorsalis communis or propria. C D

22 **Rami dorsales phalangium proximalium**. Branches of V. interdigitalis (II, III, IV) which ramify on the adjacent dorsal aspect of Phalanges proximales. D

23 **Vv. digitales palmares propriae**. Three pairs of veins, arisen by the bifurcation of Vv. digitales palmares communes. Vv. digitales palmares propriae III and IV abaxiales originate from the corresponding Vv. digitales dorsales propriae. C D

24 **Plexus ungularis**. Around Facies parietalis phalangis distalis. This network extends also on the solear surface. The plexus is defined as the dense venous network in Dermis ungulae.

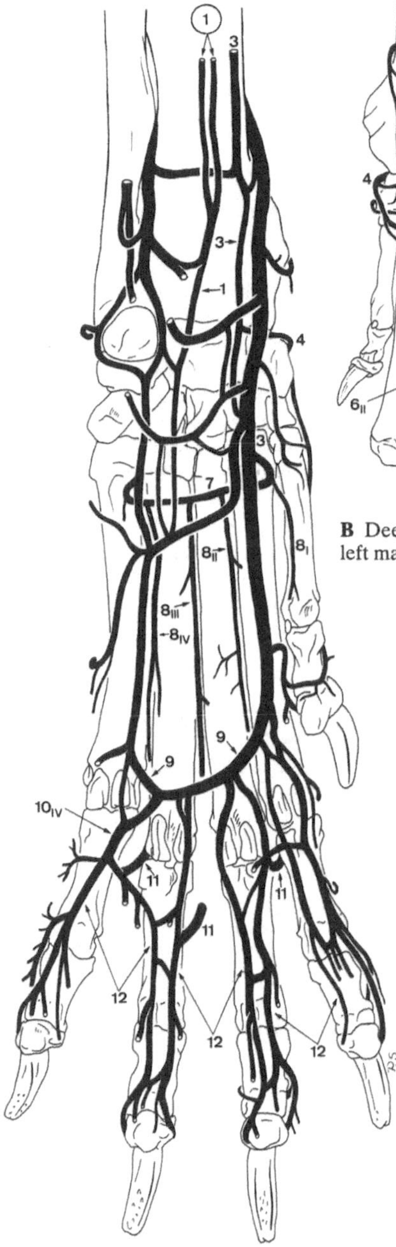

A Veins of left manus, palmar aspect (ca)

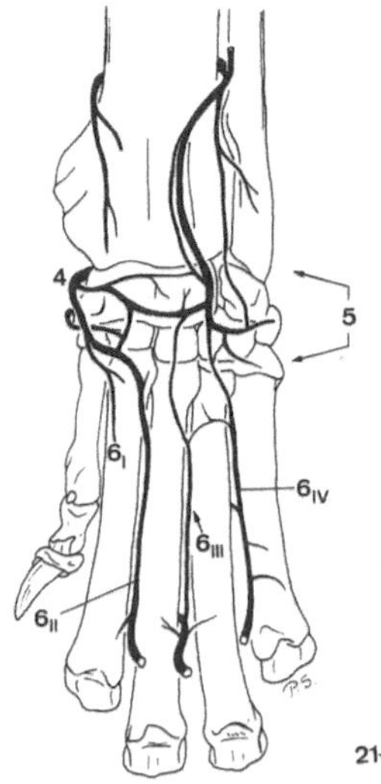

B Deep dorsal veins of the left manus (ca)

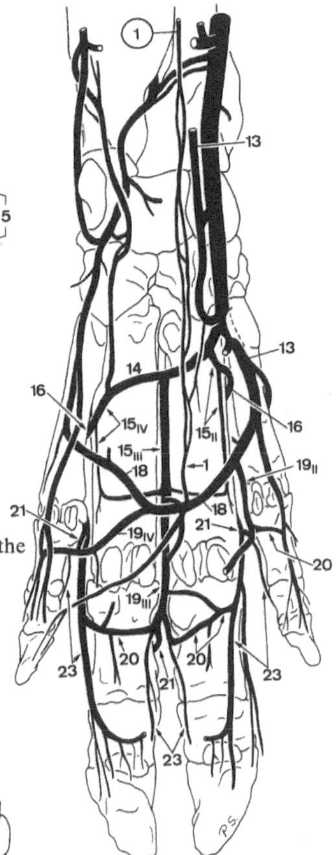

C Veins of left manus, palmar aspect (su)

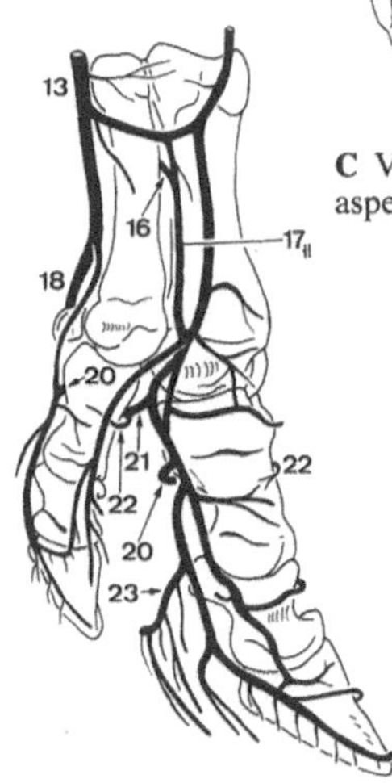

D Veins of left manus, medial aspect (su)

RUMINANTIA

1 ***V. profunda antebrachii***. Accompanies corresponding artery.

2 ***V. radialis***. Accompanies corresponding artery. A

3 *Ramus superficialis*. Variable superficial branch, joins V. mediana in the middle third of metacarpus (bo, sometimes cap). A

4 *Ramus carpeus dorsalis*. Accompanies corresponding artery. A B

5 **Rete carpi dorsale**. Network on the dorsal aspect of carpus. B

6 **V. metacarpea dorsalis III**. Inconstant branch of Rete carpi dorsale, accompanies corresponding artery. B

7 *Arcus palmaris profundus*. Connection between V. radialis and Ramus palmaris of V. interossea cranialis. A

8 **Vv. metacarpeae palmares II–IV**. Accompany corresponding arteries. Generally, V. metacarpea palmaris II, the continuation of V. radialis, is prominent. A

9 **Arcus palmaris profundus distalis**. Distal connection of Vv. metacarpeae palmares II–IV deep to M. interosseus. A

10 **Ramus perforans distalis III**. Branch of Arcus palmaris profundus distalis through Canalis metacarpi distalis, joins V. metacarpea dorsalis III (bo). A

11 **V. digitalis palmaris communis II**. Superficial branch of Arcus palmaris profundus distalis. A

12 **V. digitalis palmaris propria II axialis**. To the medial dew claw. A

13 **V. digitalis palmaris propria III abaxialis**. Continuation of V. digitalis palmaris communis II. A

14 **V. digitalis palmaris communis IV**. Superficial branch of Arcus palmaris profundus distalis. A

15 **V. digitalis palmaris propria IV abaxialis**. Continuation of V. digitalis palmaris communis IV. A

16 **V. digitalis palmaris propria V axialis**. To the lateral dew claw. A

17 ***V. digitalis palmaris communis III***. Continuation of V. mediana distal to the connection with V. digitalis palmaris communis II (Ru) s. IV (ov, cap). Double in bo. A

18 *V. interdigitalis*. Accompanies corresponding artery, joins V. digitalis dorsalis communis III (bo), arises in ov from Vv. digitales palmares propriae III or IV axiales and is double. A

19 *Vv. digitales palmares propriae III et IV axiales*. Accompany corresponding arteries. A

20 **V. coronalis**. Superficial connection of Vv. digitales palmares propriae axialis and abaxialis in the Corona ungulae. A

EQUUS

21 ***Ramus palmaris***. Accompanies corresponding artery. C

22 *Ramus superficialis [V. digitalis palmaris communis III]*. Runs along the lateral surface of the deep digital flexor tendon. C

23 **V. digitalis [palmaris propria III] lateralis**. Continuation of Ramus superficialis of Ramus palmaris of V. mediana distal to Arcus palmaris profundus distalis. Accompanies corresponding artery dorsally. C

24 **V. coronalis**. Superficial branch of V. digitalis lateralis, curves dorsally, proximal to Corona ungulae. Its distal branches form the network in the corium of the hoof (Plexus ungularis). C

25 **Arcus terminalis**. Accompanies corresponding artery. C

26 *Ramus profundus*. Accompanies corresponding artery. C

27 ***V. radialis***. Receives V. cephalica, accompanies corresponding artery. C (There is an innominate palmar carpal branch of V. radialis, which connects the Ramus palmaris v. medianae with V. radialis, and is highly significant in the Proximal check ligament desmotomy.)

28 *Arcus palmaris profundus*. Accompanies corresponding artery. C

29 **Vv. metacarpeae palmares II et III**. Accompany corresponding arteries. Pierce between the branches of M. interosseus medius, join Arcus palmaris profundus distalis. C

30 **Arcus palmaris profundus distalis**. Connection between Ramus superficialis of Ramus palmaris of V. mediana and Ramus palmaris superficialis of V. radialis in the distal third of metacarpus, between M. interosseus medius and the deep digital flexor tendon. C

31 *Ramus palmaris superficialis [V. digitalis palmaris communis II]*. Accompanies corresponding artery. C

32 **V. digitalis [palmaris propria III] medialis**. Continuation of Ramus palmaris superficialis of V. radialis distal to Arcus palmaris profundus distalis. Accompanies corresponding artery dorsally. C D

33 **V. coronalis**. Superficial branch of V. digitalis medialis, curves dorsally, proximal to Corona ungulae. Its distal branches form the network in the corium of the hoof. C D

34 **Plexus ungularis**. Around Facies parietalis phalangis distalis. This network extends also on the solear surface. The plexus is defined as the dense venous network in Dermis ungulae. D

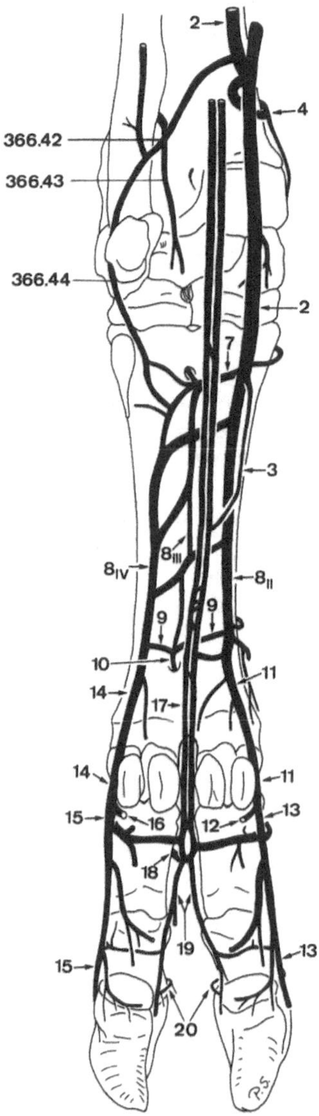

A Veins of left thoracic limb, palmar aspect (bo)

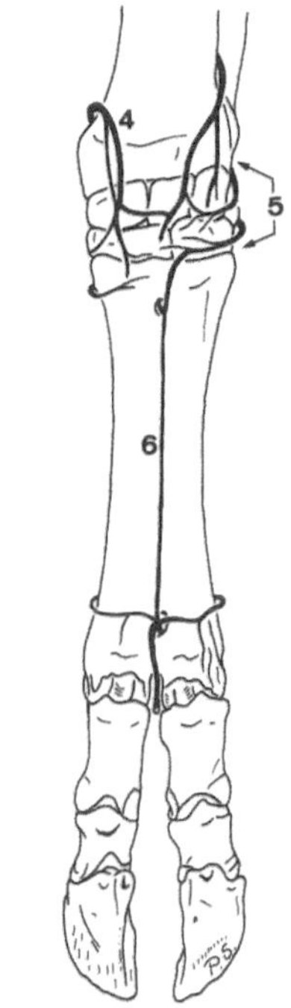

B Veins of left manus, dorsal aspect (bo)

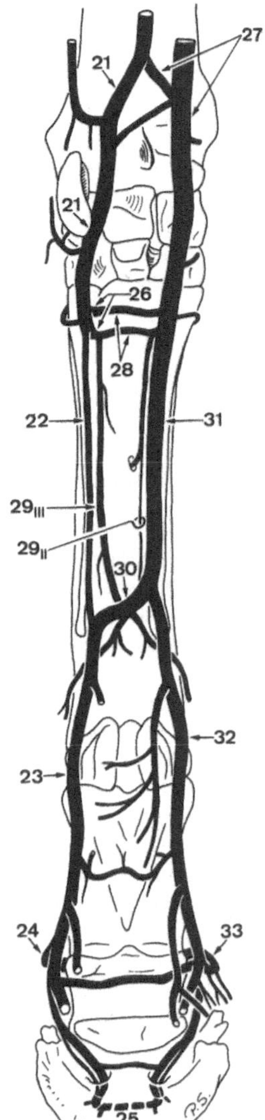

C Veins of left thoracic limb, palmar aspect (eq)

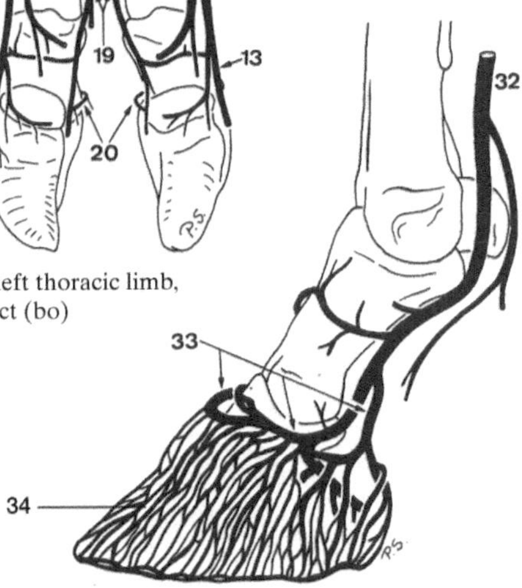

D Veins of right digit, medial aspect (eq)

TERMINI COMMUNES

1 **VENA CAVA CAUDALIS.** Leaves Sinus venarum cavarum of Atrium dextrum, courses in Plica venae cavae and pierces through Foramen venae cavae of Diaphragma into Cavum abdominis, courses along Sulcus venae cavae of the liver and continues at the right side of Aorta abdominalis. A B F

2 ***Vv. phrenicae craniales.*** Left and right, course laterally in Centrum tendineum towards Partes (lumbalis, costalis, and sternalis) of Diaphragma. A

3 ***V. phrenica caudalis.*** Bilateral, arises with V. abdominalis cranialis (Car) or from V. azygos sinistra (su). A

4 *Rami adrenales [supra-] craniales* (Car). Into Gl. adrenalis. A

5 ***V. abdominalis cranialis.*** Bilateral, arises with V. phrenica caudalis (Car) from V. cava caudalis (or, su: right side) s. V. renalis sinistra (or, su: left side), ramifies in the craniolateral abdominal wall. Double in su. A

6 ***Vv. lumbales.*** Often initially fused, segmental, accompany corresponding arteries. B

7 *Ramus dorsalis.* To Plexus vertebralis externus dorsalis. B

8 **V. intervertebralis.** Through Foramen intervertebrale, connects Plexus vertebrales externi and internus. B

9 ***V. circumflexa ilium profunda*** (Car). Accompanies corresponding artery. A

10 ***Vv. hepaticae.*** Intrahepatic, join V. cava caudalis in Sulcus venae cavae of the liver.

11 *V. hepatica dextra.* In the right part of the liver. A

12 *V. hepatica media.* In the central segments, esp. Lobus quadratus, of the liver. A

13 *V. hepatica sinistra.* In the left part of the liver. A

14 ***V. renalis.*** To the Hilus renalis, the left vein crosses Aorta abdominalis ventrally. A B

15 *Ramus adrenalis [supra-] caudalis* (Ru, eq). To Gl. adrenalis. B

16 *V. testicularis sinistra* (Car). Accompanies corresponding artery. C

17 **Plexus pampiniformis.** Network around A. testicularis. C

18 *V. ovarica sinistra* (Car). Accompanies corresponding artery. A

19 ***Vv. adrenales [supra-]*** (bo, eq). To Gl. adrenalis. B

20 ***V. testicularis dextra.*** Accompanies corresponding artery. D F

21 *V. vesicalis cranialis* (cap). In Ligamentum vesicae laterale to Vesica urinaria. F

22 *Plexus pampiniformis.* Network around A. testicularis. D

23 ***V. testicularis sinistra*** (su, cap, eq). Accompanies corresponding artery. B E F

24 *V. vesicalis cranialis* (cap). In Ligamentum vesicae laterale to Vesica urinaria. F

25 *Plexus pampiniformis.* Network around A. testicularis. E

26 ***V. ovarica dextra.*** Accompanies corresponding artery. A

27 *V. uterina* (su). Main vein of the uterus. 389 B

28 **V. vesicalis cranialis.** To Vesica urinaria. 389 B

29 *V. vesicalis cranialis* (cap). To Vesica urinaria.

30 ***V. ovarica sinistra*** (su, ov, eq). Courses in Mesovarium to the right Ovarium, Tuba uterina and Cornu uteri. B

31 *V. uterina* (su). See 27

32 **V. vesicalis cranialis.** See 28

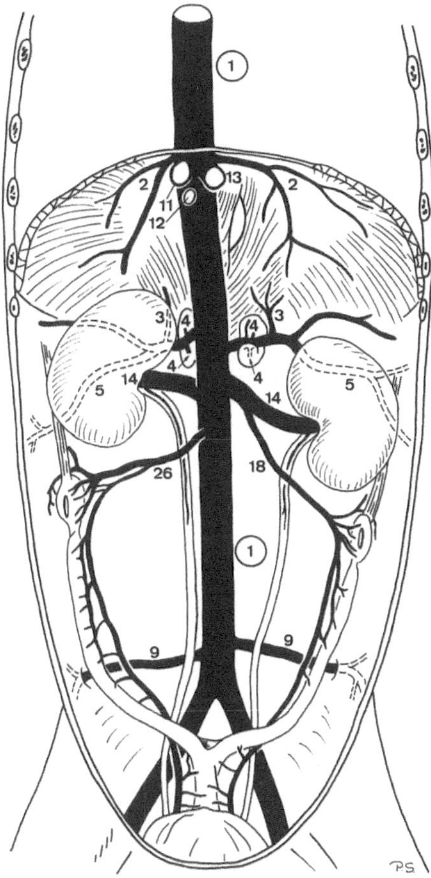

A V. cava caudalis, ventral aspect (ca fem)

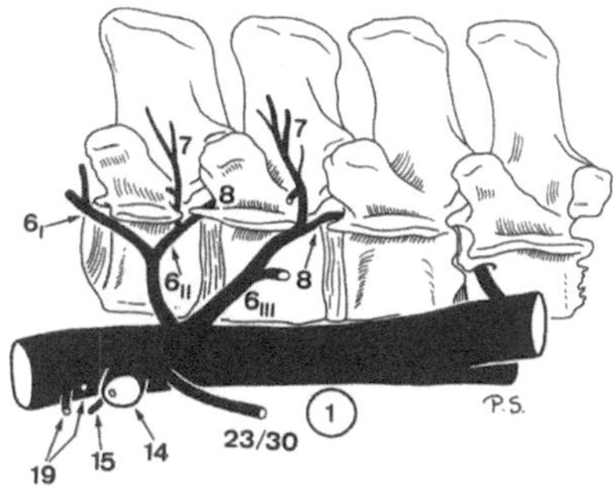

B Veins in relation to Vertebrae lumbales II–V, left lateral aspect (eq)

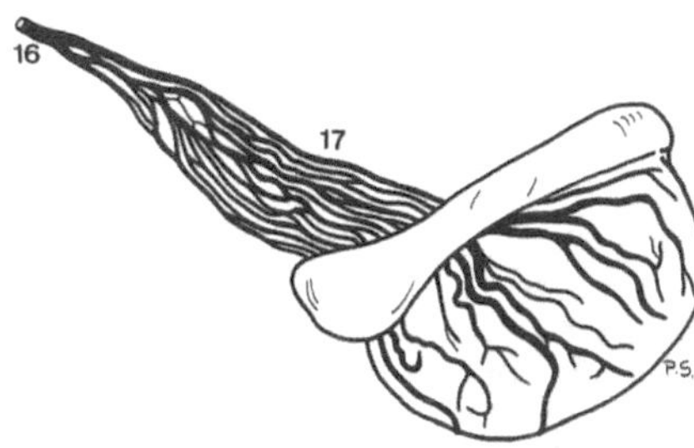

C Veins of the left testis, lateral aspect (ca)

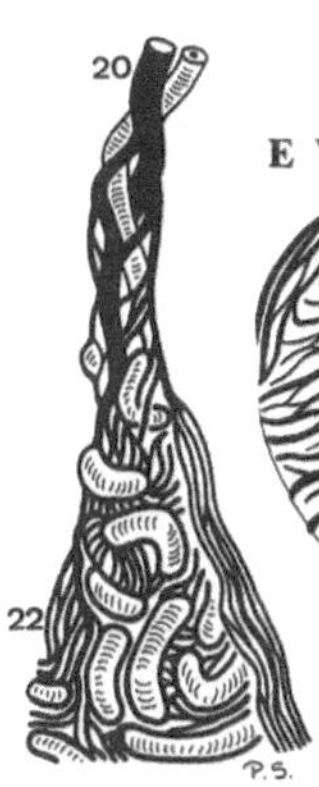

D Right Plexus pampiniformis, lateral aspect (bo)

E Veins of left testis, medial aspect (su)

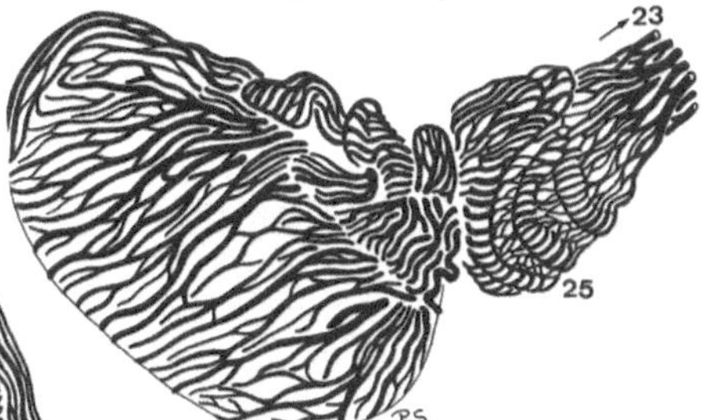

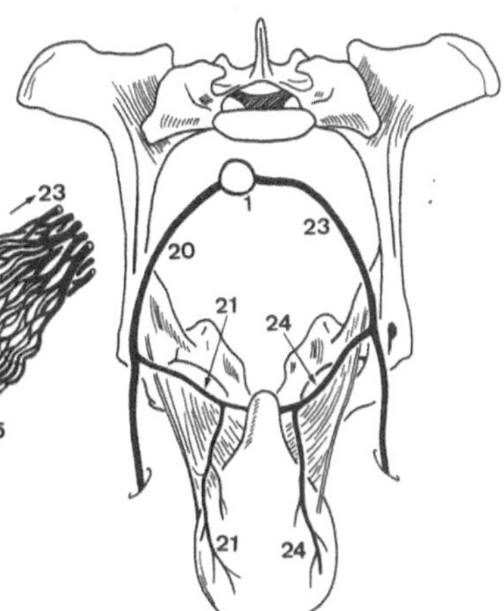

F Veins of pelvis and urinary bladder, cranial aspect (cap masc)

1 **V. PORTAE**. Unpaired vein, transports blood from the gastrointestinal tract (except the caudal segment of the rectum and the anal canal), the pancreas, and the spleen into the liver. Extends from Porta hepatis in the Omentum minus, pierces through Incisura (Car, Ru) s. Anulus (su, eq) pancreatis to the right surface of A. mesenterica cranialis. A B C

2 ***Ramus dexter***. In Lobus hepatis dexter (lateralis) and Processus caudatus. A

3 ***Ramus sinister***. In the left and central hepatic segments, including Lobus hepatis dexter medialis (Car, su, eq) s. the central segment of Lobus hepatis dexter (Ru). A

4 *Pars transversa*. Initial segment of Ramus sinister, coursing transversely to the left (Car, su, eq) s. ventrally (Ru) in Porta hepatis. A

5 *Pars umbilicalis*. Sagittal (Car, su, eq) s. transversal (Ru) continuation of Ramus sinister in Lobus hepatis sinister (medialis) towards Fissura lig. teretis. Derived from the intrahepatic segment of V. umbilicalis. A

6 **Ductus venosus** (ont) [1)]. Intrahepatic shunt connecting V. umbilicalis with V. cava caudalis. Perinatally still present in Car and Ru.

7 **V. umbilicalis** (ont) [1)]. Unpaired, conveys blood from the Placenta via Funiculus umbilicalis (where it is paired in Car and Ru), into the liver. Discharges into V. cava caudalis via Ductus venosus or via the hepatic portal venous system.

8 **Ligamentum teres hepatis**. Fibrous remnant of V. umbilicalis in Ligamentum falciforme hepatis. C

9 ***Vv. cysticae***. Drain the wall of Vesica fellea (and adjacent hepatic segments). A

10 ***V. gastrica dextra*** (ca). Accompanies corresponding artery. A

11 ***V. gastrica sinistra parietalis*** (eq). To Facies parietalis of the stomach. C

12 ***Rami pancreatici*** (eq). Into pancreas. C

13 **V. gastroduodenalis**. Unpaired affluent to V. portae, except in bo, where it joins one of its intrahepatic rami. Courses towards Flexura duodeni cranialis. A B C

14 ***V. gastrica dextra*** (fe, Un). Accompanies corresponding artery. B C

15 ***V. gastroepiploica dextra***. Accompanies corresponding artery. A B C

16 ***V. pancreaticoduodenalis cranialis***. Accompanies corresponding artery. A B C

17 **V. lienalis**. Unpaired affluent to V. portae. Accompanies corresponding artery. A B C

CARNIVORA, SUS, EQUUS

18 ***Vv. pancreaticae***. Accompany corresponding arteries. A B C

19 ***V. gastrica sinistra*** (Car, su). Accompanies corresponding artery. A B

20 *Vv. diverticuli* (su). Ramify at Diverticulum ventriculi. B

21 ***V. gastrica sinistra visceralis*** (eq). To Facies visceralis of the stomach. C

22 *Rami pancreatici*. Drain Lobus pancreatis sinister. C

23 ***Vv. gastricae breves***. Accompany corresponding arteries. A B C

24 ***V. gastroepiploica sinistra***. Accompanies corresponding artery. A B C

1) These structures were omitted from the 5th edition of the N. A. V., because they are ontogenetic terms.

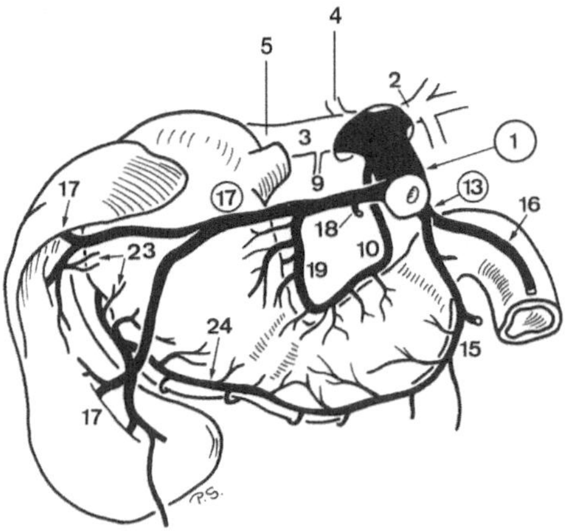

A Veins of stomach and spleen, caudal aspect (ca)

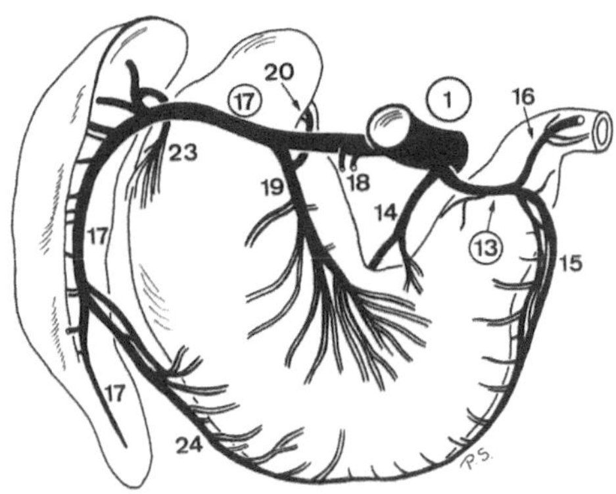

B Veins of stomach and spleen, caudal aspect (su)

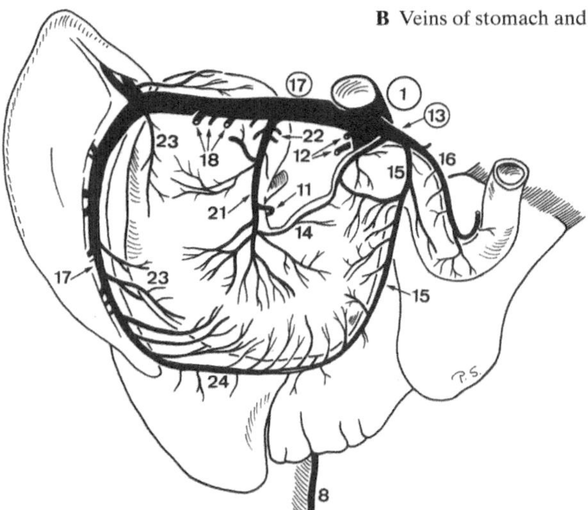

C Veins of spleen, stomach and liver, caudoventral aspect (eq)

RUMINANTIA

1 ***Vv. pancreaticae***. Into Lobus pancreatis sinister. A

2 ***Ramus epiploicus***. Accompanies corresponding artery.

3 ***V. ruminalis dextra***. Accompanies corresponding artery. A

4 *Ramus collateralis*. Courses parallel to V. ruminalis dextra. A

5 ***V. reticularis***. Accompanies corresponding artery. A

6 ***V. ruminalis sinistra***. Accompanies corresponding artery. A

7 *V. esophagea [oesophagea] caudalis*. Drains the caudal segment of Esophagus. A

8 ***V. gastrica sinistra***. Accompanies corresponding artery. A

9 *V. gastroepiploica sinistra*. Accompanies corresponding artery. A

TERMINI COMMUNES

10 **V. mesenterica cranialis**. Unpaired, major terminal tributary to V. portae. Drains most of the intestinal tract: from Pars descendens of duodenum to Colon transversum. Courses in mesenterium at the right aspect of A. mesenterica cranialis. B C D

11 ***V. pancreaticoduodenalis caudalis***. Accompanies corresponding artery. B C D

12 ***Vv. jejunales***. Accompany corresponding arteries. B C D

12a *Rami colici dextri* (ov, cap). [1]

13 ***Ramus collateralis*** (bo). Courses caudoventrally in mesojejunum, parallel to the terminal segment of V. mesenterica cranialis, gives rise to Vv. jejunales. Contributes to the jejunal venous arcades. D

14 ***Vv. ilei***. Variably arising branches (from V. mesenterica cranialis, V. ileocolica, and V. cecalis) for ileum. B C D

15 ***V. ileocolica***. Accompanies corresponding artery. B C D

16 *Ramus colicus*[1]. Accompanies corresponding artery in Car, su, eq. B C

17 *Rami colici*[1] . Accompany corresponding arteries in Ru. D

18 *Vv. colicae dextrae*[1]. Accompany corresponding arteries in Ru. D

19 *V. cecalis [caecalis]*. Accompanies corresponding artery in Car, su, Ru. C D

20 *V. cecalis [caecalis] medialis* (eq). Accompanies corresponding artery. B

21 *V. cecalis [caecalis] lateralis* (eq). Accompanies corresponding artery. B

22 ***V. colica dextra***[1]. Branch of V. ileocolica (Car, su) or Ramus colicus (eq). Accompanies corresponding artery. B C

23 ***V. colica media*** (Car, su) [1]. Arises from V. ileocolica, accompanies corresponding artery, joins V. mesenterica caudalis. C

[1] For species specific details see the homologous arteries, branches of the A. mesenterica cranialis.

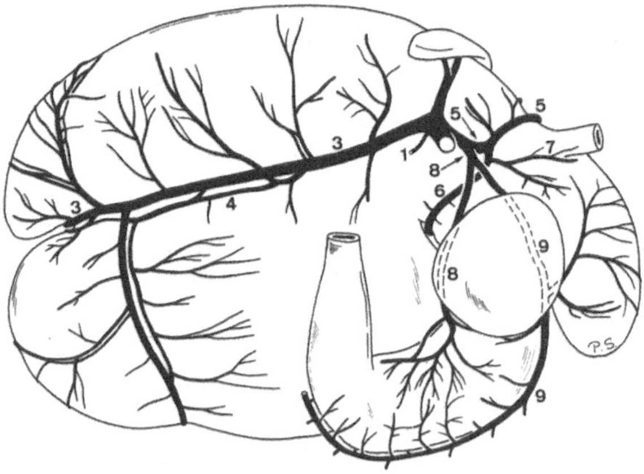

A Veins of the stomach, right lateral aspect (bo)

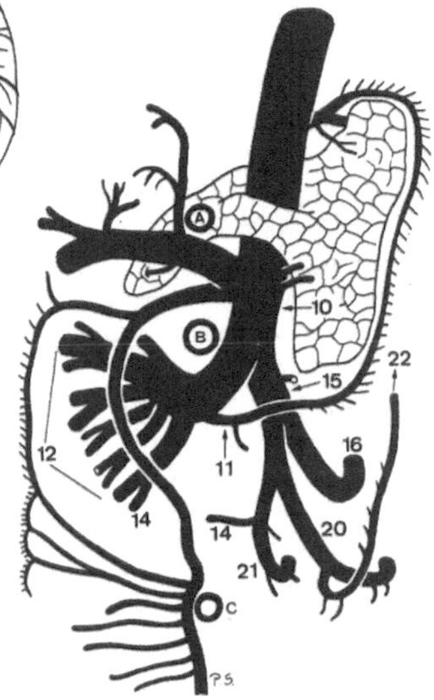

B V. portae in relation to pancreas and A. celiaca (A), A. mesenterica cranialis (B) and A. mesenterica caudalis (C), dorsal aspect (eq)

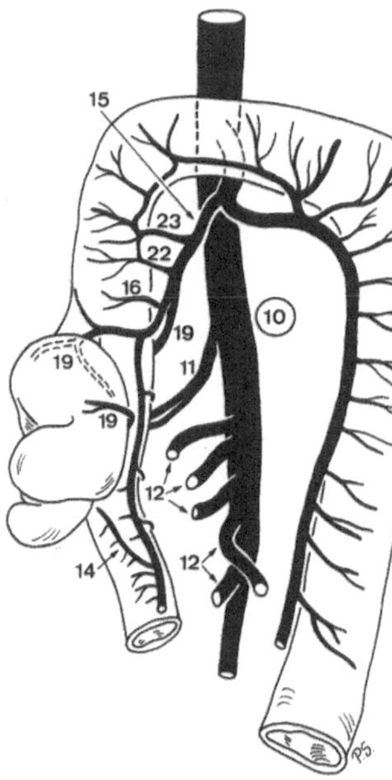

C Veins of cecum and colon, ventral aspect (ca)

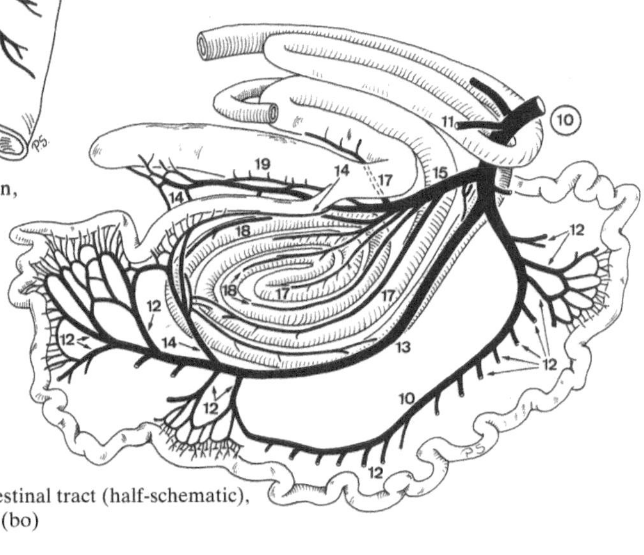

D Veins of the intestinal tract (half-schematic), right lateral aspect (bo)

1 **V. mesenterica caudalis**. Unpaired, smaller terminal tributary to V. portae. Courses in mesenterium towards Colon descendens. A

2 *V. colica media* (Ru, eq). Drains Colon transversum and courses in Mesocolon transversum to the right in order to join V. colica dextra. A

3 *V. colica sinistra*. Continuation of V. mesenterica caudalis in Mesocolon descendens close to Colon descendens, except in eq where it continues caudally in the dorsal part of mesocolon. A

4 *Vv. sigmoideae*. Accompany corresponding arteries. A

5 *V. rectalis cranialis*. Continuation of V. colica sinistra along the dorsal surface of the rectum. Anastomoses with V. rectalis (media and) caudalis. A

6 **V. ILIACA COMMUNIS**. Terminal branch of V. cava caudalis, courses caudolaterally to the medial aspect of Os ilium, splits in V. iliaca externa and V. iliaca interna. Exceptionally, V. iliaca communis sinistra is absent in cap. B E

7 *V. lumbalis V* (eq), *VI* (Un), *VII* (Car). Variably fused segmental veins. Accompany corresponding arteries. B E

8 *V. circumflexa ilium profunda* (Un). Accompanies corresponding artery. B E

9 *V. iliolumbalis* (eq). Accompanies corresponding artery. B

10 *V. testicularis sinistra* (bo, ov). Accompanies corresponding artery. D E

11 *Plexus pampiniformis*. Network around A. testicularis. D

12 *V. ovarica sinistra* (bo, cap). Courses across the dorsal aspect of aorta (bo) into mesovarium, accompanies corresponding artery. C E

13 *V. vesicalis cranialis* (cap). To Vesica urinaria.

14 **V. sacralis mediana** (Car, su, Ru). Courses along Facies pelvina of Os sacrum. Usually paired in su, sometimes (locally) in Car, cap, bo. E

15 *Rami sacrales*. Often initially fused, course into the corresponding Foramen sacrale ventrale, emerge from the Foramen sacrale dorsale, joining Plexus vertebralis externus dorsalis. The last pair pierces between Os sacrum and Vertebra caudalis I. E

16 *V. intervertebralis*. Connects the Ramus sacralis with Plexus vertebralis internus ventralis. E

17 **(V. sacralis mediana)** (eq). Accompanies corresponding artery. B

18 **V. caudalis [coccygea] mediana** (Car, su, Ru). Variably developed continuation of V. sacralis mediana (except eq), accompanies corresponding artery. Paired in Car, su, and sometimes cap. E

19 *Rami caudales [coccygei]*. Accompany corresponding arteries. E

20 *V. intervertebralis*. Passes medially between Vertebrae caudales and connects Plexus vertebrales externi (and internus). E

21 *V. caudalis [coccygea] ventrolateralis*. Accompanies corresponding artery. Contributes to Plexus vertebralis externus ventralis. E

22 *V. caudalis [coccygea] dorsolateralis*. Accompanies corresponding artery. Contributes to Plexus vertebralis externus dorsalis. E

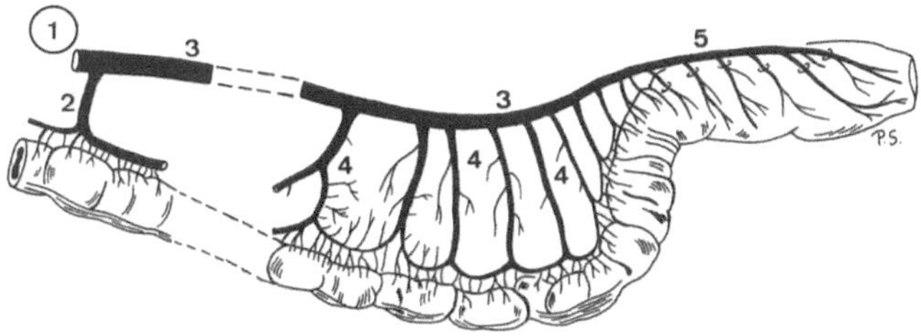

A Veins of Colon tenue and Rectum, left lateral aspect (eq)

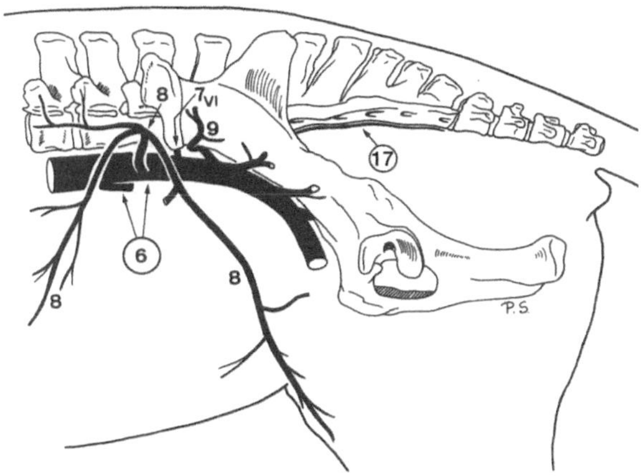

B Branches of V. iliaca communis, left lateral aspect (eq)

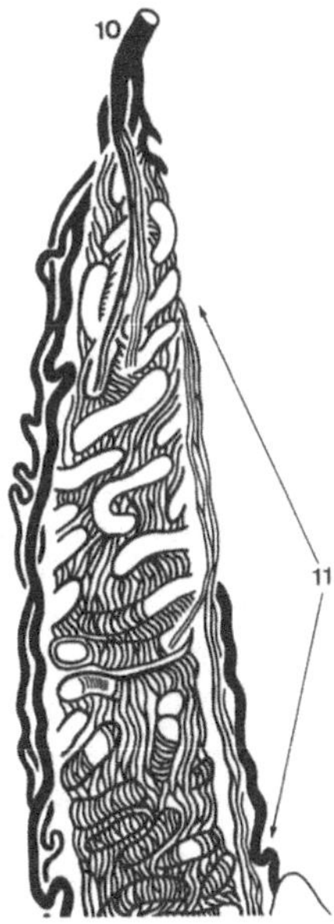

D Corrosion cast of the left V. testicularis, craniomedial aspect (bo)

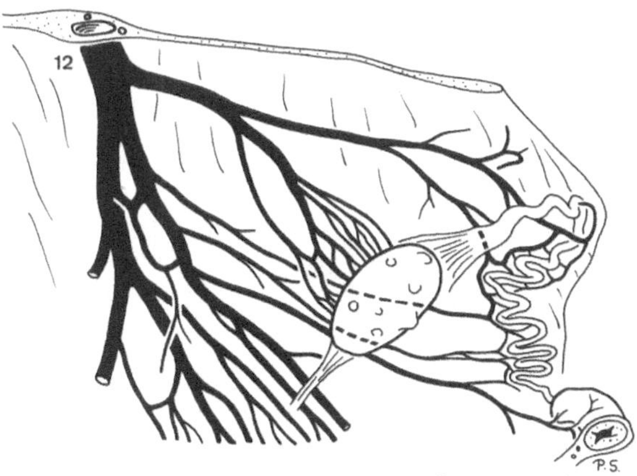

C Veins of left Ovarium, tuba uterina, and Cornu uteri, medial aspect (bo)

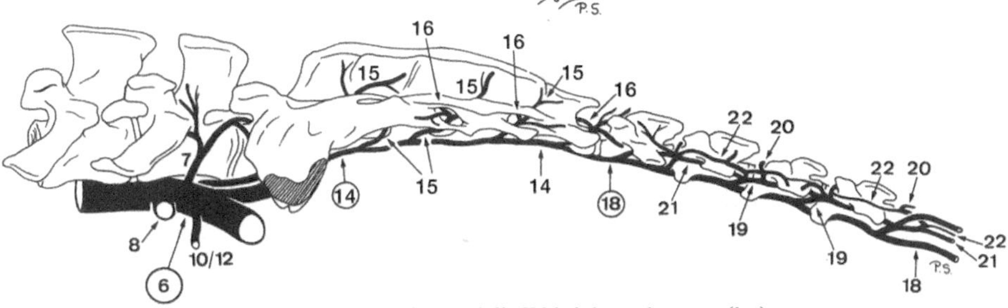

E Veins in relation to Vertebrae lumbalis V–caudalis IV, left lateral aspect (bo)

TERMINUS COMMUNIS

1 **V. ILIACA INTERNA.** Medial terminal branch of V. iliaca communis, courses into Cavum pelvis. Accompanies corresponding artery. A C

CARNIVORA

2 ***V. iliolumbalis.*** Accompanies corresponding artery. A C

3 ***V. obturatoria.*** Branch of V. iliaca interna (fe) s. V. glutea caudalis (ca) towards Foramen obturatum. A C

4 ***V. prostatica.*** To Prostata. C

5 *V. ductus deferentis.* To Ductus deferens. C

6 **V. vesicalis caudalis.** Drains the venous plexus of Vesica urinaria. C

7 *V. rectalis media.* To rectum. C

8 ***V. vaginalis.*** To the lateral wall of the vagina. A

9 *V. uterina.* Accompanies corresponding artery. A

10 **V. vesicalis caudalis.** Drains the venous plexus of Vesica urinaria. A

11 *V. rectalis media.* To rectum. A

12 ***V. glutea [glutaea] cranialis.*** Accompanies corresponding artery. A C

13 ***V. caudalis [coccygea] lateralis.*** Accompanies corresponding artery. A B C

14 *V. caudalis [coccygea] dorsalis* (fe). Unpaired, formed by tributaries from the left and right Vv. caudales laterales, located at the dorsal surface of the tail. B

15 ***V. glutea [glutaea] caudalis.*** Accompanies corresponding artery. A C

16 *V. perinealis dorsalis.* Drains the dorsal part of perineum. A

17 ***V. pudenda interna.*** Accompanies corresponding artery. A C

18 *V. urethralis.* Drains the pelvic part of the urethra. A C

19 *V. dorsalis penis.* Accompanies corresponding artery. The left and right are united for a short distance at Arcus ischiadicus. C

20 *V. dorsalis clitoridis.* Accompanies corresponding artery. The left and right veins are fused for a short distance at Arcus ischiadicus. A

21 *V. perinealis ventralis.* To perineum and anus. A C

22 **V. rectalis caudalis.** Accompanies corresponding artery, often accompanied by a branch of V. pudenda interna (ca). A C

23 **V. scrotalis dorsalis.** Often accompanied by branches of V. penis. C

24 **V. labialis dorsalis.** Accompanies corresponding artery (ca). A

25 *V. penis.* Accompanies corresponding artery. Common trunk for V. bulbi penis and V. profunda penis. C

26 **V. bulbi penis.** Accompanies corresponding artery. C

27 **V. profunda penis.** Accompanies corresponding artery. C

28 *V. clitoridis.* Accompanies corresponding artery. Common trunk for V. bulbi vestibuli and V. profunda clitoridis. A

29 **V. bulbi vestibuli.** Drains Bulbus vestibuli. A

30 **V. profunda clitoridis.** Fuses with its counterpart (ca), drains Corpus cavernosum clitoridis with several branches. A

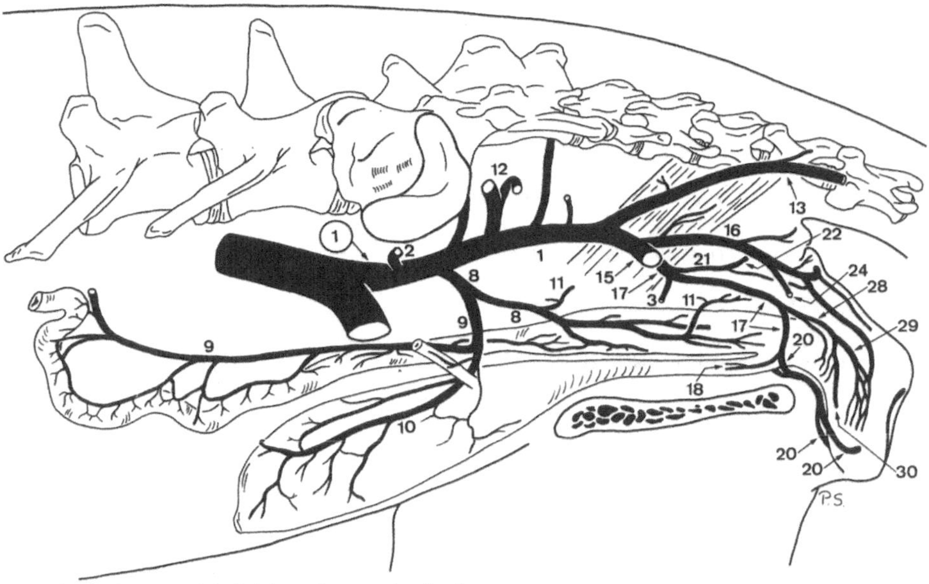

A Veins in Cavum pelvis, left lateral aspect (ca fem)

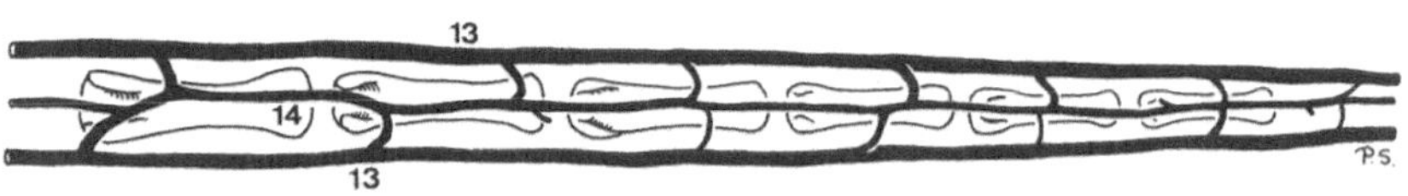

B Veins in relation to Vertebrae caudales XII–XVII, dorsal aspect (fe)

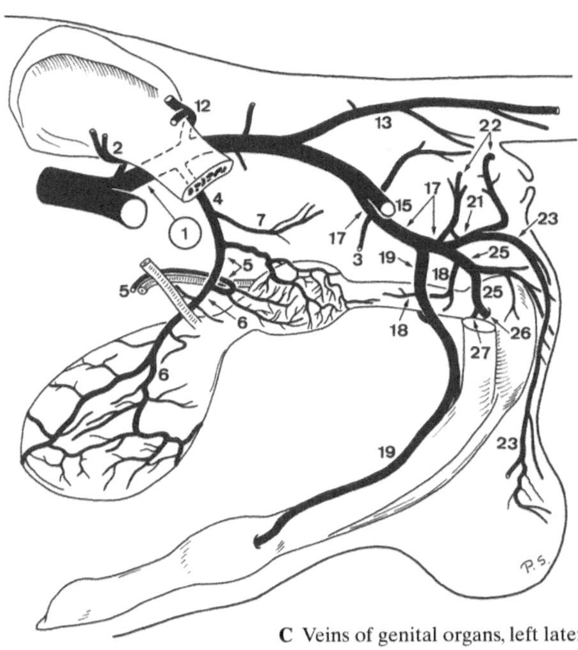

C Veins of genital organs, left lateral aspect (ca masc)

SUS

1 ***V. iliolumbalis***. Accompanies corresponding artery. A B

2 ***V. glutea [glutaea] cranialis***. Accompanies corresponding artery. A B

3 ***V. prostatica***. Accompanies corresponding artery. A

4 *V. vesicalis caudalis*. Accompanies corresponding artery. A

5 ***V. vaginalis***. Accompanies corresponding artery. B

6 *Ramus uterinus*. Accompanies corresponding artery. B

7 *V. vesicalis caudalis*. Accompanies corresponding artery. B

8 ***V. obturatoria***. Accompanies corresponding artery. Usually connected with V. profunda femoris and V. penis s. clitoridis. A B

9 ***V. glutea [glutaea] caudalis***. Accompanies corresponding artery. A B

10 *V. perinealis dorsalis*. Branch of V. iliaca interna and/or V. caudalis dorsolateralis to perineum. A B

11 **V. rectalis caudalis**. Drains Canalis analis. A B

12 ***V. pudenda interna***. Accompanies corresponding artery. A B

13 *V. perinealis ventralis*. Passes to perineum. A B

14 **V. scrotalis dorsalis**. Drains the dorsal segment of scrotum. Accompanied by branches of V. bulbi penis. A

15 **V. labialis dorsalis**. Drains Labium pudendi. Accompanied or replaced by branches of V. perinealis dorsalis. B

16 *V. penis*. At Arcus ischiadicus connected with its counterpart by a large cranial branch, which continues into V. obturatoria and V. profunda femoris. A

17 **V. bulbi penis**. Drains Corpus spongiosum penis. A

18 **V. profunda penis**. Drains Corpus cavernosum penis. A

19 **V. dorsalis penis**. Accompanies corresponding artery. Usually bilaterally asymmetrical or only unilaterally represented in its initial segment. A

20 *V. clitoridis*. Accompanies corresponding artery. At Arcus ischiadicus connected with its counterpart by a large cranial branch, which continues into V. obturatoria and V. profunda femoris. B

21 **V. bulbi vestibuli**. Courses to Bulbus vestibuli. B

22 **V. profunda clitoridis**. Drains Corpus cavernosum clitoridis. B

23 **V. dorsalis clitoridis**. Variably developed, along the ventral surface of Corpus clitoridis. B

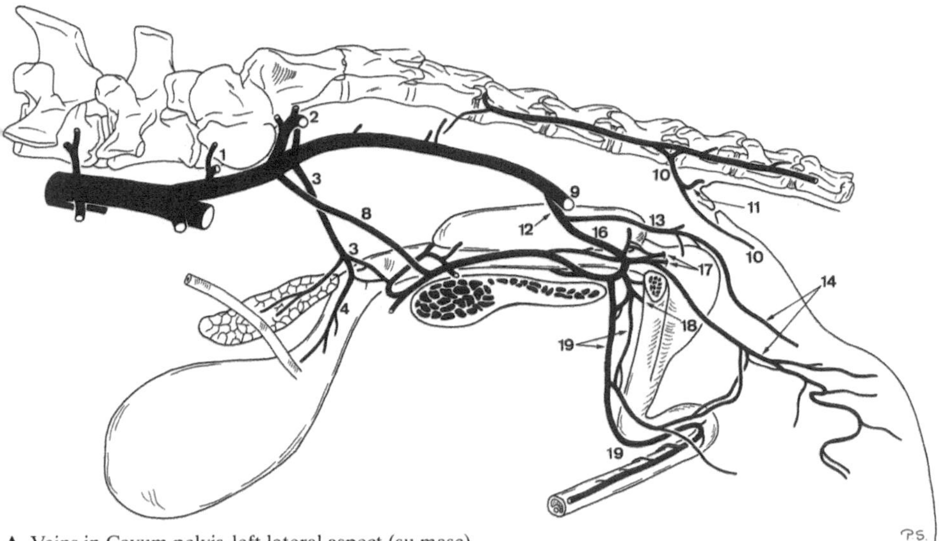

A Veins in Cavum pelvis, left lateral aspect (su masc)

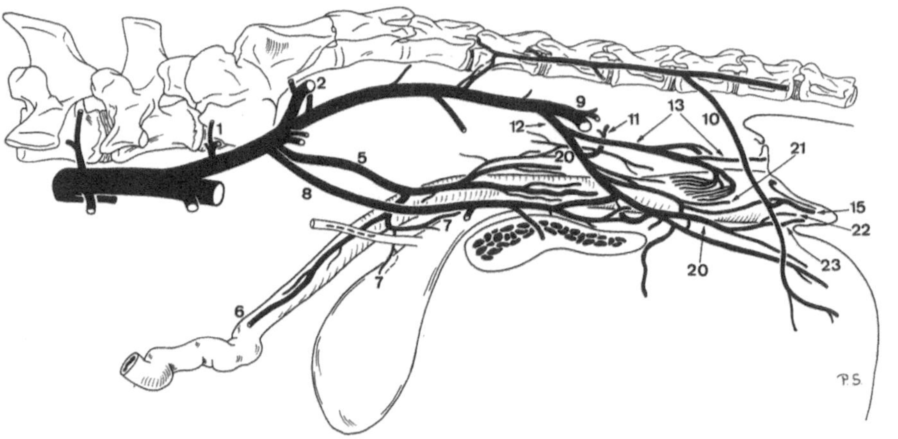

B Veins in Cavum pelvis, left lateral aspect (su fem)

RUMINANTIA

1 ***V. uterina*** (bo). Slender, inconstant, accompanies A. uterina into the uterine venous network. B

2 ***V. iliolumbalis***. Accompanies corresponding artery. A B

3 ***V. glutea [glutaea] cranialis***. Accompanies corresponding artery. A B

4 ***V. obturatoria***. Courses to Foramen obturatum. May be double and arise from V. pudenda interna (bo). A B

5 ***V. vaginalis accessoria*** (bo). Often double, to vagina. B

6 ***V. prostatica***. Accompanies corresponding artery. A

7 *V. ductus deferentis*. Accompanies corresponding artery. A

8 **V. vesicalis caudalis**. Drains the venous plexus of Vesica urinaria. A

9 ***V. vaginalis***. Accompanies corresponding artery. B

10 *Ramus uterinus*. Accompanies corresponding artery, contributes to the uterine venous network. Plexiform in bo. B

11 **V. vesicalis caudalis**. Drains the venous plexus of Vesica urinaria. B

12 *V. rectalis media*. To the rectum (bo, cap) (branch of V. prostatica in the male). Often unilaterally absent. B

13 *V. perinealis dorsalis*. To perineum (branch of V. prostatica in the male). B

14 **V. rectalis caudalis** (bo fem, cap). Accompanies corresponding artery. Variable in shape and origin. B

15 **V. labialis dorsalis**. Accompanies corresponding artery. B

16 ***V. glutea [glutaea] caudalis***. Accompanies corresponding artery. A B

17 ***V. pudenda interna***. Accompanies corresponding artery. Connected with its counterpart at Arcus ischiadicus in the female. A B

18 *V. rectalis caudalis* (bo masc, ov). Accompanies corresponding artery. Variable in shape and origin. A

19 *V. vestibularis* (bo). Accompanies corresponding artery. B

20 *V. perinealis ventralis*. To perineum. A B

21 **V. labialis dorsalis et mammaria**. Accompanies corresponding artery, joins V. labialis ventralis [mammaria caudalis]. May fuse with its counterpart, or be absent unilaterally (bo). B

22 *V. penis*. Accompanies corresponding artery. Joins or anastomoses with its counterpart at Arcus ischiadicus. A

23 **V. bulbi penis**. Drains Corpus spongiosum penis. A

24 **V. profunda penis**. Drains Corpus cavernosum penis. A

25 **V. dorsalis penis**. Unpaired on Dorsum penis. Especially in ov and cap reinforced at Flexura sigmoidea penis by a large unpaired branch of V. pudenda externa. The unpaired caudal portion of V. dorsalis penis may be lacking (cap). A

26 ***V. clitoridis***. Accompanies corresponding artery. B

27 *V. bulbi vestibuli* (ov, cap). Drains Bulbus vestibuli.

28 *V. profunda clitoridis*. Drains Corpus cavernosum clitoridis. B

29 *V. dorsalis clitoridis*. Along the ventral border of Corpus clitoridis. B

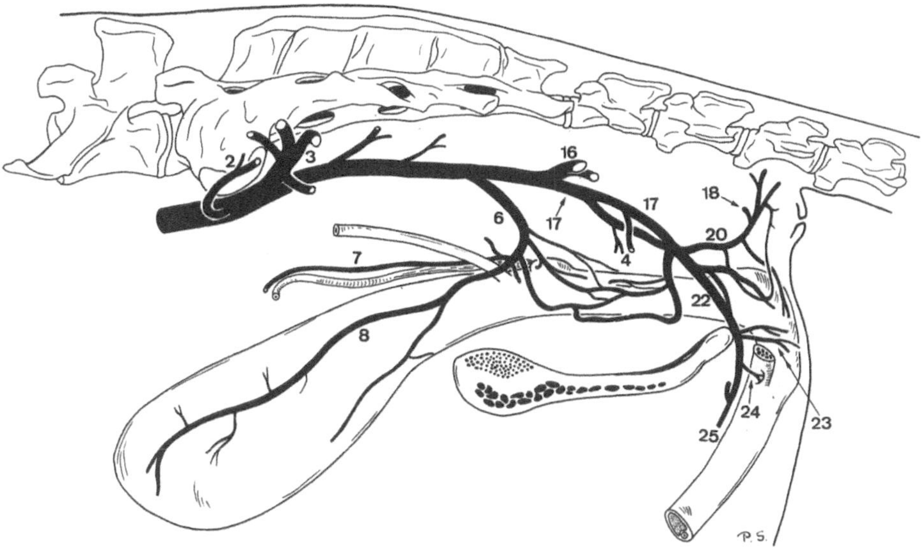

A Veins in Cavum pelvis, left lateral aspect (bo masc)

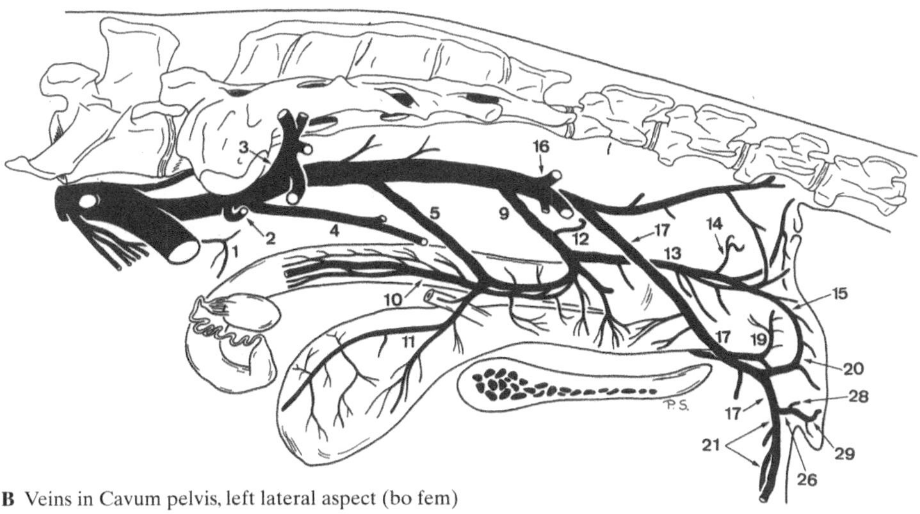

B Veins in Cavum pelvis, left lateral aspect (bo fem)

EQUUS

1 ***V. glutea [glutaea] caudalis.*** Accompanies corresponding artery. A B

2 *V. glutea [glutaea] cranialis.* Accompanies corresponding artery. A B

3 *Rami sacrales.* Course into each Foramen sacrale ventrale, emerge from the corresponding Foramen sacrale dorsale, joining Plexus vertebralis externus dorsalis. Ramus sacralis I arises from V. iliaca interna. A B

4 **V. intervertebralis.** Arises in Canalis sacralis, connects Ramus sacralis with Plexus vertebralis internus ventralis. A

5 *V. caudalis [coccygea] mediana.* Unpaired, arises from the left or right V. glutea caudalis or is formed by the fusion of asymmetrical branches of both Vv. gluteae caudales. Seldom given off by V. sacralis mediana. A

6 *V. caudalis [coccygea] ventrolateralis.* Accompanies corresponding artery. Contributes to Plexus vertebralis externus ventralis. A B

7 **Rami caudales [coccygei].** Accompany corresponding arteries. A

8 **V. intervertebralis.** Medial branch of Ramus caudalis, passes between Vertebrae caudales, connects the Plexus vertebrales externi with internus ventralis. A

9 **V. caudalis [coccygea] dorsolateralis.** Accompanies corresponding artery. Contributes to Plexus vertebralis externus dorsalis. A

10 ***V. pudenda interna.*** Accompanies corresponding artery. The caudal segment is usually accompanied by a parallel vein which courses along the lateral surface of Ligamentum sacrotuberale latum and joins the main vein again at Foramen ischiadicum minus. A B

11 *V. prostatica.* To Prostata. A

12 **Ramus ductus deferentis.** Accompanies corresponding artery. A

13 **V. vesicalis caudalis.** Arises from Ramus ductus deferentis and drains the venous plexus of Vesica urinaria. A

14 **V. rectalis media.** To the rectum. A

15 *V. vaginalis.* Accompanies corresponding artery. B

16 **Ramus uterinus.** To Cervix et Corpus uteri. B

17 **V. vesicalis caudalis.** Arises from Ramus uterinus, drains the venous plexus of Vesica urinaria. B

18 **V. rectalis media.** Arises from V. vesicalis caudalis or V. vaginalis, to the rectum. B

19 *V. perinealis ventralis.* To the perineum. A B

20 **V. rectalis caudalis.** To the rectum. A B

21 *V. penis.* To Radix penis. A

22 ***V. bulbi penis.*** Enters Bulbus penis, drains Corpus spongiosum penis. A

23 ***V. profunda penis.*** Drains Corpus cavernosum penis. A

24 ***V. dorsalis penis.*** Very slender, along the caudal segment of Dorsum penis. Reinforced by V. penis media, continues upon Dorsum penis, and, receiving the multiple V. penis cranialis forms a complex of large coiled veins that drain Corpora spongiosa penis and glandis and Corpus cavernosum penis. A

25 *V. clitoridis.* Continuation of V. pudenda interna. B

26 ***V. bulbi vestibuli.*** Drains Bulbus vestibuli. B

27 ***V. profunda clitoridis.*** Drains Corpus cavernosum clitoridis. B

28 ***V. dorsalis clitoridis.*** Curves along the ventral border of Corpus clitoridis. B

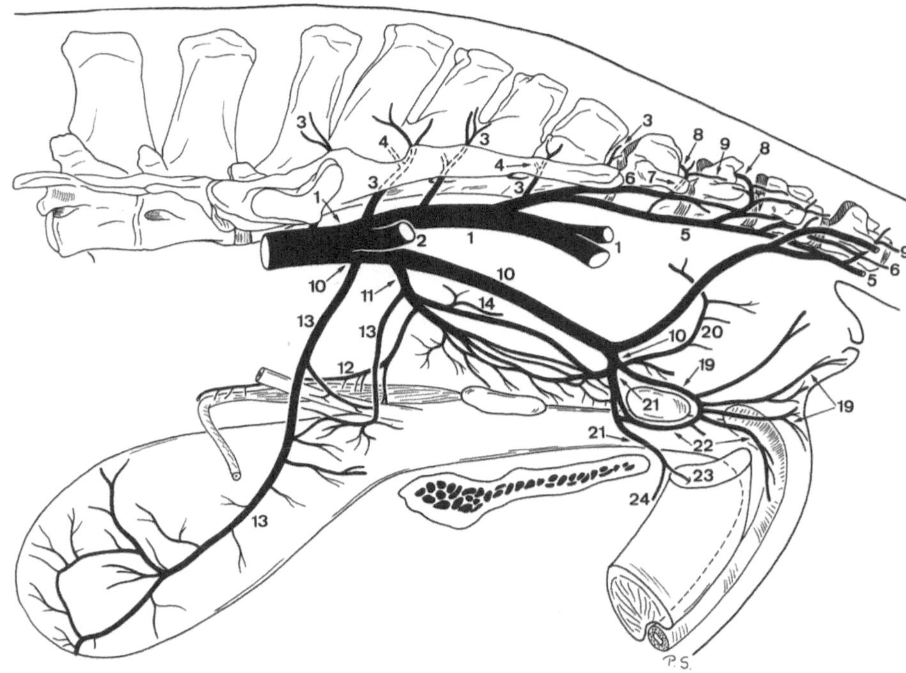

A Veins in Cavum pelvis, left lateral aspect (eq masc)

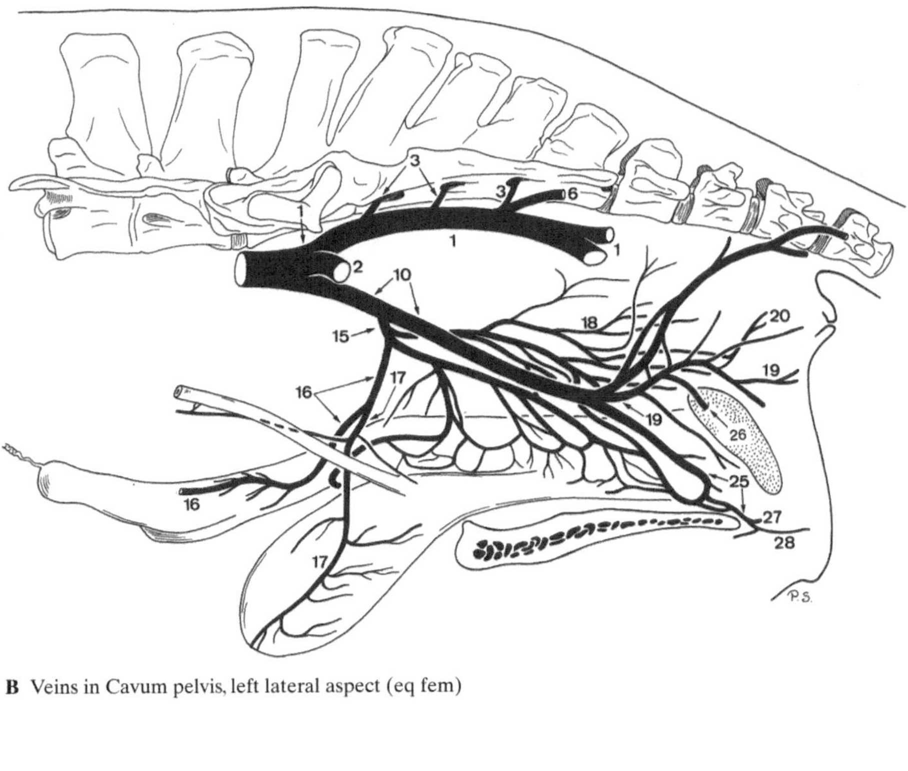

B Veins in Cavum pelvis, left lateral aspect (eq fem)

TERMINUS COMMUNIS

1 **V. ILIACA EXTERNA.** Lateral terminal branch of V. iliaca communis, courses to Lacuna vasorum along the cranial aspect of Corpus ossis ilium. A B

CARNIVORA

2 ***V. abdominalis caudalis.*** Courses into the caudolateral abdominal wall. A

3 ***V. pudendoepigastrica.*** Trunk for V. pudenda externa and V. epigastrica caudalis. A

4 *V. epigastrica caudalis.* Accompanies corresponding artery. A

5 *V. pudenda externa.* Accompanies corresponding artery. A

6 **V. vesicalis media** (fe). Courses in Ligamentum vesicae laterale to Vesica urinaria. May arise from V. epigastrica caudalis or from a muscular branch of V. iliaca externa. A

7 **V. scrotalis ventralis.** Drains scrotum. A

8 **V. labialis ventralis.** To Labium pudendi, drains also the inguinal mamma.

9 **V. epigastrica caudalis superficialis.** Accompanies corresponding artery, anastomoses by inosculation with V. epigastrica cranialis superficialis. Drains Mammae abdominales and inguinalis. A (see 306.15)

10 ***V. profunda femoris.*** Courses along the medial surface of M. iliopsoas. A

11 *V. circumflexa femoris medialis.* Continuation of V. profunda femoris. Accompanies corresponding artery. A

SUS

12 ***V. ductus deferentis.*** Drains the terminal segment of Ductus deferens.

13 *V. vesicalis cranialis.* To Vesica urinaria.

14 ***V. profunda femoris.*** Trunk for V. pudendoepigastrica and V. circumflexa femoris medialis. B

15 *V. pudendoepigastrica.* Double trunk for V. pudenda externa and V. epigastrica caudalis. B

16 **V. epigastrica caudalis.** Accompanies corresponding artery. B

17 **V. pudenda externa.** Accompanies corresponding artery. B

18 **V. scrotalis ventralis.** Double branch of V. pudenda externa along the corresponding artery.

19 **V. labialis ventralis.** Branch of V. pudenda externa along the corresponding artery. B

20 **V. epigastrica caudalis superficialis.** Subcutaneous branch of V. pudenda externa, accompanies corresponding artery. Drains the caudal mammae s. preputium. B

21 *V. circumflexa femoris medialis.* Double continuation of V. profunda femoris. Accompanies corresponding artery. B

22 **V. saphena lateralis** [parva]. Courses between M. biceps femoris and M. semitendinosus, along the caudal aspect of M. gastrocnemius to the craniolateral surface of Tendo calcaneus communis. B C

23 **Ramus cranialis.** Superficial branch of V. saphena lateralis, courses across the lateral aspect of tarsus, joins the branches of Ramus cranialis of V. saphena medialis at Collum tali, continues along the dorsal surface of tarsus and the proximal half of metatarsus. B C

24 **Vv. digitales dorsales communes II–IV.** Superficial branches of Ramus cranialis of V. saphena lateralis. Connected with the respective Vv. metatarseae dorsales. C

25 **Vv. digitales dorsales propriae.** Arise from the bifurcation of Vv. digitales dorsales communes II–IV. Accompany corresponding arteries. C

26 **V. coronalis.** Branch of Vv. digitales dorsales propriae III et IV (axiales et abaxiales), course in the dorsal segment of Corona ungulae. C

26a **Plexus ungularis.** Around Facies parietalis phalangis distalis. This network extends also on the solear surface. The plexus is defined as the dense venous network in Dermis ungulae

27 **Ramus caudalis.** Continuation of V. saphena lateralis along the lateroplantar aspect of tarsus, joins V. plantaris lateralis. B C

28 **Ramus anastomoticus cum v. saphena mediali [magna].** Branch of V. saphena lateralis or Ramus caudalis, courses across the plantar aspect of M. flexor digitorum profundus, joins Ramus caudalis of V. saphena medialis at Sustentaculum tali. B C

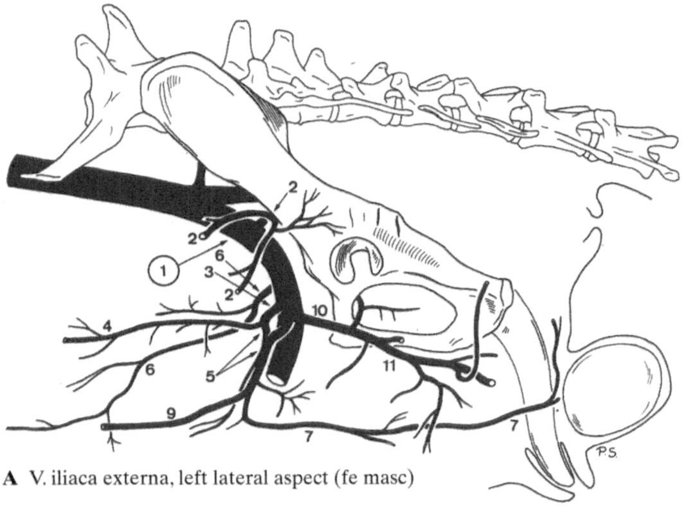

A V. iliaca externa, left lateral aspect (fe masc)

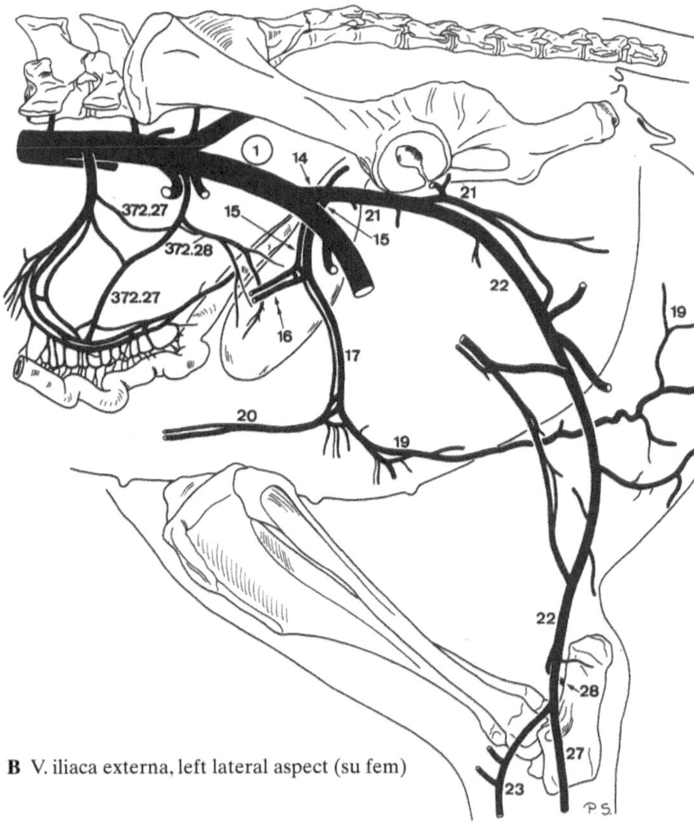

B V. iliaca externa, left lateral aspect (su fem)

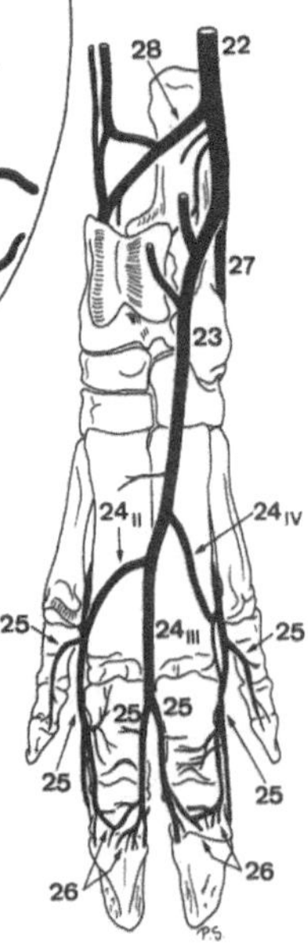

C Veins of left pes, dorsal aspect (su)

RUMINANTIA

1 ***V. profunda femoris***. Accompanies corresponding artery. A

2 *V. pudendoepigastrica*. Trunk for V. pudenda externa and V. epigastrica caudalis. A

3 **V. abdominalis caudalis**. Accompanies corresponding artery. A

4 **V. epigastrica caudalis**. Accompanies corresponding artery. A

5 **V. cremasterica**. Arises variably, accompanies corresponding artery. A

6 **V. pudenda externa**. Accompanies corresponding artery. A C

7 **V. scrotalis ventralis**. To scrotum. A

8 **V. labialis ventralis [mammaria caudalis]**. Branch of V. pudenda externa on the lateral surface of the udder, continues in Regio supramammaria towards Labium pudendi. C

9 **V. epigastrica caudalis superficialis [mammaria cranialis]**. Branch of V. pudenda externa on the craniolateral aspect of the udder in the female, continues in the ventral abdominal wall, and anastomoses by inosculation with V. epigastrica cranialis superficialis. A C (see 306.15)

10 *V. circumflexa femoris medialis*. Accompanies corresponding artery. A

11 **V. saphena lateralis [parva]**. Courses between M. gluteobiceps and M. semitendinosus along the caudal aspect of M. gastrocnemius to the craniolateral surface of Tendo calcaneus communis. A

12 **Ramus cranialis**. Branch of V. saphena lateralis across the lateral aspect of tarsus, receives a branch of V. tibialis cranialis, continues along the dorsal surface of tarsus and metatarsus. B

13 **Vv. digitales dorsales communes (II) III et IV**. Branches of Ramus cranialis of V. saphena lateralis (II-IV bo, III et IV ov, cap), II et IV join Arcus plantaris profundus distalis, III joins V. metatarsea dorsalis III et V. interdigitalis. B

14 **Vv. digitales dorsales propriae**. Arise from the bifurcation of V. digitalis dorsalis communis III, course along the axial tendons of M. extensor digitorum longus. B

15 **V. coronalis**. Branch of V. digitalis dorsalis propria, courses in Sulcus coronalis of ungula. B

15a **Plexus ungularis**. Around Facies parietalis phalangis distalis. This network extends also on the solear surface. The plexus is defined as the dense venous network in Dermis ungulae.

16 **Ramus caudalis**. Continuation of V. saphena lateralis over the lateroplantar surface of tarsus, joins V. plantaris lateralis. B

17 **Ramus anastomoticus cum V. saphena mediali [magna]**. Branch of Ramus caudalis of V. saphena lateralis, courses across the dorsal aspect of Tuber calcanei, joins V. saphena medialis. B

EQUUS

18 ***V. ductus deferentis***. To the abdominal part of Ductus deferens.

19 ***V. uterina***. Accompanies A. uterina.

20 ***V. iliacofemoralis***. Courses along the cranial aspect of Corpus ossis ilium. Usually double. D E

21 ***V. obturatoria***. Courses along the medial aspect of Corpus ossis ilium, passes through Foramen obturatum. D E

22 *V. penis media*. To the caudal part of Dorsum penis, joins V. dorsalis penis. E

23 *V. clitoridis media*. Anastomoses with its counterpart at the ventral aspect of Arcus ischiadicus, pierces between Crura clitoridis, drains Corpus cavernosum clitoridis. D

24 ***V. profunda femoris***. Accompanies corresponding artery. D E

25 *V. pudendoepigastrica*. Inconstant trunk for V. pudenda externa and V. epigastrica caudalis. D E

26 **V. epigastrica caudalis**. Double. Accompanies corresponding artery. D E

27 **V. pudenda externa**. The equine V. pudenda externa accompanying the A. pudenda externa is small. D E

27a *V. pudenda externa accessoria*. Large vein that is complementary to the small V. pudenda externa. It connects the dorsal venous plexus of the penis or udder directly with the V. profunda femoris through a foramen in the tendon of origin of M. gracilis. E

28 **V. scrotalis ventralis**. Branch of V. pudenda externa or its inguinal network to the scrotum. E

29 **V. penis cranialis**. Branches of V. pudenda externa and its complementary vein to Dorsum penis. E

30 **V. labialis ventralis [mammaria caudalis]**. Branch of V. pudenda externa and the complementary vein, to Regio supramammaria and Labium pudendi. D

31 **V. epigastrica caudalis superficialis [mammaria cranialis]**. Branch of V. pudenda externa to Regio abdominis caudalis, anastomoses by inosculation with V. epigastrica cranialis superficialis. D E

32 *V. circumflexa femoris medialis*. Accompanies corresponding artery. D E

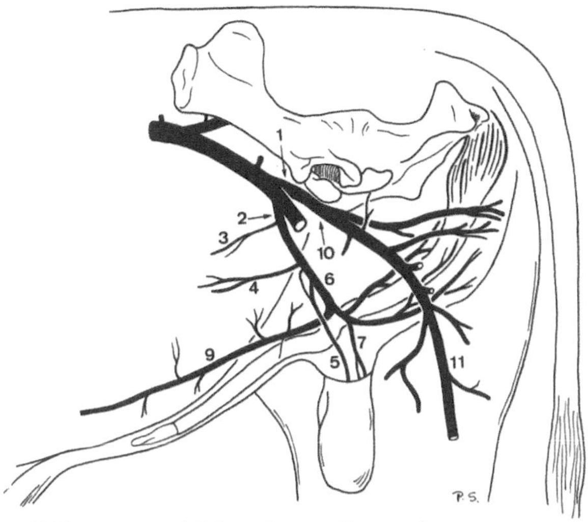

A V. iliaca externa, left lateral aspect (bo masc)

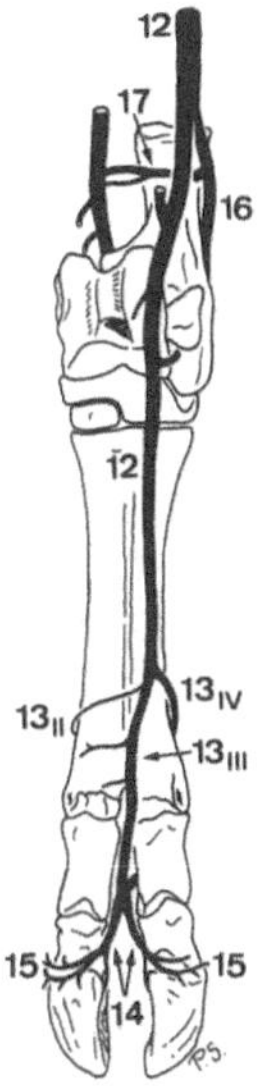

B Veins of left pes, dorsal aspect (bo)

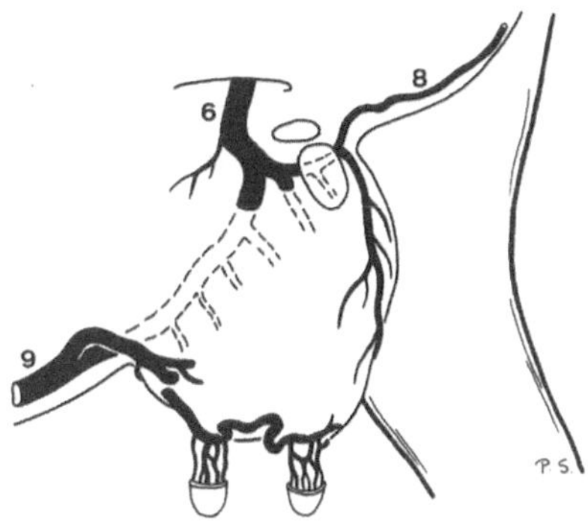

C Superficial veins of the udder, left lateral aspect (bo)

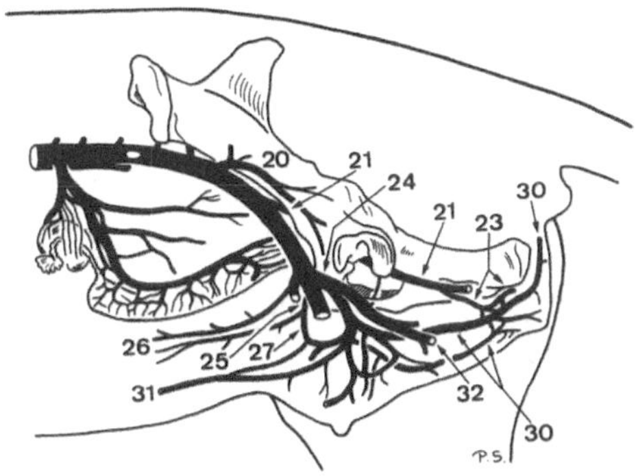

D V. iliaca externa, left lateral aspect (eq fem)

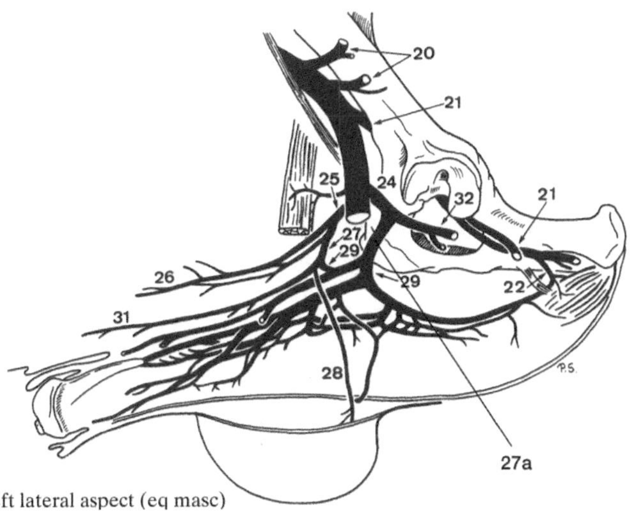

E V. iliaca externa, left lateral aspect (eq masc)

CARNIVORA

1 **V. femoralis**. Continuation of V. iliaca externa beyond Lacuna vasorum. Courses caudal to A. femoralis. A

2 ***V. circumflexa ilium superficialis*** (ca). Accompanies corresponding artery. A

3 ***V. circumflexa femoris lateralis.*** Accompanies corresponding artery. A

4 ***V. caudalis femoris proximalis.*** Accompanies corresponding artery. A

5 ***V. saphena medialis [magna].*** Accompanies A. saphena. A

6 *Ramus cranialis*. Accompanies corresponding artery, joins Ramus cranialis of V. saphena lateralis or its Ramus anastomoticus, continues at the dorsomedial surface of tarsus, anastomoses with V. dorsalis pedis. Continues dorsal to Os metatarsale II as V. digitalis dorsalis communis II (fe), or as the medial root of Arcus dorsalis superficialis (ca). A B C

7 **V. tarsea medialis** (ca). Curves to the medial and plantar aspect of tarsus, where it ramifies. Sends the V. plantaris medialis (see 7a). A B

7a **V. plantaris medialis.** Runs along the medioplantar surface of metatarsus to Arcus plantaris superficialis. B

8 **V. digitalis dorsalis communis II** (fe). Dorsal common digital V. II. C

9 **Vv. digitales dorsales propriae.** Arise from the bifurcation of V. digitalis dorsalis communis II. C

10 *Ramus caudalis*. Accompanies corresponding artery. Ramifies at the medioplantar aspect of tarsus. A D

11 **V. plantaris medialis** (fe). Courses along the medioplantar surface of metatarsus into Arcus plantaris superficialis. D

12 ***V. genus descendens.*** Accompanies corresponding artery. A

13 *Ramus articularis genus*. Drains Articulatio genus and Corpus adiposum infrapatellare. A

14 ***V. caudalis femoris media.*** Accompanies corresponding artery. A

15 ***V. caudalis femoris distalis.*** Accompanies corresponding artery. A

16 *V. saphena lateralis [parva]*. Courses along M. gastrocnemius, becomes subcutaneous by piercing between M. biceps femoris and M. semitendinosus, continues in Regio cruris lateralis. A

17 **Ramus cranialis.** Courses across Regio cruris lateralis and the dorsal surface of tarsus and metatarsus. A B C

18 **Ramus anastomoticus cum v. saphena mediali [magna].** Branch of Ramus cranialis of V. saphena lateralis, joins Ramus cranialis of V. saphena medialis. A B C

19 **V. digitalis dorsalis V abaxialis** (ca). Branch of Ramus cranialis of V. saphena lateralis along the abaxial border of Os metatarsale V. B

20 **V. tarsea lateralis** (ca). Branch of Ramus cranialis of V. saphena lateralis to the lateral and dorsal aspect of tarsus, anastomoses with Ramus caudalis of V. saphena lateralis. A B

21 **Arcus dorsalis superficialis** (ca). Variably shaped connection between Ramus cranialis of Vv. saphenae lateralis and medialis. B

22 **V. digitalis dorsalis II abaxialis.** Branch of Arcus dorsalis superficialis. B

23 **Vv. digitales dorsales communes II–IV.** Branches of Arcus dorsalis superficialis, accompany corresponding arteries. B

24 **Vv. digitales dorsales propriae.** Accompany corresponding arteries. B

25 **Vv. digitales dorsales communes III et IV** (fe). Branches of Ramus cranialis of V. saphena lateralis. Accompany corresponding arteries. C

26 **Vv. digitales dorsales propriae.** Arise from the bifurcation of Vv. digitales dorsales communes III et IV. Accompany corresponding arteries. C

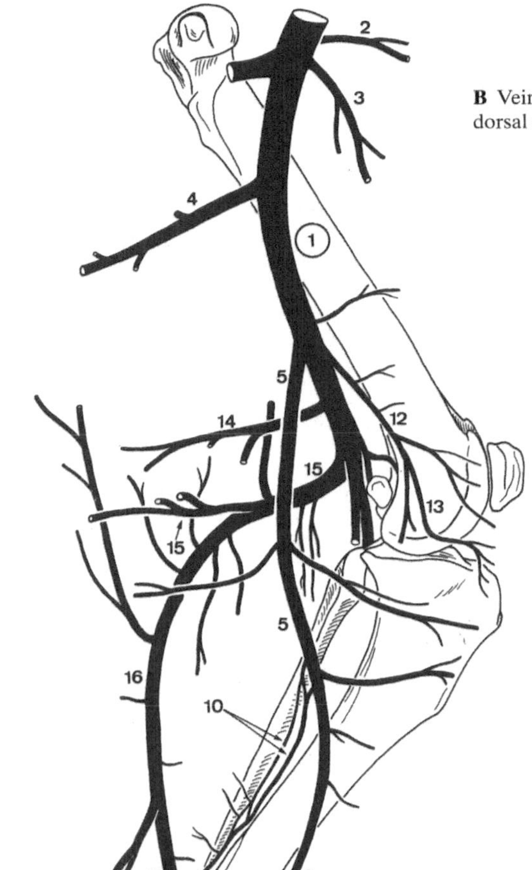
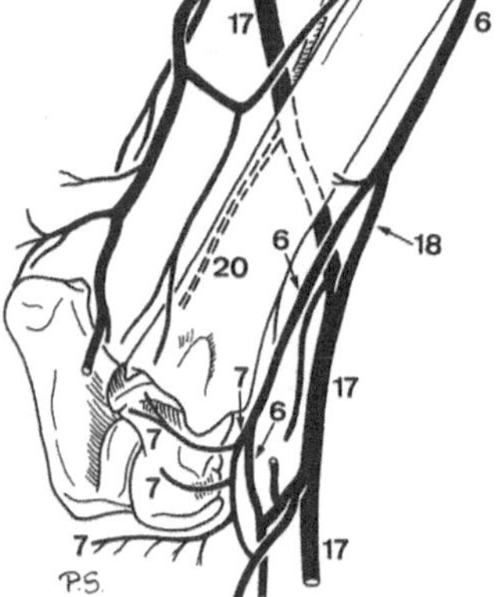

A Veins of left pelvic limb, medial aspect (ca)

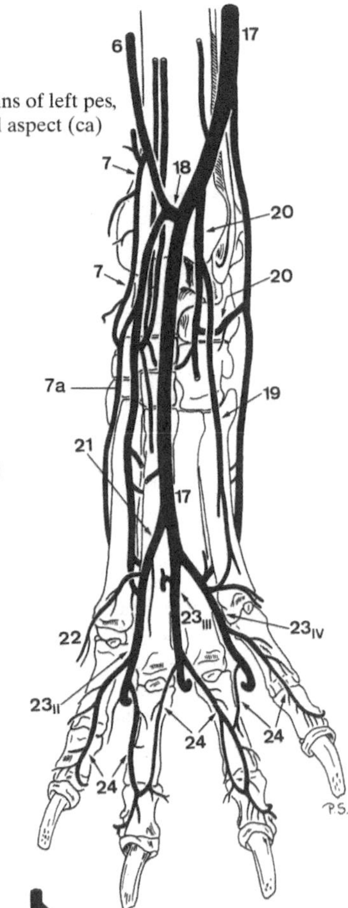

B Veins of left pes, dorsal aspect (ca)

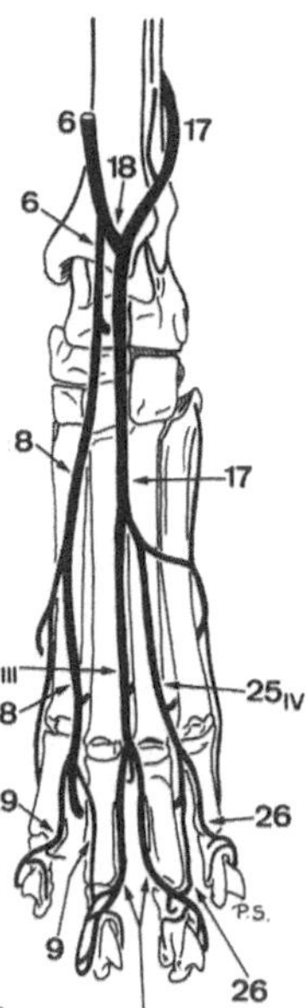

C Veins of left pes, dorsal aspect (fe)

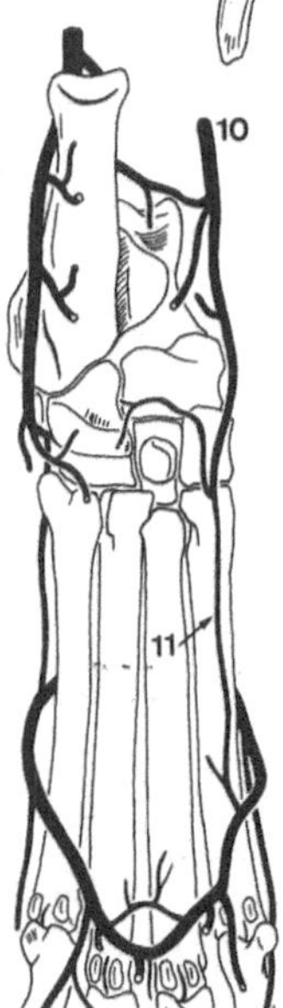

D Veins of left pes, plantar aspect (fe)

1 **Ramus caudalis**. Courses in Regio cruris lateralis to the lateroplantar surface of tarsus and metatarsus. A C

2 **Ramus anastomoticus cum v. saphena mediali [magna]**. Branch of Ramus caudalis of V. saphena lateralis, joins Ramus caudalis of V. saphena medialis. A C

3 **Arcus plantaris profundus**. Medial branch of Ramus caudalis of V. saphena lateralis which courses transversely across the plantar (fe) or dorsal (ca) aspect of Mm. interossei, joins V. plantaris medialis (ca, sometimes fe) and the proximal perforating branch of V. metatarsea dorsalis II. A C

4 **Vv. metatarseae plantares II–IV**. Branches of Arcus plantaris profundus, plantar (fe) or dorsal (ca) to Mm. interossei, join Arcus plantaris superficialis. A C

5 **Arcus plantaris superficialis**. Medial branch of Ramus caudalis of V. saphena lateralis, curves across the plantar aspect of the tendons of the digital flexor muscles in the distal third of metatarsus, and joins V. plantaris medialis (fe) or the distal branch of V. tarsea medialis (ca). A C

6 **V. digitalis plantaris II abaxialis** (fe). Arises from the connection between Arcus plantaris superficialis and V. digitalis dorsalis communis II. A

7 **Vv. digitales plantares communes II et IV (fe), II–IV** (ca). Distal branches of Arcus plantaris superficialis. Accompany corresponding arteries. A C

8 **V. interdigitalis**. Branch of V. digitalis plantaris communis or one of Vv. digitales plantares propriae. Joins the corresponding V. digitalis dorsalis communis or propria. A C

9 **Vv. digitales plantares propriae**. Accompany corresponding arteries. A C

10 **V. digitalis plantaris V abaxialis** (fe). Branch of Arcus plantaris superficialis. A

11 **V. poplitea**. Continuation of V. femoralis beyond the origin of V. caudalis femoris distalis. Accompanies corresponding artery. D

12 ***Vv. genus***. Variably developed, drain Articulatio genus. D

13 ***V. tibialis cranialis***. Craniodistal continuation of V. poplitea, accompanies corresponding artery. B D

14 *V. dorsalis pedis*. Continuation of V. tibialis cranialis distal to Articulatio tarsocruralis at the dorsal aspect of tarsus. Anastomoses (fe) or fuses (ca) with Ramus cranialis of V. saphena medialis halfway the tarsus. B

15 **V. tarsea medialis** (fe). To the medial and plantar aspect of tarsus. B

16 **V. tarsea lateralis** (fe). To the lateral and plantar aspect of tarsus, anastomoses with Ramus caudalis of V. saphena lateralis. B

17 **Arcus dorsalis profundus**. Courses across the dorsal surface of Ossa metatarsalia III et IV. Arises from V. dorsalis pedis in fe, from Ramus cranialis of V. saphena medialis in ca, but may be an arcuate branch of Ramus caudalis of V. saphena lateralis. B

18 **Vv. metatarseae dorsales II–IV (ca), II (III) IV** (fe). Branches of Arcus dorsalis profundus. Vv. metatarseae dorsales III et IV join the corresponding V. digitalis dorsalis communis in ca. Vv. metatarseae dorsales II (Car) and IV (fe) are rudimentary beyond the origin of the proximal perforating branch. B

19 ***V. tibialis caudalis***. Accompanies corresponding artery. Usually accompanied (ca) or replaced by a branch of V. caudalis femoris distalis. D

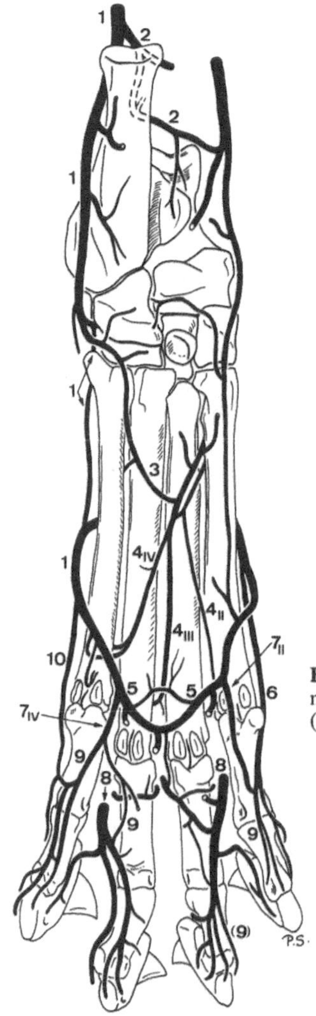

A Veins of left pes, plantar aspect (fe)

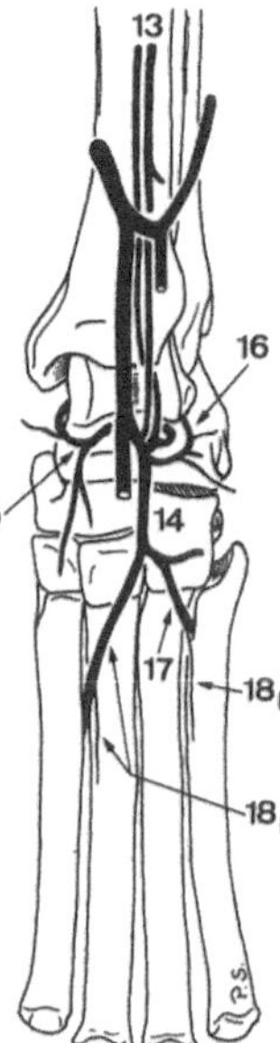

B Veins of left tarsus and metatarsus, dorsal aspect (fe)

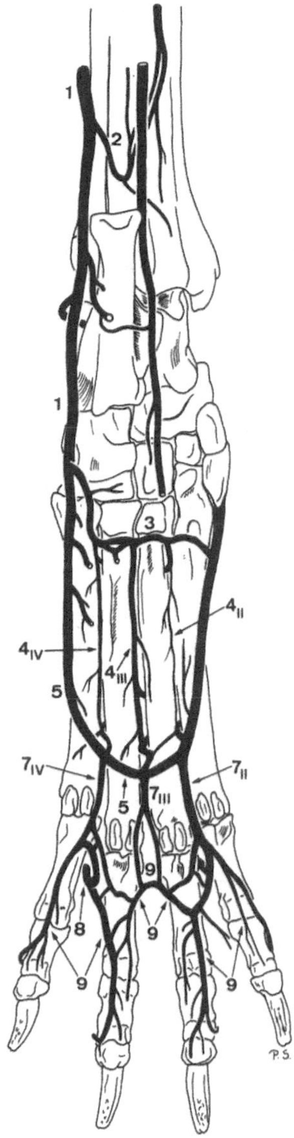

C Veins of left pes, plantar aspect (ca)

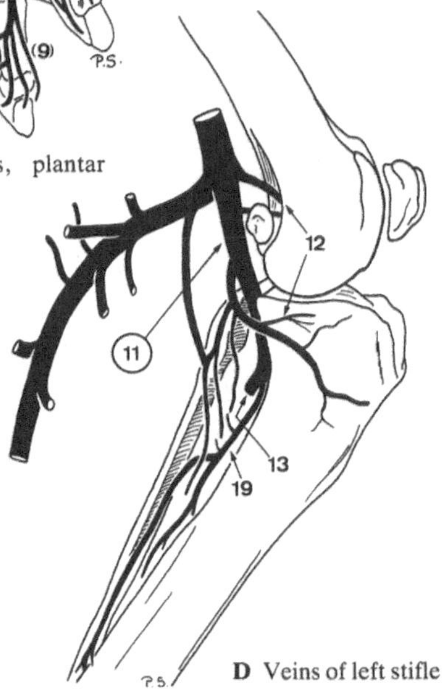

D Veins of left stifle, medial aspect (ca)

SUS

1 **V. femoralis**. Continuation of V. iliaca externa beyond Lacuna vasorum. Courses caudal to A. femoralis. A

2 ***V. circumflexa femoris lateralis***. Accompanies corresponding artery. A

3 ***V. saphena medialis [magna]***. Double vein along A. saphena. A

4 *Ramus cranialis*. Accompanies corresponding artery. Receives an anastomosis from V. epigastrica caudalis superficialis. A

5 **Ramus medialis**. May arise directly from V. saphena medialis, pursues a variable, subcutaneous course to the dorsomedial aspect of tarsus. A C

6 **Ramus lateralis**. Arises from the anastomosis between Ramus cranialis of V. saphena medialis and V. epigastrica caudalis superficialis, pursues a coiled, subcutaneous course towards Collum tali, joins Ramus cranialis of V. saphena lateralis. A C

7 *Ramus caudalis*. Superficial double continuation of V. saphena medialis along the border of Corpus tibiae, reinforced by Ramus anastomoticus of Ramus caudalis of V. saphena lateralis. Splits at the medioplantar aspect of tarsus into Vv. plantares medialis and lateralis. A B

8 **V. plantaris medialis**. Double continuation of Ramus caudalis, accompanies corresponding artery. A B

9 **Ramus profundus**. Branch of V. plantaris medialis, accompanies corresponding artery. A B

10 **Ramus superficialis**. Double continuation of V. plantaris medialis, accompanies corresponding artery. A B

11 **Vv. digitales plantares communes II–IV**. Branches of Ramus superficialis of V. plantaris medialis. Accompany corresponding arteries. B

12 **Vv. digitales plantares propriae**. Arise from the variably shaped bifurcation of Vv. digitales plantares communes II, III and IV. B D

13 **V. interdigitalis**. Accompanies corresponding artery. B D

14 **V. plantaris lateralis**. Accompanies corresponding artery. Joins Ramus caudalis of V. saphena lateralis. A B D

15 **Arcus plantaris profundus**. Connection between V. plantaris lateralis and Ramus profundus of V. plantaris medialis, accompanies corresponding artery. B D

16 **Vv. metatarseae plantares II–IV**. Arise from Arcus plantaris profundus, accompany corresponding arteries. B

17 **Rami perforantes proximales II et IV**. Branches of Vv. metatarseae plantares, accompany corresponding arteries. B C D

18 **Vv. metatarseae dorsales II et IV**. Continuations of Rami perforantes proximales accompany corresponding arteries, join V. digitalis dorsalis. C D

19 **Ramus perforans distalis III**. Connects V. metatarsea plantaris with its dorsal counterpart. B C

20 ***V. genus descendens***. Accompanies corresponding artery. A

21 ***Vv. caudales femoris***. Accompany corresponding arteries. A

22 **V. poplitea**. Continuation of V. femoralis in poples. Accompanies corresponding artery. A

23 ***Vv. genus***. Drain Articulatio genus. A

24 ***V. tibialis cranialis***. Continuation of V. poplitea. It accompanies corresponding artery as a double vein. A C

25 *V. interossea cruris*. Accompanies corresponding artery. B C

26 *V. dorsalis pedis*. Extension of V. tibialis cranialis distal to Articulatio tarsocruralis. Double vein along A. dorsalis pedis. C

27 **V. tarsea lateralis**. Accompanies corresponding artery. C

28 **V. tarsea perforans proximalis**. Branch of V. tarsea lateralis, accompanies corresponding artery. C

29 **V. tarsea medialis**. Accompanies corresponding artery. C

30 **V. tarsea perforans distalis**. Connects V. dorsalis pedis and Arcus plantaris profundus via Canalis tarsi. C

31 **V. metatarsea dorsalis III**. Double continuation of V. dorsalis pedis, accompanies corresponding artery. C

32 ***V. tibialis caudalis***. To the caudal musculature of crus. A

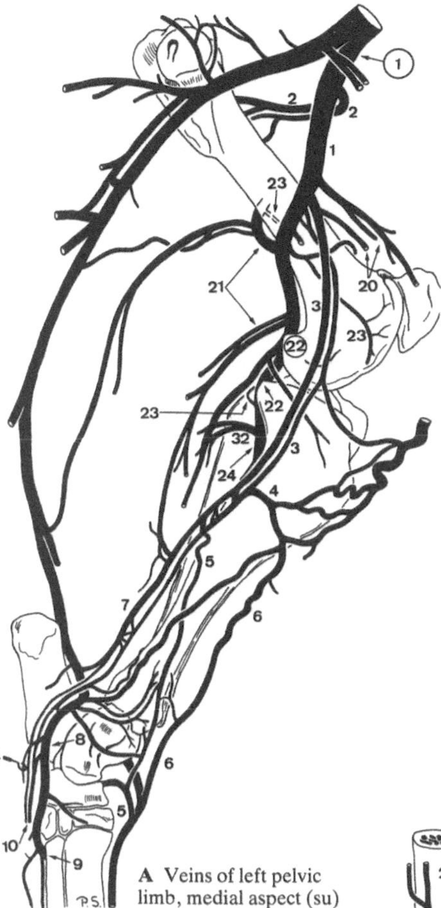

A Veins of left pelvic limb, medial aspect (su)

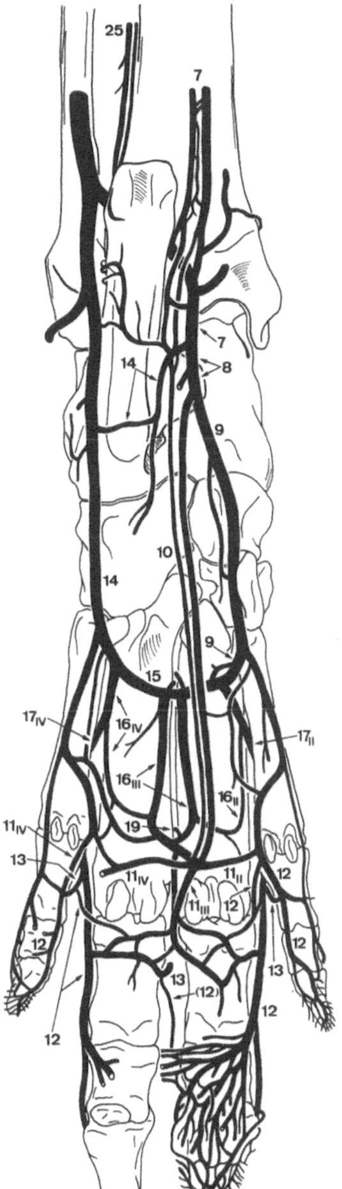

B Veins of left pes, plantar aspect (su)

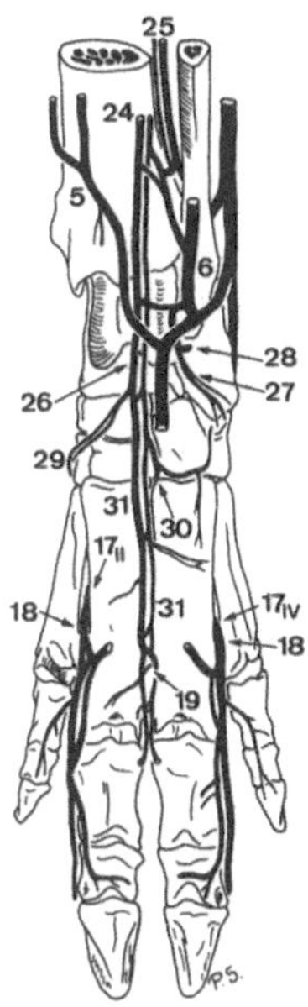

C Veins of left pes, dorsal aspect (su)

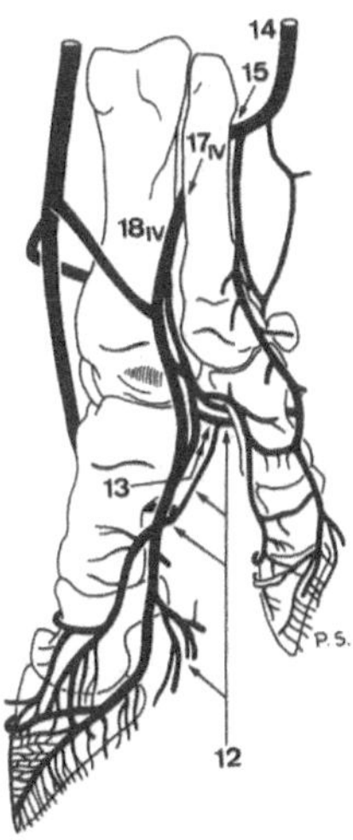

D Veins of left pes, lateral aspect (su)

RUMINANTIA

1 **V. femoralis**. Continuation of V. iliaca externa, accompanies corresponding artery. A

2 ***V. circumflexa femoris lateralis***. Accompanies corresponding artery. A

3 ***V. saphena medialis [magna]***. Pierces between M. sartorius and M. gracilis, courses superficially towards Articulatio genus and continues caudodistally along the caudomedial border of Corpus tibiae. A

4 *Ramus caudalis*. Continuation to the medioplantar aspect of tarsus. A B

5 **V. plantaris medialis**. Accompanies corresponding artery. A B

6 **Ramus profundus**. Accompanies corresponding artery. A B

7 **Ramus superficialis** (bo). Accompanies corresponding artery. A B D

8 **V. digitalis plantaris communis II**. Medial continuation of Ramus superficialis of V. plantaris medialis, reinforced by a large connection with Arcus plantaris profundus distalis. Accompanies corresponding artery. A B D

9 **V. digitalis plantaris propria II axialis**. Accompanies corresponding artery. A B

10 **V. digitalis plantaris propria III abaxialis**. Continuation of V. digitalis plantaris communis II. Accompanies corresponding artery. A B D

11 **V. coronalis**. Branch of V. digitalis plantaris propria III abaxialis, curves dorsally in the abaxial segment of Corona ungulae. A B

12 **V. digitalis plantaris communis III**. Lateral continuation of Ramus superficialis of V. plantaris medialis. Accompanies corresponding artery. A B D

13 **V. interdigitalis**. Connects V. digitalis plantaris communis III and its dorsal counterpart. B D

14 **Vv. digitales plantares propriae III et IV axiales**. Arise from the bifurcation of V. digitalis plantaris communis III, accompany corresponding arteries. B D

15 **V. coronalis**. Branch of V. digitalis plantaris propria in the axial segment of Corona ungulae. B D

16 **V. plantaris lateralis**. Accompanies corresponding artery. A B

17 **Arcus plantaris profundus**. Connection between V. plantaris lateralis and Ramus profundus of V. plantaris medialis. Accompanies corresponding artery. B

18 **Vv. metatarseae plantares III–IV**. Branches of Arcus plantaris profundus. Accompany corresponding arteries. A B D

19 **Arcus plantaris profundus distalis**. Variably shaped connection between Vv. metatarseae plantares II–IV, located distally between Os metatarsale III et IV and M. interosseus. B D

20 **Ramus perforans distalis III**. Branch of Arcus plantaris profundus distalis through Canalis metatarsi distalis, joins V. metatarsea dorsalis III. B

21 **Vv. digitales plantares communes IV (bo), II–IV** (ov, cap). Arise usually from Arcus plantaris profundus distalis, accompany corresponding arteries in the distal third of metatarsus. B D

22 **Vv. digitales plantares propriae**. Arise from the bifurcation of Vv. digitales plantares communes. Accompany corresponding arteries. B

23 ***V. genus descendens***. Accompanies corresponding artery. A

24 ***Vv. caudales femoris***. Variably arising, to the musculature in the poples. A

25 **V. poplitea**. Continuation of V. femoralis, accompanies corresponding artery. A

26 ***Vv. genus***. Variably developed, drain Articulatio genus. A

27 ***V. tibialis cranialis***. Continuation of V. poplitea. Usually represented by two anastomosing veins bordering A. tibialis cranialis. A C

28 *V. dorsalis pedis*. Continuation of V. tibialis cranialis distal to Articulatio tarsocruralis. A C

29 **V. tarsea perforans**. Accompanies corresponding artery, joins Arcus plantaris profundus. A C

30 **V. metatarsea dorsalis III**. Continuation of V. dorsalis pedis, accompanies corresponding artery. It courses proximally and represents the strong cranial root (branch) of the V. saphena lateralis* on the dorsolateral aspect of the distal crus. After a caudodorsal oblique route, it joins the caudal root. A C (The V. saphena lateralis is not listed in the 5th edition of the N. A. V., even though it is an obvious structure known as such by all anatomists and clinicians. It has a cranial branch and a medial branch, and is highly important in clinics as choice for blood samples and/or I. V. injections, and in large ruminants for indirect nerve block anesthesia.)

31 ***V. tibialis caudalis***. To the musculature at the caudal aspect of crus. Actually replaced by one of the V. caudalis femoris. A

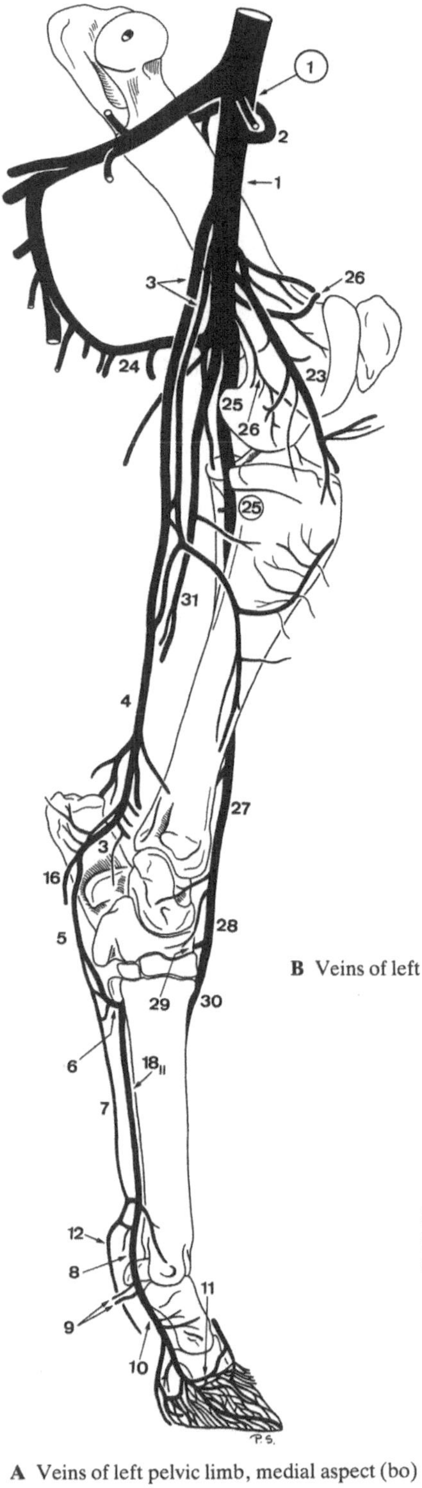

A Veins of left pelvic limb, medial aspect (bo)

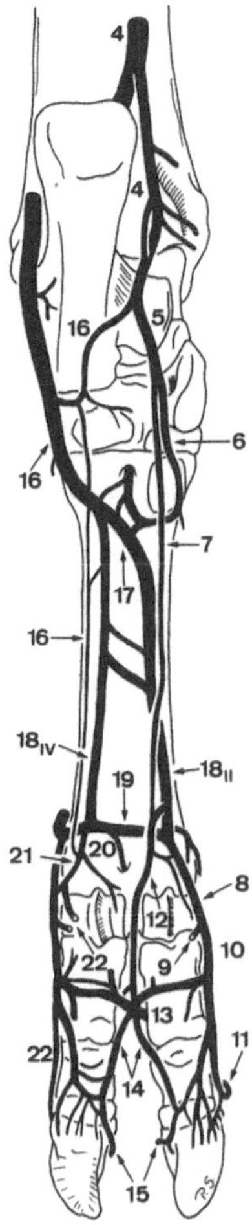

B Veins of left pes, plantar aspect (bo)

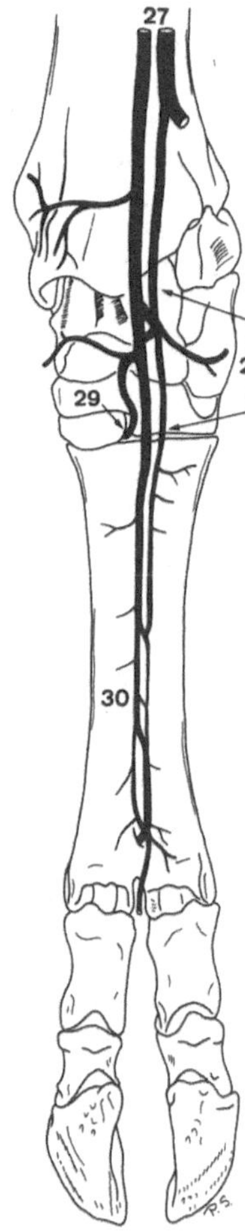

C Veins of left pes, dorsal aspect (bo)

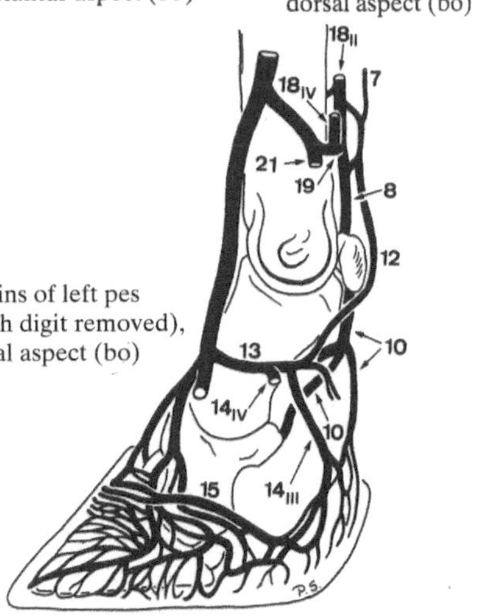

D Veins of left pes (fourth digit removed), abaxial aspect (bo)

EQUUS

1 **V. femoralis**. Continuation of V. iliaca externa. Accompanies corresponding artery. A

2 ***V. circumflexa femoris lateralis***. Accompanies corresponding artery. A

3 ***V. saphena medialis [magna]***. Courses superficially over the medial surface of the thigh, bifurcates in the proximal segment of Regio cruris medialis. A

4 *Ramus cranialis*. Courses to Facies medialis of Corpus tibiae, continues to the dorsomedial surface of tarsus, where it is connected with V. dorsalis pedis by a large anastomosis. A C

5 **V. digitalis dorsalis communis II**. Continuation of Ramus cranialis of V. saphena medialis, curves to the plantar aspect of metatarsus, joins Ramus superficialis of V. plantaris medialis. Largest vein of the equine metatarsus. A B C

6 *Ramus caudalis*. Accompanies corresponding artery, receives a large anastomosis from V. tibialis caudalis, bifurcates into Vv. plantares medialis and lateralis. A B

7 **V. plantaris medialis**. Accompanies corresponding artery. A B

8 **Ramus profundus**. Deep branch of V. plantaris medialis, accompanies corresponding artery. A

9 **Ramus superficialis [V. digitalis plantaris communis II]**. Continuation of V. plantaris medialis, accompanies corresponding artery, joins Arcus plantaris profundus distalis. A B

10 **V. digitalis [plantaris propria III] medialis**. Continuation of Ramus superficialis of V. plantaris medialis. Accompanies corresponding artery. A B

11 **V. coronalis**. Branch of V. digitalis medialis, curves proximal to Corona ungulae, and joins its counterpart. Its distal branches form the venous network of the corium of the hoof. A B

11a **Plexus ungularis**. Around Facies parietalis phalangis distalis. This network extends also on the solear surface. The plexus is defined as the dense venous network in Dermis ungulae. A

12 **Arcus terminalis**. Arch inside Canalis solearis, formed by the union of Vv. digitales lateralis and medialis. B

13 **V. plantaris lateralis**. Accompanies corresponding artery. A B

14 **Arcus plantaris profundus**. Connection between V. plantaris lateralis and Ramus profundus of V. plantaris medialis. Accompanies corresponding arterial arch. B

15 **Vv. metatarseae plantares II et III**. Branches of Arcus plantaris profundus. Accompany corresponding arteries. A B

16 **Arcus plantaris profundus distalis**. Connection between Rami superficiales of Vv. plantares lateralis and medialis plantar to M. interosseus medius in the distal third of metatarsus. Receives Vv. metatarseae plantares II et III. B D

17 **Ramus superficialis [V. digitalis plantaris communis III]**. Continuation of V. plantaris lateralis, accompanies corresponding artery along the lateral border of the tendon of M. flexor digitalis profundus and joins Arcus plantaris profundus distalis. B D

18 **V. digitalis [plantaris propria III] lateralis**. Continuation of Ramus superficialis of V. plantaris lateralis. Accompanies corresponding artery. B D

19 **V. coronalis**. Branch of V. digitalis lateralis, curves proximal to Corona ungulae, joins its medial counterpart. Its distal branches form the network of the corium of the hoof. B D

20 ***V. genus descendens***. Accompanies corresponding artery. A

21 ***V. caudalis femoris***. Accompanies corresponding artery. A

22 *V. saphena lateralis [parva]*. Courses along the M. gastrocnemius. A

23 **Ramus caudalis**. Continuation along the craniolateral border of Tendo calcaneus communis. A B

24 **V. poplitea**. Continuation of V. femoralis. Accompanies corresponding artery. A

25 ***Vv. genus***. Drain Articulatio genus. A

26 ***V. tibialis cranialis***. Continuation of V. poplitea, accompanies corresponding artery. C

27 *V. dorsalis pedis*. Variably developed continuation of V. tibialis cranialis distal to Articulatio tarsocruralis. C

28 **V. tarsea perforans**. Accompanies corresponding artery, joins Arcus plantaris profundus. B C

29 **V. metatarsea dorsalis II**. Continuation of V. dorsalis pedis over Facies dorsalis of Os metatarsale III. C

30 ***V. tibialis caudalis***. Accompanies corresponding artery, anastomoses with Ramus caudalis of V. saphena medialis. A B

31 *V. malleolaris caudalis lateralis*. Accompanies corresponding artery. A B

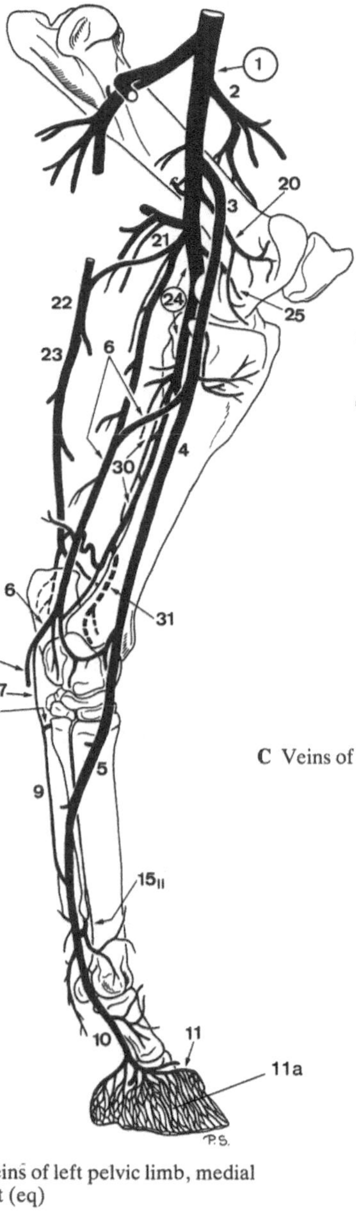

A Veins of left pelvic limb, medial aspect (eq)

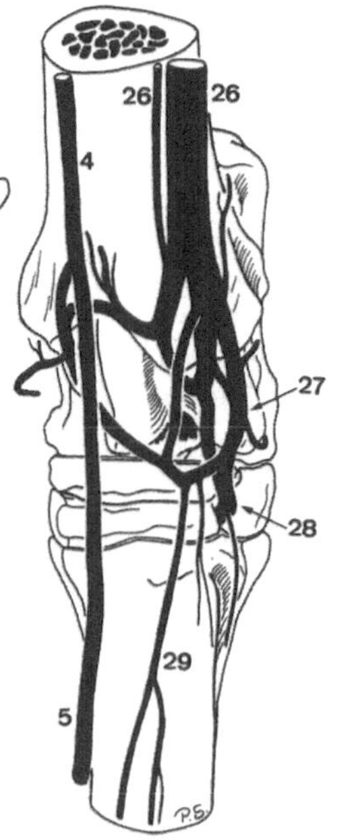

C Veins of left tarsus, dorsal aspect (eq)

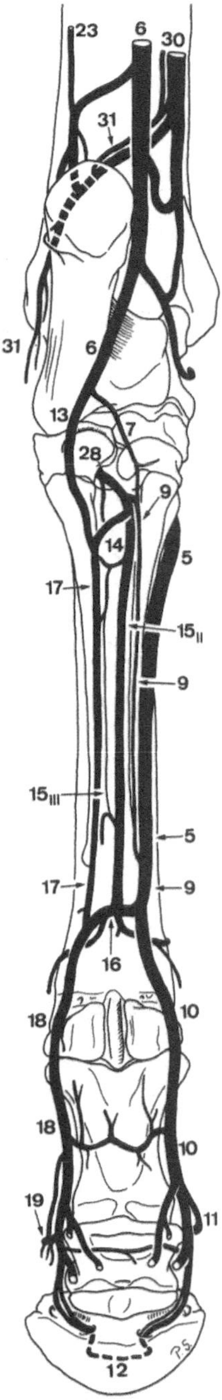

B Veins of left pes, plantar aspect (eq)

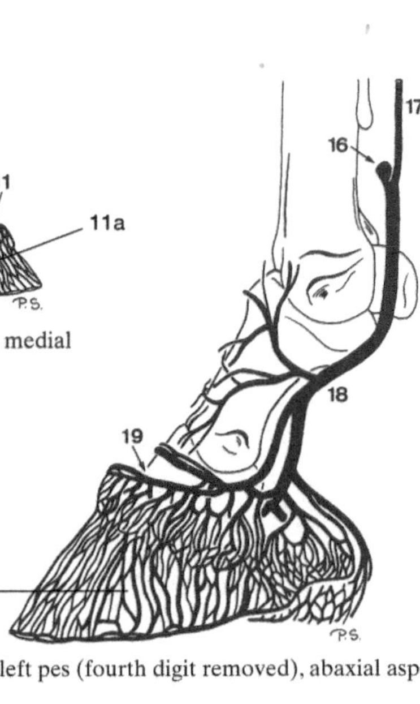

D Veins of left pes (fourth digit removed), abaxial aspect (bo)

1 **SYSTEMA LYMPHATICUM**. System of lymphatic organs (Lymphonodi, Lymphonoduli, Tonsillae, Lien, and Thymus) and lymphatic vessels.

2 ***Lymphonodus [Nodus lymphaticus].*** Organized lymphatic organ provided with a capsule. A B C D

3 ***Lymphonodus hemalis [haemalis].*** Spleen-like organization, contains lymphatic tissue with blood circulating in the sinuses. Occur in su and Ru.

4 ***Vas lymphaticum.*** Thin-walled vessel with valves which contains lymph. A B C D

5 *Vas lymphatica superficialia.* Cutaneous and subcutaneous lymphatic vessels. A

6 *Vasa lymphatica profunda.* Lymphatic vessels beneath the fasciae. A

7 ***Valvula lymphatica.*** Valve of one or two leaflets in lymphatic vessels. D

8 ***Plexus lymphaticus.*** Network of lymphatic vessels.

9 ***Lymphocentrum.*** A lymph node or a group of lymph nodes that occurs constantly in the same region and receives vessels from the same region in all species. A

10 **DUCTUS THORACICUS**. Starts near (Ru) or in Hiatus aorticus, courses along the right-dorsal (occasionally left-dorsal) side of Aorta thoracica, then at the level of the 6th thoracic vertebra to the left in Mediastinum craniale. It empties into V. cava cranialis near the point of origin of V. jugularis sinistra (interna, externa, or both) or V. subclavia sinistra. The point of entry is called left venous angle and can be identified at Apertura thoracis cranialis. May locally be plural. A C

11 ***Truncus trachealis [Truncus jugularis].*** Bilateral lymphatic duct along the trachea. Conveys lymph from head and neck. Usually the right duct ends in Ductus lymphaticus dexter (except cap), the left in Ductus thoracicus. A B

12 ***Ductus lymphaticus dexter.*** Lymphatic vessel in the right-caudal part of the neck, collecting lymph from cervical, thoracic and axillary lymph nodes and Truncus trachealis dexter. It empties at the right venous angle. May be absent. B

13 **CISTERNA CHYLI**. Lymphatic sac dorsal to Aorta abdominalis. Collects lymph from Truncus visceralis (or Truncus celiacus and Truncus intestinalis) and Trunci lumbales. Discharges into Ductus thoracicus. C

14 ***Trunci lumbales.*** Paired, collect lymph from pelvic limbs and pelvis to Cisterna chyli. May be plexiform (ca, su). C

15 ***Truncus visceralis.*** Unpaired, collects lymph from Truncus celiacus and Truncus intestinalis. May be absent (eq, sometimes cap) or plexiform (Car). C

16 ***Truncus celiacus [coeliacus].*** Collects lymph from Lymphocentrum celiacum, empties in Truncus visceralis (Car, su, Ru) or Cisterna chyli (eq). C

17 ***Truncus intestinalis.*** Collects lymph from Lymphocentrum mesentericum craniale, empties in Truncus visceralis (Car, su, Ru) or Cisterna chyli (eq, sometimes cap). May be plexiform (Car). C

18 ***Truncus colicus.*** Collects lymph from Lymphonodi colici, empties in Truncus intestinalis or Truncus visceralis (sometimes bo). May be plural (Car, su). C

19 ***Truncus jejunalis.*** Collects lymph from Lymphonodi jejunales, empties in Truncus intestinalis. May be plural (Car). C

20 ***Truncus gastricus.*** Collects lymph from the gastric lymph nodes, empties in Truncus celiacus or Cisterna chyli (Ru), sometimes Truncus intestinalis (cap). C

21 ***Truncus hepaticus.*** Collects lymph from Lymphonodi hepatici and hepatici accessorii. Joins Truncus celiacus or Truncus intestinalis (Ru). C

22 **LYMPHONODI [NODI LYMPHATICI]**. See 2

23 ***Vasa lymphatica afferentia.*** Lymphatic vessels which enter the convex surface (Car, Ru, eq) or the Hilus (su). D

24 ***Sinus lymphaticus.*** Subcapsular and medullary network of spaces. D

25 ***Vasa lymphatica efferentia.*** Leave the Lymphonodus through the Hilus (Car, Ru, eq) or at the periphery (su). D

26 ***Capsula.*** Capsule, contains some elastic and smooth muscle fibers. D

27 ***Cortex.*** Peripheral (Car, Ru, eq) or central (su) zone containing Lymphonoduli. D

28 ***Trabecula.*** Connective tissue cord. D

29 ***Medulla.*** Central (Car, Ru, eq) or peripheral (su) zone with lymphatic tissue organized in medullary cords. D

30 ***Hilus.*** Indentation for the entry of arteries, nerves, and Vasa afferentia (su) and the exit of veins and the Vasa efferentia (Car, Ru, eq). D

31 ***Lobulus.*** Segment incompletely separated by Trabeculae. D

32 ***Lymphonodulus [Nodulus lymphaticus].*** Small cell-rich mass of lymphatic tissue with no lumen. D

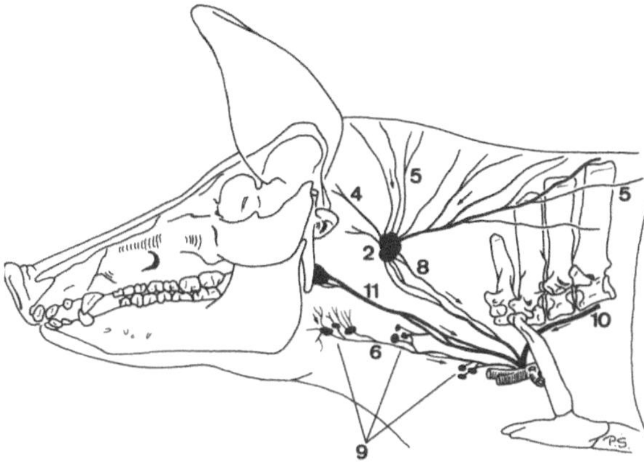

A Cervical lymph nodes, left lateral aspect (su)

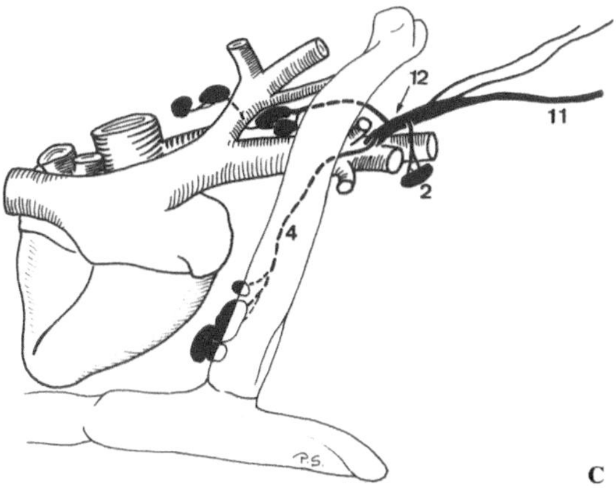

B Ductus lymphaticus dexter, right lateral aspect (su)

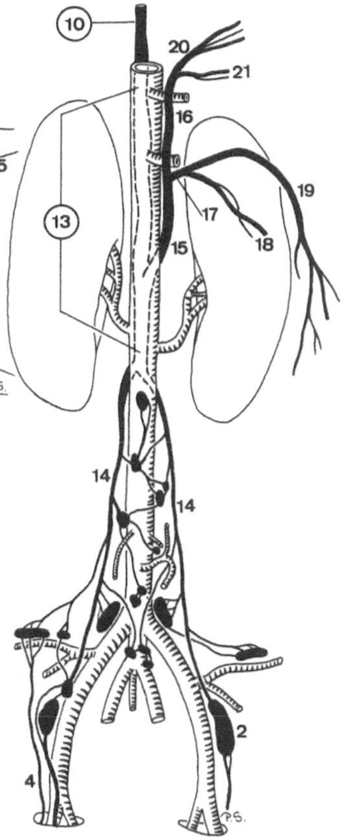

C Lymph vessels in relation to Aorta abdominalis, ventral aspect (su)

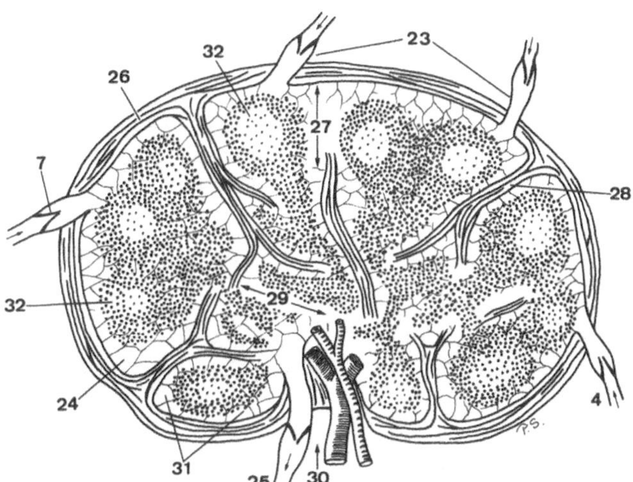

D Section of a lymph node (schematic)

1 **Lymphocentrum parotideum**. Near Gl. parotis. Drains the cranial regions. (This lymphocenter also includes Lymphonodi parotidei accessorii [Constantinescu et al. 1988], alternatively designated as Lymphonodi temporales [Casteleyn et al. 2008], which are frequently present in the temporal region of the ox.)

2 ***Lymphonodi parotidei superficiales*** (Car, su, bo, ov)*. Rostral to Gl. parotis. A

3 ***Lymphonodi parotidei profundi***. In or medial to Gl. parotis. A

4 **Lymphocentrum mandibulare**. In the caudal half of Regio intermandibularis. Drains the facial regions.

5 ***Lymphonodi mandibulares****. Near Angulus mandibulae (Car, su) or Incisura vasorum facialium (Ru, eq). A

6 ***Lymphonodi mandibulares accessorii*** (or, fe, su). At the bifurcation of V. jugularis externa, medial to Gl. parotis. A

6a ***Lymphonodus buccalis*** (or, ca). Occurs constantly in the rabbit, inconstant in the dog.

7 ***Lymphonodus pterygoideus*** (bo). Inconstant, near the rostral border of Ramus mandibulae, rostromedial to M. pterygoideus medialis. Drains Palatum durum. B

8 **Lymphocentrum retropharyngeum**. In Fossa retromandibularis. Drains the deep structures of the head, including nasal structures, larynx and pharynx.

9 ***Lymphonodi retropharyngei mediales****. On the dorsomedial pharyngeal wall. A B

10 ***Lymphonodi retropharyngei laterales****. Ventral to Ala atlantis at the caudomedial aspect of Gl. mandibularis (bo) and Gl. parotis. A B

11 ***Lymphonodus hyoideus rostralis*** (bo). Inconstant, at the lateral aspect of Thyrohyoideum. Drains Apex linguae. B

12 ***Lymphonodus hyoideus caudalis*** (bo). Inconstant, at Angulus stylohyoideus. Drains Mandibula. B

13 **Lymphocentrum cervicale superficiale**. Receives the cervical Vasa lymphatica superficialia and drains thoracic limb and thoracic wall.

14 ***Lymphonodi cervicales superficiales*** (ca, Ru, eq)*. Craniodorsal to Articulatio humeri, medial to M. cleidocephalicus, M. omotransversarius and M. trapezius (eq). C D E

15 ***Lymphonodi cervicales superficiales dorsales*** (fe, su). At the medial aspect of M. trapezius and M. omotransversarius. A

16 ***Lymphonodi cervicales superficiales medii*** (or, su). Medial to M. cleidocephalicus. A

17 ***Lymphonodi cervicales superficiales ventrales*** (or, fe, su). Along the dorsal border of V. jugularis externa (or), between M. cleidocephalicus and V. jugularis externa (fe), Gl. parotis (su). Drain also thoracic mammae (su). A

18 ***Lymphonodi cervicales superficiales accessorii*** (bo, ov.). Medial to M. trapezius and M. omotransversarius. Receive lymph from Regio nuchalis. C D

19 **Lymphocentrum cervicale profundum**. Chain of lymph nodes along trachea, draining the deep cervical structures.

20 ***Lymphonodi cervicales profundi craniales*** (abs. or). Along the cranial portion of trachea. Drain also lymph from the head. B

21 ***Lymphonodi cervicales profundi medii***. Along the middle third of trachea. C

22 ***Lymphonodi cervicales profundi caudales***. Near trachea cranial to the first rib. Drain also Lymphocentrum axillare (bo, eq) and Truncus trachealis (eq). C

23 ***Lymphonodus costocervicalis*** (Ru). At the craniomedial aspect of the first rib near Truncus costocervicalis. C

24 ***Lymphonodus subrhomboideus*** (bo). Inconstant, at the ventromedial aspect of M. rhomboideus cervicis. Drains muscles of the neck and shoulder. C

25 **Lymphocentrum axillare**. Receives the deep lymphatic vessels from the thoracic limb and the lateral thoracic wall.

26 ***Lymphonodi axillares***[1]. Collective term for all lymph nodes caudomedial to Articulatio humeri.

27 ***Lymphonodi axillares proprii*** (abs. su). Caudomedial to Articulatio humeri. Absent in su and sometimes ov. C D E

28 ***Lymphonodi axillares primae costae*** (fe, su, Ru). Lateral to the first rib near V. axillaris. Sometimes absent in fe, bo. C

29 ***Lymphonodus axillaris accessorius*** (or, Car, bo, ov). At the dorsal border of M. pectoralis profundus. Often absent, described also in eq. C

30 ***Lymphonodi pectorales***[1]. Not described in domestic mamals.

31 ***Lymphonodi subscapulares***[1]. Not described in domestic mamals.

32 ***Lymphonodi cubitales*** (ov, eq). Medioproximal to Articulatio cubiti. Inconstant in ov. E

33 ***Lymphonodus infraspinatus*** (bo). Inconstant, at the caudal border of M. infraspinatus. D

1) These terms were omitted from the 5th edition of the N. A. V.

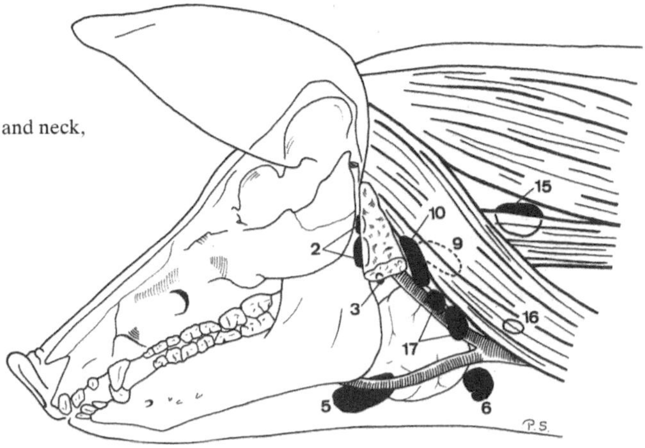

A Lymphocentres of head and neck, left lateral aspect (su)

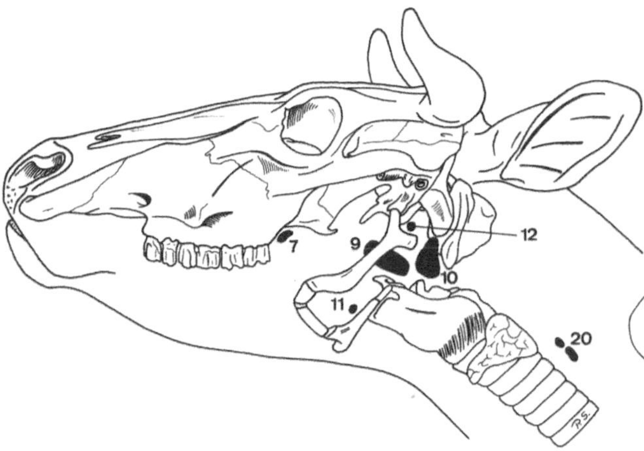

B Lymphocentrum retropharyngeum, left lateral aspect (bo)

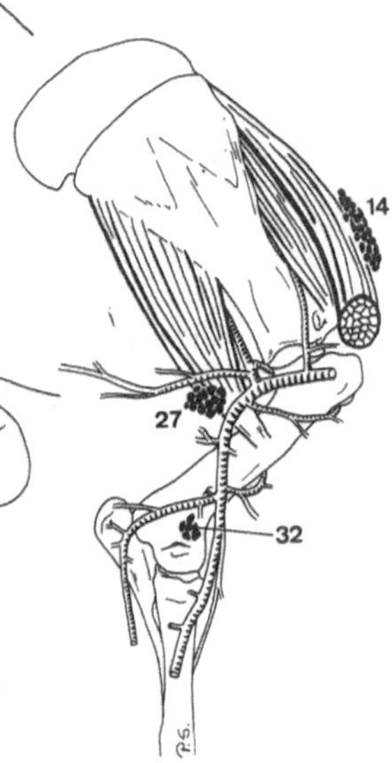

E Cervical and axillary lymph nodes, left medial aspect (eq)

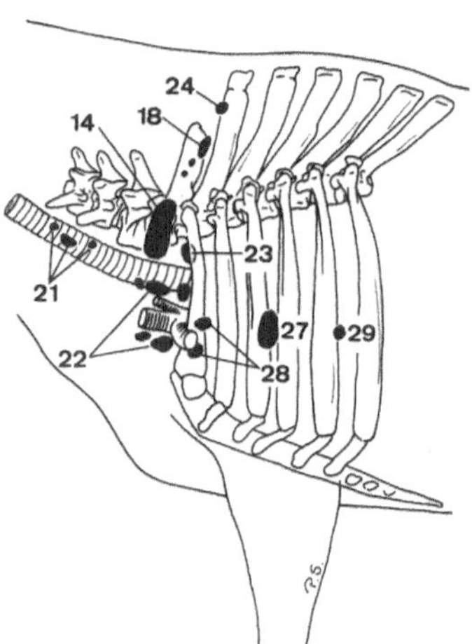

C Cervical and axillary lymphocentres, left lateral aspect (bo)

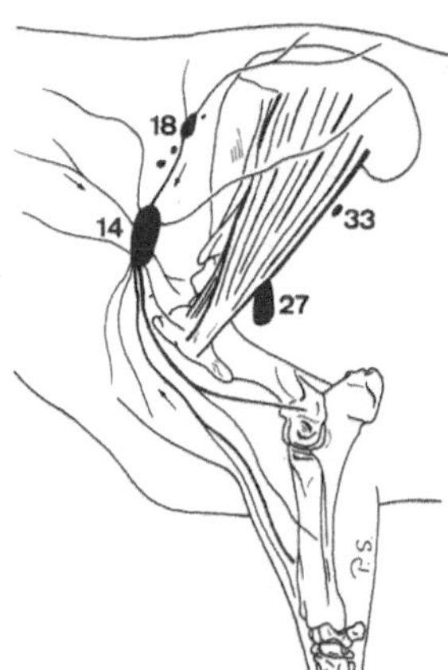

D Cervical and axillary lymph nodes, left lateral aspect (bo)

1 **Lymphocentrum thoracicum dorsale**. Along the dorsal aspect of Aorta thoracica. Primarily draining the dorsal and lateral parts of the thoracic wall, Diaphragma and Mediastinum.

2 ***Lymphonodi thoracici aortici*** (abs. ca). At the dorsolateral side of Aorta thoracica. Absent sometimes also in fe. A

3 ***Lymphonodi intercostales*** (abs. or). In Spatia intercostalia near Capita costarum, covered by pleura and Fascia endothoracica. May be absent in Car, su. A

4 **Lymphocentrum thoracicum ventrale**. Along the dorsal aspect of sternum. Primarily draining the ventral and lateral thoracic wall, Diaphragma and Mediastinum.

5 ***Lymphonodi sternales***. Located upon the dorsal aspect of sternum. (These structures were omitted from the 5th edition of the N. A. V.)

6 ***Lymphonodi sternales craniales***. Near the dorsal aspect of Manubrium sterni. Rarely absent (ca, eq). A C

7 ***Lymphonodi sternales caudales*** (abs. ca, su). Along A. and V. thoracica interna, dorsal and ventral (ov, bo) or caudal (eq) to M. transversus thoracis, inconstant in fe, eq. C

7a ***Lymphonodus epigastricus cranialis superficialis*** (or, fe). Lies along A. et V. epigastrica cranialis superficialis near Processus xiphoideus.

8 ***Lymphonodi phrenici*** (fe, bo, eq). Near Foramen venae cavae (fe, eq – very small and rarely present in fe) or Pars sternalis of Diaphragma (bo, eq). Usually single or absent in eq. C

9 **Lymphocentrum mediastinale**. Located in mediastinum. Drains thoracic walls and organs.

10 ***Lymphonodi mediastinales craniales***. In Mediastinum craniale. A

11 ***Lymphonodi mediastinales medii*** (Ru, eq). In Mediastinum medium near Basis cordis at the right aspect of Arcus aortae. Absent sometimes in eq. A

12 ***Lymphonodi mediastinales caudales*** (abs. Car). In Mediastinum caudale along esophagus. Absent sometimes also in eq. A

13 ***Lymphonodus nuchalis*** (eq). Near A. and V. cervicalis profunda on the medial surface of M. longissimus cervicis. Occasionally absent. A

14 **Lymphocentrum bronchale**. Drains lungs, heart, pericardium, parts of trachea, esophagus and mediastinum.

15 ***Lymphonodi tracheobronchales [bifurcationis] dextri*** (abs. ov). At the right aspect of trachea near Bifurcatio tracheae. Inconstant in cap, bo. B

16 ***Lymphonodi tracheobronchales [bifurcationis] sinistri***. At the left aspect of trachea near Bifurcatio tracheae. A B

17 ***Lymphonodi tracheobronchales [bifurcationis] medii*** (abs. or, ov). At the caudodorsal aspect of Bifurcatio tracheae. Inconstant in cap, bo. A B

18 ***Lymphonodi tracheobronchales craniales*** (su, Ru). Ventral to the initial part of Bronchus trachealis. B

19 ***Lymphonodi pulmonales***. Inconstant, inside (fe, cap, bo, eq) or at (ca) the lung tissue near Bronchi principales. B

20 **Lymphocentrum lumbale**. Along Aorta abdominalis and V. cava caudalis. Drains the deep layers of the dorsal abdominal wall and organs of Regio lumbalis.

21 ***Lymphonodi lumbales aortici***. Located along Aorta abdominalis and V. cava caudalis. D E

22 ***Lymphonodi lumbales proprii*** (bo). Inconstant, near Foramina intervertebralia between Vertebra thoracica XIII and Vertebrae lumbales. E

23 ***Lymphonodi renales***. Near A. et V. renalis at Hilus renalis. Difficult to distinguish from Lnn. lumbales aortici in Car. D

24 ***Lymphonodus phrenicoabdominalis*** (su). Inconstant, at the lateral border of M. psoas major, caudal to A. and V. abdominalis cranialis. D

25 ***Lymphonodus ovaricus*** (eq). Inconstant, in Ligamentum suspensorium ovarii, drains Ovarium.

26 ***Lymphonodus testicularis*** (su). Inconstant, variably along A. and V. testicularis. May be plural. Drains testis and epididymis. D

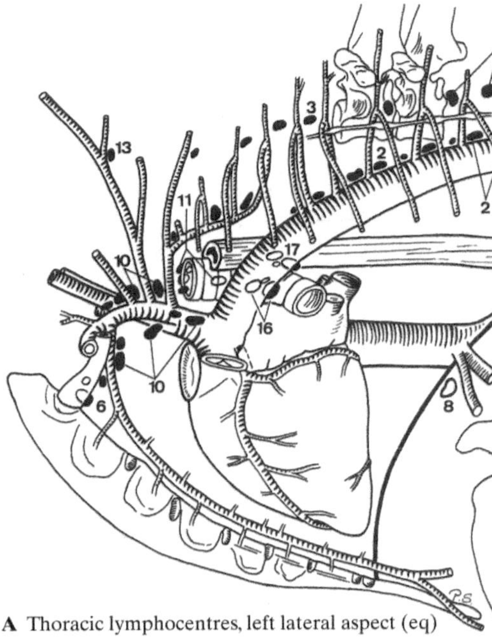

A Thoracic lymphocentres, left lateral aspect (eq)

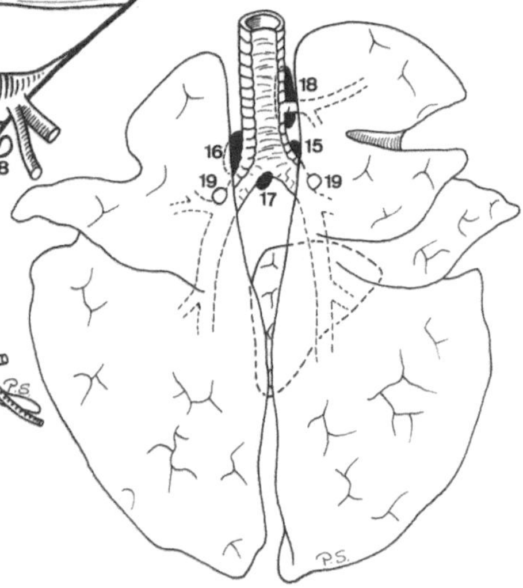

B Lymphocentrum bronchale, dorsal aspect (cap)

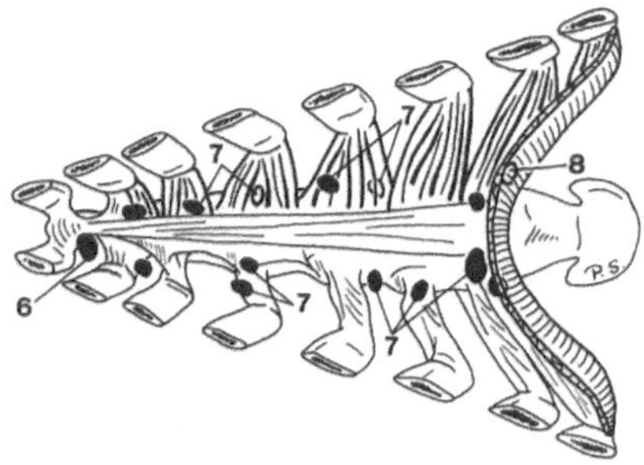

C Lymphocentrum thoracicum ventrale, dorsal aspect (bo)

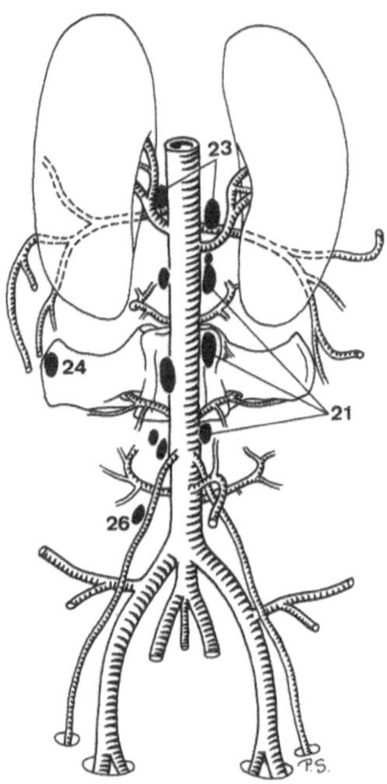

D Lymphocentrum lumbale, ventral aspect (su)

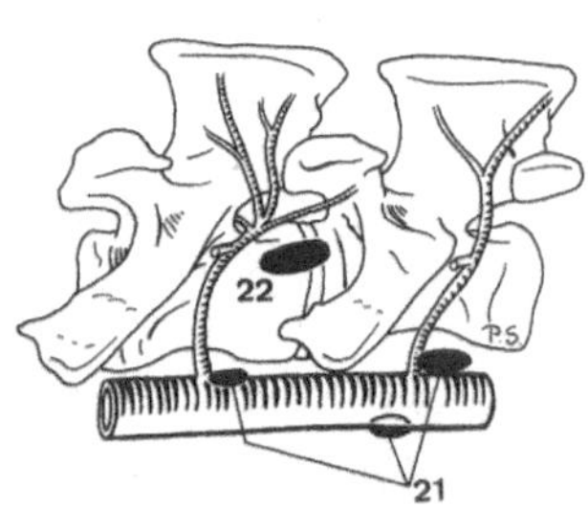

E Lymph nodes in relation to lumbar vertebrae IV and V, left lateral aspect (bo)

1 **Lymphocentrum celiacum [coeliacum].** Along A. celiaca and its branches. Drains the intrathoracally located abdominal organs. Receives lymph also from thoracic organs (ca, su, eq).

2 ***Lymphonodi celiaci [coeliaci]*** (Un). Along A. celiaca. Hard to differentiate from the adjacent lymph nodes (Lnn mesenterici craniales in Ru). Their efferent lymphatic vessels form the Truncus celiacus. A

3 ***Lymphonodi lienales*** (abs. or). Along A. and V. lienalis near Hilus lienis (Car, su, eq) or upon Atrium ruminis (Ru). May be absent (fe). A C

4 ***Lymphonodi gastrici.*** At A. gastrica sinistra near Curvatura ventriculi minor. May be absent (Car) or single (Car, su), in Ru divided into specific groups. A

5 ***Lymphonodi ruminales dextri*** (Ru). In Sulcus longitudinalis dexter of rumen. May be absent or single (cap). C

6 ***Lymphonodi ruminales sinistri*** (bo, ov). In Sulcus longitudinalis sinister of rumen. May be absent. D

7 ***Lymphonodi ruminales craniales*** (bo, cap). Deep in Sulcus cranialis of the rumen. Usually absent in ov, cap. C

8 ***Lymphonodi reticulares*** (Ru). On reticulum. May be absent. C

9 ***Lymphonodi omasiales*** (Ru). Along A. et V. gastrica sinistra near Curvatura omasi. C

10 ***Lymphonodi ruminoabomasiales*** (Ru). Between the cranioventral border of rumen and the initial segment of abomasum. May be absent (ov). D

11 ***Lymphonodi reticuloabomasiales*** (bo, cap). In the angle between rumen, reticulum, omasum, and abomasum. May be absent in cap. C D

12 ***Lymphonodi abomasiales dorsales*** (Ru). Along Curvatura minor of abomasum. C

13 ***Lymphonodi abomasiales ventrales*** (Ru). Along the caudal part of Curvatura major of abomasum. May be absent.

14 ***Lymphonodi hepatici [portales].*** Near Porta hepatis. A B

15 ***Lymphonodi hepatici accessorii*** (bo). Along Margo dorsalis of the liver near V. cava caudalis. B

16 ***Lymphonodi pancreaticoduodenales.*** At Pars descendens of duodenum and pancreas. A

17 ***Lymphonodi omentales*** (or, eq). In Omentum majus near Curvatura ventriculi major. A

18 **Lymphocentrum mesentericum craniale.** Along A. mesenterica cranialis and its branches. Drains the intestinal organs supplied by those arteries.

19 ***Lymphonodi mesenterici craniales*** (abs. Car). At A. mesenterica cranialis. Inconstant in su, cap. Hard to differentiate from the adjacent lymph nodes (esp. Ru). E

20 ***Lymphonodi jejunales.*** In mesenterium near Aa. et Vv. jejunales. More or less concentrated near the root (Car, eq) or near the intestinal attachment (su, bo) of mesenterium. In bo between the Jejunum and the last centrifugal coil of the Ansa spiralis coli. In ov, cap located between the first centripetal coil and the last centrifugal coil of Ansa spiralis coli. E

20a ***Lymphonodi ileocecales [ileocaecales]*** (abs. or, ca, cap). Located within Plica ileocecalis. E

21 ***Lymphonodi ileocolici*** (su, ov, cap). Positioned at the ileocolic junction near Ostium ileale. In su located within the Mesoileum and the most proximal part of the Mesocolon, whereas in ov, cap against the intestinal wall.

22 ***Lymphonodi cecales [caecales]*** (eq). In Plica ileocecalis (eq) and along Teniae medialis, lateralis and dorsalis of cecum (eq). Described also in fe, ov, cap.

23 ***Lymphonodi colici*** (abs. or). All lymph nodes that are located along the various segments of the colon, except those that lie directly at the ileocolic junction are called Lymphonodi colici. E

24 **Lymphocentrum mesentericum caudale.** At A. mesenterica caudalis and its branches, draining Colon descendens and rectum.

25 ***Lymphonodi mesenterici caudales.*** In Mesocolon descendens and sigmoideum and Mesorectum near A. mesenterica caudalis and its branches. E

26 ***Lymphonodi vesicales*** (eq). Occasionally single, in Ligamentum vesicae laterale. Drain Vesica urinaria (and Prostata).

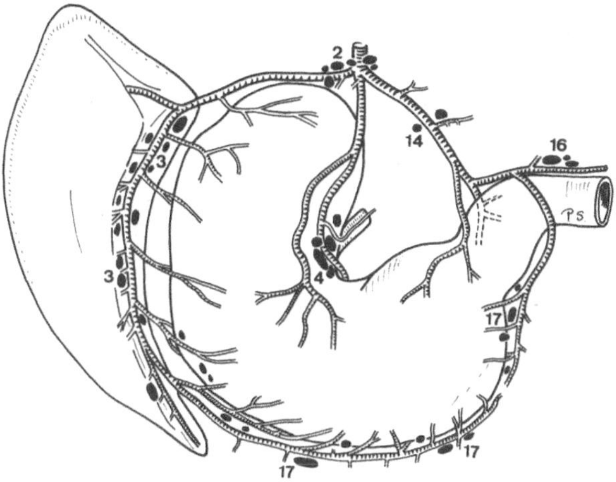

A Lymphocentrum celiacum, caudal aspect (eq)

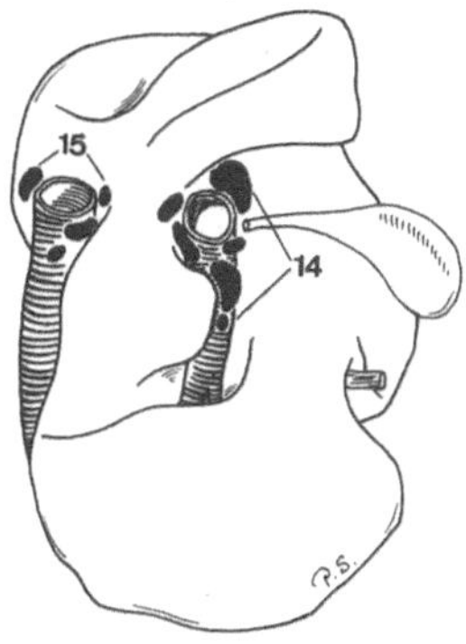

B Lymph nodes on the visceral surface of the liver (bo)

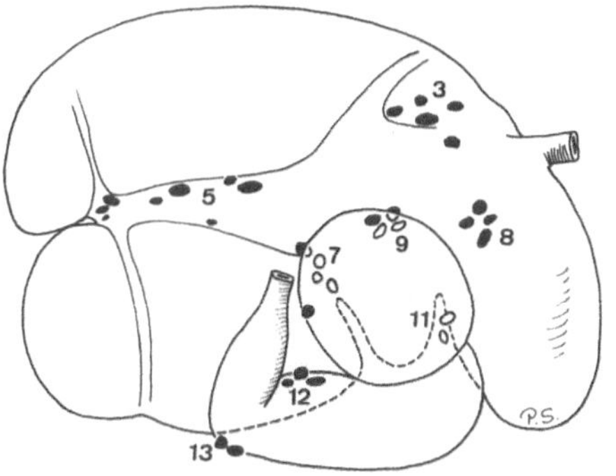

C Lymph nodes on the stomach, right aspect (bo)

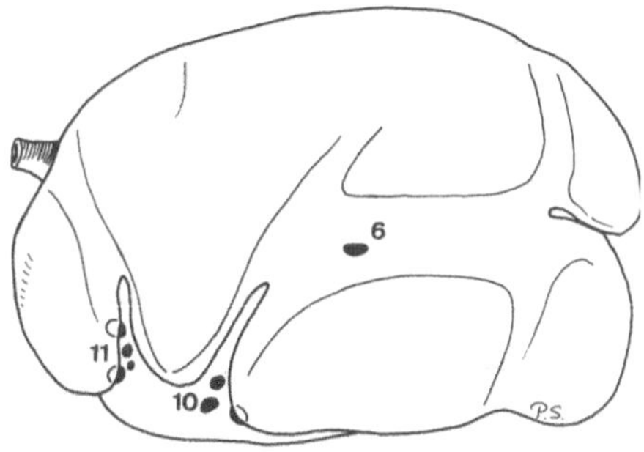

D Lymph nodes on the stomach, left aspect (bo)

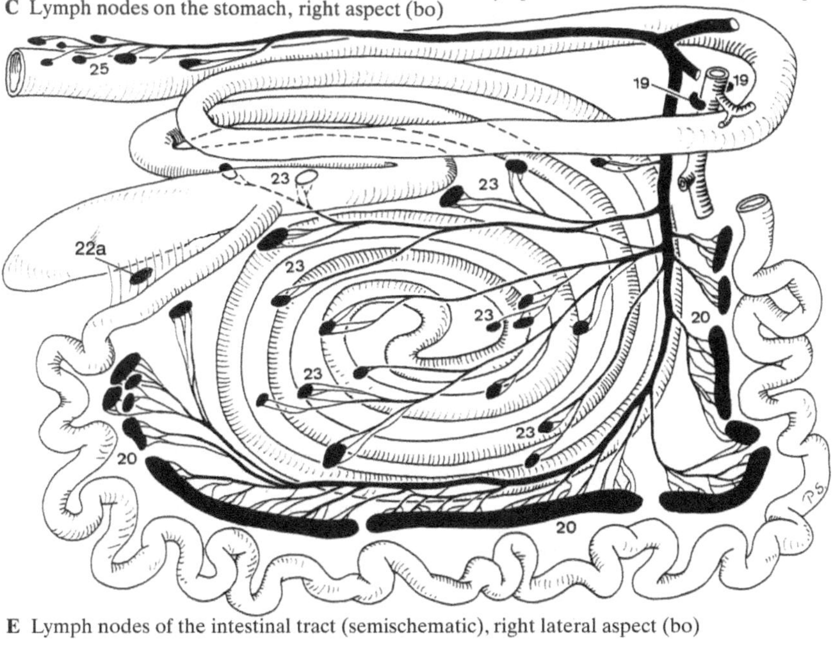

E Lymph nodes of the intestinal tract (semischematic), right lateral aspect (bo)

1 **Lymphocentrum iliosacrale**. At Facies pelvina of Os sacrum and the terminal segments of aorta and V. cava caudalis. Drains the pelvic wall, pelvic organs and Lymphocentra iliofemorale, inguinofemorale, ischiadicum and popliteum.

2 ***Lymphonodi iliaci mediales***. Along A. iliaca communis (or), or the terminal segment of aorta (Car, Un) and V. iliaca communis. A B D

3 ***Lymphonodi sacrales*** (abs. eq). Unpaired, variably developed, at the origin of A. et V. sacralis mediana. A B

4 ***Lymphonodi iliaci laterales*** (su, bo, ov, eq). Along A. et V. circumflexa ilium profunda. B

5 ***Lymphonodi iliaci interni***. Near A. et V. iliaca interna and variably its branches. Formerly lymphonodi hypogastrici. A D

6 ***Lymphonodi anorectales*** (Un). Retroperitoneally upon the dorsolateral surface of rectum (su, Ru, eq) and Canalis analis (bo, eq). Absent sometimes in su, ov. D

7 ***Lymphonodus uterinus*** (su, eq). In Ligamentum latum uteri. Often absent (su, eq) or plural (su). D

8 ***Lymphonodus obturatorius*** (eq). Occasional, at the initial segment of A. et V. obturatoria. D

9 **Lymphocentrum iliofemorale**. The former alternative term Lymphocentrum inguinale profundum has been deleted because many of the lymph nodes of this lymphocenter lie not in the inguinal region but at the entrance of the pelvic cavity along A. et V. iliaca externa.

10 ***Lymphonodi iliaci externi*** (abs. eq). At the cranial aspect of Corpus ossis ilii along A. et V. iliaca externa . A B

10a ***Lymphonodi femorales***. A collective term for the lymph nodes that lie in the Canalis femoralis along A. et V. femoralis.

10b *Lymphonodi femorales proximales [inguinalis profundi]* (eq). Large lymph nodes that lie in the Canalis femoralis along A. et V. femoralis.

11 *Lymphonodus femoralis distalis* (Car). Inconstant lymph node that lies distally in the Canalis femoralis of Car. A

12 ***Lymphonodus epigastricus caudalis profundus*** (bo). Inconstant. Along A. et V. epigastrica caudalis near Pecten ossis pubis. Drains the ventral abdominal wall.

13 **Lymphocentrum inguinofemorale**. In Regiones abdominalis lateralis and caudalis. Drains the abdominal and ventral pelvic walls, the superficial parts of thigh and the external genital organs. The former alternative term Lymphocentrum inguinale superficiale has been deleted because several lymph nodes of this lymphocenter are remote from the proper inguinal region.

14 ***Lymphonodi inguinales superficiales****. Superficially in Regio pubica.

15 *Lymphonodi scrotales**. Along the dorsolateral aspect of penis (except fe) cranial (Car, su, eq) and/or caudal (su, Ru, eq) to Funiculus spermaticus. Drain penis and scrotum. C

16 *Lymphonodi mammarii**. At the caudodorsal (Car, su, Ru) or dorsal (eq) aspect of the inguinal mammae. Often accompanied by intramammary lymph nodes in bo. Drain mammae and Pudendum femininum. D

17 ***Lymphonodi subiliaci****. Located in Plica lateralis halfway between Tuber coxae and patella. Usually absent in Car. C

17a ***Lymphonodi epigastrici caudales superficiales*** (or, fe). Lie on the homonymous blood vessels.

18 ***Lymphonodus coxalis*** (bo, ov, eq). Near the ventral aspect of Tuber coxae, medial to M. tensor fasciae latae. May be absent (esp. eq). C

19 ***Lymphonodus coxalis accessorius*** (bo). Inconstant, inside of, or lateral to, M. tensor fasciae latae. C

20 ***Lymphonodi fossae paralumbalis*** (bo)*. Inconstant, often single, subcutaneous, in the center of Fossa paralumbalis. C

21 **Lymphocentrum ischiadicum**. In Regiones glutea, clunis and tuberis ischiadici at the lateral aspect of Ligamentum sacrotuberale latum. Drains the regional musculature and skin.

22 ***Lymphonodi ischiadici*** (abs. ca). At Incisura ischiadica minor, lateral to the Ligamentum sacrotuberale latum, near A. et V. glutea caudalis. Absent sometimes in su, ov, cap. C

23 ***Lymphonodus gluteus [glutaeus]*** (su, bo, ov). Near Incisura ischiadica major, lateral to Ligamentum sacrotuberale latum. C

24 ***Lymphonodus tuberalis*** (Ru). Inconstant, subcutaneous, dorsomedial to Tuber ischiadicum. C

25 **Lymphocentrum popliteum**. In Regio poplitea, drains the distal parts of the pelvic limb.

26 ***Lymphonodi poplitei***. In poples.

27 *Lymphonodi poplitei profundi* (Un). Deep in poples, caudoproximal to M. gastrocnemius. May be absent (su). C

28 *Lymphonodi poplitei superficiales* (or, Car, su)*. Superficially in Fossa poplitea, exceptionally absent in su.

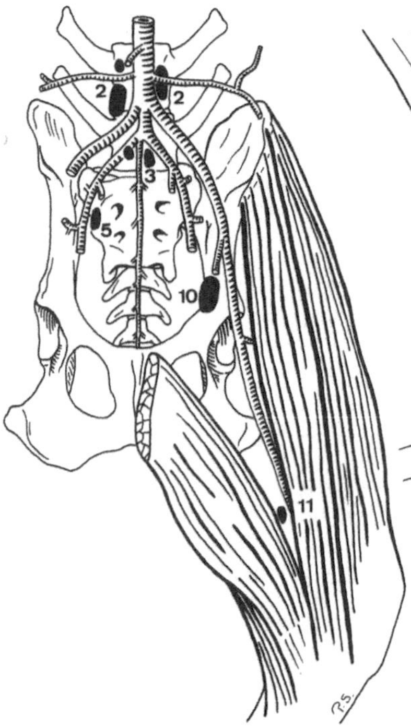

A Iliosacral and -femoral lymphocentres, ventral aspect (ca)

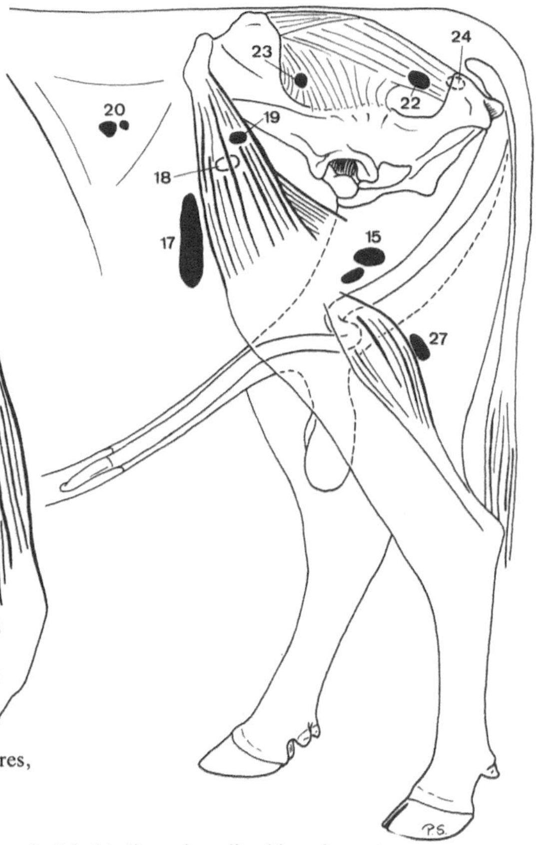

C Inguinal, ischiadic, and popliteal lymphocentres, left lateral aspect (bo masc)

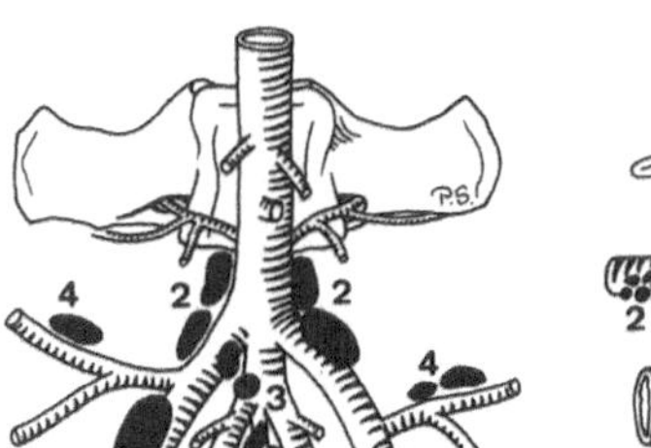

B Lymph nodes in relation to the terminal branches of Aorta abdominalis, ventral aspect (bo)

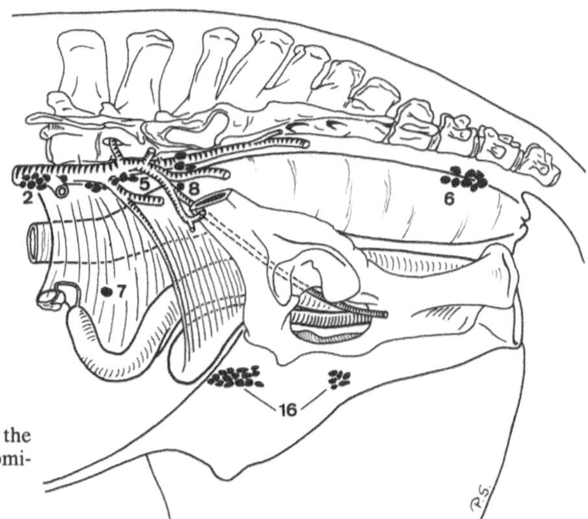

D Iliosacral and inguinal lymphocentres, left lateral aspect (eq fem)

1 **LIEN [SPLEN]**. Large abdominal lymphatic organ incorporated into the circulatory system. Variably shaped: falciform (Car, eq), elongated elliptical (su, bo), palm-shaped or triangular (ov, cap). A B C

2 ***Facies parietalis [diaphragmatica]***. Convex lateral surface, facing Diaphragma (Ru, eq) and the left-cranial abdominal wall. A C

3 ***Facies visceralis***. Concave medial surface. Contains hilus. Largely free of Tunica serosa in Ru. B

4 *Facies renalis*. Dorsal part of Facies visceralis facing the left kidney. Absent in Ru. B

5 *Facies gastrica*. Cranial part of Facies visceralis, faces the stomach. In Ru the entire Facies visceralis. B C

6 *Facies intestinalis*. Caudal segment of Facies visceralis, faces portions of jejunum and colon. Absent in Ru. B C

7 ***Extremitas dorsalis***. Dorsal extremity. A B

8 ***Extremitas ventralis***. Ventral extremity. A B

9 ***Margo cranialis***. Cranial border. A B C

10 ***Margo caudalis***. Caudal border. A B C

11 ***Hilus lienis***. Longitudinal ridge (Car, su, eq) or round depression (Ru) at Facies visceralis for entrance of nerves and arteries, for exit of veins and lymphatic vessels. B C

12 ***Tunica serosa***. Peritoneal layer covering the spleen, except at the Hilus and the larger portion of Facies visceralis (Ru). C

13 ***Capsula***. Thick capsule. Consists of collagen, elastic and smooth muscle fibers. C

14 ***Trabeculae lienis***. Centripetal cords of collagen, elastic and smooth muscle fibers which leave the capsule. Contain arteries, veins, nerves, and lymph vessels. C

15 ***Pulpa lienis rubra***. Red pulp. System of sinuses formed by reticular connective tissue, filled with blood cells. C

16 ***Pulpa lienis alba***. White pulp. Accumulations of cell-rich lymphatic tissue which surround the initial segments of the intraparenchymatous Rami lienales arteriae lienalis, forming periarterial lymphatic sheaths of larger Lymphonoduli. C

17 ***Rami lienales [arteriae lienalis]***. Branches of A. lienalis, enter capsule and trabeculae, continue in Pulpa lienis alba and then through Pulpa lienis rubra, and finally ramify brush-like into pulp arterioles. B C

18 ***Lymphonoduli [Noduli lymphatici] lienales***. Spherical accumulations of cell-rich lymphatic tissue, surround the intraparenchymatous Rami lienales arteriae lienalis locally. C

19 ***(Lien accessorius)***. Occasional small island of additional splenic tissue, described also in Ligamentum gastrolienale of su.

20 **THYMUS**. Variably shaped primary lymphatic organ which undergoes involution in the postfetal life. D

21 ***Lobus cervicalis [dexter et sinister]***. Cervical portion of thymus extending cranially along both sides of trachea. Size in young animals: large (su, Ru), variably but usually small (fe, eq), absent (ca). D

22 ***Lobus intermedius***. Bridge of thymic tissue through Apertura thoracis cranialis, connecting Lobi cervicales with Lobus thoracicus. Bilateral in su. D

23 ***Lobus thoracicus [dexter et sinister]***. Intrathoracic portion of thymus, located in the ventral (Car, su, eq) or dorsal (Ru) part of Mediastinum craniale. Left and right lobes are apparently fused. D

24 ***Lobuli thymici***. Lobules of thymus, incompletely separated by thin strands of connective tissue. D

25 *Cortex*. Peripheral part of the lobule.

26 *Medulla*. Central part of the lobule.

27 ***(Noduli thymici accessorii)***. Occasional clusters of additional thymic tissue, described also in bo.

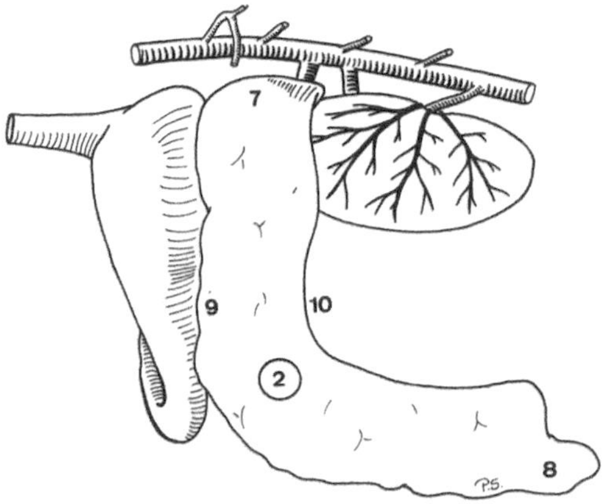

A Topography of the spleen, left/lateral aspect (fe)

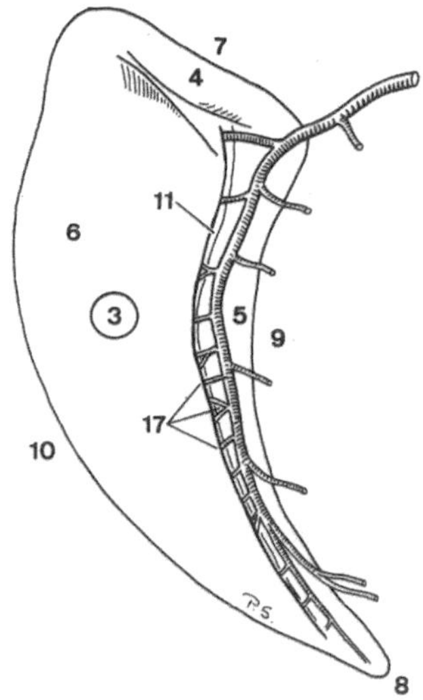

B Spleen, right/medial aspect (eq)

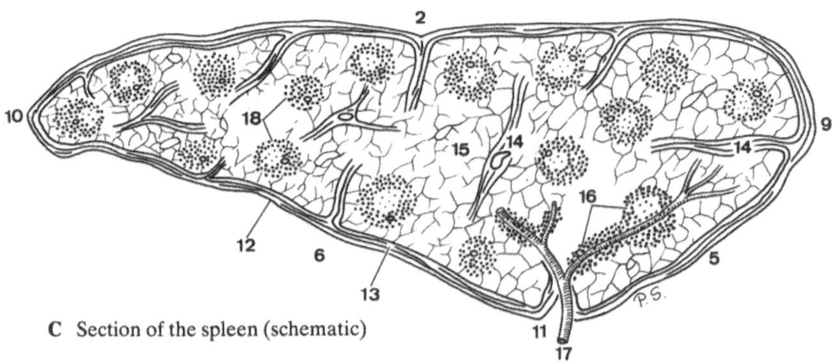

C Section of the spleen (schematic)

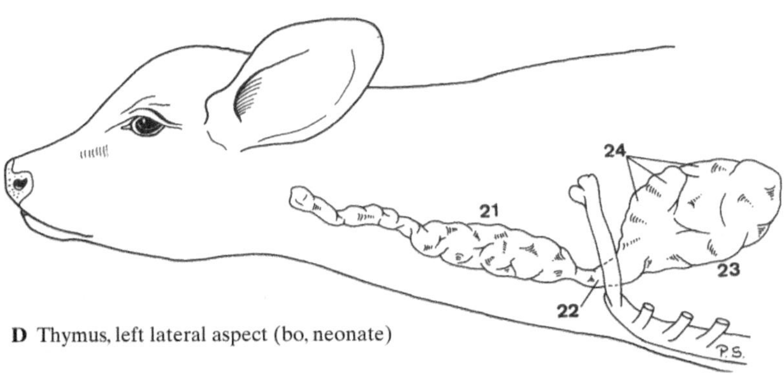

D Thymus, left lateral aspect (bo, neonate)

1 **SYSTEMA NERVOSUM CENTRALE.** Central nervous system.

2 **MEDULLA SPINALIS.** Spinal cord, extends from the first pair of Nervi cervicales to the Filum terminale. A

3 ***Pars cervicalis.*** Cervical part, corresponds to the apparent origin of Nn. cervicales. A

4 ***Intumescentia cervicalis.*** Cervical enlargement between C6 and T2. A

5 ***Pars thoracica.*** Thoracic part, corresponds to the apparent origin of Nn. thoracici. A

6 ***Pars lumbalis.*** Lumbar part, corresponds to the apparent origin of Nn. lumbales. A

7 ***Intumescentia lumbalis.*** Lumbar enlargement, between L4 and S2. A

8 ***Pars sacralis.*** Sacral part, corresponds to the apparent origin of Nn. sacrales. A

9 ***Pars caudalis.*** Caudal part, corresponds to the apparent origin of Nn. caudales. A

10 ***Conus medullaris.*** Medullary cone, the end of Medulla spinalis, that continues as the Filum terminale. A

11 ***Filum terminale.*** Thin filament of glial and ependymal cells. A C

12 ***Sulcus medianus [dorsalis].*** Groove between the Funiculi dorsales. B

13 ***Sulcus lateralis dorsalis.*** Groove between Funiculus dorsalis and lateralis. B

14 ***Sulcus intermedius dorsalis.*** Groove in the middle of the Funiculus dorsalis, corresponding to the limit between the Fasciculus gracilis, medially, and the Fasciculus cuneatus, laterally. B

15 ***Fissura mediana [ventralis].*** Median (ventral) fissure, deep longitudinal groove between the Funiculi ventrales. B

16 ***Sulcus lateralis ventralis.*** Groove between Funiculus ventralis and lateralis. B (This sulcus corresponds to the exit line [apparent origin] of the ventral roots of the spinal nerves. In many mammals it is less distinct than the Sulcus lateralis dorsalis, or even absent.)

17 ***Funiculi medullae spinalis.*** Funiculi of spinal cord, three paired columns of white matter, surounding gray matter. B

18 *Funiculus dorsalis.* Column between Cornu dorsale and Septum medianum dorsale. B

19 *Funiculus lateralis.* Column between Cornu dorsale and Cornu ventrale. B

20 *Funiculus ventralis.* Column between Fissura mediana and Cornu ventrale. B

21 **Sectiones medullae spinalis.** Cross sections of the spinal cord.

22 ***Canalis centralis.*** Central canal. B C D

23 ***Ventriculus terminalis.*** Terminal ventricle, enlargement of Canalis centralis in the Conus medullaris. C

24 ***Septum medianum dorsale.*** Thickening of the subarachnoid connective tissue within the dorsal median sulcus. Separates the Funiculi dorsales. B

25 ***Commissura grisea.*** Gray commissure, numerous non-myelinated fibers passing and crossing in the Substantia grisea, particularly dorsal to Canalis centralis. B

26 ***Commissura alba.*** White commissure, myelinated fibers crossing and passing between Fissura mediana and Substantia grisea. Albeit these fibers are extremely variable in number, there is always a continuity of the Substantia alba between the two Funiculi ventrales, as opposed to the Funiculi dorsales, which are totally separated by the Septum medianum dorsale. B

27 ***Substantia grisea.*** Gray matter, H- or butterfly-shaped central substance. D

28 *Cornu dorsale.* Dorsal horn. B D

29 *Cornu laterale.* Lateral horn. B D

30 *Cornu ventrale.* Ventral horn. B D

31 *Apex cornus dorsalis.* Apex or tip of dorsal horn. B D

32 *Substantia gelatinosa.* Rolando's substance. B D (A list of eponyms for this chapter is provided at the end of the book.)

33 *Nucleus thoracicus.* Stilling-Clarke's nucleus in C8–L2–3. D (This N.A. term replaces the term Nucleus tractus spinocerebellaris dorsalis listed in the 2nd edition. Formerly it was called the Nucleus dorsalis.)

34 *Substantia intermedia centralis.* Substantia grisea that surrounds the Canalis centralis. It is extended laterally by the Substantia intermedia lateralis and includes the Commissura grisea and other neuronal and glial elements. D

35 *Substantia intermedia lateralis.* Substantia grisea that unites the Cornu dorsale and ventrale, and adjoins the Cornu laterale. D

36 *Nucleus cervicalis lateralis.* Lateral to Cornu dorsale, in C1–C3, well developed in Car and Un. D

37 *Nucleus motorius n. accessorii.* In the dorsal region of Cornu ventrale in C1–C6–7. D

38 *Nucleus tractus spinalis n. trigemini.* Continuation with Substantia gelatinosa, in many species in C1–C5–6. D

39 *Formatio reticularis.* Mixture of white and gray matter between Cornu dorsale and laterale. B

* Reminder: The structures followed by an asterisk are landmarks for physical examination and/or clinical approach.

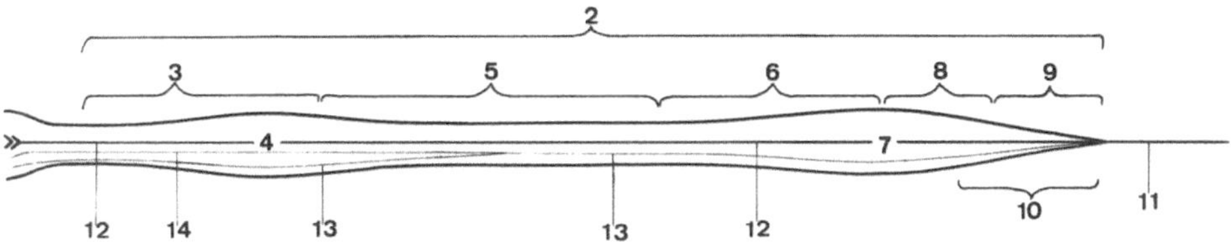

A Spinal cord, schematic dorsal aspect

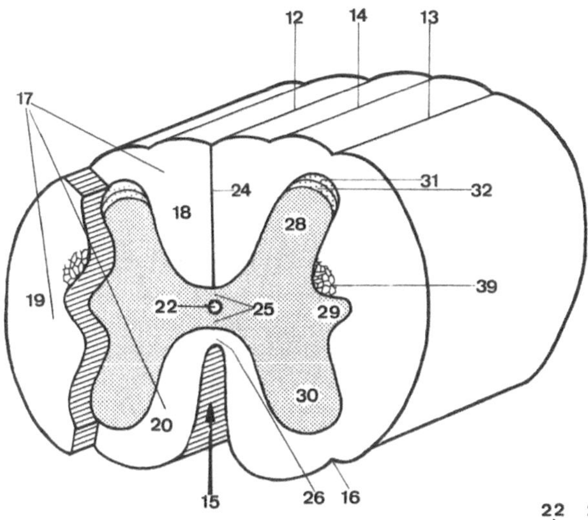

B Spinal cord, schematic transverse section

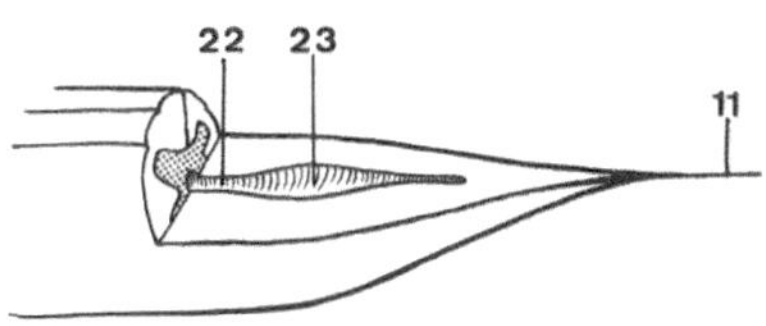

C Spinal cord, ventral half of caudal end

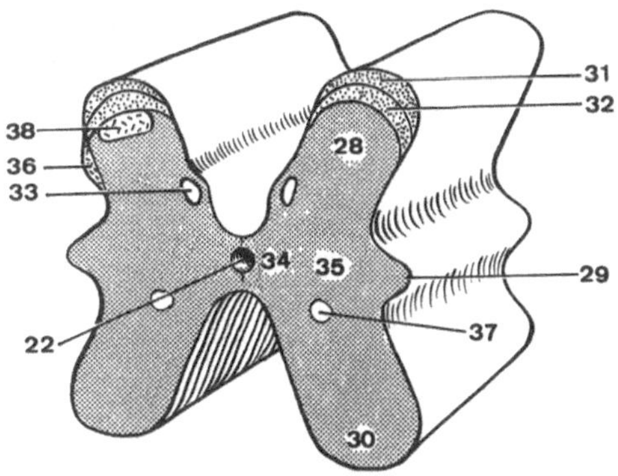

D Spinal cord, gray substance, schematic transverse section of cervical part (ca)

1 ***Substantia alba***. White matter, represented by three paired peripheral funiculi.

2 **Funiculus dorsalis**. Conducts ascending pathways. A

3 ***Fasciculus gracilis***. Goll's tract, medial segment of Funiculus dorsalis. A

4 ***Fasciculus cuneatus***. Burdach's tract, lateral segment of Funiculus dorsalis. A

5 ***Tractus pyramidalis [corticospinalis] dorsalis***. Dorsal pyramidal (corticospinal) tract. A trace of it appears in Un and or in the cranial cervical segments.

6 ***Fasciculi proprii***. Proper fascicles, connect adjacent segments. A

7 **Funiculus lateralis**. Conducts descending and ascending pathways. A

8 ***Tractus pyramidalis [corticospinalis] lateralis***. Lateral pyramidal (corticospinal) tract, lateral to the tip of Cornu dorsale. A

9 ***Tractus spinocerebellaris ventralis***. Ventral spinocerebellar or Gower's tract, on the lateroventral aspect of Funiculus lateralis. A

10 ***Tractus spinocerebellaris dorsalis***. Dorsal spinocerebellar or Flechsig's tract, on the laterodorsal aspect of Funiculus lateralis. A

11 ***Tractus spinotectalis***. Spinotectal tract, ventral to Tractus spinocerebellaris ventralis. A

12 ***Fibrae tectospinales laterales***. Lateral tectospinal fibers medial to, and between the tractus spinocerebellaris dorsalis and ventralis. There are also tectospinal fibers in the Funiculus ventralis. A

13 ***Tractus spinothalamicus***. Spinothalamic tract. Between Tractus spinocerebellaris ventralis and Fasciculi proprii. Although direct spinothalamic fibers may be too rare to justify their designation as a tract, there does exist a polyneural system between Medulla spinalis and thalamus for which is useful a collective term. A

14 ***Tractus reticulospinalis lateralis***. Lateral reticulospinal tract. Between Tractus pyramidalis lateralis and Tractus rubrospinalis. A

15 ***Tractus rubrospinalis***. Rubrospinal or Monakow's tract, connects Nucleus ruber to Cornu ventrale. Lateral to Cornu laterale. A

16 ***Tractus dorsolateralis***. Dorsolateral or Lissauer's tract, short fibers between Substantia gelatinosa and surface of the Medulla spinalis. A

17 ***Fasciculi proprii***. Proper fascicles, connect adjacent segments. Lateral to cornu ventrale. A

18 **Funiculus ventralis**. Conducts descending pathways. A

19 ***Fasciculus longitudinalis medialis***. Medial longitudinal fascicle, particularly well-developed in Un. It is in part a continuation of Fasciculus longitudinalis medialis of the brainstem and is made up of a mixture in variable proportions of several types of fibers. They have been designated by the five following terms. A

20 *Pars commissurospinalis*. Starting from Nucleus prestitialis, formerly Nucleus commissurae posterioris. A

21 *Pars interstitiospinalis*. Origin in Nucleus interstitialis of mesencephalon. A

22 *Pars tectospinalis*. Starting from Tectum mesencephali. A

23 *Pars vestibulospinalis*. Starting from Nuclei vestibulares. A

24 *Pars reticulospinalis*. Origin in Formatio reticularis of Tegmentum mesencephali. A

25 ***Tractus pyramidalis [corticospinalis] ventralis***. Ventral pyramidal (corticospinal) tract, homolateral fibers extending to Pars thoracica. The most medial tract. A

26 ***Tractus spinoolivaris***. Termination in Nucleus olivaris. The most lateral tract. A

27 ***Tractus spinothalamicus***. Spinothalamic tract, see 13. Intermediate tract between Pars tectospinalis fasciculi longitudinalis medialis – laterally –, and Tractus spinoolivaris – medially. A

28 ***Fasciculi proprii***. Proper fascicles, connect adjacent segments. Ventromedial to Cornu ventrale. A

29 **ENCEPHALON**. Brain, consisting of myelencephalon, metencephalon, mesencephalon, diencephalon and telencephalon.

30 **RHOMBENCEPHALON**. Hindbrain, consists of myelencephalon and metencephalon. B

31 **Myelencephalon**. Medulla oblongata, extends from the first pair of Nervi cervicales to pons. B

32 **Medulla oblongata**. Same as myelencephalon. B

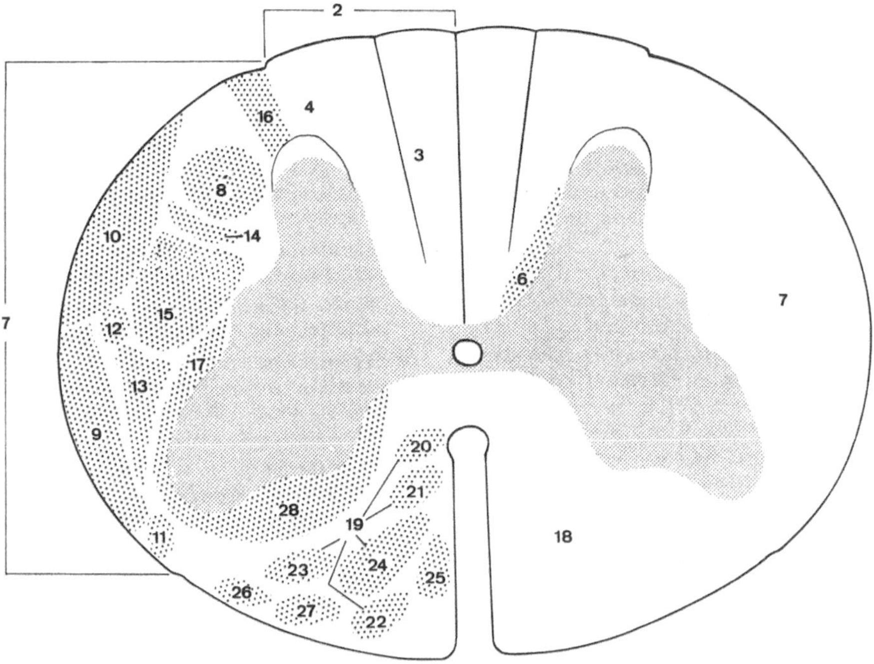

A Spinal cord, schematic cross section (only the white matter is labeled)

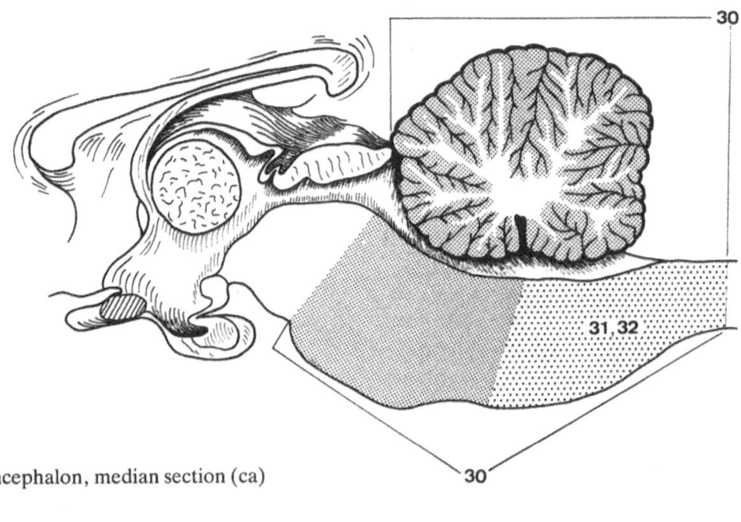

B Rhombencephalon, median section (ca)

1 ***Fissura mediana [ventralis]***. Median (ventral) fissure, groove continuing Fissura mediana [ventralis] of Medulla oblongata. A

2 ***Pyramis [medullae oblongatae]***. Pyramid of medulla oblongata, longitudinal paired prominence. A

3 ***Decussatio pyramidum***. Pyramidal decussation, visible on the ventral surface of the Medulla oblongata, can also be seen in cross sections. A

4 ***Sulcus lateralis ventralis***. Ventral lateral sulcus, groove lateral to the pyramid, exit of Nn. hypoglossus and abducens. A

4a ***Tuberculum faciale***. External prominence on the ventral aspect of Medulla oblongata at the caudal border of Corpus trapezoideum. A (This is the Tuberculum faciale ventrale. The Tuberculum faciale dorsale, not listed in the 5th edition of the N. A. V., can be seen on the floor of the Fossa rhomboidea, at the level of the Eminentia medialis [see 430.16].)

5 ***Sulcus lateralis dorsalis***. Dorsal lateral sulcus, extends along the dorsal aspect of Medulla oblongata toward the Recessus lateralis ventriculi quarti. B

5a ***Tuberculum trigeminale***. External prominence on the lateral aspect of Medulla oblongata, just cranial to glossopharyngeal nerve

6 ***Sulcus intermedius dorsalis***. Dorsal intermediate sulcus, separates Fasciculus gracilis from Fasciculus cuneatus. B

7 ***Oliva***. Olive, does not exist as external prominence in many species. (This structure was omitted from the 5th edition of the N. A. V.)

8 ***Pedunculus cerebellaris caudalis***. Caudal cerebellar peduncle, connection of medulla oblongata to cerebellum. B

9 *Corpus restiforme*. Restiform body, lateral main part of Pedunculus cerebellaris caudalis, contains largely tracts of afferent fibers. B

10 *Corpus juxtarestiforme*. Juxtarestiform body, medial smaller part of Pedunculus cerebellaris caudalis, contains Tractus vestibulocerebellaris and cerebellovestibularis. B

11 ***Funiculus lateralis***. Continuation of Funiculus lateralis medullae spinalis. A B

12 ***Faciculus cuneatus***. Burdach's tract, continuation of the corresponding tract of Medulla spinalis, lateral to Faciculus gracilis. B

13 ***Tuberculum nuclei cuneati***. Cuneate tubercle, prominence at the level of Nucleus cuneatus. B

14 ***Fasciculus gracilis***. Goll's tract, continuation of the corresponding tract of Medulla spinalis, medial to Fasciculus cuneatus. B

15 ***Tuberculum nuclei gracilis***. Gracilis tubercle or clava, prominence at the level of Nucleus gracilis. B

16 ***Fibrae arcuatae superficiales***. Superficial arcuate fibers from Nuclei cuneatus lateralis and arcuatus to cerebellum. B

17 ***Sulcus medianus [dorsalis]***. Groove continuing Sulcus medianus of Medulla spinalis up to obex. B

18 **Sectiones medullae oblongatae**. Sections (most transverse) through medulla oblongata.

19 ***Raphe [Rhaphe]***. Suture-like median wall, mainly by crossing fibers. D

20 ***Tegmentum rhombencephali***. Area ventral to Canalis centralis and Ventriculus quartus, dorsal to olives and pyramids, contains nuclei of V–XII. D

21 ***Nucleus motorius n. hypoglossi***. Caudal to the Nucleus prepositus n. hypoglossi (C) and in the most medial position (D). C D

22 ***Nucleus intercalatus***. Staderini's nucleus, probably provides reflex connections to Nucleus motorius n. hypoglossi. Between Nucleus motorius n. hypoglossi and Nucleus parasympaticus n. vagi. C D

23 ***Nucleus prepositus [prae-] n. hypoglossi***. Marburg's nucleus, probably provides reflex connections to Nucleus motorius n. hypoglossi. Rostral to Nucleus motorius n. hypoglossi. C

24 ***Nucleus ambiguus [Nucleus motorius nn. vagi et glossopharyngei]***. The most lateral nucleus, deep in the Tegmentum rhombencephali, ventral to Tractus solitarius and its nucleus. C D

25 ***Nucleus parasympathicus n. vagi***. Between Nucleus intercalatus and Tractus solitarius with its nucleus, and caudal to Nucleus parasympaticus n. glossopharyngei. C D

26 ***Nucleus parasympathicus n. glossopharyngei***. Rostral to the previous nucleus. C

27 ***Nucleus motorius n. accessorii***. The most caudal nucleus in figure C, caudal to Nucleus ambiguus, and at the same deep level. C

28 ***Tractus solitarius***. Gustatory fibers of nn. VII and IX, sensory fibers of nn. IX and X, ending in Nucleus tractus solitarii. In a dorsolateral position in the cross section D. C D

29 ***Nucleus tractus solitarii***. Condensation of nervous cell bodies, associated with Tractus solitarius. The most lateral position of the dorsal row formed by previous nuclei. C D

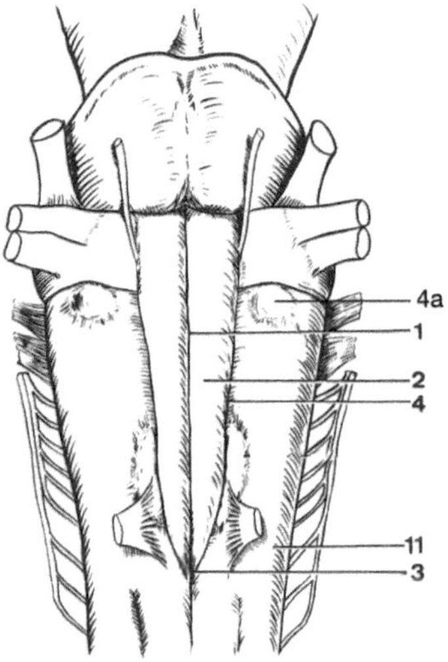

A Medulla oblongata and pons, ventral aspect (ca)

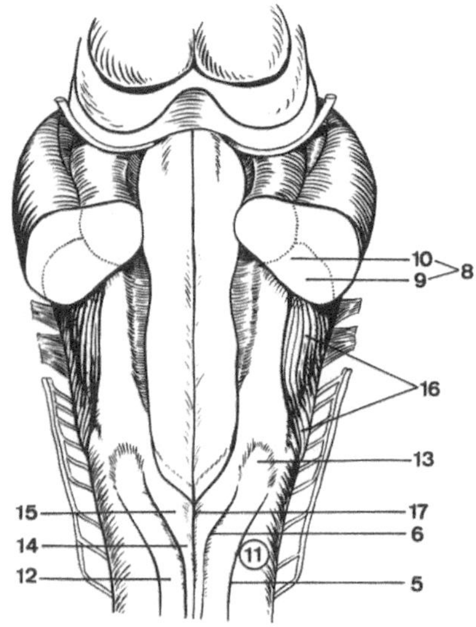

B Medulla oblongata and pons, dorsal aspect (ca)

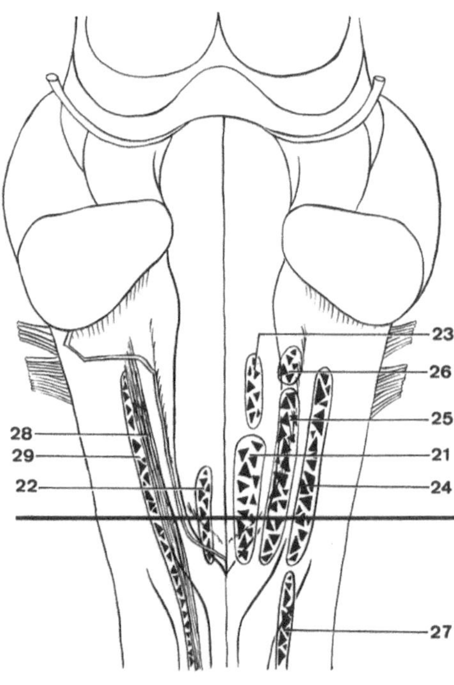

C Medulla oblongata, dorsal aspect (ca), schematic representation of some nuclei

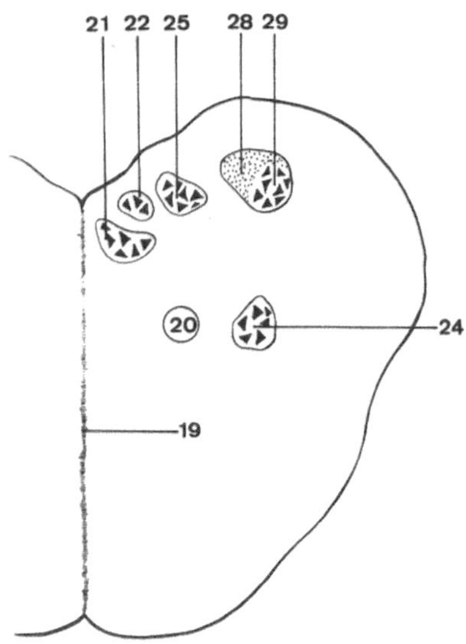

D Medulla oblongata, transverse section (ca), schematic representation of nuclei shown in C

1 ***Tractus spinalis n. trigemini***. Tract descending into the Medulla spinalis, contains pain and temperature fibers of N. trigeminus. A B C D E

2 ***Nucleus tractus spinalis n. trigemini***. Nucleus for the fibers of Tractus spinalis n. trigemini. Consists of 3 morphologically different parts. A

3 *Pars caudalis*. A D E

4 *Pars interpolaris*. Part between Pars caudalis and rostralis. A

5 *Pars rostralis*. A B C

6 ***Nucleus motorius n. trigemini***[1]. In some species located in pons. A

7 ***Nucleus cochlearis ventralis***[1]. Ventral nucleus of the cochlear part of N. vestibulocochlearis. In some species located in pons. A C

8 ***Nucleus cochlearis dorsalis [Tuberculum acusticum]***[1]. Dorsal nucleus of the cochlear part of N. vestibulocochlearis. In some species located in pons. A C

9 ***Nuclei vestibulares***[1]. Four nuclei of the vestibular part of N. vestibulocochlearis in the ventrolateral wall of Ventriculus quartus. In some species all or some of them located in pons. A

10 *Nucleus vestibularis rostralis*. Bechterew's nucleus. A B

11 *Nucleus vestibularis medialis*. Triangular or Schwalbe's nucleus. A

12 *Nucleus vestibularis lateralis*. Deiter's nucleus. A C

13 *Nucleus vestibularis caudalis [descendens]*. Spinal or Roller's nucleus. A C

14 ***Nucleus motorius n. facialis***[1]. In some species located in pons. A C

15 ***Nucleus parasympathicus n. facialis***. Origin of preganglionic fibers for Ggl. pterygopalatinum. In some species located in pons. A

16 ***Genu n. facialis***[1]. Loop of fibers from Nucleus motorius n. facialis dorsal to Nucleus motorius n. abducentis. B

17 ***Nucleus parasympathicus n. intermedii***[1]. Origin of preganglionic fibers for Ggl. mandibulare and Ggl. sublinguale (Car). In some species located in pons. A C

18 ***Nucleus motorius n. abducentis***[1]. In some species located in pons. A B

19 ***Nucleus gracilis***. Nucleus of Goll's tract, origin of Fibrae arcuatae profundae to Decussatio lemniscorum medialium. A E

20 ***Nucleus cuneatus medialis***. Medial nucleus of Burdach's tract, origin of Fibrae arcuatae profundae to Decussatio lemniscorum medialium. A D E

21 ***Nucleus cuneatus lateralis***. Lateral nucleus of Burdach's tract, origin of Fibrae arcuatae superficiales to cerebellum. A D E

22 ***Nucleus funiculi lateralis***. Origin of Fibrae arcuatae superficiales to cerebellum. D E

23 ***Nucleus olivaris***. Olivary nucleus, formerly Nucleus olivaris inferior, but inferior is no longer necessary because the term Nucleus olivaris superior has been changed to Nucleus dorsalis corporis trapezoidei. Has connections to Medulla spinalis and cerebellum. A D E

24 *Hilus nuclei olivaris*. It is distinct in or, Car, and Un. D

25 ***Nucleus olivaris accessorius medialis***. A D E

26 ***Nucleus olivaris accessorius dorsalis***. A D

27 ***Nucleus dorsalis corporis trapezoidei***. Origin of a part of Lemniscus lateralis. A B

28 ***Nuclei ventrales corporis trapezoidei***. Origin of a part of Lemniscus lateralis. A B

1) These structures whose location varies between the Medulla oblongata and the Pons according to species, have been listed in both places.

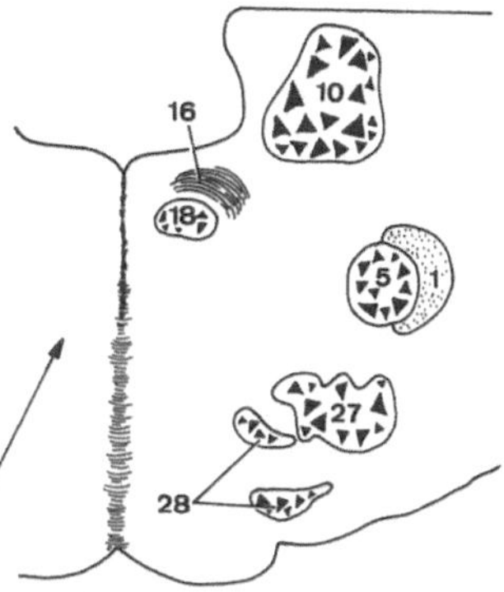

B Medulla oblongata, transverse section (ca), schematic representation of some nuclei

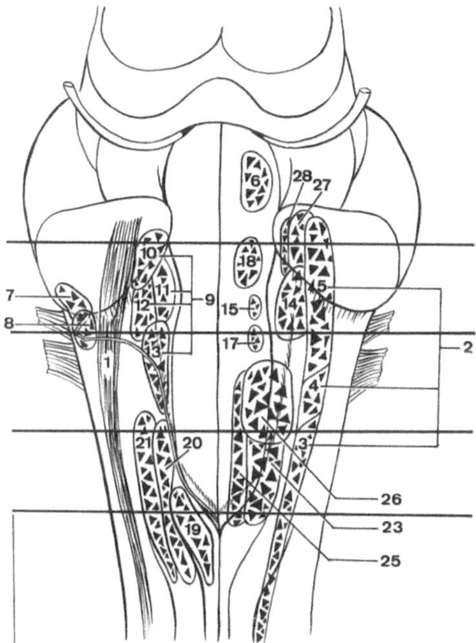

A Medulla oblongata, dorsal aspect (ca), schematic representation of some nuclei

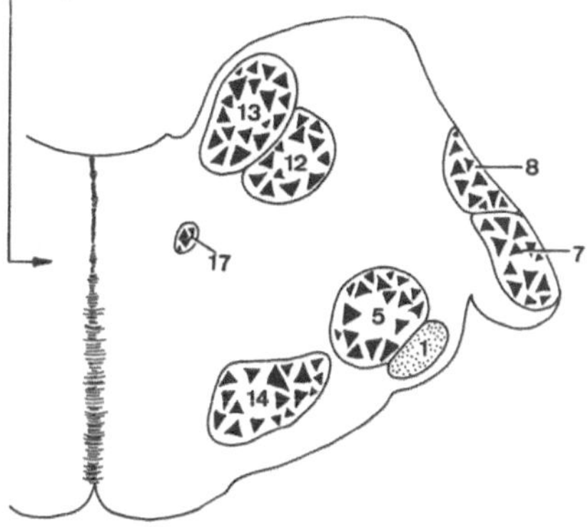

C Medulla oblongata, transverse section (ca), schematic representation of some nuclei

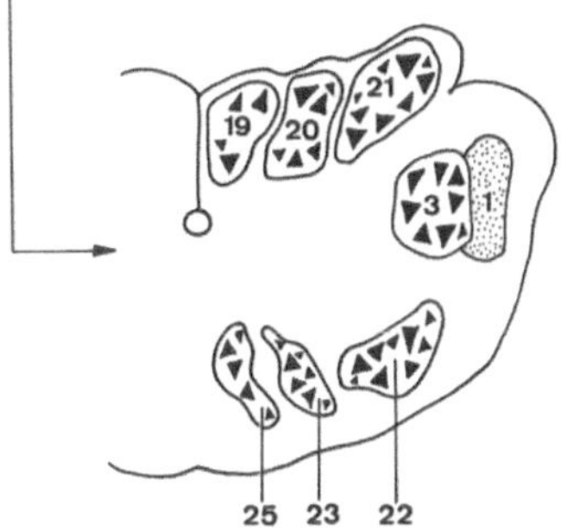

E Medulla oblongata, transverse section (ca), schematic representation of some nuclei

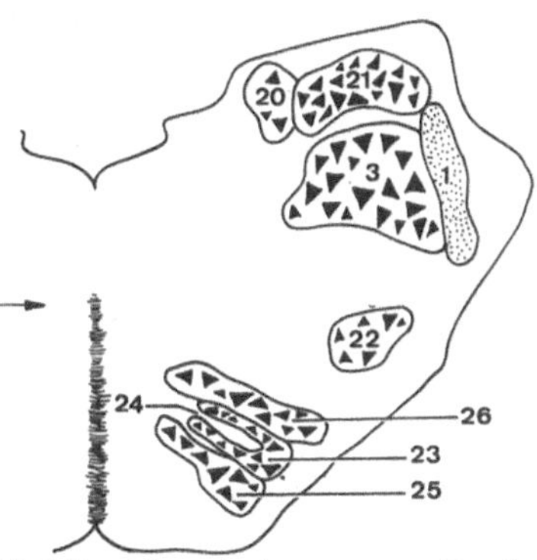

D Medulla oblongata, transverse section (ca), schematic representation of some nuclei

1 ***Nucleus arcuatus***. Origin of a part of Fibrae arcuatae superficiales. Synapse for cerebro-pontine-cerebellar tracts. C D

2 ***Fibrae arcuatae profundae***. Deep arcuate fibers, originate in Nucleus gracilis and Nucleus cuneatus medialis, form the Decussatio lemniscorum medialium. D

3 ***Formatio reticularis***. Scattered neuron cells and fibers in Tegmentum rhombencephali. C D

3a ***Nucleus reticularis lateralis***. Included in Formatio reticularis

3b ***Nuclei raphe***. See Raphe medullae oblongatae 418.19.

4 ***Fasciculus gracilis***. Goll's fascicle between Sulcus medianus [dorsalis] and Sulcus intermedius dorsalis. A D

5 ***Fasciculus cuneatus***. Burdach's fascicle, between Sulcus intermedius dorsalis and Sulcus lateralis dorsalis. A D

6 ***Tractus spinothalamici***. See 416.13. C D

7 ***Tractus reticulospinalis lateralis***. Between Formatio reticularis medullae oblongatae and Medulla spinalis. D

8 ***Tractus spinotectalis***. Between Medulla spinalis and Tectum mesencephali. D

9 ***Lemniscus medialis***. Continuation of second order neurons from Decussatio lemniscorum medialium to thalamus. C D

10 ***Decussatio lemniscorum medialium***. Formed by Fibrae arcuatae profundae from Nuclei gracilis and cuneatus medialis. D

11 ***Pedunculus cerebellaris caudalis***. Connects Medulla oblongata to cerebellum. A C

12 ***Tractus spinocerebellaris dorsalis***. Flechsig's tract, connects the same side of Medulla spinalis to cerebellum via Pedunculus cerebellaris caudalis. D

13 ***Tractus spinocerebellaris ventralis***. Gower's tract, connects the contralateral side of Medulla spinalis to cerebellum via Pedunculus cerebellaris rostralis. C D

14 ***Tractus olivocerebellaris***. Fibers from Oliva to cerebellum via Pedunculus cerebellaris caudalis. D

15 ***Fibrae arcuatae superficiales***. From Nuclei arcuatus, funiculi lateralis, and cuneatus lateralis to cerebellum, the ventral part after decussation. A B D

16 ***Corpus trapezoideum***. Trapezoid body. Sheet of transversely running fibers from the Nuclei cochleares, part of auditory pathway. B C (see footnote on page 420)

17 ***Tractus pyramidalis***. Corresponds to Pyramis and contains the following three types of fibers. C D (Because many of the fibers go no further than the Medulla oblongata, where some end in nuclei and others in the reticular formation, appropriate subdivisions have been listed under Tractus pyramidalis at this level.)

18 *Fibrae corticonucleares*. Fibers from Cortex cerebri to motor Nuclei nervorum cranialium.

19 *Fibrae corticospinales*. Fibers from Cortex cerebri to Medulla spinalis.

20 *Fibrae corticoreticulares*. Fibers from Cortex cerebri to Formatio reticularis of Medulla oblongata and Medulla spinalis.

21 ***Decussatio pyramidum***. Crossing fibers of Tractus pyramidales. B D

22 ***Tractus rubrospinalis***. Monakow's tract. From Nucleus ruber to Medulla spinalis. C D

23 ***Fibrae tectospinales laterales***. Fibers from Tectum mesencephali to Medulla spinalis. C D

24 ***Fasciculus longitudinalis medialis***. Consists of the following five parts. C D

25 *Pars commissurospinalis*. Starting from Nucleus prestitialis, formerly Nucleus commissurae posterioris of mesencephalon.

26 *Pars interstitiospinalis*. Starting from Nucleus interstitialis of mesencephalon.

27 *Pars tectospinalis*. From Tectum mesencephali.

28 *Pars vestibulospinalis*. From Nuclei vestibulares.

29 *Pars reticulospinalis*. From Formatio reticularis.

30 ***Tractus vestibulospinalis***. From Nucleus vestibularis lateralis to Medulla spinalis. C D

31 ***Tractus tegmenti centralis*** [Car]. Connects Pallidum, Zona incerta subthalami, and Nucleus ruber to Nucleus olivaris. C

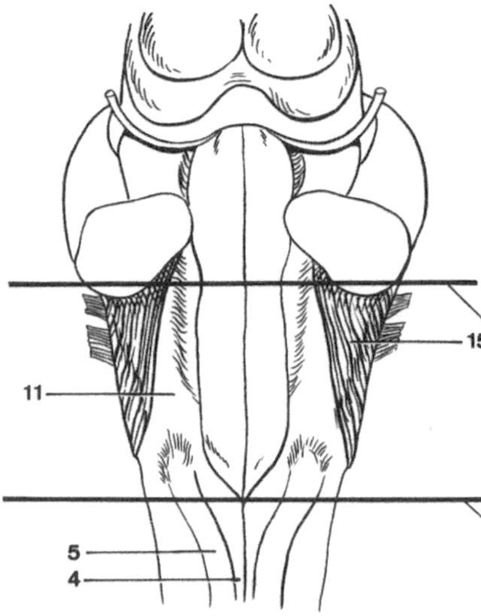

A Medulla oblongata and pons, dorsal aspect (ca)

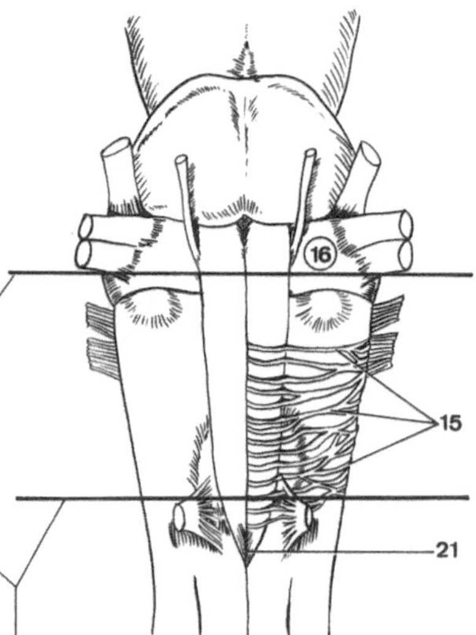

B Medulla oblongata and pons, ventral aspect (ca)

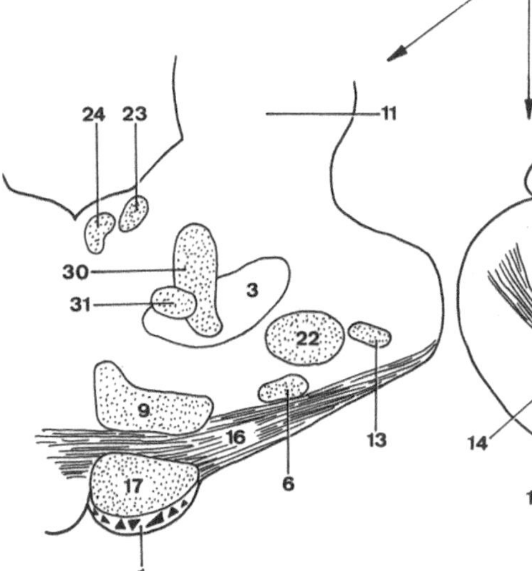

C Medulla oblongata, rostral transverse section (ca), schematic representation of some nuclei

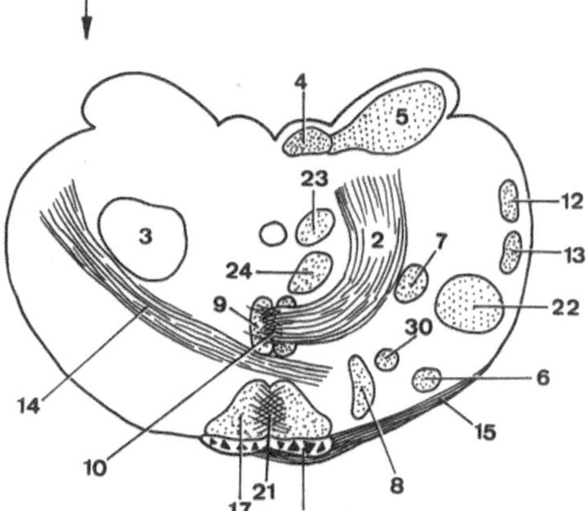

D Medulla oblongata, caudal transverse section (ca), schematic representation of some nuclei

1 **Metencephalon**. Rostal part of Rhombencephalon, consisting of pons and cerebellum. A

2 **Pons**. Prominent transversal bridge between mesencephalon and medulla oblongata. Consists of transverse fibers and cell groups belonging to cerebrocerebellar pathways of the rostral part of Tegmentum rhombencephali. A B

3 ***Sulcus basilaris***. Median groove, produced by right and left pyramidal tracts. B

4 ***Pedunculus cerebellaris medius [Brachium pontis]***. Middle cerebellar peduncle, fiber communication between pons and cerebellum. A B D

5 **Sectiones pontis**. Cross sections through pons. D E

6 **Pars dorsalis pontis [Tegmentum pontis]**. Floor of the rostral half of Ventriculus quartus with deep adjacent structures. D E

7 ***Raphe [Rhaphe]***. Median suture-like structure, mainly crossing fibers. D E (There is a similar Raphe within the Myelencephalon [see 418.19].)

8 ***Formatio reticularis***. Similar to Formatio reticularis medullae oblongatae. D E

8a ***Nuclei raphe***. Nuclei within Raphe.

9 ***Nucleus motorius n. abducentis***[1]. In some species located in medulla oblongata. C E

10 ***Nucleus motorius n. facialis***[1]. In some species located in medulla oblongata. C E

11 ***Genu n. facialis***[1]. Loop of fibers from Nucleus motorius n. facialis, dorsal to Nucleus motorius n. abducentis. C E

12 ***Nucleus motorius n. trigemini***[1]. C D

13 ***Nucleus sensibilis pontinus n. trigemini***[1]. Origin of fibers forming after decussation of the Lemniscus trigeminalis. C D

14 ***Tractus mesencephalicus n. trigemini***. Fibers to Nucleus tractus mesencephalicus n. trigemini. C

15 ***Nucleus tr. mesencephalici n. trigemini***. Rostral sensory trigeminal nucleus. C

16 ***Nucleus ceruleus [coeruleus]***. Bluish columnar cell group. D

17 ***Tractus spinalis n. trigemini***. Tract descending into the Medulla spinalis, contains pain and temperature fibers of N. trigeminus. C E

18 ***Nucleus tractus spinalis n. trigemini***. Nucleus for the fibers of Tractus spinalis n. trigemini. E

19 ***Nuclei n. vestibulocochlearis***. In some species some of them located in medulla oblongata. C

20 *Nucleus cochlearis ventralis*. Ventral nucleus of the cochlear part of N. vestibulocochlearis. In some species located in medulla oblongata. C E

21 *Nucleus cochlearis dorsalis [Tuberculum acusticum]* [1]. Dorsal nucleus of the cochlear part of N. vestibulocochlearis. In some species located in medulla oblongata. C E

22 *Nucleus vestibularis rostralis*. Bechterew's nucleus[1]. C

23 *Nucleus vestibularis medialis*. Triangular or Schwalbe's nucleus[1]. C E

24 *Nucleus vestibularis lateralis*. Deiter's nucleus[1]. C E

25 *Nucleus vestibularis caudalis [descendens]*[1]. Spinal or Roller's nucleus. C

26 ***Stria acustica***. Fibers from Nucleus cochlearis dorsalis which pass over Pedunculus cerebellaris caudalis and course medially into the floor of Ventriculus quartus. C

27 ***Corpus trapezoideum***[1]. Trapezoid body. Sheet of transversaly running fibers from the Nuclei cochleares, part of auditory pathway. B E

28 *Nucleus dorsalis corporis trapezoidei*. Formerly Nucleus olivaris superior. Origin of a part of Lemniscus lateralis. C E

29 *Nuclei ventrales corporis trapezoidei*. Origin of a part of Lemniscus lateralis. C E

30 ***Pedunculus cerebellaris rostralis [Brachium conjunctivum]***. Connects cerebellum to mesencephalon . C D

[1] Because many of the fibers go no further than the Medulla oblongata, where some end in nuclei and others in the reticular formation, appropriate subdivisions have been listed under Tractus pyramidalis at this level.

A Encephalon with emphasis on rhombencephalon, left lateral aspect (ca)

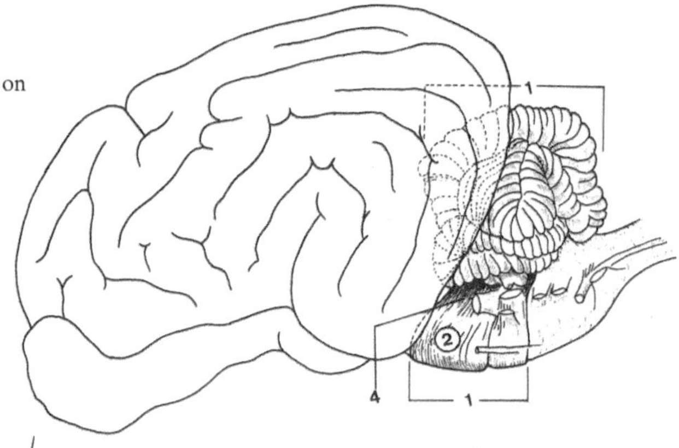

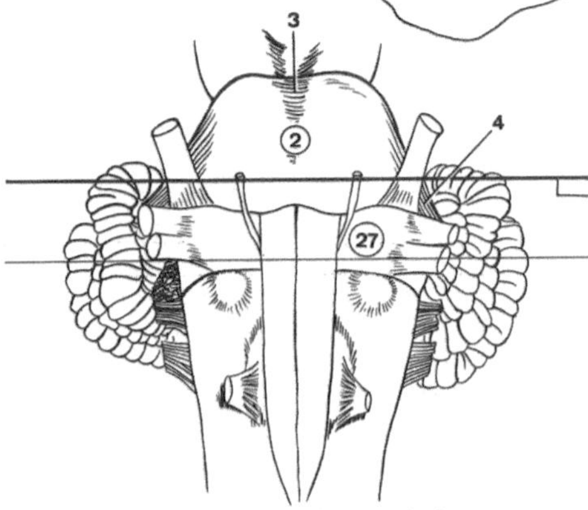

B Rhombencephalon, ventral aspect (ca)

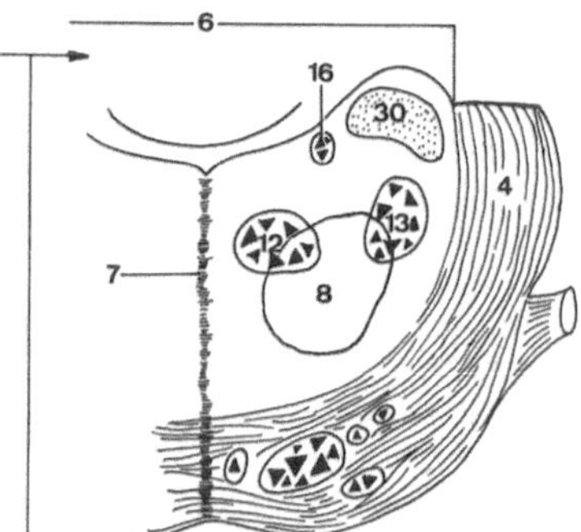

D Pons, rostral transverse section (ca), schematic representation of some nuclei

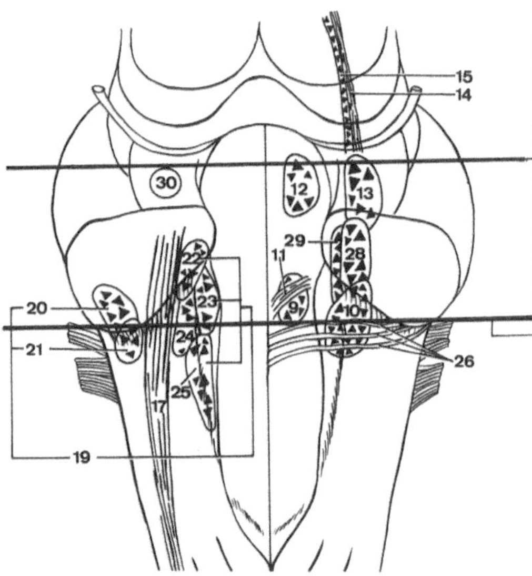

C Medulla oblongata and pons dorsal aspect (ca), schematic representation of some nuclei

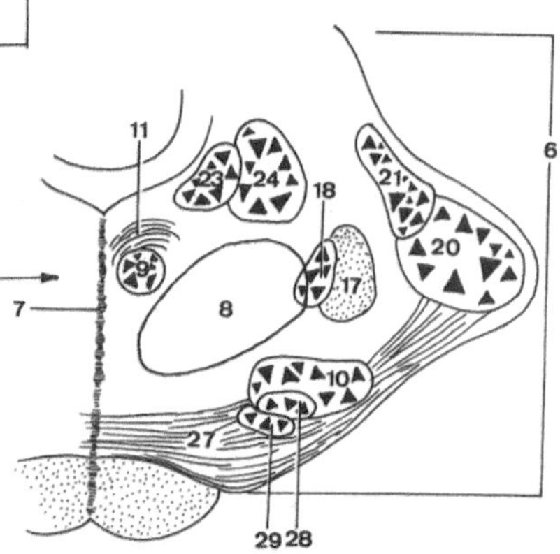

E Pons, caudal transverse section (ca), schematic representation of some nuclei

1 ***Tractus spinothalamici***. See 416.13. A

2 ***Lemniscus medialis***. Crossed fibers connecting Nuclei gracilis and cuneatus medialis to thalamus. A

3 ***Lemniscus trigeminalis***. Crossed fibers connecting Nucleus sensibilis pontinus n. trigemini to thalamus. A

4 ***Lemniscus lateralis***. Partially crossed fibers connecting Nuclei cochleares to Colliculus caudalis and Corpus geniculatum mediale. A

5 *Nucleus lemnisci lateralis*. Small groups of neurons associated to Lemniscus lateralis synapsing with some of the lemniscal fibers. A

6 ***Tractus rubrospinalis***. Monakow's tract, connects Nucleus ruber with Medulla spinalis. A

7 ***Tractus tectospinalis***. Connects Tectum mesencephali with Medulla spinalis. A

8 ***Tractus tegmenti centralis***. Connects Pallidum, Zona incerta subthalami, and Nucleus ruber to Nucleus olivaris (Car). A

9 ***Fasciculus longitudinalis medialis***. Consists of the following four parts. A

10 *Pars commissurospinalis*. Starting from Nucleus prestitialis, formerly Nucleus commissurae posterioris.

11 *Pars interstitiospinalis*. Origin in Nucleus interstitialis of mesencephalon.

12 *Pars tectospinalis*. Starting from Tectum mesencephali.

13 *Pars reticulospinalis*. Origin in Formatio reticularis of Tegmentum mesencephali.

14 ***Fasciculus longitudinalis dorsalis***. Schütz's bundle, starts from Nucleus periventricularis caudalis hypothalami, to Substantia grisea centralis mesencephali and Medulla spinalis. A

15 **Pars ventralis pontis**. A

16 ***Tractus pyramidalis***. Consists of the following three kinds of fibers. A

17 *Fibrae corticonucleares*. Fibers from Cortex cerebri to Nuclei nervorum cranialium.

18 *Fibrae corticospinales*. Fibers from Cortex cerebri to Medulla spinalis.

19 *Fibrae corticoreticulares*. Fibers from Cortex cerebri to Formatio reticularis of Medulla oblongata and Medulla spinalis.

20 ***Tractus corticopontinus***. Connects Cortex frontalis, temporalis, and occipitalis to Nuclei pontis.

21 ***Nuclei pontis***. Pontine nuclei, related to Tractus corticopontinus. A

22 *Fibrae pontis transversae*. Transverse pontine fibers, from Nuclei pontis to cerebellum. A

23 **Cerebellum**. Part of metencephalon dorsal to Fossa rhomboidea. For the nomenclature the subdivisions established by Larsell have been adopted, however the classical names of the lobules have been retained. B C D (The equivalents of the classical names of the lobules in the nomenclature of Larsell are listed on page 152 in the 5th edition of the N. A. V. They are also listed within parentheses in the next page.)

24 ***Folia cerebelli***. Cerebellar folia, gracile gyri separated by fissures. B C

25 ***Fissurae cerebelli***. Cerebellar fissures, deep and narrow grooves between Folia cerebelli. B C

26 ***Sulci cerebelli***. Cerebellar sulci, grooves between Vermis and Hemispherium and between parts of the Hemispherium. B C

27 ***Vallecula cerebelli***. Large ventral depression. D

28 ***Corpus cerebelli***. Cerebellar body, made up of Lobus rostralis and caudalis, separated from Lobus flocculonodularis by Fissura uvulonodularis (Fiss. posterolateralis of N.A.). B D

29 *Lobus rostralis*. B C D

30 *Fissura prima*. Between Lobus rostralis and Lobus caudalis B C

31 *Lobus caudalis*. B C D

32 ***Fissura uvulonodularis***. Separates Uvula from Nodulus. It corresponds to Fasciculus dorsolateralis [posterolateralis] of N.A. D

33 ***Lobus flocculonodularis***. Fusion of Flocculi of hemispheres and Nodulus vermis. C D

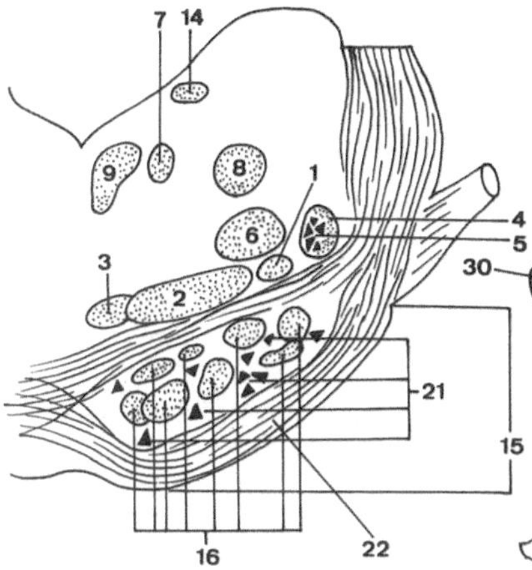

A Pons, transverse section (ca), schematic representation of some nuclei

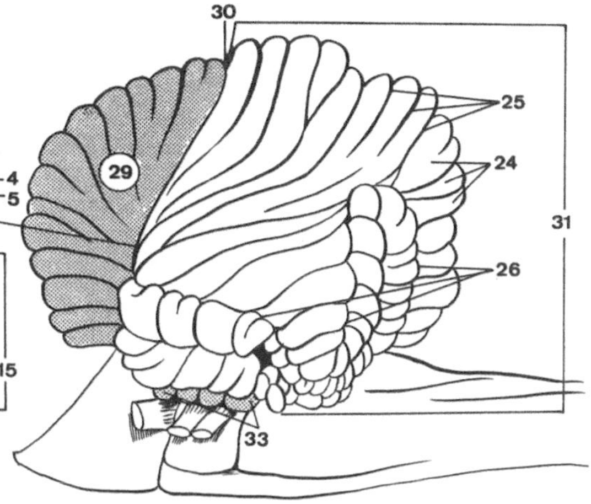

C Rhombencephalon, left lateral aspect (ca)

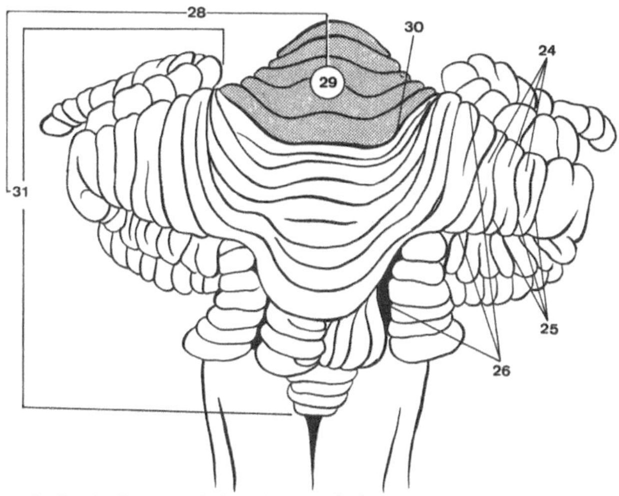

B Cerebellum, caudodorsal aspect (ca)

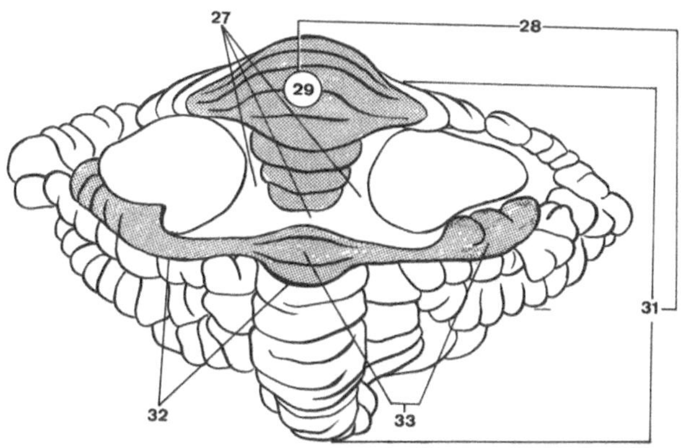

D Cerebellum, ventral aspect (ca)

1 ***Vermis***. Unpaired major component of cerebellum consisting of 10 lobules, as follows. A B D

2 *Lingula cerebelli*. (Lob. I Larsell). Corresponds to Vinculum lingulae hemispherii. A D

3 *Lobulus centralis*. (Lob. II Larsell). Corresponds to Ala lobuli centralis hemispherii. A B D

4 *Culmen*. Corresponds to Lobulus quadrangularis hemispherii. A B C

5 **Pars rostralis**. (Lob. III Larsell). A B C

6 **Pars caudalis**. (Lob. IV et V Larsell). A B C

7 *Declive*. (Lob. VI Larsell). Corresponds to Lobulus simplex hemispherii. A B C

8 *Folium vermis*. (Lob. VII A Larsell). Corresponds to Crus rostrale lobuli ansiformis hemispherii. A B C

9 *Tuber vermis*. (Lob. VII B Larsell). Corresponds to Crus caudale lobuli ansiformis hemispherii. A B C

10 *Pyramis [vermis]*. (Lob. VIII A et VIII B Larsell). Corresponds to Lobulus paramedianus and Paraflocculus dorsalis hemispherii. A B C D

11 *Uvula [vermis]*. (Lob. IX Larsell). Corresponds to Paraflocculus ventralis hemispherii. A B D

12 *Nodulus*. (Lob. X Larsell). Corresponds to Flocculus hemispherii. A D

13 ***Hemispherium [Hemisphaerium] cerebelli***. Consisting of 10 lobules, as follows. D

14 *Vinculum lingulae*. (Lob. H. I Larsell). Corresponds to Lingula cerebelli. D

15 *Ala lobuli centralis [Prolatio aliformis]*. (Lob. H. 2 Larsell). Corresponds to Lobulus centralis vermis. D

16 *Lobulus quadrangularis*. Corresponds to Culmen vermis. B C

17 **Pars rostralis**. (Lob. H. III Larsell). B C

18 **Pars caudalis**. (Lob. H. IV et H. V Larsell). B C

19 *Lobulus simplex*. (Lob. H. VI Larsell). Corresponds to Declive vermis. B C

20 *Lobulus ansiformis*. Corresponds to Folium vermis and Tuber vermis. B C

21 **Crus rostrale**. (Lob. H. VII A Larsell). Corresponds to Folium vermis. B C D

22 **Crus caudale**. (Lob. H. VII B Larsell). Corresponds to Tuber vermis. B C D

23 *Lobulus paramedianus*. (Lob. H. VIII A Larsell). Corresponds to a part of Pyramis vermis. B C D

24 *Paraflocculus*. B C D

25 **Paraflocculus dorsalis**. (Lob. H. VIII B Larsell). Corresponds to a part of Pyramis vermis. B C D

26 **Paraflocculus ventralis**. (Lob. H. IX Larsell). Corresponds to Uvula vermis. B C D

27 *Flocculus*. (Lob. H. X Larsell). Corresponds to Nodulus vermis. B D

28 **Pedunculus flocculi**. Connecting bridge to Nodulus. D

29 **Sectiones cerebelli**. A

30 ***Corpus medullare***. Central white matter, with myelinated fibers. A

31 ***Arbor vitae***. Branching of white matter, resembling a "tree of life". A

32 ***Laminae albae***. White laminae, penetrating as digitations into Folia cerebelli. A

33 ***Cortex cerebelli***. Cerebellar cortex. A

34 *Stratum moleculare*. Molecular layer, external cortical layer consisting of dendrites of Purkinje cells and basket-like cells with their axons and dendrites. A

35 *Stratum neuronorum piriformium*. Layer of piriform neurons, new term that indentifies the layer of Purkinje cells. A

36 *Stratum granulosum*. Granular layer, deepest cortical layer with abundant cells, axons, and dentrites of granular neurons.

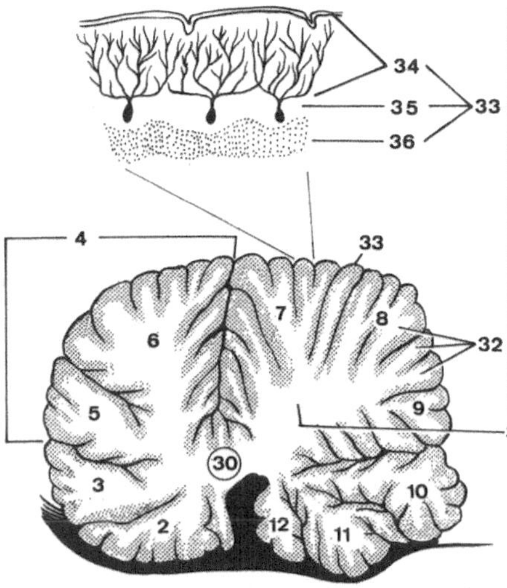

A Cerebellum, median section through vermis, right half medial aspect (ca)

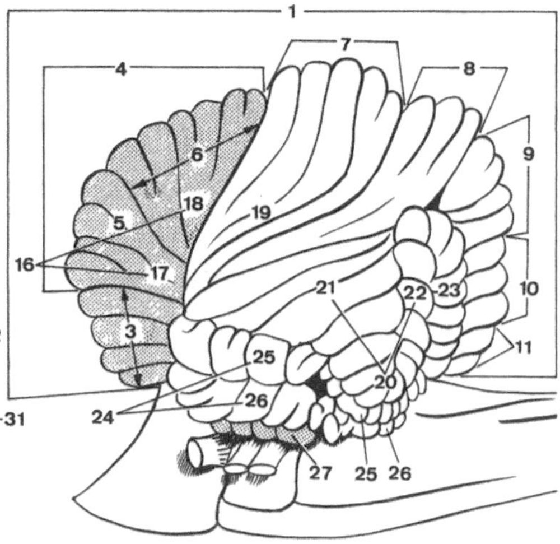

B Cerebellum, left lateral aspect (ca)

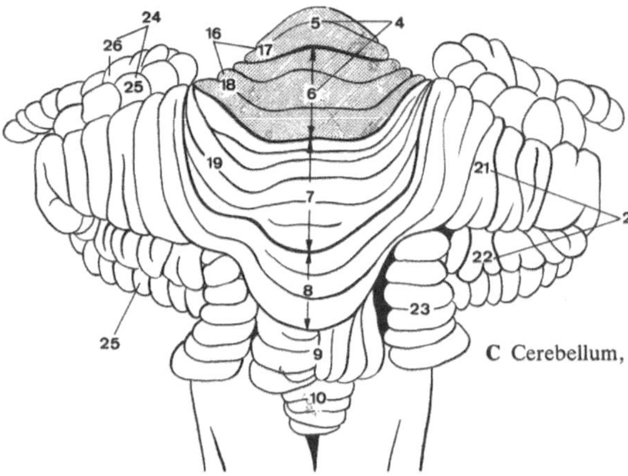

C Cerebellum, dorsal aspect (ca)

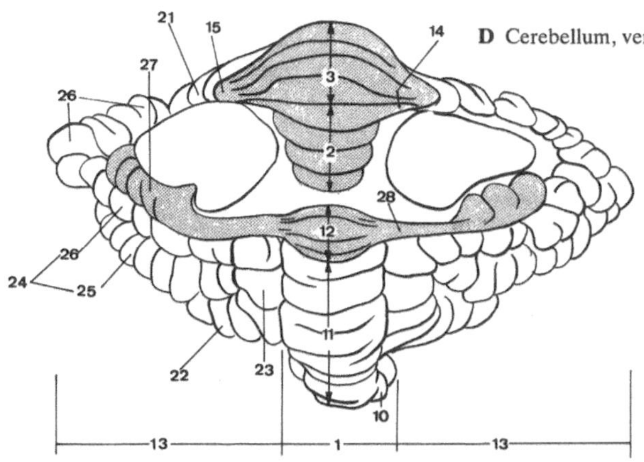

D Cerebellum, ventral aspect (ca)

1 ***Nucleus lateralis cerebelli [Nucleus dentatus]***. Lateral nucleus of cerebellum, the largest, located lateroventrally within Corpus medullare. A

2 ***Nuclei interpositi cerebelli***. Intercalated cerebellar nuclei, between Nucleus lateralis cerebelli and Nucleus fastigii. A

3 *Nucleus interpositus lateralis cerebelli [Nucleus emboliformis]*. A

4 *Nucleus interpositus medialis cerebelli [Nucleus globosus]*. A

5 ***Nucleus fastigii***. Fastigial nucleus, most medial within Corpus medullare. A

6 **Ventriculus quartus**. Fourth ventricle, belongs to rhombencephalon as a whole. A

7 ***Fossa rhomboidea***. Floor of Ventriculus quartus, becomes visible after removal of cerebellum and Tegmen ventriculi quarti. B

8 ***Sulcus medianus***. Longitudinal median groove. A B

9 ***Recessus lateralis ventriculi quarti***. Lateral recess of fourth ventricle, ends at Apertura lateralis ventriculi quarti. B C

10 ***Sulcus limitans***. Groove parallel to Sulcus medianus, separating Eminentia medialis from the rest of Fossa rhomboidea. A B

11 *Fovea caudalis*. Shallow groove at the rostral tip of Trigonum n. vagi. B

12 *Fovea rostralis*. Rostral depression of Sulcus limitans. B

13 ***Trigonum n. hypoglossi***. Medial and caudal to Trigonum n. vagi, covering Nucleus motorius n. hypoglossi. B

14 ***Striae medullares ventriculi quarti***. Medullary striae of fourth ventricle, not discernible in most mammals. The same structure is also listed as Stria acustica (424.26).

15 ***Eminentia nuclei vestibularis medialis***. Rostral to Recessus lateralis ventriculi quarti, on the lateral side of Fossa rhomboidea. A B

16 ***Eminentia medialis***. Between Sulcus medianus and Sulcus limitans. B

17 ***Trigonum n. vagi***. Vagal trigone, lateral to Trigonum n. hypoglossi. B

18 ***Area postrema***. Area with a specific histologic structure. B

19 ***Locus ceruleus [caeruleus]***. Bluish columnar cell group in lateral wall of Ventriculus quartus. B

20 ***Tegmen ventriculi quarti***. Roof of fourth ventricle. C (The summit of the fourth ventricle's roof is the so-called "Fastigium", not listed in the 5th edition of the N. A. V., albeit this term is used in the anatomical literature, and moreover, the Nucleus "fastigii" is listed at p. 430.5.)

21 *Velum medullare caudale*. Plate of white matter between right and left Pedunculus cerebellaris caudalis, Nodulus and Tela choroidea ventriculi IV. C

22 *Velum medullare rostrale*. Lamina of white matter between right and left Pedunculus cerebellaris rostralis and Lingula cerebelli. C

23 **Frenulum veli medullaris rostralis**. Thin band-like structure connecting Velum medullare rostrale to Lamina tecti mesencephali. C

24 ***Tenia [Taenia] ventriculi quarti***. Tenia of fourth ventricle, cut edge of roof of the caudal part of Ventriculus quartus. B

25 *Obex*. Unpaired transverse structure at the caudal extent of the roof of Ventriculus quartus that ends Sulcus medianus medullae oblongatae. B C

26 ***Tela choroidea [chorioidea] ventriculi quarti***. Layer of pia mater and ependyma between Velum medullare caudale and Tenia ventriculi quarti. C

27 ***Aperturae ventriculi quarti***. Openings of fourth ventricle. C

28 *Aperturae laterales ventriculi quarti*. Luschka's foramina, correspond to Recessus laterales ventriculi quarti. C

29 *(Apertura mediana ventriculi quarti)*. Magendie's foramen, unpaired opening rostral to obex, not present in Car, uncertain presence in other domestic mammals. C

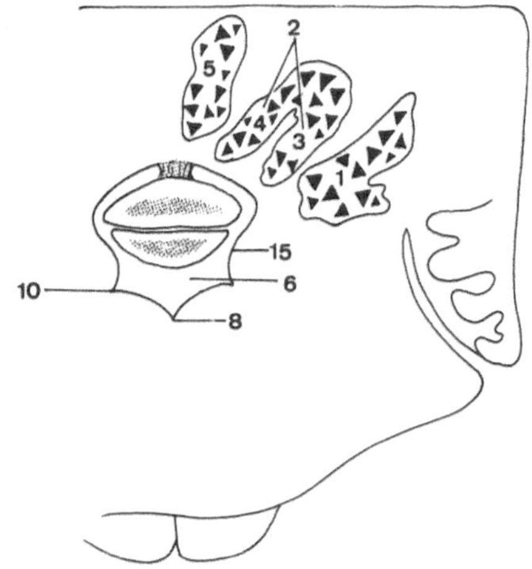

A Cerebellum, transverse section (ca), schematic representation of some nuclei

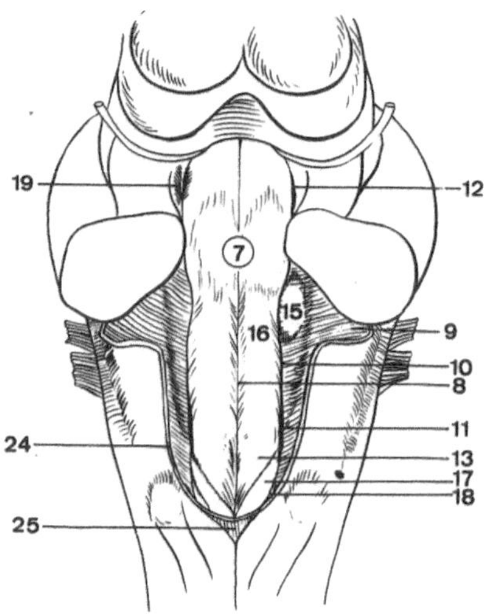

B Fossa rhomboidea (ca)

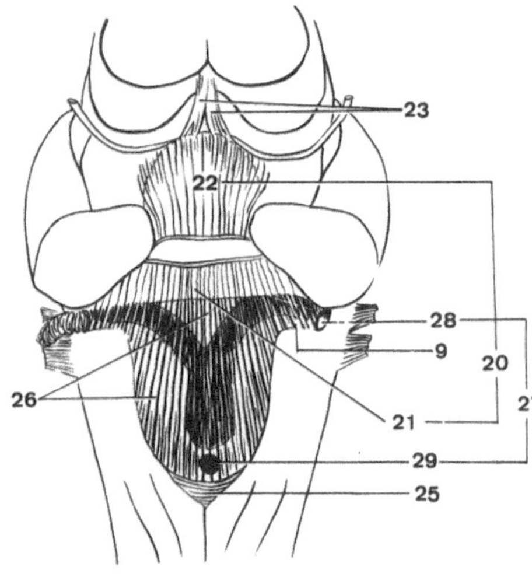

C Tegmen ventriculi quarti (ca)

1 **MESENCEPHALON.** Midbrain, part of brain that contains the Aqueductus mesencephali, between pons and diencephalon, made up of Pedunculi cerebri and Tectum. A B C D E

2 ***Pedunculus cerebri*.** Cerebral peduncle, consists of a ventral part, Crus cerebri, and a dorsal part, Tegmentum, separated by Substantia nigra. D F

3 **Crus cerebri.** Cerebral crus, carries pyramidal and pontine tracts. A B E F

4 ***Fossa interpeduncularis*.** Interpeduncular fossa, space between Crura cerebri, caudal to Corpus mamillare. A

5 ***Substantia perforata caudalis*.** Caudal perforated substance, floor of Fossa interpeduncularis allowing the passage of blood vessels. A

6 ***Tractus cruralis transversus*.** Transverse crural tract, starting from Sulcus medialis cruris cerebri, ending at Lamina tecti (eq), or near Glandula pinealis (Car, su, Ru). It constitutes the optic accessory root A B

7 ***Sulcus medialis cruris cerebri*.** Medial sulcus of cerebral crus, apparent origin of N. oculomotorius. A F (There is also a Sulcus lateralis mesencephali, not listed in the 5th edition of the N. A. V., but obviously shown as 7a in figures A B E F.)

8 **Tegmentum mesencephali.** Dorsal part of Pedunculus cerebri, separated from Crus cerebri by Substantia nigra, overlapped by Tectum mesencephali. E F

9 ***Trigonum lemnisci*.** Triangular area on the lateral aspect of Pedunculus cerebri, corresponding to Lemniscus lateralis. B

10 **Tectum mesencephali.** Roof of midbrain, dorsal to tegmentum. E F

11 ***Lamina tecti*.** Tectal lamina. E F

12 ***Colliculus rostralis*.** Rostral colliculus, hemispherical prominence, related to the visual pathway. Former Colliculus opticus. B C D E F

13 ***Colliculus caudalis*.** Caudal colliculus, lower than the previous one, related to the auditory pathway. Former Colliculus acusticus. B C D

14 ***Brachium colliculi rostralis*.** Arm of rostral colliculus, connecting Colliculus rostralis to Corpus geniculatum laterale, less evident in domestic mammals. B C

15 ***Brachium colliculi caudalis*.** Arm of caudal colliculus, connecting Colliculus caudalis to Corpus geniculatum mediale. B C

16 **Sectiones mesencephali.** Sections (most transverse) through midbrain. D E F

17 ***Tegmentum mesencephali*.** See 8. E F

18 ***Substantia grisea centralis*.** Central gray matter, surrounding Aqueductus mesencephali. E F

19 ***Aqueductus [Aquae-] mesencephali [Aqueductus cerebri]*.** Mesencephalic aqueduct (of Sylvius), canal between Ventriculus tertius and Ventriculus quartus. D E F

20 ***Formatio reticularis*.** Continuation of the same structure from Medulla spinalis, myelencephalon and pons. E

21 ***Tractus tegmenti centralis*** (Car). Connects Pallidum, Zona incerta subthalami, and Nucleus ruber to Nucleus olivaris. E

22 ***Fasciculus longitudinalis medialis*.** Medial longitudinal fascicle. See 416.19. E F

23 *Fibrae commissurospinales.* Fibers from Nucleus prestitialis, formerly Nucleus commissurae posterioris, to Medulla spinalis.

24 *Fibrae interstitiospinales.* Fibers from Nucleus interstitialis of mesencephalon to Medulla spinalis.

25 *Fibrae vestibulocommissurales.* Fibers from Nuclei vestibulares to the contralateral Nucleus prestitialis, formerly Nucleus commissurae posterioris.

26 *Fibrae vestibulotectales.* Fibers from Nuclei vestibulares to Tectum mesencephali.

27 *Fibrae vestibulothalamicae.* Fibers from Nuclei vestibulares to thalamus.

28 ***Tractus tectospinalis*.** Fibers from Tectum mesencephali to Medulla spinalis. E

29 ***Fasciculus longitudinalis dorsalis*.** Connections to hypothalamus, tegmental and many other nuclei. E F

30 ***Tractus mesencephalicus n. trigemini*.** Fibers to Nucleus tractus mesencephalici n. trigemini. E

31 ***Nucleus tr. mesencephalici n. trigemini*.** Rostral sensory trigeminal nucleus. E

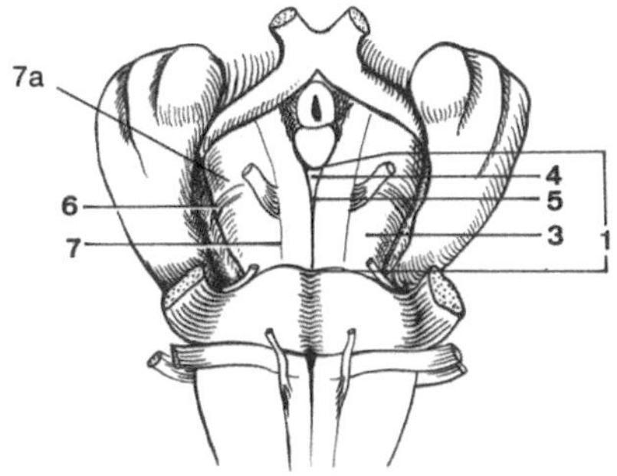

A Mesencephalon, ventral aspect (eq)

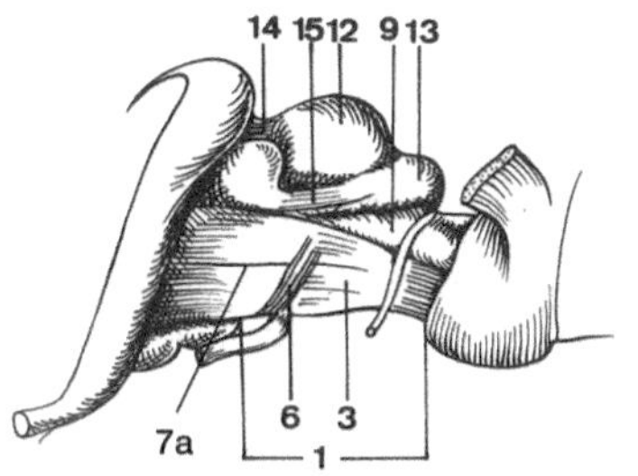

B Mesencephalon, left lateral aspect (eq)

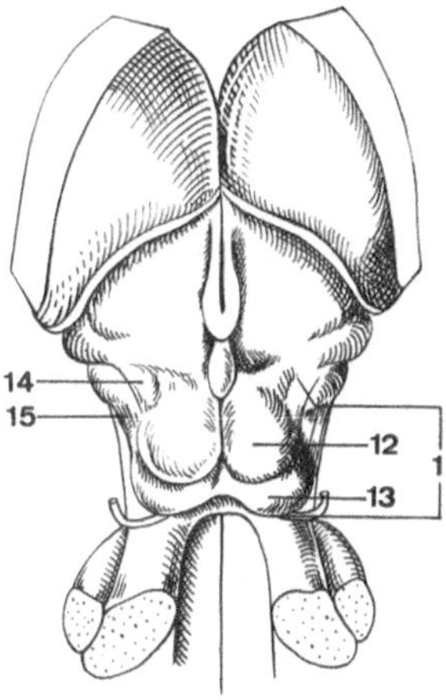

C Mesencephalon, dorsal aspect (eq)

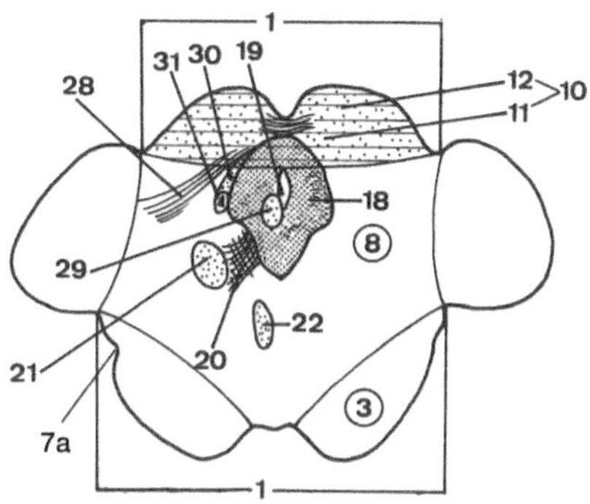

E Mesencephalon, transverse section through Colliculi rostrales (ca)

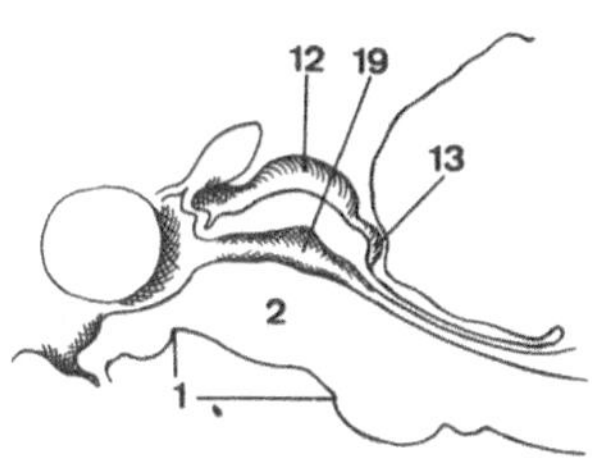

D Mesencephalon, median section, right medial aspect (eq)

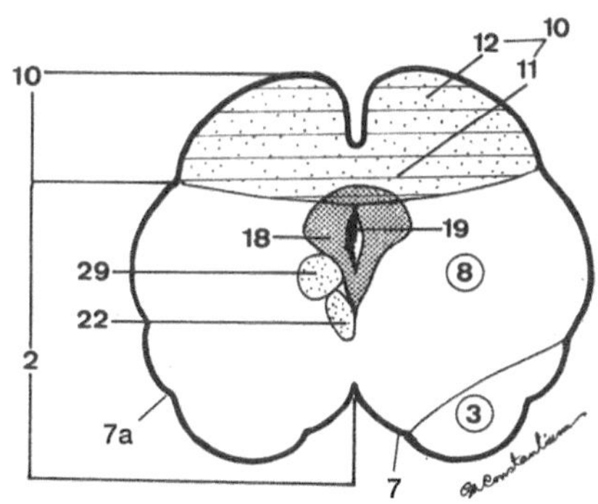

F Mesencephalon, transverse section through Colliculi rostrales (ov)

1 ***Nucleus motorius n. oculomotorii.*** Motor nucleus of N. oculomotorius. A

2 ***Nucleus motorius n. trochlearis.*** Caudal to Nucleus motorius n. oculomotorii. B

3 ***Nuclei parasympathici n. oculomotorii.*** Edinger-Westphal's nucleus, dorsomedial to Nucleus motorius n. oculomotorii. A

4 ***Nucleus interpeduncularis.*** Related to the olfactory pathway. A

5 ***Nuclei tegmenti.*** Tegmental (Gudden's) nuclei, located in Formatio reticularis, give fibers to the Fasciculus longitudinalis medialis. A

6 *Nucleus interstitialis.* Cajal's nucleus, fibers from Nuclei vestibulares, Pallidum, and Stratum griseum colliculi rostralis. A

7 *Nucleus prestitialis [prae-].* Former Nucleus commissurae posterioris.

8 *Nucleus precommissuralis [prae-].* Rostral to Commissura caudalis.

9 ***Nucleus ruber.*** Red (Stilling's) nucleus, afferent fibers from Cerebellum and cortex, origin of Tractus rubrospinalis. A

10 *Pars magnocellularis.* Phylogenetically older caudal and middle parts, predominant in domestic mammals.

11 *Pars parvocellularis.* Phylogenetically younger rostral part, predominant in man.

12 ***Decussationes tegmenti.*** Tegmental decussations. In certain cases the two decussations are intermingled and difficult to distinguish. A

13 *Decussatio dorsalis.* Meynert's decussation of Tractus tectospinales. A

14 *Decussatio ventralis.* Forel's decussation of Tractus rubrospinales and Fibrae rubroreticulares. A

15 ***Pedunculus cerebellaris rostralis [Brachium conjunctivum].*** Paired arm, anchoring Cerebellum to mesencephalon. B

16 ***Decussatio pedunculorum cerebellarium rostralium.*** In the caudal segment of Tegmentum, ventral to Fasciculus longitudinalis medialis. B

17 ***Decussatio nervorum trochlearium.*** Within the Velum medullare rostrale. 465 C

18 ***Lemniscus trigeminalis.*** Built up of crossed fibers connecting the sensory trigeminal nuclei to thalamus. B

19 ***Lemniscus medialis.*** Crossed fibers connecting Nuclei gracilis and cuneatus medialis to thalamus. B

20 ***Lemniscus lateralis.*** Partially crossed fibers of auditory pathway corresponding to Trigonum lemnisci. B

21 *Nuclei lemnisci lateralis.* Nuclei of the lateral lemniscus. B

22 ***Tractus spinothalamicus.*** Accompanies the acoustic fibers of Lemniscus lateralis. See 416.13. B

23 ***Fasciculi tegmenti.*** Tegmental fascicles, large in Un, because they contain a wide secondary dorsal tract of Wallenberg, arising from Nucleus sensibilis pontinus n. trigemini. C

24 ***Substantia nigra.*** Black (Soemmerring's) substance, separating Crus cerebri from Tegmentum, pigmented nuclear mass belonging to the extrapyramidal system. B

25 *Pars compacta.* Compact part. B

26 *Pars reticulata.* Reticulate part. B

27 ***Crus cerebri.*** See 432.3. B

28 ***Tractus pyramidalis.*** Contains fibers which end in mesencephalon or rhombencephalon, three kinds are observed. B

29 *Fibrae corticonucleares.* Connect the motor Cortex cerebri to Nuclei motorii nn. oculomotorii, trochelaris, and trigemini.

30 *Fibrae corticospinales.* End in Medulla spinalis.

31 *Fibrae corticoreticulares.* Connect Cortex cerebri to Formatio reticularis.

32 ***Tractus corticopontinus.*** Variable location within Crus cerebri, but basically lateral to Tractus pyramidalis. In certain species it has two parts, lateral and medial. B

33 *Pars frontopontina.* On the medial side of Tractus pyramidalis, greatly reduced or absent in domestic mammals. Besides, many fibers end in mesencephalon.

34 *Pars parietopontina.* On the lateral side of Tractus pyramidalis.

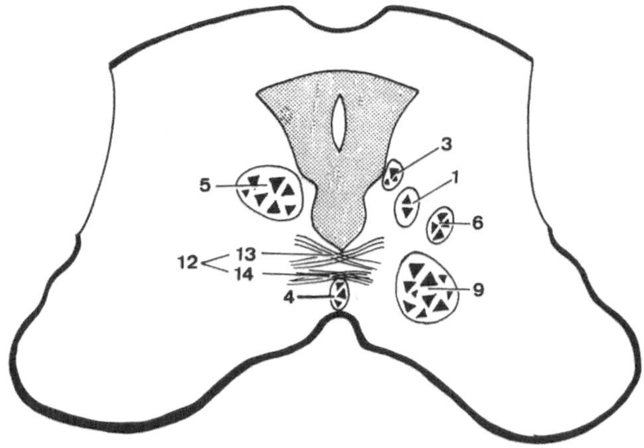

A Mesencephalon, transverse section (ca)

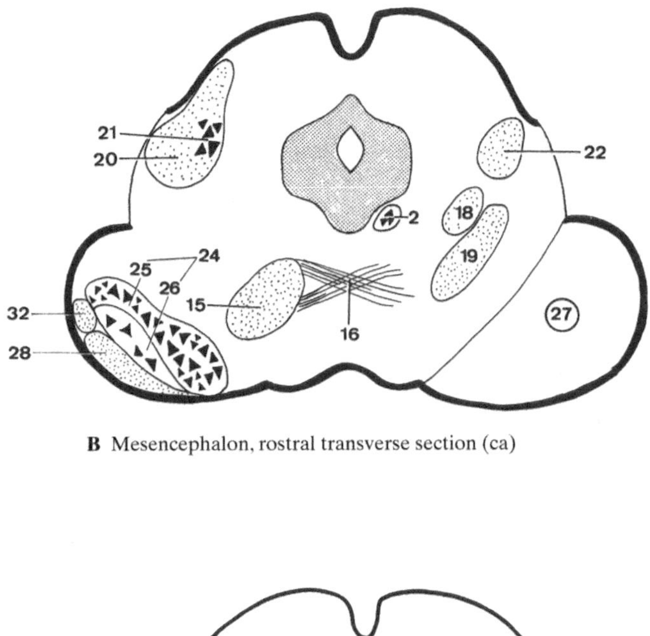

B Mesencephalon, rostral transverse section (ca)

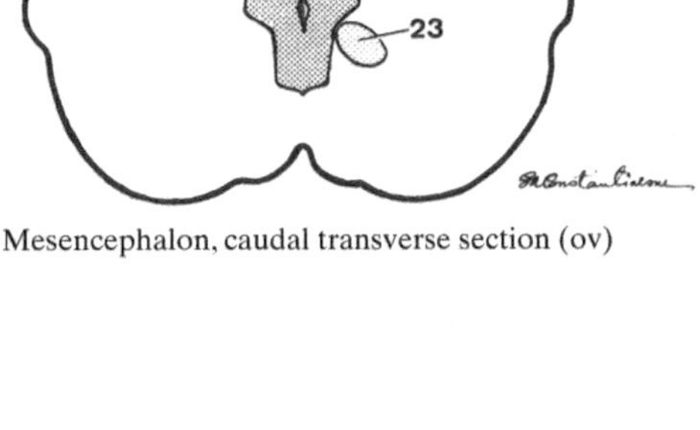

C Mesencephalon, caudal transverse section (ov)

1 ***Nucleus pretectalis [prae-].*** Between Commissura caudalis and Colliculus rostralis, receives impulses from Tractus opticus, gives fibers to Nucleus parasympathicus n. oculomotorii for light reflexes. C

2 ***Tectum mesencephali.*** Roof of midbrain, dorsal to a plane through Aqueductus mesencephali. A

3 *Stratum zonale colliculi rostralis*. External layer of rostral colliculus, made up of a very thin layer of white matter. A

4 *Stratum griseum colliculi rostralis*. Gray layer of rostral colliculus. A

4a *Stratum opticum*. Receives direct input from retinal axons. In turn, they project to the deeper layers, which also receive inputs from auditory and somatosensory systems. Main function is localization of sensory stimuli in space (G. Paxinos. The rat nervous system 3rd ed., 2004, Elsevier Academic Press). A

5 *Strata medullaria colliculi rostralis*. Medullary layers of rostral colliculus, superficial (optic), intermediate, and deep. A

6 *Commissura colliculorum rostralium*. Commissure of rostral colliculi. A

7 *Nucleus colliculi caudalis*. Nucleus of caudal colliculus. B

8 *Commissura colliculorum caudalium*. Commissure of caudal colliculi. B

9 ***Commissura caudalis.*** Caudal commissure, x-shaped bridge of decussating fibers, connecting Colliculi rostrales with the contralateral related epithalamic structures. Some authors consider it a part of epithalamus (diencephalon). C

10 ***Fasciculus retroflexus.*** Meynert's fascicle, considered by some authors as a part of diencephalon, representing the efferent fibers of Nuclei habenulares to Nucleus interpeduncularis. A

11 **PROSENCEPHALON**. Forebrain, made up of diencephalon and telencephalon. D

12 **Diencephalon**. Intermediate brain, consisting of hypothalamus, subthalamus, thalamus, metathalamus and epithalamus. C D

13 ***Ventriculus tertius.*** Third ventricle, irregular space around Adhesio interthalamica, communicating rostrally with right and left Ventriculi laterales through Foramen interventriculare and caudally with Aqueductus mesencephali. C

14 ***Tela choroidea [chorioidea] ventriculi tertii.*** Tela choroidea of third ventricle, forms the roof of Ventriculus tertius and the Recessus suprapinealis, supports the Plexus choroideus ventriculi tertii. C

15 ***Organum subfornicale.*** Subfornical organ, unpaired very small structure between Columnae fornicis. C

16 ***Commissura caudalis.*** See 9. C

17 ***Organum subcommissurale.*** Subcommissural organ, unpaired structure ventral to Commissura caudalis inside of Ventriculus tertius. It sends a slender filum (Reissner) alongside Aqueductus mesencephali, Ventriculus quartus and Canalis centralis medullae spinalis, even up to inside of Filum terminale. C

18 ***Foramen interventriculare.*** Monro's foramen, common opening of the right and left Ventriculi laterales into Ventriculus tertius. C

19 ***Sulcus hypothalamicus.*** Hypothalamic sulcus, groove alongside Ventriculus tertius, at the junction of thalamus and hypothalamus. C

20 ***Adhesio [Adhaesio] interthalamica.*** Interthalamic adhesion or intermediate mass, a connection between right and left thalami. C

21 ***Recessus opticus.*** Optic recess, an expansion of Ventriculus tertius dorsal to Chiasma opticum. C

22 ***Recessus neurohypophysialis [Rec. infundibuli].*** Neurohypophyseal recess of Ventriculus tertius, inside Infundibulum neurohypophysis. C

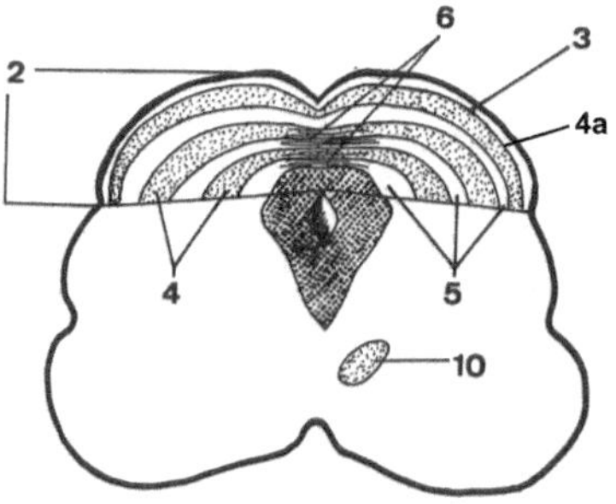

A Mesencephalon, transverse section through Colliculi rostrales (eq)

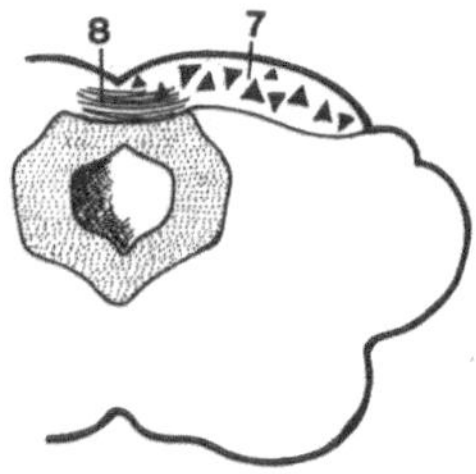

B Mesencephalon, transverse section through Colliculi caudales (eq)

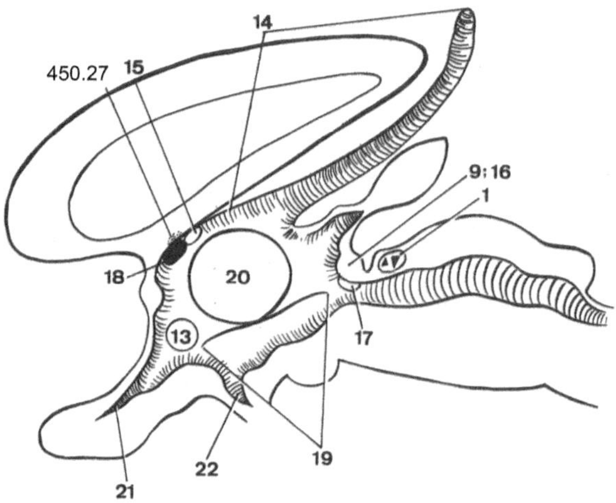

C Diencephalon, median section, right medial aspect (eq)

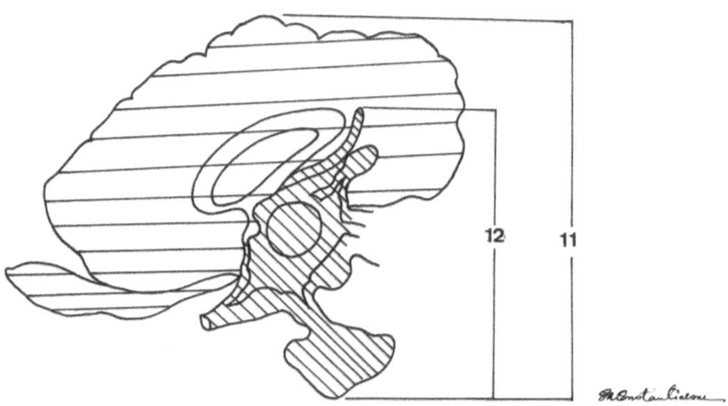

D Prosencephalon, median section, right medial aspect (eq)

1 **Hypothalamus**. The most ventral component of diencephalon, separated from thalamus by Sulcus hypothalamicus. A

2 ***Corpus mamillare***. Mamillary body, rostral to Fossa interpeduncularis, caudal to Tuber cinereum, between the two Crura cerebri. A C D

3 ***Recessus inframamillaris***. Rostral recess of Fossa interpeduncularis, caudal to (infra) Corpus mamillare. A D

4 ***Tuber cinereum***. Gray tubercle, between Chiasma opticum and Corpus mamillare. A D

5 *Pars rostralis tuberis*. Rostral to infundibulum. A

6 *Pars parainfundibularis tuberis*. On both sides of infundibulum. A

7 *Pars caudalis tuberis*. Caudal to infundibulum. A

8 *Sulcus tuberoinfundibularis*. Tuberoinfundibular groove. D

9 ***Hypophysis [Glandula pituitaria]*** (vide p. 232). C

10 ***Tractus opticus***. Part of visual pathway between Chiasma opticum and Corpus geniculatum laterale. A B C

11 *Fasciculus paraopticus*. Small bundle of nerve fibers that course along the medial border of Tractus opticus of ov. It contains the contralateral retinal projections of the accessory optic system. B

12 *Radix medialis*. Medial root, disappears beneath Corpus geniculatum mediale, terminates in Colliculus rostralis. C

13 *Radix lateralis*. Lateral root, connects Tractus opticus to Corpus geniculatum laterale. C

14 ***Chiasma opticum***. Crossing of medial fibers of Nn. optici. A F

15 ***Lamina terminalis grisea***. Gray terminal lamina, plate of gray matter closing Ventriculus tertius rostrally, dorsal to Chiasma opticum. Embriologically the rostral end of the neural tube. D

16 *Organum vasculosum laminae terminalis griseae*. Very small structure within Ventriculus tertius, dorsal to Recessus opticus. D

17 ***Organum vasculosum hypothalami***. Ependimal organ with folded surface within Ventriculus tertius, ventral to Adhesio interthalamica, dorsal to Recessus neurohypophysialis. D

18 **Sectiones hypoyhalami**. Sections through hypothalamus.

19 ***Stratum periventriculare***. Periventricular layer around Ventriculus tertius, collective term for the following groups of nuclei.

20 **Regio hypothalamica rostralis cum Reg. preoptica [prae-]**. Developmentally it doesn't belong to Diencephalon, but functionally and morphologically.

21 ***Nucleus supraopticus***. Neurosecretory fibers extend to Neurohypophysis. E

22 *Pars suprachiasmatica*. Dorsal to Chiasma opticum. E

23 *Pars postchiasmatica*. Dorsal to Tractus opticus and caudal to the previous nucleus. E

24 ***Nucleus suprachiasmaticus***. Dorsal to Chiasma opticum. F

25 ***Nucleus paraventricularis***. Between Commissura rostralis and Lamina terminalis grisea rostrally, and Adhesio interthalamica caudally. Neurosecretory fibers extend to Neurohypophysis. E

26 *Pars accessoria*. Represented by neurosecretory cells between Nuclei paraventricularis and supraopticus. E

27 ***Nucleus paraventricularis parvocellularis***. Lateral to Nucleus paraventricularis.

28 ***Nucleus hypothalamicus rostralis***. Between Commissura rostralis and Pars postchiasmatica nuclei supraoptici, lateral to Nucleus paraventricularis and Columna fornicis. F

29 ***Nucleus preopticus [prae-] medianus***. Between Chiasma opticum and Commissura rostralis. F

30 ***Nucleus preopticus [prae-] medialis***. F

31 ***Nucleus preopticus [prae-] lateralis***. F

32 ***Nucleus preopticus [prae-] periventricularis***. Between Nuclei preopticus medianus and paraventricularis. F

33 ***Nucleus periventricularis rostralis***. Between Nuclei paraventricularis and hypothalamicus dorsomedialis. E

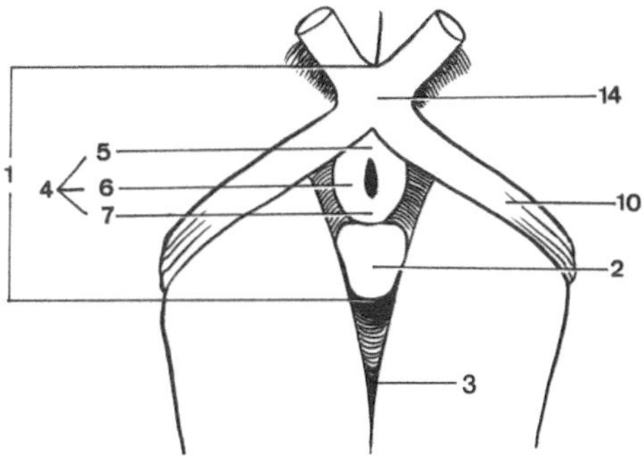

A Hypothalamus, ventral aspect (eq)

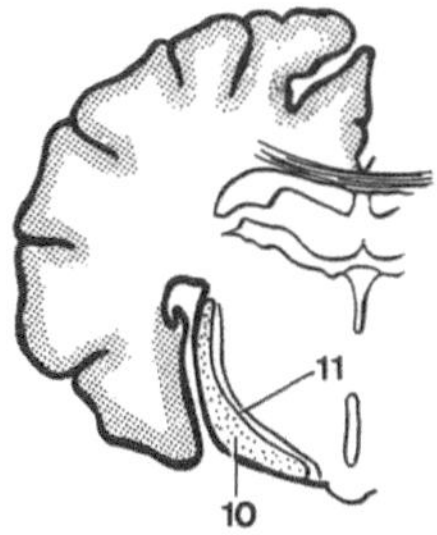

B Prosencephalon, transverse section (ov)

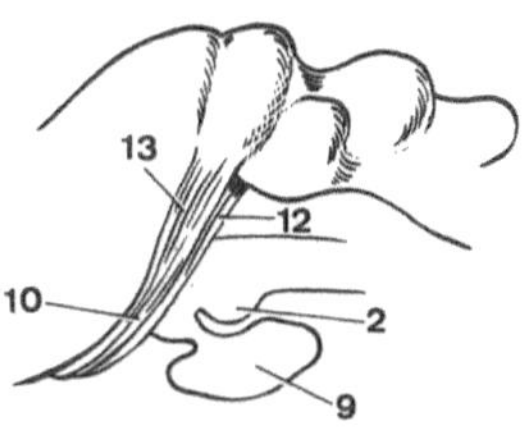

C Tractus opticus, left lateral aspect (eq)

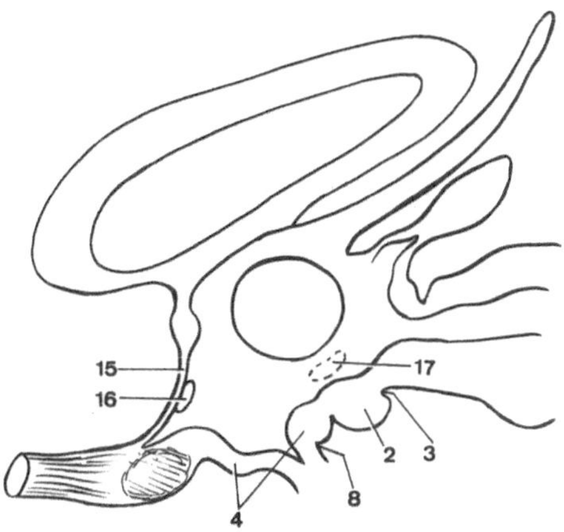

D Diencephalon, median section, right medial aspect (ov)

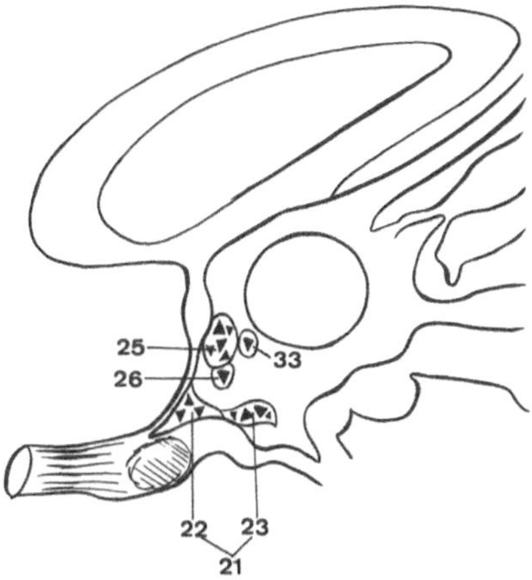

E Diencephalon, median section, right medial aspect, schematic representation of some hypothalamic nuclei (ov)

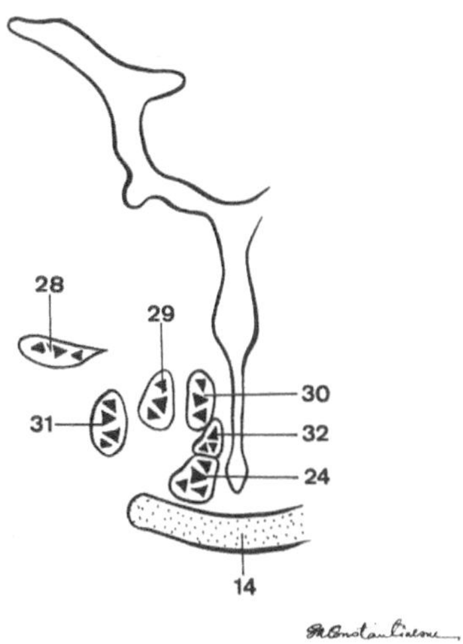

F Diencephalon, transverse section, schematic representation of some hypothalamic nuclei (fe)

1 **Regio hypothalamica intermedia [tuberalis].**

2 ***Nucleus hypothalamicus dorsomedialis.*** Between Nuclei paraventricularis and hypothalamicus ventromedialis. A

3 ***Nucleus hypothalamicus ventromedialis.*** Cajal's nucleus, between Nuclei hypothalamicus dorsomedialis and periventricularis caudalis. A

4 ***Nucleus infundibularis.*** At the origin of Infundibulum neurohypophysis. A

5 ***Area hypothalamica lateralis.*** Includes the following groups of nuclei. B

6 *Nuclei tuberis laterales.* Lateral nuclei of gray tubercle, dorsolateral to Nucleus infundibularis, in Pars parainfundibularis tuberis. B

7 *Nucleus tuberomamillaris.* In Pars caudalis tuberis and dorsal to Corpus mamillare. A

8 **Pars caudalis [Nucleus intercalatus].** Caudal extension between Corpus mamillare and Crus cerebri. A C

9 **Pars supramamillaris.** Main part of Nucleus tuberomamillaris. A (has a wrong indentation in the N. A. V.)

10 **Regio hypothalamica caudalis.** Includes Corpus mamillare.

11 ***Nucleus premamillaris [prae-].*** Between Nucleus infundibularis and Nuclei mamillares. A

12 ***Area hypothalamica dorsalis.*** Dorsal to Area hypothalamica lateralis. B

13 ***Area hypothalamica dorsocaudalis.*** Dorsocaudal to Area hypothalamica lateralis. B

14 ***Nucleus hypothalamicus lateralis.*** Located within the dorsolateral part of hypothalamus, between Ansa lenticularis and fornix. It is not related to Area hypothalamica lateralis. D

15 ***Nucleus hypothalamicus perifornicalis.*** Hypothalamic nucleus around fornix. D

16 ***Nucleus periventricularis caudalis.*** Origin of a part of Fibrae periventriculares. A

17 ***Nucleus mamillaris medialis.*** Medial nucleus of mamillary body. C

18 ***Nucleus mamillaris lateralis.*** Lateral nucleus of mamillary body. C

19 ***Nucleus mamillaris cinereus.*** Gray mamillary nucleus, between Tuber cinereum and Corpus mamillare. A

20 **Commissurae.** Commissures of white matter connecting right and left structures. D

21 ***Commissurae supraopticae.*** Transverse fiber connections dorsal to Tractus opticus and Chiasma opticum. D

22 *Commissura supraoptica dorsalis.* Ganser's commissure. D

23 *Commissura supraoptica ventralis.* Meynert's and Gudden's commissures. D

24 ***Commissura supramamillaris.*** Dorsal to Corpus mamillare.

25 ***Commissurae intrahypothalamicae.*** Within the hypothalamus.

26 **Tractus nervosi projectionis.** Projection fibers, connecting segments of Encephalon with each other and with Medulla spinalis, descending or ascending.

27 ***Fibrae periventriculares.*** Periventricular fibers, from Stratum periventriculare hypothalami to Fasciculus longitudinalis dorsalis. A

28 ***Fornix.*** Arcuate fibers connecting Hippocampus to Corpus mamillare, running in both directions. D

29 ***Fasciculus medialis telencephali.*** Medial fascicle of endbrain, connecting rhinencephalon, hypothalamus and Formatio reticularis. A

30 ***Stria terminalis.*** Bundle of myelinated fibers connecting Corpus amygdaloideum to Pars septalis rhinencephali, Nuclei habenulares, and rostral region of hypothalamus, partially crossed through Commissura rostralis. See 452.17.

31 ***Fasciculus longitudinalis dorsalis.*** Connects hypothalamus to mesencephalon, rhombencephalon, and Medulla spinalis. A

32 ***Fibrae hypothalamoretinales.*** Hypothalamoretinal fibers.

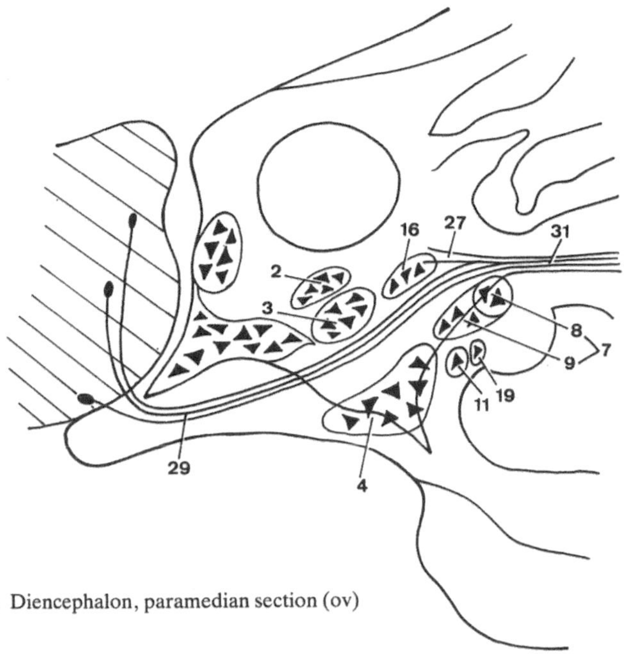

A Diencephalon, paramedian section (ov)

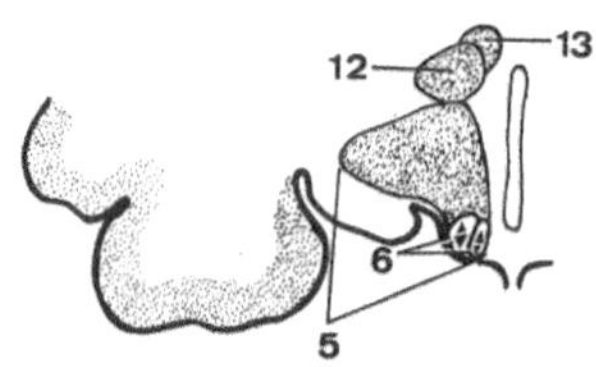

B Hypothalamus, transverse section through Tuber cinereum (fe)

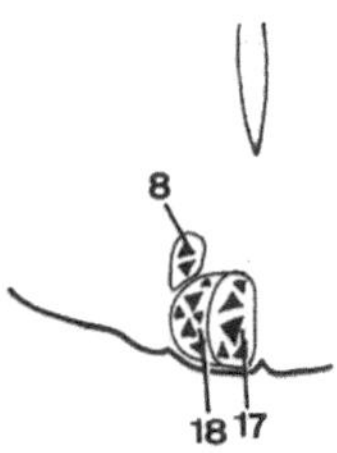

C Hypothalamus, transverse section through Corpus mamillare (fe)

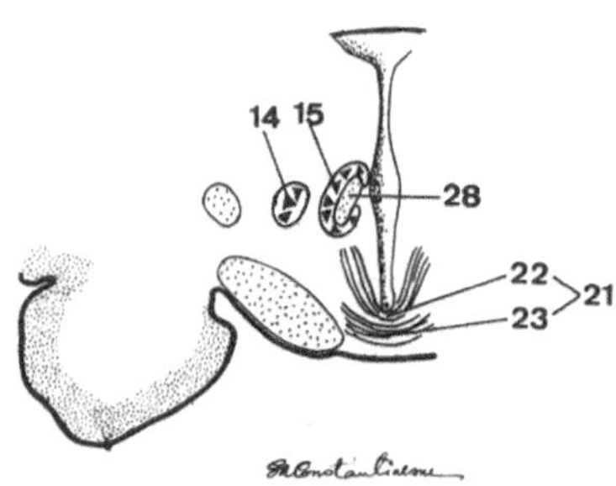

D Hypothalamus, transverse section through Commissurae hypothalami (fe)

1 ***Tractus supraopticohypophysialis***. Fibers from Nucleus supraopticus to Lobus nervosus neurohypophysis, neurosecretory. D

2 ***Tractus paraventriculohypophysialis***. Fibers from Nucleus paraventricularis to Lobus nervosus neurohypophysis, neurosecretory. D

3 ***Tractus tuberohypophysialis***. Former Tractus tuberoinfundibularis. Fibers from the parvocellular hypothalamic nuclei (Nuclei infundibularis, ventromedialis, dorsomedialis), ending around the capillary loops in the Pars proximalis neurohypophysis. D

4 ***Pedunculus mamillaris***. Fibers lateral to Fossa interpeduncularis between Corpus mamillare and mesencephalon. D

5 ***Tractus mamillotegmentalis***. Connects Corpus mamillare and nuclei in the tegmentum. D

6 ***Faciculus mamillohypothalamicus***. Connects Corpus mammilare with hypothalamus.

7 ***Tractus mamillothalamicus***. In the lateral wall of Ventriculus tertius, connects Corpus mamillare with Nuclei rostrales thalami. First short segment runs together with Tractus mamillotegmentalis as Vicq d'Azyr's bundle. A D

8 **Subthalamus**. Between Thalamus and Substantia nigra. A

9 ***Corpus subthalamicum***. Subthalamic body, the Nucleus subthalamicus and related structures lateral to it. A

10 ***Zona incerta***. Uncertain zone, between Tractus mamillothalamicus and Ansa lenticularis. A

11 **Sectiones subthalami**. Cross sections through subthalamus. A B

12 ***Zona incerta***. Uncertain zone. See 10. A

13 ***Nucleus subthalamicus***. Luys's nucleus, between Tractus mamillothalamicus, Nucleus reticulatus thalami, and Substantia nigra. A

14 ***Nucleus endopeduncularis***. Corresponds to medial portion of pallidum of primates. B (Therefore, it shouldn't be listed in the N. A. V.)

15 ***Ansa peduncularis***. Bundle of fibers ventral to Nucleus lentiformis, connecting thalamus to insula and claustrum. B

16 ***Ansa lenticularis***. Bundle of fibers connecting pallidum to thalamus, Nucleus subthalamicus, and mesencephalon. A

17 ***Pedunculus ventralis thalami***. Connecting bridge between thalamus and hypothalamus, contains also connections to telencephalon. B

18 **Thalamencephalon**. Thalamus and associated structures. C

19 **Thalamus**. On both sides of Ventriculus tertius, dorsal to Sulcus hypothalamicus. A C

20 ***Tuberculum rostrale thalami***. Rostral tubercle of thalamus. C

21 ***Tenia [Taenia] thalami***. Thalamic tenia, attachment of Tela choroidea ventriculi tertii along Stria habenularis. C

22 ***Pulvinar***. Not distinct in most domestic mammals. C

23 **Metathalamus**. Represented by Corpora geniculata. C

24 ***Corpus geniculatum mediale***. Medial geniculate body, connected to Colliculus caudalis. Part of auditory pathway. C

25 ***Corpus geniculatum laterale***. Lateral geniculate body, connected to Colliculus rostralis, end of Radix lateralis of Tractus opticus. C

26 **Epithalamus**. Consists of Glandula pinealis (Epiphysis cerebri), the two Habenulae and related structures. C D

27 ***Glandula pinealis***. Pineal gland, or Epiphysis cerebri. C D

28 *Corpus [glandulae pinealis]*. Body [of epiphysis]. D ("Cerebri" should be added, to differentiate it from the Epiphysis of the bones.)

29 *Pedunculus [glandulae pinealis]*. Rostral part, connected with right and left Habenula. D

30 *Recessus pinealis*. Extension of Ventriculus tertius into Corpus et Pedunculus glandulae pinealis. D

31 ***Recessus suprapinealis***. Caudodorsal extension of Ventriculus tertius dorsal to Glandula pinealis. D

32 ***Habenula***. White matter anchoring Glandula pinealis to thalamus. C (It should be "Habenulae", because there are two structures anchoring the Epiphysis cerebri ["Habenulae" is the nominative plural of Habenula], and as a proof, in Commissura habenularum – vide 33 –, "habenularum" is the genitive plural of "Habenula"].)

33 ***Commissura habenularum***. Decussation of fibers connecting the symmetrical Nuclei habenulares. C

34 ***Stria habenularis thalami***. Habenular or medullary stria, band of white matter, rostral continuation of Habenula. C

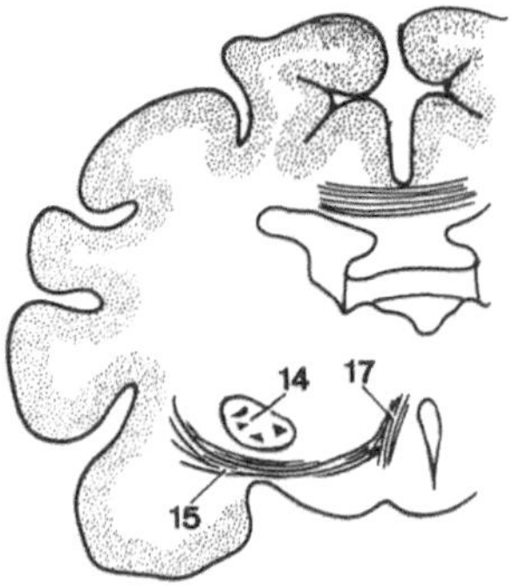

B Subthalamus, transverse section through Tuber cinereum (ca)

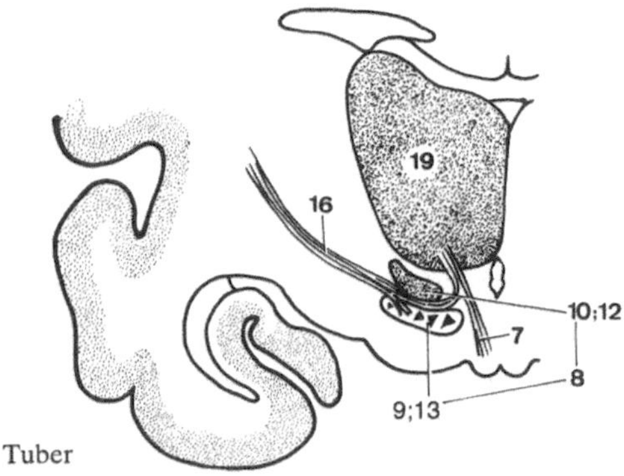

A Thalamus and subthalamus, transverse section through Corpus mamillare (ca)

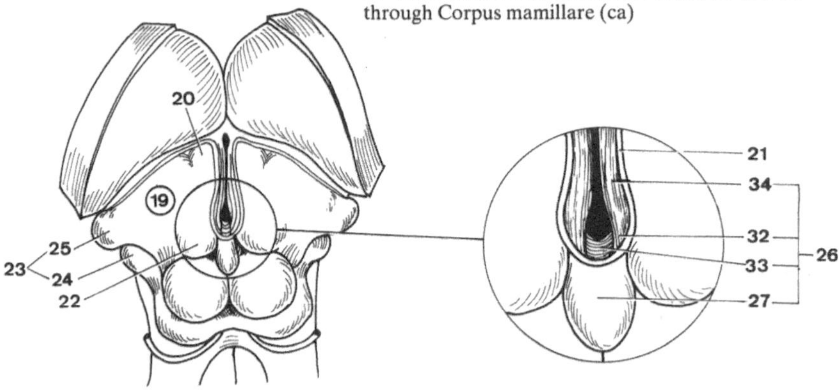

C Thalamencephalon, dorsal aspect (eq)

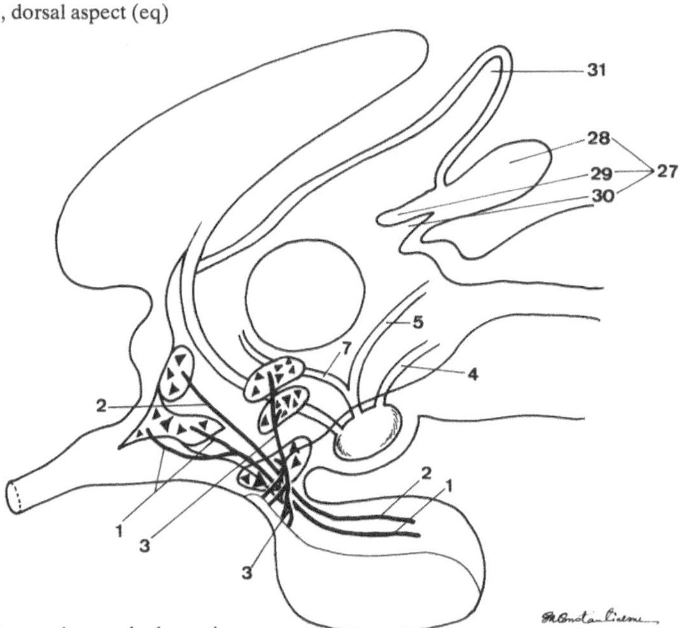

D Epithalamus, median section, and schematic representation of tracts in hypothalamus (ov)

1 **Sectiones thalamencephali.** Sections through thalamus and associated structures. A B C

2 **Sectiones thalami.** Cross sections through thalamus. A B C

3 ***Stratum zonale.*** Zonal layer, layer of white matter covering thalamus on the dorsal aspect. A B C

4 ***Nuclei rostrales thalami.*** Three rostral (anterior) thalamic nuclei, in Tuberculum rostrale thalami, at the dorsal aspect of thalamus, between Stria habenularis and Stria terminalis. Afferent pathways are represented by Tractus mamillothalamicus and fibers from Fasciculus medialis telencephali. Efferent pathways are directed to Nuclei habenulares, Gyrus cinguli and Cortex frontalis. A

5 *Nucleus rostralis dorsalis*. Dorsal rostral nucleus. A

6 *Nucleus rostralis medialis*. Medial rostral nucleus. A

7 *Nucleus rostralis ventralis*. Ventral rostral nucleus. A

8 ***Nuclei laterales thalami.*** Lateral thalamic nuclei, group of six nuclei lateral to Lamina medullaris thalami interna. A B

9 *Nucleus ventralis rostralis*. Afferent fibers from pallidum, cerebellum, and Nucleus interstitialis. Efferent connections to motor cortex. A

10 *Nucleus ventralis lateralis*. Afferent fibers from Nuclei vestibulares and cerebellum. Efferent connections to Cortex parietalis. A

11 *Nucleus ventralis caudalis*. Caudal ventral nucleus. B

12 **Pars medialis.** Medial part. Synapse between Lemniscus trigeminalis and sensory cortex. B

13 **Pars lateralis.** Lateral part. Synapse between Lemniscus medialis and sensory cortex. B

14 *Nucleus lateralis dorsalis*. Located dorsal to 9 and 10. Connections with other thalamic nuclei and Cortex temporalis. A

15 *Nucleus lateralis caudalis*. Located dorsal to 11. Connections with other thalamic nuclei and Cortex temporalis. B

16 *Nucleus pulvinaris*. Afferent fibers from other thalamic nuclei and Nuclei pretectales. Efferent connections to sensory cortex. B

17 ***Lamina medullaris thalami externa.*** External thalamic medullary lamina, thin layer of white matter separating Nucleus reticulatus from Nuclei laterales thalami. A C

18 ***Lamina medullaris thalami interna.*** Internal thalamic medullary lamina, thin layer of white matter separating Nuclei laterales thalami from Nuclei rostrales thalami. A C

19 ***Nuclei intralaminares thalami.*** Afferent fibers from cerebellum and Lemniscus medialis. Efferent connections to Corpus striatum and Nucleus dorsomedialis thalami. There are five thalamic intralaminar nuclei (20–24). C

20 *Nucleus centralis medialis*. Medial central nucleus. C

21 *Nucleus paracentralis*. Paracentral nucleus. C

22 *Nucleus centralis lateralis*. Lateral central nucleus. C

23 *Nucleus centralis thalami [Centrum medianum]*. Thalamic central (centromedian) nucleus, morphologically not strictly intralaminar, more developed in primates, easily visible also in Un. Morphologically not strictly intralaminar. C

24 *Nucleus parafascicularis*. Morphologically not strictly intralaminar, similar to the previous one. However, they are included in the group because they have similar functional characteristics. C

25 ***Nucleus dorsomedialis thalami.*** Thalamic dorsomedial nucleus. Caudal to Nucleus paraventricularis. Afferent fibers from Pedunculus ventralis thalami. Efferent connections with thalamic and hypothalamic nuclei as well as with Cortex frontalis. C

26 ***Nuclei paraventriculares thalami.*** Thalamic paraventricular nuclei, sometimes referred to as “midline nuclei”, near the median plane. They are sometimes confused with Nuclei intralaminares thalami.

27 ***Nucleus reticulatus thalami.*** Between Lamina medullaris thalami externa and Capsula interna. A

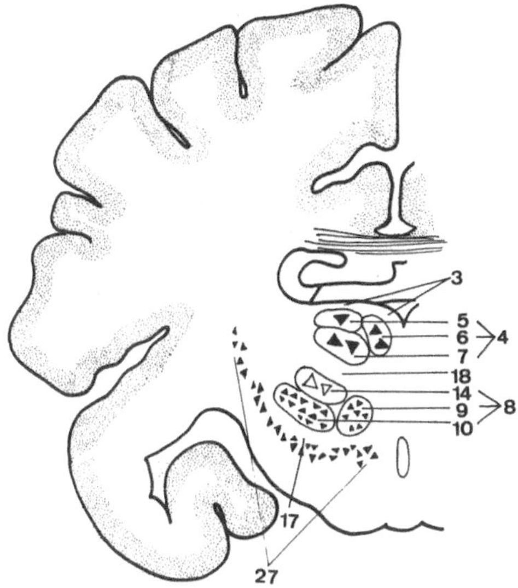

A Thalamencephalon, transverse section through Corpus mamillare (eq)

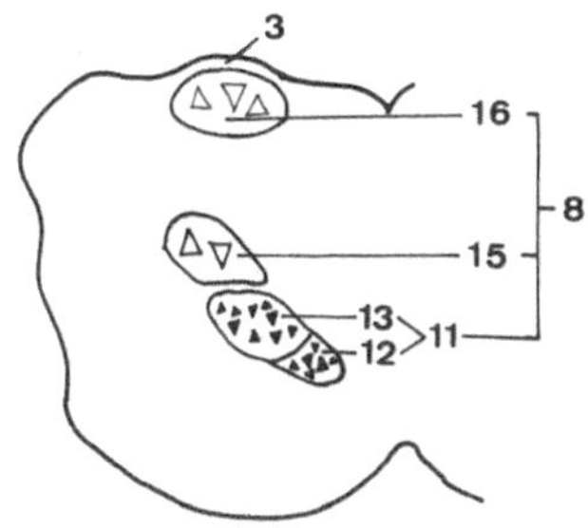

B Thalamencephalon, transverse section through Corpora geniculata and Pedunculi cerebri (eq)

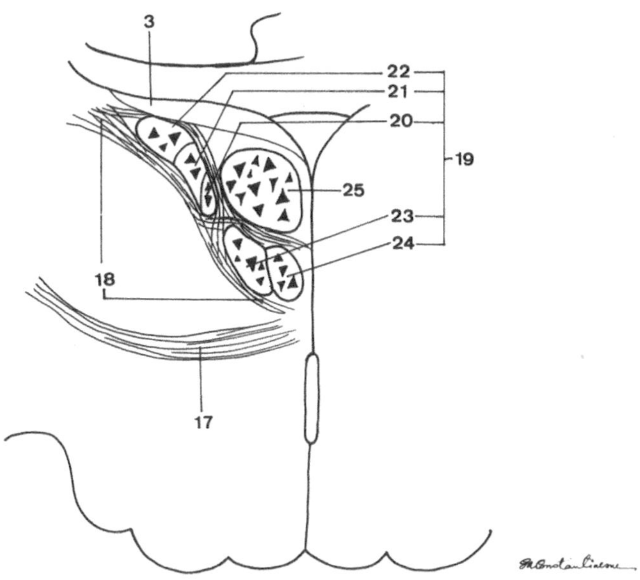

C Thalamus, transverse section, schematic representation of Nuclei intralaminares

1 **Sectiones metathalami.** Only one cross section through metathalamus is shown in fig. A. A

2 ***Nucleus geniculatus medialis.*** Cell group in Corpus geniculatum mediale, synapse in the auditory pathway. A

3 ***Nucleus geniculatus lateralis.*** Related to Corpus geniculatum laterale, in the visual pathway. A

4 *Pars dorsalis.* Dorsal (main) part. End of Radix lateralis of Tractus opticus, start of Radiatio optica to Area striata of Lobus occipitalis. A

5 *Pars ventralis.* Ventral part. A

6 **Sectiones epithalami.** Only one cross section through epithalamus is shown in fig. B. B

7 ***Nuclei habenulares.*** Related to habenula. Synapse between Stria habenularis thalami and mesencephalon. B

8 *Nucleus habenularis medialis.* Medial habenular nucleus. B

9 *Nucleus habenularis lateralis.* Lateral habenular nucleus. B

10 ***Commissura habenularum.*** Connects right and left Nuclei habenulares. B

11 ***Fasciculus retroflexus.*** Meynert's fascicle, from Nuclei habenulares to Nucleus interpeduncularis. B

12 **Telencephalon.** Endbrain, the most developed segment of Prosencephalon, its principal components are Neopallium, Rhinencephalon and Corpus striatum.

13 **Cerebrum.** The two hemispheres connected by commissures. C

14 ***Fissura longitudinalis cerebri.*** Cerebral longitudinal fissure, separating the two hemispheres. The Falx cerebri is located within it. A C D

15 ***Fissura transversa cerebri.*** Cerebral transverse fissure, between the two hemispheres and cerebellum. The Tentorium cerebelli membranaceum is located within it. C

16 ***Basis cerebri.*** Cerebral basis, corresponds to the ventral aspect of cerebrum. D

17 **Hemispherium [Hemisphaerium].** The two symmetrical and biggest segments of cerebrum. C

18 ***Facies convexa [F. dorsolateralis].*** Convex (dorsolateral) surface of each hemisphere. E

19 ***Facies medialis.*** Medial surface, separated from its fellow by Fissura longitudinalis cerebri. F

20 ***Facies basilaris.*** Basal or ventral surface. D

21 ***Margo dorsalis [dorsomedialis].*** Dorsal (dorsomedial) border, separates Facies convexa and medialis. A E F

22 ***Polus rostralis [frontalis].*** Rostral (frontal) pole. E F

23 ***Polus caudalis [occipitalis].*** Caudal (ocipital) pole. E F

24 ***Pallium.*** Cloak- or mantle-like part of the hemisphere enveloping the brainstem. D

25 *Paleopallium [Palaeo-].* Oldest part of pallium, part of the Rhinencephalon on the ventral aspect of the hemisphere between Sulcus rhinalis lateralis and Sulcus endorhinalis, includes Lobus piriformis. D

26 *Archipallium.* On the medial aspect of the hemisphere, represented by Hippocampus and associated structures (ammonic complex). A

27 *Neopallium.* Youngest part of pallium, located dorsolaterally between the two previous structures. A D

28 ***Cortex cerebri.*** Cerebral cortex, superficial gray matter overlapping the hemispheres. A

29 ***Sulci cerebri.*** Cerebral sulci, grooves separating gyri. A E F

30 ***Gyri cerebri.*** Cerebral gyri, convolutions of cerebral surface, separated by sulci. A E F

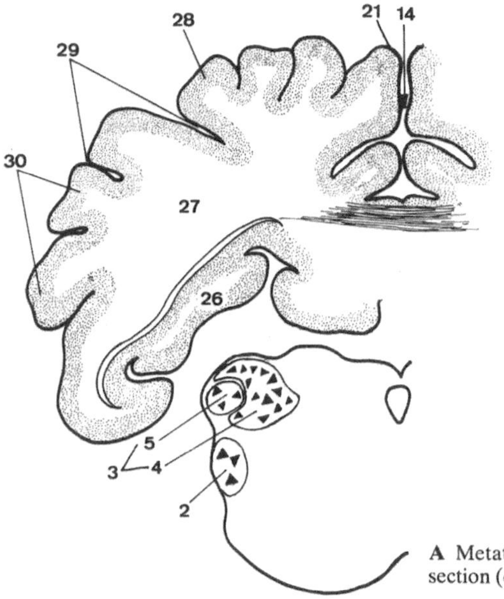

A Metathalamus and Hemispherium, transverse section (eq)

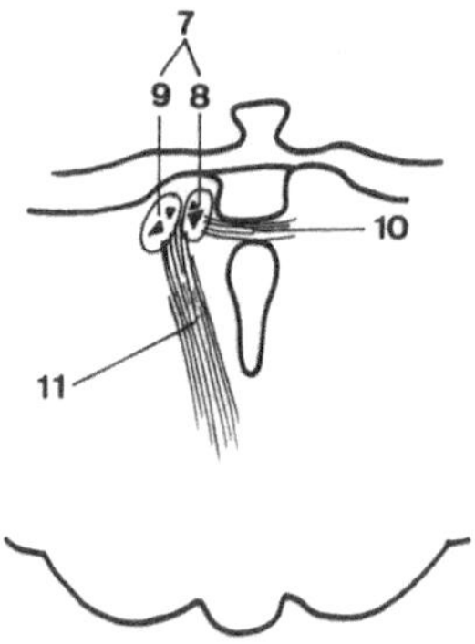

B Epithalamus, transverse section (eq)

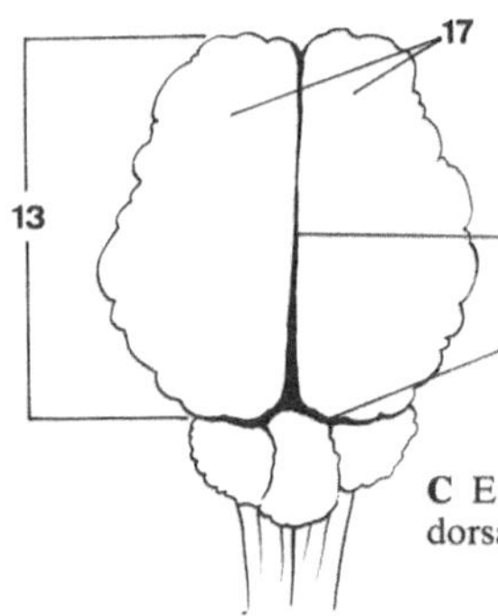

C Encephalon, dorsal aspect (eq)

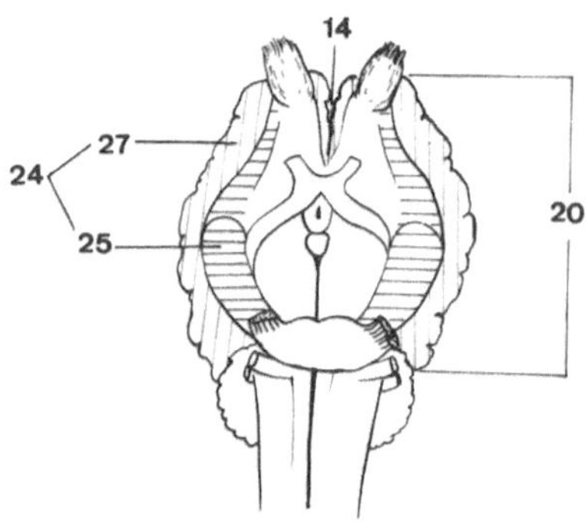

D Basis cerebri (eq)

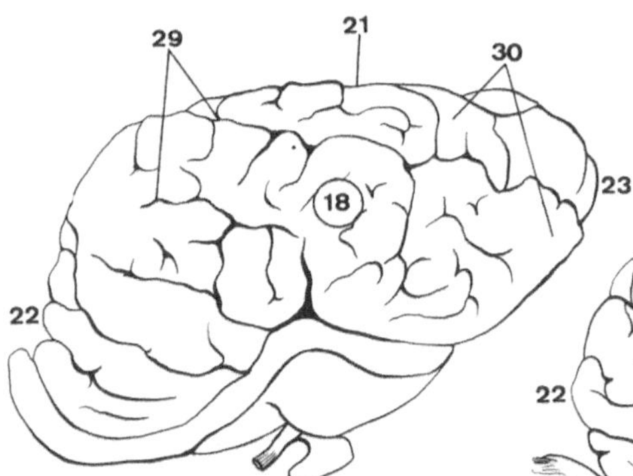

E Facies convexa (lateralis) of left hemispherium (eq)

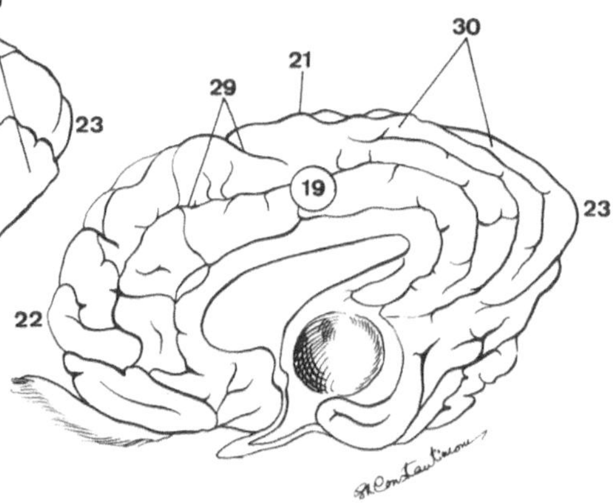

F Facies medialis of right hemispherium (eq)

1 **Rhinencephalon**. Olfactory brain, consisting of basal Telencephalon, Hippocampus and associated structures. The function is not wholly related to olfaction.

2 **Pars basalis rhinencephali.** Basal part of olfactory brain. A

3 ***Sulcus rhinalis lateralis***. Lateral olfactory groove, separates Neopallium from Rhinencephalon. A B

4 *Pars rostralis*. Rostral part. A B

5 *Pars caudalis*. Caudal part, separated from Pars rostralis by Limen insulae. A B

6 ***Sulcus rhinalis medialis***. Medial olfactory groove, separates Pedunculus olfactorius from Neopallium. A

7 ***Bulbus olfactorius***. Olfactory bulb, the most rostral part of the Rhinencephalon containing the mitral cells with their many dendrites. A B

8 ***Sulcus limitans bulbi olfactorii***. Limiting groove of olfactory bulb, separates Bulbus olfactorius from Pedunculus olfactorius. A

9 ***Bulbus olfactorius accessorius***. Accessory olfactory bulb, lateral, medial and superior to Bulbus olfactorius in Car and Un, associated with the vomeronasal system. 465 A

10 ***Pedunculus olfactorius***. Olfactory peduncle, joins Bulbus olfactorius to Hemispherium. A

11 ***Tractus olfactorius lateralis***. Lateral olfactory tract. A

12 ***Tractus olfactorius medialis***. Medial olfactory tract. A

13 ***Trigonum olfactorium***. Olfactory trigone, term applies to microsmatic mammals.

14 ***Sulcus limitans trigoni olfactorii***. Term applies to microsmatic mammals.

15 ***Lobus piriformis***. Piriform lobe, caudal to Pedunculus olfactorius, extends from Tuberculum olfactorium to Tuberculum hippocampi, caudally not clearly delimited from Neocortex. A

16 *Pars rostralis*. Rostral part. A

17 *Pars caudalis*. Caudal part, separated from Pars rostralis by Vallecula lateralis cerebri. A

18 ***Gyrus olfactorius lateralis***. Lateral olfactory gyrus, borders on Pars rostralis and the rostral part of Pars caudalis of Lobus piriformis. Term used only for microsmatic animals. A B

19 ***Limen insulae***. Limen (pole) of insula, between Pars rostralis and Pars caudalis of Sulcus rhinalis lateralis. The band of transition between the anterior portion of the gray matter of the Insula and Substantia perforata rostralis. B

20 ***Gyrus parahippocampalis***. Caudal continuation of Lobus piriformis, located lateral to Sulcus hippocampi. Formerly known as Gyrus hippocampi. It is used only for microsmatic animals. A C

21 ***Vallecula [Fossa] lateralis cerebri***. Lateral cerebral depression in lower macrosmatic mammals, and is gradually transformed into a fossa in the higher macrosmatic and the microsmatic species. It separates the two parts of Lobus piriformis and the two parts of the Sulcus rhinalis lateralis. A B

22 ***Sulcus endorhinalis***. Endorhinal groove, the lateral limit of Tuberculum olfactorium. A

23 ***Tuberculum olfactorium***. Olfactory tubercle, bordered by Tractus olfactorius medialis and Sulcus endorhinalis. A

24 ***Substantia perforata rostralis***. In general, it is only found in higher and microsmatic mammals.

25 **Pars septalis rhinencephali**. Septal part of olfactory brain, located on the medial aspect of the hemisphere. C

26 ***Area subcallosa***. Ventral to Genu and Rostrum corporis callosi. C

27 ***Gyrus paraterminalis***. Grossly visible only in microsmatic mammals. It represents the former Gyrus subcallosus (Pedunculus corporis callosi). C

28 ***Gyrus diagonalis***. Ventral part of Gyrus paraterminalis. It designates a superficial elevation, the ventral part of the Gyrus paraterminalis. C

29 ***Septum telencephali [cellulare, verum]***. Septum of endbrain. Septum telencephali is applied to all species, it connects Corpus callosum and Fornix and separates the Ventriculi laterales. The synonyms “cellulare” and “verum” are applied to lower mammals in which the thick septum contains many nerve cells and can be hardly called Septum pellucidum. C

30 ***Septum telencephali [pellucidum]***. Septum of endbrain (pellucid septum). Term applies to microsmatic mammals.

31 *Cavum septi telencephali [pellucidi]*. The cavity of telencephalic septum.

32 *Lamina septi telencephali [pellucidi]*. The lamina of telencephalic septum.

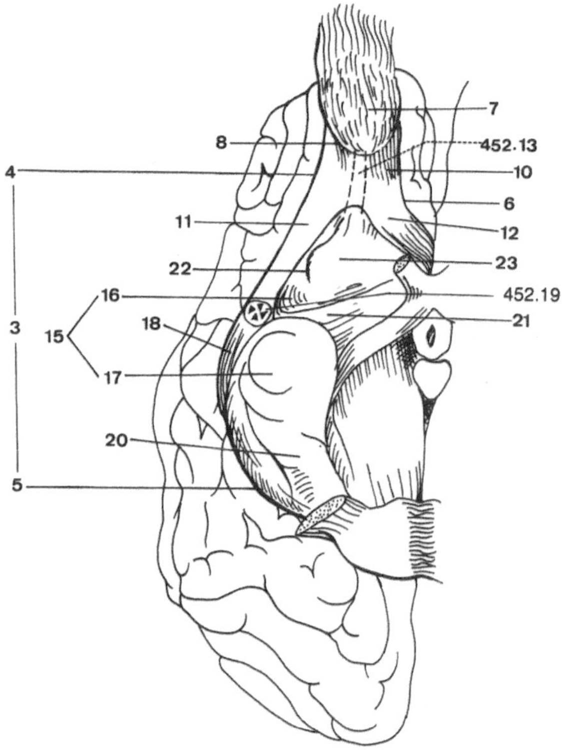

A Pars basalis rhinencephali (eq)

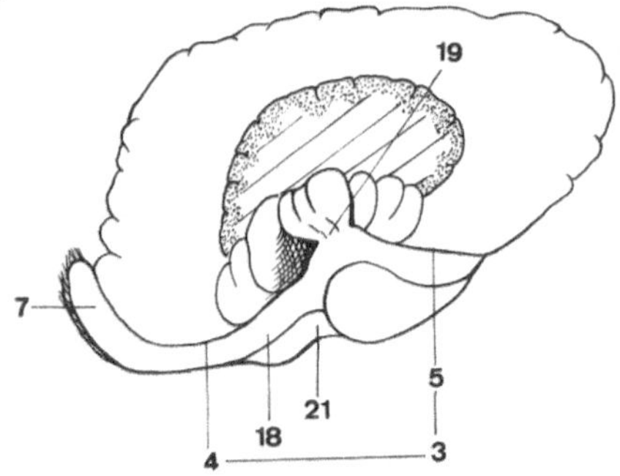

B Left insula, opercula removed (eq)

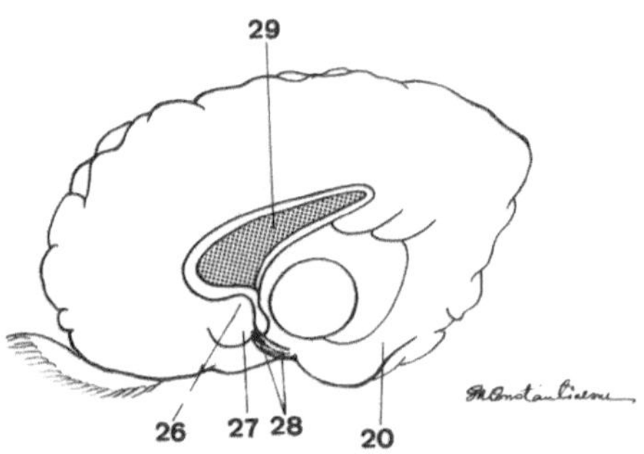

C Pars septalis rhinencephali

1 **Pars limbica rhinencephali**. Limbic (marginal) part of olfactory brain.

2 ***Hippocampus***. The Pars retrocommissuralis is the hippocampus proper, the two other parts are not so well developed.

3 *Pars precommissuralis [prae-]*. Extends rostral to Genu corporis callosi as far as the root of Pedunculus olfactorius, seldom macroscopically distinct. It can include a dorsal part of Gyrus paraterminalis. B

4 *Pars supracommissuralis [Indusium griseum]*. On Corpus callosum as a thin layer of gray matter and in Sulcus corporis callosi. B C

5 *Pars retrocommissuralis*. Hippocampus proper, elongated prominence in Pars centralis and Cornu temporale of lateral ventricle. A B C

6 ***Gyrus geniculi***. Genicular gyrus, continuation of Gyrus supracallosus below the Genu corporis callosi. B

7 ***Gyrus supracallosus***. If the Sulcus corporis callosi is not directly adjacent to the Corpus callosum, there appears a small Gyrus supracallosus. B C

8 ***Sulcus corporis callosi***. Separates Corpus callosum or Gyrus corporis callosi from Gyrus cinguli. B C

9 ***Striae longitudinales***. Longitudinal white bands on Corpus callosum. C

10 *Stria longitudinalis lateralis*. The lateral Lancisi's stria. C

11 *Stria longitudinalis medialis*. The medial Lancisi's stria. C

12 ***Pes hippocampi [Cornu ammonis]***. Ventral end of hippocampus, in man pawshaped. C

13 ***Alveus hippocampi***. Thin layer of white matter covering the internal surface of the hippocampus. A C

14 ***Fimbria hippocampi***. Free border of alveus, traveling along the border of the hippocampus parallel to Gyrus dentatus. Continues as Crus fornicis. A B C

15 ***Cornu ammonis inversum***. Inverse ammon's horn, part of ammonic complex on the extraventricular surface. In man vestiges which remain superficially form the Gyrus fasciolaris. B

15a ***Gyrus fasciolaris [Fasciola cinerea]***. A, see 15

16 ***Gyrus dentatus [Fascia dentata]***. Denticulated by virtue of numerous crenations, between Sulcus hippocampi and Sulcus fimbriodentatus. C

17 ***Sulcus hippocampi***. Ammon's horn groove, between Gyrus parahippocampalis and Gyrus dentatus. B C

18 ***Sulcus fimbriodentatus***. Groove between Fimbra hippocampi and Gyrus dentatus. B C

19 ***Sulcus dentatoammonis***. Groove between Gyrus dentatus and Cornu ammonis inversum. B

20 ***Sulcus fimbrioammonis***. Groove between Fimbria hippocampi and Cornu ammonis inversum. B

21 ***Tuberculum hippocampi***. Ammon's horn tubercle, medial to the rostral end of Gyrus parahippocampalis, corresponds to uncus of primates. B

21a ***Uncus***. The Uncus of higher primates is homologous to the Tuberculum hippocampi of other mammals[1)].

21b ***Incisura unci***. The groove between the Uncus and the Gyrus parahippocampalis [1)].

21c ***Diverticulum unci***. A recess of the temporal horn of the lateral ventricle [1)].

22 ***Fornix***. Arcuate fibers connecting Hippocampus to Corpus mamillare, running in both directions. A 22, 25 B 23–26, 28

23 *Crus fornicis*. Paired convergent structure, arises from hippocampus, fuses with the contralateral one to form the Corpus fornicis. B

24 *Corpus fornicis*. Body of fornix, unpaired structure formed by fusion of the crura. B

25 *Tenia [Taenia] fornicis*. Border of fornix to which the tela choroidea is attached. A B C

26 *Columna fornicis*. Paired structure starting from Corpus fornicis, surrounds Foramen interventriculare rostrally, runs in the wall of Ventriculus III to Corpus mamillare. B

27 *Commissura fornicis [hippocampi] ventralis [Psalterium ventrale]*. Rostroventral connection, relation to a Nucleus septi. 437 C

28 *Commissura fornicis [hippocampi] dorsalis [Psalterium dorsale]*. Caudodorsal connection of Crura fornicis, difficult to distinguish from Corpus callosum. B

29 ***Organum subfornicale***. See 436.15.

1) These are structures found only in primates, therefore they shouldn't be listed in the N.A.V.

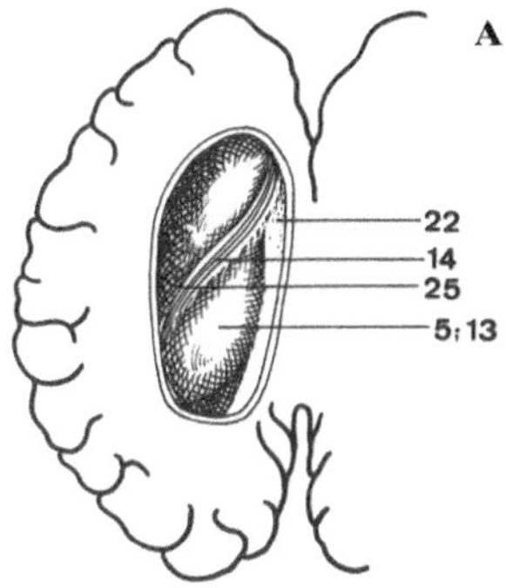

A Left ventriculus lateralis opened, dorsal aspect (eq)

B Pars limbica rhinencephali, median section right half (eq)

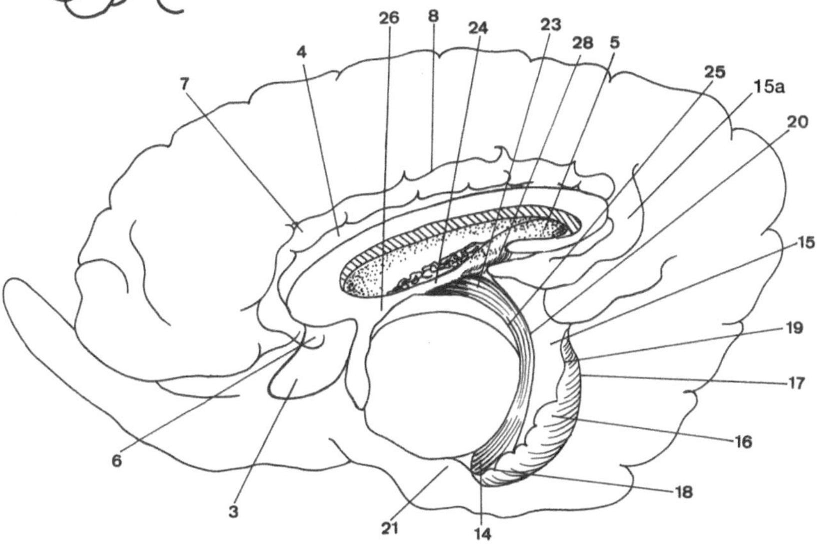

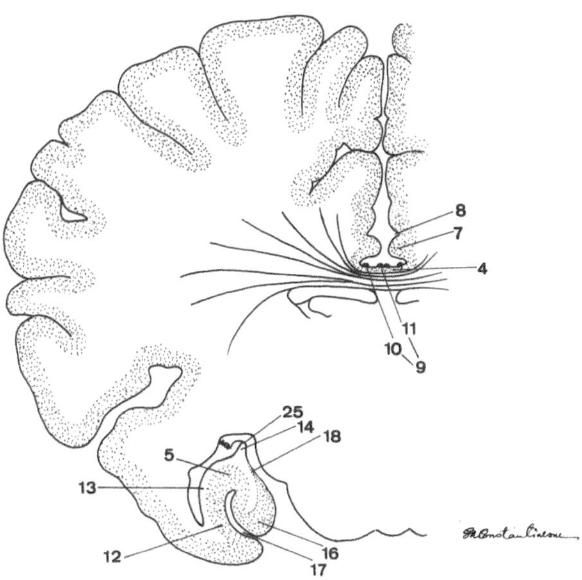

C Pars limbica rhinencephali, transverse section (eq)

1 **Sectiones rhinencephali**. Sections through the olfactory brain.

2 **Allocortex**. The rind of Paleopallium and Archipallium, covers the territories of Rhinencephalon. A

3 *Stratum moleculare*. Molecular layer, contains the end segments of pyramidal cell dendrites, a few small cell bodies and many neuroglial cells. A

4 *Stratum pyramidale*. Pyramidal layer, contains pyramidal cells of various sizes, and nerve cell endings. A

5 *Stratum granulare*. Granular layer, consists of small cell bodies of various shapes, and nerve cell endings. A

6 *Paleocortex [Palaeo-]*. Cortex of the Pars basalis rhinencephali, covers the Lobus piriformis. A

7 *Peripaleocortex [-palaeo-]*. Superficial paleocortex. A

8 *Archicortex*. Cortex of Pars septalis and Pars limbica rhinencephali (Hippocampus, Gyrus dentatus). A

9 **Subiculum**. Cortex of the dorsal part of Gyrus parahippocampalis, near Sulcus hippocampi, covered by a layer of white substance. A

10 **Pes hippocampi [Cornu ammonis]**. The cortex is made up of the same main layers described in Allocortex, with the exception of Stratum granulare which is replaced by a polymorphic or multiform lamina, similar to Stratum multiforme of Neocortex. A B

11 **Gyrus dentatus [Fascia dentata]**. The section through Gyrus dentatus shows its relationships with the very end lamina of hippocampus surrounded by a molecular layer, a pyramidal layer with very small nerve cells and a polymorphic cell layer. A

12 *Periarchicortex*. Superficial archicortex. A

13 ***Tractus olfactorius intermedius***. Intermediate olfactory tract, a penetrating mass of gray substance, which is well developed in macrosmatic mammals. In microsmatic mammals there is a progressive reduction of the gray matter and a greater development of the fibers. 449 A

14 ***Commissura rostralis***. Bridge of white matter, belonging to Paleopallium, connects right and left Rhinencephalon, located in the rostral wall of Ventriculus III, dorsal to Lamina terminalis grisea. B

15 *Pars rostralis*. Rostral part, the stronger one, runs in laterorostroventral direction to Bulbus olfactorius. B

16 *Pars caudalis*. Caudal part, more delicate, runs over Nucleus lentiformis in laterocaudoventral direction to Lobus piriformis. B

17 ***Stria terminalis***. Bundle of myelinated fibers running in Sulcus thalamocaudatus, connecting Corpus amygdaloideum to Pars septalis rhinencephali, Nuclei habenulares and the rostral region of hypothalamus, partly crossed by Commissura rostralis. D

18 ***Corpus amygdaloideum***. Amygdaloid body, although part of basal ganglion, functionally related to Rhinencephalon, contains synapses of olfactory pathway, located rostral to Cornu temporale of Ventriculus lateralis, in connection with ammonic complex and claustrum. B C

19 *Nucleus tractus olfactorii lateralis*. Located at the caudal extent of Tractus olfactorius lateralis. Afferent fibers from Bulbus olfactorius. 449 A

20 *Nucleus corticalis*. In connection with cortex. Afferent fibers from Bulbus olfactorius. C

21 *Nucleus basalis*. Same function as Nucleus lateralis. C

22 *Nucleus lateralis*. Extends most rostrally as far as claustrum. Afferent fibers from the other nuclei of Corpus amygdaloideum, efferent to Stria terminalis and olfactory cortex. C

23 *Nucleus centralis*. Afferent fibers from Bulbus olfactorius. C

24 *Nucleus medialis*. Afferent fibers from Bulbus olfactorius. C

25 ***Lamella diagonalis***. Broca's lamella, histological structure belonging to Gyrus diagonalis (see 448.28). E

26 ***Nuclei septi***. Nuclei of the septal region, protrude partly into Ventriculus lateralis from its medial wall. E

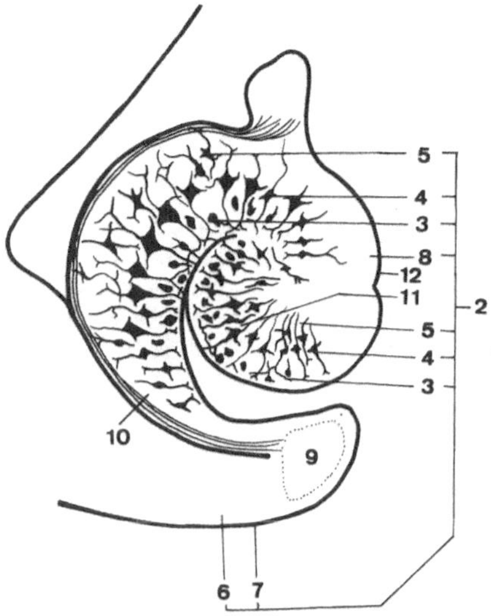

A Schematic transverse section through left temporal horn of lateral ventricle, Gyrus parahippocampalis, Hippocampus and Gyrus dentatus, caudal aspect

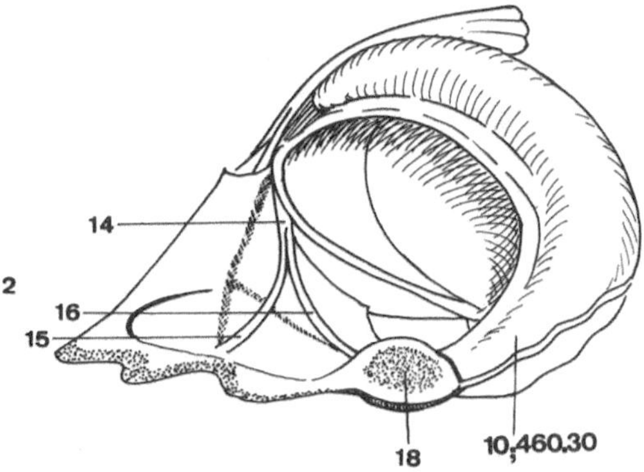

B Left ammonic complex and Commissura rostralis, lateral aspect (eq)

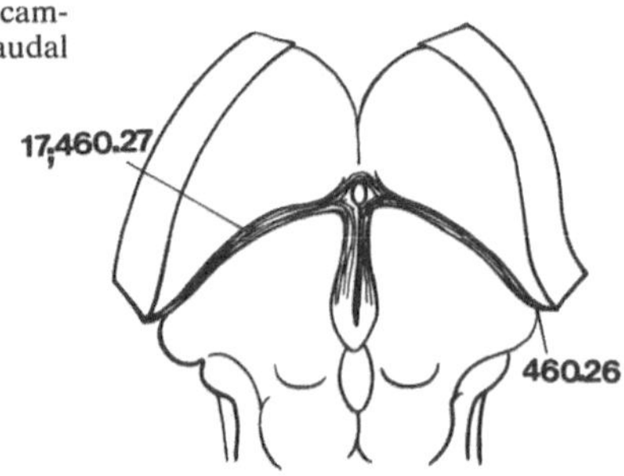

D Nucleus caudatus and thalamus, dorsal aspect (eq)

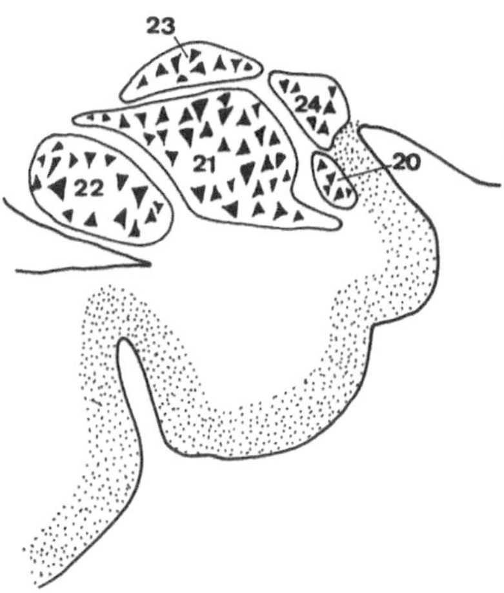

C Corpus amygdaloideum, transverse section (eq)

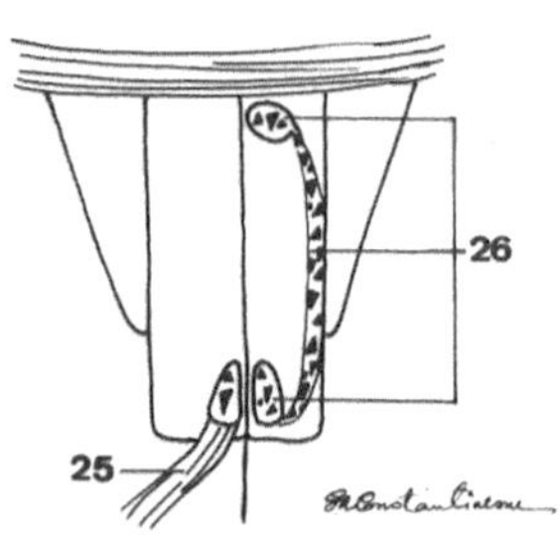

E Septum telencephali, transverse section

1 **Neopallium**. Phylogenetically the youngest part of pallium. The list of Sulci and Gyri neopalii has been reduced to the terms designating the most obvious features. The following species have been selected as types: a carnivore, Felis catus, the best known, even though the figures D – F are drawn from Canis familiaris, and an ungulate, Equus caballus.

2 ***Fissura pseudosylvia***. Pseudosylvian fissure, occurs in Car and is primitive. It is located lateral and dorsal to Lobus piriformis and joins Sulcus rhinalis lateralis at the junction of its Pars rostralis with Pars caudalis. D

3 ***Fissura sylvia [lateralis cerebri]***. Sylvian [lateral cerebral] fissure, appears in Un and Pr as a result of a process of opercularisation. Similar topographical position as Fissura pseudosylvia, but deeper. A

4 ***Sulcus ectosylvius rostralis***. Rostral ectosylvian groove, rostral and dorsal to the previous two fissures. A D

5 ***Sulcus diagonalis*** (Un). Diagonal groove, ventral to the previous. A

6 ***Sulcus ectosylvius caudalis***. Caudal ectosylvian groove. A D

7 ***Sulcus presylvius [prae-]***. Presylvian groove, ventral to Sulcus diagonalis. A D E

8 ***Sulcus proreus [orbitalis]*** (Un). Prorean groove, ventral to Sulcus presylvius. A

9 ***Sulcus suprasylvius medius***. Middle suprasylvian groove, dorsal to Gyrus ectosylvius medius. A D E

10 ***Sulcus suprasylvius rostralis***. Rostral suprasylvian groove, the rostral continuation of the previous, dorsal to Gyrus ectosylvius rostralis. A D E

11 ***Sulcus suprasylvius caudalis***. Caudal suprasylvian groove, the caudal continuation of Sulcus suprasylvius medius, dorsal or caudal to Gyrus ectosylvius caudalis. A C D E

12 ***Sulcus marginalis [sagittalis]***. Marginal [sagittal] groove. Appears on the dorsolateral aspect of the hemisphere. C D E

13 ***Sulcus ectomarginalis [ectosagittalis]***. Ectomarginal [ectosagittal] groove, on the dorsolateral aspect. A C D E

14 ***Sulcus endomarginalis [endosagittalis]***. Endomarginal [endosagittal] groove, on the dorsal aspect. May be absent in Car. B C D E

15 ***Sulcus ansatus***. Ansiform groove, in Un on both sides over the dorsal border of the hemisphere. B C D E

16 ***Sulcus postcruciatus [postcentralis]*** (Car). Postcruciate [postcentral] groove on the dorsolateral surface, between Sulcus ansatus and Sulcus cruciatus. D E

17 ***Sulcus coronalis***. Coronal groove, in Car located on the lateral aspect ventral to Gyrus precruciatus and Gyrus postcruciatus. C D E

18 ***Sulcus cruciatus [centralis]***. Cruciate [central] groove. In Car analogous to Sulcus centralis of Primates and located on both sides of the hemisphere. In the other domestic mammals visible only on the medial aspect rostral to sulcus ansatus. B C D E F

19 ***Sulcus splenialis***. Splenial groove, on the medial aspect midway between Corpus callosum and the dorsal border of the hemisphere. B F

20 ***Sulcus suprasplenialis***. Suprasplenial groove, midway between Sulcus splenialis and the dorsal border of the hemisphere. B F

21 ***Sulcus obliquus***. Oblique groove, caudal to Fissura sylvia and to Gyrus obliquus rostralis, present in most Un, best developed in eq. A C

22 ***Sulcus genualis***. Genual groove, well developed in Un, poorly in ca, and absent in fe. Rostral continuation of Sulcus splenialis. B F

23 ***Sulcus calcarinus*** (Un). Calcarine groove, caudal continuation of Sulcus splenialis. B (calcar = spur-shaped)

24 ***Sulcus rostralis internus*** (Un). Rostral internal groove, dorsal to, and parallel to Sulcus rhinalis medialis. B

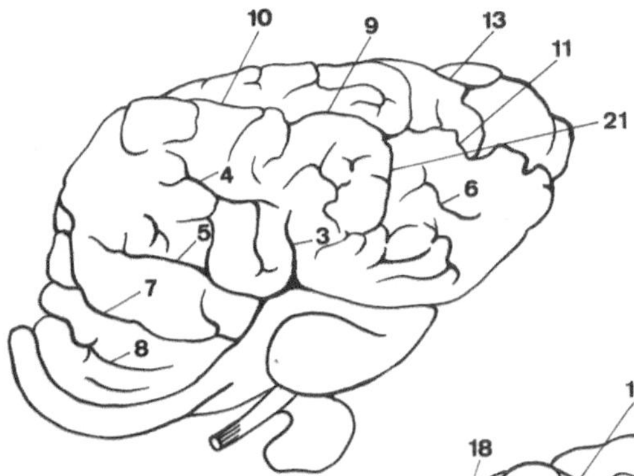

A Sulci of neopallium, left lateral aspect (eq)

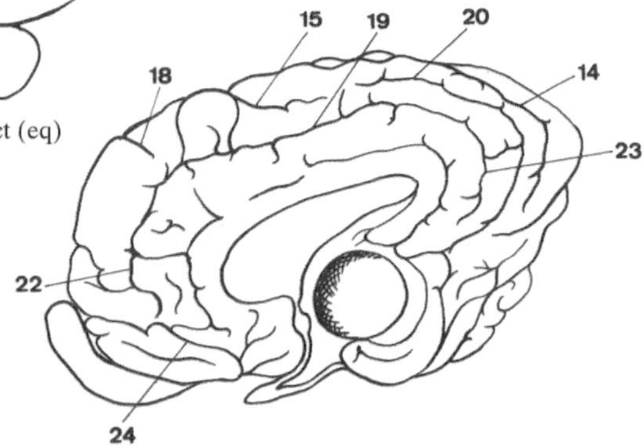

B Sulci of neopallium, medial aspect right half (eq)

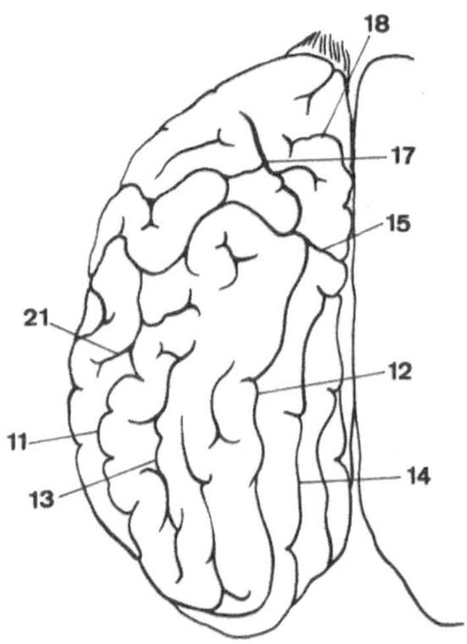

C Sulci of left neopallium, dorsal aspect (eq)

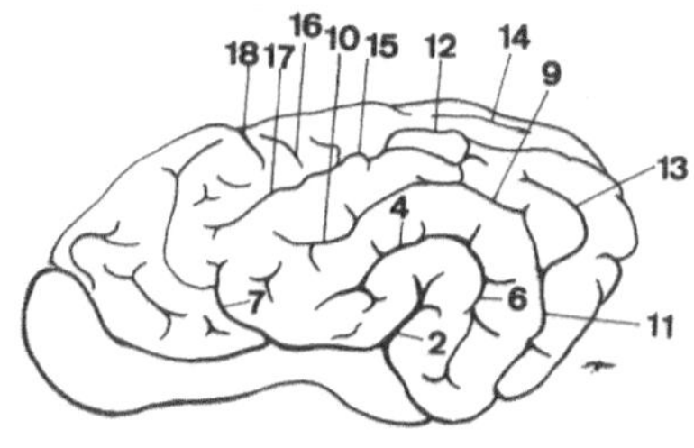

D Sulci of neopallium, left lateral aspect (ca)

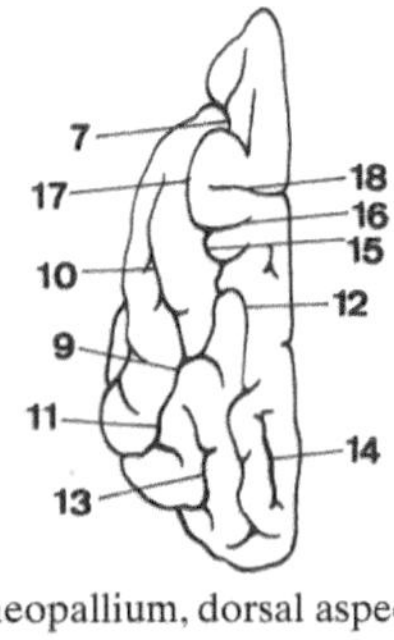

E Sulci of left neopallium, dorsal aspect (ca)

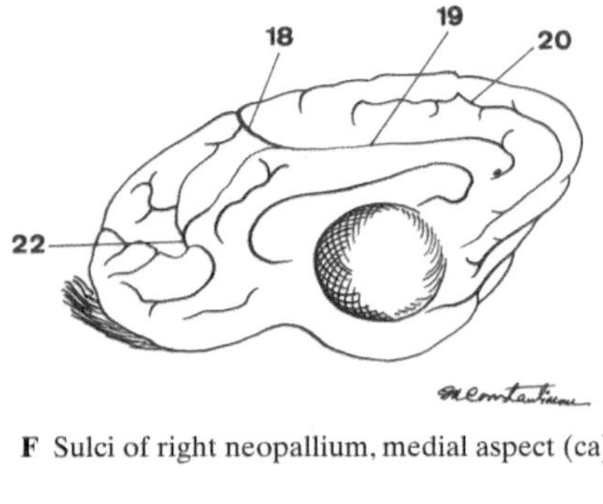

F Sulci of right neopallium, medial aspect (ca)

1 ***Gyrus sylvius rostralis***. Rostral sylvian gyrus. A D

2 ***Gyrus sylvius caudalis***. Caudal sylvian gyrus. A D

3 ***Gyrus compositus rostralis***. Rostral composite gyrus. In Car rostral to Gyrus ectosylvius rostralis and dorsal to Sulcus rhinalis lateralis, in Un the most rostrodorsal structure of the lateral aspect. A C D

4 ***Gyrus compositus caudalis***. Caudal composite gyrus, most ventrocaudal gyrus. A D

5 ***Gyrus ectosylvius medius***. Middle ectosylvian gyrus, ventral to Sulcus suprasylvius medius. A C D E

6 ***Gyrus intersylvius***. Intersylvian gyrus, formerly Gyrus felinus, occurs in Car, between Gyrus sylvius caudalis, Gyrus ectosylvius medius, Sulcus ectosylvius rostralis and caudalis. D E

7 ***Gyrus obliquus rostralis***. Rostral oblique gyrus, occurs in Un, between Fissura sylvia and Sulcus obliquus. A C

8 ***Gyrus obliquus caudalis***. Caudal oblique gyrus, occurs in Un, caudal to Sulcus obliquus and dorsal to Gyrus sylvius caudalis. A C

9 ***Gyrus ectosylvius rostralis***. Rostral ectosylvian gyrus, ventral to Sulcus suprasylvius rostralis. A C D E

10 ***Gyrus ectosylvius caudalis***. Caudal ectosylvian gyrus, ventral and rostral to Sulcus suprasylvius caudalis. A C D E

11 ***Gyrus ectomarginalis [ectosagittalis] medius***. Middle ectomarginal [ectosagittal] gyrus, dorsocaudally located on the lateral aspect, between Sulcus suprasylvius medius and Sulcus marginalis. A C D E

12 *Pars lateralis* (Un). Lateral part, lateral to Sulcus ectomarginalis. A C

13 *Pars medialis* (Un). Medial part, medial to Sulcus ectomarginalis. A C

14 ***Gyrus ectomarginalis [ectosagittalis] caudalis***. Caudal ectomarginal [ectosagittal] gyrus, between Sulcus suprasylvius caudalis and Sulcus marginalis (Car), Pars medialis gyri ectomarginalis (Un). A D E

15 ***Gyrus ectomarginalis [ectosagittalis] rostralis***. Rostral ectomarginal [ectosagittal] gyrus, between Gyrus ectosylvius rostralis and Sulcus coronalis (Car), dorsal to Sulcus suprasylvius rostralis (Un). A D

16 ***Gyrus occipitalis***. Occipital gyrus, most caudal extent of the hemisphere. B C E F

17 ***Gyrus marginalis [sagittalis]***. Marginal [sagittal] gyrus, on the dorsal border, in the middle and caudal thirds. B C E F

18 ***Gyrus postcruciatus [postcentralis]***. Postcruciate [postcentral] gyrus, caudal to Sulcus cruciatus. B C E F

19 ***Gyrus precruciatus [precentralis, prae-]***. Precruciate [precentral] gyrus, rostral to Sulcus cruciatus. B C E F

20 ***Gyrus proreus***. Prorean gyrus, most rostroventral gyrus visible from the lateral, medial, and dorsal perspectives. A C D 6 E

21 ***Gyrus cinguli***. Cingulate gyrus, dorsal and parallel to Corpus callosum. B F

22 ***Insula*** (Un). Originally superficial, during ontogenesis covered by opercula, at least to a large extent. In Car there is no opercularisation. G

23 *Gyri insulae*. Insular gyri. G

24 ***Limen insulae***. Between Pars rostralis and Pars caudalis of Sulcus rhinalis lateralis. G

25 ***Opercula insulae***. Insular opercula, part of hemisphere covering insula. G

26 **Corpus callosum**. The biggest fiber connection between the two hemispheres, in the bottom of Fissura longitudinalis cerebri. B

27 ***Splenium corporis callosi***. The caudal extent of Corpus callosum. B

28 ***Truncus corporis callosi***. Body, between Splenium and Genu corporis callosi. B

29 ***Genu corporis callosi***. Knee, the rostral extent of Corpus callosum. B

30 ***Rostrum corporis callosi***. Beak-shaped structure connecting Genu corporis callosi to Lamina terminalis grisea over Commissura rostralis. B

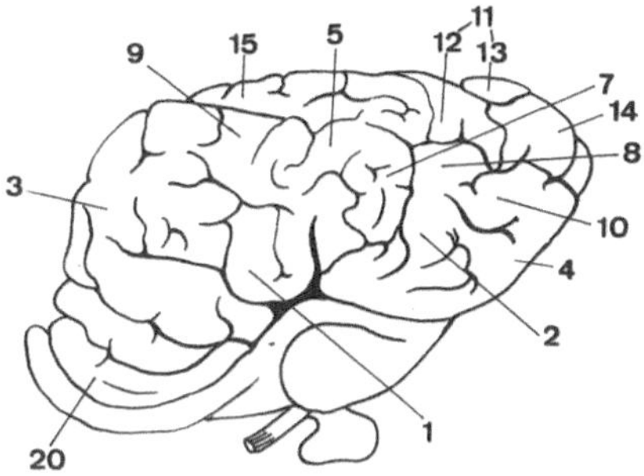

A Gyri of neopallium, left lateral aspect (eq)

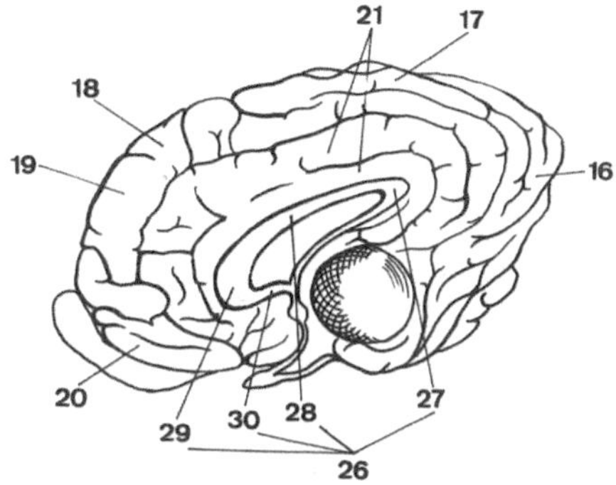

B Gyri of right neopallium, medial aspect (eq)

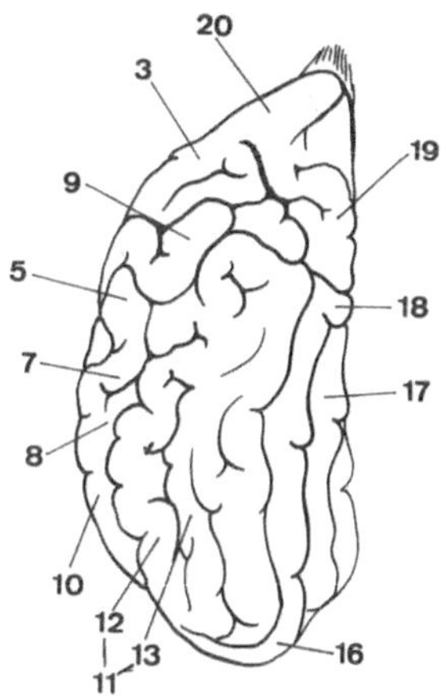

C Gyri of left neopallium, dorsal aspect (eq)

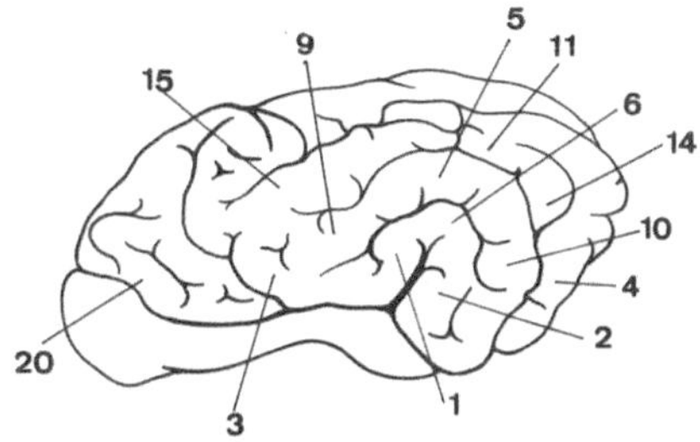

D Gyri of neopallium, left lateral aspect (ca)

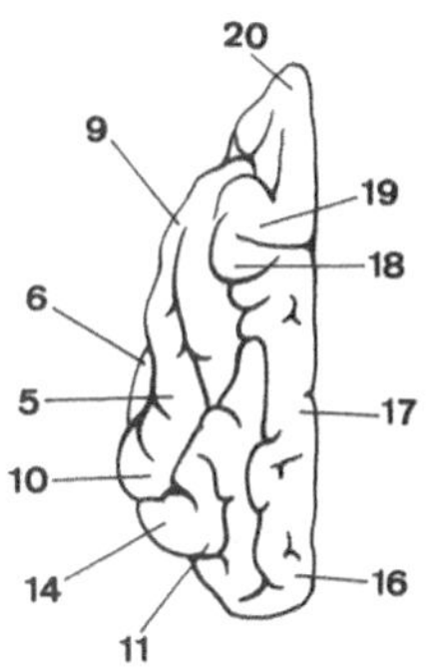

E Gyri of left neopallium, dorsal aspect (ca)

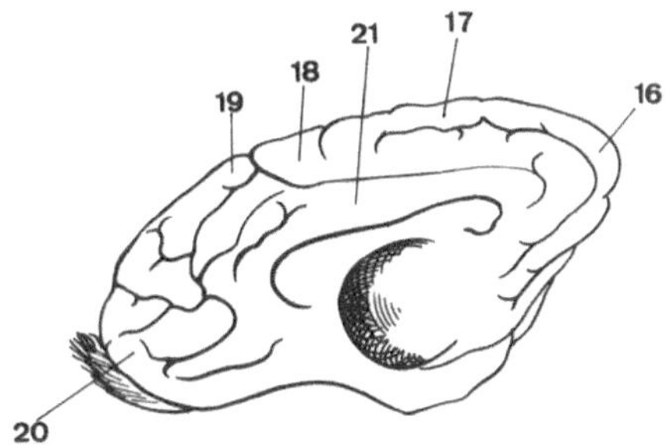

F Gyri of right neopallium, medial aspect (ca)

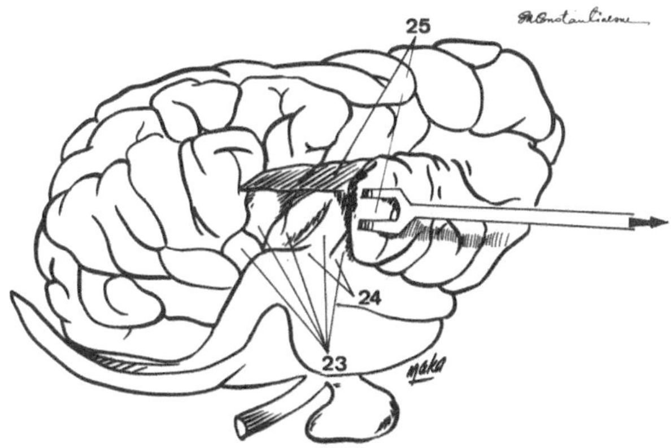

G Left insula, opercula partly removed (eq)

1 **Sectiones neopallii**. Sections through neopallium.

2 ***Neocortex [Isocortex]***. Gray matter built up by six (seven) layers of nerve cell bodies and nerve fibers. A

3 *Stratum moleculare [plexiforme]*. Molecular [plexiform] layer, consisting of ramified afferent fibers, tangential fibers, dendrite endings of pyramidal cells, glial elements, and rare nerve cell bodies. A

4 *Stratum granulare externum*. External granular layer, with small granular, stellate, and pyramidal nerve cell bodies and their dendrites. A

5 *Stratum pyramidale externum*. External pyramidal layer, with medium size and large pyramidal neurons, their dendrites, and first segment of axons. It is the thickest layer of the Neocortex. A

6 *Stratum granulare internum*. Internal granular layer, with specific thalamic afferent fibers, small granular, stellate, and pyramidal neurons. In the sensory areas these neurons are packed to form a thick layer. A

7 *Stratum pyramidale internum*. Internal pyramidal layer, consisting of medium size to very large pyramidal neurons. A

8 *Stratum multiforme*. Multiform layer, composed of a wide variety of neurons, predominantly spindle-shaped. Some small or medium size pyramidal cells might be observed. A

9 *Cortex frontalis*. Dorsal to Pars rostralis of Sulcus rhinalis lateralis, rostral to Fissura pseudosylvia (sylvia), and Sulcus cruciatus. B

10 *Cortex parietalis*. Dorsal part of Neocortex, between Cortex frontalis and occipitalis, Sulcus suprasylivius and Sulcus splenialis. B

11 *Cortex temporalis*. Dorsal to Pars caudalis of Sulcus rhinalis lateralis, ventral to Lobus parietalis and occipitalis, caudal to Lobus frontalis. B

12 *Cortex occipitalis*. Caudal part of Neocortex, caudal to Cortex parietalis, caudodorsal to Cortex temporalis. B

13 ***Centrum semiovale***. Semioval center, white matter of Neopallium. C

14 ***Fibrae arcuatae cerebri***. Arciform fibers between neighbouring gyri. C

15 ***Cingulum***. Fiber bundle located within Gyrus cinguli, connecting the Gyrus parahippocampalis to the area rostral to Commissura rostralis (so-called precommissural area). C D

16 ***Fasciculus longitudinalis superior***. Association bundle connecting Cortex frontalis, occipitalis and temporalis. E

17 ***Fasciculus longitudinalis inferior***. Smaller association bundle connecting Cortex temporalis and occipitalis. E

18 ***Fasciculus uncinatus***. Association fibers connecting Cortex frontalis and temporalis. E

19 ***Radiatio corporis callosi***. Radiation of Corpus callosum, lateral extension of fibers from Corpus callosum into the hemisphere. C D

20 ***Corona radiata***. Radiation of fibers from Capsula interna toward Cortex cerebri. 461 C

21 ***Radiatio optica***. Optic (Gratiolet's) radiation, fibers from Corpus geniculatum laterale to Cortex occipitalis (striate area). F

22 ***Radiatio acustica***. Acoustic radiation, fibers from Corpus geniculatum mediale to Cortex temporalis (acoustic area). F

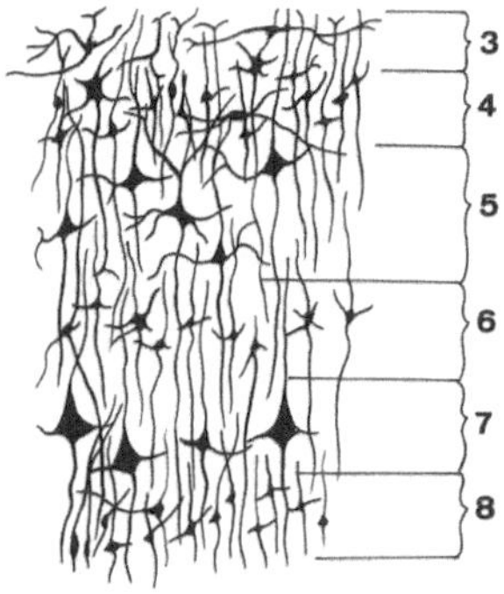

A Histological transverse section through neocortex

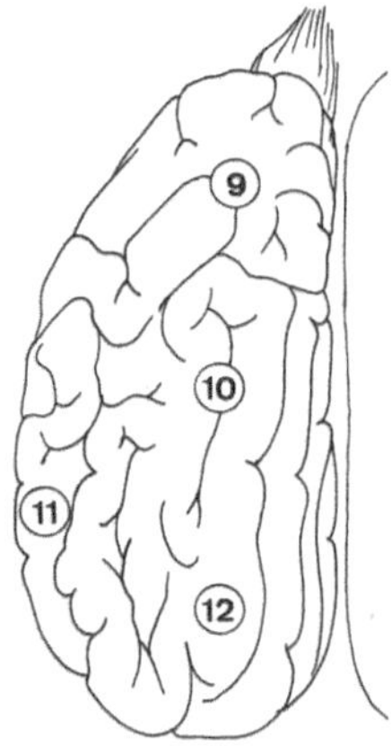

B Cortex, left hemisphere, dorsal aspect (eq)

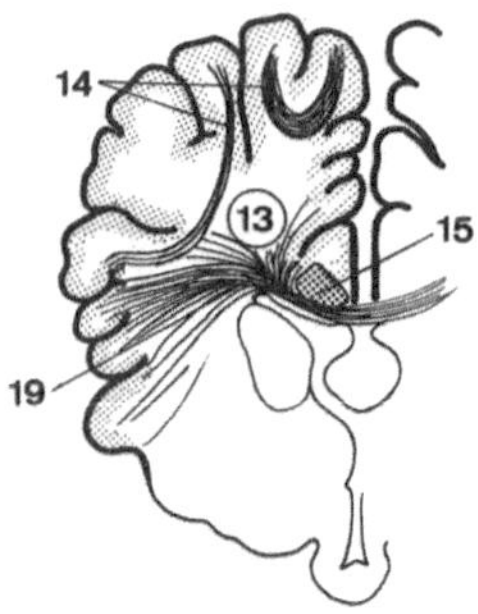

C Fiber bundles in Centrum semiovale, schematic transverse section

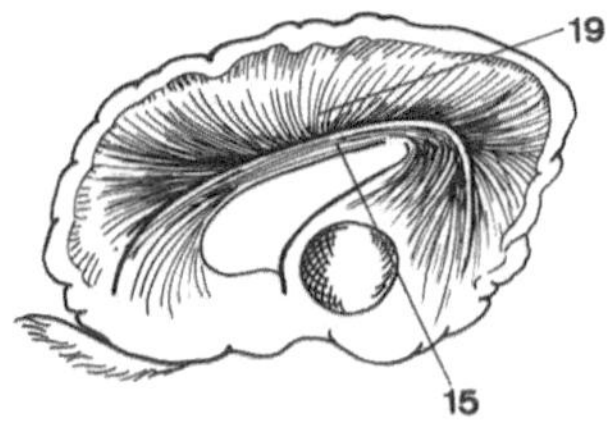

D Fiber bundles in Centrum semiovale, schematic sagittal section

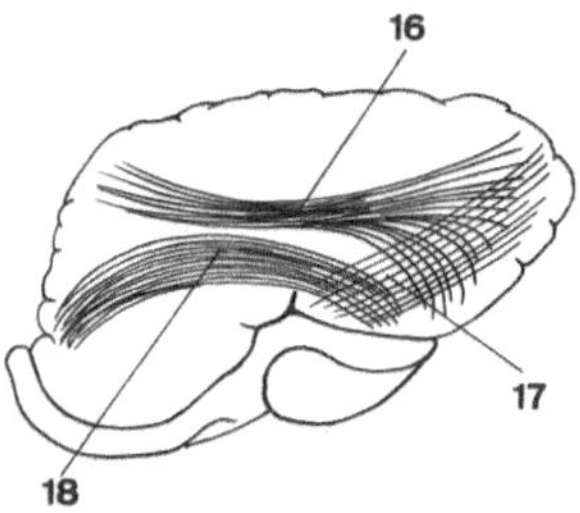

E Fiber bundles in Centrum semiovale, schematic sagittal section

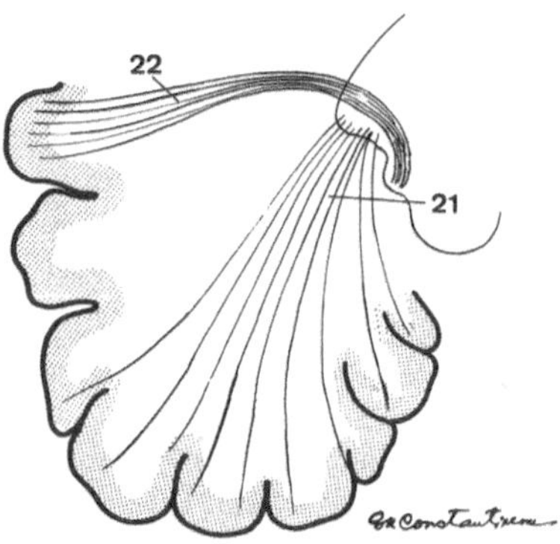

F Radiationes from Corpora geniculata to Cortex occipitalis and temporalis

1 **Corpus striatum**. Striate body, represented by basal nuclei, connected by cords of gray matter, separated by fibers from each other and the surroundings. Important extrapyramidal center. A B C

2 ***Nucleus caudatus***. Caudate nucleus, lies mediorostral and mediodorsal to Nucleus lentiformis. A B C D

3 *Caput nuclei caudati*. Head of caudate nucleus, the most rostral part. A B

4 *Corpus nuclei caudati*. Body of caudate nucleus. A

5 *Cauda nuclei caudati*. Tail of caudate nucleus, the most caudal extension. A

6 ***Nucleus accumbens***. Ventromedial to Caput nuclei caudati.

7 ***Nucleus lentiformis***. Lentiform nucleus, lense-shaped, located laterocaudal and lateroventral to Nucleus caudatus. It is divided by Lamina medullaris lateralis into putamen and pallidum. A B C

8 *Putamen*. Lateral subdivison of Nucleus lentiformis. A B C

9 *Pallidum [Globus pallidus]*. Medial subdivision of Nucleus lentiformis. B C

10 **Lamina medullaris medialis**. Medullary lamina within pallidum, much reduced in domestic mammals. C

11 **Lamina medullaris lateralis**. Sheet of white matter separating putamen from pallidum. B C

12 ***Capsula interna***. Internal capsule, a wall of white matter lateral to Nucleus caudatus and Thalamus, medial to Nucleus lentiformis, carrying the most important afferent and efferent pathways. A B C

13 *Genu capsulae internae*. Knee of internal capsule, between the two crura. B

14 *Crus rostrale capsulae internae*. Rostral limb, between Caput nuclei caudati and Nucleus lentiformis. B

15 *Crus caudale capsulae internae*. Caudal limb, between Nucleus lentiformis and thalamus. B

16 *Pars sublentiformis capsulae internae*. Sublenticular part, in the most ventral position.

17 *Pars retrolentiformis capsulae internae*. Retrolenticular part, located caudal to Nucleus lentiformis. A

18 ***Capsula externa***. External capsule, white matter separating Nucleus lentiformis from claustrum. B

19 ***Claustrum***. Long and thin lamina of gray matter, separating putamen from insula. It comes in contact with the olfactory area and Tractus olfactorius lateralis (rostrally) and with Corpus amygdaloideum (caudoventrally). B

19a *Capsula extrema*. Between Claustrum and Cortex cerebri. B (for the first time introduced in the N. A. V. [finally!])

20 **Ventriculus lateralis**. Lateral ventricle (I and II), cavity of Hemispherium, communicantes with Ventriculus III via Foramen interventriculare. C D E

21 ***Pars centralis***. Central part, between Corpus callosum (roof), Corpus nuclei caudati and hippocampus (floor). C D E

22 ***Foramen interventriculare***. Monro's foramen. Connection between Ventriculus tertius and right and left Ventriculi laterales. B D E

23 ***Cornu rostrale***. Rostral horn, extension of Ventriculus lateralis rostral to Foramen interventriculare and medial to Caput nuclei caudati, projects into Bulbus olfactorius. B D E

24 ***Cornu temporale***. Temporal horn, ventral extension of Ventriculus lateralis into Lobus piriformis. E

25 ***Nucleus caudatus***. Caudate nucleus. See 2. C D

26 ***Sulcus thalamocaudatus***. Thalamocaudate groove, separating Nucleus caudatus from thalamus. 453 D

27 ***Stria terminalis***. See 452.17. 453 D

28 ***Lamina affixa***. Floor of Ventriculus lateralis between Stria terminalis and Tenia choroidea ventriculi lateralis in man. (Therefore, it shouldn't be listed in the N. A. V.)

29 ***Tenia [Taenia] choroidea [chorioidea]***. Line of attachment of Tela choroidea ventriculi lateralis on Stria terminalis.

30 ***Pes hippocampi [Cornu ammonis]***. See 450.12 and 452.10. 453 B

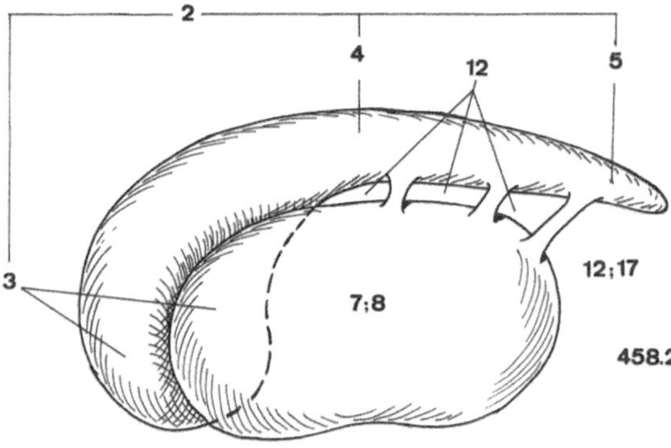

A Left Corpus striatum, lateral aspect

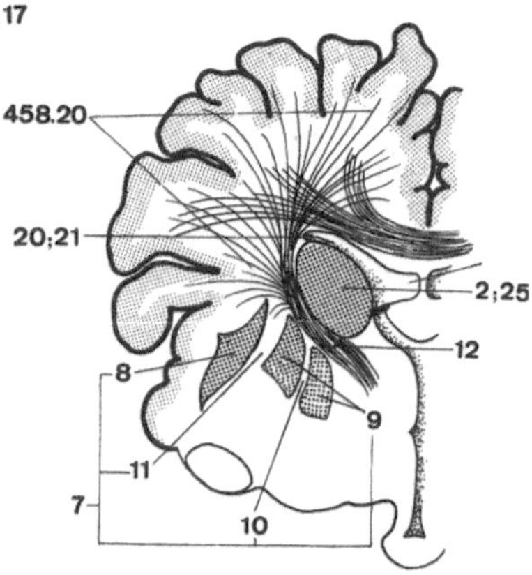

C Corpus striatum, transverse section of left hemisphere caudal aspect

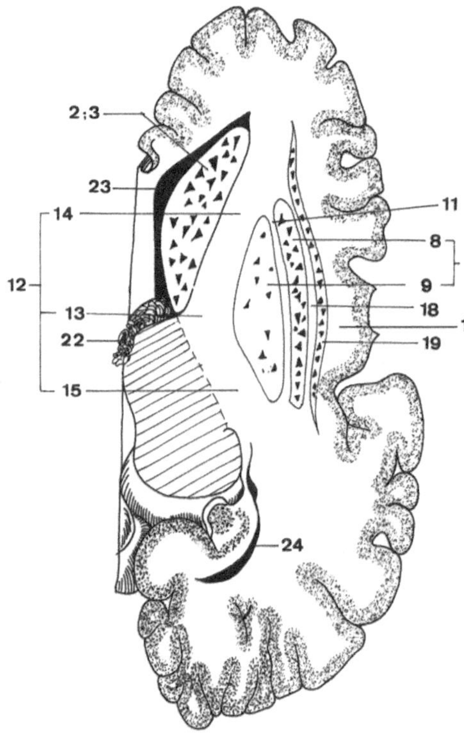

B Corpus striatum, horizontal section of right hemisphere dorsal aspect

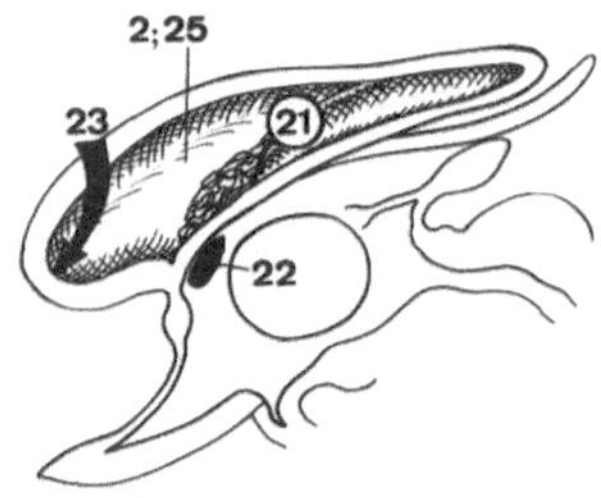

D Right Ventriculus lateralis, medial aspect

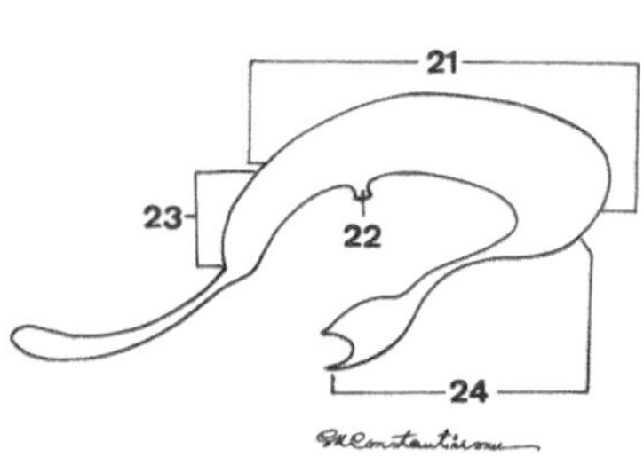

E Cast of the right Ventriculus lateralis, medial aspect (eq)

1 **MENINGES**. Three continuous membranes surrounding and protecting the Systema nervosum centrale, the Dura mater, Arachnoidea, and Pia mater.

1a **PACHYMENINX [DURA MATER]**[2].

2 **Dura mater encephali**. Pachymeninx, the outer fibrous layer of the Meninges, that protects the brain. It replaces the periosteum of cranial cavity. A C

3 ***Falx cerebri***. Sickle-shaped fibrous extension of Dura mater encephali within Fissura longitudinalis cerebri. A C

4 ***Tentorium cerebelli membranaceum***. Fibrous wall originating from Dura mater encephali on Tentorium cerebelli osseum in Car and eq (see 10.10), separating the two hemispheres from the cerebellum. A B

4a ***Falx cerebelli***. Present in man and a few wild mammals, but absent in domestic mammals[1].

5 ***Diaphragma sellae***. Horizontal extension of Dura mater encephali, partially separating hypophysis from the brain. A C

6 ***Incisura tentorii***. Tentorial notch for the passage of the brain stem. A B

7 ***Cavum trigeminale***. Meckel's cave, pouch for Ganglion trigeminale. B

8 ***Cavum subdurale***. Subdural cavity. During life Dura mater and Arachnoidea are close to each other. A C

9 **Dura mater spinalis**. Pachymeninx, protects the Medulla spinalis, separated from the wall of vertebral canal by the Cavum epidurale. A D E

10 ***Filum durae matris spinalis***. Thread-like caudal end of Dura mater spinalis. E

11 ***Cavum epidurale***. Epidural space, between Dura mater spinalis and the periosteum of Canalis vertebralis. A E

12 ***Cavum subdurale***. See 8. A E

12a **LEPTOMENINX**[2].

13 **Arachnoidea encephali**. Arachnoid of brain, component of Leptomeninx, thin nonvascular layer, connected by trabeculae with pia. A C

14 ***Cavum subarachnoideale [Cavum leptomeningeum]***. Subarachnoid space, filled with Liquor cerebrospinalis. A C

15 *Liquor cerebrospinalis*. Cerebrospinal fluid.

16 **Arachnoidea spinalis**. Spinal arachnoid. See 13. A D E

17 ***Cavum subarachnoideale [Cavum leptomeningeum]****. See 14. A E

18 *Liquor cerebrospinalis*. Cerebrospinal fluid.

19 **Cisternae subarachnoideales**. Enlargements of Cavum subarachnoideale.

20 ***Cisterna cerebellomedullaris***. Enlargement of subarachnoid space between cerebellum and medulla oblongata. A

21 ***Cisterna valleculae [fossae] lateralis cerebri***. Enlargement of subarachnoid space in Vallecula lateralis cerebri, in Un projecting into Fissura sylvia. C

22 ***Cisterna chiasmatis***. Around Chiasma opticum. A

23 ***Cisterna interpeduncularis***. Within Fossa interpeduncularis. A

24 ***Granulationes arachnoideales***. Pacchioni's granulations, villous evaginations of Arachnoidea through Dura mater into Sinus durae matris. C

25 **Pia mater encephali**. Pia mater of brain, soft vascular layer adherent to brain, penetrating into sulci. C

26 ***Tela choroidea [chorioidea] ventriculi quarti***. See 430.26. A

27 ***Plexus choroideus [chorioideus] ventriculi quarti***. Wreath-like accumulation of vascular villi attached to Tela choroidea ventriculi quarti, extending into Aperturae laterales. A

28 ***Tela choroidea [chorioidea] ventriculi tertii***. See 436.14. A

29 ***Plexus choroideus [chorioideus] ventriculi tertii***. Wreath-like accumulation of villi attached to Tela choroidea ventriculi tertii, from Foramen interventriculare to Recessus suprapinealis. A C

30 ***Plexus choroideus [chorioideus] ventriculi lateralis***. Wreath-like accumulation of vascular villi within Ventriculus lateralis from Foramen interventriculare to Cornu temporale. C

31 ***Glomus choroideum [chorioideum]***. Thickening of Plexus choroideus ventriculi lateralis, described in man[1].

32 **Pia mater spinalis**. Soft vascular internal layer of Leptomenix, adherent to spinal cord. A D E

33 ***Lig. denticulatum***. Fibrous anchors of Medulla spinalis to dura. D

34 ***Septum intermedium***. Intermediate septum, connective tissue separating Fasciculus gracilis from Fasciculus cuneatus in the cervical part of the spinal cord. F

1) Therefore, it shouldn't be listed in the N. A. V.

2) Pachymeninx [Dura mater], Cavum epidurale, Leptomeninx, Cavum subarachnoideale [Cavum leptomeningeum]. Terminology of the meninges was elaborated by adding the Greek roots Pachy- and Leptomeninx which are used in pathologic and clinical terminology dealing with meningitis. The alternative term Spatium epidurale is listed as a synonym for Cavum epidurale in the Nomina Histologica Veterinaria.

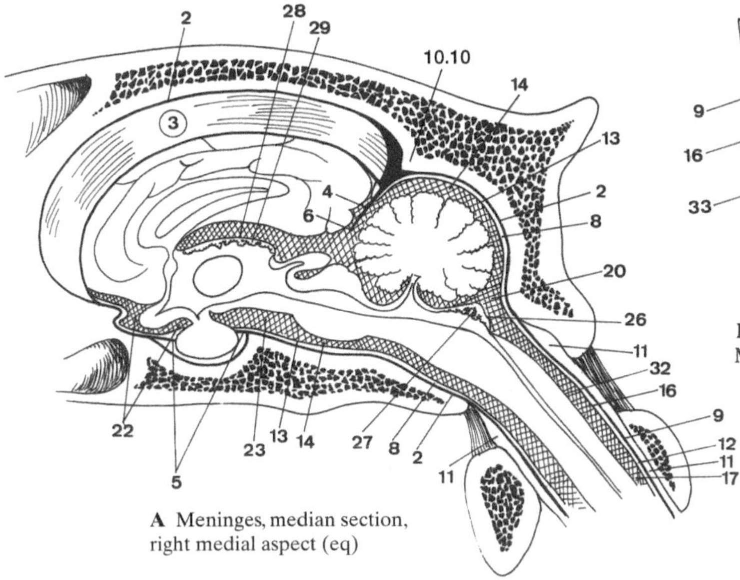

A Meninges, median section, right medial aspect (eq)

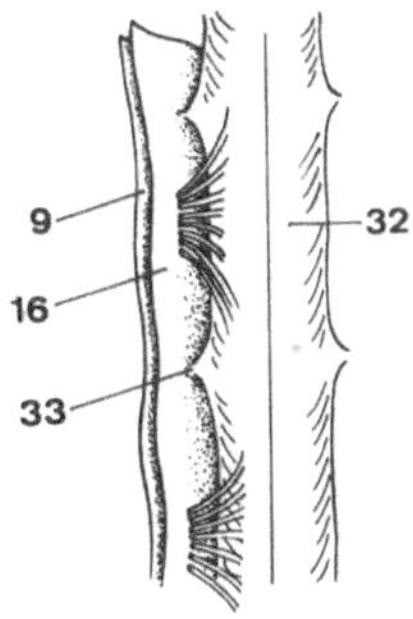

D Meninges of Medulla spinalis

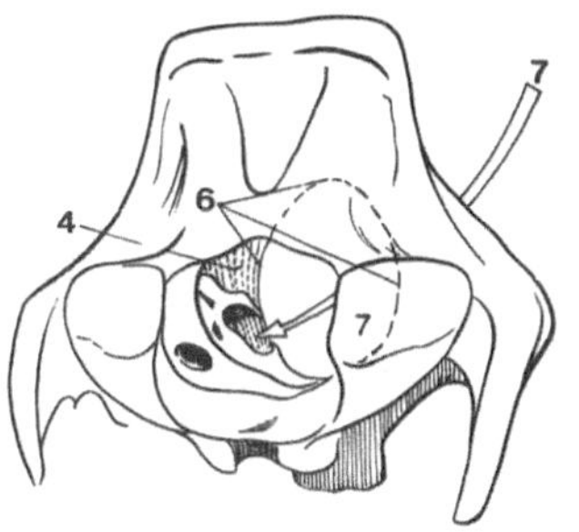

B Tentorium cerebelli membranaceum, caudal aspect (eq)

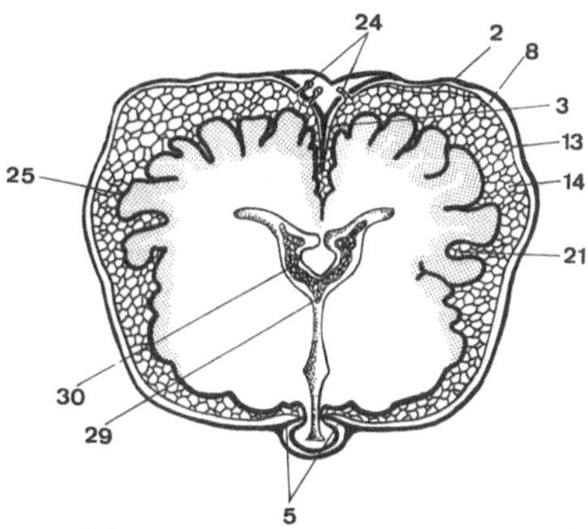

C Meninges of brain, transverse section (eq)

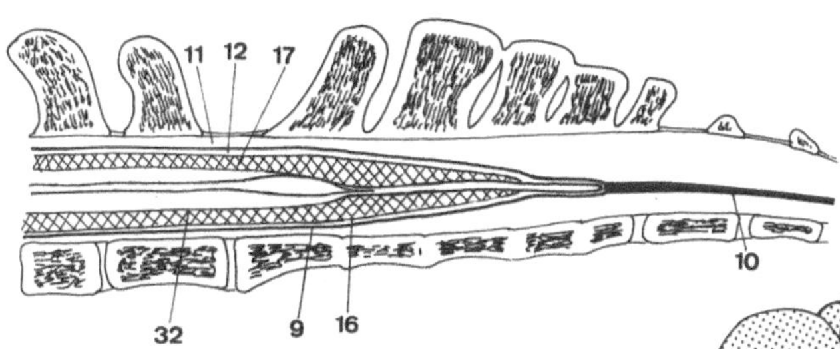

E Meninges of Medulla spinalis, median section (eq)

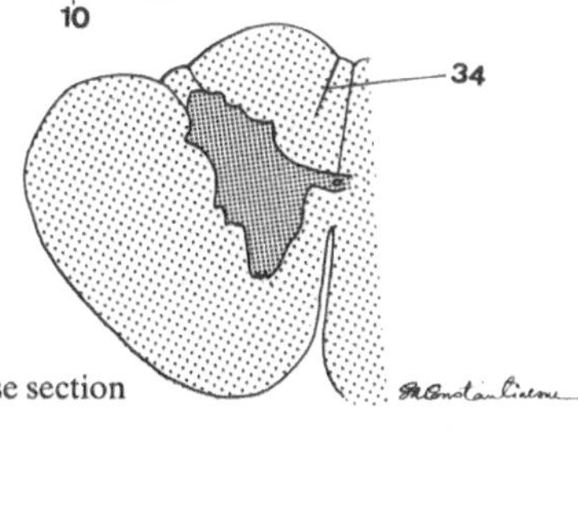

F Medulla spinalis, transverse section

1 **SYSTEMA NERVOSUM PERIPHERICUM**. Peripheral nervous system.

2 **NERVI CRANIALES**. Cranial nerves, 12 pairs (CN I–XII).

3 **Nn. olfactorii**. Olfactory nerves, or Fila olfactoria (CN I), carry the excitations from olfactory cells through Lamina cribrosa ossis ethmoidalis into Bulbus olfactorius, and represent the extranevraxial pathway of olfaction. A

4 ***N. vomeronasalis***. Vomeronasal nerve, starts from Organum vomeronasale, ends in Bulbus olfactorius accessorius. A

5 ***N. terminalis***. Terminal nerve, starts from Organum vomeronasale and adjacent mucosa of the Septum nasi, enters the Cavum cranii and joins the Pedunculus olfactorius, postfetally described in Car. A

6 *Ganglion terminale*. Terminal ganglion, sensory. A

7 **N. opticus**. Optic nerve (CN II), carries optic fibers from retina through Canalis opticus, meets with its fellow in Chiasma opticum. B

8 **N. oculomotorius**. Oculomotor nerve (CN III), somatomotor and parasympathetic, emerges from Sulcus medialis cruris cerebri, passes through Fissura orbitalis or Foramen orbitorotundum in su and Ru, together with CN IV, CN VI and CN V_1. B

9 ***Ramus dorsalis***. Dorsal branch, supplies Mm. rectus dorsalis and levator palpebrae superioris. B

10 ***Ramus ventralis***. Ventral branch, supplies Mm. rectus medialis, rectus ventralis and obliquus ventralis. B

11 **Ganglion ciliare**. Ciliary ganglion, at the origin of the branch of CN III that supplies M. obliquus ventralis. Synapses between pre- and postganglionic parasympathetic fibers. B

12 ***Radix oculomotoria***. Oculomotor root, the preganglionic parasympathetic branch of CN III. B

13 ***Nn. ciliares breves***. Short ciliary nerves, represent the postganglionic parasympathetic fibers and the sympathetic fibers (see 14) supplying posterior structures of the eye. B

14 ***(Ramus sympathicus ad ganglion ciliare)***. Slender postganglionic fibers from Plexus caroticus (sympathetic), without synapse in ganglion. B

15 ***Ramus communicans cum n. nasociliari***. Branch communicating with nasociliary nerve (Ru, eq), or ophthalmic nerve (Car, su). B

16 **N. trochlearis**. Trochlear nerve (CN IV), emerges dorsocaudally from Lamina tecti, passes through Foramen trochleare (eq, inconstant), Fissura orbitalis (Car, eq), or Foramen orbitorotundum (su, Ru), and supplies M. obliquus dorsalis following a medial superficial route under the Periorbita, medially. C

17 ***Decussatio nervorum trochlearium***. Crossing of trochlear nerves in Velum medullare rostrale. C

18 **N. trigeminus**. Trigeminal nerve (CN V). Somatosensitive fibers from skin and mucous membranes of the head and somatomotor fibers to masticatory muscles, except Venter caudalis m. digastrici. D

19 ***Radix major***. Sensory root, between pons and Ganglion trigeminale. D

20 *Ganglion trigeminale*. Trigeminal ganglion, in Cavum trigeminale of dura mater. Former ganglion of Gasser. See 463.7. D

21 ***Radix minor***. Motor root, origin in pons. Carries all motor fibers of CN V and contains also sensitive fibers. D

22 **N. ophthalmicus**. Ophthalmic nerve, first and smallest branch of N. trigeminus (CN V_1), passes through Fissura orbitalis or Foramen orbitorotundum in su and Ru, sensory for eye, eyelids, conjunctiva, skin of forehead and around the orbit, and part of nasal mucosa. C D

23 ***Ramus meningeus***. Recurrent meningeal branch, sensory, to meninges. D

24 ***N. lacrimalis****. Lacrimal nerve, one of the most superficial nerves under the Periorbita which ramifies in Glandula lacrimalis, Palpebra superior and also the skin at the Angulus oculi lateralis. C D

25 ***N. frontalis****. Frontal nerve, also superficial under the Periorbita, leaves Orbita (through Foramen supraorbitale in eq), branches into N. supraorbitalis and N. supratrochlearis. C D

26 *N. sinuum frontalium*. Frontal sinus nerve, runs dorsally between Mm. recti lateralis and dorsalis to a small foramen in the medial wall of the orbit, entering the Sinus frontalis; may originate from Ramus zygomaticotemporalis n. zygomatici (bo) before it merges from Foramen orbitorotundum. D

27 *N. supraorbitalis*. Supraorbital nerve, one of the two branches of N. frontalis, sensitive for upper eyelid and skin of the forehead. D

28 *N. supratrochlearis*. Supratrochlear nerve, the other branch of the N. frontalis ends in Palpebra superior at Angulus oculi medialis, sensitive also to the skin around the Angulus oculi medialis. D

A Nn. olfactorii, vomeronasalis, and terminalis (ca) (McCotter)

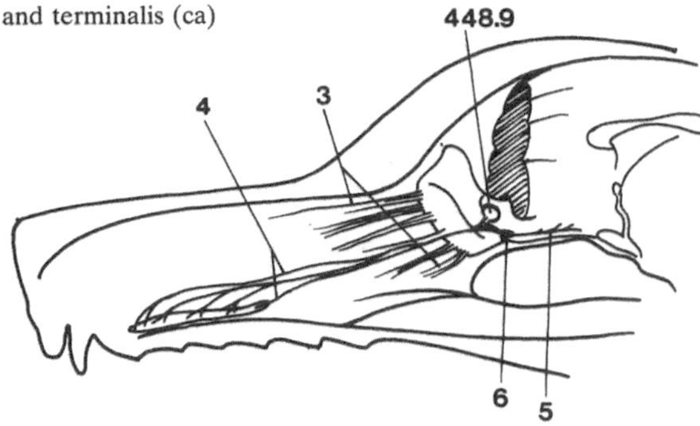

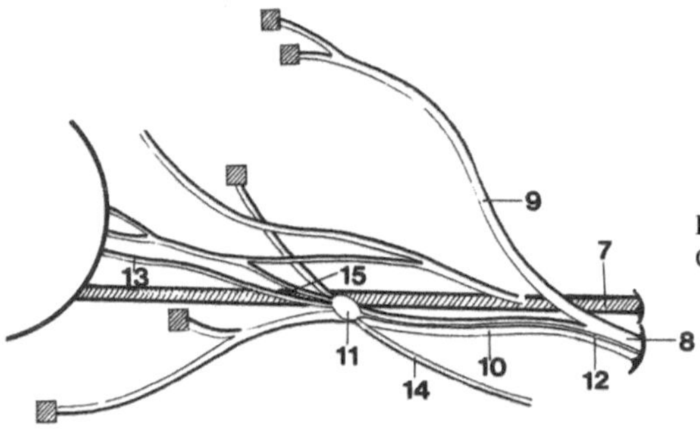

B Nervi opticus and oculomotorius in the Orbita, schematic representation

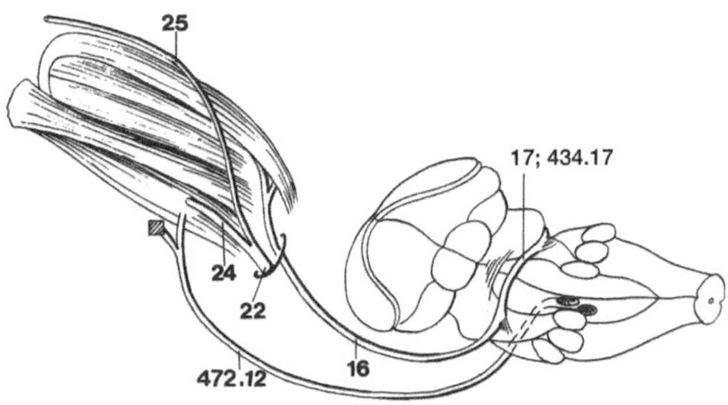

C Nn. trochlearis, ophthalmicus, and abducens left side (ca)

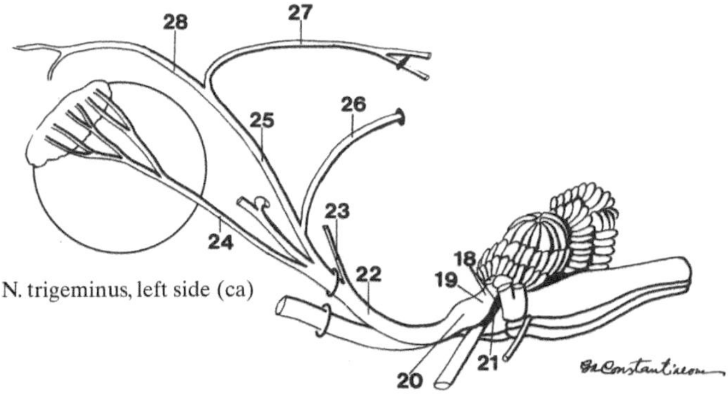

D N. trigeminus, left side (ca)

1 ***N. nasociliaris.*** Nasociliary nerve, deep between M. rectus medialis and M. obliquus dorsalis, but easy to expose deep between M. rectus lateralis and M. rectus dorsalis. A

2 *Ramus communicans cum ganglio ciliari.* Branch communicating with Ganglion ciliare. A

3 *Nn. ciliares longi.* Long ciliary nerves, supply the anterior structures of the eyeball. A

4 *N. ethmoidalis.* Ethmoidal nerve, enters the skull through Foramen ethmoidale, then pierces Os ethmoidale reaching Cavum nasi. A B C

5 **Ramus nasalis lateralis.** Lateral nasal branch, supplies Conchae nasales. B

6 **Rami sinus frontalis** (eq). Frontal sinus branches, distribution to Sinus frontalis. B

7 **Ramus nasalis medialis.** Medial nasal branch, distribution to Septum nasi. C

8 **Rami nasales externi** (Car). External nasal branches, to the skin rostral to the nasal bone. C

9 *N. infratrochlearis**. Infratrochlear nerve, to lacrimal caruncle, ducts and sac, and third eyelid, then passes through Incisura trochlearis to supply the skin around the Angulus oculi medialis. This nerve should be blocked prior to dehorning goats. A G

10 **Rami sinus frontalis** (eq). Frontal sinus branches. A

11 **Rami palpebrales.** Palpebral branches to Palpebra superior. A

12 **Rami cornuales** (cap)*. Cornual branches. G (should be blocked prior to dehorning goats)

13 **N. maxillaris.** Maxillary nerve, second branch of N. trigeminus (CN V_2), sensory, passes through Foramen rotundum (ca, eq), or Foramen orbitoritundum (su, Ru). D E F

14 ***Ramus meningeus.*** Meningeal branch, innervates a small area of Dura mater encephali. E

15 ***N. zygomaticus.*** Zygomatic nerve. D E

16 *Ramus zygomaticotemporalis**. Zygomaticotemporal branch, communicates with a branch of the N. lacrimalis, runs caudodorsally to the skin of the temporal region, and the lacrimal gland. Because of the close association of the ophthalmic and maxillary nerves, and the communicating branch between the lacrimal and zygomatic nerves, the Ramus zygomaticotemporalis was formerly described as the N. lacrimalis or as a branch of it. It may also be described as a branch of N. zygomaticus, and the interpretation agrees with that of the N.A. D

17 **Ramus cornualis** (Ru)*. Cornual branch. G (should be blocked in dehorning bo and cap)

18 *Ramus communicans cum n. lacrimali.* Branch communicating with N. lacrimalis. D

19 *Ramus zygomaticofacialis**. Zygomaticofacial branch, supplies the Palpebra inferior and the neighbouring skin. D

20 *Ramus zygomaticofacialis accessorius.* Accessory zygomaticofacial branch. D

21 ***N. pterygopalatinus.*** Ptyerygopalatine nerve, divides after a short course into three nerves. D F

22 *N. palatinus minor.* Lesser palatine nerve, innervates the mucosa of Palatum molle. D F

23 *N. palatinus major.* Greater palatine nerve, traverses Canalis palatinus, supplies mucosa of Palatum durum. The following two are its branches. D F

24 **N. palatinus accessorius.** Accessory palatine nerve, parallels N. palatinus major. D F

25 **Rami nasales caudales ventrales** (eq). Ventral caudal nasal branches, perforate Palatum durum. F

26 *N. nasalis caudalis.* Caudal nasal nerve, enters the Cavum nasi through Foramen sphenopalatinum. Supplies the mucosa of the walls and septum nasi. C D F

27 **N. nasopalatinus.** Nasopalatine nerve, continuation of the septal branch, through Fissura palatina to the muscosa of the palate. C

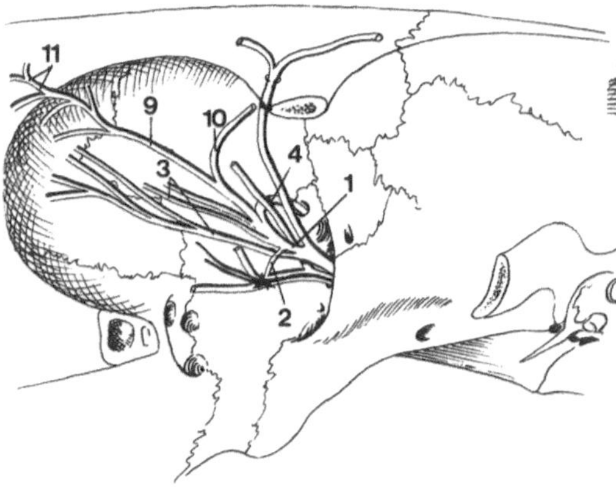

A N. nasociliaris, left orbit (eq)

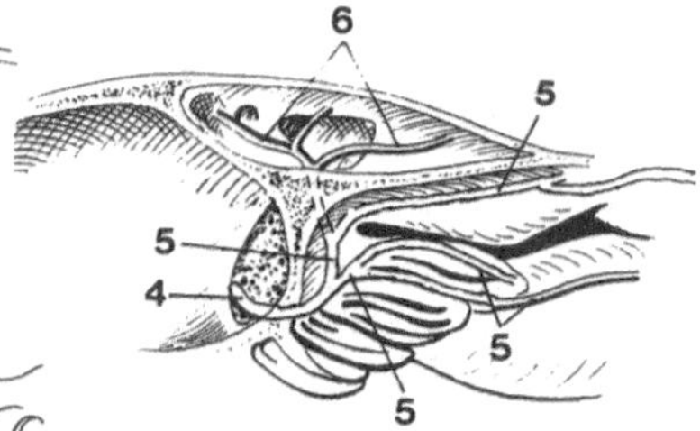

B N. ethmoidalis, left medial aspect (eq)

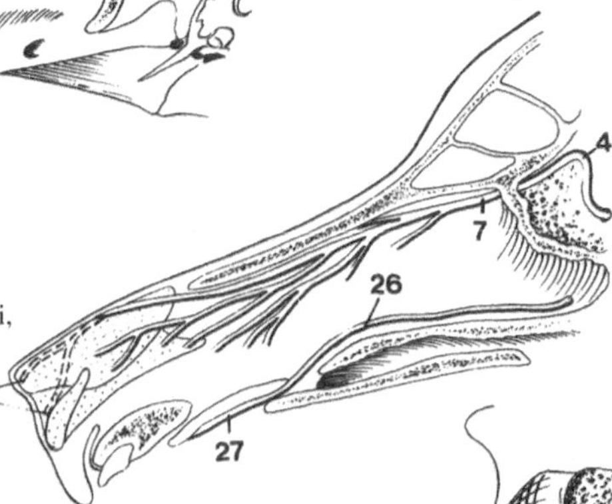

C Nerves in Cavum nasi, right medial aspect (ca)

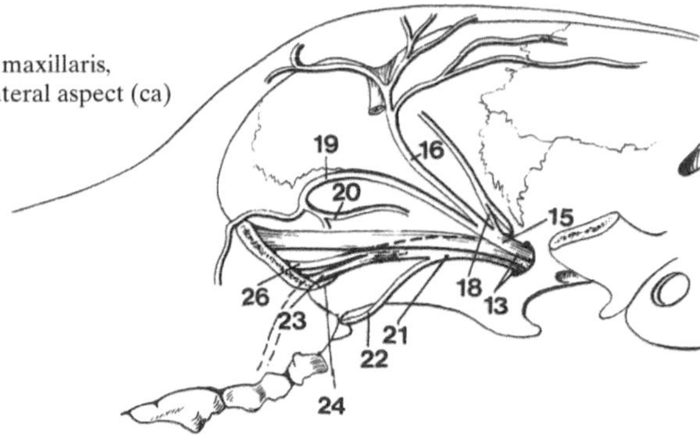

D N. maxillaris, left lateral aspect (ca)

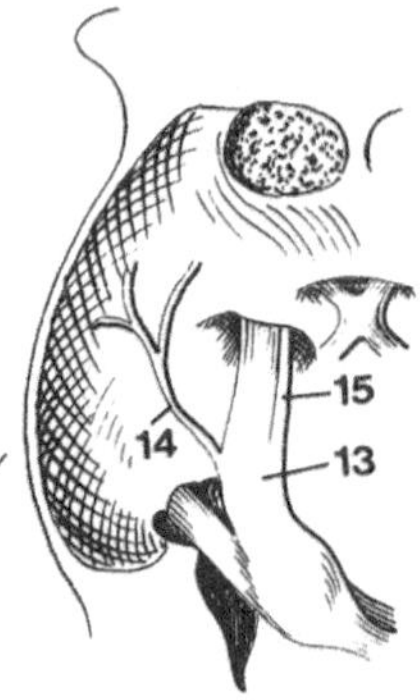

E N. maxillaris within the cranial cavity, left side (eq)

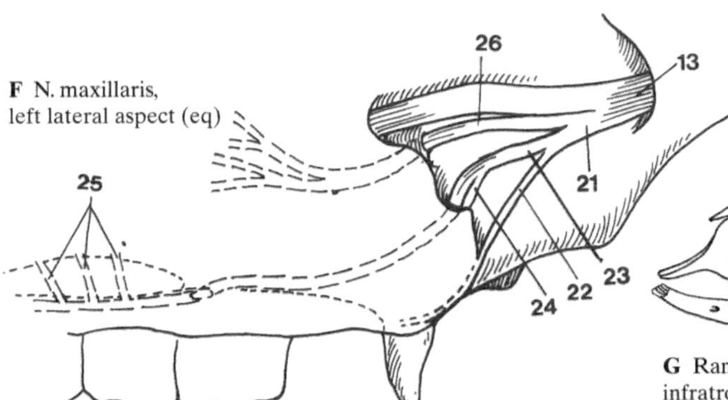

F N. maxillaris, left lateral aspect (eq)

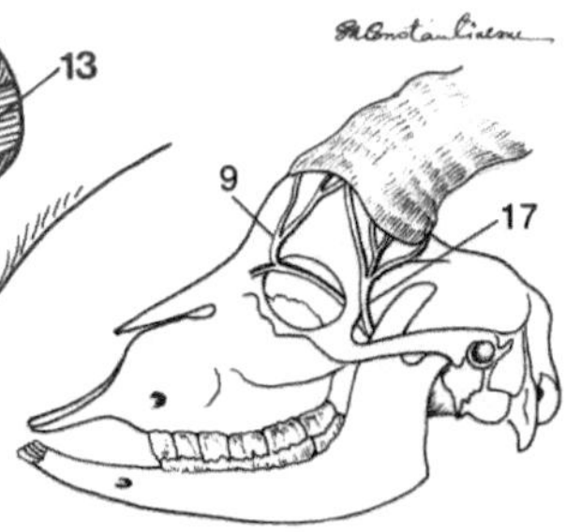

G Ramus cornualis and Ramus infratrochlearis in the goat, left lateral aspect (cap)

1 ***N. infraorbitalis****. Infraorbital nerve, continuation of N. maxillaris, passes through Canalis infraorbitalis and exits through Foramen infraorbitale. It supplies the skin outlined by the facial tubercle and commisure of the lips, ventrally, and from the facial tubercle a perpendicular line to the dorsal median line of the head, caudally. A C

2 *Rami alveolares superiores caudales*. Caudal superior alveolar branches, for last Dens molaris and the Sinus maxillaris. A

3 *Rami alveolares superiores medii*. Middle superior alveolar branches, to the rest of superior Dentes molares and premolares , Gingiva, and Sinus maxillaris. A

4 *Rami alveolares superiores rostrales*. Rostral superior alveolar branches, to Dentes caninus and incisivi. A

5 *Plexus dentalis superior*. Superior dental plexus, result of the union of Rami alveolares superiores. A

6 **Rami dentales superiores**. To the upper teeth. A

7 **Rami gingivales superiores**. Innervate the corresponding gingiva. A

8 *Rami nasales externi*. External nasal branches, supply the nasal region. B

9 *Rami nasales interni*. Internal nasal branches, innervate Vestibulum nasi. B

10 *Rami labiales superiores*. Superior labial branches, supply the skin of the rostral part of Bucca, and skin and mucosa of Labium superius. B

11 **Ganglion pterygopalatinum**. Pterygopalatine ganglion, parasympathetic, located at the N. pterygopalatinus. In Ru and eq there are more than one ganglion. C

12 ***Rami orbitales***. Orbital branches, some may innervate Glandula lacrimalis. C

13 ***N. canalis pterygoidei***. Nerve of pterygoid canal, is represented by the union of the following two nerves. C

14 *N. petrosus major*. Greater petrosal nerve, parasympathetic from N. facialis. C

15 *N. petrosus profundus*. Deep petrosal nerve, sympathetic, from Plexus caroticus internus. C

16 ***Rami communicantes cum n. palatino minore***. Branches communicating with lesser palatine nerve. C

17 ***Rami communicantes cum n. palatino majore***. Branches communicating with greater palatine nerve. C

18 ***Rami communicantes cum n. nasali caudali***. Branches communicating with caudal nasal nerve. C

19 **N. mandibularis.** Mandibular nerve, third branch of N. trigeminus (CN V_3), mixed. Passes through Foramen ovale. D

20 ***Ramus meningeus***. Meningeal branch, enters the cranial cavity through Foramen spinosum (Incisura spinosa of Foramen lacerum). E

21 ***N. masticatorius***. Masticatory nerve. D E

22 *N. massetericus*. Masseteric nerve, passes through Incisura mandibulae. D E

23 *Nn. temporales profundi*. Deep temporal nerves (caudal and middle), supply the M. temporalis. D E

24 ***N. pterygoideus lateralis***. Lateral pterygoid nerve, supplies the M. pterygoideus lateralis, may be a branch of N. buccalis (eq). D E

25 ***N. pterygoideus medialis***. Medial pterygoid nerve, supplies the M. pterygoideus medialis. D E

26 ***N. tensoris tympani***. Tensor tympani nerve, enters Cavum tympany through Canalis musculotubarius, supplies the M. tensor tympani. D

27 ***N. tensoris veli palatini***. Tensor veli palatini nerve, supplies the M. tensor veli palatini. D E

28 ***N. buccalis***. Buccal nerve, is sensory to the buccal mucosa, carries parasympathetic fibers to the buccal glands, and in Ru to the parotid gland and supplies the M. temporalis by N. temporalis profundus rostralis (eq). D E

29 ***N. auriculotemporalis****. Auriculotemporal nerve, surrounds the neck of the mandible caudally and joins the N. facialis. It brings sensory fibers which supply the skin between the base of the ear, zygomatic arch, facial crest, commissure of the lips, and, except the inferior lip and the chin, a line back to the base of the ear on, or a little bit dorsal to, the ventral line of the head. D E

30 *N. meatus acustici externi*. Nerve to external acoustic meatus. D E

31 *Ramus membranae tympani*. Branch to tympanic membrane. D E

32 *Rami parotidei*. Parotid branches. D E

A Left N. infraorbitalis (ca)

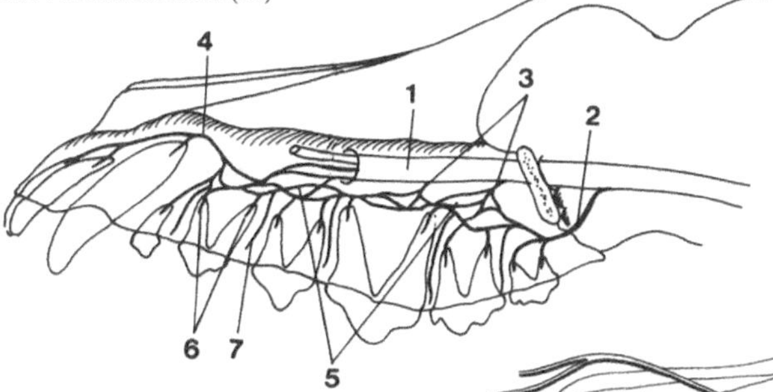

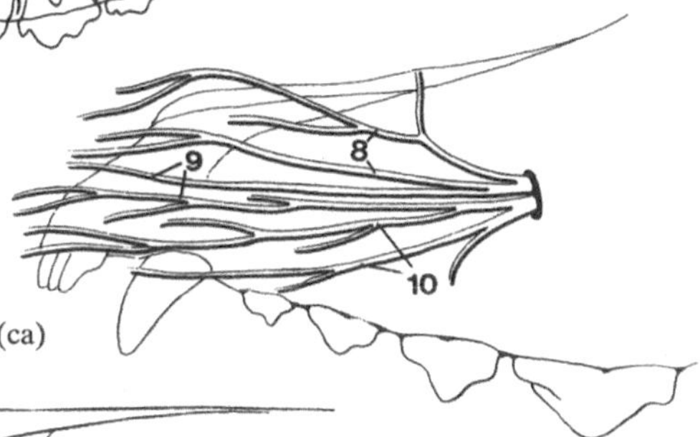

B Rami nasales and labiales superiores (ca)

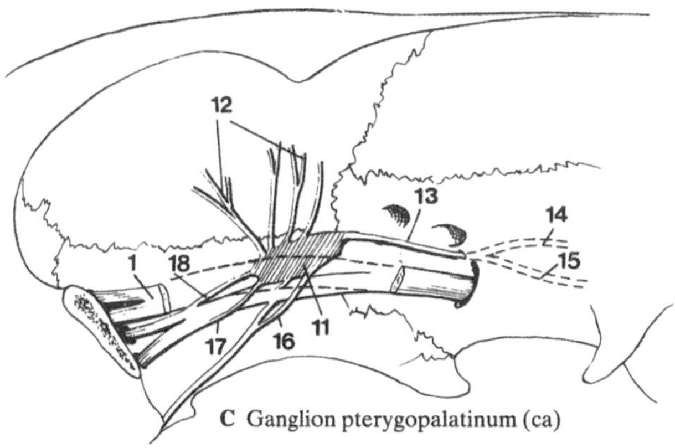

C Ganglion pterygopalatinum (ca)

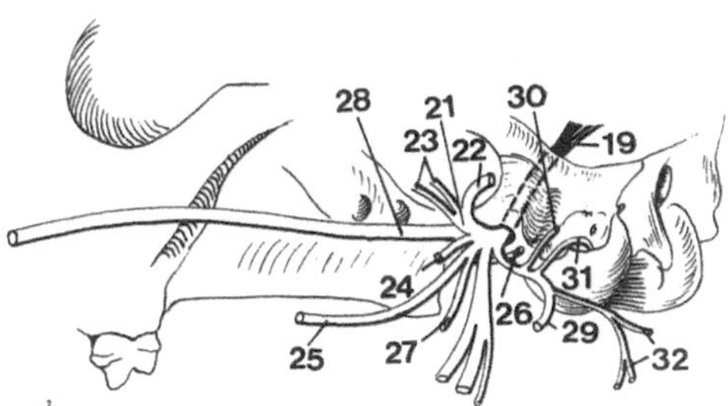

D N. mandibularis (ca)

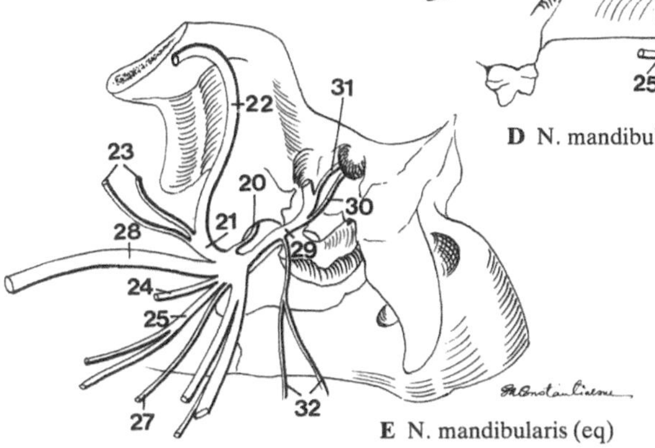

E N. mandibularis (eq)

1 *Nn. auriculares rostrales*. Rostral auricular nerves, sensory, supply the skin of the rostral (and lateral) area of the Auricula. A

2 *Ramus transversus faciei*. Transverse facial branch, parallels the transverse facial vessels, supplies the skin of the cheek. A

3 *Rami communicantes cum n. faciali*. Branches communicating with facial nerve, contribute to the formation of Rami buccales. A

4 ***N. lingualis***. Lingual nerve, arises with N. alveolaris inferior, goes to the tongue accompanying the Chorda tympani, which carries gustatory and parasympathetic fibers from the N. Intermediofacialis. B

5 *Rami isthmi faucium*. Branches to Isthmus faucium. B

6 *Ramus communicans cum chorda tympani*. Communicating branch with Chorda tympani. B

7 *N. sublingualis*. Sublingual nerve, gives off branches to Glanda mandibularis and Recessus sublingualis lateralis. B

8 *Rami linguales*. Lingual branches, supply the rostral two thirds of the lingual mucosa with sensory and taste fibers. B

9 *Rami communicantes cum n. hypoglosso*. Branches communicating with the N. hypoglossus. B

10 ***N. alveolaris inferior****. Inferior alveolar nerve, enters the Canalis mandibulae. C

11 *N. mylohyoideus*. Mylohyoid nerve, the only branch before N. alveolaris inferior enters the Canalis mandibulae. It supplies M. mylohyoideus and Venter rostralis m. digastrici, and the skin of the rostral part of the intermandibular space. C

12 *Rami alveolares inferiores caudales*[1]. Caudal inferior alveolar branches, supply Dentes molares and corresponding gingiva. C

13 *Rami alveolares inferiores medii*[1]. Intermediate inferior alveolar branches, supply Dentes premolares and corresponding gingiva. C

14 *Ramus alveolaris inferior rostralis*[1]. Rostral inferior alveolar branch, to Dentes caninus and incisivi. C

15 *Plexus dentalis inferior*[1]. Inferior dental plexus, nervous network inside Canalis mandibulae. C

16 **Rami dentales inferiores**[1]. Inferior dental branches to the lower teeth. C

17 **Rami gingivales inferiores**. Inferior gingival branches to the gingiva. C

18 *N. mentalis* (Ru, eq)*. Mental nerve, passes through Foramen mentale and supplies the chin and the lower lip. C

19 **Rami mentales**. Mental branches, supply the chin. C

20 **Rami labiales inferiores**. Inferior labial branches, supply the lower lip. C

21 *Nn. mentales* (Car, su). Mental nerves, several branches emerging from several Foramina mentalia lateralia, and Foramen mentale mediale (su). D

22 **Rami mentales**. Mental branches, supply the chin. D

23 **Rami labiales inferiores**. Inferior labial branches, supply the lower lip. D

1) By a typo mistake these branches are not listed in the 5th edition of the N. A. V. They have been reintroduced in the Revised 5th edition of the N. A. V., 2012.

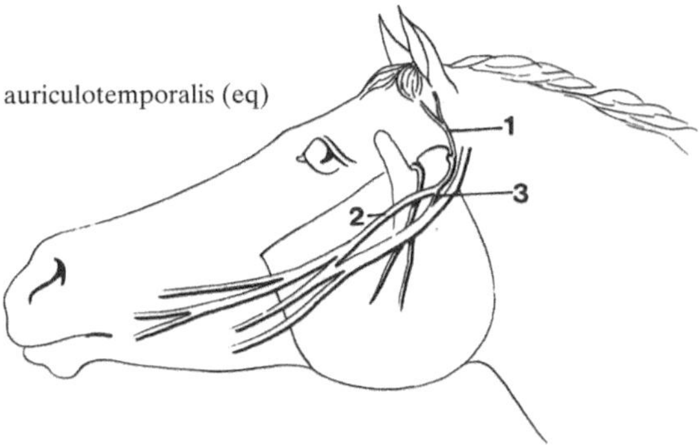

A Left N. auriculotemporalis (eq)

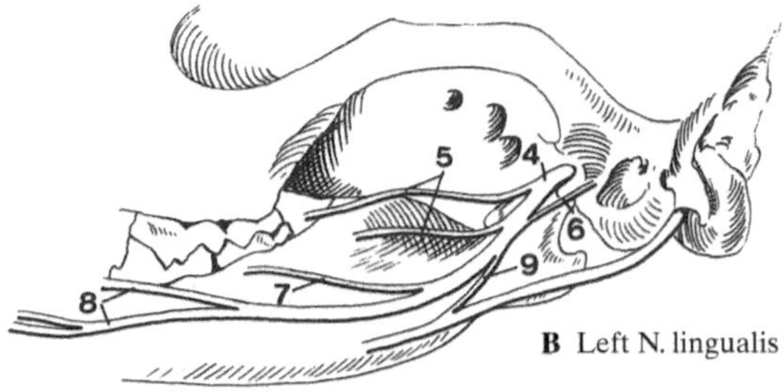

B Left N. lingualis (ca)

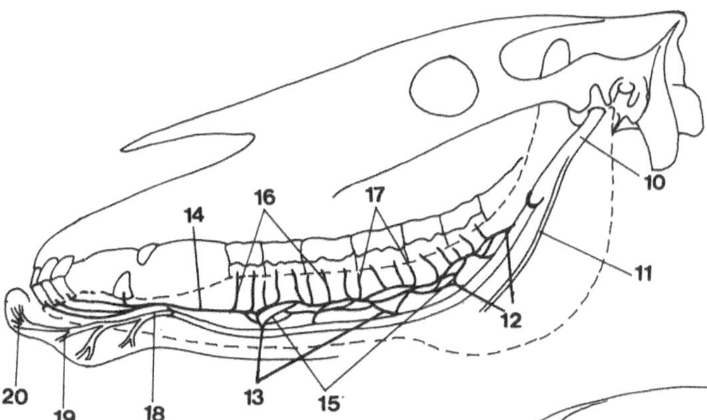

C Left N. alveolaris inferior (eq)

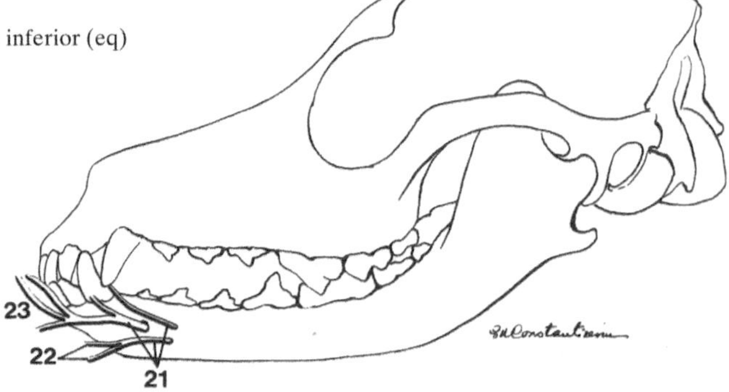

D Left Nn. mentales (ca)

1 **Ganglion oticum**. Otic ganglion, parasympathetic, at the origin of N. buccalis, gives off secretory fibers to Gl. parotis, Gll. buccales, and Gl. zygomatica (Car). A

2 ***N. petrosus minor***. Lesser petrosal nerve, preganglionic fibers. A

3 ***Rami communicantes cum n. buccali***. Communicating branches to the buccal nerve, carry parasympathetic fibers to buccal glands and Gl. zygomatica (Car). A

4 ***Rami communicantes cum n. auriculotemporali***. Communicating branches to the auriculotemporal nerve. Carry parasympathetic fibers to Gl. parotis. A

5 **Ganglion mandibulare**. Mandibular ganglion, at the origin of N. sublingualis, but in Car at the hilus of Gl. mandibularis. The preganglionic fibers proceed from Chorda tympani. A C

6 ***(Ramus sympathicus ad ganglion mandibulare)***. Sympathetic branch to mandibular ganglion from Plexus caroticus internus, without synapses in Ganglion mandibulare. A C

7 ***Rami communicantes cum n. linguali***. Communicating branches to lingual nerve. A

8 ***Rami glandulares***. Glandular branches to the Gll. sublinguales and mandibularis. A

9 **Ganglion sublinguale** (Car). Sublingual ganglion, in the angle between N. lingualis and the communicating branches of Ganglion mandibulare to N. lingualis. A

10 ***Rami communicantes cum n. linguali***. Communicating branches to the lingual nerve. A

11 ***Rami glandulares***. To Gll. sublinguales. A

12 **N. abducens**. Abducent nerve (CN VI), supplies Mm. retractor bulbi and rectus lateralis. 465 C

13 **N. facialis [N. intermediofacialis]**. Facial [intermediofacial] nerve (CN VII), carries motor, parasympathetic and taste fibers, passes through Meatus acusticus internus and Canalis facialis, exits through Foramen stylomastoideum. B C D

14 ***Geniculum n. facialis***. Genu of facial nerve, the first bend in the intraosseous course. B

15 ***Ganglion geniculi***. Geniculate ganglion (see 32). B

16 ***N. petrosus major***. Greater petrosal nerve, emerges at the genu, parasympathetic, and joins N. petrosus profundus to form the N. canalis pterygoidei (468.13). B C

17 ***N. stapedius***. Nerve to M. stapedius. B

18 ***Ramus auricularis internus****. Internal auricular branch, pierces the pinna and supplies the skin of the inner surface. Receives Ramus auricularis n. vagi (476.6) after leaving the Canalis facialis. B D

19 ***N. auricularis caudalis***. Caudal auricular nerve, supplies the caudal muscles of the ear. B D

20 ***Ramus digastricus***. Digastric branch, for Venter caudalis et Pars occipitomandibularis (in eq) m. digastrici. D

21 *Ramus stylohyoideus*. To M. stylohyoideus. D

22 ***Plexus parotideus***. Parotid plexus. D

23 ***N. auriculopalpebralis****. Auriculopalpebral nerve. D E

24 *Rami auriculares rostrales*. Rostral auricular branches, for rostral auricular muscles. D

25 *Ramus zygomaticus*. Zygomatic branch. D

26 **Rami palpebrales**. Palpebral branches, supply M. orbicularis oculi. D

27 ***Rami buccales***. Buccal branches, supply the muscles of cheek, lips, and nose. D E

28 *Rami buccolabiales*. Buccolabial branches. E

29 ***Ramus marginalis mandibulae***. Mandibular marginal branch (except eq). E (It replaces the former N. buccalis ventralis.)

30 ***Ramus colli***. Cervical branch, for Mm. parotidoauricularis and cutaneus colli. D

31 **N. intermedius**. Intermediate nerve, parasympathetic and sensory component of N. intermediofacialis. B

32 ***Ganglion geniculi***. Geniculate ganglion, similar to a spinal ganglion, located within Canalis facialis at Geniculum n. facialis. B

33 *Chorda tympani*. Passes through Fissura petrotympanica to join N. lingualis. B C

A Left Ganglia oticum, mandibulare, and sublinguale (ca)

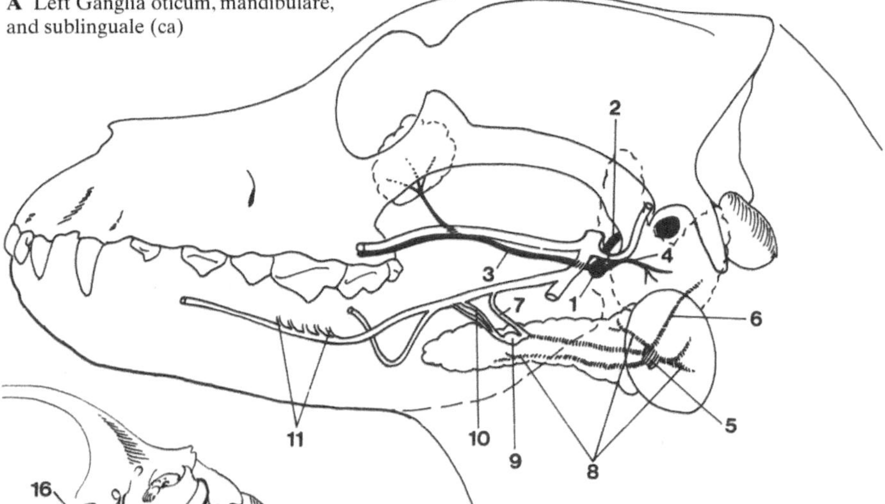

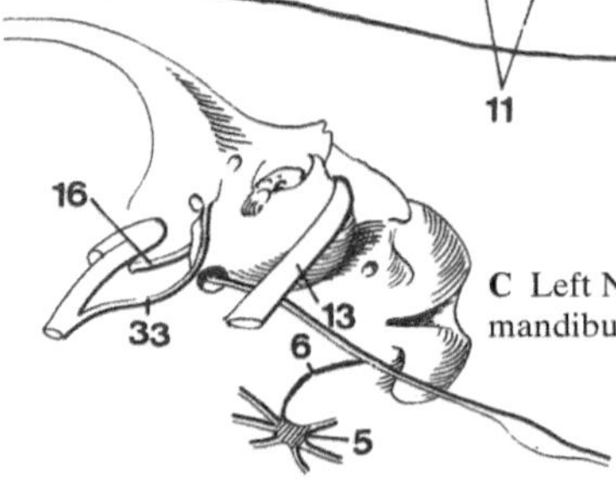

C Left N. facialis and Ganglion mandibulare (ca)

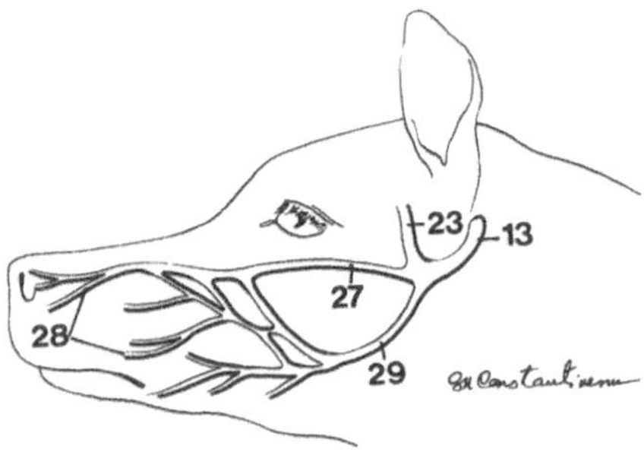

E Left N. facialis (ca)

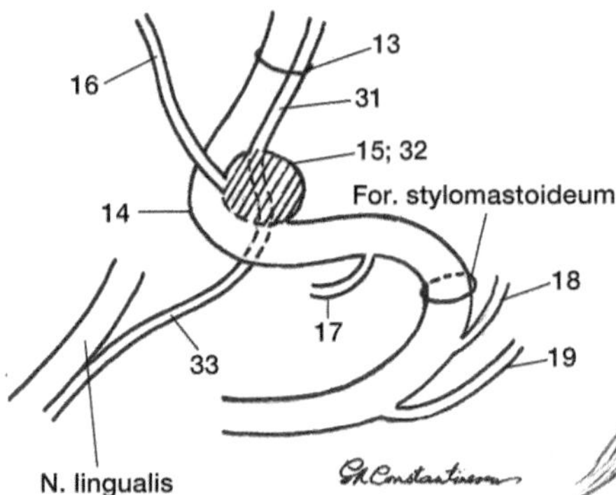

B N. intermediofacialis

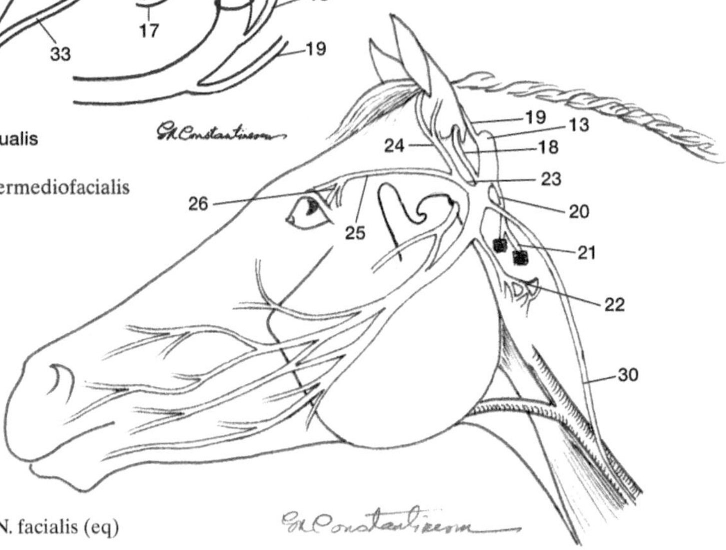

D Left N. facialis (eq)

1 **N. vestibulocochlearis.** Vestibulocochlear nerve (CN VIII), carries fibers for the sense of position of the body, and the mechanism of equilibrium (N. vestibularis) and for the sense of hearing (N. cochlearis). Former the acousticovestibular or statoacoustic nerve. A

2 ***Radix vestibularis.*** Vestibular root. A

3 ***Radix cochlearis.*** Cochlear root. A

4 ***N. vestibularis.*** Vestibular nerve, ends in Ganglion vestibulare. A

5 *Ganglion vestibulare.* Vestibular ganglion, located in the bottom of Meatus acusticus internus. A

6 **Pars superior.** Superior part, related to Ductus semicirculares anterior and lateralis, Utriculus and the anterior segment of Sacculus. A

7 **Pars inferior.** Inferior part, related to Ductus semicircularis posterior and to the posterior segment of Sacculus. A

8 **N. utriculoampullaris.** Utriculoampullary nerve, to Macula utriculi and Ampullae membranaceae anterior and lateralis. A

9 **N. utricularis.** Utricular nerve, supplies the Macula utriculi. A

10 **N. ampullaris anterior.** Anterior ampullary nerve, to Ampulla membranacea anterior. A

11 **N. ampullaris lateralis.** Lateral ampullary nerve, to Ampulla membranacea lateralis. A

12 **N. ampullaris posterior.** Posterior ampullary nerve, to Ampulla membranacea posterior. A

13 **N. saccularis.** Saccular nerve, to Macula sacculi. Two Nn. sacculares from both, Pars superior and Pars inferior of Ggl. vestibulare. A

14 ***N. cochlearis.*** Cochlear nerve, ends in Ganglion spirale cochleae. A

15 *Ganglion spirale cochleae.* Spiral ganglion, located in Modiolus along the base of Lamina spiralis ossea. See 530.13. A

16 **N. glossopharyngeus.** Glossopharyngeal nerve (CN IX), carrying motor, sensory, and parasympathetic fibers. Passes through Foramen jugulare. B C D

17 ***Ganglion proximale.*** Proximal ganglion. In the N.A. the ganglia of N. glossopharyngeus and N. vagus are designated superior and inferior. In the N. A. V. the terms proximale and distale are preferred because they are independent of the position of the animal. The proximal ganglion is located in Foramen jugulare. B C

18 ***Ganglion distale.*** Distal ganglion. This term replaces the former term Ganglion petrosum. Usually not separated from Ganglion proximale in ca and eq. B C D

19 *N. tympanicus.* Tympanic nerve, enters the tympanic cavity. C D

20 **Plexus tympanicus.** Tympanic plexus, nervous network on the surface of Promontorium. C

21 **N. petrosus minor.** Lesser petrosal nerve, arises from Plexus tympanicus and carries parasympathetic fibers to Ganglion oticum. C

22 **Nn. caroticotympanici.** Caroticotympanic nerves, arise from the sympathetic Plexus carotideus internus, become component of Plexus tympanicus. C

23 **Ramus tubarius.** Tubal branch, to Tuba auditiva. C

24 ***Ramus sinus carotici.*** Carotid sinus branch, for Sinus caroticus and Glomus caroticum. D

25 ***Ramus m. stylopharyngei caudalis.*** Branch to M. stylopharyngeus caudalis. D

26 ***Ramus pharyngeus.*** Pharyngeal branch, runs to the dorsal pharyngeal wall. D

27 *Plexus pharyngeus.* Pharyngeal plexus, made up by the intermingled fibers of Rami pharyngei of Nn. glossopharyngeus and vagus, and sympathetic fibers from Ganglion cervicale craniale. D

28 ***Ganglion lateropharyngeum*** (bo, ov). Lateropharyngeal ganglion, located medial to the rostroventral end of the stylohyoid bone.

29 ***Ramus lingualis.*** Lingual branch, supplies the mucosa of the caudal third of the tongue. D

30 *Rami tonsillares.* Tonsillar branches. D

A Right N. vestibulocochlearis, caudal aspect

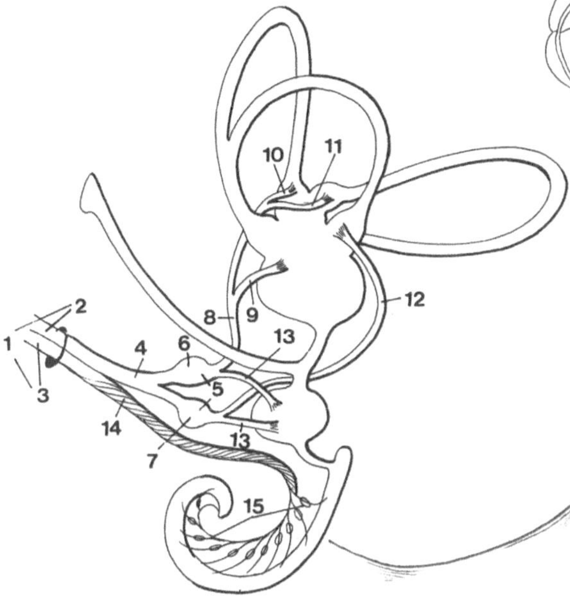

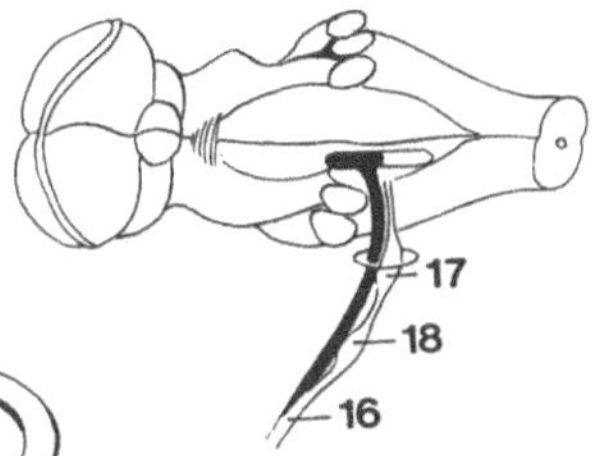

B Origin of N. glossopharyngeus from Fossa rhomboidea

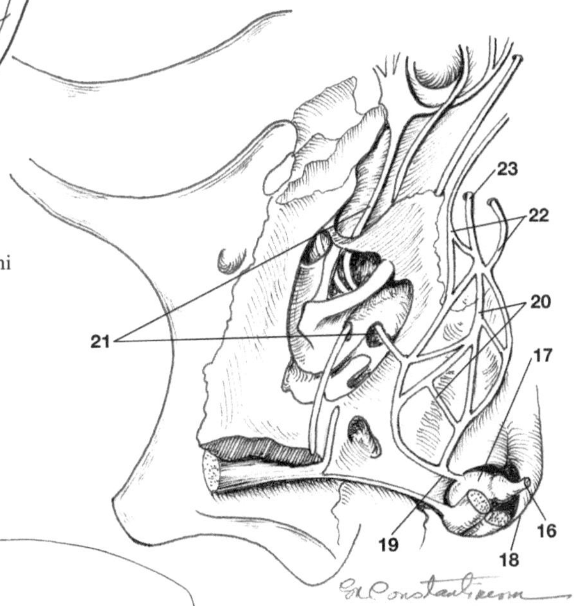

C Left N. glossopharyngeus within the tympanic cavity (Cavum tympani opened), ventral aspect (ca)

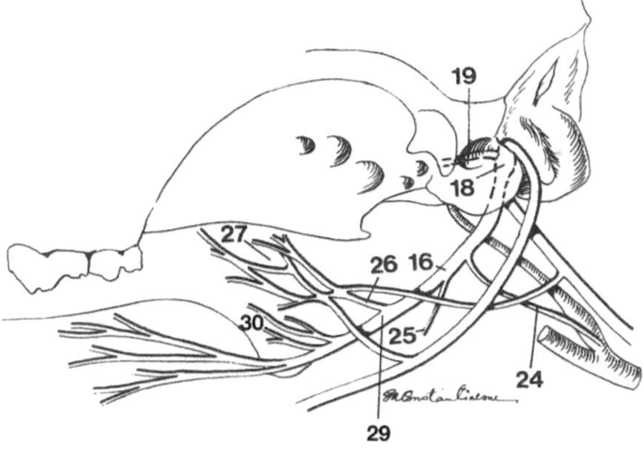

D N. glossopharyngeus (Cavum tympani opened), left ventrocaudal aspect (ca) (modified and redrawn from H. Evans)

1 **N. vagus**. Vagus nerve (CN X), carrying motor, sensory, and parasympathetic fibers, passes through Foramen jugulare. A B C D

2 ***Ganglion proximale***. Proximal ganglion, located in Foramen jugulare, was formerly named Ganglion jugulare. A B

3 ***Ganglion distale***. Distal ganglion, located caudal to A. carotis interna and Ggl. cervicale craniale, formerly named Ganglion nodosum. A

4 ***Ramus meningeus***. Meningeal branch, arises from Ganglion proximale. A

5 ***Ramus communicans cum n. glossopharyngeo***. Branch communicating with glossopharyngeal n. A

6 ***Ramus auricularis****. Auricular branch, communicates with N. facialis within Canalis facialis, supplies an area on the inner surface of the pinna. B

7 ***Rami pharyngei***. Pharyngeal branches, supply the pharynx together with Ramus pharyngeus of N. glossopharyngeus. A

8 *Plexus pharyngeus*. Pharyngeal plexus, result of the joining of Rami pharyngei nn. glossopharyngei and vagi, and sympathetic fibers. A

9 *Ramus esophageus [oesophageus]*. Esophageal branch. A

10 ***N. laryngeus cranialis***. Cranial laryngeal nerve. A

11 *Ramus externus*. External branch, supplies M. cricothyroideus. A

12 *Ramus internus*. Internal branch, supplies the mucosa in association with the N. laryngeus caudalis. A

13 ***Ramus communicans cum n. laryngeo caudali***. Branch communicating with caudal laryngeal n., inside the larynx. A

14 ***N. depressor***. Arises from N. vagus or N. laryngeus cranialis, enters the N. vagus again, distributed to pressoreceptors in aorta. A

15 ***Truncus vagosympathicus****. Vagosympathetic trunk, common course of Truncus sympathicus and N. vagus in the neck. A

16 ***Rami cardiaci***. Cardiac branches, parasympathetic fibers to the heart. C

17 ***N. laryngeus recurrens****. Recurrent laryngeal nerve: the left loops around the aorta, the right around the Truncus costocervicalis. Both run along trachea to the larynx. C D

18 *Rami tracheales*. Tracheal branches. D

19 *Rami esophagei [oesophagei]*. Esophageal branches. D

20 *N. laryngeus caudalis*. Caudal laryngeal nerve, end of N. laryngeus recurrens, supplies all laryngeal muscles, (except M. cricothyroideus), and the mucosa in association with the N. laryngeus cranialis. A C D

21 ***Rami bronchales***. Bronchial branches. C D

22 ***Plexus pulmonalis***. Pulmonary plexus. C D

23 ***Rami esophagei [oesophagei] [Plexus esophageus, oesophageus]***. Esophageal branches [plexus]. C D

24 ***Truncus vagalis ventralis***. Ventral vagal trunk, composed of the ventral branches of right and left N. vagus. C D E

25 *Rami gastrici parietales*. Parietal gastric branches, on Facies parietalis ventriculi (except Ru). C

26 *Ramus communicans*. Communicating branch, connects Trunci vagales ventralis and dorsalis, usually to left of esophagus in Ru, inclined caudodorsally or caudoventrally. E

27 *Rami atriales ruminis*. Branches to Atrium ruminis. E

28 *Rami reticulares craniales*. Branches to Facies diaphragmatica reticuli. E

29 *Ramus pyloricus*. Pyloric branch. C

30 *Rami hepatici*. Hepatic branches. One of these may arise from Truncus vagalis dorsalis in Ru. C

31 *Rami duodenales*. Branches to duodenum and pancreas. C

32 *Rami ad sulcum ventriculi*. Branches to ventricular groove in Ru. E

33 *Rami omasiales*. Omasal branches. E

34 *Rami abomasiales parietales*. Branches to Facies parietalis abomasi. E

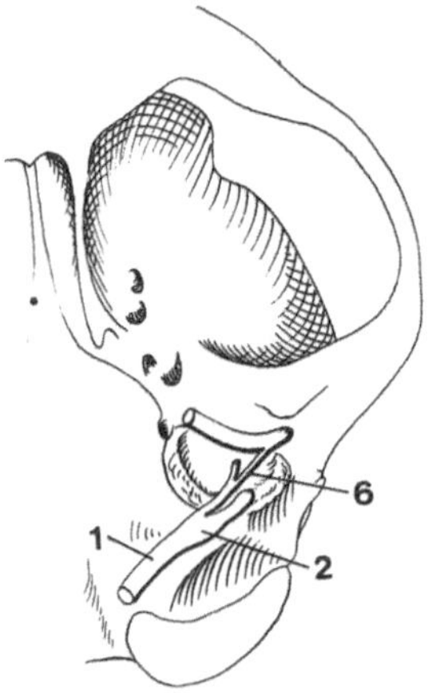

B Ramus auricularis of left N. vagus, ventrolateral view (ca)

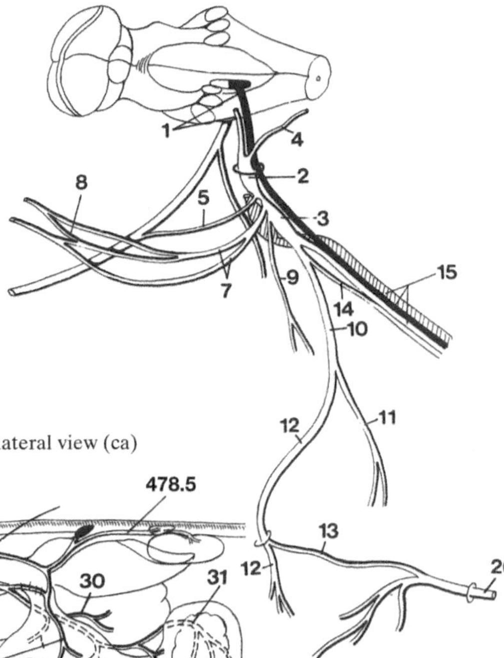

A Left N. vagus (ca)

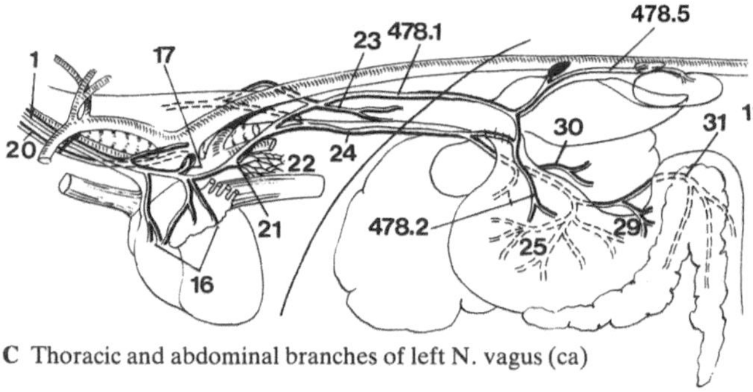

C Thoracic and abdominal branches of left N. vagus (ca)

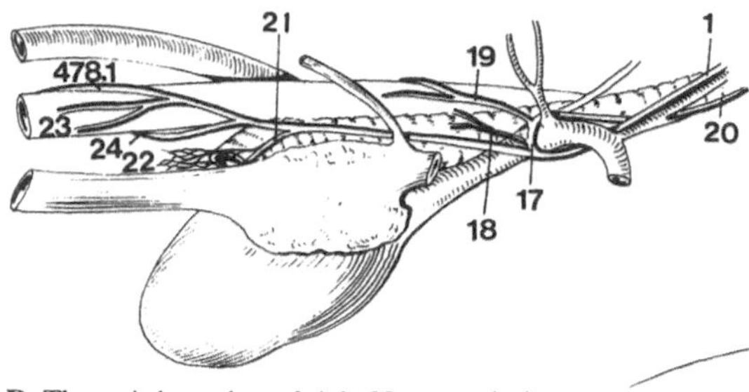

D Thoracic branches of right N. vagus (ca)

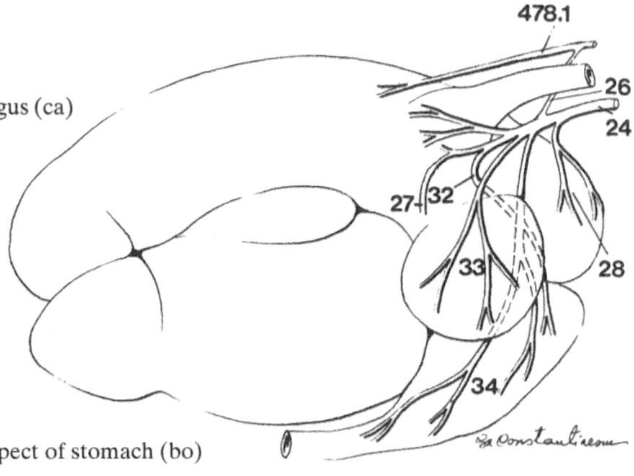

E Truncus vagalis ventralis, right aspect of stomach (bo)

1 ***Truncus vagalis dorsalis***. Dorsal vagal trunk, composed of the dorsal branches of left and predominantly right N. vagus. A, 477 C D E

2 *Rami gastrici viscerales*. Visceral gastric branches to Facies visceralis ventriculi. 477 C

3 *Rami atriales ruminis*. Branches to Atrium ruminis. A

4 *Rami celiaci [coeliaci]*. Celiac branches, to Plexus celiacus. A

5 *Rami renales*. Renal branches, supply kidneys and adrenal glands. 477 C

6 *Rami ruminales dorsales*. Dorsal ruminal branches, continuations of Truncus vagalis dorsalis to rumen, except its atrium. A

7 *Ramus ruminalis dexter*. Right ruminal branch, is the main branch of Truncus vagalis dorsalis, on the Facies visceralis ruminis. A

8 *Ramus ad sulcum cranialem*. Branch to cranial groove of rumen. A

9 *Rami ad sulcum ventriculi*. Branches to ventricular groove. A

10 *Rami reticulares caudales*. Caudal reticular branches, supply Facies visceralis reticuli. A

11 *Ramus ad curvaturam majorem abomasi*. Branch to greater abomasal curvature. A

12 *Rami omasiales*. Omasal branches to Facies visceralis omasi. A

13 *Rami abomasiales viscerales*. Visceral abomasal branches, supply Facies visceralis abomasi. A

14 **N. accessorius**. Accessory nerve (CN XI), exclusively motor, passes through Foramen jugulare. B C

15 ***Radices craniales***. Cranial roots, origin in medulla oblongata and supply the fibers of Ramus internus, which joins N. vagus. C

16 ***Radices spinales***. Spinal roots, origin in the spinal cord and supply the fibers of Ramus externus, which was formerly designated N. accessorius spinalis, or simply N. accessorius. C

17 ***Ramus internus***. Internal branch, communicates with N. vagus. C

18 ***Ramus externus***. External branch, continuation of N. accessorius which courses caudoventrally to supply muscles. B C

19 *Ramus dorsalis*. Dorsal branch, supplies the Mm. trapezius, cleidocephalicus, and omotransversarius. B

20 *Ramus ventralis**. Ventral branch, innervates M. sternocephalicus. B

21 **N. hypoglossus**. Hypoglossal nerve (CN XII), exclusively motor, supplies the musculature of the tongue and the Mm. thyrohyoideus and geniohyoideus. Passes through Canalis n. hypoglossi. D

22 ***Rami linguales***. Lingual branches, supply the muscles of the tongue. D

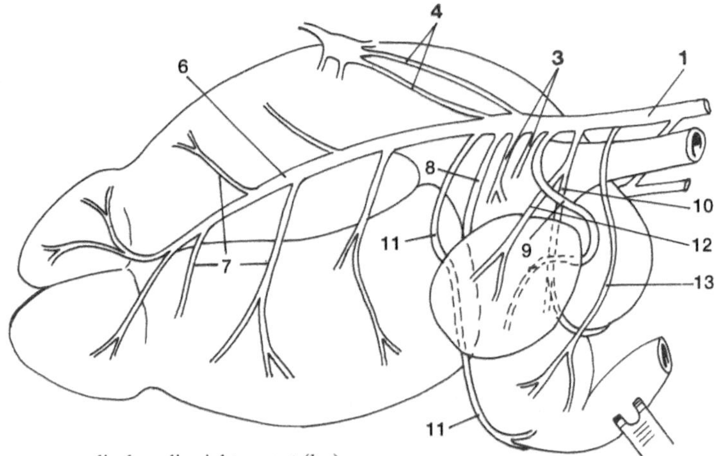

A Truncus vagalis dorsalis, right aspect (bo).
Omasum and abomasum reflected cranially to expose their visceral aspect

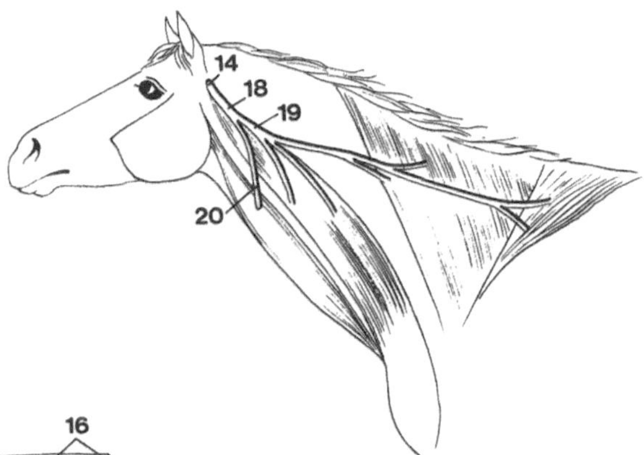

B Left N. accessorius (eq)

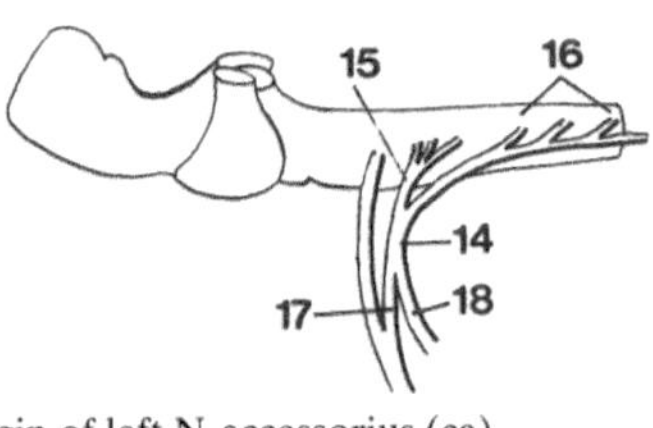

C Origin of left N. accessorius (ca)

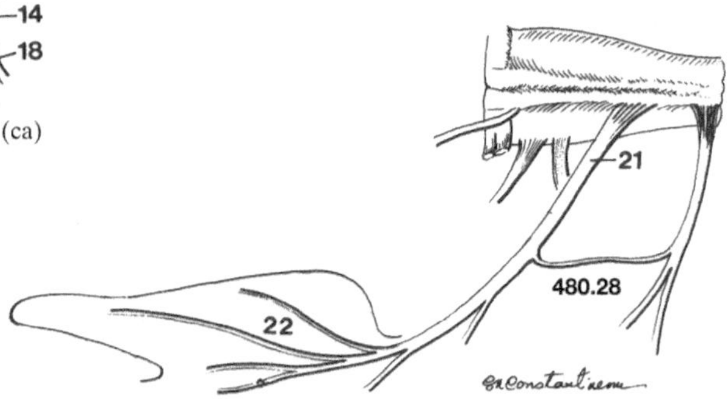

D Left N. hypoglossus (ca)

1 **NERVI SPINALES.** Spinal nerves, mixed and metameric, with a ventral and a dorsal root starting from Medulla spinalis. Exit through Foramina intervertebralia. A

2 ***Fila radicularia.*** Root filaments, represent the origin of Radix ventralis and Radix dorsalis. A

3 ***Radix ventralis.*** Ventral, motor root. A

4 ***Radix dorsalis.*** Dorsal, sensory root. A

5 *Ganglion spinale.* Spinal ganglion, located in Radix dorsalis, immediately before it joins the Radix ventralis in Canalis vertebralis. A

6 ***Ramus ventralis.*** Ventral branch, larger than dorsal branch. A

7 ***Ramus dorsalis.*** Dorsal branch, smaller than ventral branch. A

8 ***Rami communicantes.*** Communicating branches between Nn. spinales and Truncus sympathicus. A

9 ***Ramus meningeus.*** Meningeal branch, reenters the Canalis vertebralis. A

10 ***Cauda equina.*** Horse tail-shaped structure, represented by the sacral and caudal spinal nerves, surrounding the Filum terminale. B

11 ***Ansae.*** Loops, connecting neighbouring nerves.

12 **Nervi cervicales.** Cervical nerves. 8 pairs of spinal nerves originating from the cervical part of Medulla spinalis. C

13 ***Rami dorsales.*** Dorsal branches, supply muscles and skin in the dorsal part of the neck. C

14 *Ramus medialis.* Medial branch, motor and mainly sensory fibers (except C 8). C

14a **Ramus cutaneus dorsalis.** Branch of Ramus medialis only in the cervical area. C

15 *Ramus lateralis.* Lateral branch, contains only motor fibers. C

16 *N. suboccipitalis.* Suboccipital nerve, dorsal branch of the first N. cervicalis, motor supplying muscles of the cranial part of the neck, sensory – called N. occipitalis – to the medial side of Scapha of the Auris externa. C

17 *N. occipitalis major.* Greater occipital nerve, dorsal branch of the second N. cervicalis. Sensory to the Dorsum auriculae. C

18 ***Rami ventrales.*** Ventral branches, larger and more diverse than Rami dorsales. Their fibers intermingle resulting Plexus cervicalis. C

19 *N. auricularis magnus**. Great auricular nerve, from Ramus ventralis of C2. Sensory to the base of the ear and the caudal part of Dorsum auriculae. C

20 *N. transversus colli**. Transverse cervical nerve or transverse nerve of the neck, from Ramus ventralis of C2, was formerly designated Nervus cutaneus colli, but there are many cutaneous nerves of the neck, therefore the cleaner N.A. term was adopted. Sensory to the intermandibular space. C

21 **Rami craniales.** Cranial branches. C

22 **Rami caudales.** Caudal branches. C

23 *Nn. supraclaviculares.* Supraclavicular nerves, arise from Rami ventrales of Nn. cervicales III–IV (Car), IV–V (su, Ru), V–VI (eq). Sensory for the skin of the shoulder. C

24 **Nn. supraclaviculares ventrales.** Ventral supraclavicular nerves. C

25 **Nn. supraclaviculares intermedii.** Intermediate supraclavicular nerves. C

26 **Nn. supraclaviculares dorsales.** Dorsal supraclavicular nerves. C

27 **Plexus cervicalis.** Cervical plexus. Network formed by Rami ventrales of Nn. cervicales I–V.

28 ***Ansa cervicalis.*** Cervical loop, between N. hypoglossus and Ramus ventralis of C1 (esp. ca). Rami ventrales of C1 and C2 and sometimes C3 (esp. Un). Supplies Mm. sterno- and omohyoideus, and sternothyroideus C, 479 D

29 *Radix cranialis.* Cranial root. from N. hypoglossus or Ramus ventralis of C1. C

30 *Radix caudalis.* Caudal root, from Rami ventralis of C1 or C2 (sometimes additionally C3). C

31 **N. phrenicus.** Phrenic nerve, arises from Rami ventrales of Nn. cervicales V–VII and sometimes IV, to the diaphragm. C, 483 B

32 ***Rami pericardiaci.*** Pericardiac branches. C

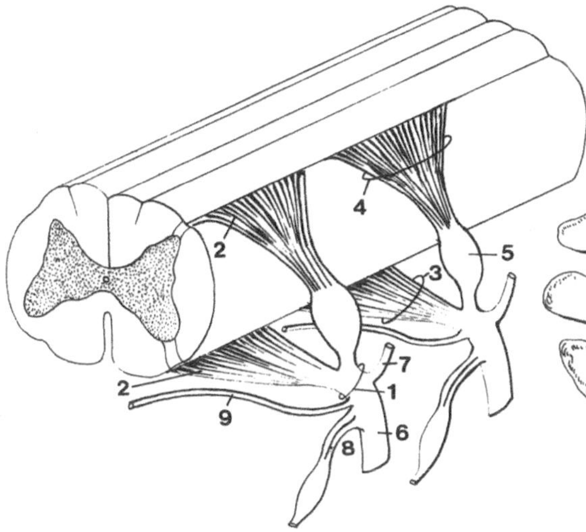

A Left nervi spinales, roots and branches

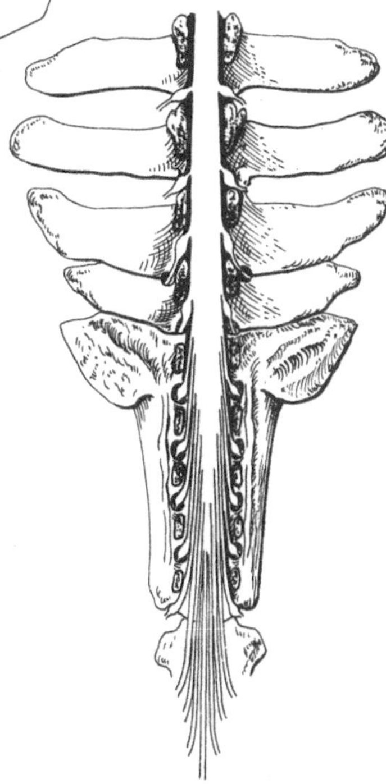

B Cauda equina (eq)

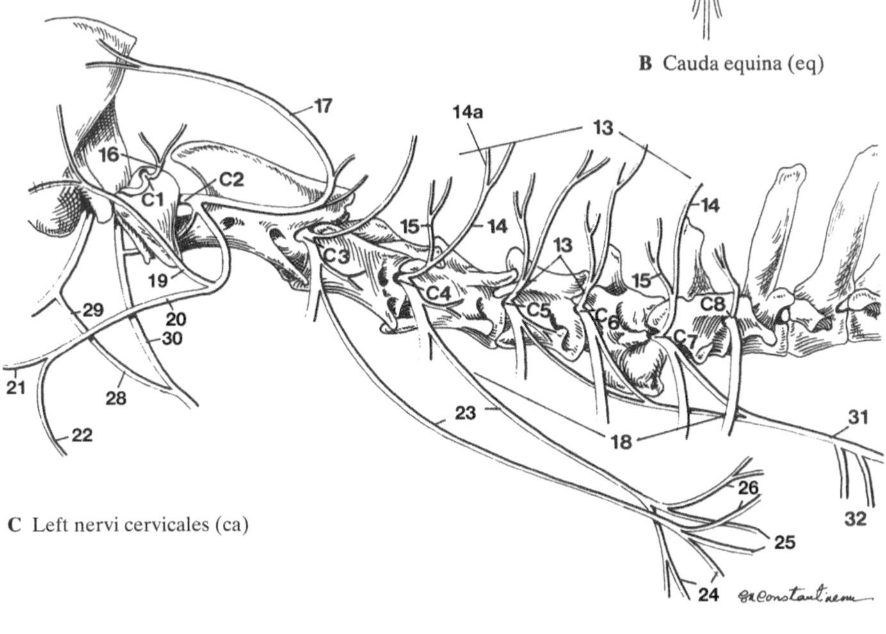

C Left nervi cervicales (ca)

1 ***Plexus brachialis***. Brachial plexus, network of Rami ventrales of Nn. cervicales V (su), VI–VIII and thoracici I, II (ca, Ru, eq), runs to the axilla, supplies the forelimb and partially the shoulder girdle (the extrinsic muscles of the thoracic limb). A B

2 **Radices plexus**. Roots of plexus, branches of the Rami ventrales that form the plexus. A

3 **Trunci plexus**. Trunks of plexus, some roots unite proximal to the plexus to form Trunci plexus. A B

4 **N. dorsalis scapulae**. Dorsal scapular nerve, small branch (usually not described in veterinary textbooks) to Mm. serratus ventralis cervicis and rhomboidei. A B

5 **N. subclavius**. Subclavian nerve, innervates M. subclavius in Un. B

6 **N. suprascapularis**. Suprascapular nerve, arising form C6–C7 (eq C8), supplies the Mm. supraspinatus and infraspinatus. A B

7 **Nn. subscapulares**. Subscapular nerves, originating from C6–C8, supply the M. subscapularis. A B

8 **N. musculocutaneus**. Musculocutaneous nerve, arises from C6 (Un), C7, C8 (Car, eq), descends medial to shoulder joint to join the N. medianus in Un. A B

9 ***Ramus muscularis proximalis***. Proximal muscular branch, supplies Mm. coracobrachialis and biceps brachii. A B

10 ***Ansa axillaris***. Axillary loop, formed by the junction of Nn. musculocutaneus and medianus, around the distal surface of the A. axillaris in Un. The Ramus muscularis distalis and the N. cutaneus antebrachii medialis n. musculocutanei separate from N. medianus in the distal part of the Brachium. The communication between Nn. musculocutaneus and medianus near the elbow in Car is not homologous to the Ansa axillaris. B

10a ***Ramus communicans cum n. mediano*** (Car). Communicating branch before the origin of Ramus muscularis distalis, on the medial aspect of the elbow joint.

11 ***Ramus muscularis distalis***. Distal muscular branch. Arises, together with N. cutaneus antebrachii medialis in the distal part of the brachium (Un), and supplies the M. brachialis. A B

12 ***N. cutaneus antebrachii medialis****. Medial cutaneous antebrachial nerve, descends on the medial side of the antebrachium, carpus, and metacarpus and can be felt through skin on the medial side of Lacertus fibrosus. A B, 491 A B

13 **N. axillaris**. Axillary nerve, arises from C6–C7 (C7–C8 eq), supplies shoulder muscles and an area of the skin of brachium and antebrachium. A B

14 ***Rami musculares***. Muscular branches, innervate the Mm. cleidobrachialis, deltoideus, teres minor, teres major, articularis humeri (fe, su, eq), and the caudal part of M. subscapularis. A B

15 ***N. cutaneus brachii lateralis cranialis****. Cranial lateral cutaneous brachial nerve, arises between Caput longum and Caput laterale of M. triceps brachii, supplies the skin on the lateral surface of the brachium, cranial to the territory of N. intercostobrachialis. A B

16 ***N. cutaneus antebrachii cranialis****. Cranial cutaneous antebrachial nerve, becomes apparent at the ventral border of deltoideus m. at its insertion on the deltoid tuberosity. It supplies the skin over the muscular part of M. extensor carpi radialis. A B

17 **Nn. pectorales craniales**. Cranial pectoral nerves, supply Mm. pectorales superficiales. A B

18 **N. thoracicus longus**. Long thoracic nerve, from C7 and/or C8, runs caudally supplying the M. serratus ventralis thoracis. B

19 **N. thoracodorsalis**. Thoracodorsal nerve, originates mainly from C8, innervates the M. latissimus dorsi. A B

20 **N. thoracicus lateralis**. Lateral thoracic nerve, arises mainly from C8 and T1, supplies the M. cutaneus trunci. Some of its fibers join in Un cutaneous branches of the 2nd and 3rd (in Ru also the 1st) intercostal nerves to form the N. intercostobrachialis. A B

21 **Nn. pectorales caudales**. Caudal pectoral nerves, innervate the M. pectoralis ascendens. A B

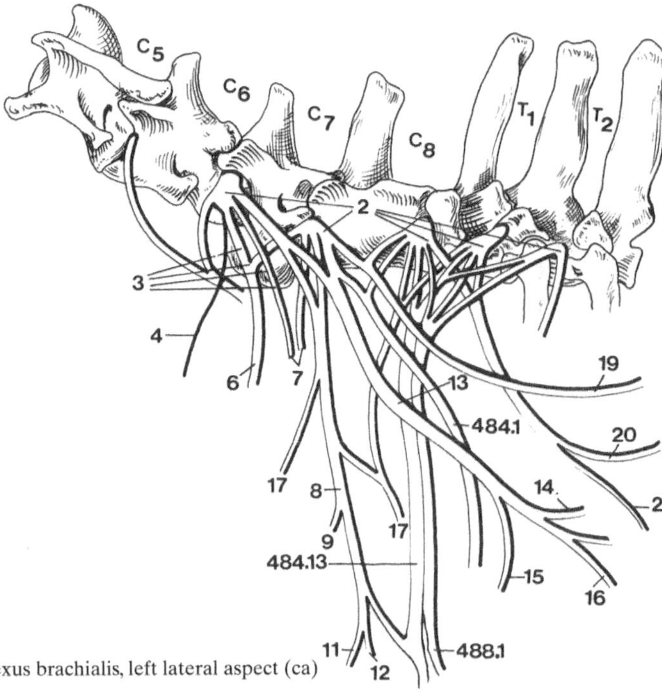

A Plexus brachialis, left lateral aspect (ca)

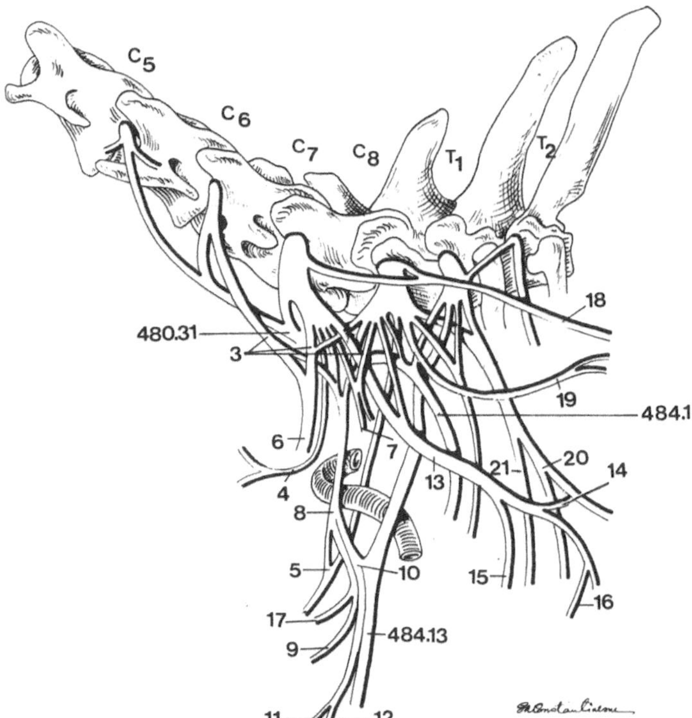

B Plexus brachialis, left lateral aspect (eq)

1 **N. radialis***. Radial nerve, arises from C7–T1, runs caudal to A. brachialis, enters the space between M. triceps brachii and humerus, accompanies the M. brachialis around the humerus in Sulcus m. brachialis. A, 483 A B

2 ***Rami musculares***. Muscular branches, for Mm. triceps brachii, tensor fasciae antebrachii, and anconeus. A

3 ***N. cutaneus brachii lateralis caudalis***. Caudal lateral brachial cutaneous nerve, supplies the skin covering the lateral head of M. triceps brachii. A

4 ***Ramus profundus***. Deep branch. A

5 ***Rami musculares***. Muscular branches to all the extensor muscles of the forearm, including the M. extensor carpi ulnaris (flexor of autopodium), and in Car also to the Mm. brachioradialis and supinator. A

6 ***Ramus superficialis***. Superficial branch, entirely sensory. A, 491 A B

7 *N. cutaneus antebrachii lateralis**. Lateral antebrachial cutaneous nerve, becomes apparent at the ventral edge of the lateral head of M. triceps brachii, supplies the skin covering the digital extensor muscles in the forearm. A

8 *Ramus lateralis* (Car, su). Lateral branch, descends to the carpus parallel with V. cephalica. A B C

9 *Ramus medialis* (Car, su). Medial branch, descends to the carpus parallel with V. cephalica. A B C

10 *Nn. digitales dorsales communes* [1]. Dorsal common digital nerves, only in Car (I, II, III, IV), su (II, III, IV), and Ru (II, III). B C, 491 A

11 **Nn. digitales dorsales proprii** [1]. Dorsal proper digital nerves, originate from the bifurcation of common digital nerves. B C, 491 A

12 *N. digitalis dorsalis I abaxialis* (Car). Dorsal abaxial digital nerve I, supplies digit I on the dorsal aspect of the abaxial side. B

13 **N. medianus**. Median nerve, originates from C8 and T1 (T2), supplies some flexor muscles of the forearm, part of the skin on the palmar aspect of carpus, metacarpus, and digits. D E, 483 A B, 487 A B C

14 ***Radix medialis***. Medial root, arises from T1 (T2). D

15 ***Radix lateralis***. Lateral root, arises from C8. D

16 ***Rami musculares***. Muscular branches, supply the following flexor muscles of the forearm: flexor carpi radialis, M. flexor digitorum/digitalis superficialis, M. flexor digitorum/digitalis profundus (caput radiale and pars of caput humerale), also the Mm. pronator teres, pronator quadratus. D

17 ***N. interosseus antebrachii***. Antebrachial interosseous nerve, for the periosteum. D

CARNIVORA

18 ***N. digitalis palmaris I abaxialis***. Abaxial palmar digital nerve I, supplies the palmar aspect of the abaxial side of the first digit. E

19 ***N. digitalis palmaris communis I***. Palmar common digital nerve I, the medial terminal branch of N. medianus, receives the corresponding N. metacarpeus palmaris from Ramus profundus of N. ulnaris. E (Nn. digitales palmares communes I, II, III are the terminal branches of N. medianus in Car. They receive the Nn. metacarpei palmares from the Ramus profundus n. ulnaris just before they divide into N. digitales proprii. N. digitalis communis IV is formed by the Ramus superficialis n. ulnaris and is joined by N. metacarpeus palmaris IV from Ramus profundus n. ulnaris.)

20 *N. digitalis palmaris proprius I axialis*. Palmar axial proper digital nerve I, supplies the palmar aspect of the axial side of digit I. E

21 *N. digitalis palmaris proprius II abaxialis*. Palmar abaxial proper digital nerve II, supplies the palmar aspect of the abaxial side of digit II. E

22 ***N. digitalis palmaris communis II***. Palmar common digital nerve II, the middle terminal branch of N. medianus, receives the N. metacarpeus II from N. ulnaris. E

23 *N. digitalis palmaris proprius II axialis*. Axial palmar proper digital nerve II. E

24 *N. digitalis palmaris proprius III abaxialis*. Abaxial palmar proper digital nerve III. E

25 ***N. digitalis palmaris communis III***. Palmar common digital nerve III, the lateral terminal branch of N. medianus, receives the N. metacarpeus III. E

26 *N. digitalis palmaris proprius III axialis*. Axial palmar proper digital nerve III. E

27 *N. digitalis palmaris proprius IV axialis*. Axial palmar proper digital nerve IV. E

28 *Ramus communicans* (fe). Communicating branch between Nn. digitales palmares communes II and III. E

[1] The superficial nerves of the metapodium are designated Nn. digitales communes; the deep nerves, Nn. metacarpei/metatarsei. Digital nerves that originate from the bifurcation of the Nn. digitales communes are called Nn. digitales proprii. Those that originate from some other source (independently) the term proprii is omitted and are simply Nn. digitales.

A N. radialis – left brachium and antebrachium, cranial aspect (ca)

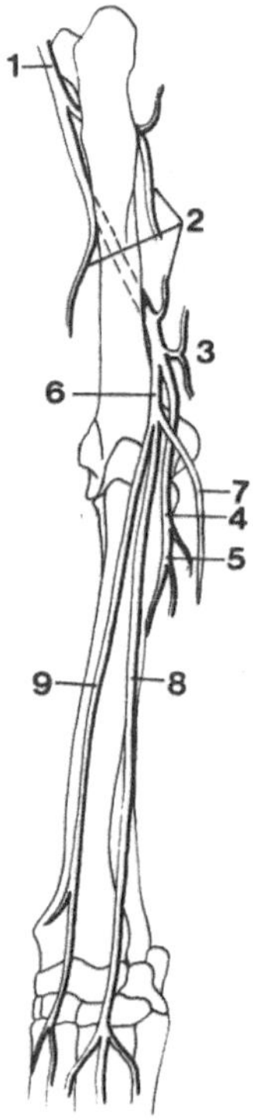

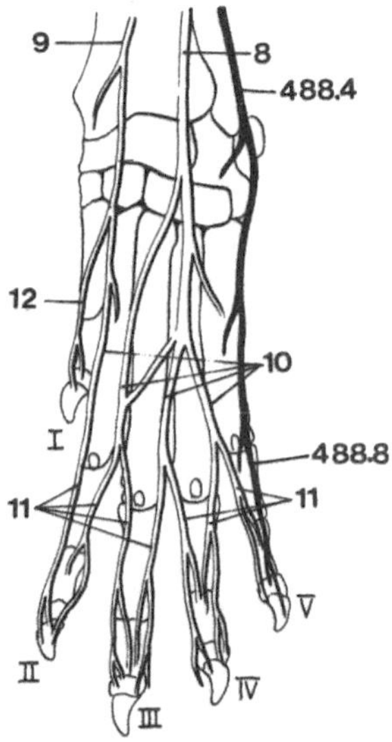

B Nn. radialis and ulnaris – left manus, dorsal aspect (ca)

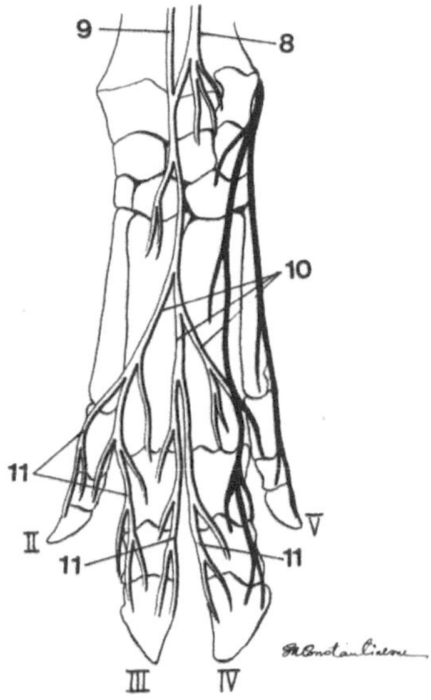

C Nn. radialis and ulnaris – left manus, dorsal aspect (su)

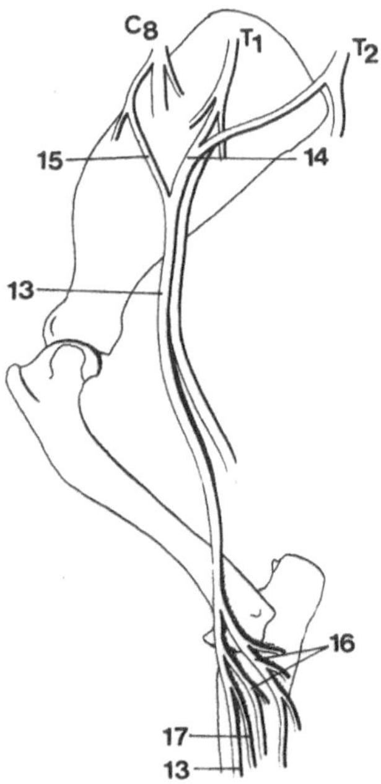

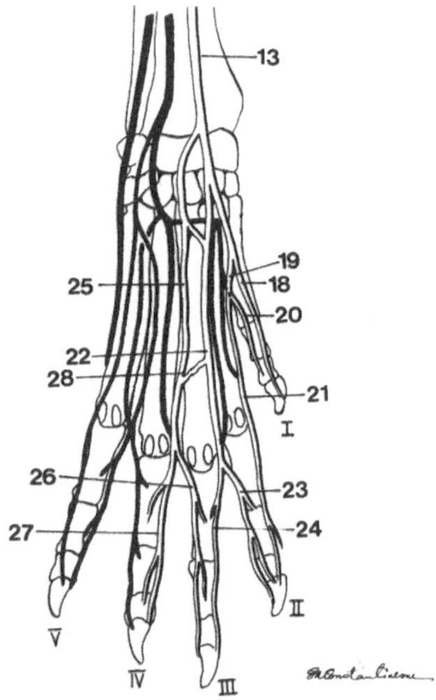

D N. medianus – right shoulder, brachium, elbow, medial aspect (ca)

E N. medianus – left manus, palmar aspect (fe)

SUS

1 ***N. digitalis palmaris II abaxialis.*** Palmar abaxial digital nerve II, arises from the medial branch of N. medianus to supply the palmar aspect of the abaxial side of digit II. A

2 ***N. digitalis palmaris communis II.*** Palmar common digital nerve II, arises from the medial branch of N. medianus. A

3 *N. digitalis palmaris proprius II axialis.* Axial palmar proper digital nerve II. A

4 *N. digitalis palmaris proprius III abaxialis.* Abaxial palmar proper digital nerve III. A

5 ***N. digitalis palmaris communis III.*** Palmar common digital nerve III. A

6 *N. digitalis palmaris proprius III axialis.* Axial palmar proper digital nerve III. A

7 *N. digitalis palmaris proprius IV axialis.* Axial palmar proper digital nerve IV. A

8 *Ramus communicans.* Communicating branch between N. digitalis palmaris communis III and N. digitalis palmaris communis IV (from N. ulnaris). A

RUMINANTIA

9 ***N. digitalis palmaris communis II.*** Palmar common digital nerve II, arises from the medial branch of N. medianus. B

10 *N. digitalis palmaris proprius II.* Palmar proper digital nerve II, a very short branch, in bo only. B

11 *N. digitalis palmaris proprius III abaxialis.* Palmar abaxial proper digital nerve III, the continuation of N. digitalis communis II on the abaxial side of digit III. B

12 ***N. digitalis palmaris III axialis.*** Palmar axial digital nerve III, arises from the medial branch of N. medianus and lies on the axial side of digit III (bo, ov). In cap there is a N. digitalis palmaris communis III continued by Nn. digitales palmares proprii III and IV axiales. B

13 ***N. digitalis palmaris IV axialis.*** Palmar axial digital nerve IV, lateral branch of N. medianus, descends on the axial side of digit IV (bo, ov). In cap it arises from N. digitalis palmaris communis III. The Nn. digitales palmares III and IV axiales often reunite in bo for a short distance, forming a N. digitalis palmaris communis III as they pass into the interdigital space, but they separate again immediately. B

14 *Ramus communicans.* Communicating branch, connects the lateral branch of N. medianus with the palmar branch of N. ulnaris. B

EQUUS

15 ***N. palmaris medialis [N. digitalis palmaris communis II]****. Medial palmar nerve, descends through Canalis carpi and along the medial border of the tendon of M. flexor digitalis profundus. C D (A branch of it unofficially [yet] called the Medial sesamoidean nerve supplies the medial proximal sesamoid bone [Cornelissen BPM et al. 1997].)

16 *Ramus communicans.* Communicating branch between Nn. palmares in the middle of metacarpus, on the surface of the tendon of M. flexor digitalis superficialis. C D

17 *N. digitalis palmaris [proprius] medialis**. Palmar [proper] medial digital nerve, continuation of N. palmaris medialis in the digital area, along the tendons of the digital flexors. C D

18 **Ramus dorsalis.** Dorsal branch, arises at the level of Articulatio metacarpophalangea and runs obliquely towards the Facies dorsalis of the digit. In some individuals it gives off an intermediate branch. In others, N. digitalis palmaris medialis gives off the intermediate branch (D18a). C D

19 ***N. palmaris lateralis [N. digitalis palmaris communis III]****. Lateral palmar nerve, accompanies the tendon of M. flexor digitalis profundus on the lateral side of the metacarpus after receiving the Ramus palmaris of N. ulnaris. C (A branch of it unofficially [yet] called the Lateral sesamoidean nerve supplies the lateral proximal sesamoid bone [op. cit.].)

20 *Ramus profundus**. The Ramus profundus of the lateral palmar nerve contains fibers from the median nerve as well as from the ulnar nerve. Therefore, it is listed under both nerves. C 490.15

21 **N. metacarpeus palmaris medialis.** Medial palmar metacarpal nerve. C 490.16

22 **N. metacarpeus palmaris lateralis.** Lateral metacarpal nerve. C 490.17

23 **Rami articulares carpi.** Supply the carpal joints.

24 **N. interosseous medius***. Supplies the M. interosseus medius. C 490.19

25 *N. digitalis palmaris [proprius] lateralis**. Lateral palmar (proper) digital nerve, continuation of N. palmaris lateralis. C 490.20

26 **Ramus dorsalis.** Dorsal branch, arises at the level of Articulatio metacarpophalangea and runs obliquely towards the Facies dorsalis of the digit. C 490.21

A Nn. medianus and ulnaris – left manus, palmar aspect (su)

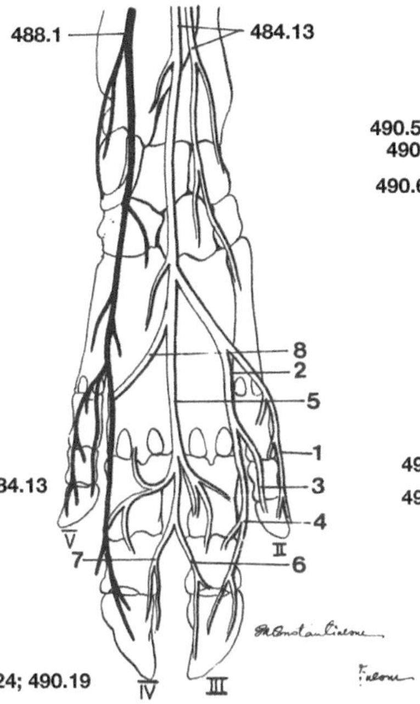

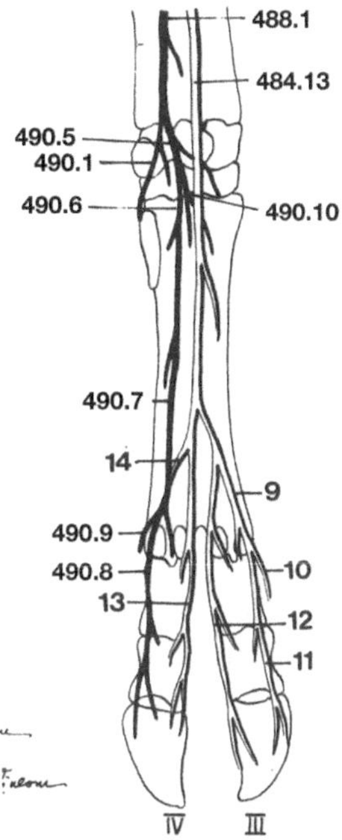

B Nn. medianus and ulnaris – left manus, palmar aspect (bo)

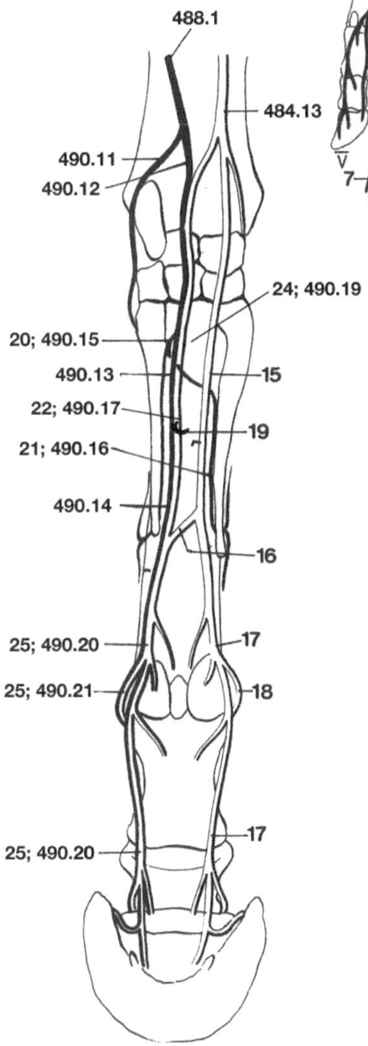

C Nn. medianus and ulnaris – left manus, palmar aspect (eq)

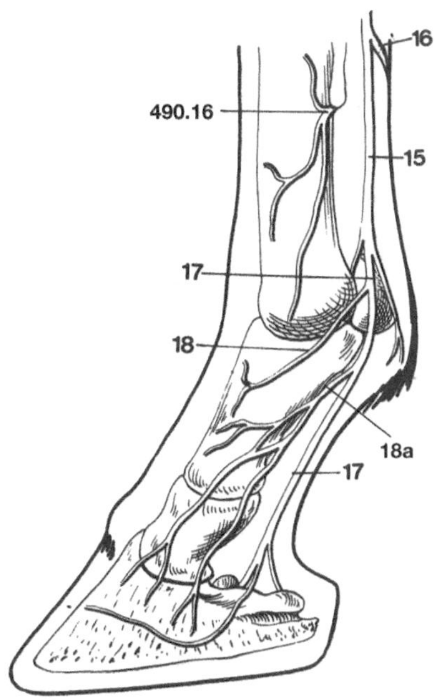

D N. medianus, right digit, medial aspect (eq)

TERMINI COMMUNES

1 **N. ulnaris**. Ulnar nerve, originates from C8, T1 (T2 bo, eq, sometimes ca, ov, cap), runs caudal to N. medianus, supplies the Mm. flexor carpi ulnaris, flexor digitalis superficialis (eq), flexor digitorum/digitalis profundus (caput ulnare and parts of caput humerale), and skin of the caudal side of forearm and the lateral side of manus. A, 483 A, 487 A B C

2 ***N. cutaneus antebrachii caudalis****. Caudal cutaneous antebrachial nerve, becomes apparent on the caudal border of the olecranon. A

3 ***Rami musculares***. Muscular branches, to M. flexor carpi ulnaris, M. flexor digitorum/digitalis superficialis (eq, sometimes bo), and M. flexor digitorum/digitalis profundus (caput ulnare and parts of caput humerale). A

CARNIVORA

4 ***Ramus dorsalis***. Dorsal branch. A B C, 485 B

5 *N. digitalis dorsalis communis IV* (fe). Dorsal common digital nerve IV. B

6 **N. digitalis dorsalis proprius IV abaxialis** (fe). Abaxial dorsal proper digital nerve IV, runs on the dorsal aspect of the abaxial side of digit IV. B

7 **N. digitalis dorsalis proprius V axialis** (fe). Axial dorsal proper digital nerve V, runs on the dorsal aspect of the axial side of digit V. B

8 *N. digitalis dorsalis V abaxialis*. Abaxial dorsal digital nerve V, on the dorsal aspect of abaxial side of digit V. B, 485 B

9 ***Ramus palmaris***. Palmar branch. A C

10 *Ramus superficialis*. Superficial branch. C

11 **N. digitalis palmaris communis IV**. Palmar common digital nerve IV, receives N. metacarpeus palmaris IV. C

12 **N. digitalis palmaris proprius IV abaxialis**. Abaxial palmar proper digital nerve IV, runs on the palmar aspect of the abaxial side of digit IV. C

13 **N. digitalis palmaris proprius V axialis**. Axial palmar proper digital nerve V, runs on the palmar aspect of the axial side of digit V. C

14 **N. digitalis palmaris V abaxialis**. Abaxial palmar digital nerve V, runs on the palmar aspect of the abaxial side of digit V. C

15 *Ramus profundus*. Deep branch. C

16 **Nn. metacarpei palmares** (ca). Palmar metacarpal nerves I, II, III, IV, reinforce the Nn. digitales palmares communes at the Articulatio metacarpophalangea. C

SUS

17 ***Ramus dorsalis***. Dorsal branch, turns on the dorsal surface of the carpus and bifurcates immediately. D E

18 *N. digitalis dorsalis communis IV*. Dorsal common digital nerve IV, results from union of a branch of Ramus superficialis n. radialis and the medial branch of Ramus dorsalis n. ulnaris. D

19 **N. digitalis dorsalis proprius IV abaxialis**. Abaxial dorsal proper digital nerve IV, runs on the dorsal aspect of the abaxial side of digit IV. D

20 **N. digitalis dorsalis proprius V axialis**. Axial dorsal proper digital nerve V, runs on the dorsal aspect of the axial side of digit V. D

21 *N. digitalis dorsalis V abaxialis*. Abaxial dorsal digital nerve V, continuation of the lateral branch of Ramus dorsalis on the dorsal aspect of the abaxial side of digit V. D

22 ***Ramus palmaris***. Palmar branch, continuation of N. ulnaris. E

23 *Ramus superficialis*. Superficial branch. E

24 **N. digitalis palmaris communis IV**. Palmar common digital nerve IV, continuation of Ramus superficialis. E

25 **N. digitalis palmaris proprius IV abaxialis**. Abaxial palmar proper nerve IV, continuation of N. digitalis palmaris communis IV on the palmar aspect of the abaxial side of digit IV. E

26 **N. digitalis palmaris proprius V axialis**. Axial palmar proper digital nerve V, runs on palmar aspect of the axial side of digit V. E

27 **N. digitalis palmaris V abaxialis**. Abaxial palmar digital nerve V, runs on the palmar aspect of the abaxial side of digit V. E

28 *Ramus profundus*. Deep branch. E

A N. ulnaris – right shoulder, brachium, antebrachium, medial aspect (ca)

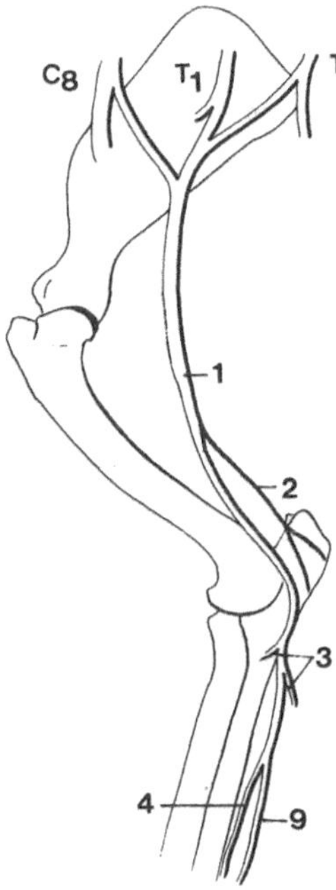

B N. ulnaris – left manus, dorsal aspect (fe)

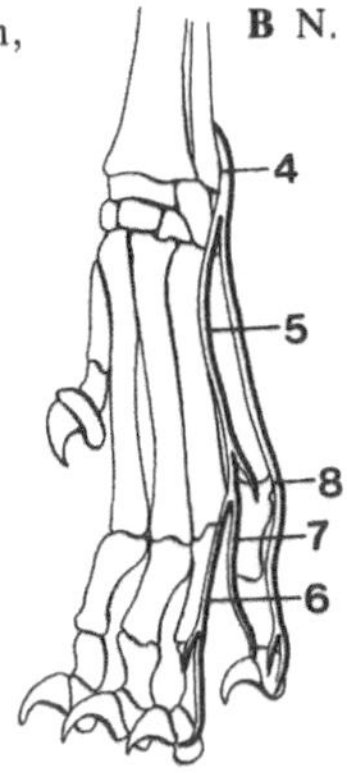

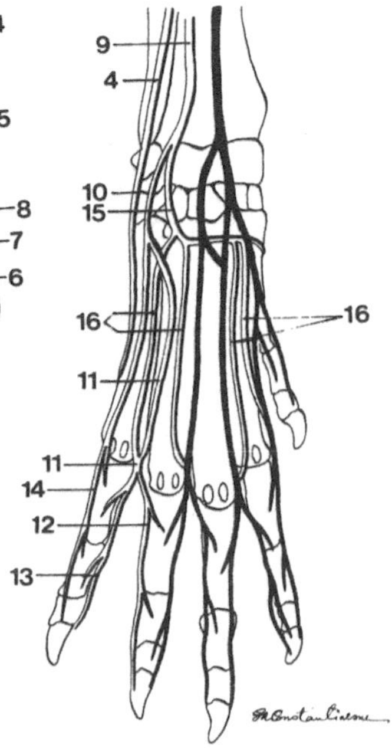

C N. ulnaris – left manus, palmar aspect (ca)

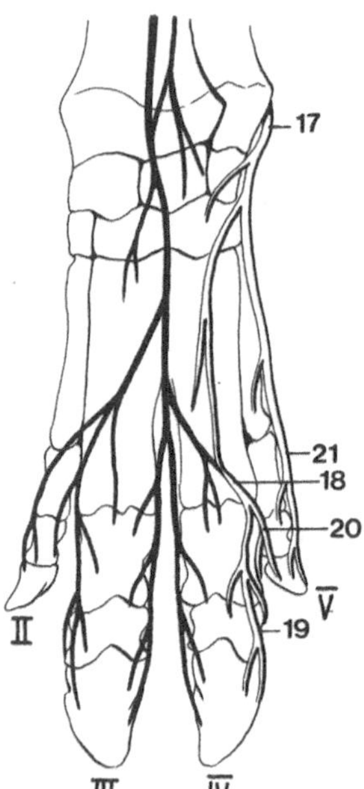

D Nn. ulnaris and radialis – left manus, dorsal aspect (su)

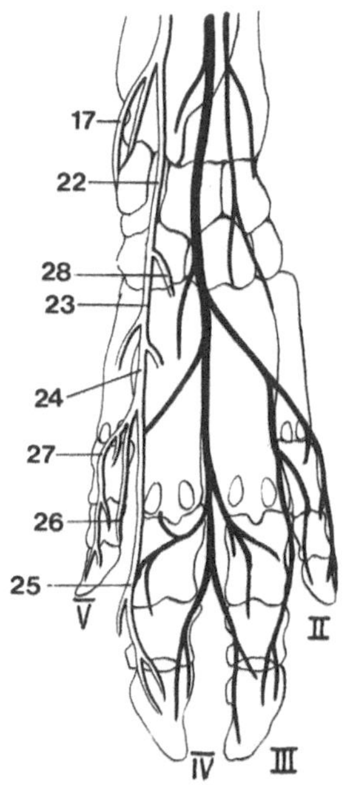

E Nn. ulnaris and medianus – left manus, palmar aspect (su)

RUMINANTIA

1 ***Ramus dorsalis***. Dorsal branch of N. ulnaris, turns to the dorsal aspect of the metacarpus. A, 487 B

2 *N. digitalis dorsalis communis IV.* Dorsal common digital nerve IV. On the dorsal aspect of the lateral side of Os metacarpale IV. A

3 **N. digitalis dorsalis proprius IV abaxialis**. Abaxial dorsal proper digital nerve IV. Continuation of N. digitalis dorsalis communis IV on the abaxial side of digit IV. A

4 **N. digitalis dorsalis proprius V.** Dorsal proper digital nerve V. On the dorsal aspect of the digit V. A

5 ***Ramus palmaris***. Palmar branch. 487 B

6 *Ramus superficialis.* Superficial branch. 487 B

7 **N. digitalis palmaris communis IV.** Palmar common digital nerve IV. Receives Ramus communicans from N. digitalis palmaris IV axialis. 487 B

8 **N. digitalis palmaris proprius IV abaxialis**. Abaxial palmar proper digital nerve IV. Continuation of N. digitalis palmaris communis IV. 487 B

9 **N. digitalis palmaris proprius V.** Palmar proper digital nerve V. On the palmar aspect of digit V. 487 B

10 *Ramus profundus.* Deep branch. 487 B

EQUUS

11 ***Ramus dorsalis***. Dorsal branch of N. ulnaris, turns to the laterodorsal aspect of the carpus and metacarpus. B, 487 C

12 ***Ramus palmaris***. Palmar branch, continuation of N. ulnaris, exchanges fibers with N. palmaris lateralis. 487 C

13 *Ramus superficialis.* Superficial branch, in the horse represented only by fibers of the ulnar nerve that continue in N. palmaris lateralis distal to the carpal communication between Ramus palmaris n. ulnaris and N. palmaris lateralis. 487 C

14 **N. palmaris lateralis [N. digitalis palmaris communis III]**. See 486.19, 487 C (A branch of it unofficially [yet] called the Lateral sesamoidean nerve supplies the lateral proximal sesamoid bone [op. cit.].)

15 *Ramus profundus**. Deep branch, innervates Mm. interossei and lumbricales laterales and gives off Nn. metacarpei palmares. It contains fibers from the ulnar nerve as well as from the median nerve. 487 C

Nn. metacarpei palmares. [These nerves were omitted from the 5th edition of the N. A. V., because they are listed individually at 16 (see also 486.21) and 17 (see also 486.22).]

16 **N. metacarpeus palmaris medialis.** Medial palmar metacarpal nerve. 487 D

17 **N. metacarpeus palmaris lateralis.** Lateral palmar metacarpal nerve. 487 C

18 **Rami articulares carpi**. Carpal articular branches.

19 **N. interosseous medius***. Supplies the M. interosseus medius. 487 C

20 **N. digitalis palmaris [proprius] lateralis**. See 486.25. 487 C

21 **Ramus dorsalis**. See 486.26. 487 C

TERMINI COMMUNES

22 **Nn. thoracici**. Thoracic nerves, 13–18 pairs, depending on species. C

23 ***Rami dorsales***. Dorsal branches are the thinner ones. C

24 *Ramus medialis.* Medial branch, supplies epaxial musculature. C

25 *Ramus lateralis.* Lateral branch, mixed, supplies M. iliocostalis and skin. C

26 **Ramus cutaneus medialis**. Medial cutaneous branch, a small twig running towards the dorsal median line. C

27 **Ramus cutaneus lateralis**. Lateral cutaneous branch, runs ventrally as far as the middle of the costal wall. C

28 ***Rami ventrales [Nn. intercostales]***. Ventral branches [intercostal nerves] are the thicker branches of the Nn. thoracici. C

29 *Ramus cutaneus lateralis [pectoralis et abdominalis].* Lateral cutaneous branch [pectoral and abdominal], perforates Mm. intercostales in the middle of the thoracic wall, supply the skin and are directed ventrally. C

30 **Rami mammarii laterales**. Lateral mammary branches, only in Car and su. C

31 *N. intercostobrachialis.* Intercostobrachial nerve, results from fusion of a branch of N. thoracicus lateralis with branches of the 1st (Ru), 2nd and 3rd (Car, Ru, eq) Nn. intercostales; the nerve is sensory for Regio tricipitalis in all species, and motor for the M. cutaneus omobrachialis in Ru and eq. D

32 *Ramus cutaneus ventralis [pectoralis et abdominalis].* Ventral cutaneous branch [pectoral and abdominal]. C

33 **Rami mammarii mediales**. Medial mammary branches, only in Car and su. C

34 *N. costoabdominalis.* Costoabdominal nerve, the ventral branch of the last N. thoracicus, called costoabdominal and not intercostal, because it does not course between two ribs.

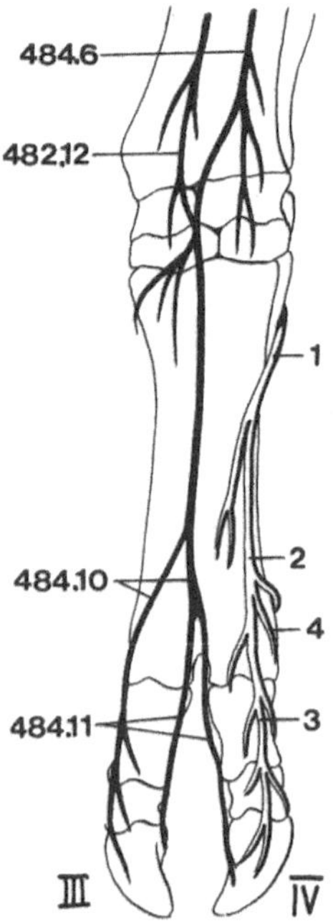

A Nerves of left manus, dorsal aspect (bo)

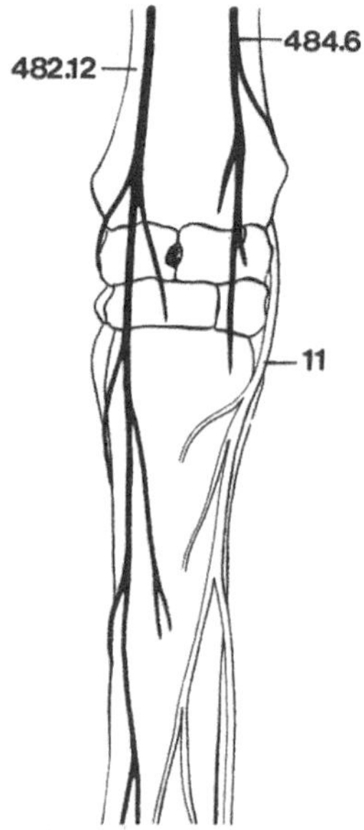

B Nerves of left carpus and metacarpus, dorsal aspect (eq)

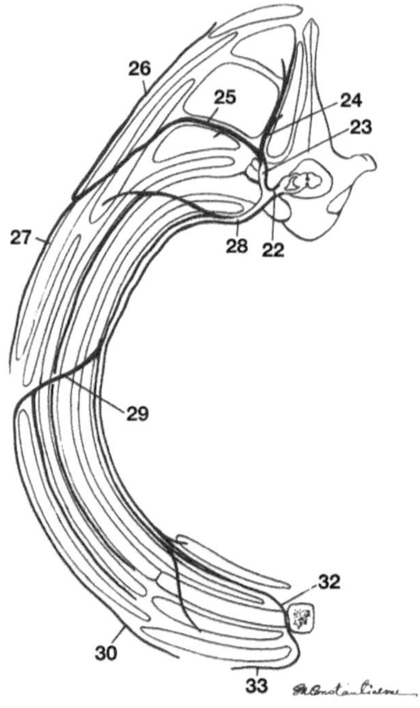

C N. thoracicus VIII – transverse section of thorax (ca)

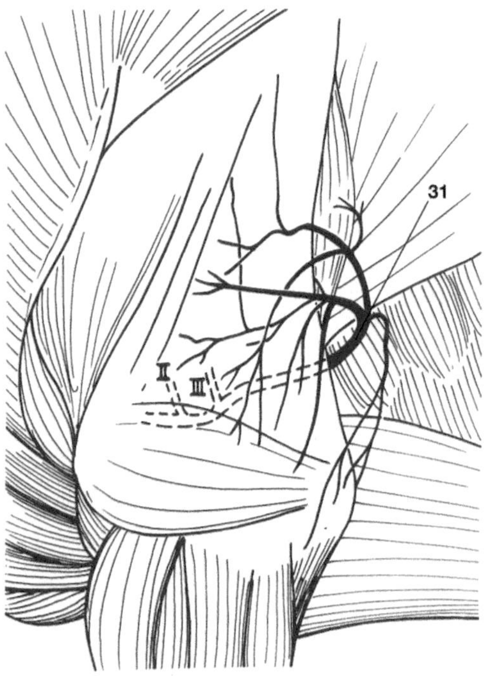

D Left N. intercostobrachialis (bo) (Schaller)

1 **Nn. lumbales, sacrales et caudales [coccygei].** Lumbar, sacral and caudal [coccygeal] nerves.

2 **Nn. lumbales.** Lumbar nerves, number depends on species and even breeds (the Arabian horse has only 5 lumbar vertebrae for example). A B D E

3 ***Rami dorsales.*** Dorsal branches, supply the epaxial musculature and the skin of the lumbar and the gluteal regions. A B E

4 *Ramus medialis.* Medial branch, motor for the epaxial musculature. A B

5 *Ramus lateralis.* Lateral branch, passes between Mm. longissimus and iliocostalis becomes subcutaneous and bifurcates immediately. A B E

6 **Ramus cutaneus medialis.** Medial cutaneous branch. A B E

7 **Ramus cutaneus lateralis.** Lateral cutaneous branch. A B E

8 **Nn. clunium craniales.** Cranial clunial nerves, innervate the skin of the gluteal region and over M. tensor fasciae latae (esp. Ru and eq). C

9 ***Rami ventrales.*** Ventral branches, contribute to form the Plexus lumbalis. A B E

10 **Nn. sacrales.** Sacral nerves. A

11 ***Rami dorsales.*** Dorsal branches. A

12 *Ramus medialis.* Medial branch, innervates the epaxial musculature of the tail (Mm. sacrocaudalis dorsalis, intertransversarii dorsales). A

13 *Ramus lateralis.* Lateral branch, mainly cutaneous. A

14 **Nn. clunium medii.** Middle clunial nerves, supply the skin over M. gluteus superficialis and the cranial part of M. biceps femoris, corresponding to Regio clunis. C

15 ***Rami ventrales.*** Ventral branches contribute to form the Plexus sacralis, and innervates the hypoaxial musculature of the tail (Mm. sacrocaudalis ventralis, intertransversarii ventrales). A

16 **Plexus lumbosacralis.** Lumbosacral plexus, includes lumbar and sacral plexuses, and Truncus lumbosacralis.

17 **Radices plexus.** Roots of the plexus, parts of the Rami ventrales that form the plexus. E

18 **Trunci plexus.** Trunks of the plexus, formed by the union of the roots, proximal to the plexus. E

19 **Plexus lumbalis.** Lumbar plexus, supplies the cranial and medial muscles of the thigh and the skin on the medial aspect of thigh, crus, tarsus, and metatarsus. D E

20 **N. iliohypogastricus***. Iliohypogastric nerve, Ramus ventralis of L1 in species with six lumbar vertrebrae, supplies abdominal muscles and skin. E

21 ***Ramus cutaneus lateralis.*** Lateral cutaneous branch. E

22 ***Ramus cutaneus ventralis.*** Ventral cutaneous branch.

23 **N. iliohypogastricus cranialis.** Cranial iliohypogastric nerve, Ramus ventralis of L1 in species with seven lumbar vertebrae. D

24 ***Ramus cutaneus lateralis.*** Lateral cutaneous branch. D

25 ***Ramus cutaneus ventralis.*** Ventral cutaneous branch. D

26 **N. iliohypogastricus caudalis.** Caudal iliohypogastric nerve, Ramus ventralis of L2 in species with seven lumbar vertebrae. D

27 ***Ramus cutaneus lateralis.*** Lateral cutaneous branch. D

28 ***Ramus cutaneus ventralis.*** Ventral cutaneous branch. D

29 **N. ilioinguinalis***. Ilioinguinal nerve, Ramus ventralis L2 or L3 depending on species. D E

30 ***Ramus cutaneus lateralis.*** Lateral cutaneous branch. D E

31 ***Ramus cutaneus ventralis.*** Ventral cutaneous branch. D E

32 **N. genitofemoralis***. Genitofemoral nerve, arises from L2 (Ru, eq), L3 and L4. D E

33 ***Ramus genitalis.*** Genital branch, passes through Canalis inguinalis, supplies M. cremaster, Preputium, Scrotum, Mammae. D E

34 ***Ramus femoralis.*** Femoral branch. D E

35 **N. cutaneus femoris lateralis***. Lateral cutaneous femoral nerve, arises from L3, L4 (L5), supplies the skin on the craniomedial aspect of the thigh. D E

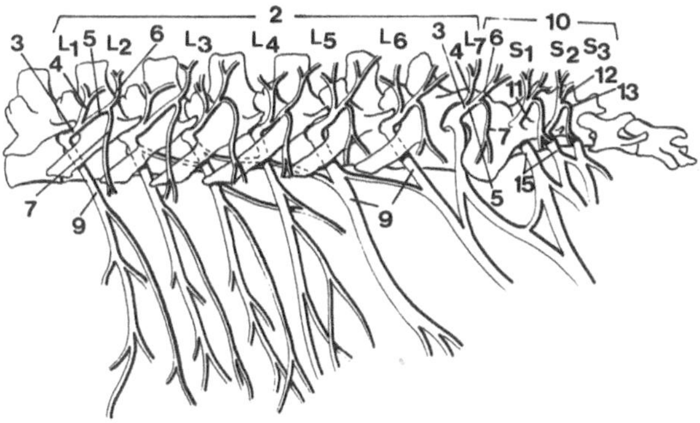

A Plexus lumbosacralis, left side (ca)

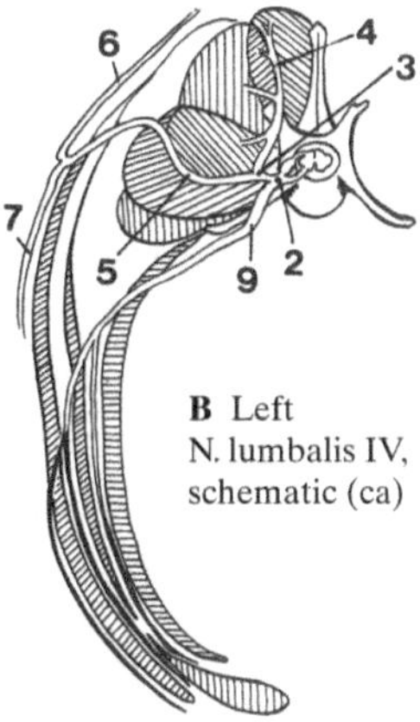

B Left N. lumbalis IV, schematic (ca)

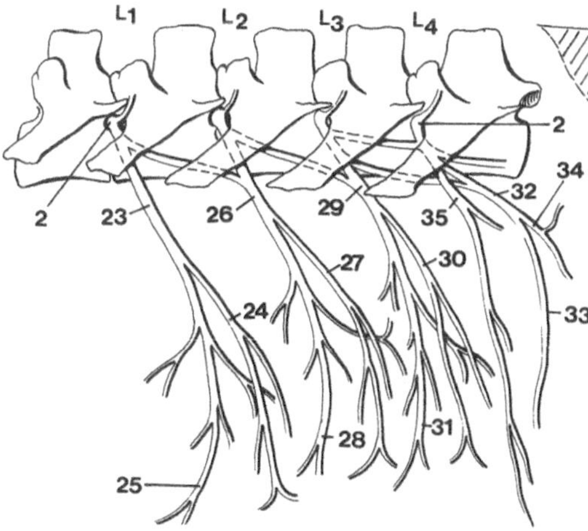

D Plexus lumbalis, left side (ca)

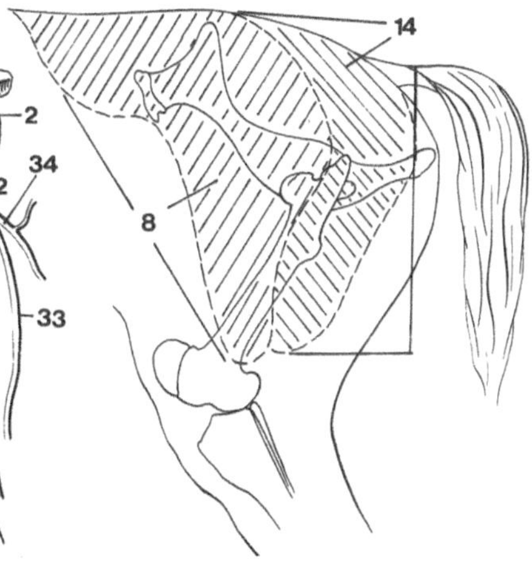

C Nn. clunium craniales and medii, left side (eq)

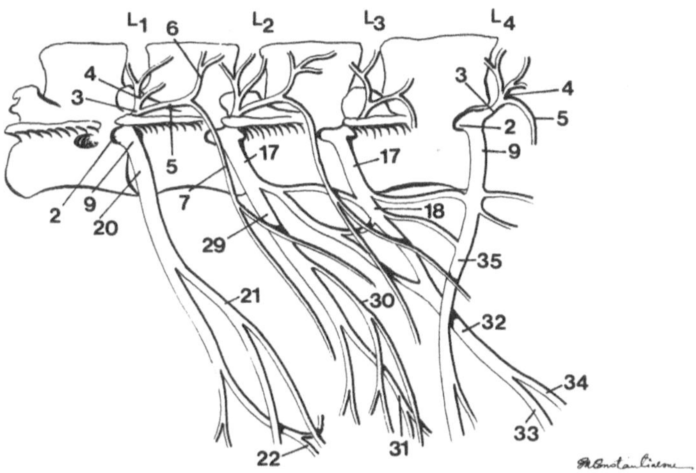

E Plexus lumbalis, left side (bo)

1 **N. femoralis**. Femoral nerve, arises from L3–L6 depending upon species. Is the thickest nerve of Plexus lumbalis. A

2 ***Rami musculares***. Muscular branches, supply Mm. iliopsoas, psoas minor, quadriceps femoris, sartorius and part of pectineus. A

3 ***N. saphenus***. Saphenous nerve, mixed (in ca only sensory), given off in the Canalis femoralis. A, 497 A B C D

4 *Rami musculares*. Muscular branches, supply parts of Mm. sartorius, gracilis, and pectineus (except ca).

5 *Rami cutanei**. Cutaneous branches, distributed on the skin of the medial aspect of crus, tarsus, and metatarsus. A

6 **N. obturatorius***. Obturator nerve, arises from L4–S1. A B C

7 ***Ramus cranialis***. Cranial branch, supplies some adductor muscles of the thigh. A B

8 ***Ramus caudalis***. Caudal branch, supplies adductor muscles and M. obturatorius externus. A B

9 **Plexus sacralis**. Sacral plexus, gives off nerves supplying the caudal muscles of the thigh and of entire crus and pes as well as the corresponding skin. A

10 **Truncus lumbosacralis**. Lumbosacral trunk, is represented by the branch from Plexus lumbalis that reinforces the Plexus sacralis. A

11 **N. gluteus [glutaeus] cranialis**. Cranial gluteal nerve, originates from L5–S1, supplies the Mm. gluteus medius, profundus, and tensor fasciae latae, and in eq the cranial part of M. gluteus superficialis. A

12 **N. gluteus [glutaeus] caudalis**. Caudal gluteal nerve, originates from S1–S2, supplies the M. gluteus superficialis (exc. cranial part in eq) and proximal parts of Mm. biceps femoris and semitendinosus. A

13 **N. cutaneus femoris caudalis**. Caudal cutaneous femoral nerve, originates from S1–S3 and supplies the skin on the lateral and caudal aspects of hip and thigh. A, 501 C

14 ***Nn. clunium caudales***. Caudal clunial nerves, supply a skin area in the vicinity of Tuber ischiadicum. A

15 **N. ischiadicus**. Sciatic nerve, the thickest nerve of the body, arises from L6–S2. Exits from the pelvic cavity through Foramen ischiadicum majus, passes around the Articulatio coxae and terminates by giving rise to Nn. fibularis communis and tibialis. A C D

16 ***Rami musculares***. Muscular branches, to the Mm. gemelli, quadratus femoris, the caudal thigh muscles and in Car and eq also M. obturatorius internus. C D

17 **N. fibularis [peron(a)eus] communis***. Common fibular [peroneal] nerve, runs parallel to N. tibialis within the space medial to the M. biceps femoris, then obliquely crossing Caput laterale m. gastrocnemii. On the lateral side of the proximal end of crus, it terminates in Nn. fibularis superficialis and profundus. C D E

18 ***N. cutaneus surae lateralis***. Lateral cutaneous sural nerve, penetrates the M. biceps femoris between its cranial and caudal divisions to supply the skin on the caudolateral aspect of stifle and crus. C D

19 ***Rami musculares***. Muscular branches, only in Car, to M. abductor cruris caudalis. D

20 **N. fibularis [peron(a)eus] superficialis**. Superficial fibular nerve. D E, 497 A B C D

21 ***Rami musculares***. Muscular branches, to Mm. extensor digitorum/digitalis lateralis, fibularis longus and in Car fibularis brevis. E

22 ***Rami cutanei****. Cutaneous branches, supply the dorsolateral aspect of the distal part of crus, tarsus and metatarsus. 497 C

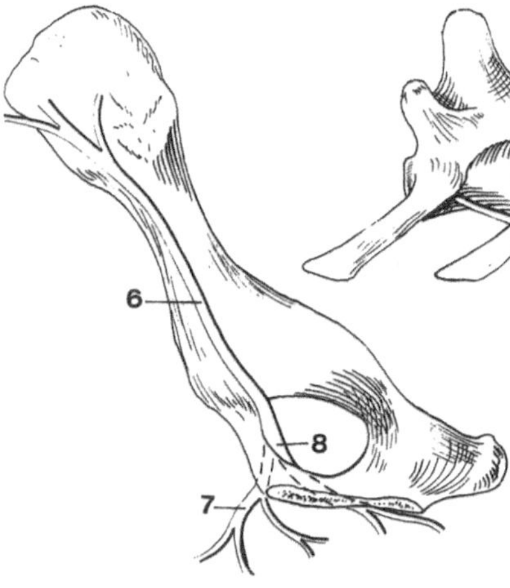

B Right N. obturatorius (ca)

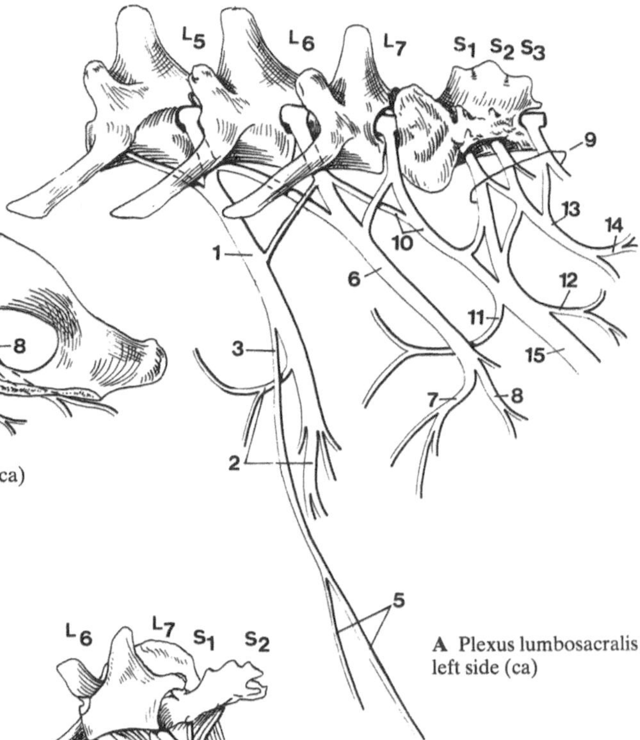

A Plexus lumbosacralis, left side (ca)

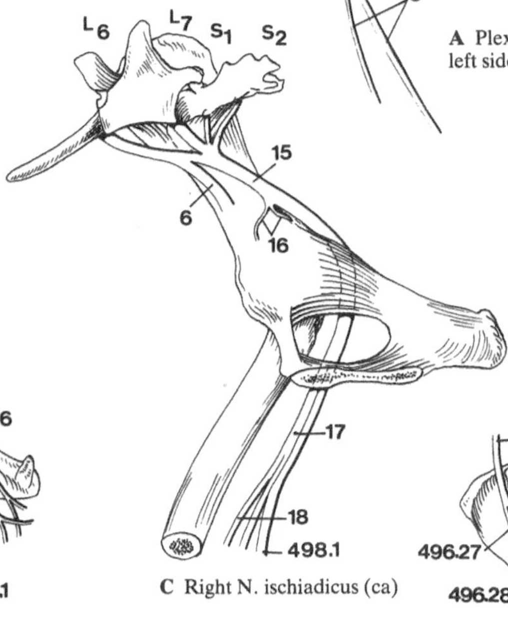

C Right N. ischiadicus (ca)

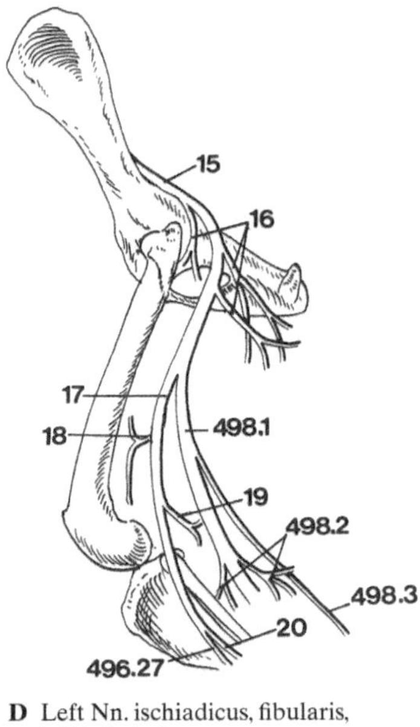

D Left Nn. ischiadicus, fibularis, and tibialis (ca)

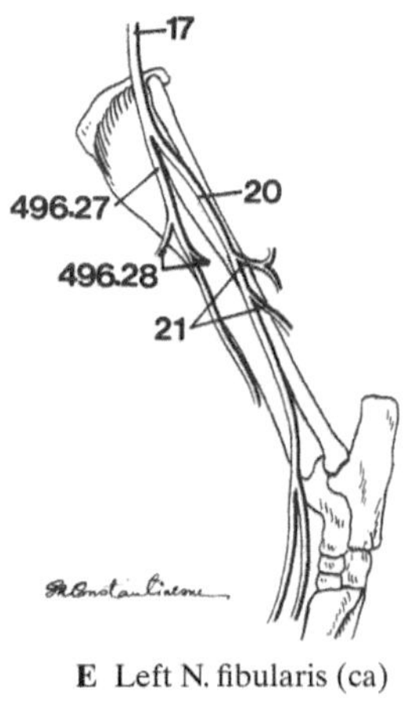

E Left N. fibularis (ca)

CARNIVORA, SUS

1 ***N. digitalis dorsalis II abaxialis***. Abaxial dorsal digital nerve II. A B

2 ***N. digitalis dorsalis communis II***. Dorsal common digital nerve II. A B

3 *N. digitalis dorsalis proprius II axialis*. Axial dorsal proper digital nerve II. A B

4 *N. digitalis dorsalis proprius III abaxialis*. Abaxial dorsal proper digital nerve III. A B

5 ***N. digitalis dorsalis communis III***. Dorsal common digital nerve III. A B

6 *N. digitalis dorsalis proprius III axialis*. Axial dorsal proper digital nerve III. A B

7 *N. digitalis dorsalis proprius IV axialis*. Axial dorsal proper digital nerve IV. A B

8 ***N. digitalis dorsalis communis IV***. Dorsal common digital nerve IV. A B

9 *N. digitalis dorsalis proprius IV abaxialis*. Abaxial dorsal proper digital nerve IV. A B

10 *N. digitalis dorsalis proprius V axialis*. Axial dorsal proper digital nerve V. A B

11 ***N. digitalis dorsalis V abaxialis***. Abaxial dorsal digital nerve V. A B

RUMINANTIA

12 ***N. digitalis dorsalis communis II***. Dorsal common digital nerve II. C

13 *Rami cutanei*. Cutaneous branches. C

14 *N. digitalis dorsalis proprius II axialis*. Axial dorsal proper digital nerve II. C

15 *N. digitalis dorsalis proprius III abaxialis*. Abaxial dorsal proper digital nerve III. C

16 ***N. digitalis dorsalis communis III***. Dorsal common digital nerve III. C

17 *Rami cutanei*. Cutaneous branches. C

18 *Ramus communicans cum n. metatarseo dorsali III*. Branch communicating with the dorsal metatarsal nerve III. C

19 *N. digitalis dorsalis proprius III axialis*. Axial dorsal proper digital nerve III. C

20 *N. digitalis dorsalis proprius IV axialis*. Axial dorsal proper digital nerve IV. C

21 ***N. digitalis dorsalis communis IV***. Dorsal common digital nerve IV. C

22 *Rami cutanei*. Cutaneous branches. C

23 *N. digitalis dorsalis proprius IV abaxialis*. Abaxial dorsal proper digital nerve IV. C

24 *N. digitalis dorsalis proprius V axialis*. Axial dorsal proper digital nerve V. C

EQUUS

25 ***Ramus dorsalis***. Dorsal branch. D

26 ***Ramus lateralis***. Lateral branch. D

TERMINI COMMUNES

27 **N. fibularis [peron(a)eus] profundus**. Deep fibular nerve. A B C D, 495 D E

28 ***Rami musculares***. Muscular branches to the craniolateral muscles of the crus, except Mm. extensor digitorum/ digitalis lateralis, fibularis longus, and in Car fibularis brevis. 495 E

CARNIVORA, SUS

29 ***N. metatarseus dorsalis II*** (Car). Dorsal metatarsal nerve II. A

30 ***N. metatarseus dorsalis III***. Dorsal metatarsal nerve III. A B

31 ***N. metatarseus dorsalis IV*** (Car). Dorsal metatarsal nerve IV. A

RUMINANTIA

32 ***N. metatarseus dorsalis III***. Dorsal metatarsal nerve III. C

33 *Ramus communicans cum n. digitali plantari proprio III axiali*. Branch communicating with the axial plantar proper digital nerve III, passes across the interdigital space. C

34 *Ramus communicans cum n. digitali plantari proprio IV axiali*. Communicating branch to the axial plantar proper digital nerve IV, passes across the interdigital space. C

EQUUS

35 ***N. metatarseus dorsalis II****. Dorsal metatarsal nerve II, the medial cutaneous branch of the deep fibular nerve. D

36 *N. digitalis dorsalis III medialis*. Medial dorsal digital nerve III. D

37 ***N. metatarseus dorsalis III****. Dorsal metatarsal nerve III, the lateral cutaneous branch of the deep fibular nerve. D

38 *N. digitalis dorsalis III lateralis*. Lateral dorsal digital nerve III. D

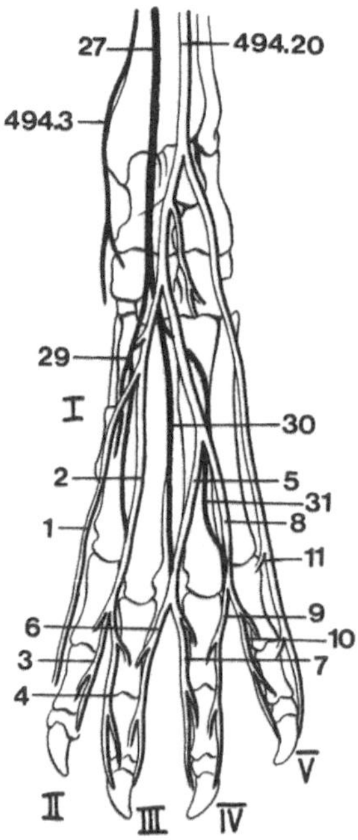

A Nn. fibulares superficialis and profundus – left pes, dorsal aspect (ca)

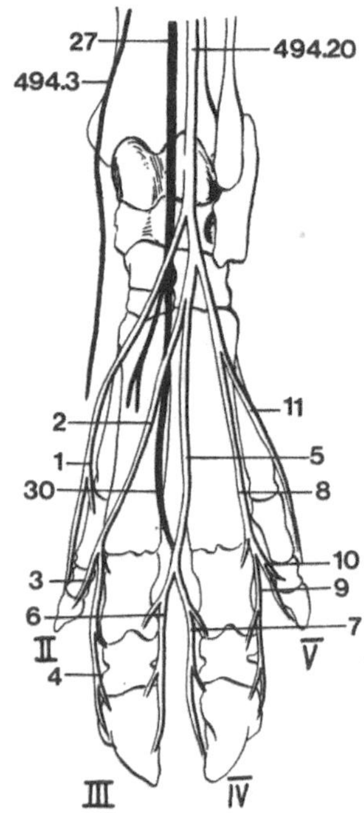

B Nn. fibulares superficialis and profundus – left pes, dorsal aspect (su)

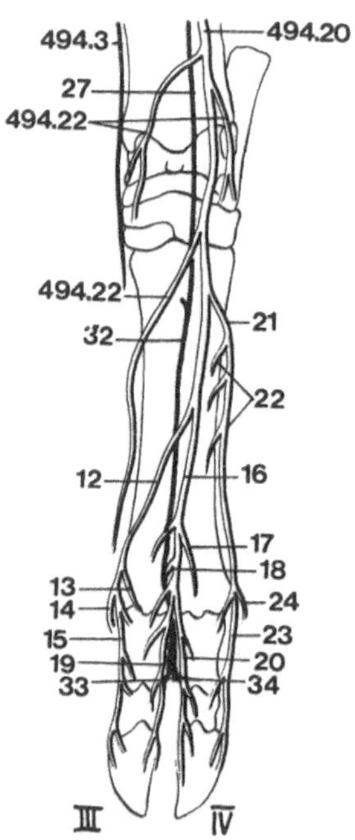

C Nn. fibulares superficialis and profundus – left pes, dorsal aspect (bo)

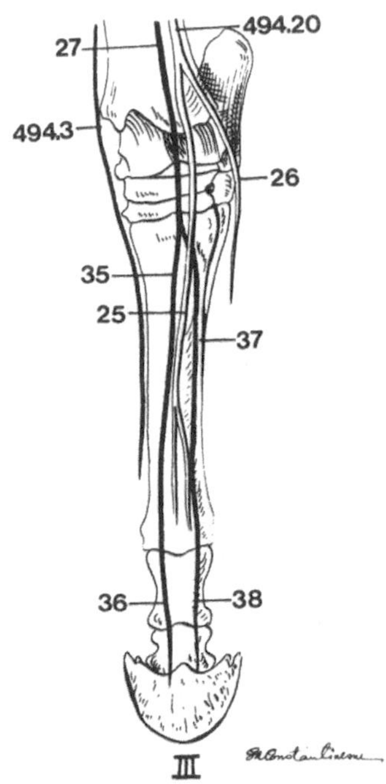

D Nn. fibulares superficialis and profundus – left pes, dorsal aspect (eq)

TERMINI COMMUNES

1 **N. tibialis.** Tibial nerve, runs parallel to N. fibularis communis, then dips between the two heads of M. gastrocnemius and runs between the deep digital flexor muscles and Tendo calcaneus communis. A B C D, 495 C D, 501 A

2 ***Rami musculares.*** Muscular branches, to all caudal muscles of the crus. 495 D

3 ***N. cutaneus surae caudalis****. Caudal cutaneous sural nerve. A B C D, 495 D, 501 A

3a *N. cutaneus surae caudalis proximalis* (Car). Proximal caudal cutaneous sural nerve.

3b *N. cutaneus surae caudalis distalis* (Car). Distal caudal cutaneous sural nerve.

4 ***Rami cutanei [Ramus cutaneus tarsalis medialis (eq)].*** Cutaneous branches [medial tarsal cutaneous branch, eq]. 501 A

CARNIVORA, SUS

5 ***N. plantaris medialis.*** Medial plantar nerve. A B

6 *N. digitalis plantaris II abaxialis.* Abaxial plantar digital nerve II. A B

7 *N. digitalis plantaris communis II.* Plantar common digital nerve II. A B

8 **N. digitalis plantaris proprius II axialis.** Axial plantar proper digital nerve II. A B

9 **N. digitalis plantaris proprius III abaxialis.** Abaxial plantar proper digital nerve III. A B

10 *N. digitalis plantaris communis III.* Plantar common digital nerve III. A B

11 **Ramus communicans cum n. digitali plantari communi IV** (su). Branch communicating with the plantar common digital nerve IV. B

12 **N. digitalis plantaris proprius III axialis.** Axial plantar proper digital nerve III. A B

13 **N. digitalis plantaris proprius IV axialis.** Axial plantar proper digital nerve IV. A B

14 *N. digitalis plantaris communis IV* (Car). Plantar common digital nerve IV. A

15 **N. digitalis plantaris proprius IV abaxialis** (Car). Abaxial plantar proper digital nerve IV. A

16 **N. digitalis plantaris proprius V axialis** (Car). Axial plantar proper digital nerve V. A

17 ***N. plantaris lateralis.*** Lateral plantar nerve, gives branches to the skin. A B

18 *Ramus profundus.* Deep branch, trunk of Nn. metatarsei plantares, supplies the Mm. interossei. A B

19 **Nn. metatarsei plantares** (Car). Plantar metatarsal nerves (II, III, IV). A

19a **N. digitalis plantaris communis IV** (su). Plantar common digital nerve IV. B

19b **N. digitalis plantaris proprius IV abaxialis** (su). Abaxial plantar proper digital nerve IV. B

19c **N. digitalis plantaris proprius V axialis** (su). Axial plantar proper digital nerve V. B

20 *N. digitalis plantaris V abaxialis.* Abaxial plantar digital nerve V. A

RUMINANTIA

21 ***N. plantaris medialis.*** Medial plantar nerve, runs in the groove between M. interosseus medius and the digital flexor tendons. C

22 *N. digitalis plantaris communis II.* Plantar common digital nerve II. C

23 **N. digitalis plantaris proprius II.** Plantar proper digital nerve II. C

24 **N. digitalis plantaris proprius III abaxialis.** Abaxial plantar proper digital nerve III. C

25 **Ramus communicans cum n. digitali dorsali proprio III abaxiali.** Branch communicating with the abaxial dorsal proper digital nerve III. C

26 *N. digitalis plantaris communis III.* Plantar common digital nerve III. C

27 **N. digitalis plantaris proprius III axialis.** Axial plantar proper digital nerve III. C

28 **N. digitalis plantaris proprius IV axialis.** Axial plantar proper digital nerve IV. C

29 ***N. plantaris lateralis.*** Lateral plantar nerve, gives branches to the skin. D

30 *Ramus profundus.* Deep branch, to Mm. interossei. D

31 *N. digitalis plantaris communis IV.* Plantar common digital nerve IV, continuation of N. plantaris lateralis. D

32 **N. digitalis plantaris proprius IV abaxialis.** Abaxial plantar proper digital nerve IV. D

33 **Ramus communicans cum n. digitali dorsali proprio IV abaxiali.** Branch communicating with the abaxial dorsal proper digital nerve IV. D

34 *N. digitalis plantaris proprius V.* Plantar proper digital nerve V. D

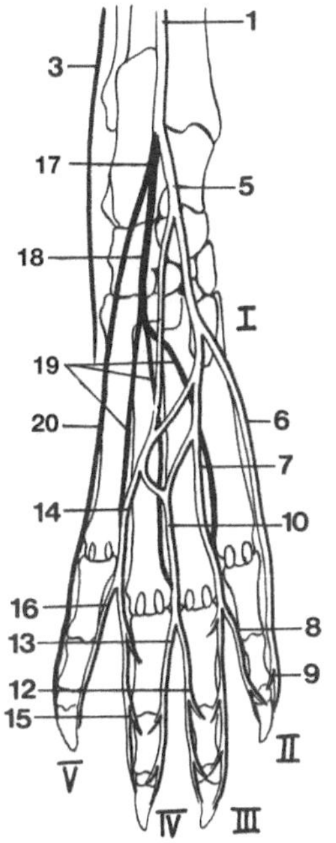

A Nerves of left pes, plantar aspect (ca)

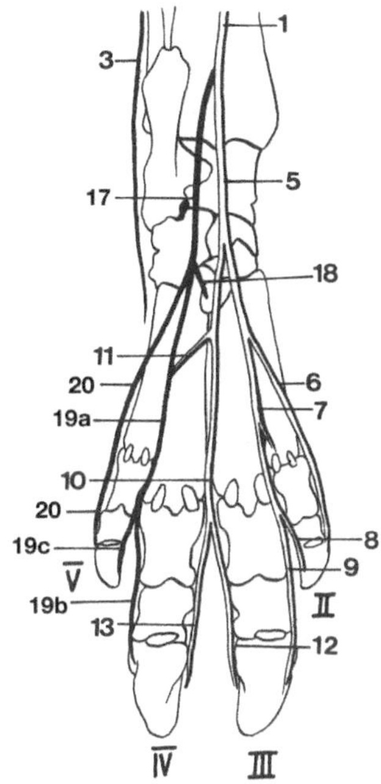

B Nerves of left pes, plantar aspect (su)

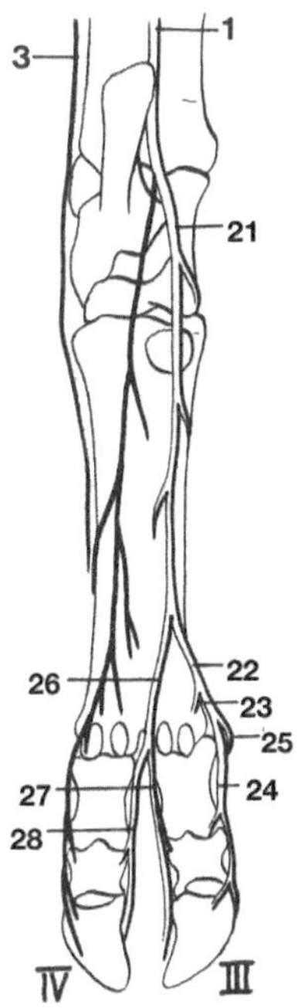

C Nerves of left pes, plantar aspect (bo)

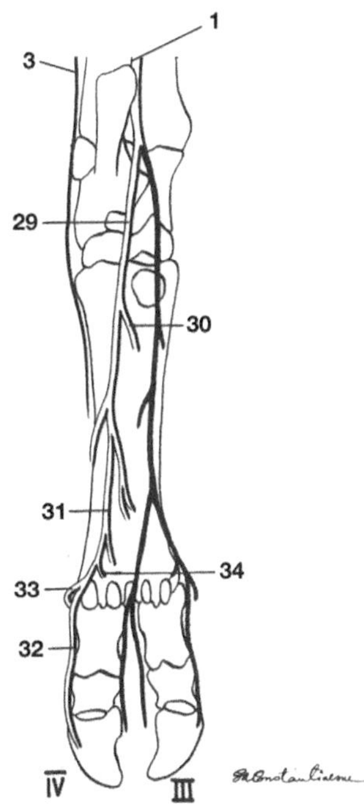

D Nn. plantares, left pes (bo)

EQUUS

1 ***N. plantaris medialis [N. digitalis plantaris communis II]****. Medial plantar nerve, runs in the groove between M. interosseus medius and the digital flexor tendons. A

2 *Ramus communicans*. Branch communicating with N. plantaris lateralis, crosses flexor tendons superficially. A

3 *N. digitalis plantaris [proprius] medialis**. Medial plantar [proper] digital nerve. A

4 **Ramus dorsalis. Dorsal branch. A**

5 ***N. plantaris lateralis [N. digitalis plantaris communis III]****. Lateral plantar nerve, runs in the groove between M. interosseus medius and the digital flexor tendons. B

6 *Ramus profundus**. Deep branch, supplies the M. interosseus medius. B

7 **Nn. metatarsei plantares**. Plantar metatarsal nerves (II, III), course between M. interosseus medius and the corresponding splint bones. B

8 *N. digitalis plantaris [proprius] lateralis**. Lateral plantar [proper] digital nerve. B

9 **Ramus dorsalis**. Dorsal branch. B

TERMINI COMMUNES

10 **Ramus musculi coccygei**. Branch for the M. coccygeus. Originates in ca from Nn. sacrales directly, in su and eq combined with Nn. rectales caudales, in bo usually combined with Ramus m. levatoris ani and N. pudendus or N. rectalis caudalis. The latter combination was formerly called N. haemorrhoidalis medius. C

11 **Ramus musculi levatoris ani**. Branch for m. levator ani, has the same relationships as Ramus musculi coccygei (see 10). C

12 **N. pudendus***. Pudendal nerve, arises from S1–S2 (S3) (ca), S2–S3 (fe, su), S2–S4 (Ru), S3–S4 (eq), carries motor, sensor, and parasympathetic fibers. C

13 ***Rami cutanei***. Proximal and distal cutaneous branches in su and Ru, innervate approximately the same area as N. cutaneus femoralis caudalis of other species, the distal also supplies the N. perinealis superficialis in su and Ru. C

14 ***Ramus communicans cum n. cutaneo femoris caudali***. Communicating branch with the N. cutaneus femoris caudalis. C

15 ***N. perinealis profundus***. Deep perineal nerve, arises by common trunk with N. perinealis superficialis in eq, independently as the last pelvic branch of the pudendal nerve in bo, and as a series of branches in ca. Innervates perineal muscles. C

16 ***N. perinealis superficialis***. Arises together with N. perinealis profundus in eq, is supplied by the distal cutaneous branch of N. pudendus in su and Ru. C

17 *Nn. scrotales dorsales*. Dorsal scrotal nerves. C

18 *Nn. labiales*. Labial nerves.

19 ***Ramus preputialis [prae-] et scrotalis***. Preputial and scrotal branch. Terminal branch of N. pudendus in bo and eq, represented by a series of branches of N. dorsalis penis in other species. C

20 ***Ramus mammarius***. Mammary branch, for the Mammae inguinales.

21 ***N. dorsalis penis****. Runs on the dorsal surface of the penis to Glans penis and Lamina interna preputii. C

22 ***N. dorsalis clitoridis***. Dorsal nerve of the clitoris.

23 **Nn. rectales caudales***. Caudal rectal nerves, one or two from S3–S5. In ca the single nerve arises from N. pudendus. D E

24 ***Ramus communicans cum n. pudendo***. Communicating branch with the N. pudendus. E

25 ***Rami musculares***. Muscular branches, supply Mm. sphincter ani externus, retractor penis (clitoridis), bulbospongiosus, in eq also a part of M. semimembranosus. D E

26 ***Rami cutanei***. Cutaneous branches, supply the skin around the anus. D E

27 **Nn. caudales [coccygei]**. Caudal [coccygeal] nerves, 5–8 pairs depending on species. D

28 ***Rami dorsales***. Dorsal branches. Form Plexus caudalis dorsalis. D

29 *Plexus caudalis [coccygeus] dorsalis*. Gives off branches for the dorsal muscles of the tail and the corresponding skin. D

30 ***Rami ventrales***. Form Plexus caudalis ventralis. D

31 *Plexus caudalis [coccygeus] ventralis*. Gives off branches to the ventral muscles of the tail and corresponding skin. D

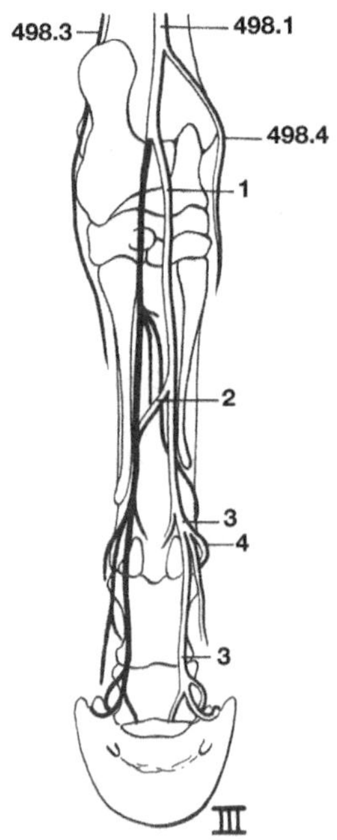

A Nerves of left pes, plantar aspect (eq)

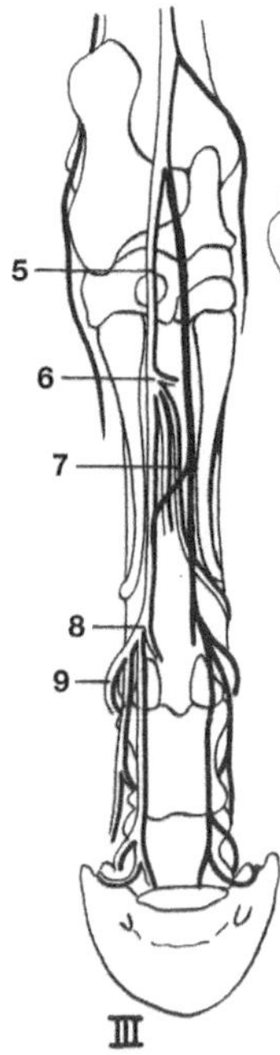

B N. plantaris lateralis, left pes (eq)

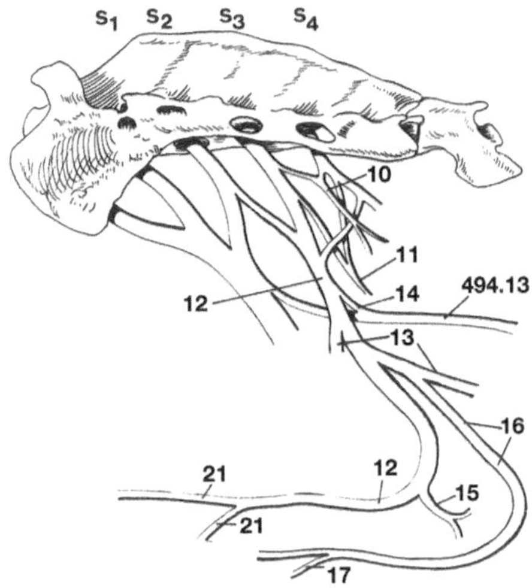

C Left N. pudendus (bo masc)

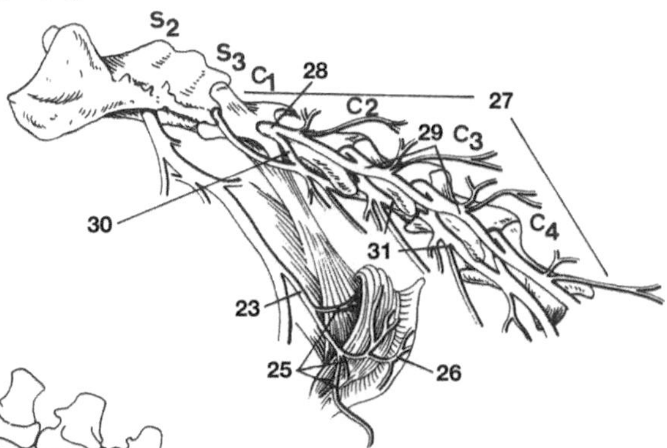

D Nn. rectales and caudales, left side (ca masc)

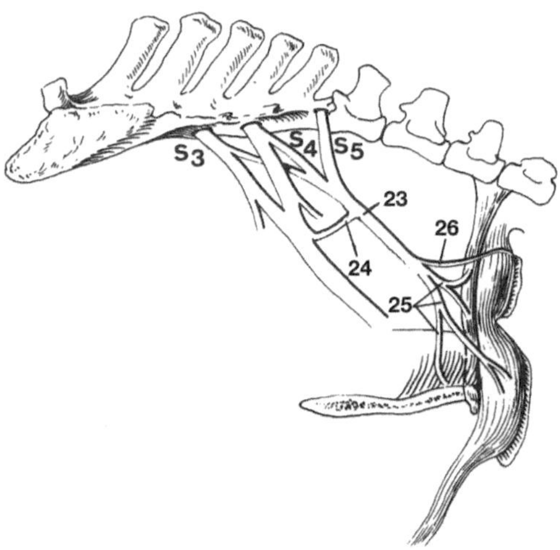

E Nn. rectales and caudales, left side (eq fem)

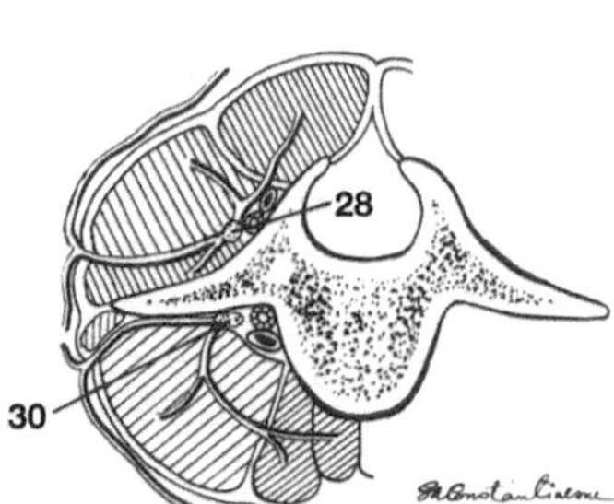

F Cauda, transverse section (eq)

1 **SYSTEMA NERVOSUM AUTONOMICUM.** Autonomic nervous system, consisting of Plexus autonomici, Ganglia plexuum autonomicorum, and Ganglia autonomica.

2 **Plexus aorticus thoracicus.** Thoracic aortic plexus, network surrounding Aorta ascendens, Arcus aortae, and Aorta thoracica, with branches of Truncus sympathicus, and parasympathetic fibers from N. vagus. A

3 ***Plexus cardiacus.*** Cardiac plexus, network of sympathetic fibers from Ganglia cervicothoracicum, cervicale medium, and thoracica, and parasympathetic fibers from N. vagus.

4 ***Ganglia cardiaca.*** Cardiac ganglia. A

5 ***Plexus esophageus [oesophageus].*** Esophageal plexus, with sympathetic and parasympathetic fibers (N. vagus), lies on the thoracic part of the esophagus. A

6 ***Rami pulmonales.*** Pulmonary branches. A

7 *Plexus pulmonalis.* Pulmonary plexus, contains sympathetic and parasympathetic fibers. A

8 **Plexus aorticus abdominalis.** Abdominal aortic plexus, on Aorta abdominalis.

9 ***Plexus celiacus [coeliacus].*** Celiac plexus, network on A. celiaca. B C

10 ***Ganglia celiaca [coeliaca].*** Celiac ganglia, paired, on both sides of A. celiaca, connected by communicating branches. B C

11 ***Plexus mesentericus cranialis.*** Cranial mesenteric plexus. B C

12 ***Ganglion mesentericum craniale.*** Cranial mesenteric ganglion, non paired, located at the origin of A. mesenterica cranialis. B C

13 ***Plexus intermesentericus.*** Intermesenteric plexus, connecting Plexus mesentericus cranialis and caudalis. B C

14 ***Plexus mesentericus caudalis.*** Caudal mesenteric plexus, network surrounding A. mesenterica caudalis. B C

15 ***Ganglion mesentericum caudale.*** Caudal mesenteric ganglion, unpaired, located at the origin of A. mesenterica caudalis. B C

16 ***Ganglia aorticorenalia.*** Aorticorenal ganglia, paired, located at the level of A. renalis. B C

17 ***Ganglia phrenica.*** Phrenic ganglia (su, Ru), in a network that surrounds A. phrenica caudalis.

18 ***Plexus hepaticus.*** Hepatic plexus, from Plexus celiacus, accompanies A. hepatica to the liver. D

19 ***Plexus lienalis.*** Splenic plexus, from Plexus celiacus, accompanies A. lienalis. D

20 ***Plexus gastrici.*** Gastric plexuses. Fibers from Plexus celiacus accompanying the branches of gastric arteries. D

21 ***Plexus ruminalis dexter.*** Right ruminal plexus, from Plexus celiacus, contains also fibers from N. vagus, esp. its dorsal trunk. E

22 ***Plexus ruminalis sinister.*** Left ruminal plexus, from Plexus celiacus, contains also fibers from N. vagus, esp. its dorsal trunk, arising on the right side, passing to the left in Sulcus cranialis ruminis. E

23 ***Plexus reticularis.*** Reticular plexus. E

24 ***Plexus pancreaticus.*** Pancreatic plexus, from Plexus celiacus, accompanying pancreatic arteries. D

25 ***Plexus adrenalis [suprarenalis].*** Adrenal [suprarenal] plexus, formed by Nn. splanchnici and Plexus celiacus, contains preganglionic fibers for the adrenal medulla.

26 ***Plexus renalis.*** Renal plexus, surrounds A. renalis with fibers from Plexus mesentericus cranialis and Nn. splanchnici. B C

27 ***Ganglia renalia.*** Renal ganglia, may be observed in the Plexus renalis.

28 ***Plexus uretericus.*** Ureteric plexus, accompanies the ureters with fibers from Plexus renalis and aorticus abdominalis.

A Systema nervosum autonomicum, thoracic part – left side (ca)

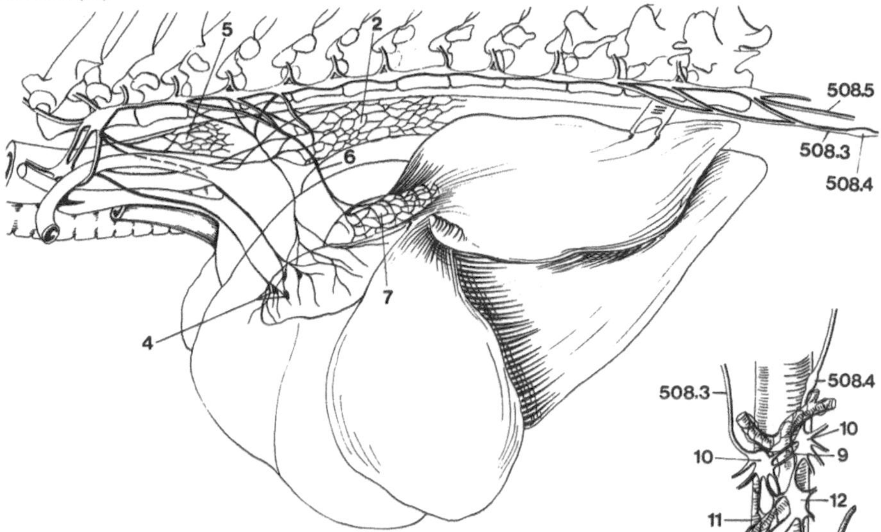

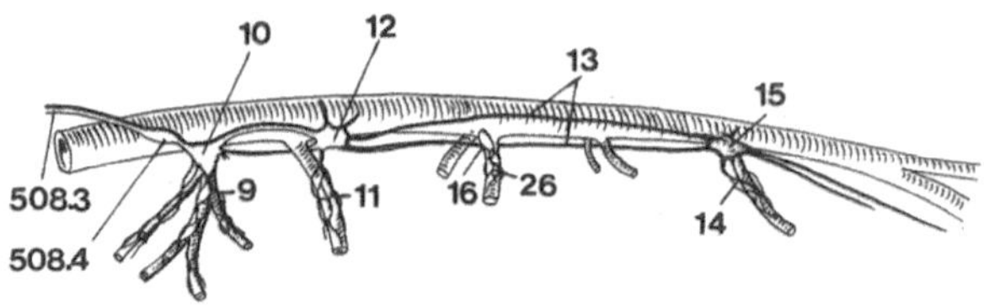

B Plexus aorticus abdominalis, left aspect (ca)

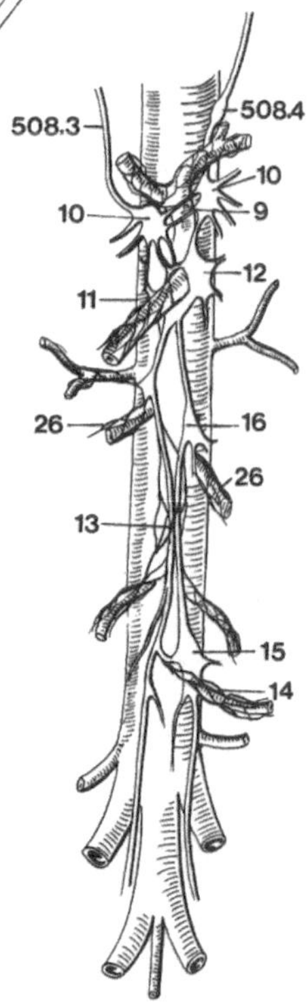

C Plexus aorticus abdominalis, ventral aspect (ca)

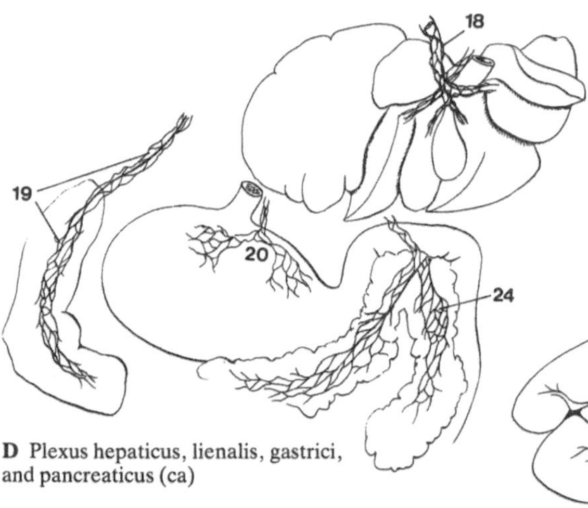

D Plexus hepaticus, lienalis, gastrici, and pancreaticus (ca)

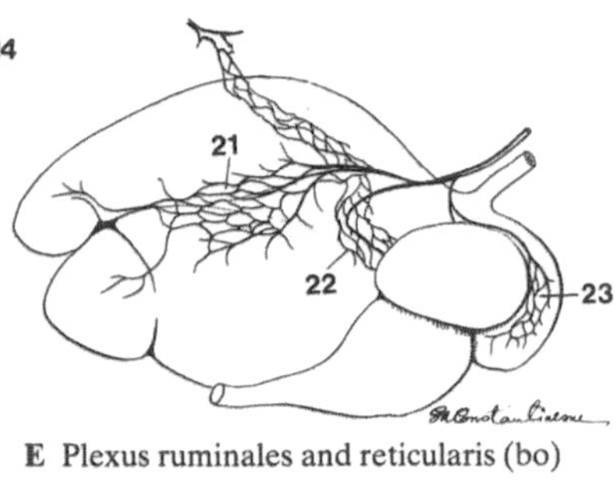

E Plexus ruminales and reticularis (bo)

1 ***Plexus testicularis.*** Testicular plexus, receives fibers from Plexus abdominalis aorticus, Plexus mesentericus caudalis, and Nn. splanchnici lumbales, innervates testis and epididymis. A

2 ***Plexus ovaricus.*** Ovarian plexus, receives fibers from Plexus aorticus abdominalis, Plexus mesentericus caudalis, and Nn. splanchnici lumbales, accompanies A. ovarica and can be divided into ovarian, tubal, and cranial uterine plexuses. B

3 ***Plexus colicus.*** Colic plexus, occurs in eq. It connects the Plexus mesentericus cranialis and caudalis by passing through the dorsal part of the Mesenterium. Its connection with Rami celiaci trunci vagalis dorsalis provides a pathway for parasympathetic fibers to Colon descendens. It follows the A. colica sinistra. C

4 ***Plexus rectalis cranialis.*** Cranial rectal plexus, follows A. rectalis cranialis. C

5 ***Plexus entericus.*** Enteric plexus, general term for the autonomic nervous network supplying the intestinal wall. D

6 *Plexus subserosus*. Subserosal plexus, network deep to the serosa of the intestine. D

7 *Plexus myentericus**. Myenteric or Auerbach's plexus, between the two muscular layers of the intestinal wall; provided with microganglia. D

8 *Plexus submucosus**. Submucosal or Meissner's plexus, located in the submucosa; provided with microganglia. D

9 ***Plexus iliaci.*** Iliac plexuses, continuation of Plexus aorticus abdominalis, following the right and left external and internal iliac arteries. C

10 ***Plexus femoralis.*** Femoral plexus, continuation of Plexus iliacus on A. femoralis. C

11 ***N. hypogastricus.*** Hypogastric nerve (right and left), arises from Plexus mesentericus caudalis, runs to Plexus pelvinus. E F

12 ***Plexus pelvinus.*** Pelvic plexus, contains sympathetic fibers from N. hypogastricus and sacral parasympathetic fibers, is located at the lateral wall of rectum, extraperitoneally, contains pelvic ganglia. E F

13 ***Plexus rectales medii.*** Middle rectal plexuses, continuations of Plexus pelvinus into the retroperitoneal portion of the rectum along A. rectalis media. E

14 ***Plexus rectales caudales.*** Caudal rectal plexuses, continuations of Plexus pelvinus to the caudal portion of the rectum along A. rectalis caudalis. E

15 ***Plexus prostaticus.*** Prostatic plexus, located chiefly on the dorsal surface of the prostate body, extends along the pelvic part of urethra. E

16 ***Plexus deferentialis.*** Deferential plexus, from Plexus pelvinus, accompanying the Ductus deferens. E

17 ***Plexus uterovaginalis.*** Uterovaginal plexus, basically located in the parametrium, sending branches to vagina and uterus. F

18 *Nn. vaginales*. Vaginal nerves. F

19 ***Plexus vesicales.*** Vesical plexuses. The cranial one (a) accompanies Aa. vesicales craniales in Lig. versicae laterale to Vertex vesicae, the caudal one (b) extends to Corpus and Cervix vesicae. E

20 ***Nn. corporis cavernosi penis.*** Nerves of Corpus cavernosum penis, from Plexus prostaticus. E

21 ***Nn. corporis cavernosi clitoridis.*** Nerves of Corpus cavernosum clitoridis, from Plexus uterovaginalis. F

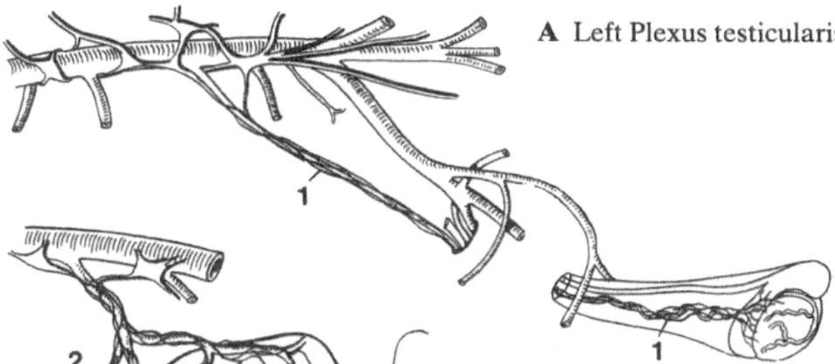

A Left Plexus testicularis, lateral aspect (ca)

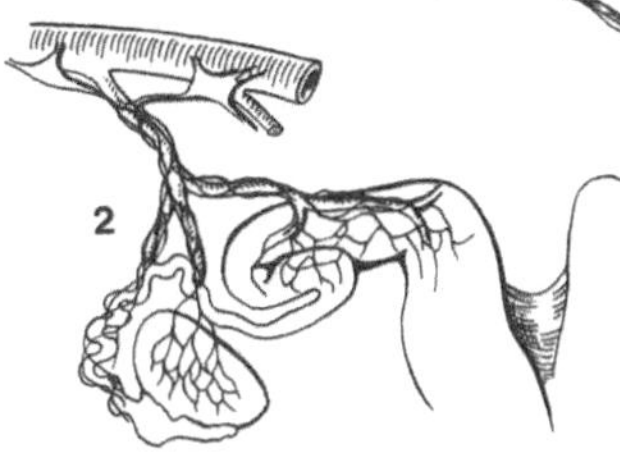

B Left Plexus ovaricus, lateral aspect (bo)

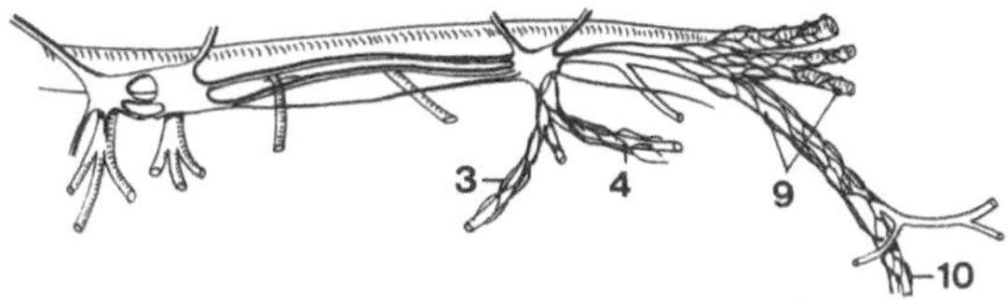

C Plexus colicus, rectalis cranialis and iliaci (ca)

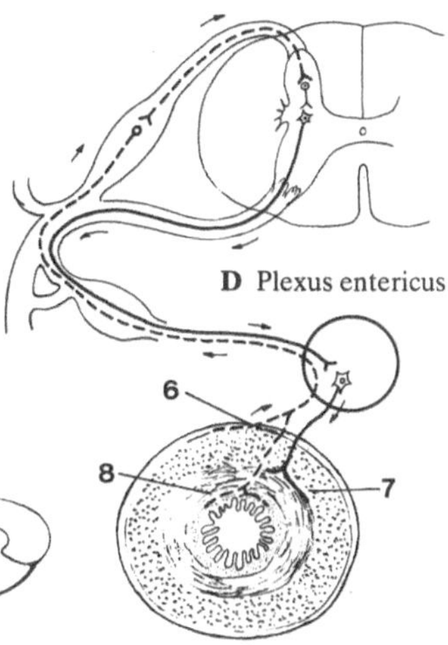

D Plexus entericus

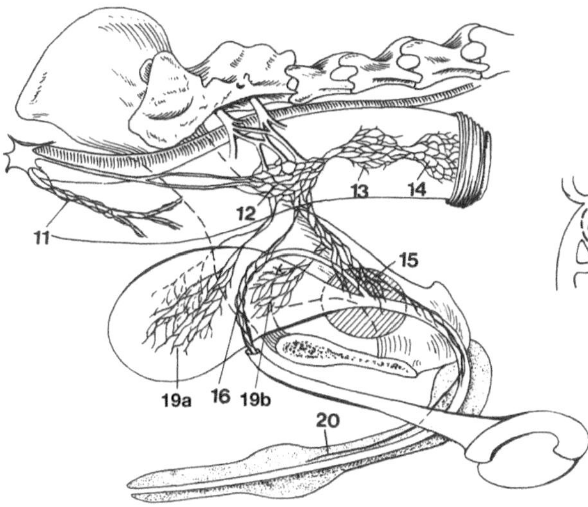

E N. hypogastricus and Plexus pelvinus, left side (ca masc)

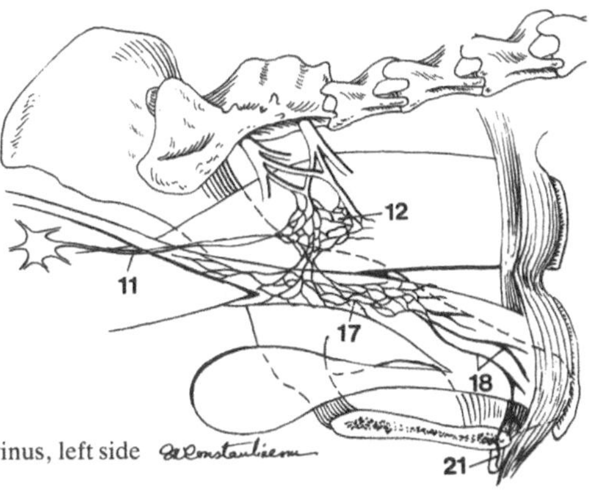

F N. hypogastricus and Plexus pelvinus, left side (ca fem)

1 **Pars sympathica**. Sympathetic part of Systema nervosum autonomicum. Its origin in Medulla spinalis is between (T1) T2 and L2–4, its extent into the lumbar part depending on species.

2 **Truncus sympathicus**. Sympathetic trunk, paired ganglionic chain ventrolateral to the vertebral column from the first thoracic to the 4th–7th caudal vertebra, only the cervical part runs with N. vagus in the Vagina carotica. B

3 ***Ganglia trunci sympathici***. Sympathetic trunk ganglia. In these ganglia, composed of multipolar nerve cells, preganglionic neurons synapse with postganglionic neurons. A B

4 ***Ganglia intermedia***. Intermediate ganglia, most commonly found in the Rami communicates of the lumbar region and in the Rami interganglionares. A

5 ***Rami interganglionares***. Interganglionic branches, connect the Ganglia trunci sympathici of the homolateral chain, in some cases also the paired ganglia. B

6 ***Rami communicantes***. Communicating branches, connections between Truncus sympaticus and Nn. spinales, contain preganglionic fibers from Medulla spinalis or postganglionic fibers to the periphery. A B

7 ***Ganglion cervicale craniale***. Cranial cervical ganglion, most cranial condensation of nerve cells in which preganglionic sympathetic neurons synapse with postganglionic neurons, located close to A. carotis interna, between it and A. occipitalis. C

8 *N. jugularis*. Jugular nerve. Branch communicating with Nn. glossopharyngeus and vagus. C

9 *N. caroticus internus*. Internal carotid nerve, forms Plexus caroticus internus. C

10 *Plexus caroticus internus*. Internal carotid plexus, in the wall of A. carotis interna, gives off N. petrosus profundus and branches to the ear and the eye. C

11 *Nn. carotici externi*. External carotid nerves, descending branches to Plexus caroticus externus. C

12 *Plexus caroticus externus*. External carotid plexus, network surrounding the A. carotis externa. C

13 *Plexus caroticus communis*. Common carotid plexus, surrounds A. carotis communis. C

14 *Rami laryngopharyngei*. Laryngopharyngeal branches.

15 ***Ganglion cervicale medium***. Middle cervical ganglion, inconstant grossly in eq, located in the thoracic inlet. D

16 *N. cardiacus cervicalis*. Cervical cardiac nerve from the middle cervical ganglion. D

17 ***Ganglion cervicothoracicum [stellatum]***. Cervicothoracic [stellate] ganglion, results from the fusion of the Ganglion cervicale caudale with one or more Ganglia thoracica, lateral to the thoracic part of M. longus colli in the first intercostal space. D

18 *Ansa subclavia*. Loop around A. subclavia, between Ganglion cervicothoracicum and Ganglion cervicale medium. D

19 *Plexus subclavius*. Subclavian plexus, network in the wall of A. subclavia. D

20 *N. vertebralis*. Vertebral nerve, connection of nerve fibers from Ganglion cervicothoracicum to C8–C2, accompanies A. vertebralis into the vertebral canal. Sometimes a vertebral ganglion is present. D

21 *Plexus vertebralis*. Vertebral plexus, surrounds A. vertebralis. D

22 ***Nn. cardiaci cervicales***. Cervical cardiac nerves, named according to the ganglion of origin, in this case they arise from Ganglion cervicale caudale (cervicothoracicum). D

A Ganglion lumbale and Ganglion intermedium

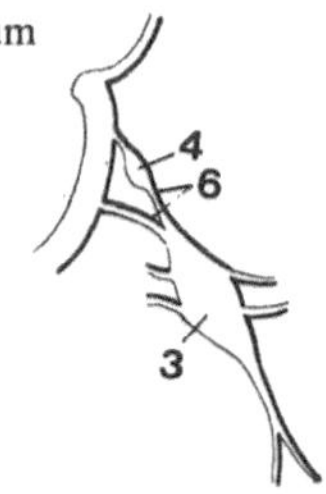

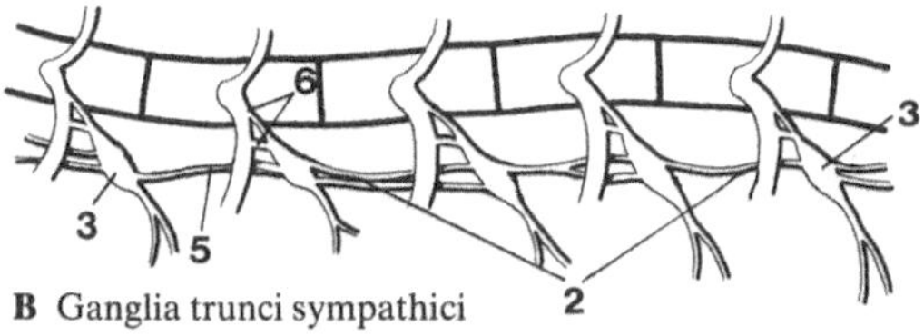

B Ganglia trunci sympathici

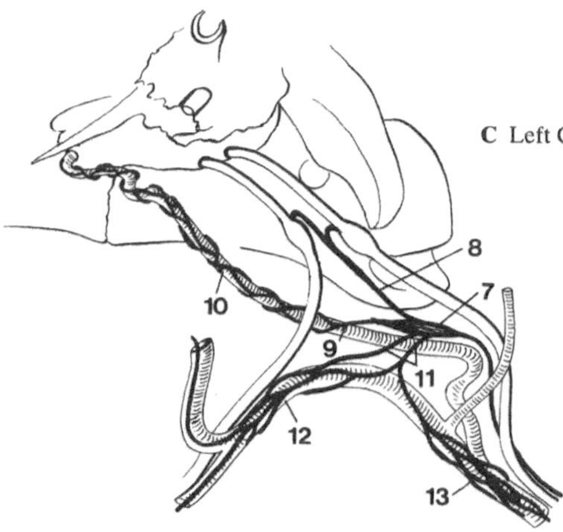

C Left Ganglion cervicale craniale (eq)

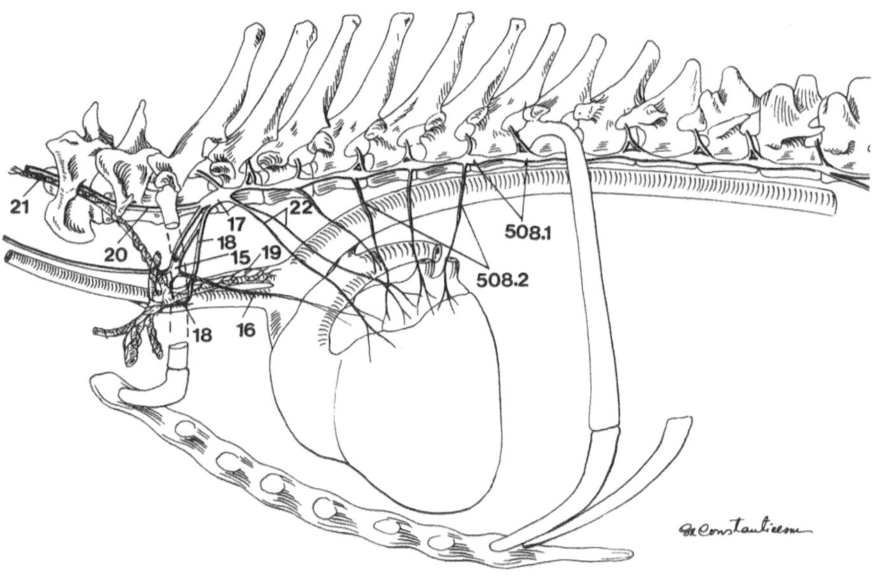

D Left Ganglia cervicale medium and cervicothoracicum (ca)

1 ***Ganglia thoracica.*** Thoracic ganglia, 13–18 depending on species; they lie in the thoracic segment of Truncus sympathicus. 507 D

2 *Nn. cardiaci thoracici.* Thoracic cardiac nerves, named according to the ganglion of origin; start from the first 5–6 Ganglia thoracica. 507 D

3 *N. splanchnicus major.* Greater splanchnic nerve, derives from Ganglia thoracica except the first 5–7 and the last 2–3 depending on species, and runs between the crus of the diaphragm and the M. psoas minor into Cavum abdominis, ends in Ganglion celiacum and medulla of Gl. adrenalis. 503 A B C

4 *Ganglion splanchnicum.* Splanchnic ganglion, occurs in ca and eq, at the end of the course of N. splanchnicus major. 503 A B C

5 *N. splanchnicus minor.* Lesser splanchnic nerve, arises from the last 2–3 Ganglia thoracica (eq) or first 1–3 Ggl. lumbalia, ends in Plexus celiacus and Plexus renalis. 503 A

6 *Ramus renalis.* Renal branch, a communicating branch from N. splanchnicus minor to Plexus renalis and adrenalis.

7 *(N. splanchnicus imus).* The most caudal (lowest in humans) splanchnic nerve, occasionally present, branch of last Ganglion thoracicum to Plexus renalis.

8 ***Ganglia lumbalia.*** Lumbar ganglia, variable in number, usually 5–7 pairs, lying in the lumbar part of Truncus sympathicus. A

9 *Nn. splanchnici lumbales.* Lumbar splanchnic nerves from Ganglia lumbalia, running towards Plexus celiacus and mesentericus cranialis. A

10 ***Ganglia sacralia.*** Sacral ganglia, 3–5 pairs, in the sacral part of Truncus sympathicus. A

11 *Nn. splanchnici sacrales.* Sacral splanchnic nerves, 0–4 small nerves which contribute to Plexus pelvinus. A

12 ***Ganglia caudalia [coccygea].*** Caudal [coccygeal] ganglia, in variable number, very small, located in the tail. A B

13 ***Ganglion impar.*** The last and unpaired sympathetic ganglion, located in the tail. B

14 **Pars parasympathica.** Parasympathetic part, antagonist to Pars sympathica of the Systema nervosum autonomicum. Its outflow from the central nervous system comes from the brainstem and the sacral part of Medulla spinalis.

15 ***Ganglion ciliare.*** Ciliary ganglion, with its Radix oculomotoria, Nn. ciliares breves, Ramus sympathicus ad ganglion ciliare, and Ramus communicans cum n. nasociliari is described on page 464. C

16 ***Ganglion pterygopalatinum.*** Pterygopalatine ganglion, with its Rami orbitales, the other nerves and communicating branches are described on page 468. C

17 ***Ganglion oticum.*** Otic ganglion, described with N. petrosus minor and its communicating branches on page 472. C

18 ***Ganglion mandibulare.*** Mandibular ganglion, described with its branches on page 472. C

19 ***Ganglion sublinguale.*** Sublingual ganglion, described with its branches on page 472. C

20 ***Nn. pelvini.*** Pelvic nerves, Nn. splanchnici pelvini (Nn. erigentes) in the N.A. These nerves contain efferent and afferent fibers for the pelvic viscera and are in relation not solely to erectile tissue. They originate in S2–S3 (4). With N. hypogastricus they form the Plexus pelvinus. B

21 ***Ganglia pelvina.*** Pelvic ganglia, embedded in Plexus pelvinus. B

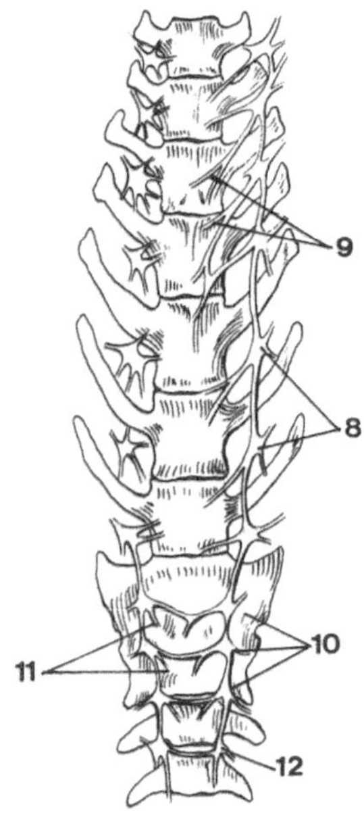

A Ganglia lumbalia, sacralia, and caudalia, ventral aspect (ca)

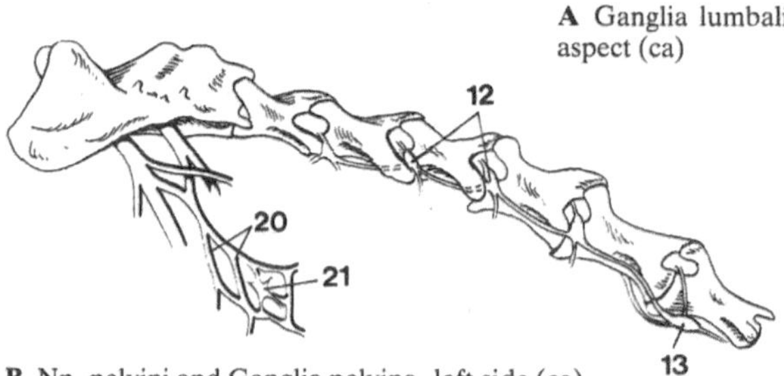

B Nn. pelvini and Ganglia pelvina, left side (ca)

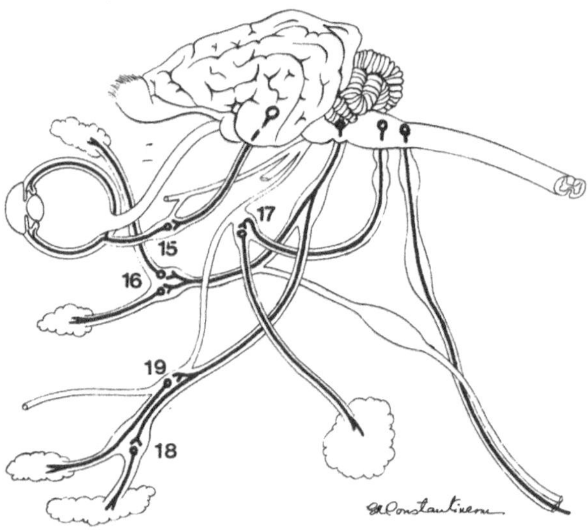

C Parasympathetic ganglia of the head, left side (ca)

1 **ORGANUM VISUS**. The organ of vision.

2 **OCULUS**. Eye. A

3 ***N. opticus***. Optic nerve, CN II, actually a tract of the central nervous system enveloped by extensions of the meninges. Extends from the Chiasma opticum to the Bulbus oculi, radiates in the retina. In fact, it send to the cerebral cortex the visual information to be processed into visual sensation. A C

4 ***Vagina externa n. optici***. External sheath of the optic nerve, extension of the dura mater united with the arachnoid (Nickel et al. 1992). C

5 ***Vagina interna n. optici***. Internal sheath of the optic nerve, extension of pia mater, deep to the Vagina ext. n. optici. C

6 *Spatia intervaginalia*. Intervaginal spaces, the subarachnoid space (Cavum leptomeningicum), a capillary space between the vagina externa and interna surrounding the optic nerve. C

7 **Bulbus oculi**. Eyeball, comprising cornea and sclera and the structures and spaces enclosed. B

8 ***Polus anterior***. Anterior pole, the highest point of the cornea. B

9 ***Polus posterior***. Posterior pole, the highest point on the posterior hemisphere of the eyeball, opposite to the anterior pole. B

10 ***Equator [Aequator]***. The largest circumference of the eyeball between anterior and posterior poles. B

11 ***Meridiani***. Meridians, lines encircling the eyeball and passing through anterior and posterior poles. B

12 ***Axis bulbi externus***. External axis of eyeball, line connecting anterior and posterior poles. A

13 ***Axis bulbi internus***. Internal axis of eyeball, the segment of the external axis of the eyeball from the posterior surface of the cornea to the anterior surface of the retina. A

14 ***Axis opticus***. Optic axis, line through the optical centers of cornea, lens and Corpus vitreum, usually coincident with the external axis of the eyeball connecting the two poles. A

15 ***Vesicula ophthalmica*** (ont) [1].

16 ***Caliculus ophthalmicus*** (ont) [1].

17 **Tunica fibrosa bulbi**. Fibrous coat of eyeball, the outer wall consisting of cornea and sclera. A

18 **Sclera**. The bluish-white protective layer covering the eyeball except for the anterior portion which is covered by the cornea. It consists of dense fibrous connective tissue. Close to, and around the cornea it is covered by Bulbar conjunctiva. A C E

19 ***Sulcus sclerae***. Scleral groove, the shallow groove at the junction of sclera and cornea. B

20 ***Anulus sclerae***. Scleral ring, the circular ridge on the inner surface of the sclera near the Limbus corneae to which the ciliary muscle is attached. E

21 ***Sinus venosus sclerae***. Venous sinus of the sclera, following the Limbus corneae and in communication with the spaces of the iridocorneal angle through which aqueous humor leaves the anterior chamber. E

22 ***Plexus venosus sclerae***. Venous plexus of the sclera, formed by the often double or multiple Sinus venosus sclerae. E

23 ***Lamina episcleralis***. Episcleral lamina, a thin layer of loose connective tissue on the external surface of the sclera between the latter and the Vagina bulbi. E

24 ***Substantia propria sclerae***. Proper substance of the sclera, consisting mainly of interwoven collagenous and some elastic fibers. E

25 ***Lamina fusca sclerae***. Dark lamina of the sclera, the innermost layer of the sclera consisting of less dense connective tissue and pigmented cells. C

26 ***Area cribrosa sclerae***. Cribriform area of the sclera, the fine holes in the wall of the sclera through which the fiber bundles of the optic nerve leave the interior of the eyeball. D

1) These structures were omitted from the 5th edition of the N. A. V., because they are ontogenetic terms.

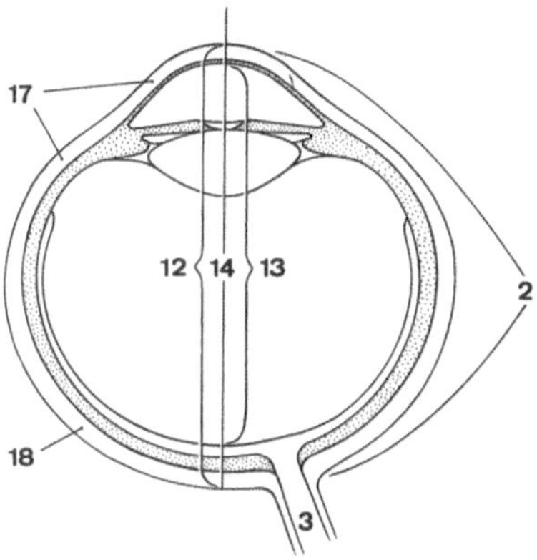

A Eyeball, meridional section, schematic (ca)

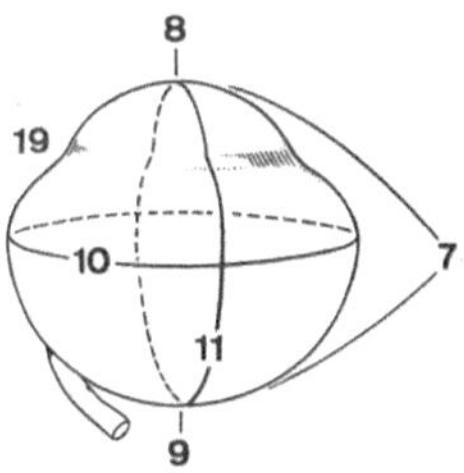

B Right eyeball, medial aspect (eq) (Sack and Habel)

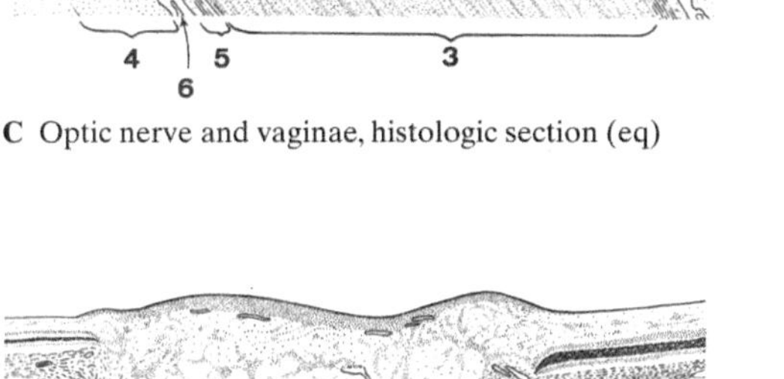

C Optic nerve and vaginae, histologic section (eq)

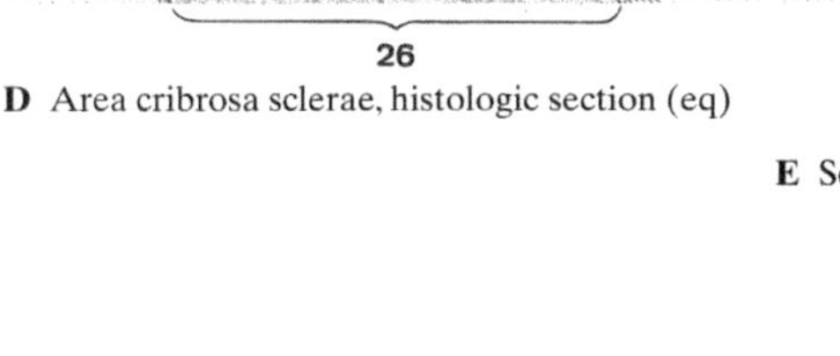

D Area cribrosa sclerae, histologic section (eq)

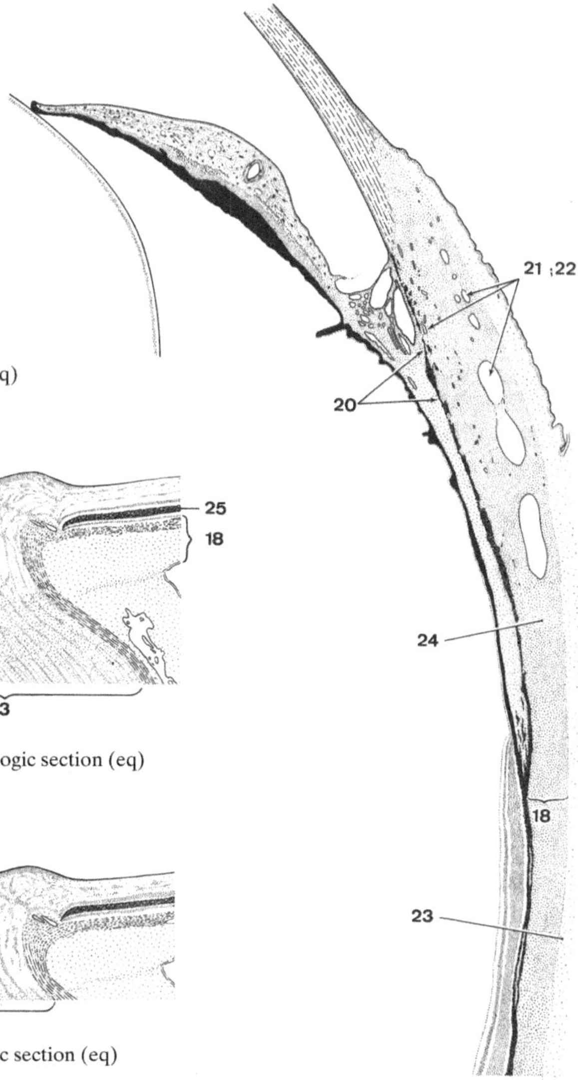

E Sclera, iris, ciliary body, meridional section (fe)

1 **Cornea**. Avascular translucent anterior wall of the eyeball, more strongly curved than the sclera. A

2 ***Anulus conjunctivae***. Conjunctival ring, the junction of the anterior epithelium of the cornea with the epithelium of the conjunctiva. A

3 ***Limbus corneae***. Corneal limbus, the edge of the cornea where it is continuous with the sclera at Sulcus sclerae. A

4 ***Vertex corneae***. The highest part of the cornea. A

5 ***Facies anterior***. Anterior surface of the cornea. A

6 ***Facies posterior***. Posterior surface of the cornea. A

7 ***Epithelium anterius corneae***. Anterior corneal epithelium, about 5–12 layers of cells which do not cornify and remain soft and nucleated. B

8 ***Lamina limitans anterior***. Anterior limiting membrane, thin, nearly homogeneous, not very distinct, between anterior epithelium and Substantia propria. B

9 ***Substantia propria corneae***. Proper substance of cornea, connective tissue lamellae of interweaving fibrils; the cementing substance contains flat cells connected by cytoplasmic processes. B

10 ***Lamina limitans posterior***. Descemet, posterior limiting membrane, fairly thick, homogeneous; between Substancia propria and posterior epithelium. B

11 ***Epithelium posterius corneae***. Posterior corneal epithelium, single layer of flat cells on the posterior surface of the cornea in contact with the aqueous humor. B (The correct and clinically proven name of it after birth is "Endothelium posterius corneae", bathed by the aqueous humor similar to the vascular endothelium bathed by blood.)

12 **Tunica vasculosa bulbi [uvea]**. Vascular tunic of the eyeball, consisting of Choroidea, Corpus ciliare and Iris. A

13 **Choroidea [Chorioidea]**. Choroid, part of the Tunica vasculosa bulbi between sclera and Pars optica retinae. A C (Actually, the retina is one undivided structure [see foot note p. 516].)

14 ***Lamina suprachoroidea [-chorioidea]***. Suprachoroid layer, outermost layer of the choroid, composed of elastic fibers and pigmented connective tissue cells that form loosely connected lamellae. C

15 ***Spatium perichoroideale [chorioideale]***. Perichoroid space, interlamellar spaces in the Lamina suprachoroidea, contain lymph, blood vessels, and nerves. C

16 ***Lamina vasculosa***. Vascular layer, thickest layer of the choroid containing the branches of Aa. ciliares posteriores longae et breves and of Vv. vorticosae. C

17 ***Tapetum lucidum***. In Ru and eq fibrous, in Car cellular, avascular layer deep to the Lamina vasculosa that gives the luster to the eyes of some animals. C

18 ***Lamina choroidocapillaris [chorioideo-]***. Choroidocapillary layer on the inner surface of Lamina vasculosa or Tapetum lucidum. C

19 ***Complexus basalis***. Basal layer, transparent innermost layer of the choroid lying next to the Stratum pigmentosum. It replaces the former term Lamina basalis in conformity with most human and veterinary anatomical textbooks and the terminology used in the Nomina Histologica Veterinaria. C

20 **Corpus ciliare**. Ciliary body, thick annular part of the Tunica vasculosa between choroid and iris. A D

21 ***Corona ciliaris***. Ciliary crown, raised portion of the ciliary body adjacent to the iris, bearing the ciliary processes. D

22 ***Processus ciliares***. Ciliary processes, radially arranged fibroelastic ridges on the inner surface of the Corona ciliaris which secrete the aqueous humor. D

23 ***Plicae ciliares***. Ciliary folds, microscopic folds on, and between, the ciliary processes. D

24 ***Orbiculus ciliaris***. Ciliary ring, peripheral flat portion of the ciliary body continuous with the choroid. D

25 ***M. ciliaris***. Ciliary muscle, ring of smooth muscle fibers in the ciliary body; it functions in the accomodation of the lens. E

26 *Fibrae meridionales*. Meridian fibers, forming the bulk of the ciliary muscle. E

27 *Fibrae circulares*. Circular fibers, parallel to the free margin of the iris and posterior to the Fibrae meridionales. E

28 ***Lamina basalis***. Basal layer, the innermost layer of the ciliary body, lying next to the Stratum pigmentosum. E

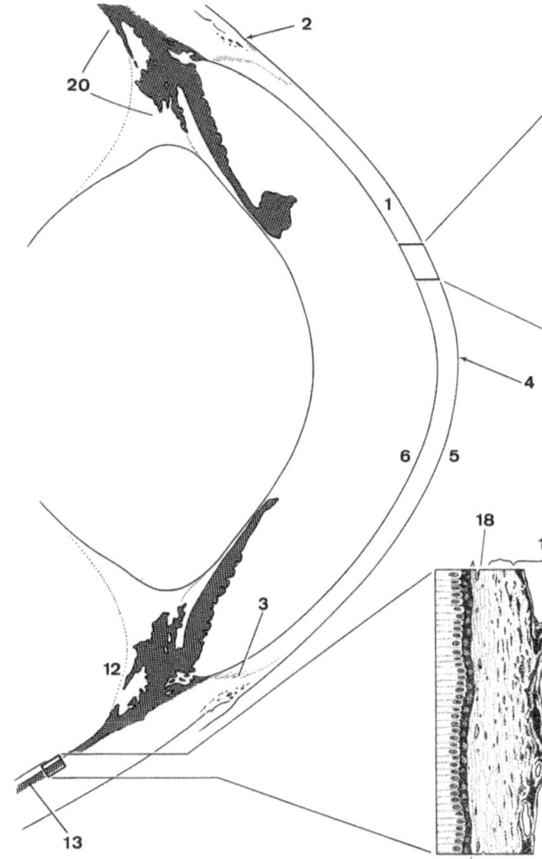

A Anterior part of the eyeball, meridional section (eq) (Sack and Habel 1982)

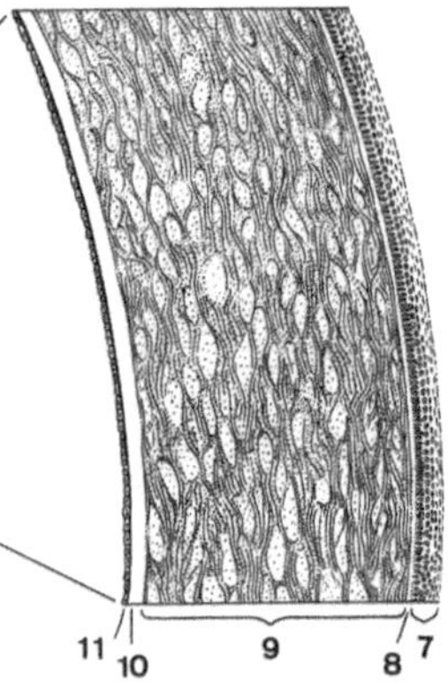

B Cornea, histologic section (eq) (Sack and Habel 1982)

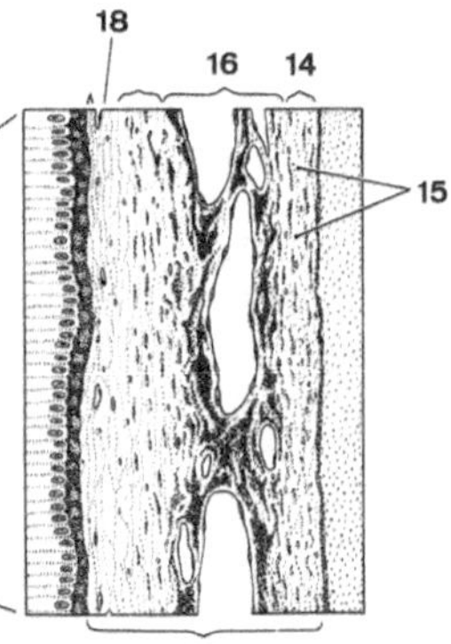

C Chorioidea, histologic section (eq)

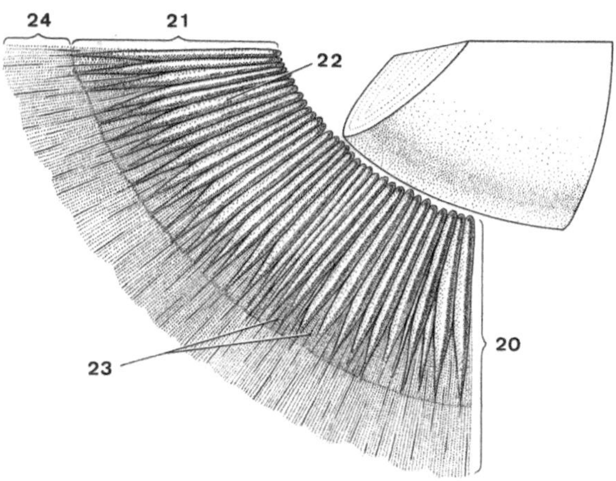

D Internal surface of ciliary body (eq) (Sack and Habel)

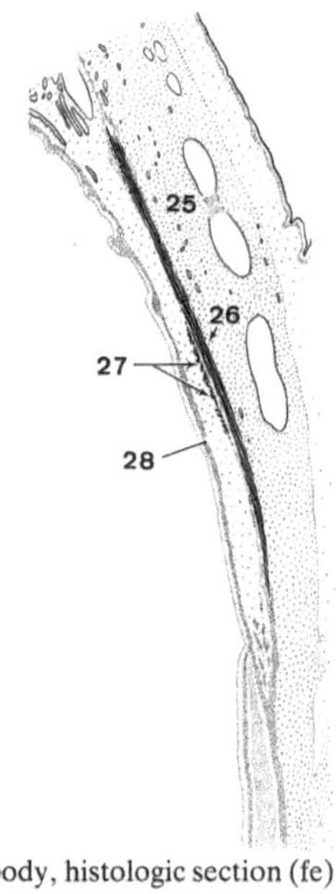

E Ciliary body, histologic section (fe)

1 **Iris**. Contractile diaphragm with a central opening (pupil) anterior to the lens; it is the most anterior part of the Tunica vasculosa bulbi and regulates the amount of light admitted into the fundus of the eye. A

2 ***Margo pupillaris***. Pupillary margin, central margin of the iris surrounding the pupil. A

3 *Granula iridica*. Iridic granules, vascular extensions of the stroma of the iris covered on the posterior surface with pigmented epithelium of the Pars iridica retinae. A B

4 ***Margo ciliaris***. Ciliary margin, the periphery of the iris continuous with the ciliary body and attached to the inside of the Limbus corneae by the Lig. pectinatum anguli iridocornealis. A

5 ***Facies anterior***. Anterior surface, facing the cornea. A B

6 ***Facies posterior***. Posterior surface, facing the lens. B

7 ***Anulus iridis major***. Major iridic ring, the wider peripheral portion of the iris that has a relatively uneven and folded anterior surface. A B

8 ***Anulus iridis minor***. Minor iridic ring, the narrow central portion of the iris that has a relatively smooth anterior surface. A B

9 ***Plicae iridis***[1]. Folds of the iris, present on the anterior surface; they may be permanent or temporary; some are radially arranged while others run parallel to the pupillary margin. A B

10 ***Pupilla***[1]. Pupil opening, surrounded by the iris. A

11 *M. sphincter pupillae*. Band of smooth muscle fibers in the Anulus iridis minor that constricts the pupil. B

12 *M. dilator pupillae*. Nearly radially oriented smooth muscle fibers near the posterior surface of the iris that open the pupil. B

13 ***Stroma iridis***. Stroma of the iris, composed mainly of branching interconnected pigment cells and predominantly radially arranged collagenous fibers; contains the vessels of the iris. B

14 ***Epithelium pigmentosum***. Pigmented epithelium, simple squamous epithelium covering the iridic stroma anteriorly and continuous in the iridocorneal angle with the posterior epithelium of the cornea, provides the specific color of the eyes. B (This structure was omitted from the 5th edition of the N. A. V.)

15 ***Lig. pectinatum anguli iridocornealis***. Pectinate ligament of the iridocorneal angle, collagenous trabeculae covered with iridic epithelium; between the trabeculae are the Spatia anguli iridocornealis. A B

16 ***Spatia anguli iridocornealis***. Spaces of the iridocorneal angle, epithelium lined spaces between the trabeculae that form the Lig. pectinatum through which the aqueous humor reaches the Plexus venosus sclerae. B

17 ***Circulus arteriosus iridis major***. Major arterial ring of the iris near Margo ciliaris, formed by anastomosing branches of principally the Aa. ciliares posteriores longae; the ring gives rise to radial branches that pass toward the pupil in the stroma of the iris. C

18 ***Circulus arteriosus iridis minor***. Minor arterial ring of the iris, near the pupillary margin, often incomplete, formed by anastomoses of the radial branches of the Circulus arteriosus iridis major. C

19 ***Membrana pupillaris*** (ont). (This structure was omitted from the 5th edition of the N. A. V., because it is an ontogenetic term.)

1) These structures were omitted from the 5th edition of the N. A. V. However, the Pupilla should not have been omitted since eight other terms include it (see 514.1, 2, 11, 12, 17, 18 and 516.2, 5).

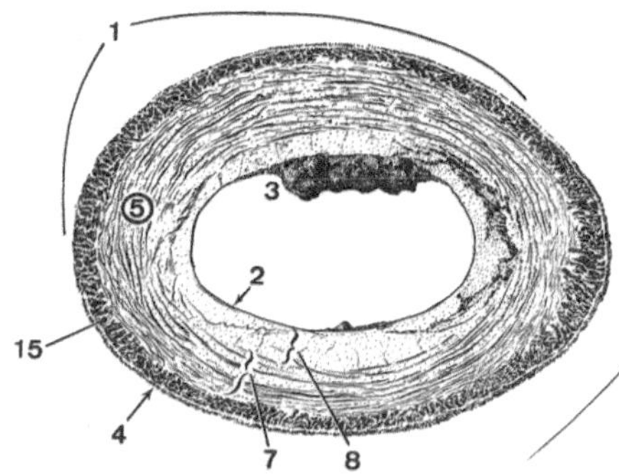

A Anterior surface of iris (eq)

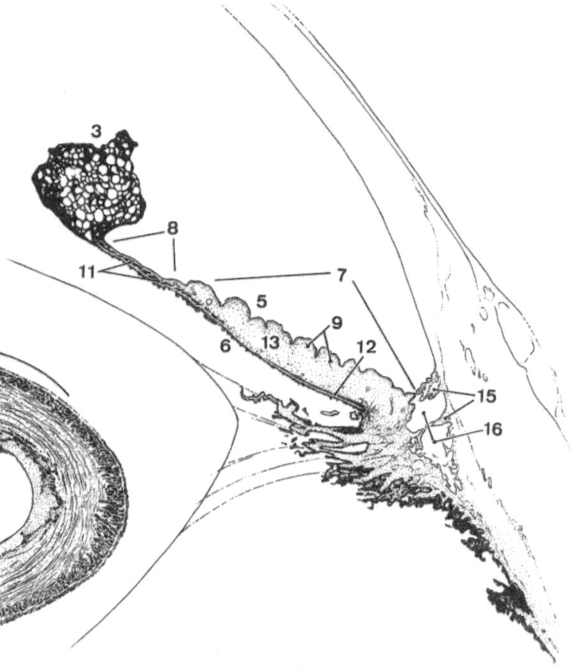

B Iris, meridional section (eq)

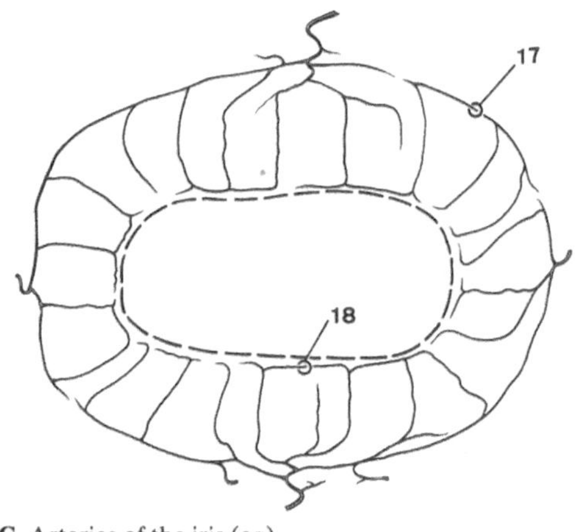

C Arteries of the iris (eq)

1 **Tunica interna bulbi**. Internal lining of the eyeball, consisting of the retina with its pigmented epithelium. A

2 **Retina**. Internal lining of the eyeball, extending from the pupil to the Discus n. optici. A

3 ***Pars optica retinae***[1]. Light sensitive part of the retina, extending from the Ora serrata to the Discus n. optici. A

4 ***Ora serrata***[1]. Edge of the Pars optica retinae, continuous with the thinner Pars ceca retinae, serrated in man. A F

5 ***Pars ceca [caeca] retinae***[1]. Light-insensitive part of the retina, extending from the pupil to the Ora serrata. A

6 *Pars ciliaris retinae* [1]. Ciliary part of the retina on the inner surface of the ciliary body. A

7 *Pars iridica retinae*[1]. Iridic part of the retina on the posterior surface of the iris. A

8 ***Fundus oculi***. Fundus of the eyeball. C

8a ***Discus n. optici***. Optic disc, beginning of the optic nerve visible on the fundus, lacks receptors. C

9 *Excavatio disci*. Central depression in the Discus n. optici. B

10 ***Macula***. Small area of the retina of higher visual acuity, faintly visible on the fundus in some species. C E

11 *Area centralis rotunda*. Round part of the macula, faintly visible in some species on the fundus, lateral on the Discus n. optici. C

12 *Area centralis striaeformis*. Additional bandlike part of the macula in Un, running mediolaterally across the retina. C

13 *Fovea centralis*. Central depression in the macula of man; absent or indistinct in domestic mammals.

14 ***Stratum pigmentosum***. Pigmented external layer of the retina, derived from the outer layer of the optic cup. F

15 *Stratum pigm. retinae*[1]. Pigmented external layer of the light-sensitive part of the retina. F

16 *Stratum pigm. corp. cil.*[1] Pigmented external layer of retina on the inner surface of the ciliary body. F

17 *Stratum pigm. iridis* [1]. Pigmented external layer of the retina on the posterior surface of the iris. F

18 ***Stratum nervosum***. The microscopic layers of Stratum nervosum of the retina have been deleted from NAV as they are hardly visible macroscopically, and are listed in detail in the Nomina Histologica Veterinaria. F

19 *Stratum neuroepitheliale*. Neuroepithelial layer, the most external layer of the Stratum nervosum, consisting of the rods and cones and their nuclei. F

20 *Stratum ganglionare retinae*. Middle layer of the Stratum nervosum, containing bipolar ganglion cells. F

21 *Stratum ganglion. n. optici*. Internal layer of the Stratum nervosum, containing multipolar ganglion cells and their unmyelinated axons, internal to the ganglion cells. F

22 **Vasa sanguinea retinae**. Retinal blood vessels.

23 ***Circulus vasculosus n. optici***. Vascular ring of the optic nerve; anastomosing branches of Aa. [Vv.] ciliares posteriores breves and A. [V.] centralis retinae. B

24 ***Rami a. [v.] centralis retinae***. Branches of the central retinal artery [vein] leaving the Discus n. optici and extending toward the periphery of the retina. D

25 ***Arteriola [Venula] lateralis retinae dorsalis***. Laterodorsal arteriole [venule] of the retina. E

26 ***Arteriola [Venula] lateralis retinae ventralis***. Ventrolateral arteriole (venule) of retina. D

27 ***Arteriola [Venula] medialis retinae dorsalis***. Dorsomedial arteriole [venule] of the retina. D

28 ***Arteriola [Venula] medialis retinae ventralis***. Ventromedial arteriole [venule] of the retina. D

29 ***Arteriola [Venula] macularis dorsalis***. Branches for the dorsal part of the macular area. E

30 ***Arteriola [Venula] macularis ventralis***. Branches for the ventral part of the macular area. E

31 ***Arteriola [Venula] medialis retinae***. Medial arteriole [venule] of the retina. E

1) If this is embriologically true, postnatally the retina continues anteriorly with the nonpigmented epithelium of the ciliary body at the level of ora serrata, therefore there is no Pars optica, Pars caeca, Pars ciliaris, and Pars iridica retinae. Only the so-called Pars optica retinae should be listed as, simply, "Retina", clinically proven the light sensitive tunic of the eyeball (Constantinescu 2002).

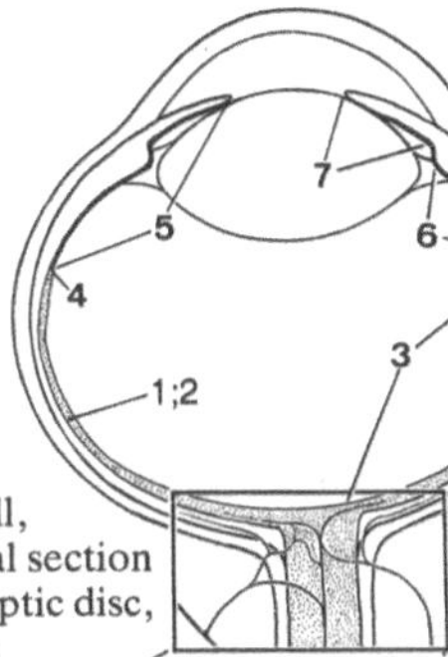

A Eyeball, meridional section through optic disc, schematic

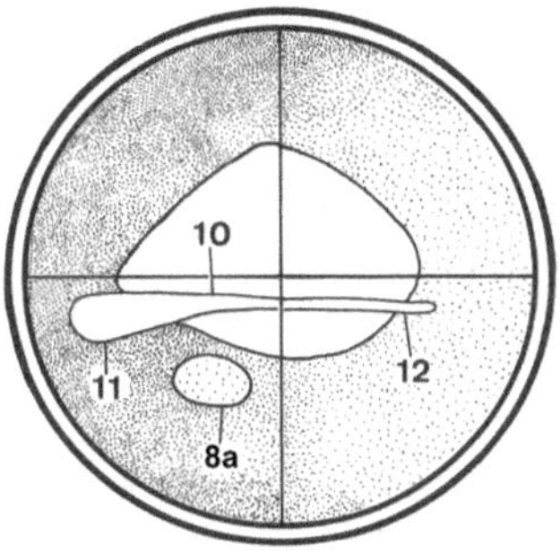

C Fundus of the eyeball, schematic (eq) (Seiferle, Hebel)

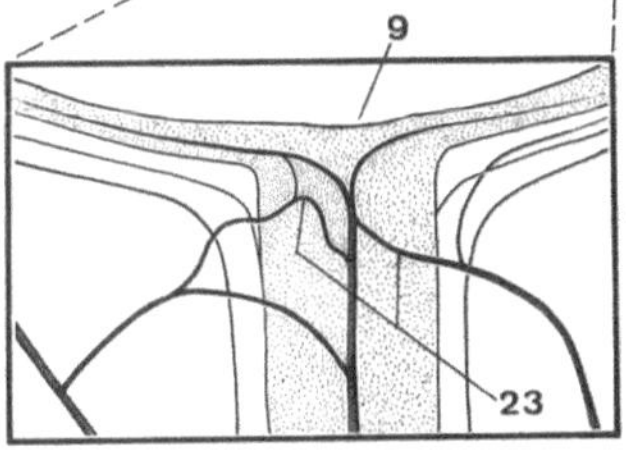

B Discus n. optici, arteries of the retina (ca)

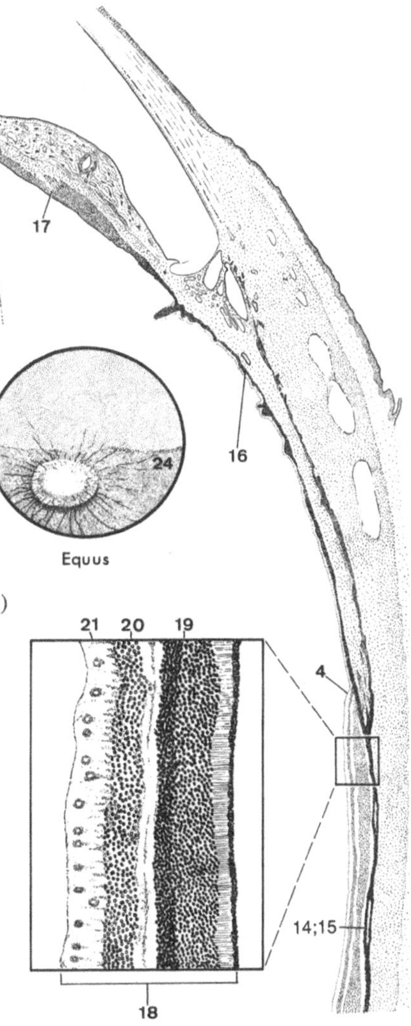

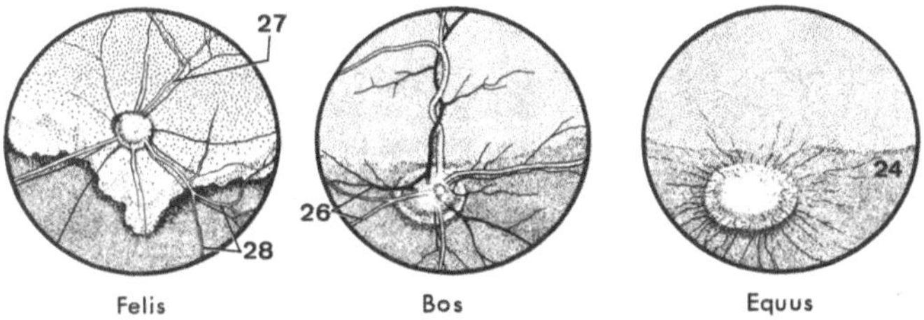

D Discus n. optici, vessels of the retina (fe, bo, eq) (Habel)

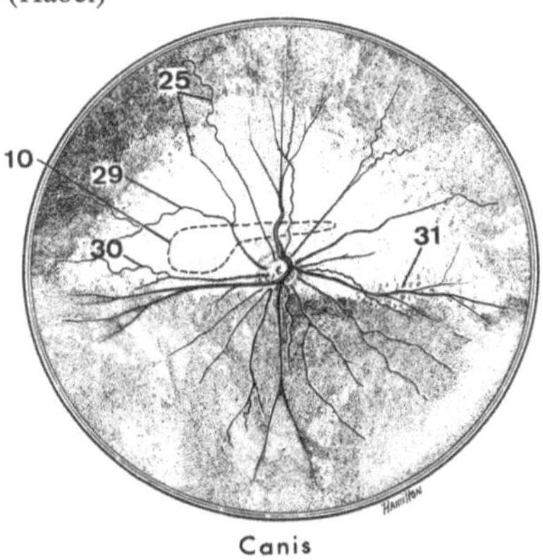

E Fundus of the eyeball (ca) (Evans and Christensen 1979)

F Retina, histologic section (fe)

1 **Camera anterior bulbi**. Anterior chamber of the eyeball, space between iris and cornea, contains aqueous humor. A

2 ***Angulus iridocornealis***. Iridocorneal angle, between iris and cornea, contains the Lig. pectinatum. A

3 ***Humor aquosus***. Aqueous humor, fluid in the anterior and posterior chambers of the eyeball.

4 **Camera posterior bulbi**. Posterior chamber of the eyeball, space between iris and lens, contains aqueous humor. A

5 ***Humor aquosus***. Aqueous humor.

6 **Camera vitrea bulbi**. Vitreous chamber of the eyeball, the space posterior to lens and ciliary body. A

7 ***Corpus vitreum***. Vitreous body, gelatinous mass filling the vitreous chamber of the eyeball. A

8 ***A. hyaloidea*** (ont). (This structure was omitted from the 5th edition of the N. A. V., because it is an ontogenetic term.)

9 ***(Processus hyaloideus)***. Remmant of the A. hyaloidea in the middle of the Discus n. optici. About 2 mm long in eq, present also in Ru. B

10 ***Canalis hyaloideus***. Hyaloid canal, condensation fibrils of the vitreous body, from the Discus n. optici to the posterior pole of the lens, contains the fetal A. hyaloidea. A

11 ***(Conus papillaris)***. Projection of minute blood vessels covered by pigmented epithelium from the Discus n. optici. In 15 to 20 percent of cap (and golden hamsters). D

12 ***Fossa hyaloidea***. Hyaloid fossa, depression on the anterior surface of the vitreous body occupied by the lens. A

13 ***Membrana vitrea***. Vitreous membrane, condensation of vitreous fibrils at the periphery of the vitreous body. A

14 ***Stroma vitreum***. Stroma of the vitreous body, framework of transparent fibrils whose meshes contain the vitreous humor.

15 ***Humor vitreus***. Vitreous humor, fluid filling the meshes of the vitreus body.

16 **Lens**. Transparent, biconvex structure focuses the light on the retina. E

17 ***Substantia lentis***. Substance of the lens.

18 ***Cortex lentis***. Cortex of the lens, outer, softer zone of the lens. C

19 ***Nucleus lentis***. Lens nucleus, the harder center of the lens. C

20 ***Fibrae lentis***. Lens fibers, transparent, constituting the substance of the lens. They are hexagonal in cross section; those close to the periphery are nucleated and have a semiliquid content. C

21 ***Radii lentis***. Lens stars, Y-shaped figures on the lens where the ends of individual lens fibers meet. E

22 ***Epithelium lentis***. Lens epithelium, a single layer of cuboidal cells on the anterior surface of the lens. C

23 ***Capsula lentis***. Lens capsule, a highly elastic covering of the lens, thicker on the anterior surface and at the equator than on the posterior surface. C

24 ***Polus anterior lentis***. Anterior pole of the lens, the highest point on the anterior surface. E

25 ***Polus posterior lentis***. Posterior pole of the lens, the highest point on the posterior surface. E

26 ***Facies anterior lentis***. Anterior surface of the lens, in Un less convex than the posterior surface. C

27 ***Facies posterior lentis***. Posterior surface of the lens, in Un more strongly curved than the anterior surface. C

28 ***Axis lentis***. Axis of the lens, passing through both poles of the lens. E

29 ***Equator [Aequator] lentis***. Equator of the lens, border of the lens. E

30 **Zonula ciliaris**. Suspensory apparatus of the lens, consisting of many fibers that extend from the ciliary processes to the lens capsule, anterior and posterior to the equator. C (Zinn zonula)

31 ***Fibrae zonulares***. Zonular fibers, fine homogeneous fibers extending from the ciliary processes to the capsule of the lens. C

32 ***Spatia zonularia***. Zonular spaces, between the Fibrae zonulares. C

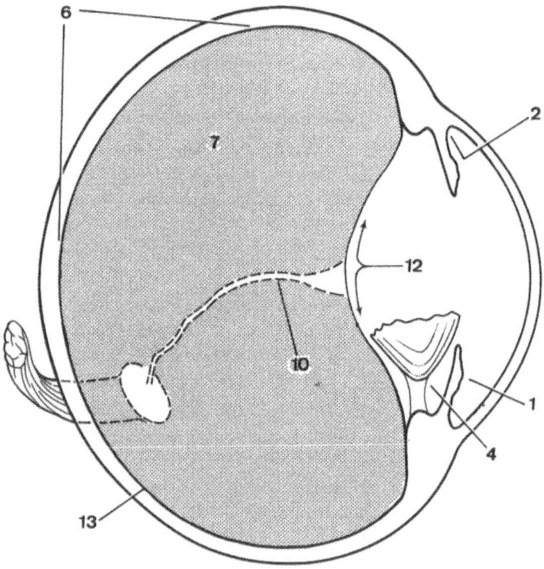

A Eyeball, meridional section (ov)

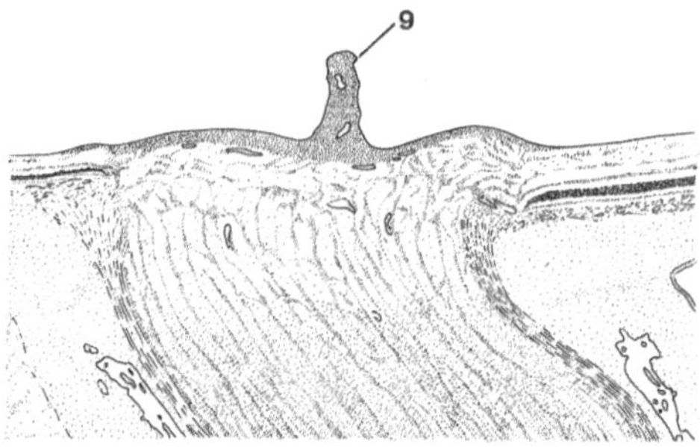

B Discus n. optici, section (eq)

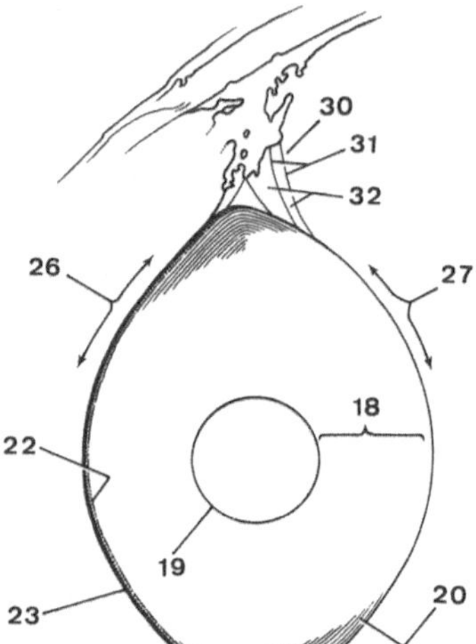

C Lens, meridional section (cap)

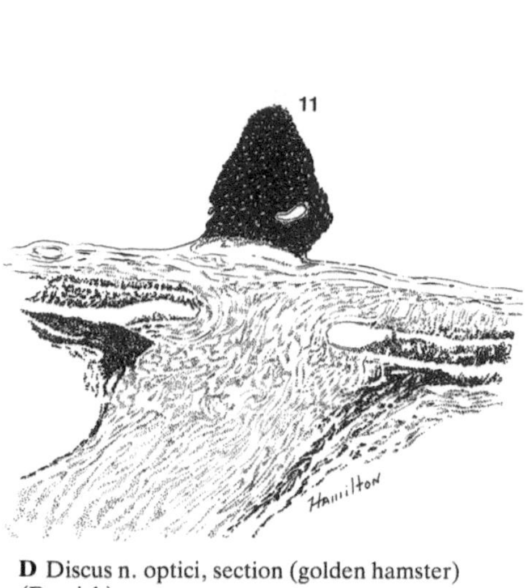

D Discus n. optici, section (golden hamster) (Bacsich)

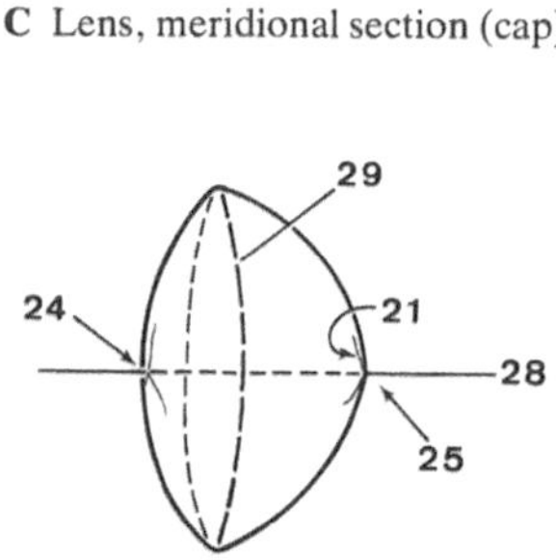

E Lens (bo)

1 **ORGANA OCULI ACCESSORIA.** Accessory organs of the eye, consisting of bulbar muscles, orbital fasciae, eyelids, conjunctiva, and lacrimal apparatus.

2 **Musculi bulbi.** Muscles of the eyeball.

3 ***M. orbitalis.*** Smooth muscle consisting of three sheets. A sheet of circular fibers in the deep part of the periorbita, protruding the eyeball; a ventral sheet with longitudinal fibers extending from the sheath of M. rectus ventralis into the lower lid and the third eyelid; and a medial sheet with longitudinal fibers extending from the sheath of M. rectus medialis and the trochlea into the upper lid and the third eyelid. Ventral and medial sheets retract the lids. A

4 ***M. rectus dorsalis.*** Dorsal rectus m., from the vicinity of the Canalis opticus to the dorsal surface of the eyeball anterior to the equator. B C D

5 ***M. rectus ventralis.*** Ventral rectus m., from the vicinity of the Canalis opticus to the ventral surface of the eyeball anterior to the equator. B C

6 ***M. rectus medialis.*** Medial rectus m., from the vicinity of the Canalis opticus to the medial surface of the eyeball anterior to the equator. B C

7 ***M. rectus lateralis.*** Lateral rectus m., from the vicinity of the Canalis opticus to the lateral surface of the eyeball anterior to the equator. B C D

8 ***M. retractor bulbi.*** Retracts the bulbus deep into the orbit. From the vicinity of the Canalis opticus (Fissura orbitalis in Car) to the eyeball posterior to the equator. It consists of four fascicles deep to the four corresponding recti muscles. B C D G

9 ***M. obliquus dorsalis.*** Dorsal oblique m. From the vicinity of the Canalis opticus, passes anteriorly on the dorsomedial wall of the orbit, passes laterally around the trochlea and is inserted near the equator deep to M. rectus dorsalis. B C G

10 *Trochlea.* Plate of cartilage on the dorsomedial wall of the orbit; deflects the M. obliquus dorsalis. B F G

11 *Vagina synovialis m. obliqui dorsalis.* Tendon sheath of the dorsal oblique m., permits frictionless passage of the M. obliquus dorsalis around the trochlea. B

12 ***M. obliquus ventralis.*** Ventral oblique m. From the medial wall of the orbit, passes laterally to the equator just ventral to the insertion of the M. rectus lateralis. C D

13 ***M. levator palpebrae superioris.*** Arises dorsal to the Canalis opticus, passes dorsal to the M. rectus dorsalis into the upper eyelid. C D E G

14 **Fasciae orbitales.** Orbital fasciae.

15 ***Periorbita.*** Cone-shaped fibrous membrane enclosing the eyeball and its muscles, vessels, and nerves. It is attached with its base to the bony rim of the orbit fusing with the periosteum, and is thicker and free caudally where the orbit is deficient. D E G

16 ***Septum orbitale.*** Orbital septum, two semilunar fibrous membranes extending from the margin of orbit to the tarsi in the eyelids. G

17 ***Fasciae musculares.*** The superficial fascia is loose and fatty and envelopes the M. levator palpebrae superioris and the lacrimal gland, the deep is fibrous, arises from the lids and Limbus corneae, envelopes the eyeball (Vagina bulbi) and reflects around the bulbar muscles and the optic nerve. E

18 ***Vagina bulbi.*** The part of the deep fascia, that envelopes the eyeball and the M. retractor bulbi. E (called also fascia of Tenon)

19 ***Spatium episclerale.*** Episcleral space between the Vagina bulbi and the sclera. E (called also spaces of Tenon)

20 ***Corpus adiposum orbitae.*** Orbital fat inside and outside the periorbita.

21 *Corpus adiposum intraperiorbitale.* Orbital fat inside the periorbita, filling the spaces between eyeball, muscles, vessels and nerves. G

22 *Corpus adiposum extraperiorbitale.* Orbital fat outside the periorbita. D G

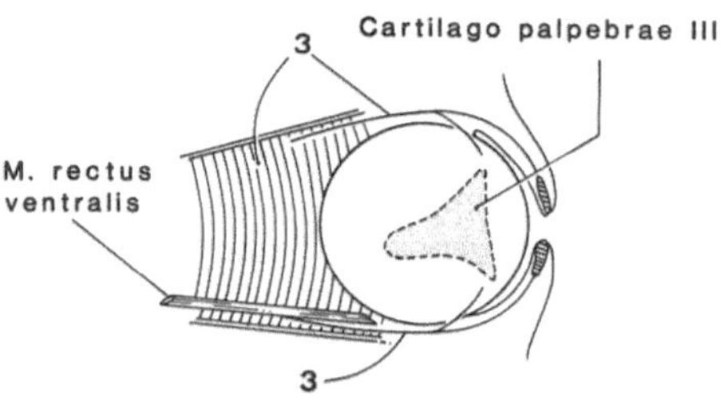

A M. orbitalis, schematic (fe) (Acheson)

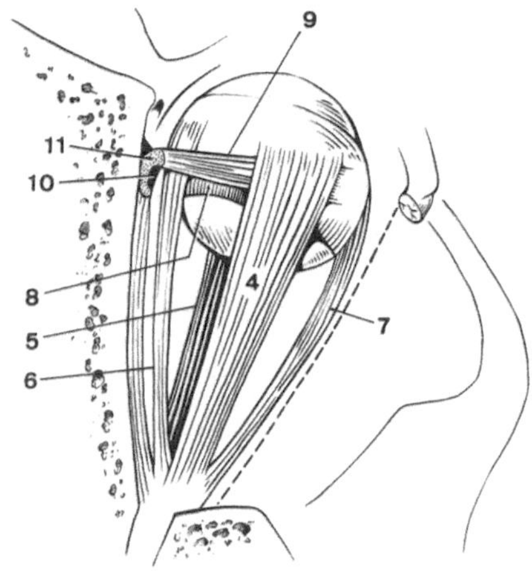

B Muscles of the right eyeball, dorsal aspect (fe)

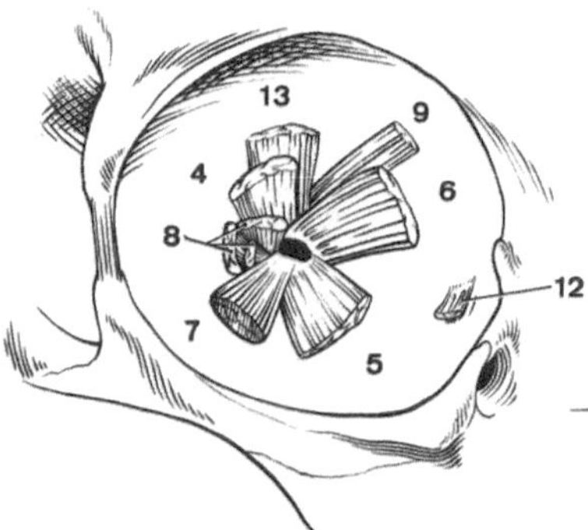

C Proximal stumps of Musculi bulbi in right orbit (fe)

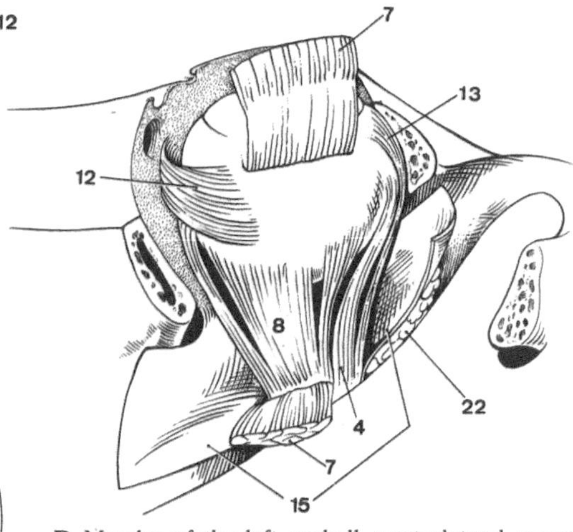

D Muscles of the left eyeball, ventrolateral aspect (eq)

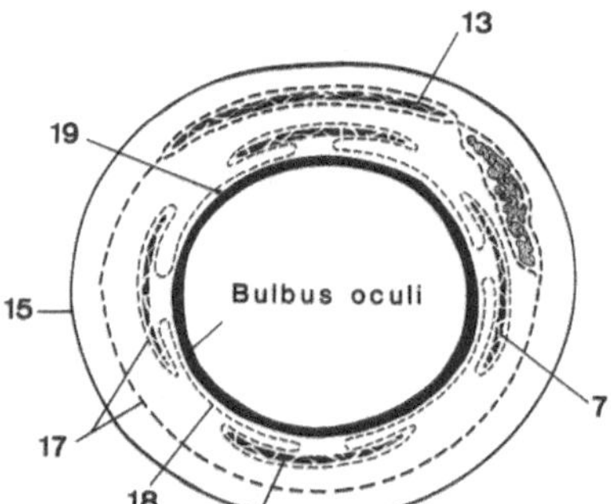

E Fasciae orbitales, schematic (Sack and Habel)

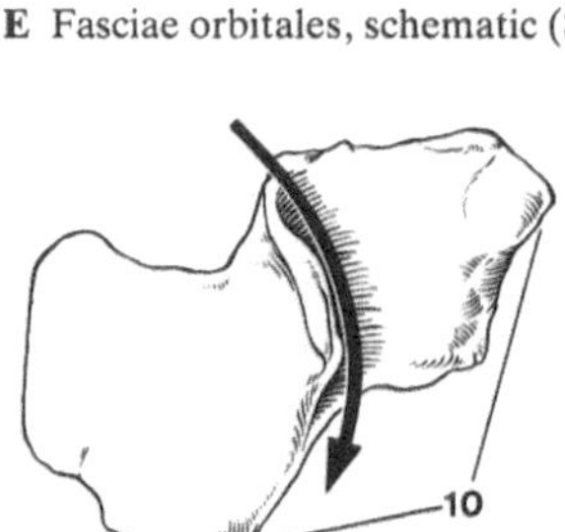

F Right trochlea, dorsal surface (bo)

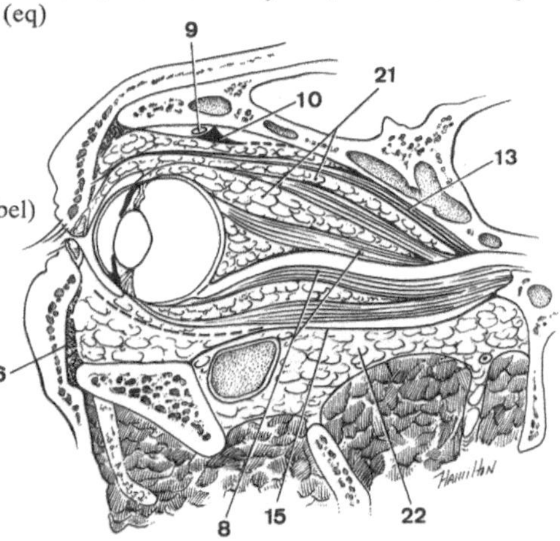

G Right orbit, longitudinal section (bo)

1 **Palpebrae**. Eyelids.

2 ***Palpebra superior***. Upper eyelid. B

3 ***Palpebra inferior***. Lower eyelid. B

4 ***Facies anterior palpebrarum***. Anterior surface of the eyelids formed by skin. A

5 ***Facies posterior palpebrarum***. Posterior surface of the eyelids formed by the palpebral conjunctiva. A

6 ***Rima palpebrarum***. Palpebral fissure, the space between upper and lower eyelids. B

7 ***Commissura palpebrarum lateralis***. Lateral palpebral commissure, the lateral union of upper and lower eyelids. B

8 ***Commissura palpebrarum medialis***. Medial palpebral commissure, the medial union of upper and lower eyelids. B

9 ***Angulus oculi lateralis***[1]. Lateral angle/corner of the eye, the lateral end of the Rima palpebrarum. B

10 ***Angulus oculi medialis***[1]. Medial angle/corner of the eye, the medial end of the Rima palpebrarum. B

11 ***Limbi palpebrales anteriores***. The anterior edges of the free borders of the eyelids associated with the cilia. A

12 ***Limbi palpebrales posteriores***. The posterior edges of the free borders of the eyelids associated with the openings of the tarsal glands. A

13 ***Cilia***. Specialized hairs arising from the anterior edges of free borders of the eyelids. They may be absent on the lower lid of Car and su. C

14 ***Glandulae ciliares***. Ciliary glands, sudoriferous glands associated with the cilia. A (called also Moll glands)

15 ***Glandulae sebaceae***. Sebaceous glands, found near the roots of the cilia. A (called also Zeis glands)

16 ***Tarsus superior***. Upper tarsus, plate of dense collagenous fibers between M. orbicularis oculi and palpebral conjunctiva close to the free edge of the upper lid. It is best developed in su. A

17 ***Tarsus inferior***. Lower tarsus, plate of dense collagenous fibers between M. orbicularis oculi and palpebral conjunctiva close to the free edge of the lower lid. It is best developed in su. C

18 ***Ligamentum palpebrale mediale***. Medial palpebral ligament, a fibrous connection between the medial commissure of the eyelids and the medial margin of the orbit. It, together with the Lig. palpebrale laterale, assures that the palpebral fissure, when narrowed by the M. orbicularis oculi, remains elliptical rather than becoming circular. D

19 ***Raphe [Rhaphe] palpebralis lateralis***. Lateral palpebral raphe, for the attachment of fibers of the M. orbicularis oculi. D

20 ***Ligamentum palpebrale laterale***. Lateral palpebral ligament, the fibrous connection between the lateral commissure of the eyelids and the lateral margin of the orbit (Ligamentum orbitale in Car and su). D

21 ***Glandulae tarsales***. Tarsal glands, elongated sebaceous glands in the tarsi. They stand at right angles to the free border of the lids and open near the Limbi palpebrales posteriores. Their fatty secretion causes the eyelids to repell the lacrimal fluid, keeping it on the eye for drainage through the nasolacrimal duct. A C

22 ***M. tarsalis superior***. A sheet of smooth muscle extending from the sheath of the M. rectus medialis and the trochlea into the upper lid. It attaches to the upper tarsus and is part of the M. orbitalis. A

23 ***M. tarsalis inferior***. A sheet of smooth muscle extending from the sheath of the M. rectus ventralis into the lower lid. It attaches to the lower tarsus and is part of the M. orbitalis. C

[1] In clinics they are called canthi, medial and lateral, respectively (sing. canthus).

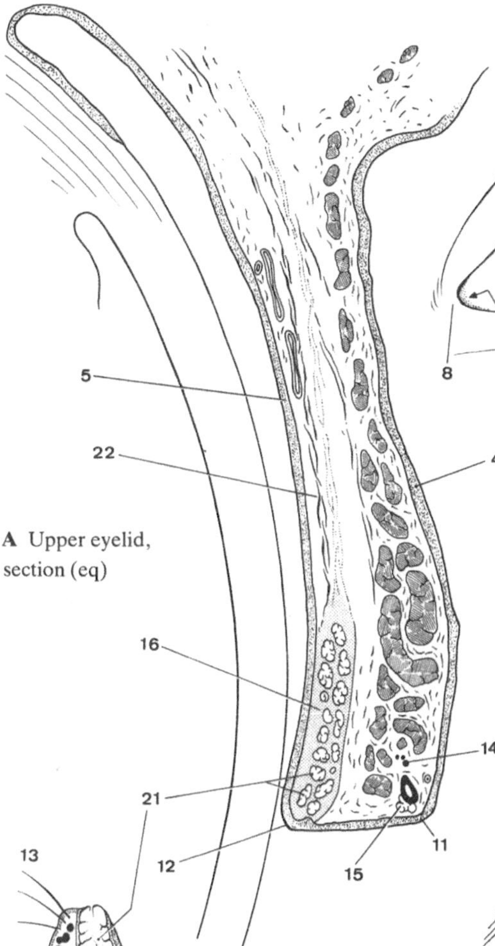

A Upper eyelid, section (eq)

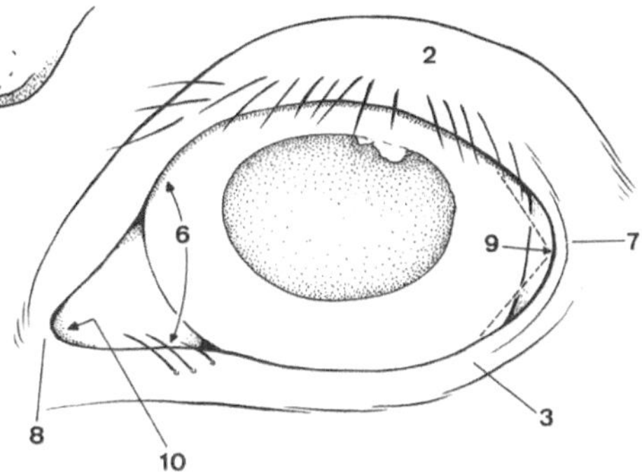

B Left eye (eq)

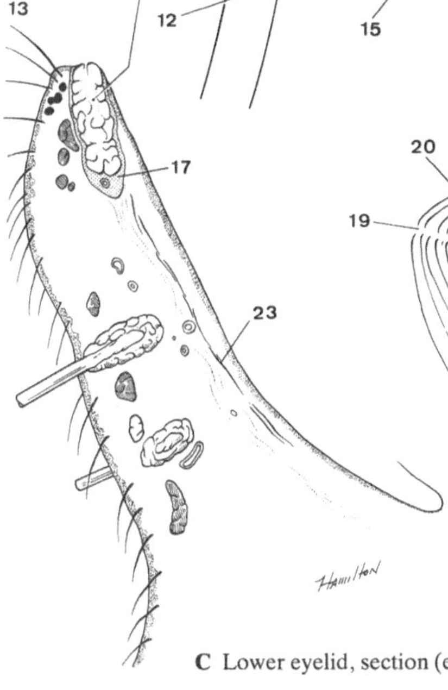

C Lower eyelid, section (eq)

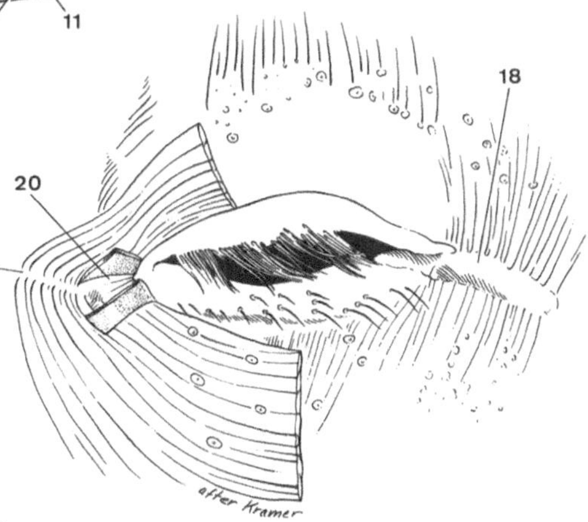

D Ligaments of right eyelids (su)

1 **Tunica conjunctiva**. Conjunctiva, the mucous membrane on the posterior surface of the eyelids, reflects itself onto the anterior surface of the eyeball to the edge of the cornea. B

2 ***Palpebra tertia***. Third eyelid, palpebra tertia or nictitating membrane is a fold of conjunctiva supported by a thin plate of cartilage in the medial angle of the eye. It slides over the eyeball when the latter is retracted. There are accumulations of lymphoid nodules on its bulbar surface. A

3 *Cartilago*. Supporting cartilage of the third eyelid, roughly T-shaped with the bar of the T in the free edge of the third eyelid and the stem between the medial wall of the orbit and the eyeball. C

4 *Glandula superficialis*. Accessory lacrimal gland surrounding the stem of the T-shaped cartilage of the third eyelid. Its secretion enters the conjunctival sac on the bulbar surface of the third eyelid. C

5 *Glandula profunda*. Deep accessory lacrimal gland in su and bo, called also the Harder's gland. C

6 ***Caruncula lacrimalis***. Lacrimal caruncle, elevation in the medial angle of the eye, bears fine hairs and contains sebaceous and sudoriferous glands. A

7 *Glandula carunculae lacrimalis*. Gland deep to the lacrimal caruncle in ca.

8 ***Tunica conjunctiva bulbi***. Bulbar conjunctiva, on the anterior surface of the eyeball except the cornea. It is loosely attached to the sclera and covered with stratified squamous epithelium. B

9 ***Tunica conjunctiva palpebrarum***. Palpebral conjunctiva, on the posterior surface of the eyelids. It is covered with a stratified columnar to cuboidal epithelium containing goblet cells near the fornix. B

10 ***Fornix conjunctivae superior***. Upper fornix, formed by the reflection of the palpebral conjunctiva onto the bulbar conjunctiva. B

11 ***Fornix conjunctivae inferior***. Lower fornix, formed by the reflection of the palpebral conjunctiva onto the bulbar conjunctiva. B

12 ***Saccus conjunctivae***. Conjunctival sac, space between bulbar and palpebral conjunctivae. B

13 ***Glandulae conjunctivales***. Conjunctival glands, small accessory lacrimal glands in the vicinity of the fornix. B

14 ***Lymphonoduli [Noduli lymphatici] aggregati conjunctivales***. Lymph nodules in the conjunctiva. B

15 **Apparatus lacrimalis**. Lacrimal apparatus.

16 ***Glandula lacrimalis***. Lacrimal gland, located dorsolateral to the eyeball. E

17 *Ductuli excretorii*. Excretory ductules, connecting the lacrimal gland with the lateral part of Fornix conjunctivae superior. E

18 ***(Gll. lacrimales accessoriae)***. Accessory lacrimal glands, especially in the vicinity of the fornices. B

19 ***Rivus lacrimalis***. The narrow space, filled with lacrimal fluid, between the free borders of the closed eyelids and the eyeball.

20 ***Lacus lacrimalis***. Lacrimal lake, the semicircular recess surrounding the lacrimal caruncle. A

21 ***Punctum lacrimale***. Lacrimal punctum (plur. Puncta – there are two Puncta), minute, slitlike opening through which the lacrimal fluid leaves the eye on the Limbus palpebralis posterior close to the medial angle of the eye. A

22 ***Canaliculus lacrimalis***. Lacrimal canaliculus, short duct connecting the Punctum lacrimale with the lacrimal sac. E

23 ***Saccus lacrimalis***. Lacrimal sac, enlargement of the proximal end of the nasolacrimal duct occupying the Fossa sacci lacrimalis. E

24 *Fornix sacci lacrimalis*. Dorsal recess of the lacrimal sac in ov.

25 ***Ductus nasolacrimalis***. Nasolacrimal duct, connects the lacrimal sac with the nasal cavity. It opens on the floor of the nostril on Limen nasi, but may have accessory openings farther caudally. E

26 ***Plica lacrimalis***. Lacrimal fold, at the opening of the nasolacrimal duct in some species. D

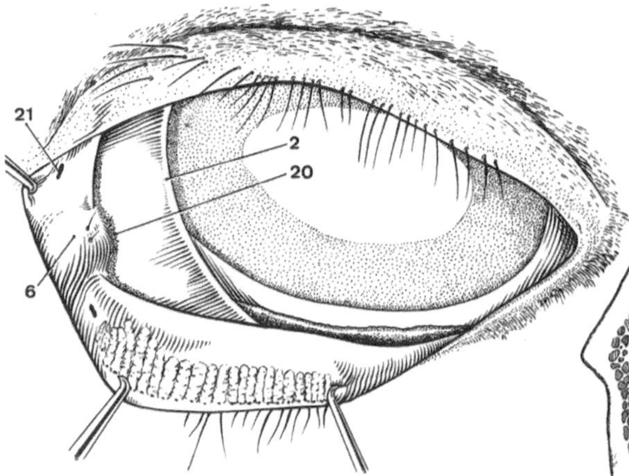

A Left eye (eq)

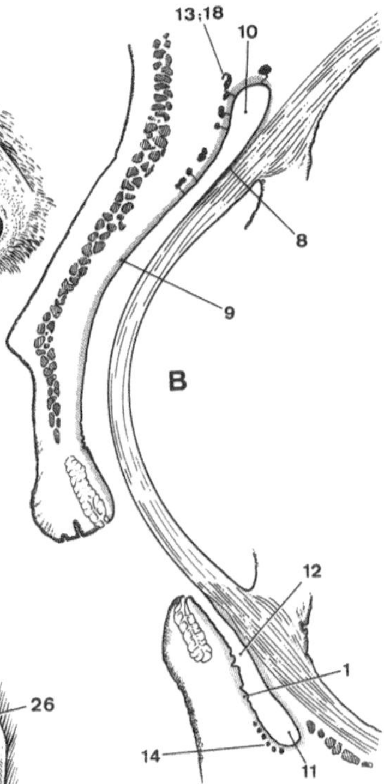

B Anterior portion of the eye, section (eq)

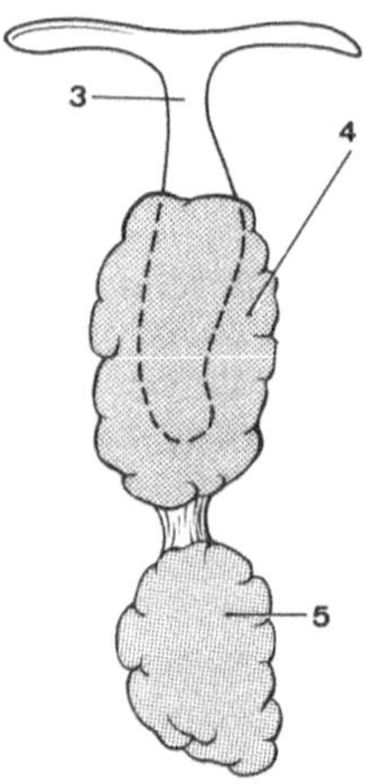

C Cartilage of third eyelid (su) (Ellenberger and Baum)

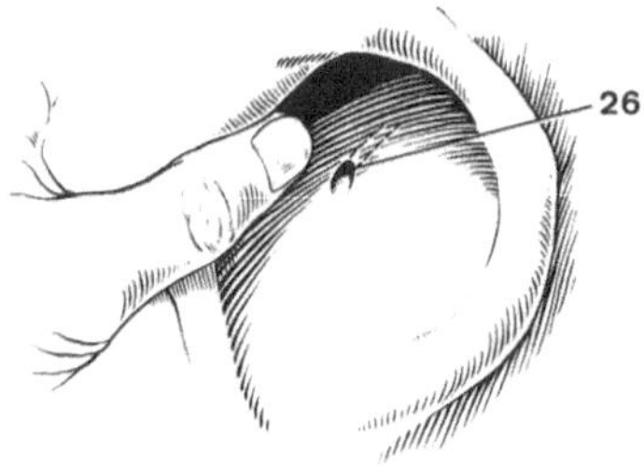

D Opening of nasolacrimal duct in the left nostril (eq)

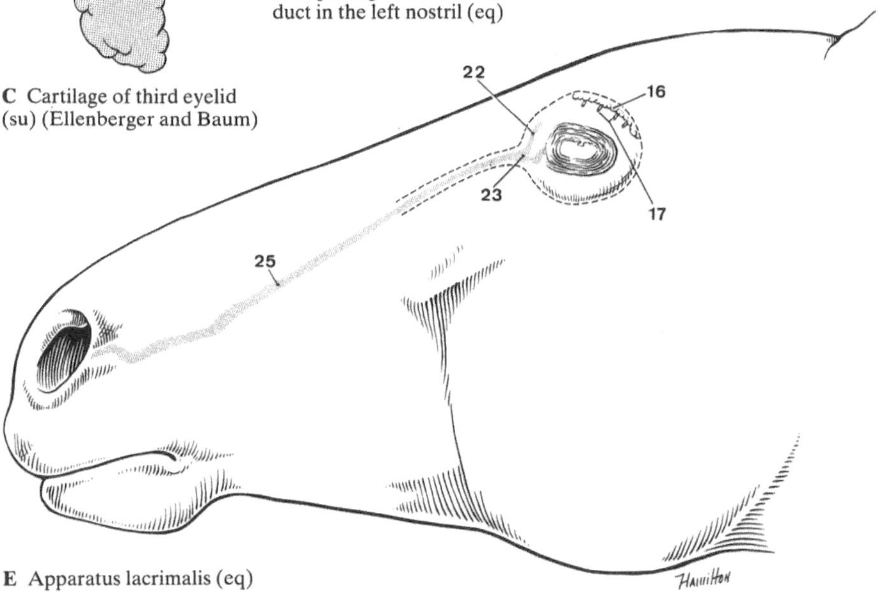

E Apparatus lacrimalis (eq)

1 **ORGANUM VESTIBULOCOCHLEARE [AURIS]**. Vestibulocochlear organ (ear). Sense organ receptive to sounds, gravity and changes in the position of the head and body in general.

2 **AURIS INTERNA**. Internal ear, located in the petrosal bone, converts the mechanical stimuli of sound and positional changes into nerve impulses.

3 **Labyrinthus membranaceus**. Membranous labyrinth, closed system of membranous ducts and cavities, contains endolymph, is located in the osseous labyrinth. A

4 ***Ductus endolymphaticus***. Endolympathic duct, in the Aqueductus vestibuli from the Sacculus to the Dura mater. A

5 ***Saccus endolymphaticus***. Endolymphatic sac, the slightly enlarged end of the Ductus endolymphaticus. A

6 ***Ductus utriculosaccularis***. Utriculosaccular duct, short connection between the saccular end of the Ductus endolymphaticus and the Utriculus. A

7 ***Utriculus***. Enlargement of the membranous labyrinth that gives rise to the three semicircular ducts. It occupies the Recessus ellipticus of the Vestibulum. A B

8 ***Ductus semicirculares***. Semicircular ducts, membranous, originating and ending at the Utriculus. They are oriented at nearly right angles to each other. C

9 *Ductus semicircularis anterior*. Anterior semicircular duct, the plane of its circle relative to the base of the skull faces rostromedially. A

10 *Ductus semicircularis posterior*. Posterior semicircular duct, the plane of its circle relative to the base of the skull faces rostrolaterally and slightly dorsally. A

11 *Ductus semicircularis lateralis*. Lateral semicircular duct, the plane of its circle relative to the base of the skull faces dorsally and slightly caudally. A

12 ***Membrana propria ductus semicircularis***. Propria mucosae of the semicircular duct, external layer of the wall. C

13 ***Membrana basalis ductus semicircularis***. Basal membrane of the semicircular duct, thin layer between propria mucosae and epithelium. C

14 ***Epithelium ductus semicircularis***. Epithelium of the semicircular duct, simple squamous cells lining the interior of the duct. Along the concave surface of the duct is a strip of columnar cells that extends into the ampulla. C

15 ***Ampullae membranaceae***. Membranous ampullae, spindle-shaped enlargements of the semicircular ducts near their junction with the Utriculus, one for each duct.

16 *Ampulla membranacea anterior*. Enlargement of the anterior semicircular duct. A

17 *Ampulla membranacea posterior*. Enlargement of the posterior semicircular duct. A

18 *Ampulla membranacea lateralis*. Enlargement of the lateral semicircular duct. A

19 ***Crista ampullaris***. Semilunar crest projecting into the membranous ampulla, consists of connective tissue and nerve fibers, covered with neuroepithelium from which tufts of sensory hair project into the overlying cupula. B

20 ***Cupula***. Tall, gelatinous layer on the Crista ampullaris, bell-shaped in cross section, consists of fibrillar columns alternating with endolymphatic spaces for the sensory hairs of the neuroepithelium. B

21 ***Crura membranacea***. Ends of the semicircular ducts where they join the Utriculus.

22 *Crus membranaceum simplex*. Single nonampullated end of the lateral semicircular duct. A

23 *Crura membranacea ampullaria*. Junctions between the ampullated ends of the semicircular ducts and the Utriculus. A

24 *Crus membranaceum commune*. Common junction of the non-ampullated ends of the anterior and posterior semicircular ducts with the Utriculus. A

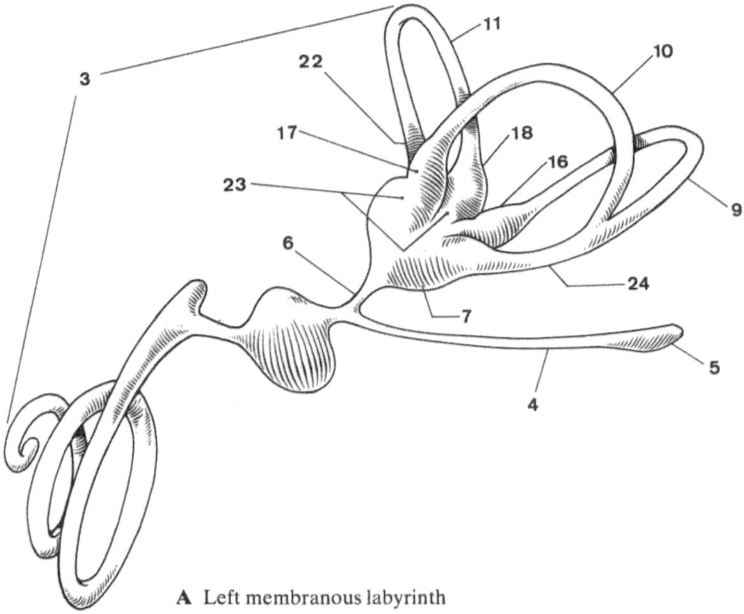

A Left membranous labyrinth

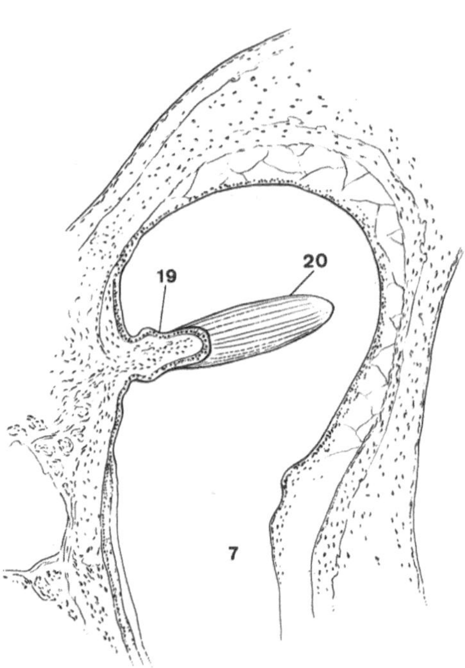

B Ampulla, section (guinea pig)

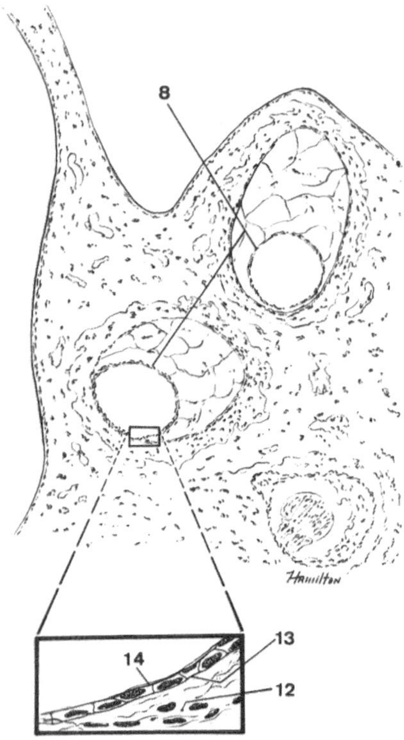

C Canales semicirculares, section (guinea pig)

1 ***Ductus reuniens***. Short duct connecting the Sacculus with the Ductus cochlearis. B

2 ***Sacculus***. Enlargement of the membranous labyrinth occupying the Recessus sphericus of the Vestibulum. B

3 ***Maculae***. Oval areas of neuroepithelium in the wall of the membranous labyrinth monitoring the position of the head. B

4 *Macula utriculi*. Macula in the medial wall of the Utriculus. B

5 *Macula sacculi*. Macula in the medial wall of the Sacculus. A B

6 *Statoconia*. Minute calcium carbonate rods in the surface of the Membrana statoconiorum. A

7 *Membrana statoconiorum*. Gelatinous layer covering the neuroepithelial cells of the macula. It contains the statoconia and the sensory hairs of the neuroepithelial cells. A

8 ***Endolympha***. Endolymph, fluid in the membranous labyrinth.

9 ***Perilympha***. Perilymph, fluid in the spaces between the membranous and osseous labyrinths.

10 ***Spatium perilymphaticum***. Perilymphatic space, between membranous and osseous labyrinths, subdivided by fine trabeculae, except in the scalae. A

11 *Scala vestibuli*. Perilymphatic space on the cupular surface of the Ductus cochlearis. C

12 *Scala tympani*. Perilymphatic space on the basilar surface of the Ductus cochlearis. C

13 *Ductus perilymphaticus*. Perilymphatic duct, connecting the perilymphatic space in the vicinity of the base of the cochlea to the subarachnoid space. B

14 **Ductus cochlearis**. Cochlear duct, the spiral part of the membranous labyrinth, triangular in cross section, that occupies the cochlea. B C

15 ***Cecum [Caecum] cupulare***. Blind end in the cupula of the cochlea. B

16 ***Cecum [Caecum] vestibulare***. Blind beginning in the Vestibulum near the Sacculus. B

17 ***Paries tympanicus ductus cochlearis [Membrana spiralis]***. Wall of the cochlear duct facing the Scala tympani. C

18 ***Organum spirale***. Spiral organ, complex neuroepithelium in the Paries tympanicus ductus cochlearis, transforming sound waves to nerve impulses. C

19 ***Lamina basilaris***. Basilar lamina, connective tissue components of the Paries tympanicus ductus cochlearis, extending from the Lamina spiralis ossea to the Lig. spirale cochleae. C

20 ***Crista spiralis [Ligamentum spirale]***. Spiral ligament of the cochlea, condensation of periosteum, triangular in cross section, extending from the periphery of the cochlea inward to the Lamina basilaris. C

20a ***Paries internus ductus cochlearis***. This term was introduced in analogy to the Nomina Histologica Veterinaria to indicate the internal wall of the cochlear duct formed by the Limbus laminae spiralis osseae and the protruding Membrana tectoria which border the Sulcus spiralis internus.

21 ***Foramina nervosa***. Foramina in the Lamina basilaris for nerve fibers going to the Organum spirale. C

22 ***Limbus laminae spiralis osseae***. Dense connective tissue on the vestibular surface of the Lamina spiralis ossea, extending peripherally and ending in two lips between which is the Sulcus spiralis internus. C

23 ***Labium limbi vestibulare***. Lip of the Limbus laminae spiralis osseae on the vestibular side of the Sulcus spiralis internus, continued peripherally by the Membrana tectoria. C

24 ***Labium limbi tympanicum***. Lip of the Limbus laminae spiralis osseae on the tympanic side of the Sulcus spiralis internus, continued by the Lamina basilaris. C

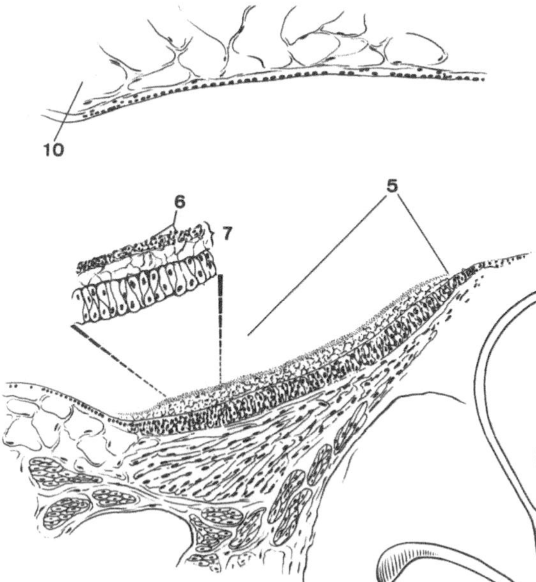

A Sacculus, section (guinea pig)

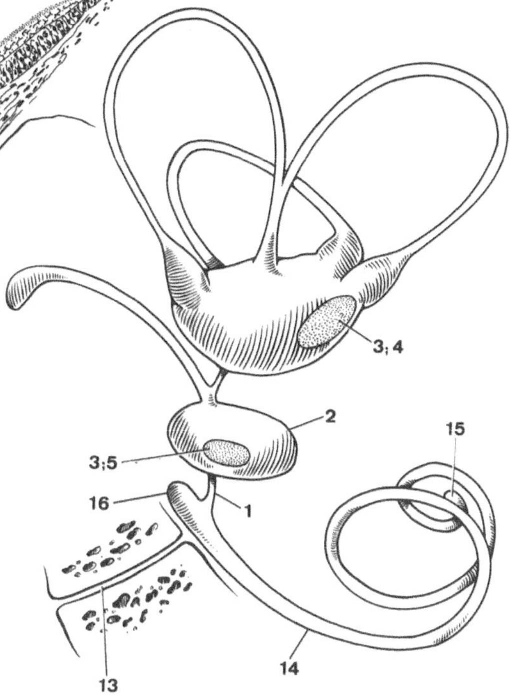

B Left membranous labyrinth, medial aspect

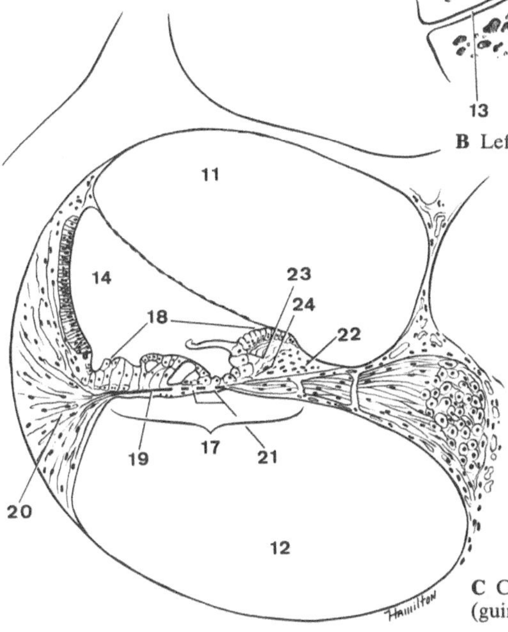

C Canalis spiralis cochleae, transverse section (guinea pig)

1 ***Membrana tectoria***. Tectorial membrane, continuation of the Labium limbi vestibulare overlying the Organum spirale and the Sulcus spiralis internus. A

2 ***Dentes acustici***. Tooth-like ridges on the vestibular surface of the Labium limbi vestibulare, caused by slightly projecting rows of cells. A

3 ***Sulcus spiralis internus***. Internal spiral sulcus, the groove between the two lips of the Limbus laminae spiralis osseae, covered by the Membrana tectoria. A

4 ***Sulcus spiralis externus***. External spiral sulcus, the groove on the peripheral end of the Organum spirale, at the junction of tympanic and external walls of the cochlear duct. A

5 ***Membrana reticularis***. Reticular membrane, covering the sensory cells of the Organum spirale, formed by the processes of the deeper lying phalangeal cells. Through its meshes project the sensory hairs of the sensory cells. A

6 ***Vas spirale***. Small vein under the Organum spirale on the tympanic side of the Lamina basilaris. A

7 ***Paries vestibularis ductus cochlearis [Membrana vestibularis]***. Vestibular wall of the cochlear duct, thin membrane between Scala vestibuli and Ductus cochlearis. A B

8 ***Paries externus ductus cochlearis***. External wall of the cochlear duct, lying against the Lig. spirale. A B

9 ***Crista basilaris***. Basilar crest of the Lig. spirale where it is continuous with the Lamina basilaris. A

10 ***Prominentia spiralis***. Spiral prominence in the external wall of the cochlear duct above the Sulcus spiralis externus. A

11 ***Vas prominens***. Small blood vessel in the Prominentia spiralis. A

12 ***Stria vascularis***. Thick layer of pigmented epithelium invaded by capillaries; it is thought to secrete endolymph. A

13 ***Ganglion spirale cochleae***. Spiral ganglion, cord-like accumulation of bipolar nerve cells in the modiolus of the cochlea. The dendrites come from the sensory cells in the Organum spirale, the axons form the N. cochlearis. A B See 474.15

14 **Vasa auris internae**. Vessels of the internal ear.

15 ***A. labyrinthi***. Labyrinthine artery, branch of A. basilaris or A. cerebelli caudalis, passes through the internal acoustic meatus into the petrosal bone to supply the internal ear. D

16 *Rami vestibulares*. Vestibular branches, for the supply of Utriculus, Ductus semicirculares, and Sacculus. D

17 *Ramus cochlearis*. Cochlear branch, passes into the center of the cochlea and supplies the cochlear duct and adjacent structures. D

18 *Glomerula arteriosa cochleae*. Glomus-type arteriovenous anastomoses between branches of Ramus cochlearis and Vas spirale. In bo and ov, they range from 0.5–2 mm in diameter, have also been seen in the Vestibulum. D

19 ***Vv. labyrinthi***. Labyrinthine veins, draining the internal ear, through Canaliculus cochleae (mainly) and Aqueductus vestibuli. There is no satellite vein to the A. labyrinthi in domestic mammals. C (Therefore, the Vv. labyrinthi should not be listed in the N. A. V.)

20 *V. spiralis modioli*. Spiral vein in the center of the cochlea. C

21 *Vv. vestibulares*. Vestibular veins, draining Utriculus, Ductus semicirculares, and Sacculus. C

22 *V. aqueductus [aquae-] vestibuli*. Vein in the Aqueductus vestibuli, draining Utriculus and Ductus semicirculares. C

23 *V. canaliculi cochleae*. Vein in the canaliculus cochleae, principal drainage of the internal ear. C

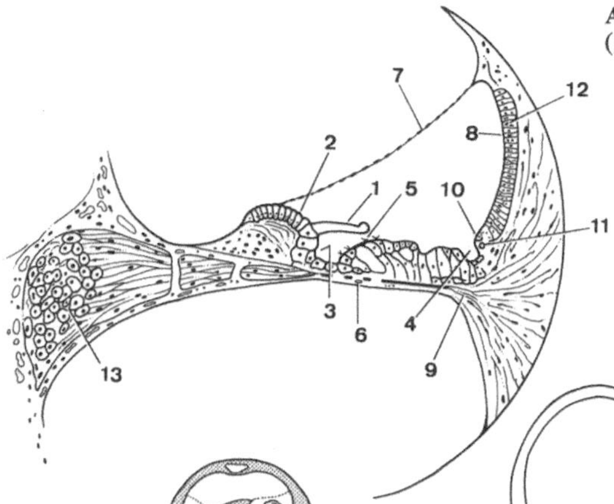

A Ductus cochlearis, transverse section (guinea pig)

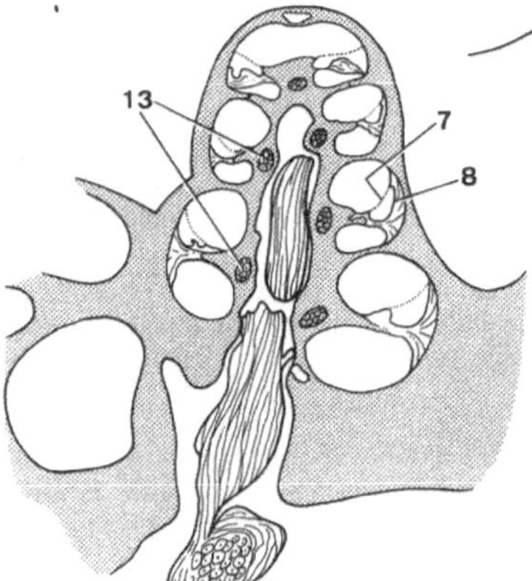

B Cochlea, longitudinal section (guinea pig)

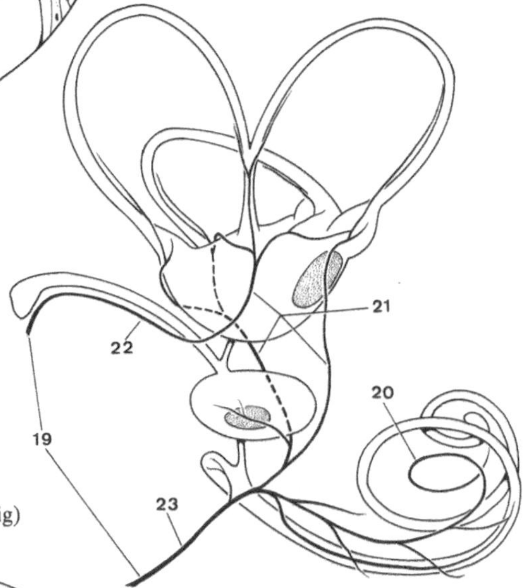

C Veins of the left membranous labyrinth, medial aspect (ca) (Shambaugh)

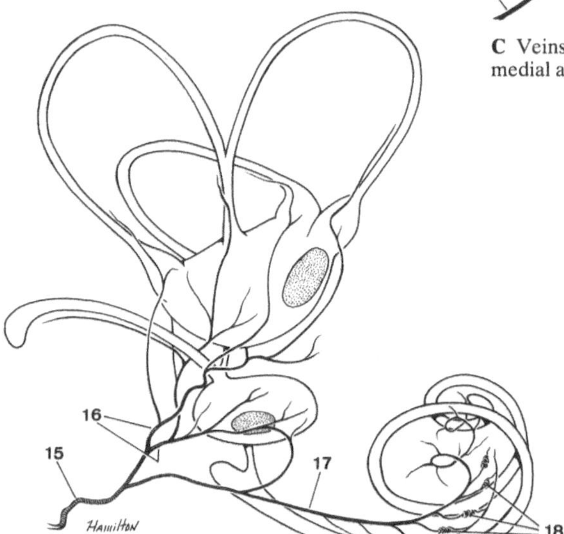

D Arteries of the left membranous labyrinth, medial aspect (ov) (Lewin)

1 **Labyrinthus osseus.** Osseous labyrinth, excavation in the petrosal bone, houses the membranous labyrinth. A

2 **Vestibulum**. Vestibule, contains Utriculus and Sacculus. B

3 ***Recessus sphericus [sphaericus].*** Spherical recess, in the anterior part of the Vestibulum containing the Sacculus. B

4 ***Recessus ellipticus.*** Ellipitcal recess, in the posterior part of the Vestibulum containing the Utriculus. B

5 ***Crista vestibuli.*** Vestibular crest, in the medial wall of the Vestibulum between Recessus sphericus and ellipticus. B

6 ***Recessus cochlearis.*** Cochlear recess, recess in the rostroventral wall of the Recessus sphericus for the Cecum vestibulare of the cochlear duct. B

7 ***Maculae cribrosae.*** Cribriform areas in the medial wall of the Vestibulum for the passage of the fibers of the N. vestibularis. B (These structures are omitted from the 5th edition of the N. A. V.)

8 **Canales semicirculares.** Osseous semicircular canals, 0.2–0.5 mm in diameter, containing the Ductus semicirculares. A

9 ***Canalis semicircularis anterior.*** Anterior semicircular canal, for the Ductus semicircularis anterior. D

10 ***Canalis semicircularis posterior.*** Posterior semicircular canal, for the Ductus semicircularis posterior. D

11 ***Canalis semicircularis lateralis.*** Lateral semicircular canal, for the Ductus semicircularis lateralis. D

12 ***Ampullae osseae.*** Osseous ampullae, fusifrom excavations at one end of the three semicircular canals for the Ampullae membranaceae.

13 *Ampulla osseae anterior.* Anterior osseous ampulla. D

14 *Ampulla ossea posterior.* Posterior osseous ampulla. D

15 *Ampulla ossea lateralis.* Lateral osseous ampulla. D

16 ***Crura ossea.*** The junctions of the osseous semicircular canals with the Vestibulum.

17 *Crus osseum commune.* The combined non-ampullated ends of the osseous anterior and posterior semicircular canals. D

18 *Crus osseum simplex.* The simple non-ampullated end of the lateral semicircular canal. D

19 *Crura ossea ampullaria.* The ampullated ends of the semicircular canals at the Vestibulum. D

20 **Cochlea.** Pyramidal excavation of the petrosal bone, similar in shape to a snail's shell. A

21 ***Cupula cochleae.*** Apex of the cochlea. C E

22 ***Basis cochleae.*** Base of the cochlea. C

23 ***Canalis spiralis cochleae.*** Spiral canal of the cochlea, winding around the modiolus in 1¼ to 4 turns. C D E

24 ***Modiolus.*** Cone-shaped osseous center of the cochlea. E

25 *Basis modioli.* Base of the modiolus, the center of the base of the cochlea. E

26 *Lamina modioli.* The spiral shelf passing around the modiolus between adjacent turns of the spiral canal of the cochlea. E

27 *Canalis spiralis modioli.* Spiral canal of the modiolus, space for the Ganglion spirale cochleae in the base of the Lamina spiralis ossea. E

28 *Canales longitudinales modioli.* Longitudinal canals of the modiolus, containing the fibers of the N. cochlearis. E

29 ***Lamina spiralis ossea.*** Osseous spiral lamina, shelf projecting from the modiolus into the Canalis spiralis cochleae. E

30 *Hamulus laminae spiralis.* Hook-like end of the Lamina spiralis ossea in the Cupula cochleae. E

31 ***Helicotrema.*** Opening by which Scala vestibuli and Scala tympani communicate in the Cupula cochleae. E

32 ***Lamina spiralis secundaria.*** Projects from the outer wall of Canalis spiralis cochleae, opposite to Lamina spiralis ossea, attachment of Lamina basilaris, present only in the basal turn. E

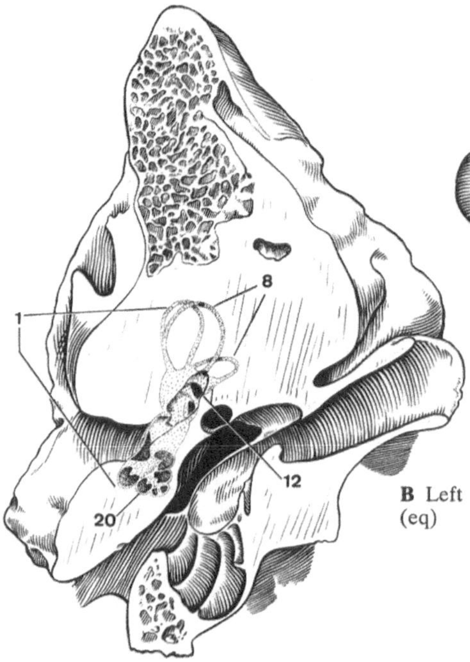

A Left petrosal bone, transverse section, rostral aspect (eq)

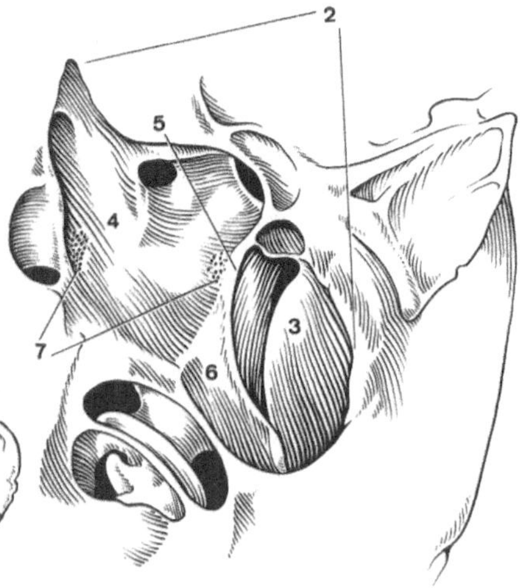

B Left osseous labyrinth, opened, ventral aspect (eq)

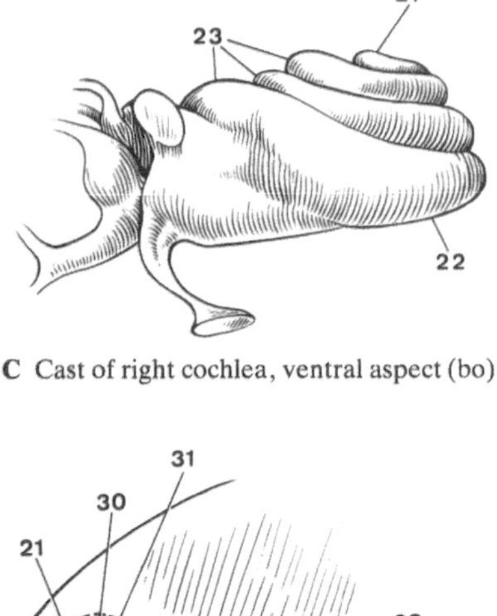

C Cast of right cochlea, ventral aspect (bo)

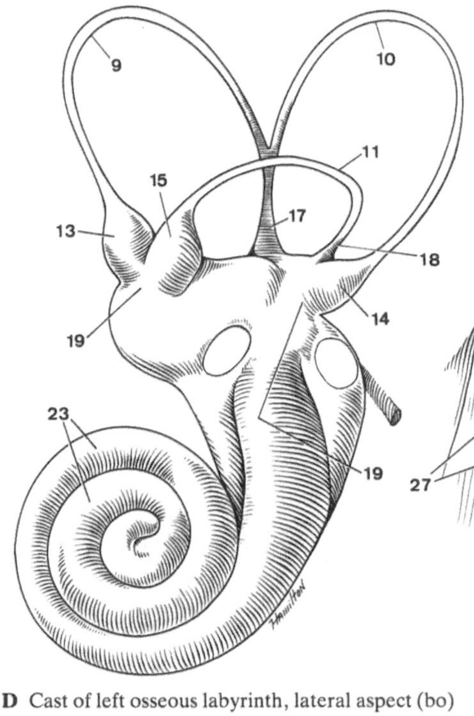

D Cast of left osseous labyrinth, lateral aspect (bo)

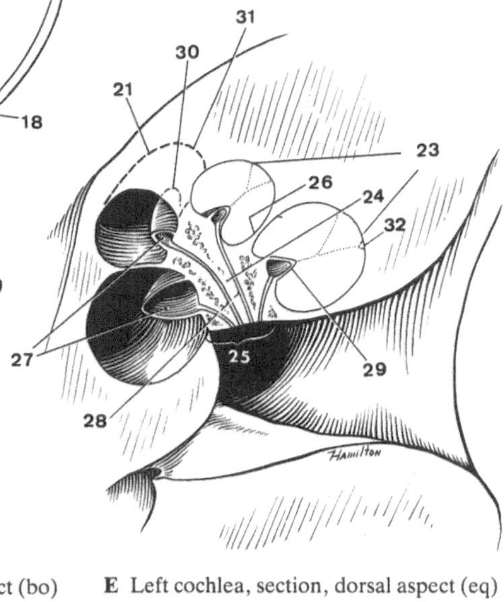

E Left cochlea, section, dorsal aspect (eq)

1 **Meatus acusticus internus**. Internal acoustic meatus, passage in the medial surface of the petrosal bone for N. facialis and N. vestibulocochlearis. A

2 ***Porus acusticus internus***. The orifice of the internal acoustic meatus. B

3 ***Fundus meatus acustici interni***. Fundus (floor) of the internal acoustic meatus. C

4 *Crista transversa*. Transverse crest, dividing the fundus into upper and lower parts. C

5 *Area n. facialis [intermediofacialis]*. Part of the fundus that contains the beginning of the facial nerve canal and shelters the N. facialis. C

6 *Area cochleae*. Small cribriform area, spiral in appearance, perforated by fibers of N. cochlearis. C

7 ***Tractus spiralis foraminosus***. Inward spiraling tract of minute foramina in the center of the Area cochleae. C

8 *Area vestibularis superior*. Small cribriform area perforated by fibers of the N. utriculoampullaris. C

9 *Area vestibularis inferior*. Small cribriform area perforated by fibers of the N. saccularis. C

10 *Foramen singulare*. Orifice for the N. ampullaris posterior. C

11 **AURIS MEDIA**. Middle ear, consists of tympanic cavity, tympanic membrane, auditory ossicles, and auditory tube.

12 **Cavum tympani**. Tympanic cavity, oblique space between Pars petrosa and tympanica of the temporal bone. In it the auditory ossicles transmit the vibrations of the tympanic membrane to the perilymphatic space in the internal ear. A

13 ***Paries tegmentalis***. Dorsal wall of the tympanic cavity. D E

14 *Recessus epitympanicus*. Epitympanic recess, dorsal part of the tympanic cavity, containing the auditory ossicles. E

15 *Pars cupularis*. A rounded recess in the upper part of the Recessus epitympanicus. E

16 ***Paries jugularis***. Caudoventral wall of the tympanic cavity. D

17 ***Paries labyrinthicus***. Medial wall of the tympanic cavity, formed by the petrosal bone. E

18 *Fenestra vestibuli*. Vestibular window, closed by the base of the stapes by means of which the vibrations act on the perilymph in the internal ear. E

19 *Promontorium*. Promontory, the convexity on the medial wall of the tympanic cavity caused by the basal turn of the cochlea. E

20 *Sinus tympani*. Depression posterior to the Promontorium and Fenestra cochleae of man. (Therefore, this structure should not be listed in the N. A. V.)

21 *Fenestra cochleae*. Cochlear window, round foramen in the medial wall of the tympanic cavity, communication to the Scala tympani, closed by the Membrana tympani secundaria. E

22 *Membrana tympani secundaria*. Secondary tympanic membrane, closing the Fenestra cochleae.

23 ***Paries mastoideus***. Caudodorsal wall of the tympanic cavity. D

24 *Annexae mastoideae*. This term was introduced in the NA for the clinically important airspaces in the human mastoid. Similar spaces are present in su and bo.

25 *Cellulae tympanicae*. The subdivisions of the ventral part of the tympanic cavity, not present in Car. D

26 *Apertura tympanica canaliculi chordae tympani*. Tympanic opening of the canal for the Chorda tympani. D

27 ***Paries caroticus***. Rostral wall of the tympanic cavity. D E

28 ***Paries membranaceus***. Lateral wall of the tympanic cavity, formed mainly by the tympanic membrane. D

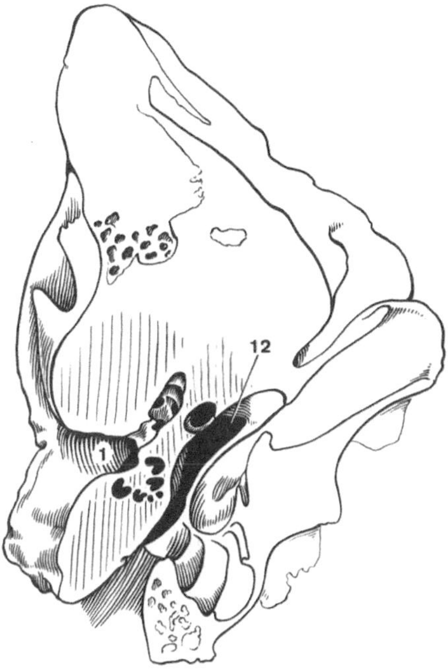

A Petrous and tympanic parts of left temporal bone, transverse section, rostral aspect (eq)

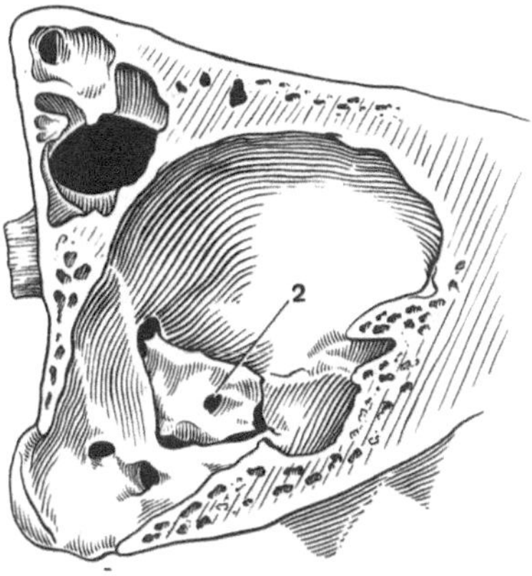

B Cranial cavity, medial aspect (bo)

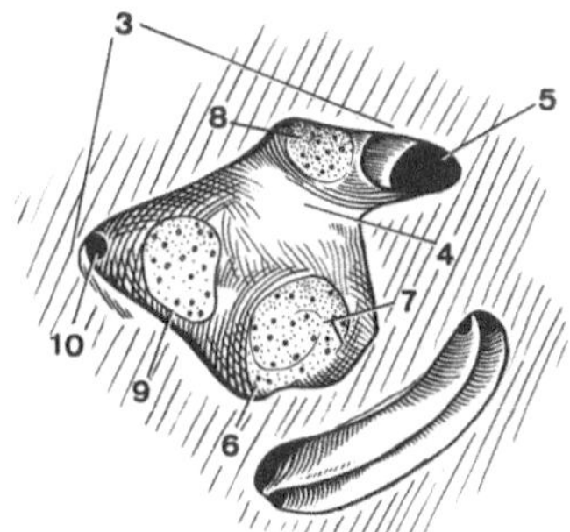

C Fundus of left internal acoustic meatus (eq)

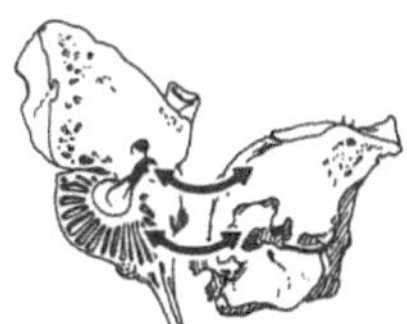

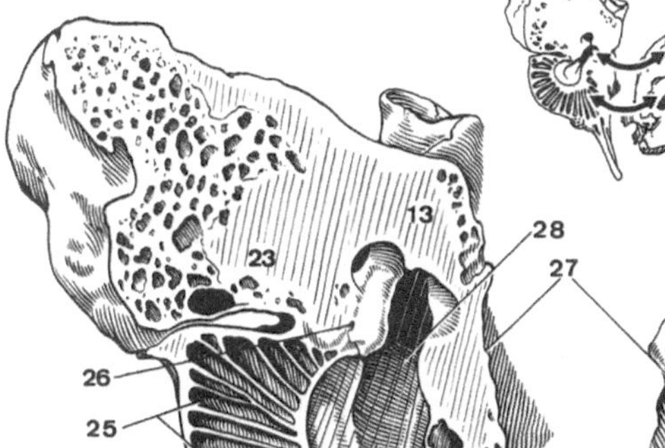

D Petrous and tympanic parts of left temporal bone, sagittal section, medial aspect (eq)

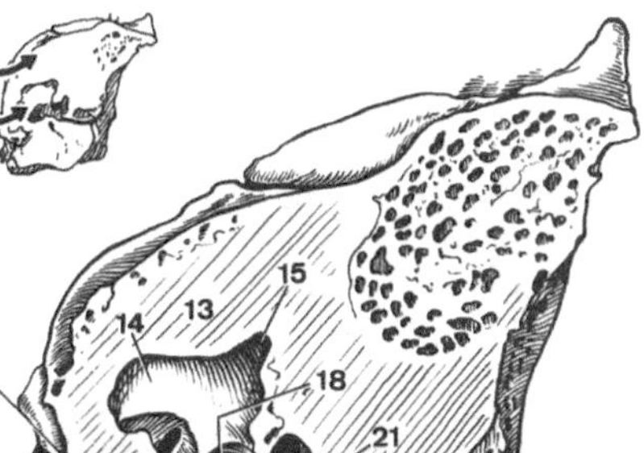

E Petrous and tympanic parts of left temporal bone, sagittal section, lateral aspect (eq)

1 **Membrana tympani**. Tympanic membrane, obliquely placed at the medial end of the external acoustic meatus. B

2 ***Pars flaccida***. Flaccid part, dorsal to the Pars tensa, closes the notch in the dorsal wall of the external acoustic meatus. A B (the only part of the tympanic membrane suited for myringotomy [paracentesis of the tympanic membrane])

3 ***Pars tensa***. Tense part, the large functional part attached to the Anulus tympanicus. A B

4 ***Plica mallearis rostralis***. Rostral fold attaching the proximal part of the Manubrium mallei to the Anulus tympanicus. B

5 ***Plica mallearis caudalis***. Caudal fold attaching the proximal part of the Manubrium mallei to the Anulus tympanicus. B

6 ***Prominentia mallearis***. Elevation of the tympanic membrane caused by the Processus lateralis mallei. A

7 ***Stria mallearis***. Light strip on the tympanic membrane caused by the Manubrium mallei. A

8 ***Umbo membranae tympani***. The apex of the tympanic membrane, projecting into the tympanic cavity caused by the distal end of the Manubrium mallei. B

9 ***Anulus fibrocartilagineus***. The fibrocartilaginous ring by means of which the tympanic membrane is attached to the osseous Anulus tympanicus. B D

10 **Ossicula auditus**. Auditory ossicles, three articulating bones, that transmit the vibrations of the tympanic membrane across the tympanic cavity to the perilymph in the Scala vestibuli. C

11 ***Stapes***. Most internal auditory ossicle, articulates with the incus and closes the Fenestra vestibuli. C

12 *Caput stapedis*. Head of stapes, articulates with the incus through the interposed Os lenticulare. C

13 *Crus rostrale*. Limb of stapes, connecting head and base rostrally. C

14 *Crus caudale*. Limb of stapes, connecting head and base caudally. C

15 *Basis stapedis*. Base of stapes, closes the Fenestra vestibuli. C

16 ***Incus***. Middle auditory ossicle, articulates with stapes and malleus. C

17 *Corpus incudis*. Body of incus, articulates with the malleus. C

18 *Crus longum*. Long process, articulates with the stapes. C

19 **Processus lenticularis**. Lenticular process, the end of the Crus longum which articulates with the stapes in man and occasionally ca. C

20 **Os lenticulare**. Minute accessory ossicle in the articulation between incus and stapes. C

21 *Crus breve*. Short process, attached to the wall of the Recessus epitympanicus. C

22 ***Malleus***. Most external auditory ossicle, articulates with the incus, its manubrium is embedded in the tympanic membrane. C

23 *Manubrium mallei*. Handle-like process of the malleus which is embedded in the tympanic membrane. C

24 *Caput mallei*. Head of malleus, articulates with the incus. C

25 *Collum mallei*. Indistinct constriction between head and manubrium of the malleus. C

26 *Processus lateralis*. Short lateral process at the proximal end of the manubrium. C

27 *Processus rostralis*. Long rostral process, connected to the vicinity of the Anulus tympanicus. C

28 *Processus muscularis*. Muscular process, attachment of the M. tensor tympani. C

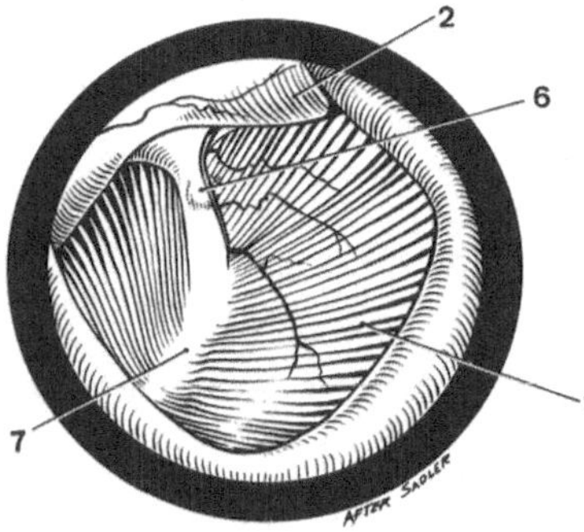

A Left tympanic membrane as seen through the otoscope (ca) (de Lahunta and Habel)

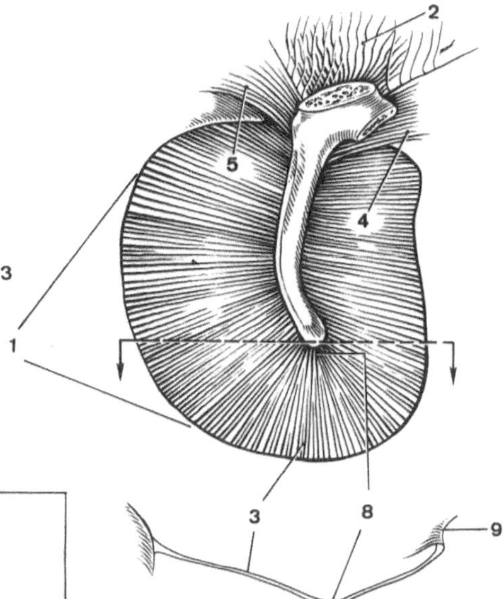

B Left tympanic membrane, internal surface (ca) (Spreull)

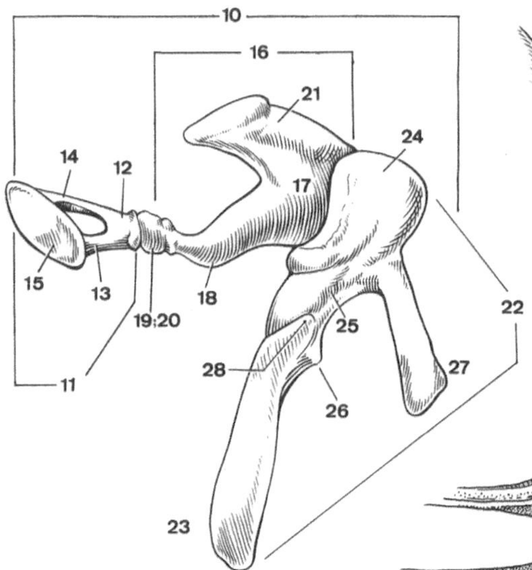

C Left auditory ossicles, rostromedial aspect (eq) (Holz)

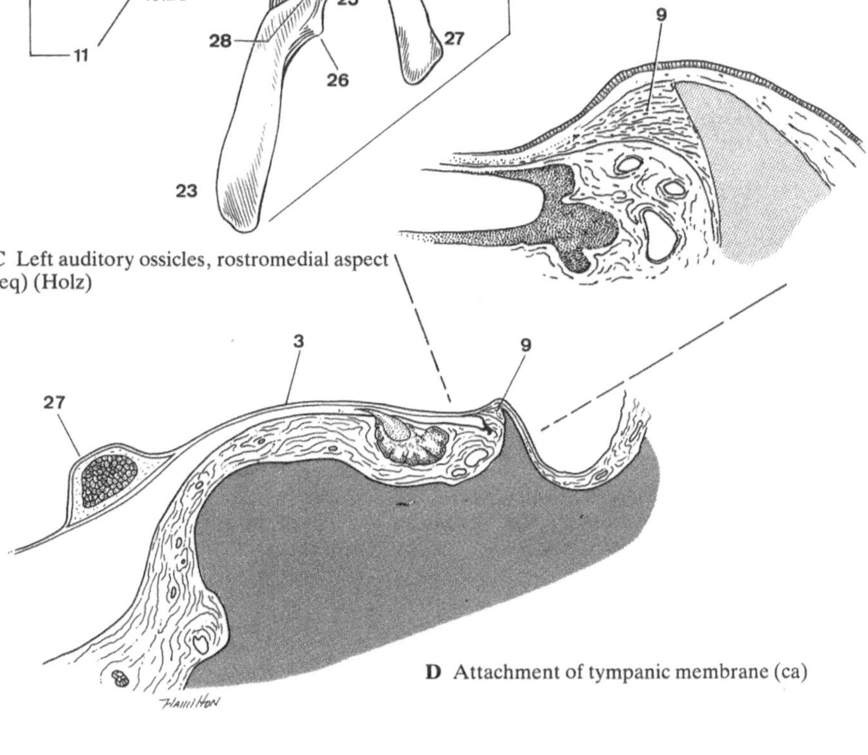

D Attachment of tympanic membrane (ca)

1 ***Articulationes ossiculorum auditus.*** Articulations of the auditory ossicles.

2 *Articulatio incudomallearis.* Articulation between the body of incus and the head of malleus. A

3 *Articulatio incudostapedia.* Articulation between the Crus longum of the incus, the Os lenticulare, and the head of stapes. A

4 *Syndesmosis tympanostapedia.* Attachment of the base of stapes to the margin of Fenestra vestibuli by the Lig. anulare stapedis. A

5 ***Ligg. ossiculorum auditus.*** Ligaments that attach the auditory ossicles to the walls of the tympanic cavity.

6 *Ligg. mallei.* Ligaments associated with the malleus. A

7 *Ligg. incudis.* Ligaments associated with the incus. A

8 *Membrana stapedis.* Stapedial membrane, closing the space between crura and base of stapes. D

9 *Lig. anulare stapedis.* Anular ligament of stapes, attaching the base of stapes to the margin of the Fenestra vestibuli. A D

10 ***Mm. ossiculorum auditus.*** Muscles associated with the auditory ossicles.

11 *M. tensor tympani.* Arises from the wall of the tympanic cavity, ends on the Processus muscularis of the malleus. A B

12 *M. stapedius.* Arises from the wall of the tympanic cavity, ends on the head of stapes, slowing the vibrations of the ossicles. A

13 **Tunica mucosa cavi tympani.** Mucous membrane lining the tympanic cavity, reflected over the auditory ossicles.

14 ***Plica mallearis caudalis.*** Caudal malleolar fold, from the Manubrium mallei to the caudal part of the Anulus tympanicus, contains the Chorda tympani. B

15 ***Plica mallearis rostralis.*** Rostral malleolar fold, from the Manubrium mallei to the rostral part of the Anulus tympanicus, contains the Chorda tympani. B

16 ***Plica mallearis tympani.*** Fold covering the Chorda tympani crossing the dorsal part of the tympanic membrane. B

17 ***Plica incudis.*** Fold reflected over the Crus breve of the incus. A

18 ***Plica stapedis.*** Fold reflected over the stapes and the M. stapedius. A

19 **Tuba auditiva.** Auditory (Eustachian, pharyngotympanic) tube, connecting the tympanic cavity with the nasopharynx. E

20 ***Ostium tympanicum tubae auditivae.*** Tympanic opening of the auditory tube. C

21 ***Pars ossea tubae auditivae.*** Osseous part of the auditory tube, the short caudal part, supported by the temporal and (in part) basisphenoid bones. C

22 *Isthmus tubae auditivae.* The constriction of the auditory tube at the junction of its osseous and cartilaginous parts. C

23 ***Pars cartilaginea tubae auditivae.*** Cartilaginous part of the auditory tube, the longer rostral part supported by cartilage. C

24 *Cartilago tubae auditivae.* Cartilage of the auditory tube, shaped like an inverted trough. C

25 **Lamina [cartilaginis] medialis.** Wider medial lamina of the cartilage. C

26 **Lamina [cartilaginis] lateralis.** Shorter lateral lamina of the cartilage. C

27 *Lamina membranacea.* The portion of the wall that is not supported by cartilage. C

28 ***Tunica mucosa.*** Mucous membrane, covered with pseudostratified ciliated epithelium containing goblet cells. C

29 *Glandulae tubariae.* Mucous or mixed glands in the wall of the auditory tube, esp. numerous in ov. C

30 ***Lymphonoduli [Noduli lymphatici] tubarii.*** Lymph nodules in the wall of the auditory tube, well developed in Ru and su, forming the tubal tonsil. C

31 ***Ostium pharyngeum tubae auditivae.*** Pharyngeal opening of the auditory tube, in the lateral wall of the nasopharynx. E

32 ***Diverticulum tubae auditivae*** (eq). Guttural pouch of eq, caudoventral enlargement of the auditory tube with a capacity of about 300 ml. E

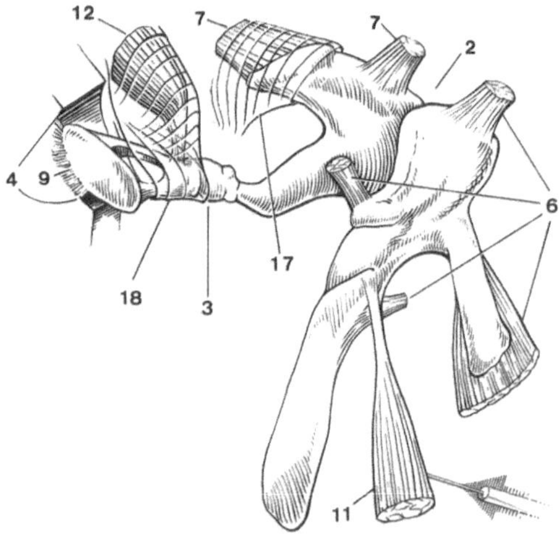

A Muscles and ligaments of the left auditory ossicles, rostromedial aspect (eq)

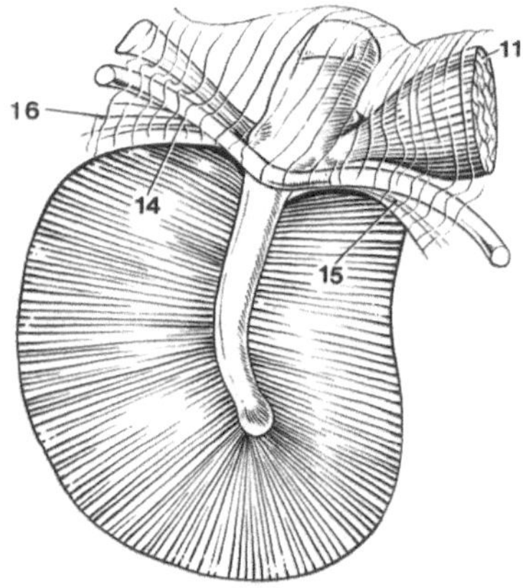

B Left tympanic membrane, internal surface (ca) (Spreull)

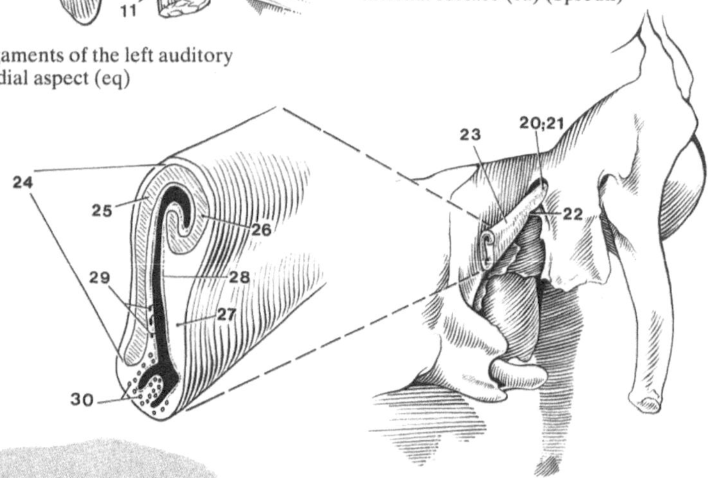

C Left auditory tube, schematic (su)

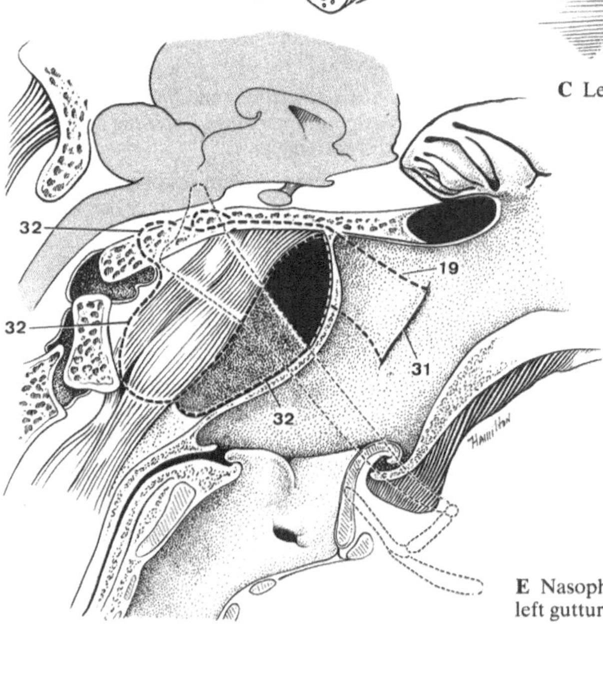

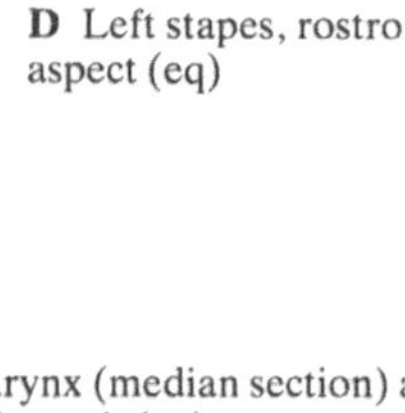

D Left stapes, rostromedial aspect (eq)

E Nasopharynx (median section) and left guttural pouch (eq)

1 **AURIS EXTERNA**. External ear, consisting of the auricle and the external acoustic meatus. B

2 **Meatus acusticus externus**. External acoustic meatus, the canal leading from the base of the auricle to the tympanic membrane. B

3 ***Porus acusticus externus***. Opening of the osseous part of the external acoustic meatus, visible on the skull. A

4 ***Meatus acusticus externus cartilagineus***. The cartilaginous part of the external acoustic meatus. B

5 *Cartilago anularis*. Anular cartilage, separate, supporting the external acoustic meatus proximal to the rolled-up part of the auricular cartilage. B D

6 **Cartilago meatus acustici**. Rolled-up proximal part of the auricular cartilage, supports the distal portion of the external acoustic meatus. B D (In the dog the cartilage is bent rostrally, showing on the caudal aspect a palpable conchal eminence, landmark in surgical procedures on the external ear.)

7 *Incisurae cartilaginis meatus acustici*. Notches in the rolled-up proximal part of the auricular cartilage. B E

8 ***Lamina tragi***. Prominent rostral portion of the rolled-up proximal part of the auricular cartilage. B E

9 **Auricula**. Auricle, the externally visible part of the ear. C

10 ***Cartilago auriculae***. Auricular cartilage, covered with skin on both sides; it gives the various shapes to the ears of the domestic mammals. E

11 ***Helix***. The free margin of the auricle passing over the apex. B E

12 ***Crus helicis mediale***. Medial crus of helix, the mediocaudal crus at the proximal end of the Margo tragicus. B E

13 ***Crus helicis laterale***. Lateral crus of helix, the laterorostral crus at the proximal end of the Margo tragicus. B E

14 ***Spina helicis***. Spine of helix, a projection in ca and su on the Margo tragicus distal to the crura. E

15 ***Cauda helicis***. Tail of helix, the proximal end of the Margo antitragicus, separated from the antitragus by a more or less distinct notch. D

16 ***Margo tragicus***. The rostromedial margin of the auricle. E

17 ***Margo antitragicus***. The caudolateral margin of the auricle. E

18 *Saccus cutaneus marginalis*. A cutaneous pouch on the Margo antitragicus in Car; only its rostral wall is supported by cartilage. C E

19 ***Scapha***. Concave internal side of the auricle. B E

20 *Plicae scaphae*. Ridges on the internal surface of the auricle. B E

21 ***Concha auriculae***. The funnel-shaped proximal part of the auricle. B

22 ***Cavum conchae***. Auricular cavity, the cavity of the funnel-shaped proximal part of the auricle. B

23 ***Antitragus***. The part of the auricle that forms the rostrolateral wall of the Cavum conchae; it is supported by a part of the auricular cartilage that is separated from the Margo antitragicus by a more or less distinct notch. E

24 *Processus antitragicus lateralis*. A process of the auricular cartilage, prominent in ca, projecting in the direction of the Margo antitragicus. D E

25 *Processus antitragicus medialis*. A ridge of the auricular cartilage passing caudally from the antitragus. E

26 *Plica antitragica*. A skin fold passing proximally from the antitragus into the Cavum conchae in ca. C

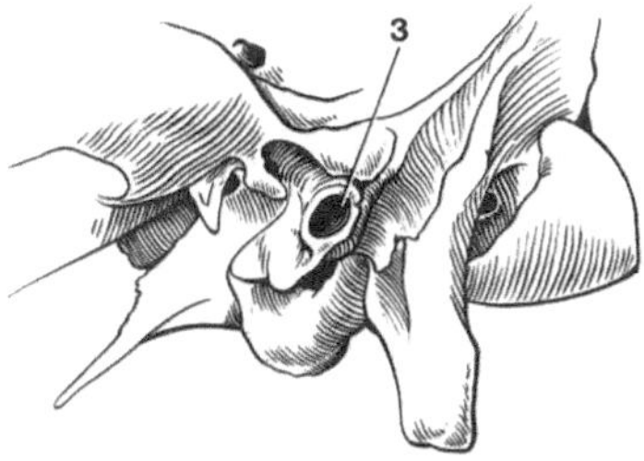

A Caudoventral part of skull, left aspect (bo)

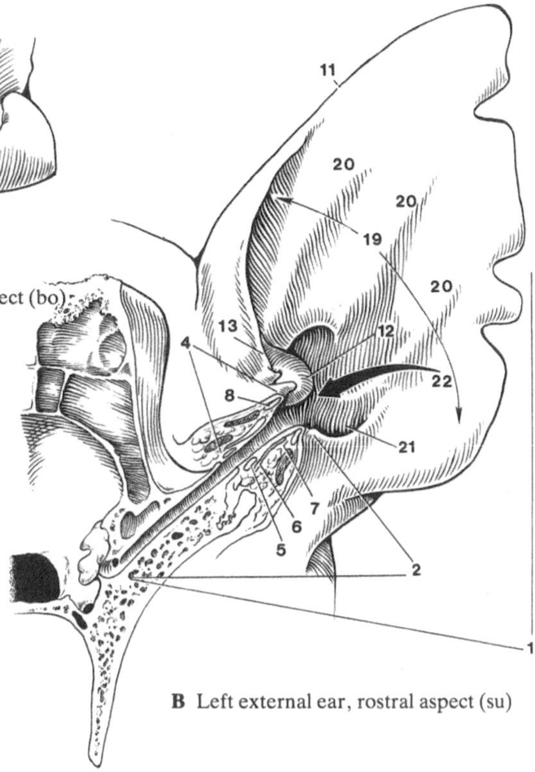

B Left external ear, rostral aspect (su)

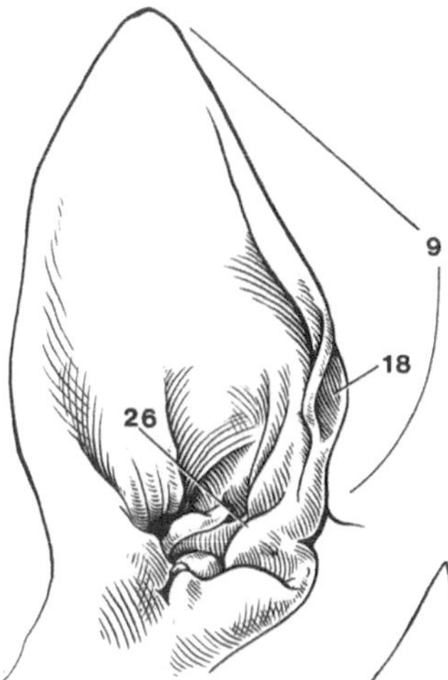

C Left auricle, shaved, rostral aspect (ca)

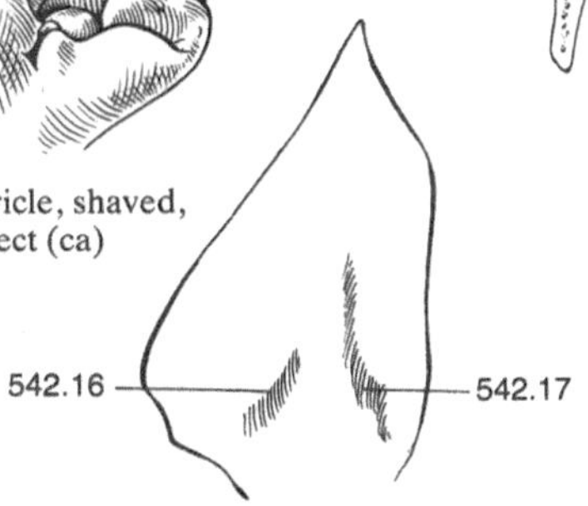

F Left auricular cartilage, caudomedial aspect (su) (Horowitz and Sack)

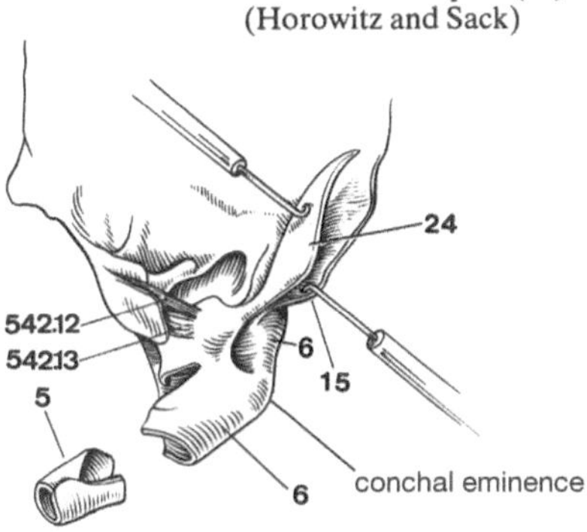

D Left Cartilagines meatus acustici and anularis, rostral aspect (ca)

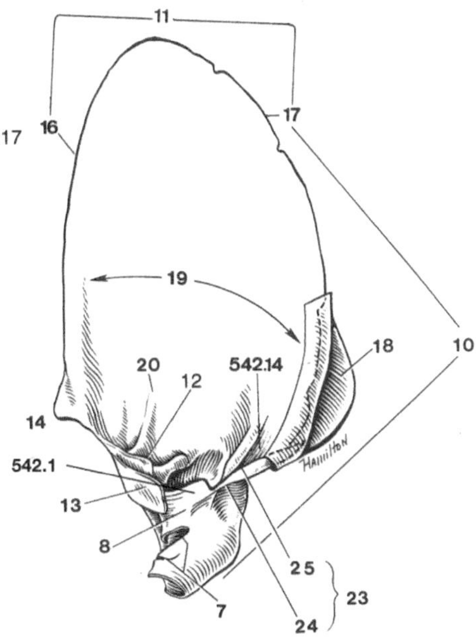

E Left auricular cartilage (ca)

1 ***Tragus***. An elongated prominence on the rostromedial border of the entrance to the Cavum conchae. A E 541 E

2 ***Incisura pretragica [prae-]***. Pretragic notch, rostromedial to the tragus, separating it from the Crus helicis laterale. A B

3 ***Incisura intertragica***. Intertragic notch, caudolateral to the tragus, separating it from the antitragus. A B E

4 ***Apex auriculae***. Tip of the auricle. A

5 ***Incisura terminalis***. Notch separating the Lamina tragi from the remainder of the auricular cartilage. E

6 ***Incisura antitragohelicina***. Antitragohelicine notch, between the antitragus and the helix. E

7 ***Processus styloideus***. Styloid process, the drawn-out proximal end of the auricular cartilage overlapping the anular cartilage caudolaterally, prominent in eq. B

8 ***Eminentia conchae***. The caudolateral bulge on the rolled-up part of the auricular cartilage indicating a change in direction of the Cartilago meatus acustici. E

9 ***Dorsum auriculae***. The convex surface of the auricle. A

10 ***Mm. auriculares***. Intrinsic auricular muscles, very small and of little importance.

11 *M. helicis*. On the Margo tragicus.

12 *M. helicis minor*. Between Crus helicis mediale and laterale, attached to Lamina tragi. 541 D

13 *M. tragicus*. Between Crus helicis laterale and Lamina tragi. 541 D

14 *M. antitragicus*. Caudal to Incisura intertragica. 541 E

15 *M. caudoantitragicus*. On the caudal surface of antitragus.

16 *M. transversus auriculae*. On the outer surface of concha. 541 F

17 *M. obliquus auriculae*. On the outer surface of concha. 541 F

18 ***Cartilago scutiformis***. Scutiform cartilage, rostromedial to the base of the auricle, lying on M. temporalis and fat. It gives attachment to several muscles that move the auricle. C

19 ***Corpus adiposum auriculare***. Auricular fat pad, surrounding the external acoustic meatus. C

20 **ORGANUM OLFACTUS**. Olfactory organ. D

21 ***Regio olfactoria tunicae mucosae nasi***. Olfactory region. The olfactory mucosa on the caudal portions of the Conchae ethmoidales and the Septum nasi. D

22 ***Glandulae olfactoriae***. Olfactory glands, serous glands deep to the olfactory epithelium. G

23 **ORGANUM VOMERONASALE**. Vomeronasal organ, former organ of Jacobson. The olfactory capability is thought to be related to sexual behavior and the recognition of kin. In some species it functions as an accessory olfactory organ. H

24 ***Ductus vomeronasalis***. Vomeronasal duct, caudally blind-ending tube of olfactory mucosa and associated olfactory glands. H

25 ***Cartilago vomeronasalis***. Vomeronasal cartilage, trough-shaped supporting the Ductus vomeronasalis. H

26 **ORGANUM GUSTUS**. Organ of taste, composed of all the taste buds.

27 ***Caliculus gustatorius***. Taste bud, spindle-shaped aggregation of sustentacular and gustatory cells of the same height as the surrounding epithelium. The gustatory cells bear microvilli with which they project through the Porus gustatorius. F

28 ***Porus gustatorius***. Taste pore, opening in the epithelium at the tip of the taste bud through which ingested substances reach the exposed ends of the gustatory cells. F

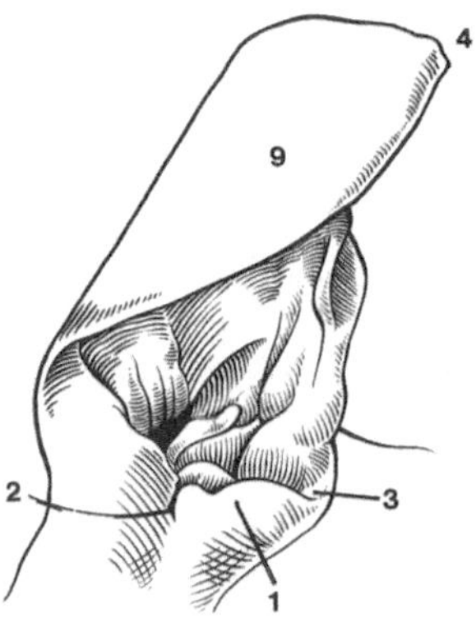

A Left auricle, shaved, rostrolateral aspect (ca)

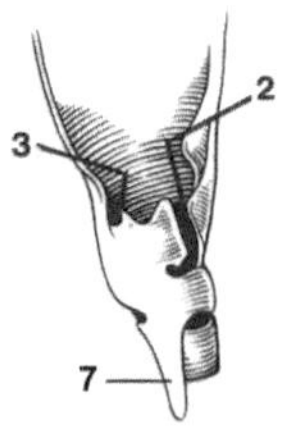

B Right Cartilagines meatus acustici and anularis, rostrolateral aspect (eq)

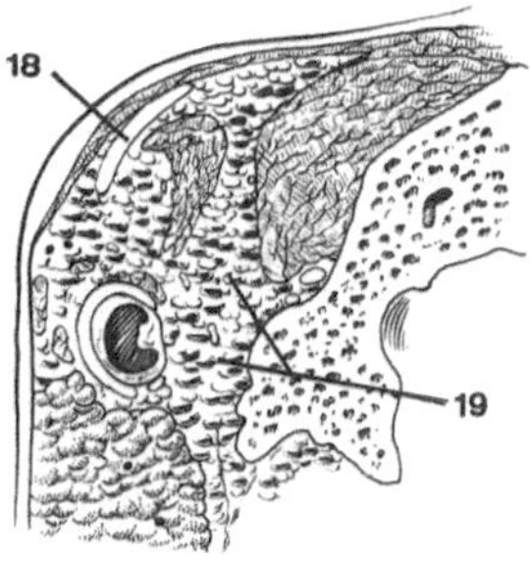

C Cartilago scutiformis and Corpus adiposum auriculare, transverse section (eq)

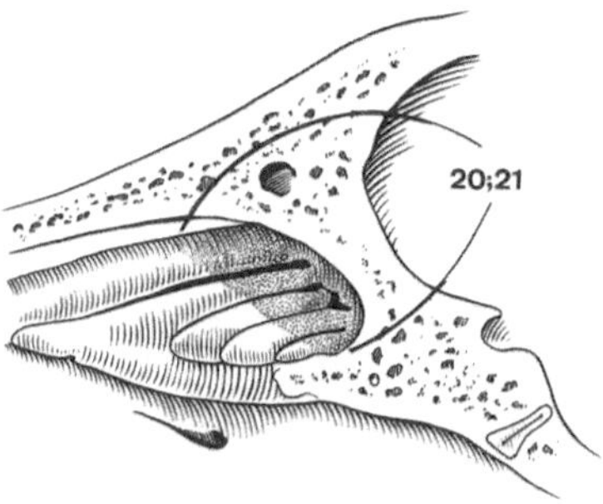

D Right nasal conchae (ov)

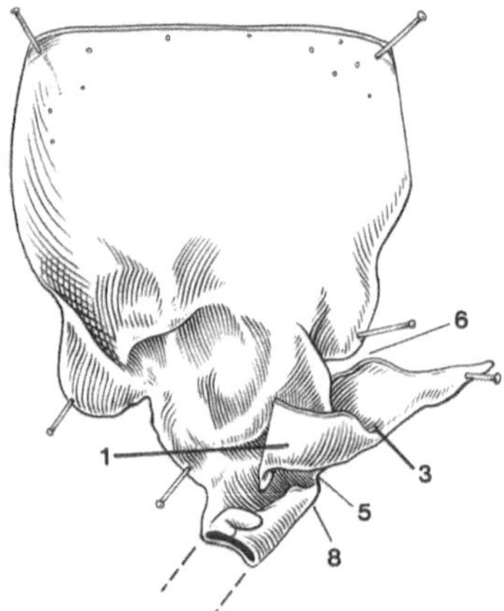

E Left auricular cartilage, rostral aspect (ca)

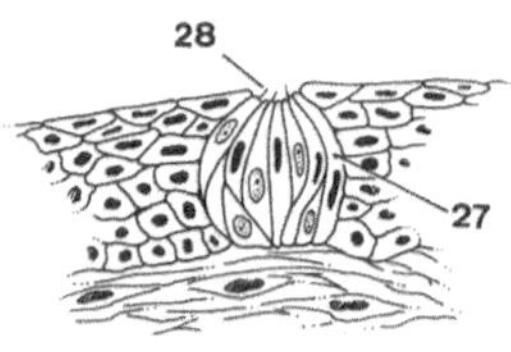

F Taste bud, histologic section

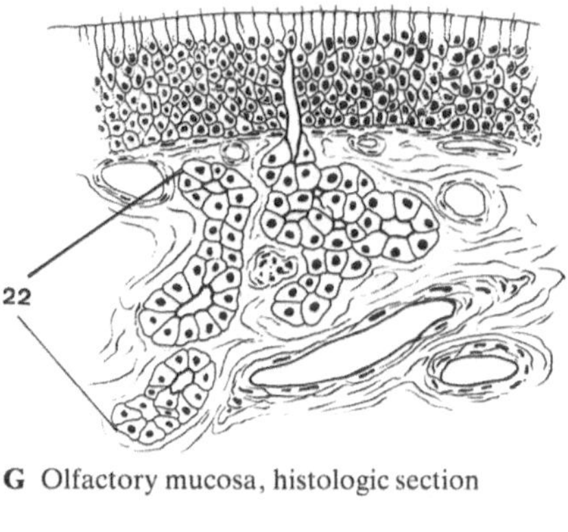

G Olfactory mucosa, histologic section

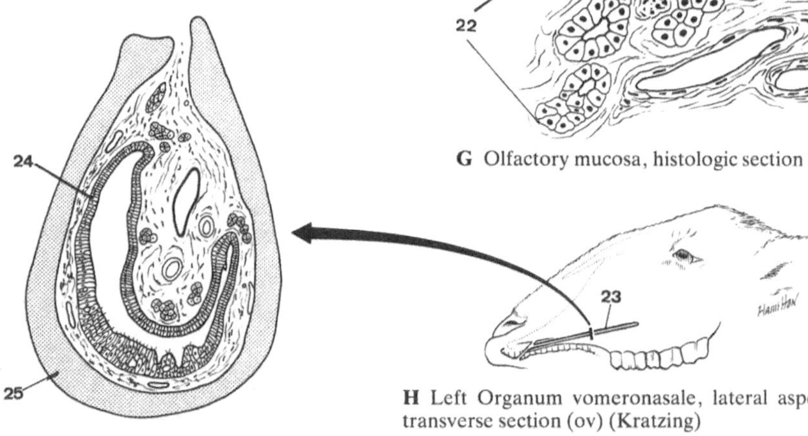

H Left Organum vomeronasale, lateral aspect and transverse section (ov) (Kratzing)

1 **CUTIS**. Skin, consisting of epidermis, dermis and tela subcutanea.

2 ***Sulci cutis***. Grooves of the skin of various depths and locations. A B

3 ***Cristae cutis***. Crests of the skin, formed by the epidermis and separated by small Sulci cutis. A

4 ***Retinacula cutis***. Strands of connective tissue attaching the skin to underlying fascia or periosteum. H

5 ***Plicae cutis***. Permanent folds of the skin in various regions. B C

6 ***Palear*** (bo). Dewlap. C

7 ***Plicae transversae colli*** (ov). Large permanent folds on the neck of Merino sheep. B

8 ***Appendices colli*** (su, ov, cap). Wattles. Cutaneous appendages on the ventral surface of the neck containing a bar of cartilage; most commonly in cap. E

9 ***Toruli tactiles*** (Car). Tactile elevations.

10 ***Sinus cutanei***. General term for various cutaneous pouches.

11 *Sinus infraorbitalis* (ov). Cutaneous pouch rostral to the eye, containing a fatty yellow secretion. B

12 *Sinus inguinalis* (ov). Cutaneous pouch in the inguinal region, containing a fatty yellow secretion. D

13 *Sinus paranalis* (Car)*. Cutaneous sac, opening into the anus and containing a fatty gray secretion with an unpleasant odor. F

14 *Sinus interdigitalis* (ov). Tubular invagination of the skin between the digits, containing a colorless waxy secretion. G

15 **Epidermis**. The stratified, squamous epithelium on the surface of the skin. H

16 **Dermis [Corium]**. The connective tissue layer of the skin deep to the epidermis, well supplied with vessels and nerves and containing the cutaneous glands. H

17 ***Papillae dermales [coriales]***. Dermal projections of various length and thickness, also branched, that are received into corresponding depressions of the epidermis. H

17a ***Cristae dermales [coriales]***. Dermal crests.

17b ***Lamellae dermales [coriales]***. The Cristae and Lamellae dermales (coriales) are two distinct basic formations of dermis

18 ***Terminationes nervorum***. Collective term for the sensory nerve endings. K

19 **Tela subcutanea [Hypodermis]**. Subcutaneous tissue consisting of collagenous and elastic fibers and fat. It merges with the overlying dermis and is loosely attached to the fascia deep to it. H

20 ***Panniculus adiposus***. Thick deposit of fat in the tela subcutanea, such as the back fat in su. I

21 ***Terminationes nervorum***. Collective term for the sensory nerve endings.

* Reminder: The structures followed by an asterisk are landmarks for physical examination and/or clinical approach.

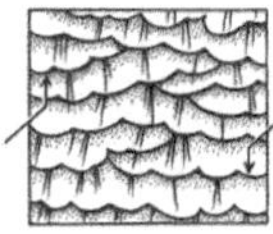

A Skin of back (ca)

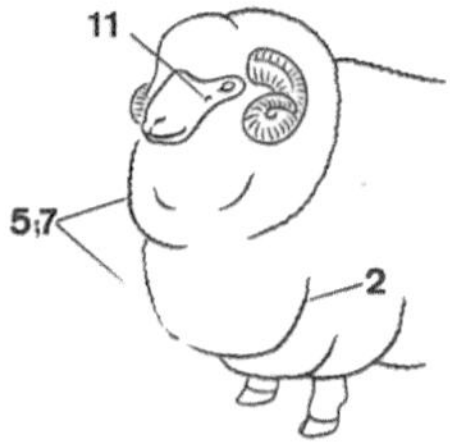

B Head and neck (ov masc, Merino)

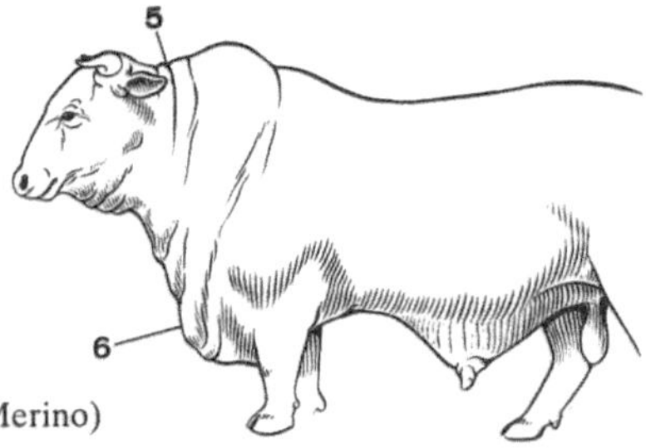

C Santa Gertrudis bull

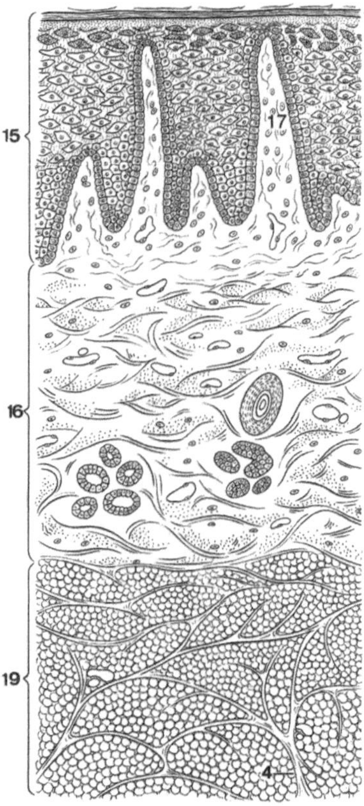

H Skin and tela subcutanea, histologic section (eq)

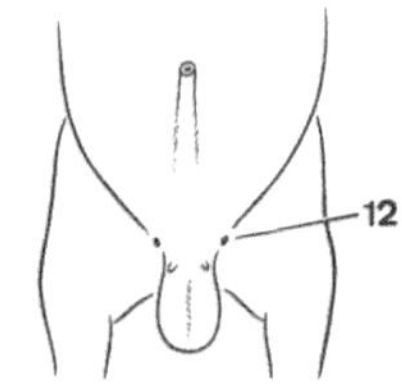

D Regio abdominis caudalis (ov masc)

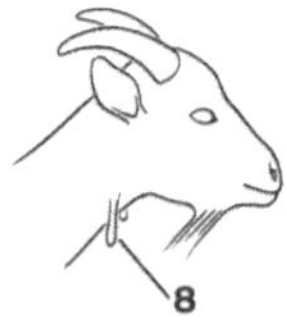

E Head (cap)

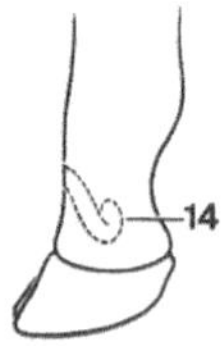

G Sinus interdigitalis (ov)

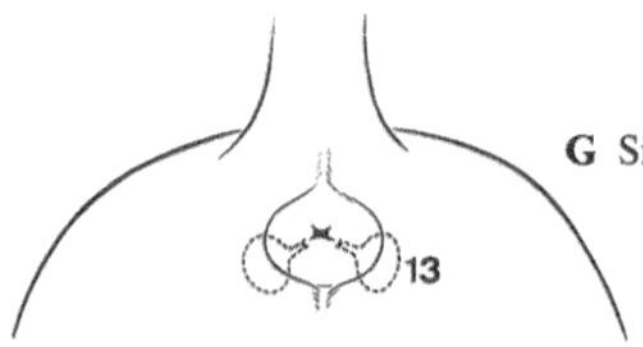

F Regio analis (ca)

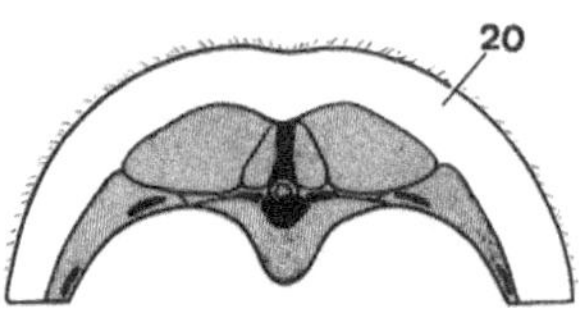

I Back, transverse section (su)

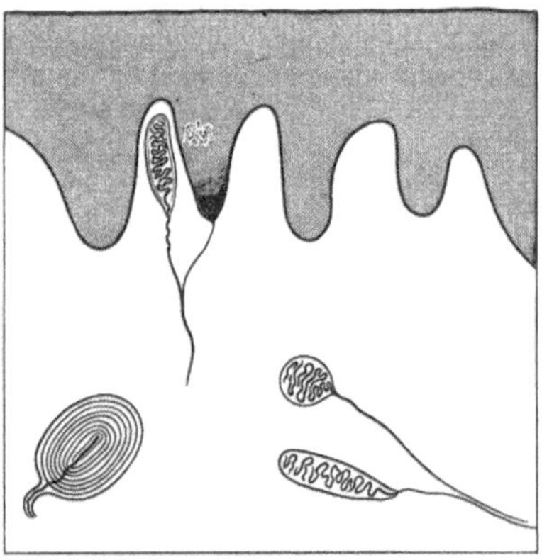
K Terminationes nervorum, histologic section (Trautmann and Fiebiger, Montagna)

1 **PILI**. Hairs. Term for all types of hair. Although the term Capilli refers to the hair of the head in man, it is employed here to designate the cover hairs of the coat as opposed to the wool hairs, the Pili lanei. The term Setae refers to the bristles of the pig.

2 ***Capilli***. The hairs of the mammal's coat, except in ov (Pili lanei) and su (mostly Setae).

3 ***Setae***. Bristles, the stiff hairs of su.

4 ***Pili lanei***. Wool hairs, comprising the fleece of ov, and forming the undercoat in other species.

5 ***Cirrus capitis***. Poll , the most cranial hairs of the mane that fall onto the forehead of eq. A

6 ***Juba***. Mane. A

7 ***Cirrus caudae***. The long hairs of the tail. C

8 ***Cirrus metacarpeus***. The tuft of long hairs on the fetlock in eq. B

9 ***Cirrus metatarseus***. The tuft of long hairs on the fetlock in eq.

10 ***Cilia***. Eye lashes. A

11 ***Barba*** (cap). Beard, the tuft of long hairs on the ventral surface of the lower jaw. D

12 *Tragi*. The hairs at the entrance to the external acoustic meatus. A

13 ***Vibrissae***. The hairs in the nostrils. A

14 ***Pili tactiles***. Tactile hairs. General term for the long stiff hairs, found mainly on the head, that are surrounded at the root by a blood sinus and numerous sensory nerve endings.

15 *Pili tact. supraorbitales*. Supraorbital tactile hairs, dorsal to the eye. D E

16 *Pili tact. infraorbitales*. Infraorbital tactile hairs, immediately ventral to the eye. A

17 *Pili tact. zygomatici*. Zygomatic tactile hairs, ventral or caudoventral to the eye. A E

18 *Pili tact. buccales*. Buccal tactile hairs, on the cheek. E

19 *Pili tact. labiales superiores*. Tactile hairs of the upper lip and around the nostrils. A

20 *Pili tact. labiales inferiores*. Tactile hairs of the lower lip. A

21 *Pili tact. mentales*. Mental tactile hairs, on the ventral surface of the lower jaw. E

22 *Pili tact. carpales* (fe). Carpal tactile hairs, on the caudomedial surface of the forearm, a short distance proximal to the carpal pad. F

23 ***Apex pili***. Tip of the hair.

24 ***Scapus pili***. Hair shaft, especially that portion that extends from the skin. G

25 ***Radix pili***. Hair root, the embedded part of the hair. G

26 ***Bulbus pili***. Bulb of the hair, the proximal enalarged part of the hair root. G

27 ***Folliculus pili***. Hair follicle, invagination of the epidermis and connective tissue enclosing the embedded part of the hair. G

28 ***Papilla pili***. Hair papilla, peg of connective tissue extending into the expanded proximal end of the hair. G

29 ***Mm. arrectores pilorum***. Thin bundles of smooth muscle extending from the side of the hair follicle to the papillary layer of the dermis. They raise the hair. G

30 ***Flumina pilorum***. Hair tracts (streams), fields of hairs pointing in one direction. H

31 ***Vortex pilorum convergens***. Converging whorl of hair. H

32 ***Vortex pilorum divergens***. Diverging whorl of hair. H

33 ***Linea pilorum convergens***. Line or crest formed between two fields of converging hairs. H

34 ***Linea pilorum divergens***. Line or trough formed between two fields of diverging hairs. H

35 ***Cruces pilorum***. Cross-shaped hair pattern formed at the intersection of two lines of converging hair. H

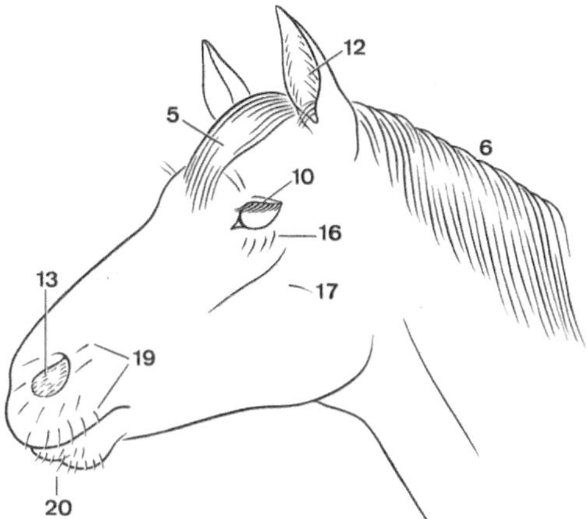

A Head and neck (eq)

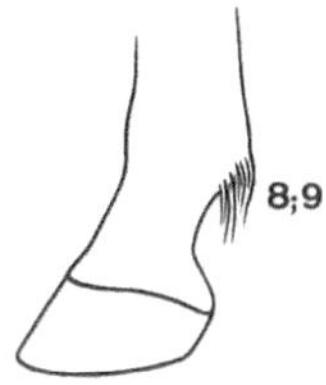

B Digit (eq)

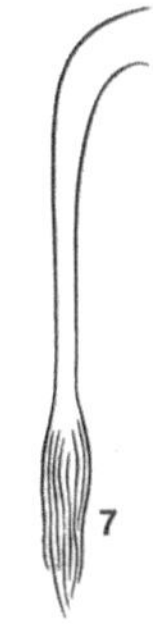

C Tail (bo)

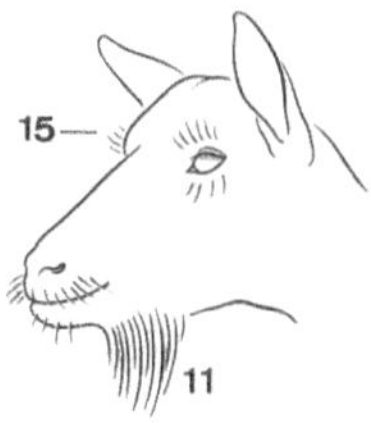

D Head (cap)

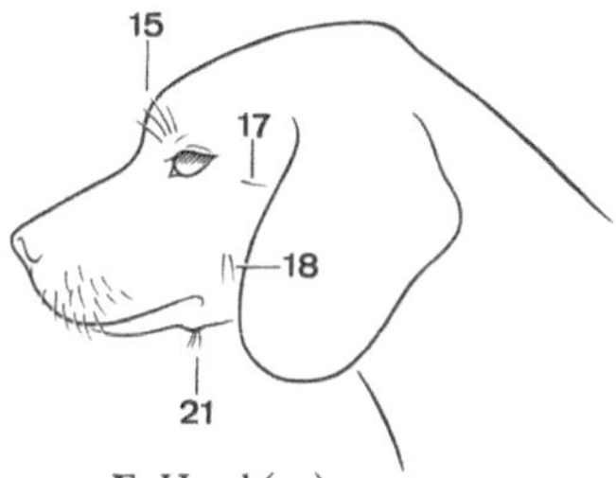

E Head (ca)

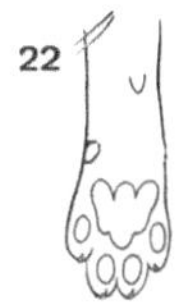

F Right manus, palmar aspect (fe)

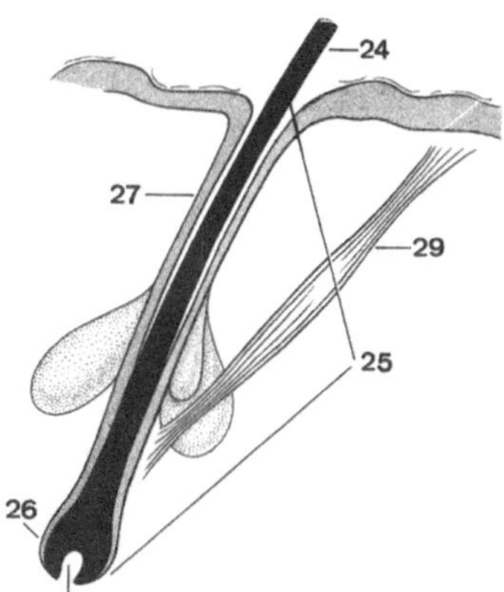

G Hair (bo)

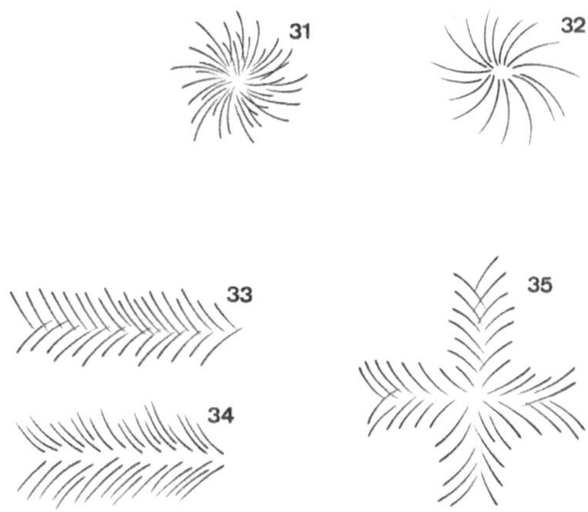

H Flumina pilorum

1 **CORNU**. The horn of Ru. A

2 ***Basis cornus***. Base of the horn, the wide proximal part. A

3 ***Corpus cornus***. Body of the horn, the elongated part between base and apex. A

4 ***Apex cornus***. The pointed tip of the horn. A

5 ***Epidermis cornus***. The epithelium of the horn, including the living cells and the cornified external part of the horn. It is homolgous to the epidermis of the skin and covers the dermis of the horn. B C

6 *Epiceras**. The zone of soft horn, the epidermis of the base of the horn. It is intermediate in character between the epidermis of the skin and that of the horn and is analogous to the Epidermis limbi (Perioplum) of the hoof. C

7 *Tubuli epidermales*. Horn tubules growing off the papillae of the dermis. They are parallel to the direction of growth of the horn and are connected by intertubular horn. B C

8 ***Dermis [Corium] cornus***. Dermis of the horn. The very vascular fibrous layer between the osseous cornual process and the epidermis of the horn. It corresponds to the dermis of the skin. B C

9 *Papillae dermales [coriales]*. Projections of the dermis of the horn which fit into conical depressions of the epidermis of the horn. The tubuli epidermales originate from the deep layers of the epidermis that cover the papillae. C

10 **TORI** (sing. Torus). The term Torus, as used in connection with the common integumentum, denotes a pad. A pad consists of a thick epidermis, dermis and a subcutaneous cushion, (Pulvinus), which may, however, be absent.

11 ***Torus carpeus****. Carpal pad. In Car on the palmar surface of the carpus. In eq it is known as the chestnut*, – on the caudomedial surface of the forearm proximal to the carpus, and it lacks a Pulvinus. D E

12 ***Torus tarseus****. Tarsal pad. Present only in eq as the chestnut* on the caudomedial surface of the tarsus. F

13 ***Torus metacarpeus****. Metacarpal pad. In Car on the palmar surface of the Regio metacarpophalangea. D

14 ***Calcar metacarpeum****. Ergot*, a rudiment of the metacarpal pad on the palmar surface of the Regio metacarpophalangea in eq. E

15 ***Torus metatarseus***. Metatarsal pad. In Car on the plantar surface of the Regio metatarsophalangea, similar to metacarpal pad.

16 ***Calcar metatarseum****. Ergot*, a rudiment of the metatarsal pad on the plantar surface of the Regio metatarsophalangea in eq, similar to the rudiment of the metacarpal pad. F

17 ***Torus digitalis****. Digital pad*, on the palmar (plantar) surface of each digit in Car. D

18 ***Torus ungulae****. Digital pad in Ru* on the Facies solearis of the hoof, palmar (plantar) to the sole. G

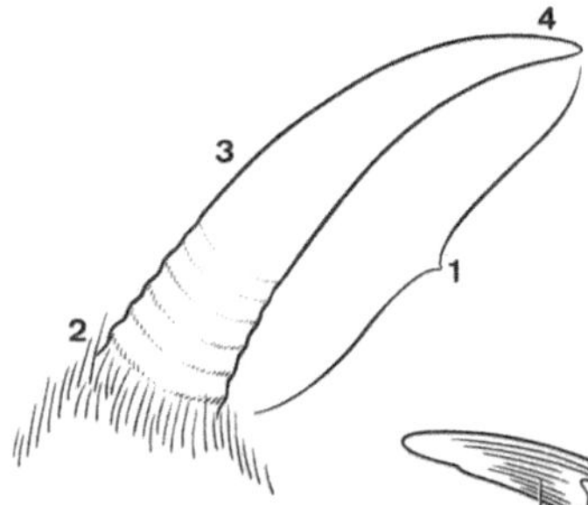

A Left horn, lateral aspect (cap)

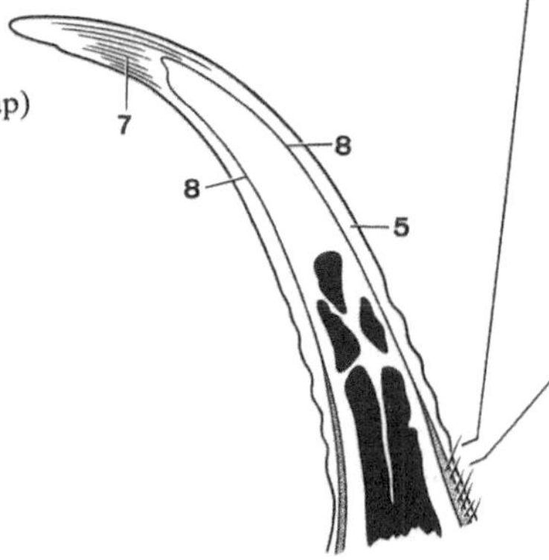

B Horn, longitudinal section (cap)

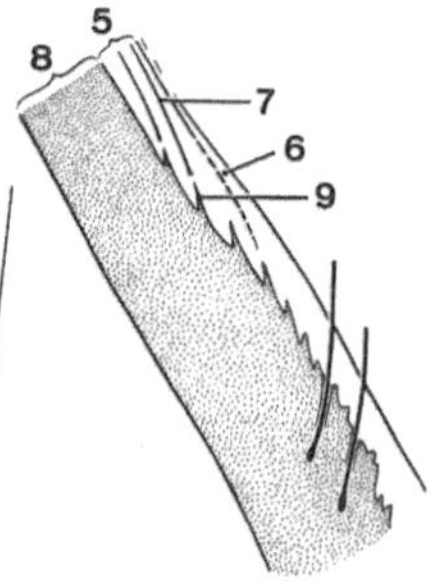

C Epiceras, schematic section (cap)

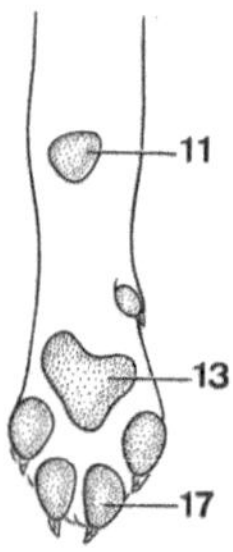

D Left manus, palmar aspect (ca)

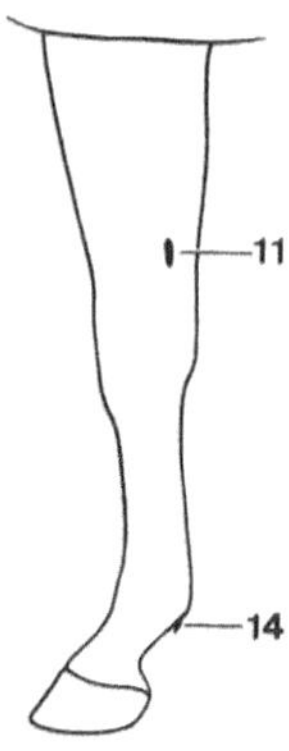

E Right thoracic limb, medial aspect (eq)

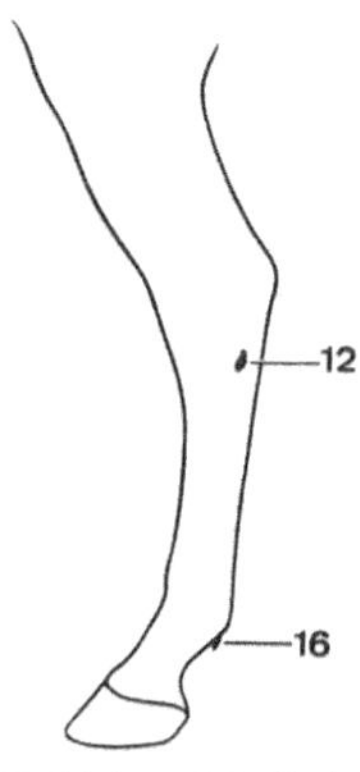

F Right pelvic limb, medial aspect (eq)

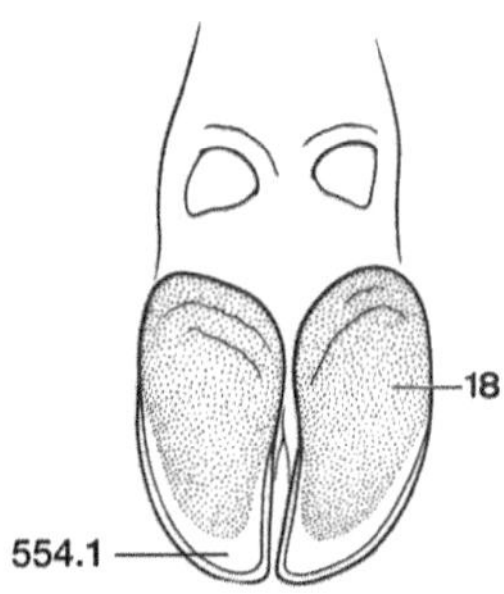

G Digits of manus, palmar aspect (bo)

1 **UNGUICULA**. Claw of Car, including the cornified epidermis, the dermis and the tela subcutanea. A

2 **UNGULA**. Hoof, including the cornified epidermis, the dermis and the tela subcutanea; in Un. C

3 **Limbus [Vallum (Car)]**. The narrow band of modified skin forming the proximal part of the claw or hoof, and including the tela subcutanea, dermis and epidermis. The latter is intermediate in character between the epidermis of the skin and that of the claw or hoof. In Car, this band and the skin proximal to it form a fold, Vallum, that partly covers the claw. In Un the transition between the skin and the hoof is called coronet. A B D (The term Limbus applies to all species. The more descriptive term Vallum may be used in Car.)

4 ***Epidermis limbi [Perioplum (Un)]***. The soft horn produced by the Limbus growing distally with the claw or hoof. The Epidermis limbi of the hoof is known as the periople and forms the Stratum externum of the horny wall of the hoof. C D (Epidermis limbi applies to all species. In Un it is known as the periople.)

5 *Tubuli epidermales* (Un). Horn tubules growing off the papillae of the Dermis limbi. They are parallel to the direction of the growth of the hoof and are connected by intertubular horn. D

6 **Dermis [Corium] limbi**. Limbic (perioplic) dermis [corium], underlying and nourishing the Epidermis limbi. It is continuous with the dermis of the skin proximally and with the Dermis coronae of the claw or hoof distally. B D

7 *Papillae dermales [coriales]*. Projections of the limbic (perioplic) dermis [corium] which fit into conical depressions of the Epidermis limbi. D

8 ***Tela subcutanea limbi [Pulvinus limbi (Un)]*** [1]. The subcutaneous tissue of the limbus which may be slightly raised to form a bandlike cushion, Pulvinus limbi. D

9 **Corona**. The bandlike proximal segment of the claw or hoof deep and distal to the limbus. It includes the tela subcutanea, dermis and epidermis. The latter grows distally over the distal phalanx and forms the middle, or thickest, layer of the horny wall. D

10 ***Epidermis coronae***. The epidermis produced by the coronary segment of the claw or hoof. It consists proximally of a thin layer of proliferating cells followed by a mass of cornified cells which form the Stratum medium of the horny wall (Lamina). D

11 *Tubuli epidermales* (Un). Horn tubules, about 160 µm in diameter, growing distally off the papillae of the coronary corium and making the epidermis much thicker and stronger. The tubules are embedded in intertubular horn; their spiral nature makes the wall of the hoof elastic to proximodistal compression. D

12 ***Dermis [Corium] coronae***. Coronary dermis [corium], a band of dermis at the proximal border of the claw or hoof nourishing the Epidermis coronae. It is continuous proximally with the Dermis limbi and distally with the Dermis parietis. D

13 *Papillae dermales [coriales]*. Projections of the coronary dermis [corium] which fit into conical depressions of the Epidermis coronae. D

14 ***Tela subcutanea coronae*** [1]. Subcutaneous tissue of the coronary segment (Corona).

15 **(Pulvinus coronae)** (Un) [1]. It bulges outward in eq to form a bandlike cushion. D

1) The term Torus cannot be applied to these cushions of the Tela subcutanea, because Torus designates the entire digital pad including the Epidermis, the Dermis and the Tela subcutanea.

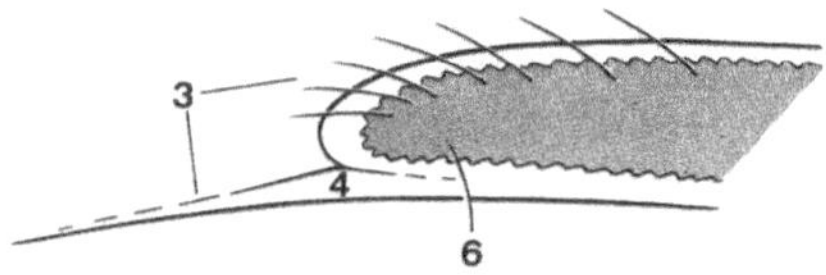

B Vallum, sagittal section (fe)

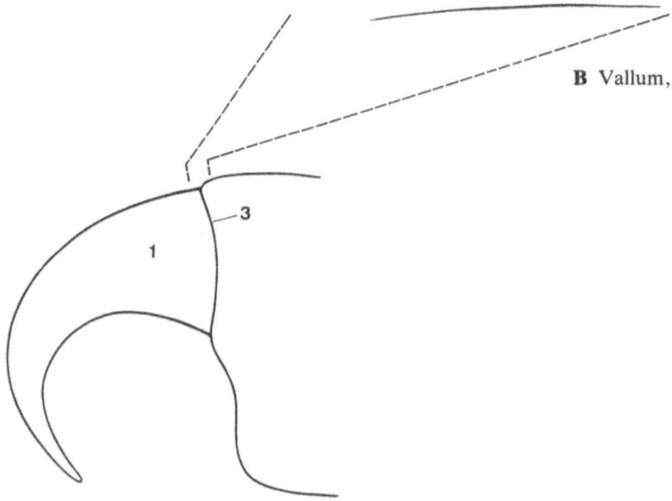

A Claw (fe)

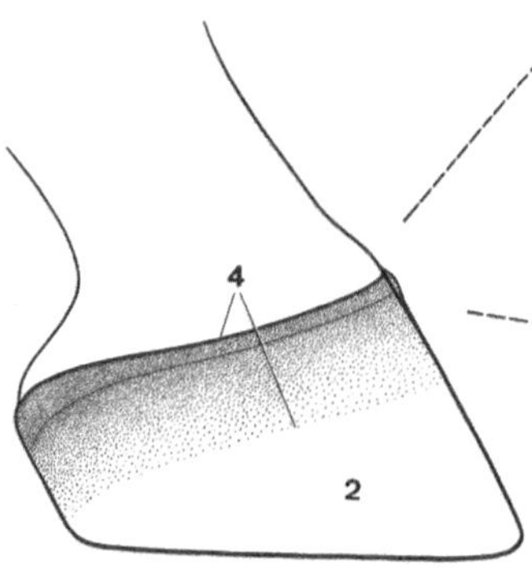

C Hoof (eq) (Sack and Habel)

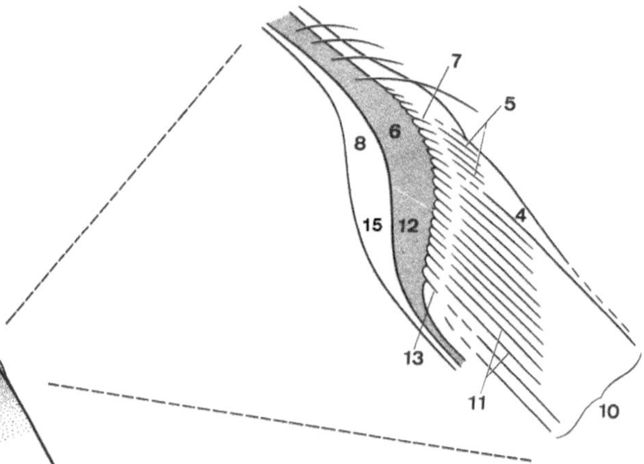

D Limbus and Corona, schematic section (eq) (Sack and Habel)

1 **Paries**. Parietal or wall segment of the claw or hoof distal to the coronary segment. It consists of the Dermis parietis and the overlying epidermis. A

2 ***Epidermis parietis***. Epidermis of the parietal segment, forming proximodistally oriented lamellae which interdigitate with the lamellae of the underlying Dermis parietis. C

3 *Lamellae epidermales* [1]. Proximodistally oriented epidermal lamellae. Their centers are cornified and form the horny lamellae on the internal surface of the horny wall (Lamina). C

3a *Tubuli epidermales* (Un). Between the Lamellae epidermales are rows of Tubuli epidermales generated above the Papillae dermales (see Zona alba).

4 ***Dermis [Corium] parietis***. Dermis [corium] of the parietal segment. It is attached to the parietal surface of the Phalanx distalis (Proc. unguicularis, Car), also to the Cartilagines ungulares (eq). C

5 *Lamellae dermales [coriales]* [1]. Lamellae formed by the dermis [corium] of paries which interdigitate with the Lamellae epidermales. In eq each lamella forms 100–200 secondary lamellae. No secondary lamellae in Ru. C

5a *Papillae dermales [coriales]*. Originate at the distal edge of each dermal lamella.

5b *Apparatus suspensorius ossis ungulae* (Un). This term includes all structures establishing the suspension of the distal phalanx within the hoof of Ungulata.

6 ***Paries corneus [Lamina]***. Horny wall consisting of cornified epidermis produced by Limbus, Corona and Paries. A F G

7 *Stratum externum*. External layer, composed proximally of the soft limbic (perioplic) horn and distally of a thin layer of glossy horn also derived from the Limbus. A G

8 *Stratum medium*. Middle layer, forming the bulk of the horny wall and composed of the cornified epidermis produced by the Corona. A E G

9 *Stratum internum*. Internal layer. In the hoof it is unpigmented and bears lamellae. A C G

10 *Zona alba sive Linea alba ungulae*. The "white zone" or the "white line" of the hoof, forming the junction between Paries corneus and Solea cornea. D E (Both terms [Zona alba and Linea alba ungulae] were adopted to avoid confusion with the Linea alba of the abdominal wall.) (Linea alba ungulae is commonly accepted by veterinarians [see white line disease].)

11 *Pars axialis*. Axial part in Car, su, Ru. H

11a **Sulcus axialis**. The oblique, irregular grove between the wall and bulb on the axial surface of the hoof of su and Ru.

11b **Incisura paraarticularis**. The slightly indented triangular area of thin horn at the proximal end of Sulcus axialis opposite the distal interphalangeal joint of su and Ru.

12 Pars abaxialis. Abaxial part in Car, su, Ru. H

12b **Sulcus abaxialis**. The oblique, irregular grove between the wall and bulb on the abaxial surface of the hoof of su and Ru.

13 Pars lateralis[2]. Pars dorsalis of the hoof (the toe) is separated from Pars lateralis (the lateral quarter) by the intersection of a line from Apex cuneus with the wall at 45° from the axial plane of the hoof. The most palmar/plantar segment of Pars lateralis is the heel with Bulbus. B

13a *Pars mobilis lateralis*. Pars lateralis is separated from pars mobilis lateralis (lateral heel) by a line across the greatest width of the hoof. B

14 *Pars medialis*[2]. Symmetrical with Pars lateralis B

14a *Pars mobilis medialis*. Symmetrical with Pars mobilis lateralis. B

15 *Margo dorsalis* (Car, su, Ru). The longitudinal ridge on the dorsal aspect of the claw or hoof, formed at the junction of the axial and abaxial parts. F H

16 *Pars dorsalis*. Dorsal part of the hoof, the toe. B

17 *Pars inflexa lateralis*. Part of the Paries corneus in eq, that extends dorsally from the Margo palmaris lateralis along the Sulcus paracunealis lateralis, known as the bar. E

18 *Pars inflexa medialis*. The part of the Paries corneus in eq, that extends dorsally from the Margo palmaris medialis along the Sulcus paracunealis medialis, known as the bar. E

19 *Margo palmaris sive plantaris lateralis*. The longitudinal ridge formed at the junction of Pars lateralis and Pars inflexa lateralis in eq. It extends from Angulus parietis lateralis to Margo coronalis. E

20 *Margo palmaris sive plantaris medialis*. The longitudinal ridge formed at the junction of Pars medialis and Pars inflexa medialis in eq. It extends from Angulus parietis medialis to Margo coronalis. E

21 ***Margo plantaris lateralis***[3]. Vide 19

21a Angulus parietis palmaris sive plantaris lateralis. Pars mobilis lateralis meets Pars inflexa lateralis. E

22 ***Margo plantaris medialis***[3]. Vide 20

22a Angulus parietis palmaris sive plantaris medialis. Pars mobilis medialis meets Pars inflexa medialis. E

23 ***Margo coronalis***. Proximal border of the Paries corneus of the claw or hoof. G

cont. p. 554 ►

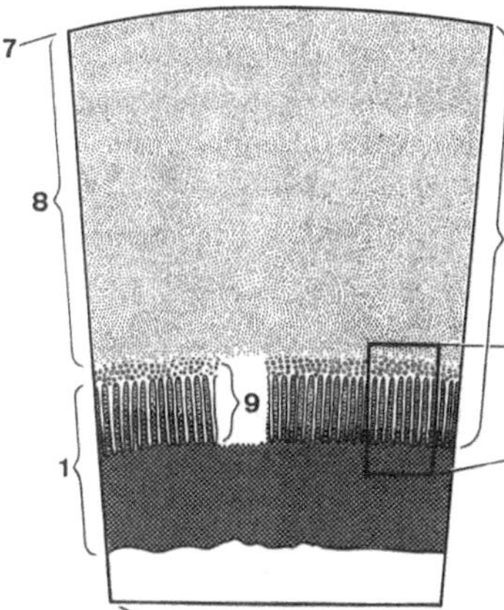

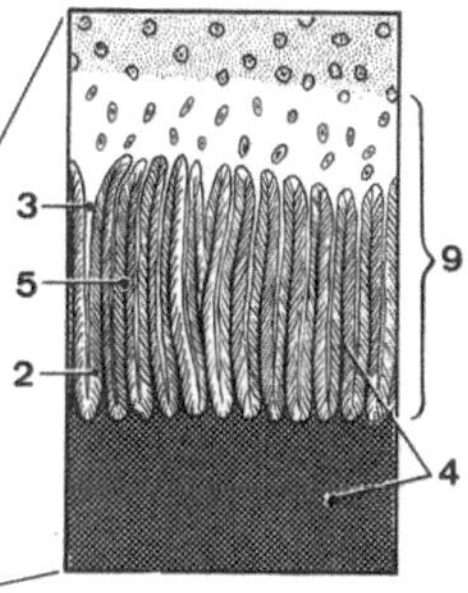

C Part of Paries ungulae, section (eq)

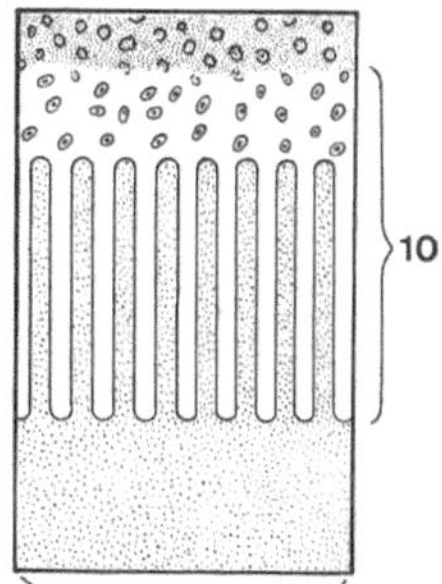

D Part of Zona alba (eq)

A Part of Lamina of hoof, section (eq)

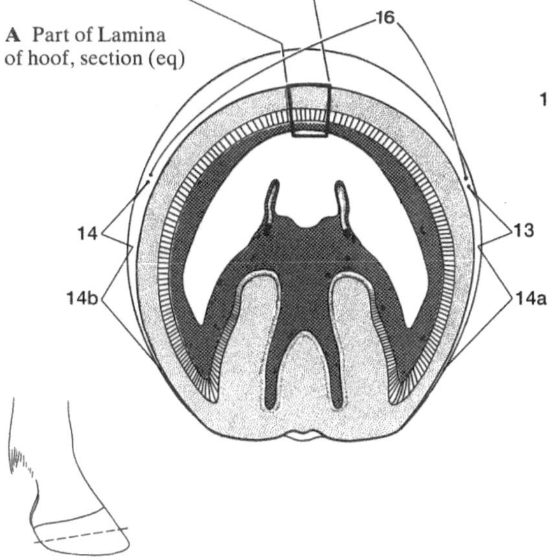

B Right hoof, transverse section, proximal side (eq)

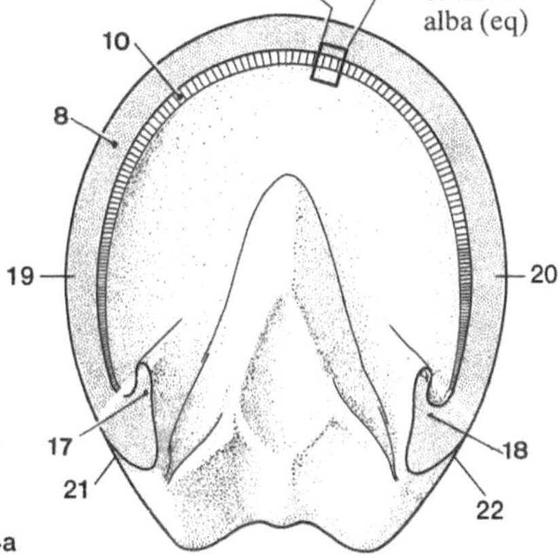

E Right hoof capsule, solear surface (eq)

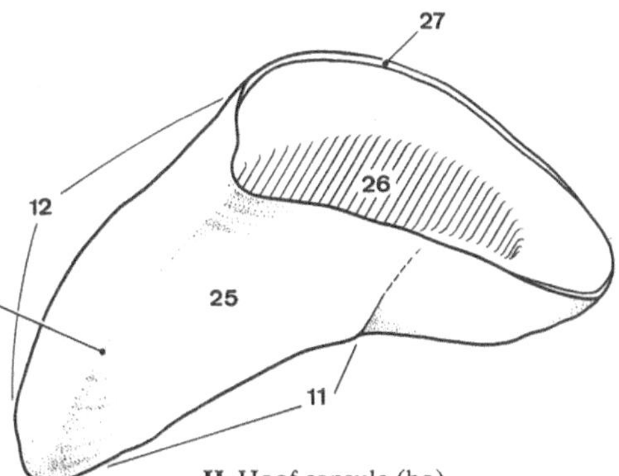

F Claw, axial aspect (ca)

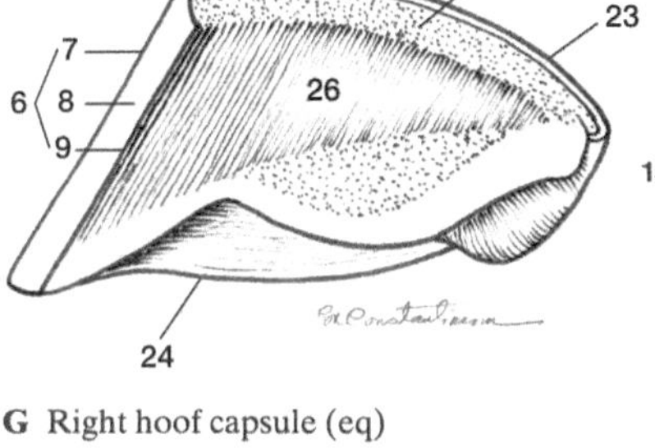

G Right hoof capsule (eq)

H Hoof capsule (bo)

24 ***Margo solearis***. Distal border of the Paries corneus of the claw or hoof, in contact with the ground in Un. G

25 ***Facies externa***. External surface of the Paries corneus. G H

26 ***Facies interna***. Internal surface of the Paries corneus. G H

27 ***Sulcus limbalis*** (Un). Narrow groove distal to Margo coronalis of the Paries corneus. It contains the Dermis limbi and the thin non-cornified layer of the Epidermis limbi. G H

28 ***Sulcus coronalis*** (Un). Groove distal to Sulcus limbalis of the Paries corneus. It contains the Dermis coronae and the thin non-cornified layer of the Epidermis coronae. G

1) There are 550–600 epidermal and dermal lamellae in eq, 1300–1500 in bo, 550–700 in ov.

2) The boundaries between the parts of Paries corneus of the horse begin at Margo solearis and extend to Margo coronalis in the direction of the horn tubules.

3) These terms were omitted from the 5th edition of the N. A. V. because they are now included in 19 and 20, respectively.

---

1 **Solea**. Sole of the claw or hoof, including tela subcutanea, dermis and epidermis. In the hoof, the sole is united with the inside of the Margo solearis of the wall. In the claw, it is concealed between the axial and abaxial free borders of the wall. B E

2 ***Epidermis soleae***. Epidermis of the sole consisting of a thin layer of proliferating cells followed by a mass of cornified cells which form the horny sole (Solea cornea). B

3 *Tubuli epidermales* (Un). Horn tubules growing distally off the papillae of the dermis of the sole. They are embedded in intertubular horn. B

4 ***Dermis [Corium] soleae***. Dermis [corium] of the sole, deep to, and nourishing the Epidermis soleae. It forms papillae, and at its periphery is continuous in the hoof with the dermis of the wall and the dermis of the torus, and in the claw with the dermis of the wall (Dermis parietis). B E

5 *Papillae dermales [coriales]*. Distally directed projections of the dermis [corium] into the epidermis of the sole. B E

6 ***Tela subcutanea soleae***. Layer of connective tissue between the dermis of the sole and the Phalanx distalis. A B

7 ***Solea cornea***. Horny sole of the claw or hoof, the cornified part of the Epidermis soleae. D F

8 *Corpus soleae*. The body or central part of the sole of the hoof, uniting the two Crura soleae. C D

9 *Crus soleae axiale*. The narrow axial part of the sole between the wall and the large Torus corneus in the hoof of su and Ru. C

10 *Crus soleae abaxiale*. See 9. C

11 *Crus soleae laterale*. The part of the sole on the lateral side of the Cuneus corneus (horny frog) in the hoof of eq. The palmar or plantar extremity of the lateral Crus is the Angulus soleae lateralis. D (In Ungulata the Apex tori or Cuneus ungulae projects into the sole, dividing it into lateral and medial Crura in the horse, and into axial and abaxial Crura in Artiodactyla.)

12 *Crus soleae mediale*. See 11. C

13 *Margo parietalis*. The border of the sole of the claw or hoof united with the wall. C D E

14 *Margo centralis*. The border of the sole of the hoof united with the Torus corneus and, specifically in eq, with the Cuneus ungulae. C D

15 *Angulus soleae axialis*. The palmarmost/plantarmost axial part of the sole of the hoof in su and Ru. C

16 *Angulus soleae abaxialis*. The abaxial part (see 15).

17 *Angulus soleae lateralis*. The palmarmost/plantarmost part of the sole of the hoof in eq, between quarter (Pars lateralis) and bar (Pars inflexa lateralis) of the wall. It is the palmar or plantar extremity of the lateral Crus. D

18 *Angulus soleae medialis*. It is the palmar or plantar extremity of the medial Crus (see 17). D

19 *Facies externa*. The external surface of the horny sole. D E

20 *Facies interna*. The internal surface of the horny sole. F

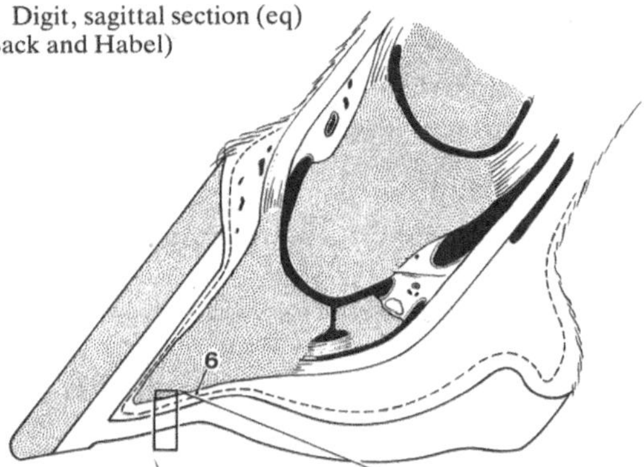

A Digit, sagittal section (eq)
(Sack and Habel)

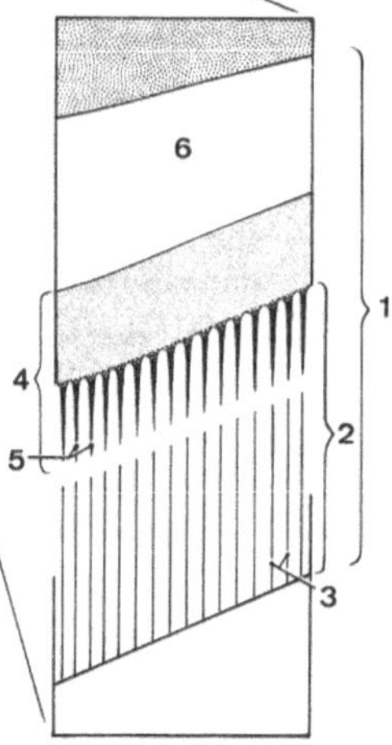

B Sole segment, histologic section (eq)
(Sack and Habel)

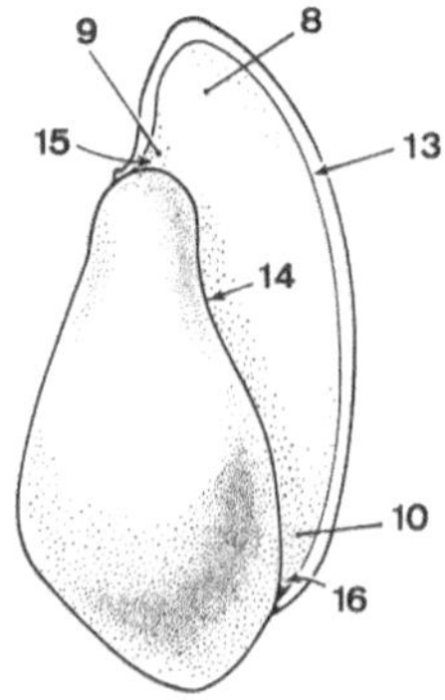

C Hoof capsule, solear surface (su)

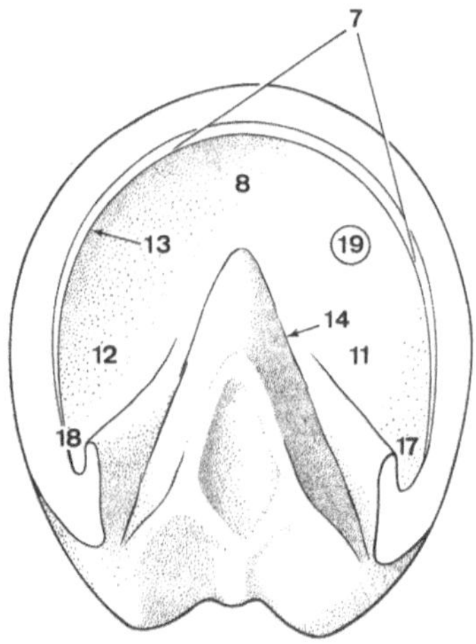

D Left hoof capsule, solear surface (eq)

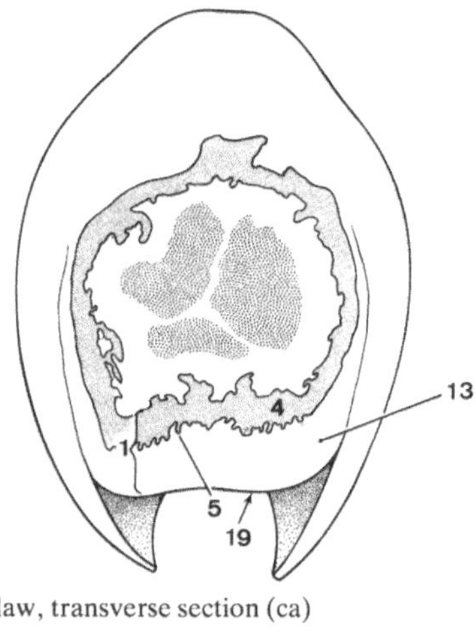

E Claw, transverse section (ca)

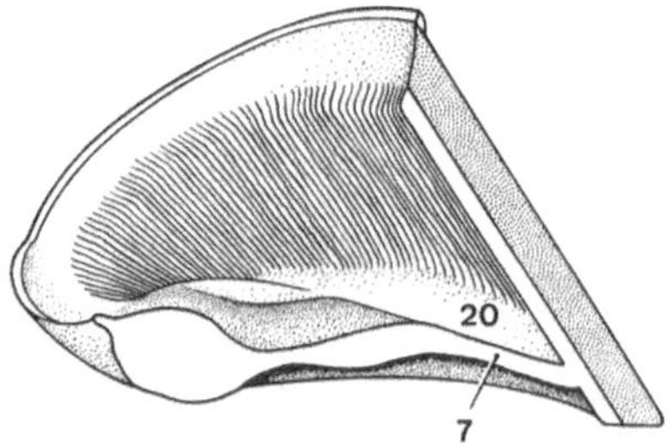

F Hoof capsule, sagittal section, inner surface (eq)

1 **Torus digitalis**. Digital pad, including tela subcutanea, dermis, and epidermis. A (The term Torus, as used in connection with the common integument, denotes a pad. It includes a thick epidermal covering, the dermis, and the subcutaneous cushion, or Pulvinus.)

2 **Torus ungulae**. Pad of the hoof, occupies the space between the borders of the wall and projects into the sole. B

3 ***Epidermis tori***. Epidermis of the digital pad, consisting of a thin layer of proliferating cells covered by a mass of cornified cells. F

4 *Tubuli epidermales* (Un). Horn tubules, growing distally off the papillae of the dermis, embedded in intertubular horn. F

5 ***Dermis [Corium] tori***. Dermis [corium] of the digital pad or pad of the hoof. F

6 *Papillae dermales [coriales]*. Distally directed projections of the dermis [corium]. F

7 ***Tela subcutanea tori [Pulvinus digitalis]***[1]. Thick layer of connective tissue deep to the dermis of the digital pad, known as the digital cushion. The Pulvinus digitalis is the digital cushion in all species. In the horse it may be divided into a Pars torica (see 8) and a Pars cunealis (see 21). C F

8 ***Pars torica pulvini digitalis***. The palmar (plantar) part of the Pulvinus digitalis in eq. E

9 ***Torus corneus***. Horny pad of the hoof. C G

10 *Pars lateralis* (eq). Lateral rounded prominence above the palmar (plantar) border of the wall (heel), known as the bulb of the heel. D

11 *Pars medialis* (eq). See 10. D

12 *Apex tori*. Apex of the digital pad which in su and Ru projects dorsally into the sole. B G

13 *Basis tori*. Palmar (plantar) part of the digital pad, in su and Ru. G

14 *Facies externa*. External surface. G

15 *Facies interna*. Internal surface. H

16 **Cuneus ungulae**. Apex tori of the hoof in eq, known as the frog. E (Cuneus ungulae, the long established term in equine anatomy for the homologue of Apex tori has been retained because of the special structure and clinical importance.)

17 ***Epidermis cunei***. Epidermis of the frog, consisting of a thin layer of proliferating cells followed by a mass of cornified cells. F

18 *Tubuli epidermales*. Horn tubules, growing distally off the papillae of the Dermis cunei, embedded in intertubular horn. F

19 ***Dermis [Corium] cunei***. Dermis [corium] of the frog. F

20 *Papillae dermales [coriales]*. Distally directed projections of the dermis [corium]. F

21 ***Tela subcutanea cunei [Pars cunealis pulvini digitalis]***. Thick layer of connective tissue of the frog, the cuneal part of the digital cushion. E F

22 ***Cuneus corneus***. Cornified part of the Epidermis cunei, the horny frog. I

23 *Apex cunei*. Apex of the wedge-shaped frog directed dorsally into the sole. I

24 *Basis cunei*. The wide part of the wedge-shaped frog between the Partes inflexae parietis (bars). I

25 *Crus cunei laterale*. Lateral crus of the frog. I

26 *Crus cunei mediale*. Medial crus of the frog. I

27 *Facies externa*. External surface. I

28 *Facies interna*. Internal surface. K

29 *Sulcus paracunealis lateralis*. Groove on the side of the frog, bounded laterally by the sole and the bar. I

30 *Sulcus paracunealis medialis*. On the medial side (see 29). I

31 *Sulcus cunealis centralis*. Central groove on the external surface of the frog. I

32 *Spina cunei*. Spine of the frog ("frog-stay"), central ridge on the internal surface of the horny frog. K

33 ***Capsula ungulae***. Horny hoof, consisting of the cornified cells of limbus, corona, wall, sole and digital pad. K

34 ***Facies solearis***. Is a composite of all structures visible on the ground surface.

35 *Facies contactus*. It includes Margo solearis, Zona alba, the peripheral zone of the sole, and Crura cunei.

36 *Facies fornicis*. Is part of Facies solearis that is not in contact with the ground.

37 ***Angulus dorsalis***. Is measured between the axial line of Pars dorsalis and Facies solearis in eq, between Margo dorsalis and Facies solearis in su and Ru.

38 ***Angulus lateralis***. Is measured between Pars lateralis (abaxialis) and Facies solearis at the greatest width of the hoof.

39 ***Angulus medialis***. Is measured between Pars medialis (axialis) and Facies solearis at the greatest width of the hoof.

40 ***Angulus palmaris sive plantaris lateralis***. Is measured between Margo palmaris sive plantaris lateralis and Facies solearis in eq.

41 ***Angulus palmaris sive plantaris medialis***. Similar with the Margo palmaris sive plantaris lateralis.

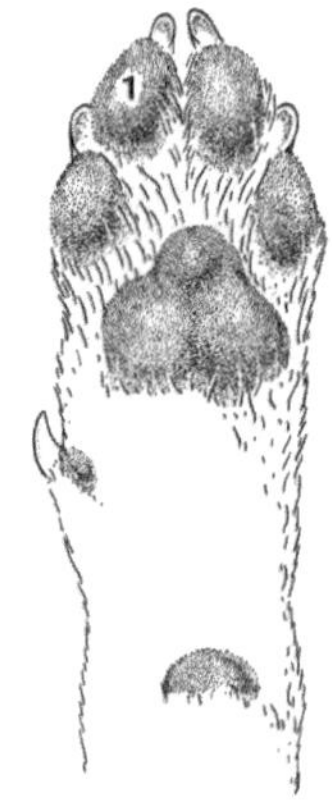

A Left manus, palmar aspect (ca)

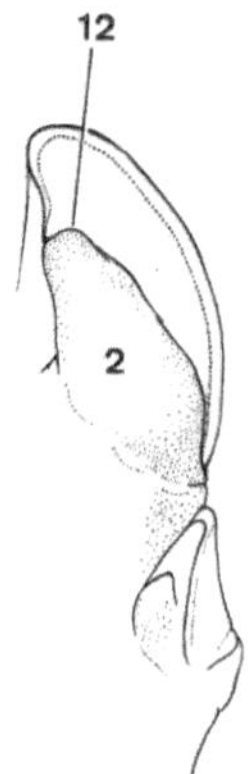

B Hoof, solear surface (su)

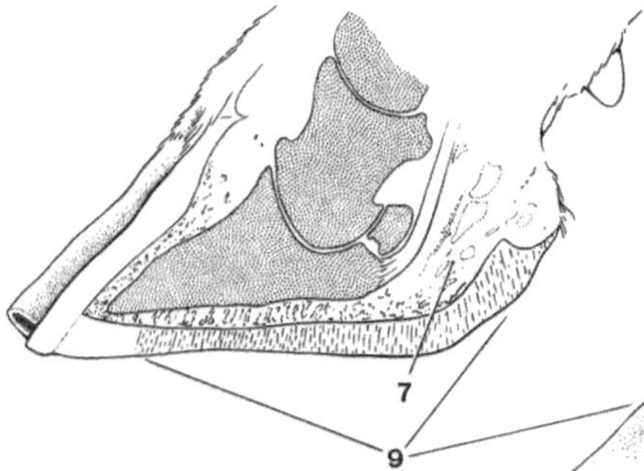

C Digit, sagittal section (bo)

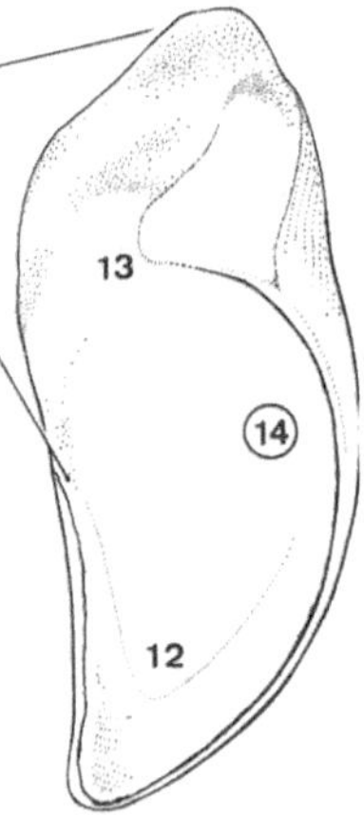

G Hoof, solear surface (bo)

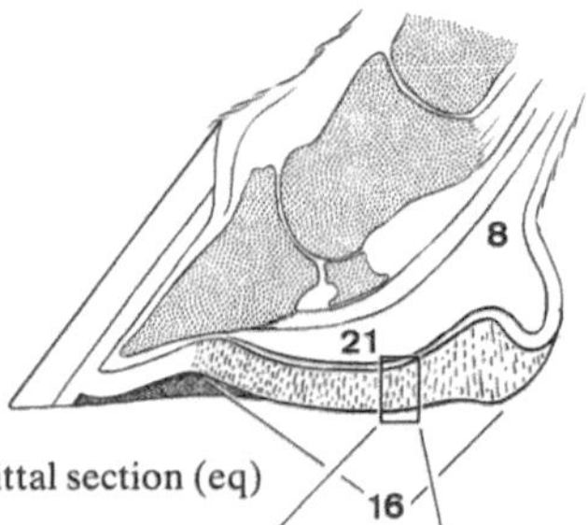

E Digit, sagittal section (eq)

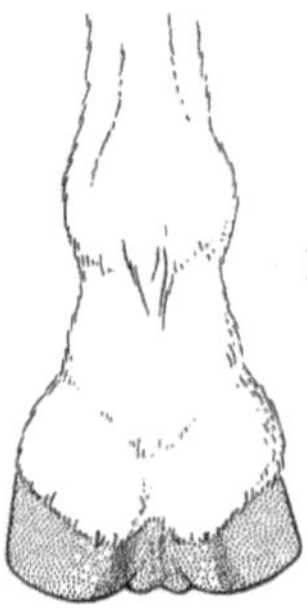

D Left digit, palmar aspect (eq)

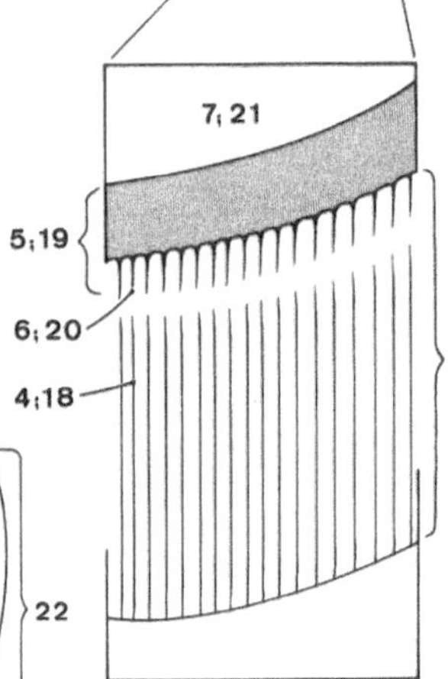

F Torus (Cuneus) ungulae, section (enlargement) (eq)

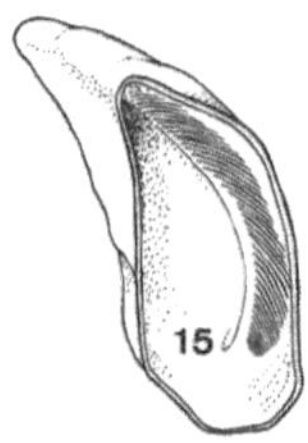

H Hoof capsule, inner surface (bo)

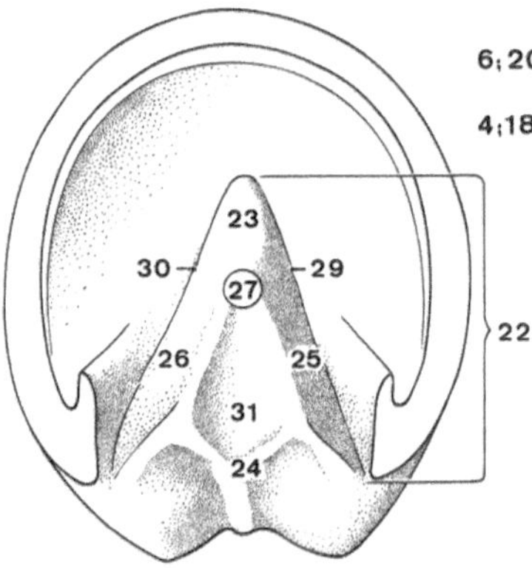

I Left hoof, solear surface (eq)

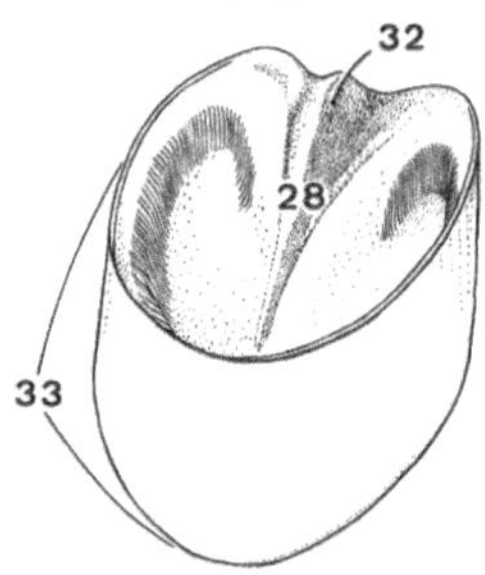

K Hoof capsule (eq)

1 **GLANDULAE CUTIS**. Glands originating from the epidermis and retaining close association with the skin. In domestic mammals most of the skin glands originate from, and discharge into, hair follicles. Glands that discharge on the surface of the epidermis are relatively rare. A

2 ***Gll. sudoriferae.*** Sweat glands. The rare eccrine glands secreting a watery sweat, e. g. through the foot pads of Car and in other glabrous areas; but also the widely distributed apocrine tubular glands discharging an albuminous sweat through the hair follicles. The latter type produces visible sweat on the body surface in eq; in the other domestic mammals, their secretion seems to be related to the characteristic odor of the species. A

3 ***Gll. sebaceae.*** Sebaceous glands. Holocrine, secreting sebum into the hair follicles deep to the orifice of the sweat glands. They occupy the middle layer of the dermis and may, in the vicinity of the genital openings for instance, be independent of hair follicles. A

4 ***Gll. ceruminosae.*** Sebaceous and modified tubular glands in the external acoustic meatus secreting a waxy substance called cerumen.

5 ***Gll. circumorales*** (fe). Large sebaceous glands in the lips, more numerous in the lower lip. B

6 ***Gll. plani rostralis.*** Tubular glands with a serous secretion in the Planum rostrale of su. C

7 ***Gll. plani nasolabialis.*** Branched tubular glands with a serous secretion in the Planum nasolabiale of bo. D

8 ***Gll. plani nasalis*** (ov). Branched tubular glands with a serous secretion in the Planum nasale. E

9 ***Gl. mentalis*** (su). Accumulation of sebaceous and tubular serous glands associated with the Pili mentales on the lower jaw. F

10 ***Gll. sinus infraorbitalis*** (ov). Large sebaceous and branched tubular glands with a fatty secretion in the wall of the Sinus infraorbitalis. H

11 ***Gl. cornualis*** (cap). Horn gland. Accumulation of sebaceous glands caudomedial to the base of the horn. G

12 ***Gll. sinus inguinalis*** (ov). Branched sebaceous and tubular glands in the wall of the Sinus inguinalis. I

13 ***Gll. circumanales*** (ca). Probably specified sebaceous glands associated with rudimentary hair follicles in the skin surrounding the anus. K

14 ***Gll. sinus paranalis*** (Car)*. Anal sac glands, tubular and sebaceous glands in the wall of the symmetrical paranal sacs. K

15 ***Gll. caudae.*** Large sebaceous and tubular glands in an oval area on the dorsal surface of the tail in Car. L

16 ***Gll. carpeae*** (su). Carpal glands, branched tubular glands with a seromucous secretion into several cutaneous invaginations on the mediopalmar surface of the carpus. M

17 ***Gll. sinus interdigitalis*** (ov). Sebaceous and tubular glands in the wall of the Sinus interdigitalis. N

18 ***Gll. tori.*** Tubular sweat glands in the pads of Car; branched tubular glands in the palmar (plantar) part of the Cuneus ungulae of eq. O

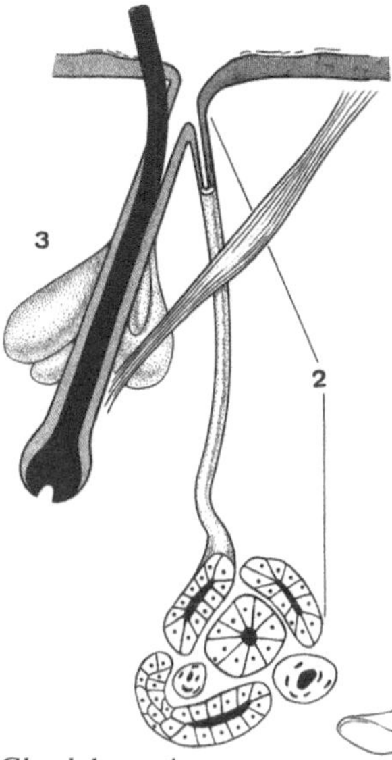

A Glandulae cutis

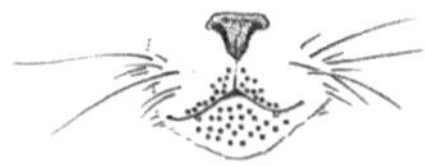
B Gll. circumorales (fe)

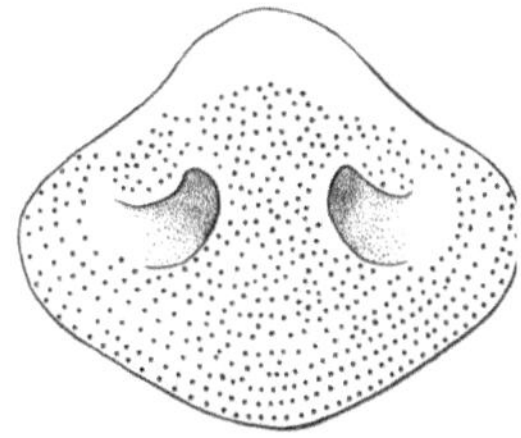
C Gll. plani rostralis (su)

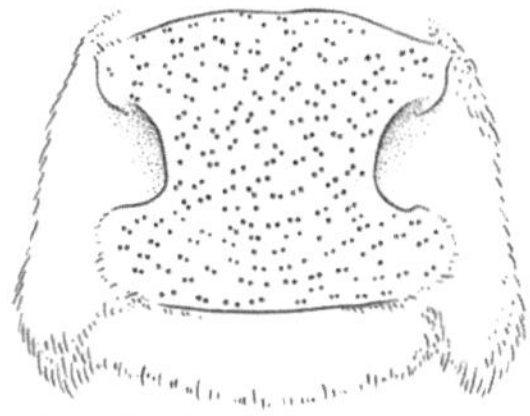
D Gll. plani nasolabialis (bo)

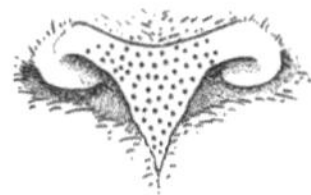
E Gll. plani nasalis (ov)

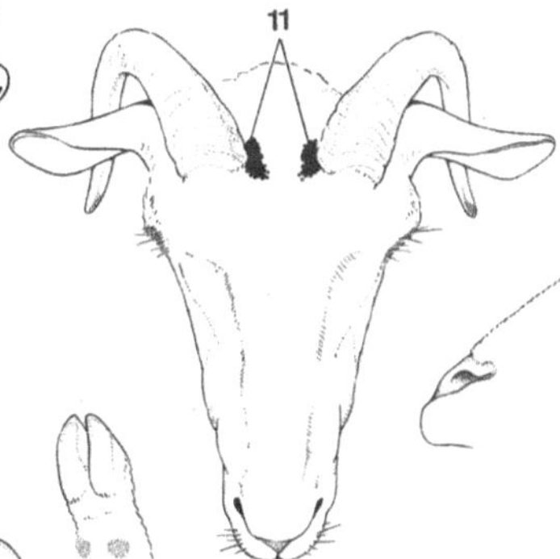

G Head (cap)

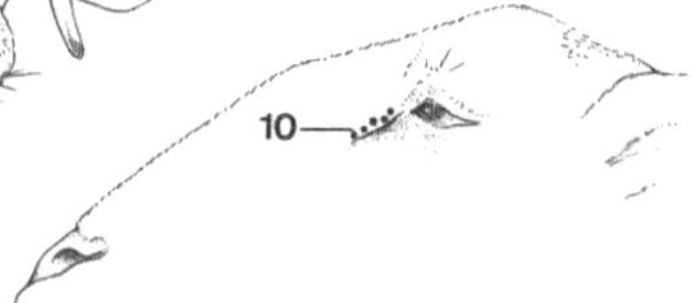

H Part of the head (ov)

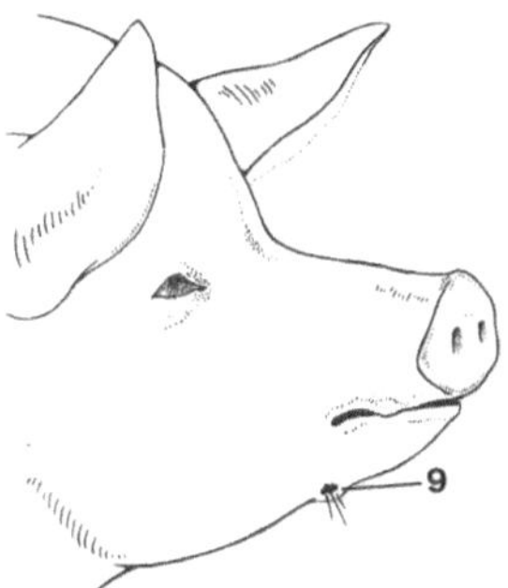

F Head (su)

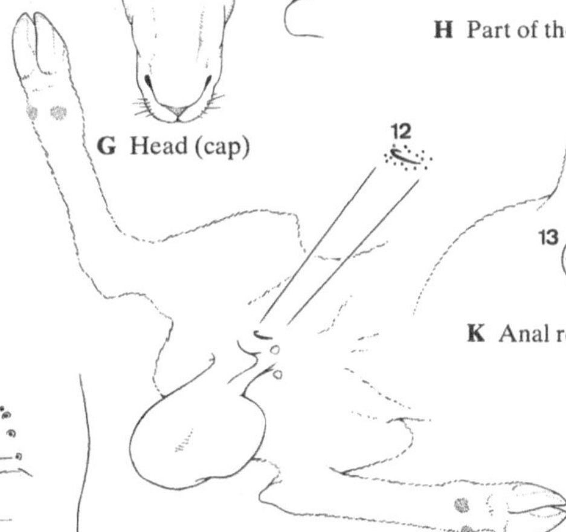

I Inguinal region (ov masc)

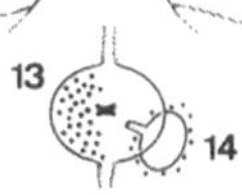

K Anal region (ca)

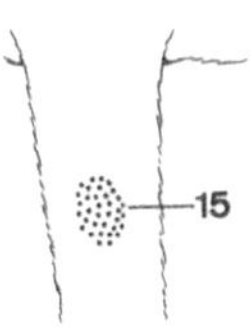

L Tail, dorsal surface (ca)

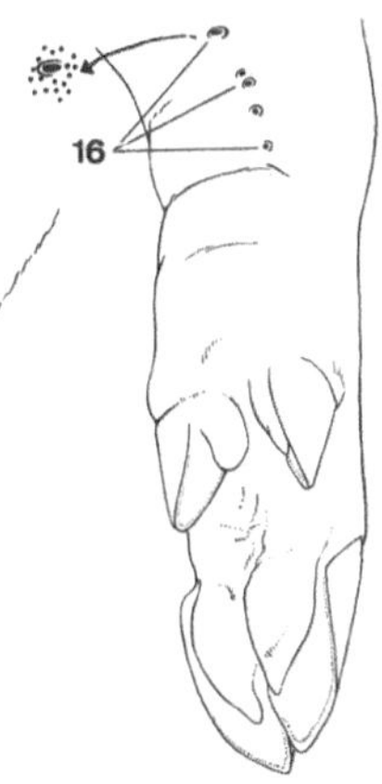

M Left manus, mediopalmar aspect (su)

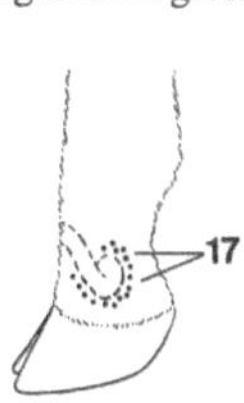

N Sinus interdigitalis (ov)

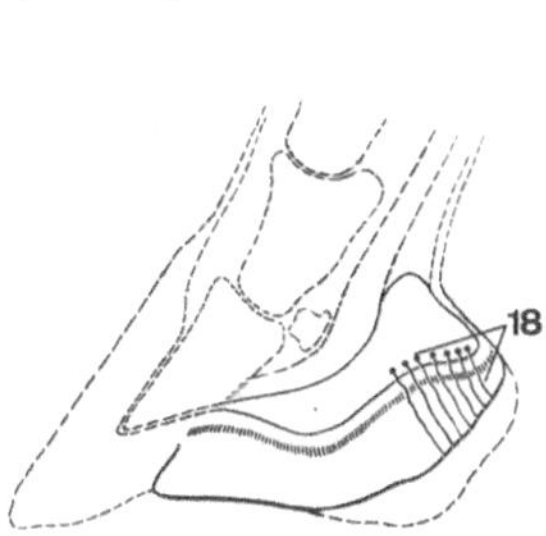

O Digit, sagittal section (eq)

1 **MAMMA**. One mammary complex consisting of one Corpus and one Papilla mammae (teat, nipple) is the homologous to one human breast. The usual number of mammae is: queen 8, bitch 10, sow 14, cow 4, ewe, goat, and mare 2. A (In Ru only the Ductus papillaris and Sinus lactifer are present in each Mamma).

2 ***Uber***. Udder, the collective term for all the mammae in Ru and eq. B

3 ***Papilla mammae***. The projection on the ventral surface of each mamma through which the milk is withdrawn; known as the nipple in Car and su, and as the teat in Ru and eq. A B C

4 *M. sphincter papillae*. Smooth muscle fibers surrounding Ductus papillaris, known as the teat sphincter in Ru. C D

5 ***Corpus mammae***. The conical body of a mamma, consisting of skin, glandular tissue and connective tissue. It is attached at its base to the ventral surface of the trunk and is continued apically by the Papilla mammae. A C

6 ***Sulcus intermammarius***. Intermammary groove, either longitudinal or transverse, separating adjacent mammae. A C

7 ***Glandula mammaria***. Single gland and associated duct system of a mamma. The usual number of glands per mamma is: fe 5–7, ca 8–14, su 2, Ru 1, eq 2. C E

8 *Lobi glandulae mammariae*. The macroscopic subdivision of the Glandula mammaria separated by connective tissue. E

9 **Lobuli glandulae mammariae**. Mammary lobule, a cluster 1 × 1.5 × 0.5 mm in size, of 150–200 (cow) alveoli secreting into a central ductule and separated from adjacent lobules by a thin layer of connective tissue. C

10 *Ductus lactiferi*. Lactiferous ducts, of various diameters, often ampullate, convey the milk to the Sinus lactifer in the ventral part of the Corpus mammae. C

11 *Sinus lactifer*. Lactiferous sinus, dilated distal part of the duct system formed by the confluence of the larger Ductus lactiferi, extending into the Papilla mammae. C

12 **Pars glandularis**. Glandular part, in the ventral end of the Corpus mammae. C

13 **Pars papillaris**. Papillary part, in the papilla and usually set off from the glandular part by a constriction (a papillary sphincter surrounded by the "papillary venous circle of Fürstenberg"). C

14 *Ductus papillaris*. Papillary duct, in the tip of the Papilla mammae, connecting the Pars papillaris sinus lactiferi with the outside. Called also the streak canal, its folded mucosa in the cow is called the "rosette of Furstenberg". D E

15 *Ostium papillare*. Papillary opening of the Ductus papillaris on the tip of the Papilla mammae. D E

16 ***Apparatus suspensorius mammarius***. Suspensory apparatus, the medial and lateral sheets of collagenous and elastic tissue that originate from the body wall and suspend the mammae; especially well developed in the heavy pendulous udder of the dairy cow. F

17 *Laminae laterales*. Connective inextensible tissue sheets on the lateral surface of the mamma. They originate from the Tendo symphysialis and Lamina femoralis. C F

18 **Lamellae suspensoriae**. Suspensory lamellae, thin sheets of connective tissue originating from the Laminae laterales and entering the mamma at different levels, thus supporting the weight. C F

19 *Laminae mediales [Ligamentum suspensorium uberis]*. The elastic connective tissue sheets on the medial surface of the mamma. The laminae of each side are apposed in the median plane and form the Lig. suspensorium uberis between the right and left halves of the udder. They originate from the Tunica flava abdominis. C F

20 **Lamellae suspensoriae**. Suspensory lamellae, thin sheets of connective tissue originating from the Laminae mediales, entering the mamma at different levels, thus supporting the weight. C F

21 ***Mamma masculina***. Rudimentary mamma of the male. Since functional glandular tissue does not usually develop, a Corpus mammae is not formed and only the papilla is present. G

22 ***(Mamma accessoria)***. Supernumerary mamma, occasionally functional, either cranial or caudal to the normally existing Mammae. B

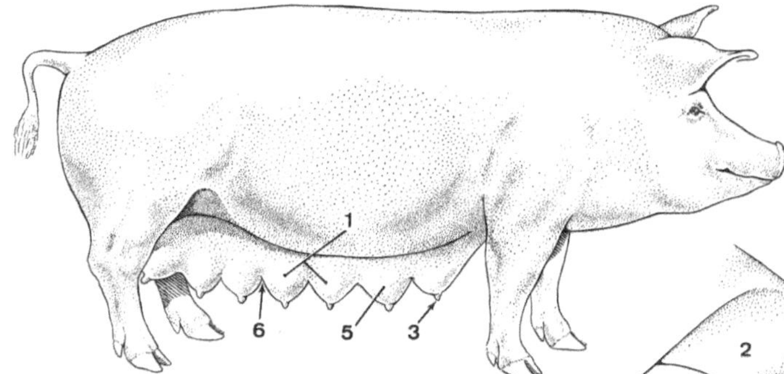

A Mammae (su)

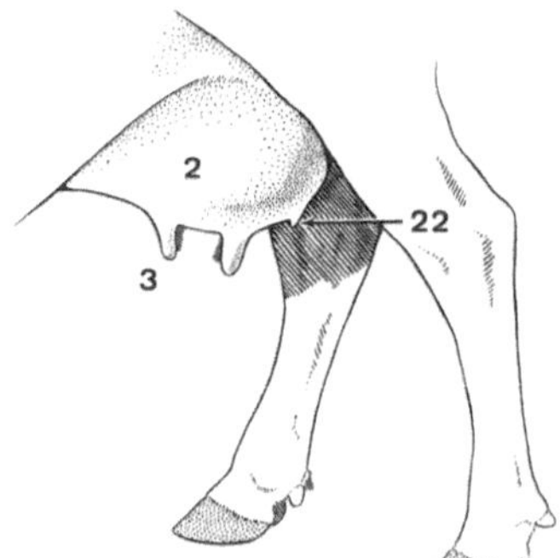

B Udder (bo)

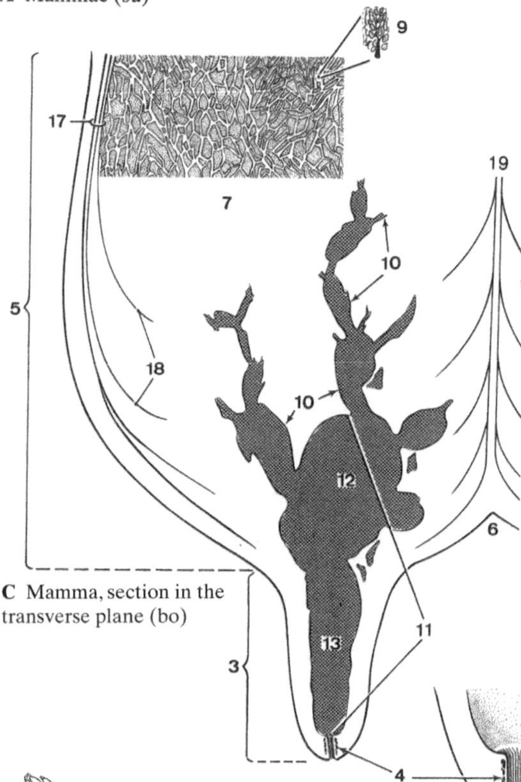

C Mamma, section in the transverse plane (bo)

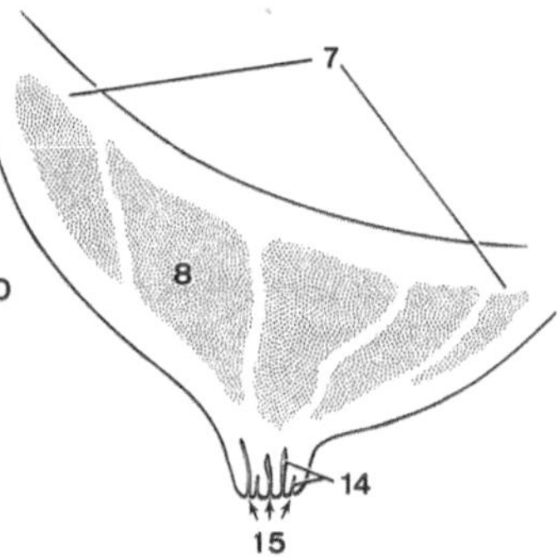

E Mamma, section in the transverse plane (ca)

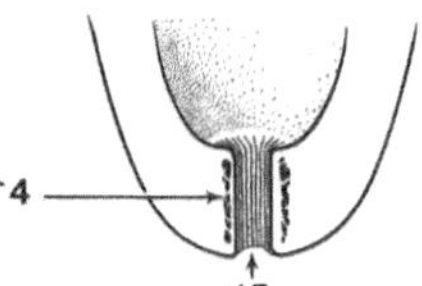

D Ductus papillaris (bo)

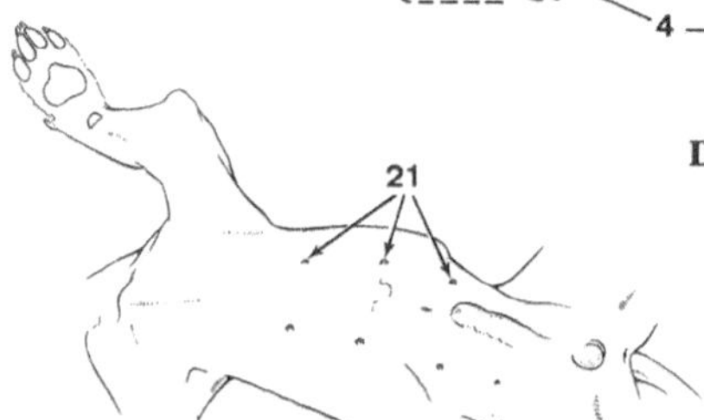

G Mammae masculinae (ca)

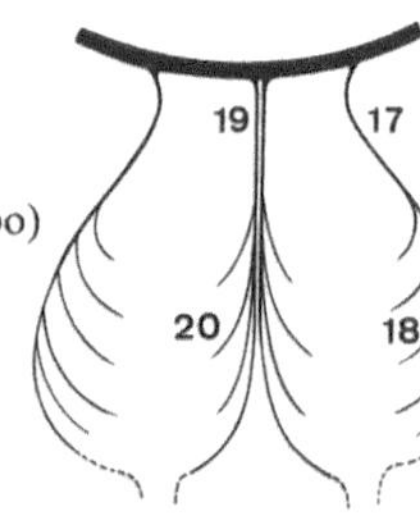

F Apparatus suspensorius mammarius, schematic (bo)

CAPUT. Head
Cranium. Skull
Vertex. Crown of the head
Sinciput. Rostral part of the cranium
Frons. Forehead
Occiput. Caudal part of the cranium
Tempora. Temples
Cornu. Horn
Auris. Ear
Auricula. Auricle
Facies. Face
Oculus. Eye
Palpebra superior. Upper eyelid
Palpebra inferior. Lower eyelid
Rima palpebrarum. Palpebral fissure
Bulbus oculi. Eyeball
Sulcus infrapalpebralis. Infrapalpebral groove
Nasus. Nose
Dorsum nasi. Bridge of the nose
Apex nasi. Apex of the nose
Ala nasi. Wing of the nose
Naris. Nostril
Planum nasale. Nasal plane
Planum nasolabiale. Nasolabial plane
Rostrum. Snout
Planum rostrale. Rostral plane
Os. Mouth (The Latin "Os" is translated either by "bone" or by "mouth". In the first case the genitive of Os is "ossis", and in the second case, "oris".)
Labium superius. Upper lip
Labium inferius. Lower lip
Rima oris. Opening of mouth
Cavum oris. Oral cavity
Lingua. Tongue
Fauces. Entrance to pharynx
Bucca [Mala]. Cheek
Mentum. Chin
Sulcus mentolabialis. Mentolabial groove
COLLUM. Neck
Cervix. Neck
Nucha. Back of the neck
Juba. Mane
Palear. Dewlap
Larynx. Between pharynx and trachea
Prominentia laryngea. Laryngeal prominence
Pharynx. Crossing of digestive and respiratory pathways in the head
Trachea. Windpipe
Esophagus [Oesophagus]. Between pharynx and stomach

TRUNCUS. Trunk
Dorsum. Back
Columna vertebralis. Vertebral column
Lumbus. Loin
Thorax. Thorax, between the neck and the abdomen
Cavum thoracis. Thoracic cavity
Pectus. Breast
Mamma thoracica[1]. Thoracic mamma
Papilla mammae. Nipple (Car, su)
Abdomen. Abdomen, between the thorax and the pelvis
Cavum abdominis. Abdominal cavity
Fossa epigastrica. Slight depression in the midline just caudal to the xiphoid process
Umbilicus. Navel
Latus. Flank
Plica lateris. Fold of the flank
Inguen. Groin
Mamma abdominalis[1]. Abdominal mamma
Papilla mammae. Nipple (Car, su)
Mamma inguinalis[1]. Inguinal mamma
Papilla mammae. Nipple (Car, su), teat (Ru, eq)
Sulcus intermammarius. Intermammary groove
Uber. Udder. All the mammae collectively in Ru and eq (Uber, the Latin term for udder, designates all the Mammae collectively in the Ruminantia and horse.)
Preputium [Praeputium]. Prepuce
Scrotum. Cutaneous pouch containing the testes
Pelvis. Pelvis, between the abdomen and the tail
Cavum pelvis. Pelvic cavity
Coxa. Hip
Nates [Clunes]. Part of the pelvis dorsal to the level of the Tuber ischiadicum on both sides, known as the croup or rump
Perineum. Under the tail and including the anus and urogenital region
Anus. Anus
Crena ani. Anal cleft
[Pudendum femininum]. Female pudendum
Vulva. Vulva
CAUDA. Tail
Radix caudae. Root of the tail
Cirrus caudae. Long hairs of the tail
MEMBRA. Limbs
Membrum thoracicum. Thoracic limb
Axilla. Between he sternum and the thoracic limb
Plica axillaris. Axillary fold

Brachium. Arm
Facies cranialis. Cranial surface
Facies caudalis. Caudal surface
Facies lateralis. Lateral surface
Facies medialis. Medial surface
Sulcus bicipitalis lateralis. Lateral bicipital groove
Sulcus bicipitalis medialis. Medial bicipital groove
Cubitus. Elbow.
Antebrachium. Forearm
Facies cranialis. Cranial surface
Facies caudalis. Caudal surface
Facies lateralis. Lateral surface
Facies medialis. Medial surface
Manus. Hand
Dorsum manus. Dorsal aspect of manus
Palma manus. Palm (palmar aspect) of manus, the inner surface of the hand
Carpus. Wrist, including carpal bones
Facies dorsalis. Dorsal surface
Facies palmaris. Palmar surface
Facies lateralis. Lateral surface
Facies medialis. Medial surface
Torus carpeus. Carpal pad (Car), chestnut (eq) (A Torus carpeus is present in Carnivora and in the horse, but in the latter it lacks a Pulvinus and is called chestnut.)
Metacarpus. Including metacarpal bones
Facies dorsalis. Dorsal surface
Facies palmaris. Palmar surface
Facies lateralis. Lateral surface
Facies medialis. Medial surface
Torus metacarpeus. Metacarpal pad (Car)
Calcar metacarpeum. Spur, ergot (eq)
Digiti manus. Digits of manus
Digitus I [Pollex]. First digit [thumb]
Digiti II–V. Second–fifth digits
Facies dorsalis. Dorsal surface
Facies palmaris. Palmar surface
Facies solearis. Solear surface
Facies lateralis. Lateral surface (eq)
Facies medialis. Medial surface (eq)
Facies axialis. Axial surface (Car, su, Ru).
Facies abaxialis. Abaxial surface (Car, su, Ru)
Paradigitus. Digit that does not reach the plane of support of other digits (Car, su, bo). Known as dewclaws in bo (no phalanges, but the structure of a hoof).
Paraungula. Horny structure without phalanx (ov, cap)
Ungula. Hoof (su, Ru, eq)
Unguicula. Claw (Car)
Membrum pelvinum. Pelvic limb
Femur. Thigh
Facies cranialis. Cranial surface
Facies caudalis. Caudal surface
Facies lateralis. Lateral surface
Facies medialis. Medial surface
Genu. Stifle
Poples. Hollow of stifle
Patella
Crus. Leg
Facies cranialis. Cranial surface
Facies caudalis. Caudal surface
Facies lateralis. Lateral surface
Facies medialis. Medial surface
Sura. Calf
Malleolus lateralis. Lateral malleolus
Malleolus medialis. Medial malleolus
Pes. Foot
Dorsum pedis. Dorsal aspect of foot
Planta pedis. Sole (plantar aspect) of foot
Tarsus. Ankle
Facies dorsalis. Dorsal surface
Facies plantaris. Plantar surface
Facies lateralis. Lateral surface
Facies medialis. Medial surface
Calx. Heel
Torus tarseus. Chestnut (eq)
Metatarsus. Including metatarsal bones
Facies dorsalis. Dorsal surface
Facies plantaris. Plantar surface
Facies lateralis. Lateral surface
Facies medialis. Medial surface
Torus metatarseus. Metatarsal pad (Car)
Calcar metatarseum. Spur, ergot (eq)
Digiti pedis. Digits of foot, toes
Digitus I [Hallux]. First digit
Digiti II–V. Second–fifth digits
Facies dorsalis. Dorsal surface
Facies plantaris. Plantar surface
Facies solearis. Solear surface
Facies lateralis. Lateral surface (eq)
Facies medialis. Medial surface (eq)
Facies axialis. Axial surface (Car, su, Ru)
Facies abaxialis. Abaxial surface (Car, su, Ru)

Paradigitus. Digit that does not reach the plane of support of other digits (ca, su, bo). Known as dewclaws in bo, they are the rudiments of digits II and V and contain small phalanges, which are not articulated with the metacarpal or metatarsal bones

(Paraunguicula). Horny structure without phalanx (ca)

Paraungula. Horny structure without phalanx, (ov, cap)

Ungula. Hoof (su, Ru, eq)

Unguicula. Claw (Car)

[1)] A Mamma is a glandular complex associated with one Papilla mammae. The sow usually has 14 Mammae, the bitch 10, the queen 8, the cow 4, the mare, ewe, and goat, 2.

TERMINI SITUM ET DIRECTIONEM PARTIUM CORPORIS INDICANTES. Terms describing location and orientation of parts of the body

Medianus. Located in the median plane

Sagittalis. Parallel to the median plane

Transversalis. Perpendicular (at right angle) to the long axis of the body or part

Medialis. Closer to the median plane

Intermedius. Intermediate

Lateralis. More distant to the median plane

Cranialis. Closer to the cranium, used on neck, trunk, and the limbs proximal to carpus and tarsus

Medius. Middle

Caudalis. Closer to the tail, used on head, neck, trunk, and the limbs proximal to carpus and tarsus

Anterior. In quadrupeds, the use is restricted to some structures of the head

Rostralis. Closer to the tip of the nose, resp. the orifice of the mouth, used on the head

Posterior. In quadrupeds, the use is restricted to some structures of the head

Dorsalis. Closer to the dorsum. This term refers to back or dorsum of the neck, trunk, and tail, to the corresponding surface of the head, dorsum of manus and pes. The dorsal plane is parallel to the dorsal surface of the body or part, and perpendicular to the median and transverse planes. It replaces the former frontal plane, because it refers to the plane of the human forehead

Ventralis. Closer to the ground in the standing position of a quadruped

Superior. In quadrupeds, the use is restricted to some structures of the head

Inferior. In quadrupeds, the use is restricted to some structures of the head

Internus. Internal

Externus. External

Dexter. Right

Sinister. Left

Longitudinalis. Longitudinal

Transversus. Transverse

Superficialis. Superficial

Profundus. Deep

TERMINI AD MEMBRA SPECTANTES. Terms related to the limbs.

Proximalis. Toward the trunk

Distalis. Toward the free end

Medialis. Closer to the median plane

Lateralis. More distant to the median plane

Axialis. Closer to the long axis of the limb, used on the digit of Car, su, Ru

Abaxialis. More distant to the long axis of the limb, used on the digits of Car, su, Ru

Dorsalis. In the limbs dorsal refers to the dorsum of manus and pes

Palmaris. Palmar, refers to the inner (caudal) surface of the palm (of manus).

Plantaris. Plantar, refers to the inner (caudal) surface of the planta (of pes).

TERMINI GENERALES. General terms, listed in a limited number, consisting of the fundamental terms used in the Veterinary Anatomy (including Veterinary Histology and Embryology)

Abducens. Abducting, moving away from the median plane

Abductor. A muscle performing the abduction

Aberrans. Abberant, deviating from what is normal

Accessorius. Accessory

Acinus. Grape-shaped structure

Acropodium. Region containing the digits

Acutus. Acute

Adductor. A muscle moving towards the median plane

Adeps, adipis. Fat

Adventitius. Adventitious. Occuring in an unusual place, or arising from an external source

Afferens. Afferent, inflowing

Affixus. Affixed, attached

Aggregatus. A mass or cluster of individual units

Albicans. Whitish

Albugineus. Resembling boiled white of egg

Albus. White

Alimentarius. Alimentary

Alveolus. Bucket

Ambiguus. Ambiguous

Ampulla. Dilation of a duct

Amygdala. Almond

Anatomia. Anatomy

Ancon, anconis. Ellbow

Ansa. Loop

Anulus. Ring

Apicalis. Apical

Appendix. Appendix

Aquosus. Aqueous

Arachne. Spider

Arcuatus. Arched

Areola. Any small area

Arrector. Raising up

Arteria. Artery

Arteriola. Arteriole

Arytena [Arytaena]. Small watering pot, ladle

Ascendens. Ascending
Asper. Rough
Associus. Associated
Atavus. Ancestor
Auditus. Sense of hearing
Autonomicus. Autonomic
Autopodium. The region including carpus/tarsus, metacarpus/metatarsus and phalanges
Azygos. Unpaired
Basalis. Basal
Basilaris. Basilar
Basipodium. The region including carpus/tarsus
Bicornis. With two horns
Bifidus. Split into two
Branchia. Gills
Brevis. Short
Bronchulus. Bronchule
Buccina. Crooked trumpet, horn
Bulbus. Bulb
Bursa. A closed sac lined with synovial membrane and containing fluid
Calix. Cup
Callosus. Callous
Calx, calcis. Heel
Canalis. Canal
Canaliculus. Small canal
Capillaris. Capillary
Capillus. Hair of head
Capitalis. Capital
Capitatus. In relation to a head
Capsula. Capsule
Cardia. Junction between esophagus and stomach
Cardiacus. Cardiac
Carneus. Fleshy
Caruncula. Caruncle, a small fleshy protuberance
Caverna. Cavern
Cavus. Hollow
Cecus [Caecus]. Blind
Celiacus [Coeliacus]. Celiac, relating to the abdominal cavity
Cella. Cell
Cellula. Cell (Hist.)
Centralis. Central
Cephalicus. Cephalic, cranial
Ceruleus [Caeruleus]. Bluish
Chroma. Color.
Chylus. Intestinal lymph
Cilium. Eyelash, a motile extension of a cell surface
Cinereus. Cinder-colored
Circumflexus. Circumflex, curving around
Clinoideus. Clinoid, resembling a four-poster bed
Clunis. Buttock
Coccyx. Tail bone(s)
Collateralis. Collateral
Collum. Neck
Comes, comitis. Companion
Communicatio. Communication
Communis. Common
Compactus. Compact
Compressor. Compressor
Condylus. Condyle
Congenitus. Congenital
Conjungatio. Conjugation
Conjunctivus. Conjunctive
Connexus. Connected
Constrictor. Constrictor
Convexus. Convex
Convolutus. Convoluted
Corniculatus. Resembling a horn
Cornu. Horn
Corpus. Body or mass
Corpusculum. Corpuscle
Cortex. The outer portion of an organ
Costa. Rib
Cotyla. Bowl
Coxa. Hip
Crassus. Thick
Cribriformis. Sieve-like
Cribrosus. Perforated
Cricoideus. Ring-shaped
Crista. Crest
Cruciatus. Crossed
Deciduus. Deciduous, not permanent, eventually falls off
Declive, declivis. Declivity
Deferens. Deferent, carrying away
Delta. Triangular-shaped
Densus. Dense
Denticulatus. Denticulate, finely dentated
Depressor. Depressor
Descendens. Descending
Digastricus. Digastric, two-bellied
Digitalis. Digital
Dilatator. Dilator
Diplois. Lying between two layers
Diverticulum. A pouch opening from a tubular organ
Ductulus. Ductule
Ductus. Duct

Durus. Hard

Efferens. Efferent, outflowing

Ejaculatorius. Ejaculatory

Elasticus. Elastic

Ellipsoideus. Ellipsoidal

Embryo. Embryo

Eminentia. Prominence

Emissarius. Emissary, relating to an outlet or drain

Endothelium. Lining of cardiovascular system

Entericus. Related to the intestine

Epigastrium. The most cranial part of abdomen

Epiphysis. 1. The extremity of a long bone. 2. The pineal body (*Epiphysis cerebri*)

Equinus. Equine, horse

Erector. Raising up

Excavatio. Excavation, depression

Extensor. Opening the angle between two parts of a limb, opposite to flexor

Extremitas. Extremity

Facies. Face, surface

Fascia. A sheet of fibrous tissue under the skin and/or surrounding muscles

Fel-felis (Latin). Gall bladder (see Vesica fellea)

Fetus. Fetus

Fibra. Fibre

Fibrilla. Minute filament

Fibrocartilago. Fibrocartilage

Fibularis. Fibular

Filamentum. Filament

Fissura. Fissure

Flavus. Yellow

Flexor. Closing the angle between two parts of a limb, opposite to extensor

Flexura. Flexure

Folliculus. Follicle

Foramen. A perforation through a bone or a membranous structure

Fossa. A depression below the level of the surface

Fovea. A natural depression on the surface of the body

Frons, frontis. Forehead

Frontalis. Frontal

Fundus. The bottom of a sac or hollow organ

Fuscus. Dark

Fusiformis. Spindle-shaped

Gallus. Chicken, fowl

Ganglion. Aggregation of nerve cell bodies

Gelatinosus. Gelatinous

Genesis. Origin

Genitalis. Genital

Germen, germinis. Germ

Germinativus. Germinative

Glandular. Relating to a gland

Globus. Globe

Glomerulum. Glomerule, a plexus of capillaries

Gluteus [Glutaeus]. Gluteal, pertaining to the buttocks

Gracilis. Slender

Granulatio. Granulation

Griseus. Gray

Gyrus. A rounded elevation of the cerebral hemispheres

Hamatus. Hamate, with a hook

Hilus. A depression where vessels and nerves enter and leave

Hyalinus. Hyalin/hyaline. A translucent albuminoid substance/glassy and transparent

Hybrida. Hybrid

Hyoideus. Hyoid, shaped like the lower case Greek letter upsilon

Hypogastrium. The most caudal part of abdomen

Hypoglossus. Hypoglossal, below the tongue

Ilia, ilium. Hip bone

Iliacus. Iliac, relating to the ilium

Impar. Unpaired

Impressio. Impression, made by pressure of one structure on another

Imus. Lowest, lowermost

Incisivus. Suitable for cutting

Incisura. Notch

Incisus. Cut open

Infundibulum. Funnel-shaped structure

Interstitium. Interstice, gap in the substance of a structure

Intestinum. Intestine

Intima. Innermost layer of a structure, lining it

Introitus. Entrance

Ischiadicus. Sciatic

Ischium. Seat, buttock

Isthmus. Constriction or narrow connection between two parts of a structure

Jugulum. Fossa between sternocephalicus, brachiocephalicus, and pectoralis descendens muscles

Labium. Lip, or lip-shaped structure

Lac, lactis. Milk

Lacer. Lacerated, torn

Lacrima. Tear

Lacuna. Small space or cavity

Lamina. Plate
Lanugo. Wool, down
Laryngeus. Laryngeal
Latissimus. Broadest
Levator. Muscle lifting up a structure
Liber. Free
Ligamentum. A fibrous tissue band connecting two or more bones or cartilages, also a fold of peritoneum
Limbus. Edge, border, or fringe of a structure
Limitans. Limiting
Linea. Line
Lobus. Lobe
Longissimus. The longest
Longus. Long
Lucidus. Clear
Lumbricus. Earth worm
Lunatus. Sichle-moon shaped
Lunula. Small half moon
Luteus. Yellow
Lympha. Lymph
Lymphaticus. Lymphatic
Lymphonodus. Lymph node
Magnus. Great, large
Major. Greater, larger
Mamilla. Nipple
Manus. Hand, the distal extremity of the thoracic limb. ("Manus" should have been listed in the 5th edition, similar to "Pes".)
Margo. Border
Masticatus. Chewed
Mastoideus. Mastoid, breast-shaped
Mater, matris. Mother
Matrix, matricis. The formative part of a structure
Meninx, meningis. Meninges
Mesothelium. Lining serous cavities
Metapodium. Region containing the metacarpal/metatarsal bones
Meatus. External opening of a canal, a passage or channel
Mediastinum. Septum or partition between two parts of an organ or a cavity
Medulla. Soft marrow-like structure
Minor. Smaller
Mitra. Miter, tall pointed hat worn by the Pope or a Roman-Catholic bishop
Mola. Millstone
Molecularis. Molecular
Mollis. Soft
Mons, montis. Mountain
Motor. A structure producing motion
Mucosus. Mucous
Mucus. Mucus
Multifidus. Split into many parts
Musculus. Muscle
Navicula. Boat
Nephros. Kidney
Nervus. Nerve
Neuron. Nerve cell
Niger. Black
Nomen, mominis. Name
Norma. Norm
Nucleolus. A small nucleus
Nutricius. Nutrient
Obliquus. Oblique
Obturator. Closing an opening of the body
Obtusus. Obtuse, blunt
Occipitalis. Occipital
Occultus. Occult, hidden from view, concealed
Olfactus. Sense of smell
Omphalos (Gr.). Umbilicus. Navel
Ophthalmicus. Ophthalmic, relating to the eye
Orbicularis. Orbicular, circular in shape
Orificium. Orifice
Os, oris. Mouth
Os, ossis. Bone
Ossiculum. Ossicle
Ostium. Orifice, small opening
Oticus. Belonging to the ear
Ovum. Egg
Pallidus. Pale
Pampiniformis. Tendril-like
Papilla. Small, nipple-like process
Paraganglion. Small body containing specific cells
Parasympathicus. Parasympathetic
Parotis, parotidis. Parotid
Pars. Part
Parvus. Small
Pedalis. Pedal
Pellis. Pelt, the skin of an animal with the fur or hair still on it
Pellucidus. Pellucid, translucent
Perforatus. Perforated
Periosteum. Double layer of connective tissue covering the bones, except articular surfaces
Peripheralis. Peripherae
Peripheria. Periphery

Permanens, permanentis. Permanent

Peroneus [Peronaeus]. Peroneal (former alternative for "fibular")

Pes. Foot, foot-like part

Petra. Rock

Petrosus. Petrous

Phallus. Penis

Pigmentum. Pigment

Pilus. Hair

Pinea. Pine cone

Pinna. Auricula, feather

Piriformis. Piriform, pear-shaped

Pisiformis. Pisiform, pea-shaped (Os pisiforme = accessory carpal bone)

Pituita. Glairy mucus, a thick nasal secretion

Pius. Tender, delicate

Planus. Plane, flat

Pneumaticus. Pneumatic

Porta. Site of entrance to an organ of the blood vessels supplying it

Primus. First

Princeps, principis. Principal

Prisma, prismatis. Prism

Processus. Projection or outgrowth

Projectio, projectionis. Projection

Prominens, prominentis. Prominent

Pronator. A muscle turning the Manus with the dorsal side forward

Proprius. Proper

Pterygma, pterygmatis. Wing

Pterygoideus. Wing-shaped, resembling a wing

Pubes. The hair on the genitals

Pudendus. Pudenal, relating to external genitalia, esp. female

Pulposus. In the condition of a soft, moist solid

Pupillaris. Pupillary

Pyramis. Pyramid

Quadratus. Quadratic, square

Quadriceps, quadricipitis. Four-headed

Radialis. Radial

Radix. Root

Ramus. Branch

Recessus. A small hollow or indentation

Rectus. Straight

Recurrens, recurrentis. Recurrent, turning back on itself

Reflexus. Reflected, bent back

Regio. Region

Renalis. Renal

Respiratio, respirationis. Respiration

Rete. Network or mesh (pl. retia)

Retinaculum. Retaining band or ligament

Retroflexus. Retroflex, bent backword

Rhis. rhinos. Nose

Rhomboideus. Rhomboid

Rotundus. Round

Ruber. Red

Rudimentum. Rudiment

Saccus[2]. Sack, pouch

Sacer. Sacred

Sacrum. Segment of the vertebral column, part of the pelvis

Saliva. Spit

Sanguis, sanguinis. Blood

Scalenus. Stairs-like

Sebaceus. Sebaceous

Sebum. Produce of the sebaceous glands

Secretum. Secretion

Semen, seminis. Seminal fluid. Secretion of the reproductive organs in the male containing spermatozoa

Sensorium. Consciousnes

Sensus. Sense

Septulum. Small septum

Septum. A wall separating a mass or cavity in two parts or spaces

Serratus. Serrate, dentate like a saw

Serum. The liquid component of the blood

Sesamoideus. Sesamoid, resembling in shape a grain of sesame

Sigmoideus. Sigmoid, S-curved

Simplex, simplicis. Simple

Singularis. Singular

Sinus. A cavity or hollow space, a dilation in a blood vessel

Solitarius. Solitary

Spatium. Space

Sperma, spermatis. Sperm, semen, spermatozoa

Sphenoidalis. Sphenoid, wedge-shaped

Spheroidalis. Spheroid, wedge-shaped

Spheroideus [Sphaeroideus]. Spherical

Sphincter. Round muscle closing a natural orifice

Spina. Spine, spinous process

Spinalis. Related to any spine or spinous process

Splanchnicus. Splanchnic, visceral

Spongiosus. Spongy

Spurius. False

Squamosus. Squamous, platelike, or resembling a scale

Status. State

Stella. Star

Stellatus. Stellate, star-shaped

Stoma, stomatis. Mouth

Stratum. One of the layers of a differentiated tissue, sheet-like mass of substance

Striatus. Striate, striped

Stylopodium. Part of the skeleton including the humerus, and the femur and patella

Stylus. Style

Succus. Juice

Sudor, sudoris. Sweat

Sulcus. Groove

Supinator. A muscle turning the Manus with the palm forward

Supinus. Turned upwards

Suspensus. Suspended

Sympathicus. Sympathetic

Symphysis. The union of two symmetrical bones by means of a fibrocartilage

Synchondrosis. The union of two bones by means of either a hyaline cartilage, or fibrocartilage

Tactilis. Tactile, touch

Tactus. Sense of touch

Tectorius. Tectorial, covering

Tempus, temporis. Temple

Tendo. Tendon

Tenia [Taenia]. Structure resembling a tapeworm

Tensor. Muscle tensing/pulling a structure

Tenuis. Thin

Teres, teretis. Round

Terminalis. Terminal

Theca. Sheath or capsule

Thorax, thoracis. Chest

Tibialis. Tibial

Tonsilla. Small rounded mass of tissue, esp. Lymphoid tissue

Tractus. Collection or bundle, esp. of nerve fibers, with the same origin and termination, and serving the same function

Trigonum. Triangle

Trochanter. One of the two-three prominences distal to the neck of the femur

Trochlea. Pulley-like articular structure

Truncus. Trunk

Tuba. A straight tube, an elongated hollow cylindrical organ

Tuber. A rounded prominence, either bony or fleshy

Tuberculum. A circumscribed, rounded, solid eminence

Tuberositas. Tuberosity

Tubulus. Tubule

Tubus. Tube

Tunica. Tunic, coat

Tympanum. Drum

Ulnaris. Ulnar

Uncinatus. Uncinate, hook-shaped

Uncus. Hook

Urina. Urine

Vagina. The genital canal in female, between uterus and vulva, also sheath

Vagus. Wandering

Valva. Valve, one leaf of a double door

Vascularis. Vascular

Vastus. Vast

Vellus. Fleece, wool, fur

Velum. Veil, courtain

Vena. Vein

Ventriculus. Ventricle

Venula. Small vein

Verus. True

Vesicalis. Vesical

Vestibularis. Vestibular

Vestigium. Vestige

Viscus, visceris. Singular of viscera, used only in plural

Visus. Sense of sight

Vita. Life

Vitellus. Yolk

Vitreus. Vitreous, glassy, resembling glass

Vocalis. Vocal

Vorticosus. Vorticose, vortex-like

Xiphoideus. Xiphoid, sword-shaped

Zeugopodium. Part of the skeleton including radius and ulna, and tibia and fibula

Zona. Zone, also girdle

Zygomaticus. Zygomatic, pertaining to zygomatic arch, connecting with

TERMINI PECULIARES. Special terms for each Chapter

OSTEOLOGIA. Osteology

Systema skeletale. Skeletal system

Pars ossea. Osseous part

Periosteum. Connective tissue layer outside the bone

Endosteum. Connective tissue layer inside the bone, lining the medullary cavity

Substantia corticalis. Cortical substance

Substantia compacta. Compact substance

Substantia spongiosa. Spongy substance, trabecular, or cancellous bone

Pars cartilaginea. Cartilaginous part

Perichondrium. Connective tissue layer outside the cartilage

Skeleton axiale. Axial skeleton

Skeleton appendiculare. Appendicular skeleton

Os longum. Long bone

Os breve. Short bone

Os planum. Flat bone

Os irregulare. Irregular bone

Os pneumaticum. Pneumatic bone

Os sesamoideum. Sesamoid bone

Diaphysis. Shaft of long bones

Metaphysis. Flared end of the diaphysis where calcified cartilage is replaced by bone

Cartilago physialis. Physial cartilage, the radiolucent plate of growing and calcifying cartilage between epiphysis and metaphysis during growth

Linea physialis. Physial line, the radioopaque lamina of dense bone in the plane of fusion of the epiphysis to the diaphysis in a mature bone, the vestige of Cartilago physialis

Epiphysis. The extremities of the long bones

Cartilago epiphysialis. Completely surrounds the Centrum ossificationis secundarium (The meaning of this term has been changed from that of the previous edition to agree with current concepts in bone research. It is histologically and functionally distinct from the Cartilago articularis and Cartilago physialis.)

Cartilago articularis (vide Articulationes)

Centrum ossificationis primarium. Primary center of ossification in the diaphysis

Centrum ossificationis secundarium. Secundary center of ossification in an epiphysis

Synostosis. Osseous connection between bones

Apophysis. Projection or bony process that lacks an independent center of ossification

Facies articularis. Articular surface

Cavum medullare. Medullary cavity

Medulla ossium flava. Yellow bone marrow[1)]

Medulla ossium rubra. Red bone marrow[1)]

Foramen nutricium. Nutrient foramen

Canalis nutricius. Nutrient canal

[1)] There is a third type of bone marrow, Medulla ossium grisea/gelatinosa, which is not listed in the 5th edition of the N. A. V. It is a normal bone marrow, fatless, found in the bones of the face and roof of the cranial cavity. In the other bones it is found in very old and/or skinny individuals [Barone 1999, p. 61].

ARTHROLIGIA. Arthrology

ARTICULATIONES. Articulations, general term for all joints – fibrous, cartilaginous, and synovial (There is another type of joint, called "Synsarcosis", which implies only soft tissue, such as muscles and/or adnexa [sarkos = flesh in Gr.], between the thoracic limbs and the body, for example.)

Articulationes fibrosae. Fibrous articulations

Syndesmosis. The opposing bony surfaces are far apart and united by ligament

Sutura. Suture

Sutura serrata. Showing deep saw-like indentations

Sutura squamosa. Scale-like and overlapping, similar to fish scales or roof shingles

Sutura foliata. Combination of the previous two types

Sutura plana. Harmonious, between bones with straight and thickened borders, smooth or rough

Schindylesis. A sharp edge (blade) of one bone into a cleft (groove) in the edge of the other

Gomphosis [Articulatio dentoalveolaris]. Implantation of the tooth in the alveolus

Periodontium. The connective tissue that surrounds the tooth root and attaches it into the alveolus

Articulations cartilagineae. Cartilaginous articulations

Synchondrosis. Two bones are united either by hyaline cartilage (primary synchondrosis, ossifies) or fibrocartilage (secondary synchondrosis, does not ossify)

Symphysis. The union between two symmetrical bones by means of a fibrocartilaginous blade (susceptible to ossify)

Articulationes synoviales. Synovial articulations, mobile joints (Articulationes synoviales replaces the former terms Diarthrosis and Articulus.)

Articulatio simplex. Simple articulation

Articulatio composita. Composite articulation, with more than two bones

Articulatio plana. Plane articulation

Articulatio spheroidea [sphaeroidea, cotylica]. Speroidal (socket) articulation, or enarthrosis

Articulatio ellipsoidea. Ellipsoidal articulation

Ginglymus. Hinge articulation, or trochlearthrosis

Articulatio condylaris. Condylar articulation

Articulatio trochoidea. Trochoid (pivoting) articulation

Articulatio sellaris. Saddle articulation

Cartilago articularis. Articular cartilage

Fossae synoviales (Un). Synovial fossae found only in Ungulates

Cavum articulare. Articular cavity

Discus articularis. Articular disk

Meniscus articularis. Articular meniscus

Labrum articulare. Articular fibrocartilaginous lip-shaped structure

Capsula articularis. Articular capsule

Stratum fibrosum. Fibrous layer

Stratum synoviale. Synovial layer

Plica synovialis. Synovial fold

Villi synoviales. Synovial villi

Synovia. Synovial fluid

Ligamenta. Ligaments

Ligg. extracapsularia. Extracapsular ligaments, with no connection to the articular capsule

Ligg. capsularia. Capsular ligaments, outside the joint capsule, thickened portions of the fibrous layer of the articular capsule

Ligg. intracapsularia. Intracapsular ligaments, within and separate from the articular capsule

MYOLOGIA. Myology, dealing with the skeletal, striated, or voluntary muscles

Musculus. Muscle

Caput. Head, the part of the belly attached to the origin of a muscle

Venter. Belly

Cauda. Tail

Endomysium. The fine connective tissue sheath surrounding only one muscle fiber

Epimysium. The fibrous connective tissue enveloping the entire muscle

Perimysium. The fibrous sheath enveloping each fascicle of a skeletal muscle fiber

Musculus fusiformis. Fusiform muscle

Musculus quadratus. Quadrate muscle

Musculus triangularis. Triangular muscle

Musculus planus. Flat muscle

Musculus unipennatus. Unipennate muscle

Musculus bipennatus. Bipennate muscle

Musculus multipennatus. Multipennate muscle

Musculus flexor. Flexor muscle

Musculus extensor. Extensor muscle

Musculus abductor. Abductor muscle

Musculus adductor. Adductor muscle

Musculus rotator. Rotator muscle

Musculus pronator. Pronator muscle

Musculus supinator. Supinator muscle

Musculus dilatator. Dilator muscle

Musculus tensor. Tensor muscle

Musculus depressor. Depressor muscle

Musculus levator. Levator muscle

Musculus retractor. Retractor muscle

Musculus protractor. Protractor muscle

Musculus sphincter. Sphincter muscle

Musculus orbicularis. Orbicular muscle, with one, or two tendons oposing each other

Musculus articularis. Articular muscle

Musculus skeleti. Skeletal muscle

Origo. Origin, the more proximal or more fixed attachment[1)]

Terminatio. Termination or insertion, the more distal or the more movable attachment[1)]

[1)] The muscles acting in propulsion, rearing, and some muscles involved in the sexual act are called muscles with reversible action, in which the origin and the insertion are interchangeable. Instead, for these muscles the terms "attachments" – proximal and distal, cranial and caudal etc. are appropriate (ex. biceps femoris, semitendinosus, semimembranosus, psoas major and minor, triceps brachii etc.).

Musculus cutaneus. Cutaneous muscle

Tendo. Tendon

Peritendineum. The continuation of perimysium

Endotendineum. The continuation of endomysium

Epitendineum. The continuation of epimysium

Aponeurosis. A flat and wide tendon

Fascia. Sheet of fibrous tissue enveloping the body under the skin, also muscles and/or groups of muscles

Intersectio tendinea. Tendinous intersection

Arcus tendineus. Tendinous arch

Vagina fibrosa tendinis. Fibrous tendon sheath

Vagina synovialis tendinis. Synovial tendon sheath

Mesotendineum. Mesotendon, the liaison between the synovial tendon sheath and the tendon. Vessels and nerves nourishing the tendon travel between its two layers.

Trochlea muscularis. Muscular trochlea

Bursa synovialis. Synovial bursa

BURSAE ET VAGINAE SYNOVIALES. Synovial bursae and sheaths

Bursa synovialis subcutanea. Subcutaneous synovial bursa

Bursa synovialis submuscularis. Submuscular synovial bursa

Bursa synovialis subfascialis. Subfascial synovial bursa

Bursa synovialis subtendinea. Subtendinous synovial bursa

Bursa synovialis subligamentosa. Subligamentous synovial bursa

Vagina synovialis tendinis. Synovial tendon sheath surrounds the tendon as double layer structure with synovial fluid in between. The two layers are connected by the Mesotendineum (see above).

SPLANCHNOLOGIA. Splanchnology

Tunica mucosa. Mucous membrane. See also pp. 150, 186

Lamina propria mucosae. Proper lamina of a mucous membrane

Lamina muscularis mucosae. Thin sheet of smooth muscle, the deepest layer of a mucous membrane. See also pp. 152, 160–164, 188

Tela submucosa. Loose connective tissue under the mucous membrane. See also pp. 150, 152, 160, 162, 164, 188, 198

Tunica muscularis. Muscular coat. See also pp. 160–164, 198, 202, 204, 210, 214, 216, 220

Tunica fibrosa. Fibrous coat. See also p. 170

Tunica albuginea. Inextensible white capsule of the testis and of the ovary. See also pp. 200, 212

Tunica adventitia. Outer coat of connective tissue. See also pp. 152, 168, 196, 202, 204, 216, 220

Tela subserosa. Layer of loose connective tissue and fat under the serous membrane. See also pp. 160, 162, 164, 170

Tunica serosa. Serous membrane. See also pp. 160–164, 170, 198, 202, 214, 216, 226, 412

Parenchyma. Specific cells, the substance of a gland or organ, supported by stroma. See also pp. 204, 230

Stroma. The framework of an organ, gland or other structure, supporting the parenchyma

Glandula. Gland. See also p. 174

Lobus. Lobe, a subdivision of an organ

Lobulus. Lobule, a small lobe or a subdivision of a lobe

Glandula mucosa. Mucous gland

Glandula serosa. Serous gland

Glandula seromucosa. Seromucous gland

ANGIOLOGIA. Angiology

Vas collaterale. Collateral vessel

Vas anastomoticum. Anastomosing vessel

Plexus vasculosus. Vascular plexus

Rete mirabile. Vascular network interrupting the continuity of an artery of vein

Arteria. Artery

Arteriola. Arteriole

Anastomosis arteriovenosa. Arteriovenous anastomosis

Arcus arteriosus. Arterial arch

Arcus venosus. Venous arch

Rete arteriosum. Arterial network

Circulus articularis vasculosus. Vascular articular circle

Vena. Vein

Vena cutanea. Cutaneous vein

Vena comitans. Accompanying vein

Venula. Venule, a small vein

Valva venosa

Valvula venosa. Venous valvule

Plexus venosus. Venous plexus

Rete venosum. Venous network

Sinus venosus. Venous sinus

Vena emissaria. Outlet or draining vein

Vas capillare [Vas haemocapillare, hemo-]. Capillary

Vas lymphocapillare

Vas lymphaticum. Lymphatic vessel

Valva lymphatica

Valvula lymphatica. Lymphatic valvule

Plexus lymphaticus. Lymphatic plexus

Lymphonodus [Nodus lymphaticus]. Lymph node

Lymphonodulus [Nodulus lymphaticus]. Lymphatic nodule

Lymphonodus hemalis [haemalis]. Hemolymph node (Ru). Spleen-like organized lymphatic tissue in sinuses of which erythrocites normally occur

Cisterna. Cavity or enclosed space serving as a reservoir

Tunica externa. External coat

Tunica media. Middle coat

Tunica intima. Intima (innermost) coat

Vasa vasorum. Small arteries distributed to the walls of blood vessels

Sanguis. Blood

Lympha. Lymph

SYSTEMA NERVOSUM. Nervous system

SYSTEMA NERVOSUM CENTRALE. Central nervous system

Substantia alba. White substance

Substantia grisea. Gray substance

Substantia gelatinosa. Gelatinous substance

Tenia [Taenia] telae. Bandlike structure along which a choroid membrane or plexus is attached to the rim of a brain ventricle

Ependyma. The cellular membrane lining the central canal of the spinal cord and the brain ventricles

Lamina epithelialis. Epethelial lamina

Sulcus limitans. Limitating groove

Lamina alaris. Alar plate of neural tube, wing plate

Lamina basalis. Basal plate of neural tube, basement membrane

Nuclei nervorum cranialium. Nuclei of the cranial nerves

Nuclei originis. Nuclei of origin

Nuclei terminationis. Nuclei of termination

SYSTEMA NERVOSUM PERIPHERICUM. Peripheral nervous system

Nervus. Nerve

Ganglion. Aggregation of nerve cell bodies outside the central nervous system, also applied to certain nuclear groups within the brain

Ramus communicans. Communicating branch

Ramus muscularis. Muscular branch

Nervus cutaneus. Cutaneous nerve

Nervus articularis. Articular nerve

Nervus vascularis. Vascular nerve

Plexus periarterialis. Periarterial plexus

Plexus nervorum spinalium. Plexus of spinal nerves

Corpuscula nervosa terminalia. Terminal nervous corpuscles (vide Nomina Histologica)

Terminationes nervorum liberae. Free nerve endings

SYSTEMA NERVOSUM AUTONOMICUM. Autonomic nervous system

Plexus autonomici. Autonomic plexuses

Ganglia plexuum autonomicorum. Ganglia of autonomic plexuses

Ganglia autonomica. Autonomic ganglia

ORGANA SENSUUM. Sense organs

INTEGUMENTUM COMMUNE. Common integument

Ammon – Sulcus hippocampi, p. 450.17
- Tuberculum hippocampi, p. 450.21, and all subsequent terms using "ammonis"

are related to the name of "Ammon" (p. 450.19, 450.20, 452.10, 460.30)

Bechterew – Nucleus vestibularis rostralis, p. 420.10, 424.22

Broca – Lamella diagonalis, p. 452.25

Burdach – Fasciculus cuneatus, p. 416.4, 418.12, 422.5
- Nucleus cuneatus medialis, p. 420.20
- Nucleus cuneatus lateralis, p. 420.21

Cajal – Nucleus interstitialis, p. 434.6
- Nucleus hypothalamicus ventromedialis, p. 440.3

Deiter – Nucleus vestibularis lateralis, p. 420.12, 424.24

Edinger-Westphal – Nuclei parasympathici n. oculomotorii, p. 434.3

Forel – Decussatio ventralis, p. 434.14

Flechsig – Tractus spinocerebellaris dorsalis, p. 416.10, 422.12

Ganser – Commissura supraoptica dorsalis, p. 440.22

Goll – Fasciculus gracilis, p. 416.3, 418.14, 422.4
- Nucleus gracilis, p. 420.19

Gowers – Tractus spinocerebellaris ventralis, p. 416.9, 422.13

Gratiolet – Radiatio optica, p. 458.21

Gudden – Nuclei tegmenti, p. 434.5
- Commissura supraoptica ventralis, p. 440.23

Lancisi – Stria longitudinalis lateralis, p. 450.10
- Stria longitudinalis medialis, p. 450.11

Larsell – Nomenclature of the subdivisions of Cerebellum, p. 426.23, 428.2–12, 428.14–23, 428.25–27

Lissauer – Tractus dorsolateralis, p. 416.16

Luschka – Aperturae laterals ventriculi quarti, p. 430.28

Luys – Nucleus subthalamicus, p. 442.13

Magendie – (Apertura mediana ventriculi quarti), p. 430.29

Marburg – Nucleus prepositus [prae-] n. hypoglossi, p. 418.23

Meynert – Decussatio dorsalis, p. 434.13
- Fasciculus retroflexus, p. 436.10, 446.11
- Commissura supraoptica ventralis, p. 440.23

Monakow – Tractus rubrospinalis, p. 416.15, 422.22, 426.6

Monroe – Foramen interventriculare, p. 436.18, 460.22

Pacchioni – Granulationes arachnoideales, p. 462.24

Purkinje – Stratum moleculare, p. 428.34
- Stratum neuronorum piriformium, p. 428.35

Reissner – Organum subcommissurale, p. 436.17

Rolando – Substantia gelatinosa, p. 414.32

Roller – Nucleus vestibularis caudalis [descendens], p. 420.13, 424.25

Schutz – Fasciculus longitudinalis dorsalis, p. 426.14

Schwalbe – Nucleus vestibularis medialis, p. 420.11, 424.23

Soemmerring – Substantia nigra, p. 434.24

Staderini – Nucleus intercalatus, p. 418.22

Stilling – Nucleus ruber, p. 434.9

Stilling-Clarke – Nucleus thoracicus, p. 414.33

Sylvius – Aqueductus [Aquae-] mesencephali [Aqueductus cerebri], p. 432.19, and all subsequent terms using "sylvian" are related to the name "Sylvius"

Vicq d'Azyr – Tractus mamillothalamicus, p. 442.7

Acheson GH. The topographical anatomy of the smooth muscle of the cat's nictating membrane. Anat Rec 1938; 71: 297

Arey LB. Developmental Anatomy. 7th ed. Philadelphia: Saunders; 1965

Backhouse KM, Butler H. The gubernaculum testis of the pig. J Anat 1960; 94: 107

Bacsich P, Chrisholm IA, Gellért A et al. On the presence of a reptilantype conus papillaris in the eye of the Golden Hamster. J Anat 1965; 99: 195

Barone R. Anatomie comparée des mammifères domestiques. Tome 3 Splanchnologie Fascicule premier Appareil Digestif – Appareil Respiratoire, Laboratoire d'Anatomie. Lyon: École Nationale Vétérinaire Lyon; 1976: 271

Barone R. Anatomie comparée des mammifères domestiques. Tome 1 Ostéologie. Paris: Vigot Frères; 1999

Barone R. Anatomie comparée des mammifères domestiques, Tome 2 Arthrologie et myologie. Paris: Vigot Frères; 1999a: 333

Barone R. Anatomie comparée des mammifères domestiques. Tome 2 Arthrologie et myologie. Paris: Vigot Frères; 2000

Blom E, Christensen NO. Cysts and cyst-like Formations in the Genitals of the Bull. Yearbook 1958. Copenhagen: Roy. Vet. and Agr. College Copenhagen; 1958: 101

Blom E, Christensen NO. The etiology of spermiostasis in the bull. Nord Vet.-Med 1960; 12: 453

Casteleyn CR, Breugelmans S, Simoens P et al. Morphological and immunological characteristics of the bovine temporal lymph node and hemal node. Vet Immunol and Immunopathol 2008; 126: 339–350

Constantinescu GM, Brown EM, McClure RC. Accessory parotid lymph nodes and hemal nodes in the temporal fossa in three oxen. Cornell Vet 1988; 78: 147–154

Constantinescu GM, Green EM, McClure RC. Block anesthesia of cranial nerves in the horse (landmarks, approaches, topographic anatomy and the technique of anesthesia). Rev Rom Med Vet 1994; 4 (1): 48–67

Constantinescu GM. Block anesthesia of cranial nerves in the ruminants. Anatomy, landmarks, and approaches. Rev Rom Med Vet 1995; 5 (3): 279–294

Constantinescu GM, Green EM. The cutaneous areas and the clinical applications of the nerve block anesthesia of the cranial nerves in the horse. Rev Rom Med Vet 1995; 5 (1): 57–66

Constantinescu GM. The Rhomboideus Atlantis M. should be listed in the Nomina Anatomica Veterinaria as a specific muscle of the pig. July 1991, Annual Meeting and Scientific Session of American Association of Veterinary Anatomists, Pullman, Washington. Anat Hist Embryol 1996; 25: 218–219

Constantinescu GM, Radu CN, Cotofan V. Retrospective and comments on the acropodial fasciae in the horse. August 1994, XXth Congress of the European Association of Veterinary Anatomists, Zurich, Switzerland. Anat Histol Embryol 1997; 26: 64

Constantinescu GM. Guide to regional ruminant Anatomy based on the Dissection of the Goat. Amos, Iowa: Iowa State University Press; 2001

Constantinescu GM. Clinical Anatomy for Small Animal Practitioners. Amos, Iowa: Iowa State Press, a blackwell Publishing Company; 2002

Constantinescu GM, Constantinescu IA. Clinical Dissection Guide for large Animals, Horse and large Ruminants. 2nd ed. Amos, Iowa: Iowa State Press, a Blackwell Publishing Company; 2004

Constantinescu GM, Wilson DA, Constantinescu IA. The anatomoclinical approach to the nerves of the pelvic limb of the horse for performing nerve block anesthesia. Wiener Tierarztliche Monatsschrift 2004; 91: 3, 63–71

Constantinescu GM, Wilson DA, Constantinescu IA et al. The anatomoclinical approach to the nerves of the thoracic limb of the horse for performing nerve block anesthesia. Wiener Tierarztliche Monatsschrift 2004; 91: 2, 30–41

Cornelissen BPM, Rijkenhuizen ABM, Kersten W et al. Nerve supply of the proximal sesamoid bone in the horse. The Veterinary Quarterly 1994; 16 (S2): 66–69. In: Cornelissen BPM. The equine proximal sesamoid bone, vascular and neural characteristics [Ph.D. thesis]. Utrecht; 1997

de Lahunta A, Habel RE. Applied Veterinary Anatomy. Philadelphia: Saunders; 1986

De Schaepdrijver L, Simoens P, Princemaille J. De glans penis en glans clitoridis by het paard: enkele morfoligische aspecten met klinisch belang. Vlaams Dierg Tijdschr 1988; 57: 72

Dyce KM, Sack WO, Wensing CJG. Textbook of Veterinary Anatomy. 3rd ed. Philadelphia: Saunders; 2002

Eichhorn EB, Boyden EA. The choledochoduodenal junction in the dog – a restudy of Oddi's sphincter. Am J Anat 1955; 97: 431

Ellenberger W, Baum H. Handbuch der vergleichenden Anatomie der Haustiere. 18. Aufl. Berlin: Springer; 1943

Evans HE. Miller's Anatomy of the Dog. 3rd ed. Philadelphia: Saunders; 1993

Evans HE, Christensen GC. Miller's anatomy of the dog. 2nd ed. Philadelphia: Saunders; 1979

Evans HE, de Lahunta A. Miller's Anatomy of the Dog. 7th ed. Philadelphia: Saunders; 2010

FCAT (Federative Committee on Anatomical Nomenclature). Terminologia Anatomica. International Anatomical Terminology. Stuttgart: Thieme; 1998: 47

Feneis H, Dauber W. Pocket Atlas of Human Anatomy based on the international Nomenclature. 4th ed. Stuttgart: Thieme; 2000

Garrett PD. Urethral recess in male goats, sheep, cattle, and swine. J Am Vet Med Ass 1987; 191: 689

Gasse H. Constantinescu GM. Simoens P et al. The Editorial Committee of ICVGAN) Nomina Anatomica Veterinaria 6th ed; 2017

Geiger G. Die anatomischen Grundlagen des „Hymenalringes" beim Rinde. Tierärztl. Umschau 1954; 9: 398

Gerisch D, Neurand K. Topographie und Histologie der Drüsen der Regio analis des Hundes. Anat Hist Emb 1973; 2: 280

Getty R. Sisson and Grossman's The Anatomy of the Domestic Animals. 5th ed. Philadelphia: Saunders; 1975

Ghetie V, Riga IT. Die funktionelle Struktur der Ligamenta collateralia am Ellbogen und Sprunggelenke des Pferdes. Anat Anz 1944/1945; 95: 271–285

Ghetie V. Anatomia Animalelor Domestice vol. I Aparatul locomotor. Ed Acad Rep Soc România 1971

Habel RE. Guide to the Dissection of Domestic Ruminants. 4th ed. Ithaca, N. Y: Published by the author; 1989

Habermehl KH. Über besondere Randpapillen an der Zunge neugeborener Säugetiere. Z Anat Entw 1952; 116: 355

Hart BL, Kitchell RL. External morphology of the erect glans penis of the dog. Anat Rec 1965; 152: 193

Hebel R. Distribution of retinal ganglion cells in five mammalian species. Anat Embryol 1976; 150: 45

Hertwig O. Entwicklungslehre des Menschen und der Wirbeltiere. Jena: Fischer; 1900

Hofmann R. Zur Topographie und Morphologie des Wiederkäuermagens in Hinblick auf seine Funktion [Dissertation]. Zbl Vet Med 1969; (Suppl. 10)

Holz K. Vergleichende anatomische und topographische Studien über das Mittelohr der Säugetiere [Dissertation]. Berlin: Freie Universität Berlin; 1931

Horowitz A, Kramer B, Sack WO. Atlas of musculoskeletal Anatomy of the Pig. Ithaca, N. Y.: Veterinary Textbooks; 1982

Int. Committe on Vet. Gross Anat. Nomenclature. Nomina Anatomica Veterinaria. 6th ed. Editorial Committee: Int. Committe on Vet. Gross Anat. Nomenclature; 2017

Krage P. Präputium der Haussäugetiere [Dissertation]. Zürich: Vet. Med. Zürich; 1907

Kratzing J. The structure of the vomeronasal organ in the sheep. J Anat 1971; 108: 247

Lewin NA. Die Venenstruktur und der venöse Abfluß im Innenohr des Rindes und des Schafes. Wien tierärztl Mschr 1963; 50: 888

McCarthy TC. Veterinary Endoscopy for the Small Animal Practitioner. Edinburgh: Elsevier Saunders; 2005: 414

McCotter RE. The connection of the vomeronasal nerves with the accessory olfactory bulb in the opossum and other mammals. Anat Rec 1912; 6: 299

McCotter RE. The Nervus terminalis in the adult dog and cat. J Comp Neurol 1913; 23: 145

Nickel R, Schummer A, Seiferle E. Lehrbuch der Anatomie der Haustiere. Vol. I. Berlin: Parey; 1954

Nickel R, Schummer A, Seiferle E. Lehrbuch der Anatomie der Haustiere. Vol. IV. Berlin: Parey; 1992

Nickel R, Schummer A, Seiferle E. Lehrbuch der Anatomie der Haustiere. Vol. IV. Berlin: Parey; 1975

Nickel R, Schummer A, Seiferle E, Sack WO. The Viscera of the Domestic Mammals. 2nd ed. Berlin: Parey; 1979

Popesko P. Atlas of topographical Anatomy of the Domestic Animals. Philadelphia: Saunders; 1971

Sack WO. Rooney's Guide to the Dissection of the Horse. 6th ed. Ithaca, N. Y.: Veterinary Textbooks; 1991

Sack WO, Habel RE. Rooney's guide to the dissection of the horse. Ithaca, N.Y.: Veterinary Textbooks; 1982

Schaller O. Der N. intercostobrachialis des Rindes. Wien tierärztl Mschr (Schreiber-Festschrift) 1960; 292

Schmaltz R. Die Geschlechtsorgane. In: Ellenberger W, Hrsg. Handbuch der vergleichenden mikroskopischen Anatomie der Haustiere. Vol. II. Berlin: Parey; 1911

Schreiber J. Der Bandapparat des Tarsus vom Schwein. Wien tierärztl Mschr 1961; 48: 602

Shambaugh GE. Bloodstream in the labyrinth of the ear of dog and man. Am J Anat 1923; 32: 189

Simoens P, De Vos NR, Lauwers H. Illustrated anatomical nomenclature of the heart and the arteries of head and neck in the domestic mammals. Gent: Medelingen Fac. Diergeneeskunde Rijksuniv. Gent; 1978; 21: 1

Simoens P, De Vos NR, Lauwers H. Illustrated anatomical nomenclature of the arteries of the abdomen, the pelvis, and the pelvic limb in domestic mammals. Gent: Medelingen Fac. Diergeneeskunde Rijksuniv. Gent; 1980; 25: II/1

Simoens P, De Vos NR, Lauwers H, Nicaise M. Illustrated anatomical nomenclature of the arteries of the thoracic limb in the domestic mammals. Gent: Medelingen Fac. Diergeneeskunde Rijksuniv. Gent; 1980; 22: 1

Spreull JSA. Treatment of otitis media in the dog. J Small Anim Pract 1964; 5: 107

Trautmann A, Fiebiger J. Fundamentals of the Histology of Domestic Animals. Ithaca, N. Y.: Comstock; 1957

Vollmerhaus B. Zur vergleichenden Nomenklatur des lymphoepithelialen Rachenringes der Haussäugetiere. Zbl Vet Med 1959; 6: 82

Waibl H, Herrmann J, Rehage J et al. Zur angewandten Anatomie des distalen „Vinculum tendinis" in der Fesselbeugesehnenscheide der Beckengliedmasse des Rindes, Dtsch Tierärztl Wschr 108, 233–280; 2001

Watson A. Vaginal ring and round ligament of the uterus in the female cat. Anat Hist Embryol 2009; 38: 319–320

Zietzschmann O, Krölling O. Lehrbuch der Entwicklungsgeschichte der Haustiere. Berlin: Parey; 1955

A

B

C

F

G

H

N

O

P

U

Z

FSC
www.fsc.org
MIX
Papier | Fördert
gute Waldnutzung
FSC® C083411

Zeitfracht Medien GmbH
Ferdinand-Jühlke-Straße 7
99095 Erfurt, Deutschland
produktsicherheit@kolibri360.de